1992 $145.00

Dr. Kevin W Morrill

Dr. Kevin W Morrill

TEMPOROMANDIBULAR DISORDERS

Diagnosis and Treatment

Andrew S. Kaplan, D.M.D., F.A.C.D., F.I.C.D.

Director, Temporomandibular Disorder/Facial Pain Clinic, The Mount Sinai Hospital

Assistant Clinical Professor, The Mount Sinai School of Medicine

Assistant Attending, The Mount Sinai Hospital

Coordinator, Department of Dentistry, The Mount Sinai Hospital

Clinical Instructor, Department of Oral Medicine, Hospital Division, New York University
College of Dentistry
New York, New York

Leon A. Assael, D.M.D.

Associate Professor and Residency Program Director, Department of Oral and Maxillofacial
Surgery, School of Dental Medicine

Associate Professor of Surgery, Department of Surgery, School of Medicine
University of Connecticut, Farmington, Connecticut

Associate Chief of Staff, John Dempsey Hospital
Farmington, Connecticut

Attending Oral and Maxillofacial Surgeon, Hartford Hospital
Hartford, Connecticut

W.B. SAUNDERS COMPANY
Harcourt Brace Jovanovich, Inc.

Philadelphia   London   Toronto   Montreal   Sydney   Tokyo

W. B. Saunders Company
Harcourt Brace Jovanovich, Inc.
The Curtis Center
Independence Square West
Philadelphia, PA 19106-3399

Library of Congress Cataloging-in-Publication Data
Temporomandibular disorders : diagnosis and treatment /
[edited by]
    Andrew S. Kaplan, Leon A. Assael.
        p.   cm.
    ISBN 0-7216-5286-7
    1. Temporomandibular joint—Diseases.   I. Kaplan,
Andrew S., 1956–   . II. Assael, Leon A.
    [DNLM: 1. Temporomandibular Joint Diseases—
    diagnosis.   2. Temporomandibular Joint Diseases—
    pathology.   3. Temporomandibular Joint Diseases—
    therapy. WU 140 T2865]
    RK470.T438   1992
    617.5′22—dc20
    DNLM/DLC
    for Library of Congress   91-21825
                                                        CIP

Editor: John Dyson
Developmental Editor: David Kilmer
Designer: W. B. Saunders Staff
Production Manager: Linda R. Garber
Manuscript Editors: Mary Anne Folcher and
                     Wendy Andresen
Illustration Specialist: Cecilia Roberts
Indexer: Nancy Weaver

Temporomandibular Disorders: Diagnosis and
Treatment   ISBN 0-7216-5286-7

Printed in the United States of America

Last digit is the print number: 9 8 7 6 5 4 3 2 1

To our wives, Sandra Kaplan and Linda Assael.

Their encouragement, support, patience, and love made it possible.

And to our children, Daniel Kaplan, Laura Kaplan, Rachel Assael, Jeanne Assael, and Julia Assael.

Their love makes it worthwhile.

CONTRIBUTORS

Leon A. Assael, D.M.D.
Associate Professor and Residency Program Director, Department of Oral and Maxillofacial Surgery; Associate Chief of Staff, John Dempsey Hospital; and Attending Oral and Maxillofacial Surgeon, Hartford Hospital; University of Connecticut School of Dental Medicine; Farmington, Connecticut.

Ronald Attanasio, D.D.S., M.S.Ed., M.S.
Associate Professor and Chairman, Department of Adult Restorative Dentistry, University of Nebraska College of Dentistry, Lincoln, Nebraska.

Michael J. Bergstein, M.D.
Clinical Instructor, Department of Otolaryngology, The Medical Center at the University of California, San Francisco, California.

Daniel Buchbinder, D.M.D.
Assistant Professor, The Mount Sinai School of Medicine; Director, Residency Training Program in Oral and Maxillofacial Surgery; and Chief, Division of Oral and Maxillofacial Surgery, The Mount Sinai Medical Center, New York, New York.

Ronald Burakoff, D.M.D., M.P.H.
Adjunct Associate Professor of Dentistry, Columbia University School of Dental and Oral Surgery; Clinical Associate Professor, New York University, College of Dentistry, New York; and Chairman, Department of Dentistry, The Long Island College Hospital, Brooklyn, New York.

Rebecca Castaneda, D.D.S.
Assistant Clinical Professor, University of California, School of Dentistry, San Francisco, California.

Paul A. Danielson, D.M.D.
Assistant Clinical Professor, University of Vermont College of Medicine; Attending in Surgery, Medical Center Hospital of Vermont; and Attending in Surgery, Fanny Allen Hospital, Burlington, Vermont.

John Dunn, B.A., P.T.
Lecturer, New York University College of Dentistry, Continuing Education, TMJ and Craniofacial Pain Program, New York; and President and Director, Community Physical Therapists, New York and New Jersey.

John E. Fantasia, D.D.S.
Chief, Division of Oral Pathology, Department of Dental Medicine, Long Island Jewish Medical Center, New Hyde Park, and Associate Professor, Department of Oral Biology and Pathology, School of Dental Medicine, State University of New York at Stony Brook, Stony Brook, New York.

Gordon Gaynor, D.D.S.
Teaching Staff, TMD/Facial Pain Clinic; Assistant Attending, Orthodontic Section, Department of Dentistry, The Mount Sinai Hospital; Assistant Clinical Professor of Dentistry, The Mount Sinai School of Medicine, New York, New York.

Michael Gelb, D.D.S., M.S.
Clinical Associate Professor, Department of Oral Medicine and Pathology and Director of the Continuing Dental Education TMJ and Craniofacial Pain Program, New York University, College of Dentistry, New York, New York.

Jay R. Goldman, D.D.S.
Clinical Instructor, Department of Oral Medicine; Staff, TMJ/Craniofacial Pain Program, New York University, College of Dentistry, New York, New York.

Leslie B. Heffez, D.M.D., M.S.
Associate Professor and Associate Head, Oral and Maxillofacial Surgery TMJ and Facial Pain Center, University of Illinois at Chicago, Chicago, Illinois.

David C. Hoffman, D.D.S.
Assistant Clinical Professor of Oral and Maxillofacial Surgery, University of Medicine and Dentistry of New Jersey (UMDNJ), New Jersey Dental School, Newark, New Jersey; Attending, The Staten Island University Hospital, Department of Dentistry; Attending, The Staten Island University Hospital, Department of Surgery; and Acting Clinical Assistant, Montefiore Hospital, Department of Dentistry, Bronx, New York.

Andrew S. Kaplan, D.M.D.
Director, TMD/Facial Pain Clinic, The Mount Sinai Hospital; Assistant Clinical Professor, The Mount Sinai School of Medicine; Assistant Attending, The Mount Sinai Hospital; Coordinator, Dental Service, The Mount Sinai Hospital; Clinical Instructor, Department of Oral Medicine, Hospital Division, New York University, College of Dentistry, New York, New York.

Steven A. King, M.D., M.S.
Clinical Associate Professor, Department of Psychiatry, University of Vermont College of Medicine, Burlington, Vermont; Director, Pain Service, Department of Psychiatry, Maine Medical Center, Portland, Maine.

Christopher Lane, D.D.S.
Chief Resident, Division of Oral and Maxillofacial Surgery, The Mount Sinai Hospital, New York, New York.

William Lawson, M.D., D.D.S.
Professor of Otolaryngology, The Mount Sinai School of Medicine, New York; Chief of Otolaryngology, Veterans Administration Hospital, Bronx, New York.

Jeffrey S. Mannheimer, M.A., P.T.
Clinical Assistant Professor and Manager of Physical Therapy Services, Center for TMJ Disorders and Orofacial Pain Management, University of Medicine and Dentistry of New Jersey, New Jersey Dental School, Newark, New Jersey; Adjunct Assistant Professor, Department of Orthopedic Surgery and Rehabilitation, Program in Physical Therapy, Hahnemann University School of Medicine, Philadelphia, Pennsylvania; and President, Delaware Valley Physical Therapy Associates, Lawrenceville, New Jersey.

Robert D. McMullen, M.D.
Assistant Professor of Psychiatry, Columbia University School of Physicians and Surgeons; Assistant Attending in Psychiatry, Columbia Presbyterian Hospital; Psychiatric Consultant, Temporomandibular Disorders—Facial Pain Clinic, Columbia University School of Dental and Oral Surgery, New York, New York.

Noshir Mehta, D.M.D.
Director, Gelb Craniofacial Pain Center and Assistant Clinical Professor, Department of Periodontology, Tufts University School of Dental Medicine; Consultant, Spaulding Rehabilitation Hospital; Active Staff, New England Medical Center, Boston; Active Staff, Newton-Wellesley Hospital, Newton, Massachusetts.

Steven G. Messing, D.M.D.
Associate Professor, Departments of Periodontics and Restorative Dentistry, University of Medicine and Dentistry of New Jersey, Newark, New Jersey; Lecturer, Graduate Program on Temporomandibular Disorders, New York University Dental School, New York; Attending, St. Peter's Hospital, Albany; Consultant, Sunnyview Hospital, Schenectady, New York.

David L. Milbauer, M.D.
Medical Director, Kips Bay Medical Imaging, New York, New York.

Richard A. Pertes, D.D.S.
Clinical Associate Professor and Acting Director, Center for TMJ Disorders and Orofacial Pain Management, University of Medicine and Dentistry of New Jersey, New Jersey Dental School, Newark, New Jersey.

Mark A. Piper, M.D., D.M.D.
Chairman, Oral and Maxillofacial Surgery, St. Anthony's Hospital, St Petersburg; Lecturer, L. D. Panky Institute, Miami, Florida.

Kurt P. Schellhas, M.D.
St. Louis Park, Missouri.

Peter Som, M.D.
Professor of Radiology and Otolaryngology, The Mount Sinai School of Medicine; Attending Radiologist, The Mount Sinai Hospital, New York, New York.

Charles B. Stacy, M.D.
Assistant Clinical Professor, Neurology, The Mount Sinai School of Medicine; Clinical Assistant Attending, The Mount Sinai Hospital; Director, Neurology Pain Clinic, Mount Sinai Hospital; Chief of Neurology, Doctors Hospital, Division of Beth Israel Hospital, New York, New York.

Steven Syrop, D.D.S.
Assistant Clinical Professor and Director, Temporomandibular Disorders—Facial Pain Clinic, Columbia University School of Dental and Oral Surgery; Attending, Columbia Presbyterian Hospital, New York, New York.

Donald Tanenbaum, D.D.S., M.P.H.
Associate Attending, Orofacial Pain/TMJ Section, Long Island Jewish Medical Center, Department of Dentistry, New Hyde Park; Assistant Attending, Beth Israel Medical Center, Department of Dentistry, New York, New York.

Mohan Thomas, D.D.S.
Director, Maxillofacial/Temporomandibular Joint Service, Hospital for Joint Diseases Orthopaedic Institute; Assistant Attending, Oral Maxillofacial Surgery, The Mount Sinai Hospital, New York, New York.

PREFACE

For several years, we have felt a need for a comprehensive text reference in temporomandibular disorders. Many excellent books have been devoted to the subject but most reflect the clinical philosophies of their authors and are therefore restricted to particular points of view. Books devoted to only a particular aspect of the field may produce a narrow perspective that can carry over into clinical practice. The clinician becomes like the haberdasher who has only one color of suit to sell. He tells the salesman, "If the man wants a blue suit, turn on the blue lights." As clinicians, we need a broad repertory of ideas and treatment regimens that will meet our patients' needs. To build that inventory, we must seek knowledge from many sources. In this multidisciplinary, carefully researched text, we feel we have given clinicians a valuable tool to develop this inventory of knowledge.

It is our goal to present a comprehensive, well-documented text encompassing the major relevant aspects of this demanding and multifaceted subject. To accomplish our goal, we have sought the participation of a wide range of expert contributors. Listening to the voices of these authors in their chapters, we heard what at first seemed a cacophony of ideas and scientific evidence. Although initially shaken by what appeared to be irreconcilable points of view, we found a common thread of scientific method. This finding supports our fundamental contention that the multidisciplinary management of temporomandibular disorders offers the best overall approach.

Nevertheless, the term temporomandibular disorders remains synonymous with controversy: controversy over diagnostic terminology, over diagnostic procedures, and over treatment. Although our text illuminates these controversies, it does not entirely resolve them. Reading this volume is akin to sitting in on one of our multidisciplinary clinic discussions when opinions are ferociously defended but always on the basis of scientific evidence.

During the preparation of this text, we have become quite familiar with the disagreements between clinicians and researchers, the unfortunate animosity between clinicians in different geographic regions, and the often vehement differences in philosophy among various professions, specialties, and factions within the field. When opinions are strongly held, the emotional investment makes them the "property" of the individual. Although it is difficult to understand the fractious differences of opinion regarding temporomandibular disorders, every student should be aware of them.

These differences need not be nearly as serious as they sometimes seem. They can be minimized if members of the professions will take the time to understand the basis of one another's point of view. That should be one of the goals of every clinician reading our text. Total agreement will not be achieved, but there will come a recognition of the common threads in many existing philosophies.

This text is designed for the serious student of temporomandibular disorders. This audience includes dentists, physicians, physical therapists, and other health care professionals involved in the multidisciplinary treatment of temporomandibular disorders. For those who already are experts in their own discipline, it will serve them well to learn more about other areas that will complement existing knowledge. This text is also a "core" reference for predoctoral students and an update for practicing clinicians.

The book is divided into five sections. The first, on basic science, contains background biomedical information that forms the foundation for the clinical aspects of the book. The second section is a description of the various pathologic states that occur, including many that are not in the lexicon of those who place all conditions into a narrower diagnostic range. The third section concerns diagnosis. It includes comprehensive information on clinical examination procedures, radiography, and diagnostic tests. The fourth section discusses nonsurgical treatment, and the last section discusses surgery.

The material in this text is carefully documented and richly referenced where possible. Clinical observations and authors' opinions are clearly shown as such.

We have been privileged to have contributions from an outstanding group of experts. They are outstanding experts in part because they are outstanding students; they have learned from their teachers, patients, and colleagues; they have learned from reading unceasingly; and they have learned as well from writing their highly researched contributions. In this way, they have become master clinicians. In this way you, the reader, can join their ranks. Enjoy this text and the knowledge it will bring you.

ANDREW S. KAPLAN, D.M.D.
LEON A. ASSAEL, D.M.D.

ACKNOWLEDGMENTS

No textbook can be written without the help of many people. A collective acknowledgment must be given to the many researchers throughout the world who have provided us with a body of research, clinical reports, and teachings in this field. It is the continuing work of these people that enables us to progress to a more rigorous scientific level in patient care.

We would like to thank the following members of the faculty of The Mount Sinai School of Medicine for their encouragement and advice: J. Gordon Rubin, D.D.S.; Daniel Buchbinder, D.M.D.; Arthur Elias, D.M.D.; and especially Jack Klatell, D.D.S., who as chairman encouraged our inquisitiveness and effort. We also thank those faculty of the University of Connecticut who through their unbending support helped us complete this project: Richard Topazian, D.D.S.; Keith Rogerson, D.D.S.; and David Shafer, D.M.D.

We are grateful to Christopher Palestro, M.D., for reviewing the section on radionuclide imaging. Michael Klein, M.D., provided important advice and assistance in preparing the photomicrographs and scanning electron micrographs in Chapters 2 and 10. Kavita Saggi was most helpful in the library research for Chapter 2. The attending staff of the Temporomandibular Disorders/Facial Pain Clinic of The Mount Sinai Hospital, Benjamin Bass, D.D.S.; Robert Pekarsky, D.D.S.; and Gordon Gaynor, D.D.S., helped free time for the completion of this project.

It has often been said that there is no such thing as writing, only rewriting. Inez Feliciano at Mount Sinai can attest to the truth of this and deserves a big thank you for typing and retyping mountains of manuscript. At the University of Connecticut, many thanks for the support of Judy Hedenberg with a little help from IBM. Our artist, Caroline Meinstein, exercised patience and expertise in drawing and redrawing the many illustrations in this text. She gained a thorough understanding of the details of this field and rendered them effectively and accurately. Theresa Dougherty and Mary Spano of Exact Photo provided us with excellent photography and reproductions.

We also wish to thank Gray Williams, whose valuable encouragement, literary advice, and friendship throughout this project helped see it through to completion. In addition, literary agent Michael Cohn must be acknowledged for his help during the preparation of this project.

We have a great respect for and gratitude to the people at W. B. Saunders Company. John Dyson is an incredibly able professional who used his unperturbed demeanor to successfully confront any and all problems during the preparation of this text. Mary Anne Folcher provided us with the highest level of meticulous attention to detail as copy editor. David Kilmer was outstanding in the editing of the chapters. Many others in design and marketing have also made invaluable contributions.

ANDREW S. KAPLAN, D.M.D.
LEON A. ASSAEL, D.M.D.

CONTENTS

SECTION III, 283
DIAGNOSIS

SECTION I

BASIC
SCIENCES

Leon A. Assael

CHAPTER 1

Functional Anatomy

The craniomandibular articulations are best considered in the context of the overall functional anatomy of the human head. The head is the most complex structure in the human body because it integrates so many different functions into a single location. It is the source of all neurologic function and houses the organs for sight, hearing, smell, and taste. As the opening of the respiratory system, it undergoes continuous interaction with the atmosphere, sensing its qualities and inspiring air on a demand basis. As the opening of the digestive system, it subjects ingested food to inspection, general and special sensory analysis, deglutition, and initial digestion.

The head is the most important structure of human communication. The human facial appearance most strongly indentifies the qualities of an individual. Through facial expression, the most important window on higher cortical brain function is obtained. The airway and masticatory structures combine to permit the mechanical aspects of speech.

With the exception of the brain, the structures that make up the masticatory apparatus occupy the largest portion of the head. These structures perform their functions in close anatomic and physiologic integration with all other functions of the head. Central to integrated masticatory function are the temporomandibular joints (TMJs) (Fig. 1–1).

OSTEOLOGY

The skeletal and muscular architecture of the masticatory system is designed to perform efficient ingestion and deglutition. The mandible is a rigid but freely movable structure. In function, force is transmitted from the teeth to the alveolar processes. The load is sustained by the symphysis and external oblique ridges. Transmission of force is then nearly in a direct line to the condylar heads. When a load is sustained by the teeth, tensile forces occur along the alveolar process and compressive forces are applied to the inferior and posterior border. These forces are neutralized along the region of the external oblique ridge.

This force is then sustained by the condylar head. Masticatory force is transmitted to the cranium via the cranial attachments of the muscles of mastication, the maxillary teeth, and the craniomandibular articulation. Although it has been said that the TMJs do not bear weight, it is clear that masticatory loads are borne by these joints. The condylar processes of the mandible are designed to sustain these major forces. The condylar neck begins to form by a thickening at the posterior border at the level of the occlusal plane. The condylar neck continues to widen superiorly for approximately 2 cm until it becomes confluent with the condylar head. The condylar head is approximately 2 cm medially to laterally and 1 cm sagittally. The anterior aspect of the condylar neck is hollowed out by the pterygoid fossae. When integrated with the slight convexity of the posterior aspect of the condylar neck, it gives the appearance of the condyle's curving forward. In its anterior aspect, the condylar neck rapidly thins out to the wafer-thin coronoid notch.

The condylar heads are remarkably symmetric, following normal growth and development. When viewed cephalad, the condylar heads are ovoid structures with their long axes only roughly transverse. The lateral pole of these ovals is slightly anterior to the medial pole. The two long axes of the condyles thus form an angle of 145 to 160 degrees. When viewed from above, the condylar head has a bilobed appearance with a thicker medial aspect (Fig. 1–2). The articulating surface is distinguished by the margins of the capsule, which form a clear circumferential ridge (Fig. 1–3). The articulating surface forms a broad flat structure approximately 2 cm by 0.5 cm,[1] from an anterior capsular margin to the superior pole, and a slightly smaller area posteriorly. The posterior aspect of the articular surface is more rounded and less broad.

The condyles articulate with the glenoid fossae and the eminentia articularis (articular eminence) of the membranous portion of the temporal bone. The anterior root of the zygomatic

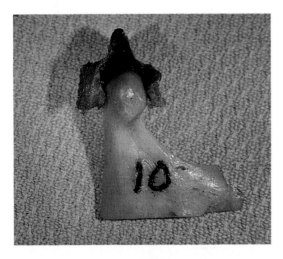

FIGURE 1–3. The condyle from the lateral view with the disc attached. Note the lateral limit of the capsule.

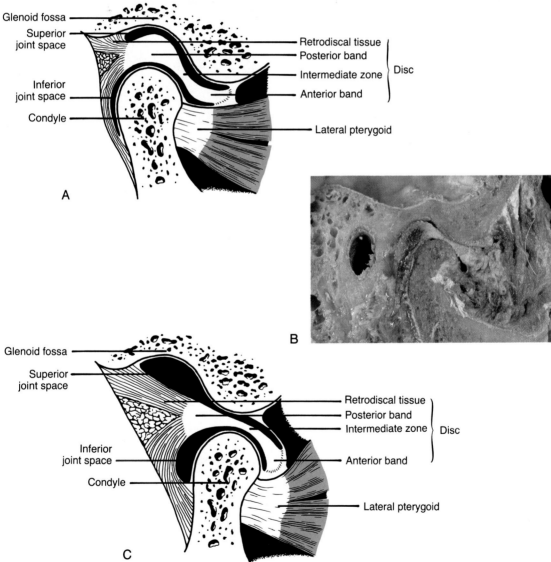

Glenoid fossa

Superior joint space

Inferior joint space

Condyle

Retrodiscal tissue

Posterior band

Intermediate zone

Anterior band

Disc

Lateral pterygoid

A

B

Glenoid fossa

Superior joint space

Inferior joint space

Condyle

Retrodiscal tissue

Posterior band

Intermediate zone

Anterior band

Disc

Lateral pterygoid

C

FIGURE 1–4. Lateral view of the temporomandibular joint. The parts of the disc and their relationship to the condyle and fossa are shown. *A,* Schematic closed view. *B,* Anatomic closed view. *C,* Schematic open view.

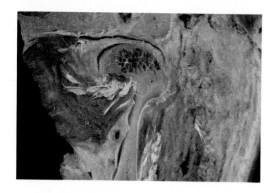

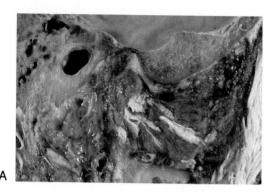

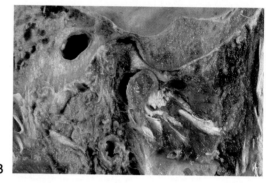

FIGURE 1–5. Coronal view of the condyle. This anatomic specimen demonstrates the capsule tightly bound to the condylar head medially and laterally. Note the attachment of the lateral pterygoid muscle in the pterygoid fossa.

A

B

FIGURE 1–6. The retrodiscal tissues during opening. Note the movement of the disc and mobility of the retrodiscal tissues during opening of the jaw. *A,* Closed view. *B,* Open view.

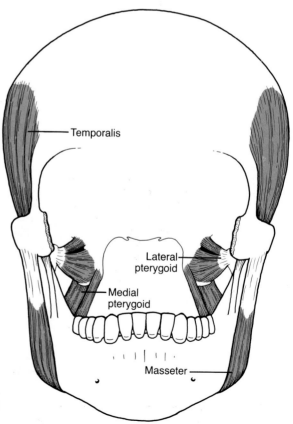

Temporalis

Lateral pterygoid

Medial pterygoid

Masseter

FIGURE 1–8. The four paired muscles of mastication: masseter, temporalis, medial pterygoid, and lateral pterygoid.

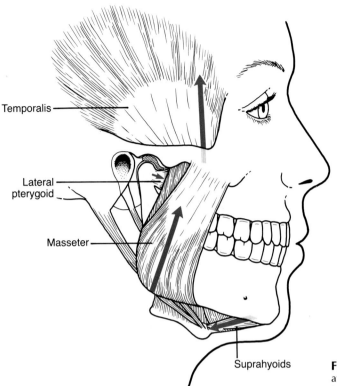

Temporalis

Lateral pterygoid

Masseter

Suprahyoids

FIGURE 1–9. Direction of force generated by the masseter, suprahyoids, and temporalis muscles.

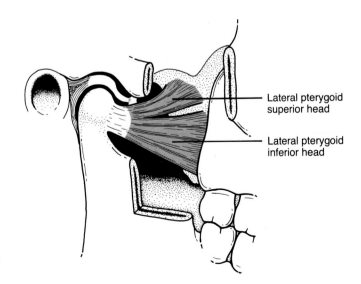

Lateral pterygoid superior head

Lateral pterygoid inferior head

FIGURE 1–10. The lateral pterygoid muscle. Two distinct heads emerge from the cranium.

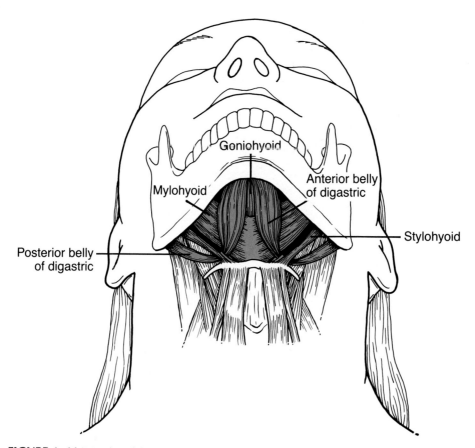

FIGURE 1–11. Muscles of the suprahyoid region: mylohyoid, geniohyoid, stylohyoid, and digastric.

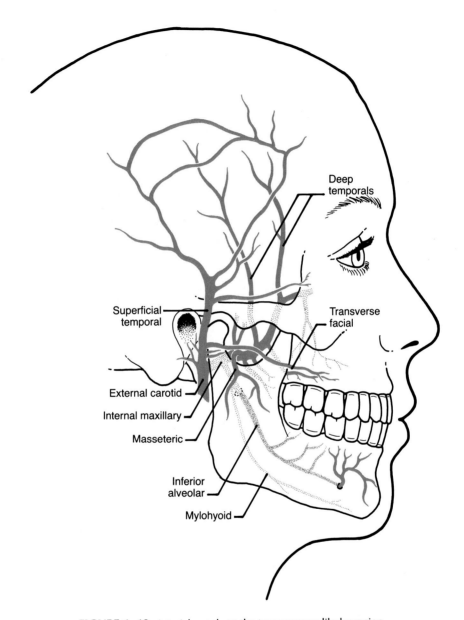

FIGURE 1–12. Arterial supply to the temporomandibular region.

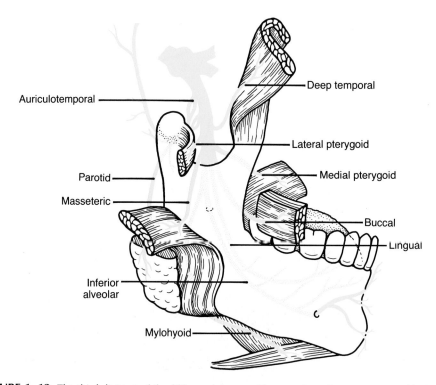

FIGURE 1–13. The third division of the fifth cranial nerve. The supply to the temporomandibular region.

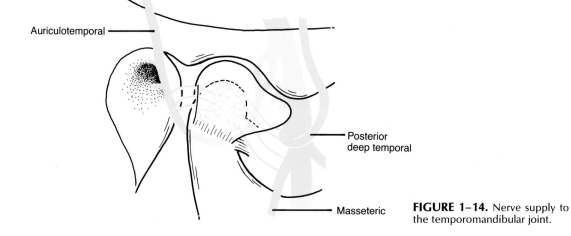

FIGURE 1–14. Nerve supply to the temporomandibular joint.

FIGURE 1-1. The temporomandibular region in its anatomic context.

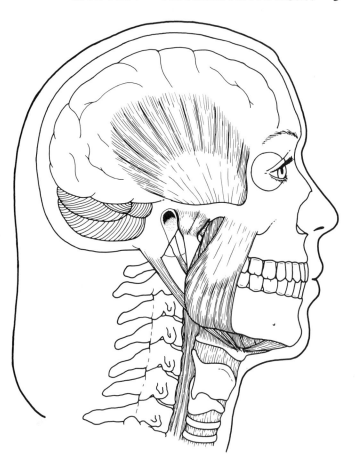

process of the temporal bone forms the eminentia articularis. The posterior slope of the eminentia articularis contacts the anterior condylar head during translation. Hence, the eminentia is concave mediolaterally.

The glenoid fossa is a thin concavity of the squamous portion of the temporal bone. The glenoid fossa separates the TMJ from the middle cranial fossa by as little as 2 mm of bone at its thinnest. The glenoid fossa is twice as wide mediolaterally than anteroposteriorly to accept the condylar head. The posterior portion of the glenoid fossa constitutes the petrous portion of the temporal bone and is separated from the main articulating surface by the glaserian fissure. The intra-articular portion of the posterior glenoid fossa is the postglenoid tubercle, which is identical to the middle root of the zygomatic arch. Posterior to the condylar head, this region includes the tympanic plate, styloid process, parotid fossa, and stylomastoid foramen. These structures are the osseous supports, in order, of the auditory canal, stylohyoid-stylomandibular ligaments, parotid tail, and facial nerve.

CRANIOMANDIBULAR ARTICULATION

The mandible forms a diarthrosis with the temporal bone. A diarthrosis is a freely movable joint in which the proximate bones are cov-

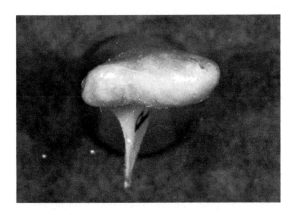

FIGURE 1-2. The condylar head as seen from the cephalad view. Note the bilobed appearance.

ered with a cartilage-like surface. They are spanned by suspensory ligaments and have a synovial lining that secretes synovial fluid. The articulation is a ginglymus, where motion occurs in a rough hinge axis along a repeatable plane supported by strong lateral ligaments. It is as well an arthrodial joint permitting gliding motion.

The suspensory ligaments of the craniomandibular articulation are those that restrain the functional movements of the mandible. The capsular ligament is circumferential and attached to the rim of the glenoid fossae. The capsular ligament is continuous with the meniscus and stabilizes its position. The lateral ligament is a distinct structure superficial to the capsular ligament. The lateral ligament is attached anteriorly and superiorly to the anterior root of the zygomatic process of the temporal bone (the tubercle of the eminentia articularis). The lateral ligament sends parallel fascicles inferiorly and posteriorly to attach to the facial surface of the condylar neck (Fig. 1–7).

The meniscus or disc of the TMJ is an intra-articular structure that separates the condylar head from the glenoid fossae. The meniscus thus divides the synovial membranes into inferior and superior joint spaces. The meniscus is a hypovascular structure of considerable resiliency and contains variable numbers of cartilage cells; hence, it is a fibrocartilage.[2] Sensory fibers of the auriculotemporal nerve do not penetrate this fibrocartilage. It is thinner in its central articulating portion (the intermediate zone) than in its periphery. The working surface of the condylar head is the region anterior to the superior pole. The posterior slope of the eminentia articularis is the working surface of the glenoid fossa. The shape of the meniscus accommodates to these functional osseous determinants. Thus, the meniscus thickens at its superior aspect (12 o'clock above the condyle in the closed position) to form a thick posterior band. The meniscus thickens medially and laterally and is tightly bound to the capsular ligaments. Just anterior to the working surface of the joint, the meniscus again thickens to form the anterior band (Fig. 1–4).

Although the meniscus is tightly bound to the capsular ligament near its attachment to the condyle medially and laterally, it is contiguous with the capsular ligament anteriorly in a looser fashion (Fig. 1–5). The medial quarter of the anterior attachment variably contains fibers of the lateral pterygoid muscle. The bulk of the disc is contained superior and posterior

to the lateral pterygoid muscle without attachment. The meniscus and the middle ear, at least in some specimens, appear to have a direct connection via the discomalleolar ligament.[3] Although it is postulated that movement of the mandible might produce movement of the malleolus, this has not been demonstrated. The function and the universal presence of this structure have not been clearly demonstrated.

Posterior to the meniscus is the retrodiscal tissue (also called bilaminar zone), which makes a loose attachment to the posterior aspect of the glenoid fossae at the junction of the tympanic plate. Inferiorly, the tissue attaches to the capsular ligament at the neck of the condyle. The retrodiscal tissue is a soft, highly areolar connective tissue with large vascular spaces, auriculotemporal nerve fibers, and loosely constructed collagen and elastin fibers. No loading of this tissue occurs during normal function. Posterior to the posterior band, comparatively free movement of the meniscus relative to the retrodiscal tissue takes place. This movement allows for the free disc translation in concurrence with condylar translation. The attachments of the retrodiscal tissue also permit the movement of the disc backward and upward when the condyle is returned to the glenoid fossae during closing. These coordinated movements of the disc and condyle can by accomplished only because of the loose but elastic nature of the retrodiscal tissue and the free movement of the disc against the glenoid fossa (Fig. 1–6).

The inferior joint space contains about 0.9 ml of synovial fluid, lies on the condylar head like a cap, drapes over all surfaces, but extends most caudad to the condylar neck in its posterior aspect. When the mandible is depressed, the inferior joint space opens to a greater extent posteriorly, giving the appearance in lateral view of a teardrop in the inferior joint space posterior to the condylar head. The anterior portion of the inferior joint space forms a small fossa, where the fibers of the capsular ligament and the anterior band of the disc form a concretion. This sling-like structure helps stabilize the disc against the condylar head during function (Fig. 1–7).

The superior joint space is larger and more anteriorly placed than the inferior joint space. This space contains about 1.2 ml of synovial fluid. Its shape in the cephalad aspect corresponds closely to the glenoid fossae. On the caudad aspect, the concavity of the intermedi-

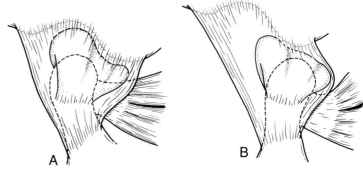

FIGURE 1–7. Stabilization of the disc by the lateral pole of the condyle and the lateral ligament. *A,* Closed view. *B,* Open view.

ate zone can be noted.[4] The separation of the retrodiscal tissue from the posterior band is clearly differentiated when viewed from the superior joint space.

The anterior fossa of the superior joint space forms a concavity in front of the condylar head. The medial fossa forms a concavity medial to the condylar head.

The sphenomandibular ligament describes a course from the spine of the sphenoid bone to the lingula of the mandible. Lateral to this ligament but medial to the mandible are the lateral pterygoid muscle, the internal maxillary artery, and the inferior alveolar artery and nerve. The stylomandibular ligament is a semirigid structure connecting the anterior inferior aspect of the styloid process to the angle of the mandible.

MUSCLES OF THE CRANIOMANDIBULAR REGION

The position of the mandible and its craniomandibular articulation in space are mainly determined by the activity of the 27 muscles that attach the jaw. These muscles can be separated into groups based on their functional activity and include the masticatory muscles, the intermaxillary muscles, the suprahyoid muscles, and the facial expression muscles.

The muscles of mastication are the paired masseter, medial pterygoid, lateral pterygoid, and temporalis (Fig. 1–8). These are the most powerful muscles acting on the mandible. With the exception of the buccinator and superior pharyngeal constrictor, these four pairs of muscles are the only ones that connect the cranium to the mandible. In their synchronous function, they are responsible for interocclusal forces and lateral, vertical, and anterior mandibular movements.

Condylar movements to the closed position

are primarily the result of function of the masseter, temporalis, and medial pterygoid muscles. Active condylar translation that produces mandibular protrusion is primarily due to the function of the lateral pterygoid muscle.

The masseter muscle is a thick and powerful muscle advantageously placed to produce maximum masticatory force in the molar region (Fig. 1–9). The fibers are directed at roughly right angles to the occlusal plane. Thus, a maximum vector of force along the long axes of the teeth can be provided during mastication. The superficial belly of the masseter forms a strong aponeurosis at the angle of the mandible. The masseter muscle attaches to the zygoma along the inferior aspect of the zygomatic body behind the malar eminence and to the zygomatic arch from the anterior slope of the eminentia articularis forward. The deep belly of the masseter forms a broader, less tendinous insertion on the lateral border of the mandible from above the angle of the mandible to the lateral aspect of the coronoid process. Attachment superiorly is to the posterior third of the medial aspect of the zygomatic arch and its whole inner portion. The parotidomasseteric fascia covers both bellies of the masseter and the parotid gland. The fascia forms the lateral limits of the masticator space. This fascia is contiguous with the superficial portion of the superficial temporal fascia covering the zygomatic arch and is continued in the neck as a portion of the deep cervical fascia.

The medial pterygoid muscle forms a dense aponeurosis at the medial aspect of the mandibular angle. This attachment extends from just posterior to the third molar to mid ramus just inferior to the lingula. The medial pterygoid attaches the cranium at the inner aspect of the lateral pterygoid plate and the maxillary tuberosity. The pterygoid's fibers are directed roughly parallel to those of the masseter muscle, joining it in a single tendinous aponeurosis at the inferior border of the mandible. These parallel formations of the masseter and the medial pterygoid muscles form a sling, which cradles the ramus of the mandible.

The lateral pterygoid muscle arises from two distinct heads in the cranium (Fig. 1–10) The inferior head is the larger of the two and forms a thick ovoid origination on the lateral pterygoid plate. The inferior head is then directed backward, laterally and upward toward the condylar neck. The superior head originates at the greater wing of the sphenoid and the pterygoid ridge, a structure that is at the junction of the temporal and zygomatic fossae. The superior head is then directed backward, laterally and inferiorly toward the condylar neck; a concrescence of these two heads fuses these fibers into a single muscle. The lateral pterygoid then inserts into the condylar neck anteromedially, at the pterygoid fossae. A small number of fibers also insert into the most anterior medial portion of the disc (see Fig. 1–5).

A debate has long continued over the functional anatomy of the two heads of the lateral pterygoid muscle. By evaluating patterns of jaw movement, electromyographic activity, and anatomic dissection, a theory of activity is stated whereby the superior head and its disc attachment are active when the jaw is being closed and the inferior head is active during opening and translation.[5] This theory gained clinical significance when a corollary promoting lateral pterygoid muscle hyperactivity as the mechanism of anterior disc displacement was promulgated. In this corollary, premature activity of the superior head of the lateral pterygoid muscle during translation was thought to produce anterior disc displacement.[6]

Carpentier and coworkers,[7,8] using fresh-frozen cadaver specimens cut along the long axis of the muscle, stated that lateral pterygoid fibers inserting on the disc could not be distinguished as originating from the superior head. Moreover, the specimens demonstrated lateral pterygoid attachment to the disc in only its most medial portion. The disc appears to be overwhelmingly stabilized by its sling-like concretion with the capsular ligament. In addition, Capentier found that the great bulk of the lateral pterygoid muscle inserting in the condyle is made up of fibers mixed from both heads. The location of this muscle tends to deflect the disc backward and upward not anteriorly. Hence, Carpentier has postulated no independent action of the two heads of the lateral pter-

ygoid muscle. The theory of asynchronous function of the two heads of the lateral pterygoid muscle and its corollary explaining disc displacement appear to be inaccurate.

The temporalis muscle is a flat, fan-shaped, broad structure with cranial and mandibular attachments (see Fig. 1–9). The muscle fills the temporal fossae with broad cranial attachments from the external angular process of the frontal bone anteriorly, the pterygoid ridge of the greater wing of the sphenoid anteriorly and inferiorly, the superior crest of the mastoid posteriorly and inferiorly, and a curved line of the parietal and temporal bones superiorly and posteriorly. From all points of this attachment, the temporalis fibers are directed in roughly a straight line to the coronoid process and the anterior aspect of the ramus of the mandible where a powerful aponeurosis is formed. An exception to this straight line occurs where the posterior fibers must bend over the anterior root of the zygomatic process of the temporal bone. This bending causes the deep portion of the posterior fibers of the temporalis to be in an intimate contact with those of the lateral pterygoid muscle. The superficial portion of the mastoid projection of the temporalis bends slightly over the external ear and is attached to the three small vestigial muscles of ear mobility.

The temporalis insertion includes the anterior and medial aspects of the coronoid and the anterior surface of the ramus on the external oblique ridge to the third or second molar. This attachment often obliterates the buccal vestibule in the third molar region where the temporalis fibers are in intimate contact with those of the buccinator and superior pharyngeal constrictor. The medial aspect of this insertion on the anterior ramus is a thick powerful attachment to the temporal crest above the occlusal plane to just anterior to the lingula.

The temporalis muscle is covered by the superficial temporal fascia. This fascia is attached superiorly at the temporal ridge and covers the temporalis thoroughly from the lateral orbit anteriorly to the zygomatic arch. The superficial temporal fascia splits about 2 cm above the zygomatic arch to enclose it. The space described by the split fascia is filled with fat. After crossing the zygomatic arch, the superficial temporal fascia is confluent with the parotidomasseteric fascia. The lingual surface of the mandible anterior to the muscles of mastication is composed of the suprahyoid region of muscles, which influences jaw position and integrates the function of the mandible with related structures (Fig. 1–11). The suprahyoid region has an important role in tongue mobility, speech, mandibular depression, manipulating boluses of food, and swallowing.

The superior pharyngeal constrictor acts to help to initiate swallowing. It is a paired muscle that originates in the medial pterygoid plate and palate. This muscle lies in close functional apposition to the tensor and levator palatini muscles. It forms an attachment to the buccinator muscle in the pterygomandibular raphe and in the midline of the retropharynx as the median raphe. The superior pharyngeal constrictor inserts on the lingual surface of the mandible posterior to the mylohyoid ridge.

The mylohyoid muscle is a paired thin membranous muscle that elevates and stabilizes the tongue, particularly when a bolus of food is retrieved from the check or when the tongue is elevated in swallowing. This muscle originates bilaterally from a broad attachment on the mylohyoid ridge of the lingual surface of the mandible. By joining in the midline as the mylohyoid raphe, it completes a membrane dividing the floor of the mouth from the neck. The mylohyoid inserts into the anterior body of the hyoid bone (see Fig. 1–11).

The genioglossus muscle originates in a firm aponeurosis on the genial tubercle of the mandible. This muscle sends fibers in the midline of the tongue from its tip to the base, which assists in protrusion, retraction, and elevation of the tongue with the force being transmitted to the mandible.

The geniohyoid muscle connects the inferior aspect of the genial tubercle to the anterior aspect of the hyoid bone. This muscle functions to elevate the hyoid bone and to stabilize the mandible posteriorly during swallowing and speech.

The digastric muscle is a paired muscle with both anterior and posterior bellies connected by a tendinous sling attached to the hyoid bone (see Fig. 1–11). The sling is composed of a round tendon that attaches the anterior and posterior bellies and a loop that acts as a pulley attached to the lateral cornu of the hyoid bone. The anterior belly attaches to the broad, ovoid digastric fossae in the parasymphysis of the lingual surface of the mandible. This belly is positioned almost directly and posteriorly to the sling. The posterior belly turns at an obtuse angle to attach to the skull at the mastoid notch. The digastric muscle acts to produce mandibular depression and retropositioning of

the mandibular symphysis. On the facial surface of the mandibular body, proximal to the mental foramen, the buccinator muscle attaches. The buccinator muscle inserts along the external oblique ridge of the mandible from behind the mental foramen to the insertion of the temporalis on the anterior ramus. In the maxilla the buccinator attaches high on the alveolar process behind the zygomatic process. The fibers of the buccinator are arranged horizontally. Anteriorly, these fibers attach to the mucosa, skin, and muscle of the lip. Posteriorly, the buccinator ends in the pterygomandibular raphe. The action of the buccinator is to stabilize the cheek when a bolus of food is being masticated.

The muscles of facial expression are attached to the labial surface of the mandible. The platysma muscle inserts into the skin of the face and neck and attaches to the labial aspect of the inferior border from the mandibular body to the mentum. The depressor anguli oris, depressor labii inferioris, orbicularis oris, and mentalis all have attachments on the labial surface of the mandibular symphysis. The fibers of these muscles insert into the soft tissues of the lower lip and chin. Their action is to provide facial expression and lip function. The contribution that the muscles of facial expression make to mandibular position is usually minor but may need to be considered in hyperactivity states.

BLOOD SUPPLY TO THE CRANIOMANDIBULAR REGION

All of the blood supply to the TMJ, mandible, mandibular muscles, and associated soft tissues is derived from the external carotid arterial system. The external carotid artery enters the craniomandibular region at the anterior aspect of the posterior belly of the digastric muscle. During its course in the superior neck, it sends two anterior branches of importance to the craniomandibular region, the lingual and facial arteries. The external carotid artery courses superiorly and posteriorly embedded in the substance of the parotid gland. At the level of the condylar neck, it bifurcates into the superficial temporal artery and the internal maxillary artery. These two arteries provide the main supply to the muscles of mastication and the TMJ (Fig. 1–12).

The lingual artery courses anteriorly from the external carotid artery into the deep surface of the hyoglossus muscle. Before entering the tongue, the lingual artery branches to form the sublingual artery, which supplies the floor of the mouth and the mylohyoid muscle. The lingual artery then courses into the parenchyma of the tongue, where it supplies the intrinsic muscles.

The facial artery may arise simultaneously with the lingual artery or superior to it on the anterior surface of the external carotid artery.[9] In the neck, the facial artery sends the ascending palatine artery to the superior constrictor. This artery then courses through the submandibular gland and over the antegonial notch anterior to the angle of the mandible. At this point, its pulse is easily palpable. The submental branch forms just beneath the antegonial notch to supply the anterior belly of the digastric muscle. Before ending at the superior lateral border of the nose, the facial artery produces the inferior and superior labial arteries, which supply the lips.

The internal maxillary artery arises from the external carotid artery just deep and posterior to the mandible at the level of the coronoid notch. This artery courses at a near right angle forward and superiorly to cross just medial to the condylar neck. As it moves medially through the parotid, the internal maxillary artery enters the infratemporal fossae. DuBrul and colleagues[10] have stated that the internal maxillary artery crosses lateral to the external pterygoid muscle in slightly greater than 50% of specimens and medial to this muscle in the remainder. In these cases, the artery is in close apposition to the inferior alveolar and lingual nerves. The internal maxillary artery exits the infratemporal fossae, according to Turvey and Fonseca[11] about 2.5 cm above the pterygomaxillary fissure. The artery then enters the pterygopalatine fossae where it forms its last branches deep and inferior to the globe.

The internal maxillary artery has branches that supply most of the deep structures of the face. These include all of the muscles of mastication and all of the facial bones and teeth. For the purpose of organization, the branches of the internal maxillary artery may be divided into three sections.[9]

The first section, the inferior alveolar artery courses at 90 degrees to the internal maxillary artery inferiorly and laterally to enter the mandible at the lingula. This completes a 180-degree turn from the direction of the external carotid artery. The inferior alveolar artery provides the entire endosteal blood supply to the mandible. Branches turn again at 180 degrees to provide the endosteal blood supply to the condyle. Anterior branches of the inferior alveolar artery include the mental artery, which exits the mental foramen, and the incisive artery, which supplies the mandibular symphysis. The mylohyoid branch of the inferior alveolar artery exits before the lingula and supplies the floor of the mouth.

The first section of the internal maxillary artery also sends two branches to the ear. The deep auricular artery and the anterior tympanic artery supply the external and middle ear. By piercing the cartilage of the external auditory canal, the deep auricular artery may supply a portion of the retrodiscal tissue of the TMJ. The middle meningeal artery exits the internal maxillary artery superiorly, passes in close apposition to the auricular temporal nerve, and supplies the dura via the foramen spinosum.

The second section of the internal maxillary artery supplies the muscle of mastication and the buccinator. The deep temporal arteries enter the temporalis muscle from the infratemporal fossae. The masseteric artery exits anteriorly and courses over the coronoid notch to supply the masseter muscle. The masseteric artery also sends branches to supply the anterior and deep aspect of the TMJ capsule. Small pterygoid branches extend both superiorly and inferiorly from the internal maxillary artery to supply the pterygoid muscles. Before leaving the infratemporal fossae, the internal maxillary artery sends the buccal artery anteriorly to supply the buccinator muscle.

The third section of the internal maxillary artery contains those branches that exit following the passage through the pterygomaxillary fissure. These branches include the posterior superior alveolar artery, the descending palatine artery, and the infraorbital artery that supply respective portions of the maxilla. The vidian artery, the pterygopalatine artery, and the sphenopalatine artery are also included and supply respective portions of the pharynx, eustachian tube, and nasal cavity.

At the source of the internal maxillary artery, the external carotid artery ends. Continuing superiorly is the superficial temporal artery, which takes a tortuous course to cross the zygomatic arch about 1.5 mm anterior to the external auditory canal. Just prior to crossing the arch, the superficial temporal artery releases the transverse facial artery anteriorly. Superior to the zygomatic arch, the middle temporal artery is formed to supply the temporalis muscle. Above the helix of the ear, the superficial temporal artery divides into branches to supply the scalp.

NERVE SUPPLY TO THE CRANIOMANDIBULAR REGION

The function of the craniomandibular articulation is controlled by communication via peripheral nerves to and from the central nervous system. These peripheral nerves may be divided as afferent sensory, efferent motor, and autonomic. Afferent sensory nerves send the brain information about the environment and status of body parts. While general afferent fibers provide pain and touch sensation, the special afferent sensory fibers communicate taste, smell, sight and hearing. The efferent motor nerves send signals that control movement of muscles. The autonomic nervous system provides information and causes visceral function to produce cardiovascular control, glandular secretion, and peristalsis in the craniomandibular region.

The trigeminal (fifth) cranial nerve provides most of the general somatic efferent motor and afferent sensory innervation to the craniomandibular region (Fig. 1–13). After exiting the foramen ovale, the third division of the fifth cranial nerve enters the infratemporal fossae. From this point, this nerve supplies motor activity for all of the masticatory muscles, the mylohyoid, and the anterior belly of the digastric muscle. The masseteric nerve branches out of the infratemporal fossae laterally over the coronoid notch to supply the masseter muscle. The posterior and anterior deep temporal nerves then leave and supply the temporalis muscle. The medial pterygoid nerve exits the third division attached to the otic ganglion in the infratemporal fossae. This nerve then supplies the medial pterygoid muscle. The lateral pterygoid nerve branches caudad from the buccal nerve.

General sensory innervation of the third division of the fifth cranial nerve is via its main branches: buccal, lingual, inferior alveolar, and auriculotemporal nerves. The buccal nerve exits first to supply the mucosa and deep tissues of the cheek. The lingual nerve descends into the submandibular triangle medial to the mandible, crosses the floor of the mouth inferior to Wharton's duct, and supplies the anterior two thirds of the tongue. The nerve carries with it fibers of the chorda tympani, which supply taste fibers to the tongue. The inferior alveolar nerve supplies the mandible distal to the lingula. The lymphohyoid nerve is a branch of the inferior alveolar nerve that supplies the floor of the mouth and the anterior belly of the digastric muscle.

The auriculotemporal nerve exits the third division in a posterior direction in the infratemporal fossae and then divides to send a branch to supply the parotid and skin over the temporal region. The nerve's other branch descends to supply the capsule of the TMJ (Fig. 1–14). This branch enters the joint posteriorly and laterally and can be seen in the retrodiscal tissue. The most anterior portion of the joint capsule is supplied by twigs of the posterior deep temporal and masseteric nerves.

The seventh cranial nerve contributes motor and deep sensory fibers to the craniomandibular region. After exiting the stylomastoid, the foramen branches extend to supply motor function to the posterior belly of the digastric muscle and the muscles of facial expression. The first branching of the supply to the muscles of facial expression occurs behind the condylar neck where the temporal ramus proceeds superiorly and anteriorly and the cervicofacial ramus exits inferiorly and anteriorly. Al-Kayat and Bramley[12] have reported that this bifurcation occurs at a mean of 3 cm inferior to the postglenoid tubercle (a structure comparable in cephalad-caudad position to the lateral pole of the condyle). Branching of the temporal ramus over the eminentia articularis produces the infraorbital, zygomatic, and temporal branches. The temporal branch crosses the zygomatic arch closest to the capsule of the TMJ, where it may be bound tightly to the temporal fascia. Al-Kayat states that its position is variable from 0.8 cm to 3.5 cm in front of the external auditory canal. The temporal branches proceed to supply the elevators of the forehead. The zygomatic and infraorbital branches supply the orbicularis oculi and expressive muscles of the midface, respectively.

The cervicofacial ramus of the seventh nerve produces the buccal branch to the buccinator and the marginal mandibular branch to the depressors of the lip. The nerve's cervical branches supply the platysma.

The autonomic nerve supply to the craniomandibular region provides visceral efferent fibers. The sympathetic nerves are postganglionic fibers from the superior cervical ganglion. Fibers destined for the craniomandibular region follow the course of the external carotid artery and its branches. The fibers supply all of the smooth muscle (arterial, salivary, and subcutaneous) of the craniomandibular region, including the TMJ. The parasympathetic nerve supply to the craniomandibular region is via preganglionic fibers that course with cranial nerves and a group of postganglionic fibers that arise in a group of extracranial ganglia deep in the head. Among these, the otic ganglion supplies the parotid and courses with the auriculotemporal nerve, innervating the TMJ.

SUMMARY

The anatomy of the craniomandibular articulation is the substance about which all conditions of the masticatory system depend. A thorough understanding of this anatomy provides the basis to reveal malfunctions and to initiate treatment. An integrated knowledge of osteology, connective tissue morphology, muscle morphology, neuroanatomy, and blood supply provides the practitioner with needed tools.

REFERENCES

1. Sarnat, B. and Laskin, D.: *The Temporomandibular Joint.* Charles C Thomas, Springfield, 1979.
2. Fried, L.: *Anatomy of the Head, Neck, Face, and Jaws.* Lea & Febiger, Philadelphia, 1980.
3. Komori, E., Masashi, S., et al: Discomalleolar ligament in the adult human. J. Craniomand. Pract. 4:299, 1987.
4. Sanders, B., Murakami, K., and Clark, G.: *Diagnostic and Surgical Arthroscopy of the Temporomandibular Joint.* W.B. Saunders Co., Philadelphia, 1989.
5. Wilkinson, T.: *The Relationship Between the Disk and the Lateral Pterygoid Muscle in the Human Temporomandibular Joint.* J. Prosth. Dent. 60:715–724, 1988.
6. McNamara, J.A.: The independent function of the two heads of the lateral pterygoid muscle. Am. J. Anat. 1387:197–206, 1973.
7. Carpentier, P., et al: Insertion of the lateral pterygoid muscle. J. Oral Maxillofac. Surg. 46:477–482, 1988.
8. Carpentier, P.: Microscopic study of the superior lateral pterygoid muscle attachment. J. Dent. Res. 65:1033, 1986.
9. Paff, G.: *Anatomy of the Head and Neck.* W.B. Saunders Co., Philadelphia, 1973.
10. DuBrul, E. and Sicher, L.: *Oral Anatomy.* C.V. Mosby Co., St. Louis, 1980.
11. Turvey, T. and Fonseca, R.: The anatomy of the internal maxillary in the pterygopalatal fossa. J. Oral Maxillofac. Surg. 38:92, 1982.
12. Al-Kayat, A. and Bramley, P.: A modified pre-auricular approach to the temporomandibular joint and malar arch. Br. J. Oral Surg. 17:91–103, 1980.

Daniel Buchbinder
Andrew S. Kaplan

C H A P T E R   2

Biology

Understanding of the temporomandibular joint (TMJ) function in health and disease requires an understanding of the different levels of its organization, including anatomy, pathology, physiology, histology, and pathophysiology. Without a familiarity with these different areas it is difficult to fully understand pathologic mechanisms.

This chapter describes the classification of joints and the development and function of diarthrodial joints. In addition, the ultrastructure of the TMJ and descriptions of the articular cartilage and the disc, synovium, and retrodiscal tissue are presented. The goals are to present the reader with a perspective as to where the TMJ fits in among the other joints in the body and to provide a basis from which an understanding of pathologic processes discussed further in this text can be built.

CLASSIFICATION OF JOINTS

An articulation is defined as a loose joining or connecting together so as to allow motion between the parts.[1] When the two objects are the bones of a skeleton, the articulation is called a joint. Joints can be classified in a number of different ways including the embryonic origin, presence or absence of movement, type of movement, size, shape, and location or the nature of the articulating surfaces.[2]

Mankin and Radin[3] divide joints into three general categories as follows:

CLASS I. Joints with bony components that are connected by a *synarthrosis* (Fig. 2–1)—an immovable union of connective tissue as seen in the sutures of the cranium.

CLASS II. Joints that allow only slight mobility. This type of joint is called an *amphiarthrosis*. This category includes the facet joints found in the spinal cord (Fig. 2–2).

CLASS III. Completely movable joints or *diarthrosis*. The shoulders, knees, and hips are included in this category as well as the TMJ.

Synarthroses can be further divided into five subgroups as follows:[3]

1. The first group includes the sutures of the skull that form a fibrous attachment. The edges of these joints interlock or overlap. Over the course of life, the bony components more closely approximate each other and eventually form a bony union called a *synostosis*.

2. A second group of joints have bony components that are adapted to each other in a way similar to the way a peg adapts to a hole. This kind of joint is called a *gomphosis*. A tooth sitting in its alveolar socket connected via its periodontal ligament is an example of this kind of joint.

3. The third group includes joints with components that are connected directly by a ligament or membrane. This joint is called a *syndesmosis*. An example is the shaft of the tibia and its connection to the shaft of the fibula (Fig. 2–3).

4. The fourth group includes joints with components that are connected by cartilage in the form of a disc, plate, or pad. This joint is termed a *symphysis*. The symphysis pubis is an example of this kind of joint (Fig. 2–4).

5. The fifth group includes joints with components that are connected by hyaline carti-

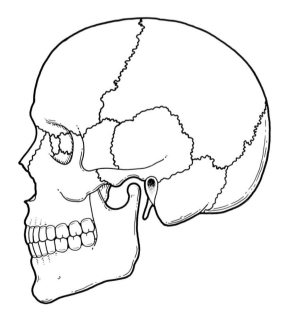

FIGURE 2–1. The sutures of the cranium are an example of synarthroses.

11

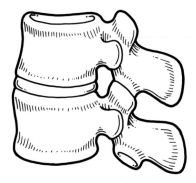

FIGURE 2–2. The facet joints of the spinal cord are examples of amphiarthroses.

lage. The joint is called a *synchondrosis*. The first sternocostal joint is an example.

DIARTHRODIAL JOINTS

Diarthrodial joints are freely movable, and the bony components are enclosed and connected to one another by a fibrous joint capsule. The capsule is lined with a synovial membrane and the joint cavity is filled with synovial fluid. For these reasons, these joints are also called *synovial joints*.[2,3]

The bony surfaces of diarthrodial joints are covered with articular cartilage and contain structures within or adjacent to the joints called plates or menisci. The fully developed diarthrodial joint is surrounded by a fibrous capsule and has associated ligamentous structures to prevent abnormal planes of movement or excessive slippage. In addition, these joints have well-developed muscle systems that not only allow for movement but protect and stabilize them from pathologic movements.

Usually, from within the connective tissue making up the capsule, thick parallel bands of

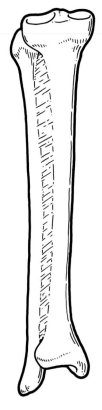

FIGURE 2–3. The connection of the tibia and fibula is an example of a syndesmosis.

collagen form the ligaments. They vary in tautness and insert on bone. The synovial lining inserts into the periosteum, extends along the margin of the articular cartilage, but does not cover functional surfaces. The nerve endings present in the synovial lining provide for proprioceptive and nociceptive inputs, which act as protective mechanisms.[4]

The collagenous covering of the articular structures allows a joint to withstand forces

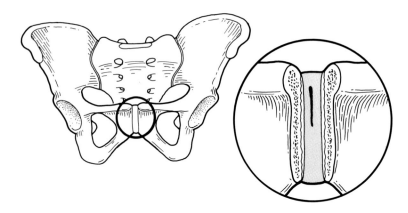

FIGURE 2–4. The pubis is an example of bones connected by a symphysis.

from both compression and movement simultaneously. Formed from chondrocytes and fibroblasts, this nonvascularized tissue must obtain its nutrition from the synovial fluid. The synovial fluid is kept in intimate contact with the functional surfaces of the joint by the capsule. Close apposition of the joint structures is maintained by a negative osmotic pressure. The inner lining or synovial membrane filters blood plasma and adds other elements to form the synovial fluid.[5]

Classification of Diarthrodial Joints

Diarthrodial joints can be subclassified, as based on the nature of their movement, into three categories: *uniaxial, biaxial,* and *triaxial.*[4,24] A uniaxial joint allows movement in one plane around a single axis and is often described as having one degree of freedom of motion.

Uniaxial joints are further subclassified into hinge and pivot types. A hinge joint is one with motion that resembles that of a door hinge (e.g., interphalangeal joint). A pivot or trochoid joint is a joint that has one component shaped like a wing and the second component shaped to articulate with the wing-shaped component (e.g., median atlantoaxial joint).[24]

Biaxial diarthrodial joints, the second subgroup, includes joints with components that can move in two planes around two axes, and these joints are often described as having two degrees of freedom. They are further subclassified into condyloid and saddle joints. The condyloid joint has a concave surface on one of its components, such that it can allow movement in two planes. A saddle joint has both convex and concave surfaces on both its bony components, and the surfaces fit together like a horse rider sitting in a saddle. The carpometacarpal joint of the thumb is an example.[24]

Triaxial diarthrodial joints, also known as multiaxial joints, have bony components free to move in three planes. These joints are said to have three degrees of motion, and movement can occur in oblique directions. Triaxial joints are further subdivided into two groups: plane joints and ball-and-socket joints. Plane joints have a gliding action between the articulating surfaces as seen in the TMJ. Ball-and-socket joints allow flexion/extension and adduction/abduction. Ball-and-socket joints are formed by a ball-like convex surface fitting into a concave socket as seen in the hip joint (Fig. 2–5).[24]

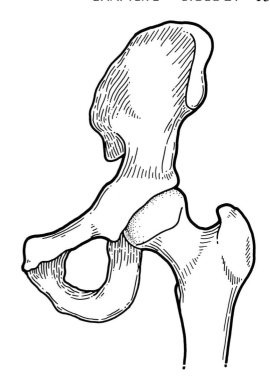

FIGURE 2–5. The hip joint is an example of a triaxial and ball-and-socket joint.

Development of Diarthrodial Joints

According to Harris,[4] O'Rahilly and Gardner[6] described the general sequence of the development of diarthrodial joints in five stages, following limb bud formation. These are briefly summarized here and in Figure 2–6).

1. *Condensation*—undifferentiated mesenchyme condenses to form a blastema.
2. *Chondrification*—the blastema divides into two components; intercellular sulfated material accumulates.
3. *Interzones (future joints)*—the space between the two components is an avascular, homogeneous, densely cellular area and secretes what is probably chondroitin sulfate, which forms an enlarged "interzone" area. This area serves as an appositional growth site.
4. *Formation of synovial mesenchyme*—the synovial tissue forms at the borders of the interzone; it is thought to originate from the blastema. Joint capsule, intracapsular ligaments, menisci, and tendons develop from the synovial mesenchyme. The synovial mesenchyme also becomes vascularized.
5. *Formation of the joint cavity*—small cavities appear by some as yet unknown mecha-

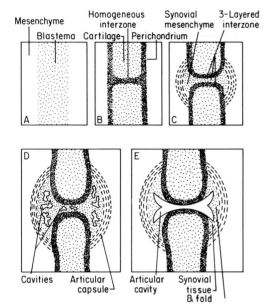

FIGURE 2–6. This diagram shows the general stages in the development of a synovial joint in utero. *A*, A single blastema forms. *B*, An interzone develops and splits the blastema into two parts and is highly cellular. *C*, A synovial mesenchyme develops around the periphery of the interzone and becomes vascularized. *D*, Cavities begin to form in the interzone and merge. *E*, The joint cavity forms, and the synovial lining differentiates. (Reprinted with permission from O'Rahilly, R. and Gardner, E.: In *The Joints and Synovial Fluid*, vol. I. Sokoloff, L. (ed.). Academic Press, New York, 1978.

Interposed between the condyle and the temporal component is a disc or meniscus also made of fibrocartilage. The disc acts to divide the joint into upper and lower compartments. The upper or superior compartment is bordered by the temporal fossa and the superior surface of the articular disc. It is in this portion of the joint that translation takes place. The lower or inferior compartment is bordered by the articulating surface of the mandibular condyle and the inferior surface of the articular disc. Rotational movement occurs in this portion of the joint.

The joint is enclosed by a fibrous capsule, which is lined by a synovial membrane. This membrane is highly vascular and is continuous with the connective tissue of the capsule and the disc. Each compartment is lined with its own synovial membrane. The synovial membrane allows diffusion of a plasma filtrate and adds components of its own to produce synovial fluid that fills both joint compartments. A passive volume in the upper compartment measures 1.2 ml and a passive volume in the lower compartment, about 0.9 ml.[8] The shape of the synovium is altered during functional movement. On opening, the superior surface of the articular disc has a sigmoid shape. The disc is firmly attached downward to the medial and lateral poles of the condylar head.

nism. These cavities coalesce and form joint spaces. As this process occurs, the joint becomes lined with either cartilage or synovium on all surfaces. The synovium secretes fluid that, in part, becomes the synovial fluid.

TEMPOROMANDIBULAR JOINT

The TMJ is considered a ginglymus diarthrodial joint, i.e., a joint with both rotational and translatory movement. The bones making up the joint are the mandibular condyle and the articular eminence (fossa) of the temporal bone. One of the features that distinguishes the TMJ from other joints in the body is that it is a bilateral diarthrosis, i.e., the left and right sides must function together. Another distinguishing feature from other diarthrodial joints is that the articulating surfaces are covered with fibrocartilage rather than hyaline cartilage. Also, the TMJ is the only joint in the human body to have a rigid endpoint of closure, that of the teeth making occlusal contact.[7]

Development of the Temporomandibular Joint

In contrast to other diarthrodial joints, the TMJ is the last joint to start development, beginning at about 7 weeks in utero.[7,9] Also, in contrast, the TMJ develops from two distinct blastemas. The first is the condylar blastema from which the condylar cartilage, the aponeurosis of the lateral pterygoid muscle, and the disc and capsule component composing the lower portion of the joint are derived. The second is the temporal blastema, which eventually forms the articular surface of the temporal component and the structures of the upper portion of the joint.[10] The condylar and temporal blastemas begin their growth at relatively distant sites but move toward each other as the joint develops.[11]

Development of the TMJ has been reviewed in several sources, the details of which are not all in agreement.[7,9–11] The general sequence of events is described here and is largely based on the work of Perry and coworkers.[11] Figure 2–7

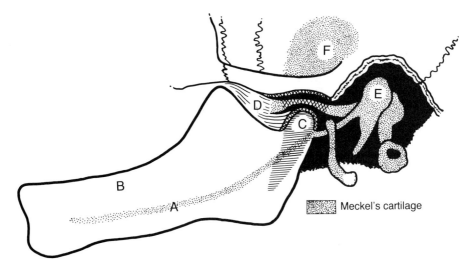

FIGURE 2–7. Diagram showing the structures involved in the formation of the temporomandibular joint. *A,* Meckel's cartilage. *B,* The developing mandible (dentary bone). *C,* Developing condyle. *D,* Lateral pterygoid and fibrous attachment extending to the malleus. *E,* Malleus. *F,* Developing temporal component. (Adapted with permission from Mohl, N.: The temporomandibular joint. In *A Textbook of Occlusion.* Mohl, N., et al (eds.). Quintessence Publishing Co., Lombard, IL., 1988.)

is a diagrammatic representation of the structures involved in the development of the TMJ.

The condylar blastema forms at the distal end of the primordium of the mandible, also called the dentary, and is seen before the temporal blastema. Both blastemas are detectable at a 38- to 45-mm crown/rump (CR) length. Lateral to the blastema is a band of cells extending to Meckel's cartilage medially. Although the temporal blastema appears after the condylar blastema, it calcifies first. Concurrent with the appearance of these blastemas is the differentiation of the muscles of mastication.

At the 45-mm CR stage the condylar blastema still is rather undifferentiated, but changes in the cellular orientation begin to take place. In addition, a cavitation develops between the condylar blastema and the band of mesenchyme connecting to Meckel's cartilage, later to become the inferior joint space. The temporal blastema shows an increase in ossification and a loss of its blastema-like character. Inferior to this region, a band of mesenchyme develops.

After formation of the inferior joint cavity, the condylar blastema begins calcification in the marginal areas. In the center of the blastema, chondrocytes differentiate and will be the site of secondary cartilage formation. The lateral pterygoid forms a fibrous attachment with the malleus in the ear (formerly the proximal portion of Meckel's cartilage), passing

through the joint space and probably contributing to the formation of the articular disc.[7]

The mesenchymal area inferior to the temporal region becomes a fibrous band. Cavitation occurs between this fibrous band and the fibrous band that formed above the developing condyle to produce the superior joint space. This process occurs at about the 70-mm CR stage. As the condyle continues to differentiate, secondary cartilage forms within the central region.[11]

After formation of the superior joint cavity, the medial and then the lateral aspects of the condyle differentiate. Interruption arteries become evident in the condylar head and are associated with new areas of calcification. By the 112-mm CR stage, chondrocytes have differentiated and show the typical organization of the postnatal condyle.[11]

Organization of the Articular Cartilage of the Condyle and Eminence of the TMJ

The ultrastructure of the articular cartilage can be divided into four zones. The following description is based on the work of de Bont and coworkers:[12–14]

ZONE I. This articular zone is found adjacent to the joint cavity and forms the outermost functional surface. Most of the collagen fibers are arranged in bundles and oriented nearly parallel to the articular surface, although some fibers are found to run obliquely. The fibers are tightly packed and are able to withstand the forces of movement (Fig. 2–8). The arrangement of the collagen, as seen on scanning electron microscopy (SEM), shows an organization of thin bands of interwoven fibrils arranged in sheets. Superimposed on this network, forming the articular surface, is a layer of coiled collagen fibrils having a cotton wool–like appearance. The articular surface is somewhat less densely packed than the layer below termed the superficial layer of the articular zone. Toward the proliferative zone, the collagen fibrils show a more oblique orientation. Figure 2–9 shows the topography of the articular surface as seen under the SEM.

ZONE II. This is also known as the proliferative zone and is mainly cellular. It is in this area that undifferentiated mesenchymal tissue is found. This tissue is pluripotent and allows for proliferation of the articular cartilage in response to new functional demands placed on it.[15] Scanning electron micrographs show the proliferative zone to be a fairly well-defined line of demarcation between the articular and fibrocartilage zones.

ZONE III. In the fibrocartilaginous zone, the collagen fibrils appear to be arranged in bundles in a crossing pattern, although some of the collagen is seen in a radial orientation. The fibrocartilage appearance with SEM is of a random orientation. This random orientation gives the fibrocartilage a three-dimensional network offering resistance against compressive and lateral forces.

ZONE IV. The calcified cartilage zone has a collagen arrangement similar to that seen in zone III. The SEM appearance is also similar, with the exception of some radially oriented fibrils.

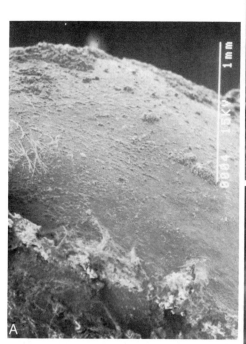
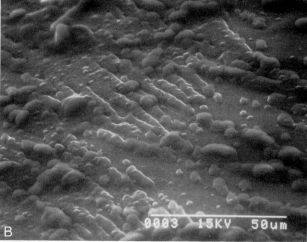
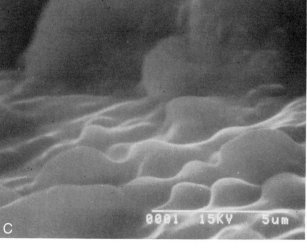

FIGURE 2–9. Scanning electron micrograph of the articular surface of the condyle. Note the texture of the articular surface probably caused by protuding collagen fibers covered with matrix. *A*, 50×. *B*, 1500×. *C*, 10,000×.

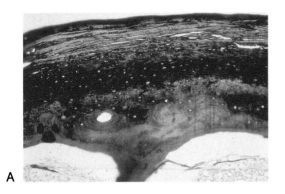

A

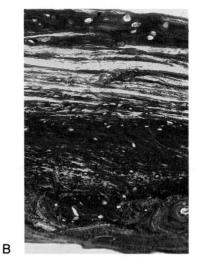

B

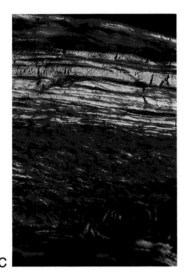

C

FIGURE 2–8. *A*, Low power light microscopic view showing structural layers. *B*, High power view showing delineation of the four zones: 1, articular zone; 2, proliferative zone; 3, fibrocartilage zone; and 4, calcified cartilage zone. *C*, Same view under polarized light.

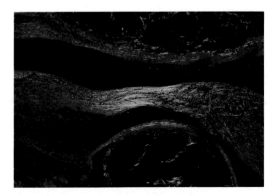

FIGURE 2–14. Light microscopic appearance under polarized light of the disc in sagittal section. Note the anterior/posterior orientation of the collagen on the superficial layers and the random orientation in the central regions.

Chondrocytes and chondroblasts are found distributed throughout the articular cartilage. Fibrocytes predominate in the articular zone, fibroblasts and chondroblasts in the proliferative zone, and chondrocytes in the deeper zones.

Organization of the Fibrocartilage in the Disc

The disc is divided into three different bands. The band sitting at 12-o'clock on the head of the condyle in the closed position is the thickest portion. The middle band sits along the articular eminence in the closed position and is the thinnest portion. The anterior band lies farthest forward and is generally of intermediate thickness (Fig. 2–10). The disc provides stability for movement of the TMJ and gives it the ability for both rotational and translatory movement.

The collagen fibers of the superficial layers of the anterior and posterior bands as well as the middle band run in an anterior/posterior direction. The fibers in the central region of the anterior and posterior bands are oriented in a random fashion. This orientation gives the disc the ability to resist forces in two directions, stretching forces in an anterior/posterior direction by the superficial layers and compressive loading by the three-dimensional network in the central region. Chondrocytes are found distributed throughout the disc, and some fibrocytes are also seen (Figs. 2–11 to 2–14).[16]

PHYSIOLOGY OF CARTILAGE

Cartilage is a highly differentiated form of connective tissue. It consists of chondrocytes embedded in a matrix composed largely of collagen fibers and proteoglycan aggregates.[3,4,12] The collagen fibers are usually oriented randomly, forming a three-dimensional network, helping the tissue maintain its shape when forces are applied to it from different directions. Proteoglycan aggregates are composed of a hyaluronic acid backbone and multiple proteoglycan monomer side chains (Fig. 2–15),[17] giving a bottle brush–like appearance.[12] The aggregates become entangled with the collagen fibers physically and probably chemically.[12] The proteoglycan molecules can bind large quantities of water giving cartilage its properties of elasticity and distensibility.

Most cartilage, but not all, found in the human body covers the articular surfaces of bone. The smooth, lubricated surfaces permit easy movement. Three forms of cartilage are found in the human body: hyaline, elastic, and fibrocartilage.[18]

HYALINE CARTILAGE. This cartilage is found on the articulating surface of long bones, in the larynx, and in some parts of the bronchial tree. Hyaline cartilage is composed of chondrocytes separated by a considerable amount of intercellular matrix. The chondrocytes lie within a lacuna, and each lacuna can contain one or a cluster of several chondrocytes. The size of the chondrocyte is dependent on its state of activ-

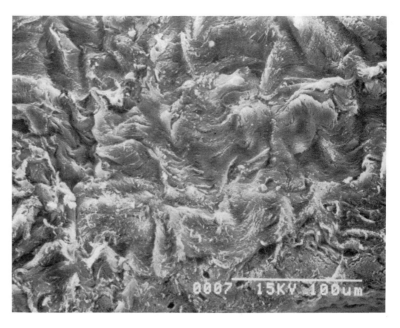

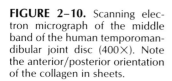

FIGURE 2–10. Scanning electron micrograph of the middle band of the human temporomandibular joint disc (400×). Note the anterior/posterior orientation of the collagen in sheets.

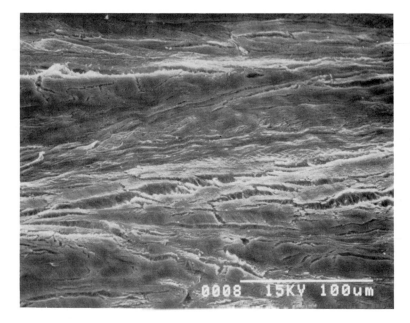

FIGURE 2–11. Scanning electron micrograph of the superficial layer of the posterior band of the disc (400×). Note the anterior/posterior orientation of the cartilage.

ity. Typically, the nucleus is large and the cell body fills the lacuna. Half of the intercellular matrix is composed of collagen fibers of variable lengths and thicknesses. The fibers are masked by a ground substance, which is thought to assist formation of larger fiber bundles during matrix synthesis.[18]

ELASTIC CARTILAGE. This cartilage is found in the larnyx, epiglottis, external ear, and symphysis pubis. Elastic cartilage is much more flexible than hyaline cartilage and exhibits properties similar to those of elastomers. This tissue easily undergoes deformation and rapidly returns to its original shape. In addition to collagen and proteoglycan aggregates, elastic cartilage contains a large number of elastic fibers present in a branching network.[18]

FIBROCARTILAGE. This cartilage has the same general properties found in hyaline cartilage but tends to be less distensible, owing to a greater proportion of dense collagen fibers. In addition, the matrix is sparse with numerous

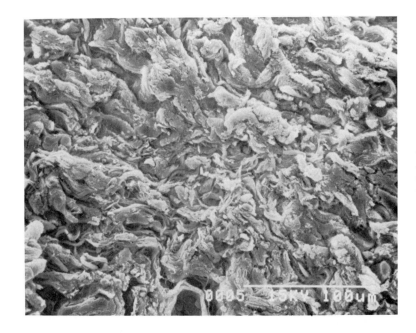

FIGURE 2–12. Scanning electron micrograph of the central area of the posterior band of the disc (400×). Note the random orientation of the collagen fibers.

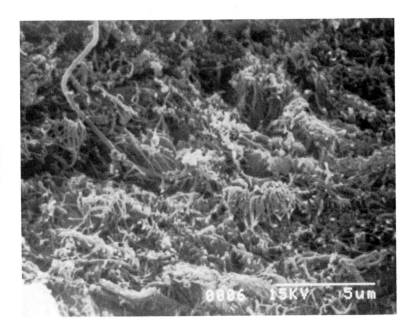

FIGURE 2–13. Scanning electron micrograph of the central area of the posterior band of the disc (6000×). Note the random orientation of the collagen fibers.

collagen fibers visible as large irregular bundles between groups of chondrocytes. The chondrocytes are arranged in rows parallel to the collagen bundles in pairs or singularly.[18]

The development of fibrocartilage reflects its intermediate nature between dense connective tissue and hyaline cartilage. During development, fibrocartilage appears first as connective tissue. The fibroblasts present in this tissue gradually transform into chondroblasts. They secrete a thin layer of matrix around themselves. The secretion, however, is limited, and the collagen bundles never become incorporated into the sparse matrix.[19] A perichondrium also fails to develop in fibrocartilaginous joints and, hence, in the TMJ.[19]

The fibrocartilage, in part, acts as a shock absorber. By providing space between bones, fibrocartilage gives the joint freedom of movement and the larger content of fibers gives the joint surface greater strength against forces in many directions.

In the TMJ, fibrocartilage covers the articular eminence and the condylar head and as noted forms the articular disc. The cartilage tends to be thickest in the functional areas of the joint, the posterior slope of the articular eminence, and the anterior slope of the condylar head. The cartilage is thinnest at the roof of the glenoid fossa where little or no function occurs in a normal joint.[15]

Fibrocartilage is an avascular, alymphatic, and aneural tissue.[12] It is normally attached firmly to the underlying bone. Healthy cartilage has a white and smooth, glistening gross appearance, although the color becomes yellow with normal aging.[4] No projections, lumps, ridges, or roughness should be evident. The thickness found in the TMJ is about 0.5 mm but varies according to the amount of function in a given area.[20] As is all cartilage, it is predominantly composed of chondrocytes, collagen fibrils, proteoglycans, and water. The collagen fibrils and the proteoglycans form the matrix. Glycoprotein and small fractions of lipids and inorganic material also can be found in the matrix.

As previously mentioned, proteoglycans are hydrophilic in nature and therefore attract water. The ground substance has been described as a hydrophilic gel that swells when infused with water present in the synovial fluid. The amount of swelling is limited by the tension exerted by the stretching collagen fibrils. Because of this mechanism, collagen fibers are under continuous stress even when the joint is not being loaded.[12]

Upon loading, the fibrocartilage has increased internal pressure as more and more force is placed on the collagen fibrils. If the internal pressure exceeds the osmotic pressure within the matrix, water squeezes out and into the synovial fluid, which is thought to assist lubrication. As subsequently discussed, this process is called "weeping lubrication." As the

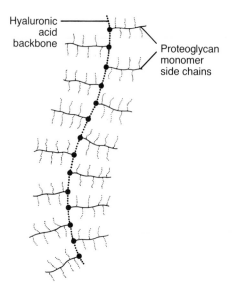

FIGURE 2–15. Proteoglycan aggregates are made up of a hyaluronic acid backbone and multiple proteoglycan monomer side chains giving the molecule a bottle brush–like appearance.

loading decreases, the osmotic pressure will exceed the hydrostatic pressure and water will again be taken up by the matrix.

The fibrocartilage, having no blood supply of its own, derives its nutrition by a double-diffusion system. Blood vessels lining the synovium and retrodiscal tissues allow diffusion of nutrients into the synovial fluid, and the synovial fluid diffuses through the dense matrix of cartilage to the chondrocytes (Fig. 2–16).

Degenerative changes result in degenerative cartilage of the posterior slope of the articular eminence and the condylar head, the functional surfaces.[21] Microscopic debris produced by this degeneration is digested by type A cells or macrophage-like cells present in the synovial membrane. Excessive particulate debris resulting from severe trauma often produces inflammation and pain and results in synovitis.[22]

SYNOVIAL TISSUE AND SYNOVIAL FLUID

The synovial tissue is a vascular connective tissue lining the fibrous joint capsule.[4] It starts at the posterior border of the disc and inserts inferiorly to the articulating surface on the condyle. It then reflects on and covers the bone to the boundaries of the articulating surfaces.[23] The largest area of the synovial tissue is on the superior and inferior retrodiscal lamina.[23] Here, the synovial tissue forms small folds or villi that stretch on translation of the condyle and disc. Both upper and lower joint compartments are lined with synovial tissue. The articulating surfaces of the temporal bone, the condyle, and the disc are not covered.

The synovial tissue can be divided into three layers.[3] The synovial lining or intima is the layer most intimate with the functional joint surfaces. It is a discontinuous layer, usually one- to four-cell layers thick, and in some areas the cells are widely spread apart. The thinnest areas are those in closest contact with movable portions of the joint. The second layer is called

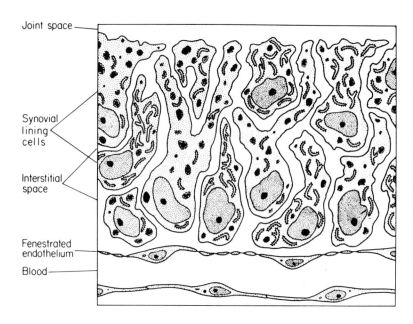

FIGURE 2–16. Diagram of synovial tissue. Diffusion of a plasma filtrate that will become a major component of the synovial fluid providing nutrients to the avascular cartilaginous components of the joint. Passage of this filtrate occurs through the microvascular endothelium of the subsynovial tissue and the interstitial spaces of the synovial lining. (Reprinted with permission from Simkin, P.: Synovial physiology. In *Arthritis and Allied Conditions,* 11th ed. D. McCarty (ed.). Lea & Febiger, Philadelphia, 1989.)

the subsynovial tissue, which is made up of cells that resemble the synovial lining but with a more developed connective tissue network. A rich supply of blood vessels is found in this layer. The third layer is the capsule, a relatively acellular layer with thick bands of collagen, which forms the outer boundary of the joint.

The cellular composition of synovial tissue includes type A cells, which resemble macrophages, type B cells, which resemble fibroblasts, and type C cells, which are intermediate in composition between type A and B. Type B cells make up about 80% of the content of the synovial lining. These cells are embedded in a connective tissue matrix called the synovial stroma. This consists of a loose network of collagen and proteoglycan aggregates. An ample supply of capillary, lymph, and nerves exists. The type B cells have a greater abundance of secretory granules and produce hyaluronic acid, a component of synovial fluid thought to be a key ingredient in providing friction-free movement.[4,23] Type A cells help keep the joint fluid free of debris.

Synovial surfaces are nonadherent. The cells on the surface bind to the underlying matrix but do not bind to the opposing tissue. Constant movement against opposing surfaces are thought to break down any forming cross links. Collagenase secretion of the synovial lining cells also helps prevent the formation of surface adhesions and ensures that fragmented collagen on the tissue surface does not activate the coagulation cascade.

The surfaces made of cartilage and synovial tissue are able to move over each other with little resistance. This movement is achieved by the surface structure of the tissues, the adsorbed macromolecules, and the synovial fluid through two complementary mechanisms:[4]

1. During movement under conditions of loading, the hydrostatic pressure exceeds the pressure within the cartilage itself, causing a squeezing out of synovial fluid. The fluid is pushed out just ahead of the contacting joint surfaces. This process is known as *weeping lubrication.*

2. During movement under conditions of little or no loading, there is thought to exist a glycoprotein that binds to the surface of the cartilage called the "lubricating protein," to keep the cartilage surfaces of a joint from actually making contact. This process is known as *boundary lubrication.*

Synovial lining in a normal joint does not get trapped between cartilage surfaces during func-

tion. It manages to maintain its surface structure and integrity of blood and lymph vessels during repeated and rapid movement. The presence of villous projections gives synovial tissue its inherent ability to deform and thus adapt to all joint movements.[5] Synovial tissue also has the ability to regenerate when damaged.

Synovial fluid is a filtrate of plasma. The plasma passes through fenestrations in the subendothelial capillaries into the intercellular spaces. Because there is no epithelium and hence no basement membrane, no barrier exists between the synovium and the fluid present in the joint spaces.[3] The movement across the synovial tissue, at least for small molecules, is mainly passive diffusion, although speculation exists that certain small and large molecules pass through via active transport and facilitated diffusion.[5]

RETRODISCAL TISSUE

The retrodiscal tissue[24] or bilaminar zone consists of a mass of soft tissue, which occupies the posterior joint space between the articular disc and posterior capsule. As its name implies, it consists of two laminae of dense connective tissue, the superior and inferior laminae, with a central layer of loose areolar, highly vascular, and well-innervated tissue.

The superior lamina originates from the posterior band of the disc and attaches to the squamotympanic fissure.[25] The superior lamina is composed mainly of loose fibroelastic tissue with a high elastin content. It has been suggested that this lamina is a remnant of the discomalleolar ligament of the fetus, which connects the lateral pterygoid tendon to the malleus through the squamotympanic fissure.[26,27] The function of the superior lamina is to counter the forward pull of the superior belly of the lateral pterygoid muscle on the articular disc. This stabilizing function is evident during the translatory phase of full mouth opening, when the condyle is displaced anteroinferiorly on the articular eminence. In this position, the retrodiscal tissue is fully stretched and exerts posterior tractive forces on the disc preventing it from dislocating anteriorly. This function also results in a posterior rotation of the meniscus allowing the thin intermediate portion of the disc to remain between the articular surfaces of the condyle and eminence. At rest, the disc occupies the most forward rotated position on the condyle that is permitted by the width of the articular space.[28] With the exception of the later phase of the translatory movement, the pterygoid muscle tonus will have a greater effect on the disc position and exceeds the elastic traction of the retrodiscal tissue.

The superior surface is covered by a synovial membrane, which is three- to four-cell layers thick. Lymphatics and venous and arterial capillaries are present in the subsynovial tissue. This is a major source of synovial fluid, important for the lubrication and nutrition of the articular surfaces.

The intermediate retrodiscal lamina is composed of loose connective tissue rich in vascular and nerve supply. The neurovascular tissue is most prominent in the posterior portion of the retrodiscal tissue, just inferior to the squamotympanic fissure. Griffin and Sharpe[29] noted the presence of both myelinated and unmyelinated nerve fibers, which appear to be closely associated with the blood vessels in this area. They also described the presence of articular arteries, probably derived from the anterior tympanic artery and internal maxillary artery. A large number of venules are also present within this lamina.

As the condyle translates forward, the volume of the retrodiscal tissue expands owing to venous distention and filling of the vacated glenoid fossa. When the condyle returns to occupy this space, the retrodiscal tissue once again returns to its former shape and size.

The inferior lamina of the retrodiscal tissue is the posteroinferior extension of the retrodiscal tissue. This lamina originates from the posterior band of the disc and inserts to the inferior margin of the posterior articular slope of the condyle. Unlike the superior lamina, the inferior lamina is composed mainly of collagenous fibers with very little elastic tissue. This histologic "wavy" appearance is characteristic of ligamentous structures.

Because of the lack of elastic fibers, the inferior lamina will not "stretch" as is the case with the superior lamina. The inferior lamina acts to stabilize the disc on top of the articular surface of the condyle. As the condyle translates forward, the disc will displace posteriorly to maintain close contact between the intermediate band of the disc and articular surface of the condyle, and the inferior lamina will not be under any tension. As is the case with the superior lamina, the inferior lamina is lined with a villous synovium with the same degree of subsynovial vascularity. The synovial fluid aids in lubrication and nutrition of the structures within the lower joint space.

Pressure changes in the retrodiscal tissue have been measured and found to be negative when the condyle translates forward and positive when the condyle is seated in the glenoid fossa.[29] A patient with a class III malocclusion tends to have higher pressures when the condyle is in its most retruded position. The normal range of pressures measured was $\pm$ 1 mm Hg.

Physiologically, the retrodiscal tissue ensures structural flexibility and stability of the intraarticular disc during function and supplies synovial fluid important in joint lubrication and nutrition. Should this tissue become damaged, its physiologic functions may become severely impaired and may lead to masticatory dysfunction and degenerative joint disease.

REFERENCES

1. *Stedman's Medical Dictionary,* 22nd ed. Williams & Wilkins, Baltimore, 1972.
2. Norkin, C. and Levangie, P.: *Joint Structure and Function.* F.A. Davis, Philadelphia, 1983.
3. Mankin, H. and Radin, E.: Structure and function of joints. In *Arthritis and Allied Conditions,* 10th ed. D. McCarty (ed.). Lea & Febiger, Philadelphia, 1985.
4. Harris, E.: Biology of the joint. In *Textbook of Rheumatology.* W.H. Kelly, E.D. Harris, S. Ruddy, and C.B. Sledge (eds.). W.B. Saunders Co., Philadelphia, 1985.
5. Simkin, P.: Synovial physiology. In *Arthritis and Allied Conditions,* 10th ed. D. McCarty (ed.). Lea & Febiger, Philadelphia, 1985.
6. O'Rahilly, R. and Gardner, E.: The development of the knee joint of the chick and its correlation with embryonic staging. J. Morphol. 98:49–88, 1956.
7. Mohl, N.: The temporomandibular joint. In *A Textbook of Occlusion,* N. Mohl, G. Zarb, G. Carlsson, and J. Rugh (eds.). Quintessence, Chicago, 1988.
8. Toller, P.: Opaque arthrography of the TMJ. Int. J. Oral Surg. 3:17, 1974.
9. Doyle, D.: Embryology and evolution. In *Diseases of the Temporomandibular Apparatus,* 2nd ed. D. Morgan, L. House, W. Hall, and S. Vamvas (eds.). C.V. Mosby, St. Louis, 1982.
10. Baume, L.J.: Embryogenesis of the human temporomandibular joint. Science 138:904, 1962.
11. Perry, H., Xu, Y., and Forbes, D.: The embryology of the temporomandibular joint. J. Craniomand. Pract. 3:2, 126, 1985.
12. de Bont, L., de Haan, P., and Boering, G.: Cartilage of the temporomandibular joint. In *Temporomandibular Joint, Articular Cartilage Structure and Function.* Druk, Van Denderen, 1985.
13. de Bont, L., Boering, G., Havinga, P., and Liem, R.: Spatial arrangement of collagen fibrils in the articular cartilage of the mandibular condyle: a light microscopic and scanning electron microcopic study. In *Temporomandibular Joint, Articular Cartilage Structure and Function.* Druk, Van Denderen, 1985.
14. de Bont, L., Liem, R., and Boering, G.: Ultrastructure of the the articular cartilage of the mandibular con-

dyle: Aging and degeneration. Oral Surg. Oral Med. Oral Path. 60:631–641, 1985.

15. Hansson, T.: TMJ changes related to dental occlusion. In *Temporomandibular Joint Problems.* W. Solberg and G. Clark (eds.). Quintessence, Chicago, 1980.

16. de Bont, L., Liem, R., Havinga, P., and Boering, G.: Fibrous component of the TMJ disc. In *Temporomandibular Joint, Articular Cartilage Structure and Function.* Druk, Van Denderen, 1985.

17. Rosenberg, L.: Structure and function of proteoglycans. In *Arthritis and Allied Conditions,* 10th ed. D. McCarty (ed.). Lea & Febiger, Philadelphia, 1985.

18. Jee, W.: The skeletal tissues. In *Histology, Cell and Tissue Biology.* L. Weiss (ed.). Elsevier Biomedical Publishers, New York, 1988.

19. Jee, W.: The skeletal tissues. In *Histology, Cell and Tissue Biology.* L. Weiss (ed.). Elsevier Biomedical Publishers, New York, 1988.

20. Hansson, T., Oberg, T., Carlsson, G., and Kopp, S.: Thickness of soft tissue layers and the articular disk of the TMJ. Acta Odont. Scand. 35:77–83, 1977.

21. Mahan, P.: The TMJ in function and pathofunction. In *Temporomandibular Joint Problems.* W. Solberg and G. Clark (eds.). Quintessence, Chicago, 1980.

22. Goldman, J.: Soft tissue trauma of the TMJ. In *Textbook of Temporomandibular Disorders.* A. Kaplan and L. Assael (eds.). W.B. Saunders Co., Philadelphia, 1991.

23. Carson, D. and Fox, R.: Structure and function of synoviocytes. In *Arthritis and Allied Conditions,* 10th ed. D. McCarty (ed.). Lea & Febiger, Philadelphia, 1985.

24. Norkin, C. and Levangie, P.: *Joint Structure and Function.* F.A. Davis, Philadelphia, 1983.

25. Rees, A.L.: The structure and function of the mandibular joint. Br. Dent. J. 96:125–133, 1954.

26. Griffin, C.J. and Sharpe, C.J.: The structure of the human temporomandibular meniscus. Aust. Dent. J. Aug.: 190–195, 1960.

27. Pinto, O.F.: A new structure related to the temporomandibular joint and and middle ear. J. Prosth. Dent. 12:95–103, 1962.

28. Coleman, R.D.: Temporomandibular joint: Relation of the retrodiskal zone to Meckel's cartilage and lateral pterygoid muscle. J. Dent. Res. 49:3 626–630, 1970.

29. Findlay, I.A.: Mandibular joint pressures. J. Dent. Res. 43:140, 1964.

Charles B. Stacy

CHAPTER 3

Synopsis of Pain

Pain is a nearly ubiquitous phenomenon—a fact of everyday life. Pain is the chief symptom that brings patients to dental or medical attention. Usually, pain serves to point toward pathology and resolves when the pathologic stimulus is addressed. Pain indicates injury, and with healing comes the subsidence of pain. The commonplace view holds that "Pain is nature's way of telling you something is wrong." Yet, behind this familiar expression lies a realm of vast complexity, which the following vignettes exemplify.

Mr. A. notices an ache in his jaw, especially while eating. It worsens daily, and soon he is able to recognize that this pain emanates from one of his molars that is tender when he is biting down. The surrounding gingival tissue is swollen and sore. He takes aspirin with some immediate benefit and visits his dentist, who diagnoses an abscessed tooth. The expected increase in pain while the dentist treats the tooth is followed by a gradual reduction, abetted by the use of mild narcotics. Eventually, everything returns to normal.

Mr. B. goes to his dentist for a gradually increasing ache in his jaw, thinking he has a problem with his teeth. Instead, cancer is found in the floor of his mouth. Despite local excision, the pain continues to grow. Even with the assistance of mild narcotics, he is unable to sleep, loses weight, and feels constantly fatigued. The cancer is now invading the jaw, and a radical excision is performed. Once he heals, the pain abates, only to start again several months later. He becomes depressed, anorexic, exhausted, and irritable. Radiotherapy produces some temporary relief. Eventually, he requires a regimen of oral morphine at high doses, amitriptyline, hydroxyzine, and ibuprofen. With a tolerable level of comfort, but with increasing sedation, his final days are spent in a hospice.

Mr. C., who is an innocent victim in a street fight, is shot through the jaw. He is astounded that he feels no pain, although he realizes he has no control of his jaw, which is mangled and bleeding. In the emergency room, the surgeon manually examines Mr. C.'s wounds, but this causes no discomfort. A tetanus shot in the arm is painful as usual. Shortly after, Mr. C. is admitted to the hospital and a deep throbbing pain begins to grow. The patient becomes agitated and begins to perspire heavily. Relief comes only when an injection of morphine allows him to sleep.

Mrs. D. begins to note a sensitivity on the left side of her mouth while brushing her teeth or drinking something hot. She visits her dentist, who assures her that all her teeth are healthy. Nonetheless, the pain grows. Sometimes, it is extremely sharp and jabbing, almost electric. At times, even the slightest movement or contact triggers an attack. Out of frustration, she revisits her dentist, who extracts a tooth of questionable pathology, but the pain is only worsened. Finally, a specialist diagnoses trigeminal neuralgia and treats her with carbamazepine. The pain disappears.

Ms. E. develops excruciating pains that shoot up the side of her face and temple on either side, apparently without provocation. She is convinced that she is having a stroke or suffering from a brain tumor. When questioned, she is unaware of any relationship of the pains with her activities or life events. The examination shows exquisite sensitivity to palpation of the masseters and temporalis muscles bilaterally and to a lesser extent of the muscles of the posterior neck and shoulder girdle. She is resistant to the explanation that her pain is caused by muscular tension in the jaw and elsewhere and remains convinced such severe pains must indicate a problem of tremendous gravity. Eventually, she recognizes that her distress over her son's recent arrest on drug charges might be expressing itself in muscular tension. She begins biofeedback and nortriptyline therapy with eventual resolution of the problem.

These vignettes illustrate a number of important and not so obvious aspects of pain that are addressed subsequently. They might be summarized, by number, as (1) acute pain related to curable and familiar pathology, (2) acute and progressive pain caused by serious incurable pathology, (3) inconstant and dynamic relationship of pain to pathology, (4) neuritic pain mistaken for that of tissue damage, and (5) chronic pain caused by dysfunction of which the chief cause is psychosocial. In all cases, the pains carry identifiable signatures and respond to specific treatments. The role of the clinician consists of identifying the mechanisms responsible for a given patient's pain and providing appropriate therapy.

Pain, according to the definition adopted by the International Association for the Study of Pain, is "An unpleasant sensory and emotional experience associated with actual or potential tissue damage or described in terms of such damage."[1] Pain is not strictly a sensation, such as cold or heat or sharpness, for sensation lacks that inherent motivating power and insistence that characterize pain. In addition, pain is not simply emotional, as we all recognize the distinction between somatic pain arising from a particular part of the body and purely emotional pain from loss or disappointment. The relationship of pain to tissue damage is both physical and metaphoric. When describing or imaging pain, bodily harm is the coin: "My head is being crushed in a vise"; "like an ice pick jabbed into the eye socket"; or "being ripped by red-hot pincers." Complaints of pain in the absence of any identifiable noxious stimuli are problematic. However, it would be inconsistent and lead to great difficulties not to treat these phenomena as pain. The source of the complaint may be psychologic rather than physical, but pain is ultimately a psychologic phenomenon and, therefore, we must rely on the subjective report.

A phenomenon as complex as pain neither can be described by a single variable nor is the physiology of pain encompassed by a single reaction. It would be useful to obtain an overview from three perspectives: pain as a temporal sequence, pain as a hierarchic process in the body, and pain as a multiplicity of psychophysical expressions.

PAIN: THREE PERSPECTIVES

Time is a dimension of great importance in pain. Immediately following certain injuries, pain may be astonishingly absent. The seminal study of Beecher[2] indicated that up to 70% of wounded soldiers reported no pain at the time they first received medical attention. Later studies indicated that over one third of patients seen in an emergency department following traumatic injuries reported an initial period free of pain.[3] In the case of the soldiers, speculations have been made that the recognition of a wound afforded immediate relief from further danger. Others have opined that the intense emotion or the "shock" following injury suppresses pain from awareness. This reason seems unlikely both because many such patients are perfectly rational and calm at the time that they feel no pain, and they are not analgesic for other stimuli during this same period. At any rate, this phenomenon of a pain-free interval is exceptionally variable and suggests complexity in pain mechanisms.

The second phase following acute injury is characterized by the development of pain accompanied by agitation, anxiety guarding, and intense preoccupation with the disorder. Patients are characteristically able to give a precise description of the qualities of the pain and appear to respond in a predictable fashion to analgesics and other interventions.

A third stage is characterized by behavioral withdrawal and inactivity. Sleep is prolonged, appetite is reduced, vigilance is restricted to areas of immediate relevance to the pain, and movement of the affected part is kept at a minimum. This situation would seem ideal to promote healing. Indeed, this stage melds into that of recovery, during which the pain diminishes progressively; a sense of well-being is restored; and normal activities are gradually resumed.

Implicit in this model is the close temporal association of pain with an episode of injury.[4] It is a description of acute pain following injury and applies less well to pains that grow gradually but persist for long periods of time, such as pain due to progressive cancer. This model does not apply at all to chronic pain. Defined as pain that persists for longer than 6 months, chronic pain bears little relationship to the sequence of injury and healing. Many obvious biologic advantages exist in the response to acute pain, but none are evident in cases of persistent or chronic pain. The outpouring of sympathetic nervous system activity in the acute phase is blunted or nonexistent in the chronic phase. Instead there is the emergence of vegetative signs and symptoms. Sleep is disturbed, and fatigue is ever present. Patients are irritable and frequently overtly depressed. They are less tolerant of incidental pains or other unpleasant events. They eventually develop alterations in personality and thought processes. They develop behavioral patterns of invalidism. They may adopt a "sick role," which is self-perpetuating and reinforcing. Chronic pain is quite obviously much more complex at the psychosocial end of the spectrum than acute pain. For reasons that are not altogether clear, patients with cancer-related pain seem to fare better in this respect than patients with benign or indefinable conditions.

Pain may also be viewed from a hierarchic perspective. This view highlights the anatomy and physiology of pain-processing systems and reveals considerable complexity in pain responses. At the periphery of the nervous system, nerve endings in tissues react to stimuli adequate for tissue damage. They transmit information about the stimulus to the central nervous system and mediate secondary changes in the tissues as well as conditioning the system for further stimuli. Thus, the first level of nociceptive response is already quite developed before the central nervous system becomes involved. At the spinal segmental level, signals trigger somatic motor reflexes, such as withdrawal, and autonomic reflexes, such as altered vasomotor tone or sweating. Intersegmental spinal reflexes allow coordinated motor responses, whereas at the supraspinal level complex reflexive movements are achieved. Brain stem and thalamic mechanisms integrate behavioral responses, such as arousal, attention, and motor readiness. Limbic connections introduce emotional response patterns. Cognitive faculties are focused on the stimulus and its environmental context. Behavioral conditioning and contextual learning are powerfully reinforced. The experience of pain elicits speculation and fantasies concerning meaning, guilt, and attribution.

Viewed from a psychophysical perspective, however, the experience of pain is not hierarchic but, rather, multifaceted. Pain is not simply a single quantity—it possesses several dimensions. The primary dimension may be termed "sensory intensity." Besides this are distinct sensory qualities, such as sharp, throbbing, jabbing, burning, and so forth. Another dimension might be termed "affective," which encompasses not only the magnitude of unpleasantness but also such qualities as anxiety, distress, and depression. The experience of pain includes other distinguishing elements, such as a loss of function and a sense of physical illness (e.g., nausea, fatigue, weakness, sickness). In the evaluation and study of pain, measurement of these psychophysical variables has proved to be of the greatest importance.

MEASURING PAIN

From the point of view of the investigator attempting to measure pain, its multifaceted nature is translated into multidimensional scaling. That is, the subject can be asked to evaluate separately and independently each aspect of the experience. Much has been learned about how this can be done, and many confusing results of early investigations can be traced to the failure to recognize these distinctions.

Isolating for a moment the most obvious quality of pain, sensory intensity, it has been shown that pain can be treated just like any other sensory modality, such as vision, hearing,

or touch-pressure. In an experimental setting, one can establish a threshold value of stimulus intensity for the perception of pain. For example, heating a point on the skin, subjects report the sensation changing from "hot" to "burning" (i.e., painful) at a particular temperature. For each subject, this is fairly constant at a given spot; for a population of subjects the values vary around a mean with a normal distribution.[5] Similarly, a threshold can be determined for pressure pain or for various pain-producing chemical substances. Such thresholds are clearly of great physiologic relevance as we see subsequently.

Above threshold, a stimulus-response curve can be determined for pain intensity. Values are reproducible in an experimental setting and reflect the physiology of the transduction process.[6] However, to an extent not found in other somatosensory modalities, the stimulus-response curve is strongly conditioned by its recent history of stimulation.

Pain tolerance would appear to be an important variable to measure. Studies in this regard purported to show sexual, racial, and age-related differences in pain tolerance, such that the greatest tolerance occurred in young white males of Anglo-Saxon descent. Today, we appreciate the naiveté of these conclusions, recognizing the multitude of factors underlying the subject's responses.[7] Such factors include cultural norms of expression, the interpersonal dynamics of the subject and experimenter, and the meaning attributed to the experimental situation. Obviously, the observed responses cannot be taken as a physiologic measurement in any direct sense.

Much of the progress in pain research has resulted from the development of reliable instruments for pain measurement. As opposed to the stimulus-dependent methods that are standard in sensory research for establishment of thresholds, the most reliable instruments are response-dependent. They all assume that the patient can quantify the sensation of pain on a scale that is entirely subjective. The most widely accepted tools are categoric, such as numeric scales, about which the subject is instructed: "If zero represents no pain and ten represents the worst pain you can imagine, give the number which describes your present pain." For children, choosing among stylized faces with different expressions may prove simpler than numeric scales. Alternatives consist of analog scales. In the visual analog scale, the subject bisects a line at a point between zero and 100 representing the current pain intensity. A more direct method of scaling is that of magnitude estimation, in which the subject arbitrarily assigns some value to a stimulus and then compares other stimuli by assigning them relative values. This is actually a special case of cross-modality matching, in which the responses may be expressed in terms of the strength of handgrip, the duration of pressing a button, or the choice of descriptors among a large group of words.[8] Remarkably, when such methods are applied to populations of patients, extraordinarily reliable and reproducible results can be obtained.

In order to capture the full complexity of the pain experience, an instrument such as a "pain questionnaire" is employed. This includes separate scales for sensory and affective components of the pain as well as descriptors for the particular characteristics of the subject's pain, such as location, time course, and different sensory qualities.[9] In order to investigate the complex relationships between pain and personality, psychometric instruments such as the Minnesota Multiphasic Personality Inventory (MMPI), depression rating scales, illness behavior quotients, and coping strategy measurements have all been applied.

Pain measured in an experimental setting is quite different from pain in the clinical setting.

The first is far more reproducible because the strength of the stimulus is fully determined and extraneous variables can be controlled. Experimental pain excludes most of the important factors that make pain problematic. It is precisely the lack of control, as well as the associated meaning of the damaging stimulus, that gives pain its full force.

ANATOMY AND PHYSIOLOGY
The Periphery

The perception of pain depends under normal circumstances on the excitation of specific receptors (nociceptors) in the periphery (Fig. 3–1).[10] This does not mean that activation of nociceptors is always painful or that other receptors play no role in pain perception. The adequate stimulus is typically capable of producing tissue damage and can be classified as mechanical, thermal, or chemical. Whereas the remainder of somatosensory modalities rely on morphologically specialized receptors with great sensitivity and selectivity, nociceptors have high thresholds, are relatively stimulus nonspecific, and consist of bare nerve endings. Because of their lack of morphologic identity, nociceptors must be categorized by their response characteristics and the conduction velocities of their parent nerve fibers.

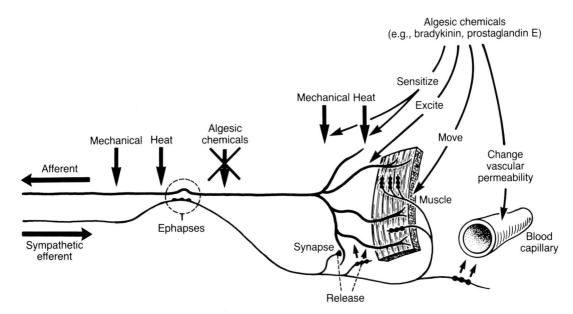

FIGURE 3–1. The nociceptor, in this case innervating muscle. The free nerve endings respond to mechanical, thermal, and chemical stimuli and can be sensitized by chemicals released from tissue injury. Sympathetic efferents affect the nociceptor directly and indirectly through effects on surrounding tissues. Following injury to the nerve, it too responds to stimuli and may develop abnormal connections.

Under normal circumstances, stimuli capable of exciting nociceptors also activate a wide variety of other receptors, endowing the sensation with many complex characteristics and probably modifying the intensity of the pain. By stimulating individual nerve fibers electrically, by selectively blocking larger or smaller fibers through ischemia or local anesthetic, or by choosing tissues endowed almost exclusively with nociceptors (tooth pulp, cornea), the psychophysical properties of these receptors can be appreciated.

Nociceptors in the skin have been studied most extensively. C-fibers responding to mechanical and heat stimuli (CMHs) are the most prevalent,[11] but there are also A-delta fibers responsive to mechanical and heat stimuli that form two subtypes (AMH-I and AMH-II).[12] All of these are capable of responding to chemical stimuli; therefore, they are often termed "polymodal nociceptors." In addition to these major categories, small numbers of C-fibers signal cold pain. These are less well characterized. The CMHs respond monotonically to increasing stimulus intensity into the noxious range, a pattern that exactly parallels pain perception.[13] If C-fiber function is blocked by anesthetics, or if C-fibers are missing as in patients with congenital insensitivity to pain, thermal pain perception threshold is altered.[14] Also, the perception of thermal pain is delayed in accord with the slow conduction rate of C-fibers, around 0.5 m/sec. The CMH responses adapt within seconds to continued heat stimulation. Type I AMHs have lower mechanical and higher thermal thresholds than CMHs. Conduction velocity is greater than 30 m/sec. The type I AMHs are prevalent on the palmar surfaces of the hands among other areas. They respond in an increasing fashion to sustained heat stimuli—a pattern that parallels heat pain perception.[15] Type II AMHs occur only on hairy skin and are much more heat sensitive than type I. They are thought to signal "first pain," the initial pricking sensation that follows sudden heat stimulation, whereas CMHs mediate "second pain," the burning that appears at an interval after heat stimulation.[16]

The mechanical threshold for CMHs is well below that for mechanically induced pain. Whereas C-fiber discharges as low as 2/sec correspond to intense heat pain, discharges at 10/sec to mechanical stimuli are not felt as painful.[17] Therefore, a central process, such as spatial summation or inhibition by coactivated A-fibers, must be invoked to explain the discrepancy.

Because most serious pains involve injury to tissues, it is important to assess changes in receptor properties caused by the injury. It is common experience that injury lowers pain thresholds so that previously innocuous stimuli become noxious. An increase in the painfulness of normally noxious stimuli also occurs, in addition to spontaneous pain. These characteristics correspond to three aspects of receptor sensitization: decreased firing threshold, increased suprathreshold firing rate, and spontaneous firing. In the case of a burn to the palm (Fig. 3–2), primary hyperalgesia in the area of injury occurs both for heat and for mechanical stimuli. The former corresponds to sensitization of type I AMHs, but the latter may depend on central changes. Secondary hyperalgesia in the surrounding area occurs only for mechanical stimuli, is not mediated by sensitization of nociceptors, and may rely on central changes as well.[18]

Receptor sensitization is chemically mediated, partly by injury-induced degranulation of tissue mast cells that release histamine, prostaglandins, and enzymes, leading to bradykinin

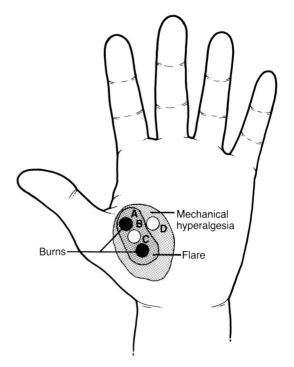

FIGURE 3–2. Cutaneous hyperalgesia. Following burns to areas A and C on the palm, they are surrounded by a "flare" mediated by the efferent actions of C-fibers. Sites A and D alone demonstrate thermal hyperalgesia, owing to sensitization of type I AMHs. Sites B and C show only mechanical hyperalgesia not caused by receptor sensitization but by central changes.

formation. Injury also induces local release of substance-P from C-fiber afferents. The interactions of these substances are complex. Some are directly excitatory to nociceptors, and some increase the responsiveness of nociceptors to other chemicals.

Tissues other than the skin are more difficult to study, but their nociceptive reactions are often quite different. Muscle pain, for instance, is felt as a deep aching, stiffness, or cramping. Stimulation in humans shows muscle pain to depend on excitation of small fiber afferents, which terminate in free nerve endings of muscles, tendons, and fascia.[19] The significant stimuli are obviously mechanical and chemical, especially related to extreme contraction and ischemia. Joints are innervated largely by unmyelinated and thinly myelinated fibers, some of which signal only noxious joint movement, while others fire with increasing frequency to movement over a wide range of force. Some of them are silent except in the arthritic joint; therefore, they must be sensitized by inflammation.[20] In the cornea, nociceptors have extremely low mechanical thresholds, appropriate to the ease of causing injury in the cornea. Thermal and chemical sensitivity are also present. The innervation is entirely by C-fibers and A-delta fibers. Tooth pulp stimulation results in one major sensation, which is pain, in response to mechanical, thermal, or chemical stimulation.[21] A-delta fibers mediate responses to drilling or scraping of dentin, whereas C-fibers react to pulpal stimulation.

The Dorsal Horn

The cell bodies of all spinal afferents are located in the dorsal root ganglia (Fig. 3–3). The central processes arising from large fibers enter the spinal cord dorsomedially. The smaller fibers enter ventrolaterally. After entering, the fibers typically bifurcate to form ascending and descending branches. Collaterals from a single fiber may spread over several adjacent spinal segments. Lissauer's tract consists chiefly of such dorsal root fibers—the majority of which come from unmyelinated afferents. Large fiber

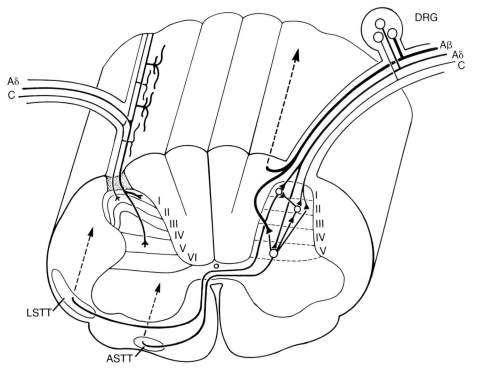

FIGURE 3–3. The dorsal horn and its connections are shown. Spinal afferents with their cell bodies in the dorsal root ganglia (DRG) approach the dorsal root entry zone, with large fibers dorsomedially and small fibers ventrolaterally. A-delta (Aδ) and C-fibers (C) bifurcate and establish numerous local branches in Lissauer's tract before entering the dorsal horn. The A-beta (Aβ) fibers ascend in the dorsal columns after sending a branch to lamina IV of the dorsal horn. A-delta fibers terminate in laminae I and V, on cells destined to form the ascending spinothalamic tracts. The C-fibers terminate in lamina II. Interneurons of lamina II connect with lamina I and IV cells. The local connections are elaborate and involve various neurotransmitters. (ASTT = anterior spinothalamic tract; LSTT = lateral spinothalamic tract.)

afferents terminate in laminae III through V of the dorsal horn or pass upward to end in the dorsal column nuclei. Collaterals from A-delta fibers terminate in laminae I and V, whereas C-fiber terminals are restricted to laminae I and II.[22] Muscle afferents end in lamina I and laminae V and VI.

The cell bodies of trigeminal afferents are located in the gasserian ganglion, with the exception of masticatory muscle spindle afferents located in the mesencephalic trigeminal nucleus. The afferents terminate in the trigeminal nuclear complex, which has four divisions: main sensory nucleus, nucleus oralis, nucleus interpolaris, and nucleus caudalis. Afferents from the entire face and oral cavity are found in each nuclear division but not equally. Nucleus oralis, for example, receives predominantly intraoral afferents. A consistent somatotopic representation occurs in all nuclear subdivisions. The ophthalmic division is ventromedial, the mandibular is dorsolateral, and a perioral to periauricular gradient runs from dorsomedial to ventrolateral.[23]

Large myelinated fibers bifurcate on entry, one branch ending in the main sensory nucleus and a descending branch sending collaterals to the other three nuclei. C-fibers do not enter the main nucleus but descend mostly to the nucleus caudalis, whose structure has given it the name "medullary dorsal horn." C-fibers terminate mostly in lamina I, whereas A-deltas terminate in lamina II, although the degree of stratification is less definite than for the spinal dorsal horn. Tooth pulp afferents, mostly A-delta fibers, are represented in all four nuclear divisions, and in laminae I, II, and V.[24] The nucleus caudalis plays a specific role in nociception. This is evident from the observation that section of the descending trigeminal tract produces analgesia on the ipsilateral face. Besides affecting pain and temperature sensibilities, lesions in this area reduce the summation effects of stimuli that produce an itch or a tickle on the face.

Synaptic transmission by primary sensory neurons includes (1) rapid excitatory actions mediated probably by glutamate or in some cases ATP and (2) slower modulating influences mediated by various peptides. Substance-P among others is released upon stimulation of high threshold afferents and exerts an excitatory postsynaptic effect.[25]

The intrinsic circuitry of the dorsal horn has proved astonishingly complex. From the point of view of nociception, this complexity consists of the lack of fixed input-output relationships among particular cells. Thus, cells that appear unrelated to the processing of noxious stimuli under certain conditions acquire such a role under other circumstances, particularly in the setting of pathology or tissue injury. Three mechanisms are responsible for these changes. The first is the "gate control" mechanism (Fig. 3–4), in which excitation of inhibitory interneurons by large fiber inputs opposes the excitation of excitory interneurons by small fiber inputs on nociceptive transmission cells. This model was originally proposed by Melzack and Wall in 1965,[26] and it has formed the heuristic basis for much pain research in subsequent years. The gate control mechanism involves rapid neurotransmission and includes inputs from descending supraspinal systems. The second mechanism, sensitivity control, consists of long latency and duration changes in excitability, probably mediated by the release of peptides from activated C-fibers originating mostly in deep tissues and from descending systems. The third mechanism, connectivity control,

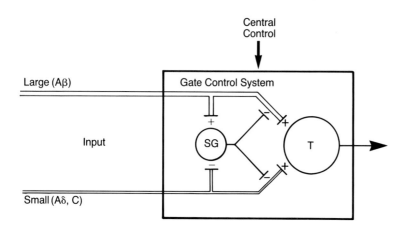

FIGURE 3–4. The hypothetic "gate control" mechanism is shown. In this model, interneurons of the substantia gelatinosa (SG) in the upper lamina of the dorsal horn are subject to opposite influences by large and small fiber inputs. The end result is that concomitant large fiber stimulation blocks the excitation of the pain transmission cell (T) by small fiber inputs. The entire mechanism is further subject to "central control."

occurs with a latency of days and may last months following damage to peripheral sensory nerves, especially C-fibers. All three mechanisms play a role in pathologic pain, but they may also provide keys to its relief.[27]

The Spinal Pathways

Nociceptive information is transmitted from the spinal cord to the brain by several pathways, the most important of which is the spinothalamic tract. The strongest evidence for the preeminence of the spinothalamic tract in pain perception is that surgical section of the anterolateral tract in humans results in immediate and profound relief of pain contralateral to the lesion beginning a few segments below. The spinothalamic tract mediates the sensory discriminative aspects of pain sensation as well as thermal sensibility. Stimulation of the tract induces pain, and spinothalamic axons are excited by noxious stimuli in their receptive fields. Nonetheless, anatomic identities of these neurons in the dorsal horn remain vague, because nociceptive afferents from the periphery do not necessarily terminate on them.[28] The spinothalamic tract terminates mostly in the thalamus, predominantly in the ventral posterior lateral and central lateral nuclei.

Several months following anterolateral cordotomy with section of the spinothalamic tract, pain sensibility inevitably returns, although appreciation of temperature may not. In this situation, the nociceptive role of other ascending pathways is uncovered. Bilateral hemisections of the cord at different levels are not sufficient to block all pain perception, so there must exist potential pathways that crisscross the cord and defy anatomic delineation. Other pathways are more clearly defined.[29] The spinoreticular tract is thought to mediate the arousal and affective-motivational aspects of pain, in addition to supraspinal motor and autonomic nocifensor reflexes. The main areas of termination pertinent to pain are the nucleus gigantocellularis of the pons and the lateral pontine tegmentum. The spinomesencephalic tract projects to the midbrain reticular formation and the periaqueductal gray matter. Stimulation in these areas evokes aversive reactions and pain, whereas lesions produce relative analgesia. Paradoxically, stimulation in the periaqueductal gray matter also produces analgesia.

Pain transmission from the trigeminal system is conveyed by the trigeminothalamic tract, which originates from all divisions of the trigeminal nuclear complex. It is unclear whether the nucleus caudalis makes mostly direct nociceptive connections with the thalamus, or whether these are mediated by connections first with the main sensory nucleus.[30] Nociceptive trigeminothalamic cells of the nucleus caudalis are functionally divided into wide dynamic range and nociceptive-specific groups. These cells terminate in ventral posterior medial and intralaminar nuclei of the thalamus.

Thalamocortical Mechanisms

It would be reasonable to assume that thalamocortical projections would be essential to the sensory-discriminative aspects of pain perception. Indeed, lesions of the thalamus in humans may abolish contralateral pain responses and produce dense anesthesia. This finding implies that no somatosensory data reach awareness without passing through the thalamus. On the one hand, partial lesions of the thalamus may result in hypesthesia and erasure of pathologic pains. On the other hand, spontaneous pains and painful dysesthesias are well-known consequences of thalamic injury (Déjérine-Roussy syndrome). These pains may be the consequence of deafferentation, which gives rise to spontaneous activity of nociceptive cells or renders them abnormally excitable.

The study of thalamocortical mechanisms is difficult because of interspecies differences and the obvious limitations of human experimentation. Nonetheless, evidence exists for neurons in the ventral posterior nuclei of the thalamus, which are excited directly by the spinothalamic tract and which respond in a graded fashion to noxious stimuli.[31] These neurons are also capable of sensitization. The intralaminar thalamic nuclei are best considered as extensions of the reticular activating system and are concerned with arousal and motor responses to pain.

The issue of cortical representation of pain is a complex one. Clinical experience has established that lesions in the somatosensory cortical areas or the white matter tracts connecting them to the thalamus do not produce long-lasting analgesia. Disturbances of contralateral sensory awareness in general are common in the acute phase of cortical damage but are not specific for pain. Rare exceptions are reported, but their rarity suggests some other explanation. Penfield and Rasmussen,[32] in their extensive stimulation studies with the cortex in awake human subjects, never found an area where activation produced the sensation of pain.

It is, therefore, surprising to discover numerous cortical neurons in the primary and secondary somatosensory areas activated by the stimulation of tooth pulp, which produces no conscious sensation other than pain itself.[33] Neurons in SI have been found that are activated specifically by noxious stimuli and whose properties reflect those of thalamic nociceptive neurons in coding stimulus strength and other features.[34] Doubtless, these are responsible for the discriminative aspects of pain perception, in contrast to its affective-motivational aspects.

No conditioner of behavior is more powerful than pain. Learning by avoidance of pain is rapid and long lasting. These observations imply powerful connections of nociceptive pathways with the limbic system and specifically with the hippocampal memory system. Some mention must be made of the so-called reward and punishment centers in the brain. The essence of punishment is aversion, and nothing is characteristically more aversive than pain. But, punishment itself often occurs without nociception and nociception without the aversive component would not be worthy of attention. It appears likely that the nociceptive system normally has a very powerful input to the punishment center.

A number of special cases are worthy of consideration. In certain trance-like states, whether induced by hypnosis or by meditative exercises, individuals subjected to highly noxious trauma report no pain and do not seem to be affected by it. The mechanism for this apparent analgesia is not known, but certain studies with hypnosis suggest that on one level the pain may be perceived but not acknowledged. Physiologic responses to acute pain are blunted but not abolished. In a condition known as "pain asymbolia," acquired in the acute and recovering phases of some cerebral lesions producing global aphasia, the subject is devoid of the usual protective mechanisms, such as withdrawal of a limb that is being struck (on the sentient side of the body) and avoidance of a blow aimed at the face. Intensely noxious stimuli elicit a full response, demonstrating basic integrity of pain pathways and suggesting that under normal circumstances, a large part of our reaction to pain, such as a pinprick, is really a learned response to the threat of pain or damage. Conversely, patients with congenital insensitivity to pain display a remarkable lack of self-preservation. They repeatedly undergo injuries and do not take the proper precautions to promote healing. They accumulate serious bodily damage as a result. Thus, the normal function of pain-related systems involves not only aspects of sensation, but also emotional and motivational states and the powerful influence of reinforcers on behavior.

ENDOGENOUS SYSTEMS FOR CONTROL OF PAIN

The existence of endogenous systems capable of modifying the perception of pain is suggested by clinical experiences showing tremendous variability in pains reported from injuries of similar magnitude, even in the same individual at different times. The gate control theory provided the first theoretic framework for such mechanisms, but the discovery of stimulation produced analgesia indicated the presence of distinct descending pain control systems.[35] In animal experiments, electrical stimulation of specific brain sites selectively and powerfully reduced responses to noxious stimuli without affecting other behaviors. Later, work in humans confirmed this finding. The discovery of the endogenous opioid peptides led to a much deeper understanding of pain modulation, both internal and external.

The opioid-mediated analgesia system involves widely distributed portions of the central nervous system (Fig. 3–5).[36] Inputs from the frontal cortex, amygdala, parafascicular nucleus of the thalamus, and hypothalamus converge on the periaqueductal gray matter, which in turn projects to the rostral ventral medulla (RVM). Both induce analgesia when electrically stimulated or when microinjected with opioids, and both contain opioids. The RVM neurons project via the dorsal lateral funiculus of the spinal cord to superficial layers of the dorsal horn, where they control transmission of nociceptive information. The system can be activated by a variety of situations, including stress, classic conditioning, and certain kinds of pain itself.

A number of opioid receptor subtypes are distributed widely through different areas of the nervous system. Through variation in location and specificity, they mediate the full spectrum of narcotic effects, including sedation, respiratory depression, and addiction, among others. Hope exists that the production of synthetic opioids will eventually allow for selective analgesia with minimal side effects.

Although the neurotransmitters involved in the descending modulation of pain are not entirely known, certain inputs are known to be prominent. The locus ceruleus is a major noradrenergic input to the periaqueductal gray matter and forms a descending spinal pathway. Serotonin-containing neurons project to the RVM from the midbrain, and from the RVM (i.e., raphe magnus) to the dorsal horn.

In the dorsal horn, opioid-releasing cells play a major role in the modulation of nociceptive transmission. Spinal injections of opioids produce profound segmental analgesia, and iontophoresis shows the site of action to be the superficial dorsal horn.[37] Evidence has been found for opioid receptors both on the terminals of primary afferent fibers and on the cells destined for the spinothalamic system. Descending control systems presumably act on opioid interneurons that mediate their effects.

Not all endogenous pain modulation is opioid mediated. For example, certain kinds of "stress" or painful conditioning stimulation induce analgesia that is blocked by naloxone, an opioid inhibitor; the analgesia from other forms of stimulation is naloxone independent.[38] The analgesia from acupuncture and that from high-intensity, low-frequency transcutaneous electrical nerve stimulation (TENS) is reversed by naloxone, whereas that of low-intensity, high-frequency TENS is not. A complexity to the endogenous pain control mechanisms concurrently defies elucidation. The hope is that eventually it will provide a multiplicity of solutions.

COGNITIVE AND EMOTIONAL ASPECTS OF PAIN

It is at the psychologic end of the nociceptive hierarchy that the largest gaps in our knowledge persist along with the greatest uncertainties in diagnosis and treatment. The impression of clinicians is that some patients claim vastly exaggerated levels of pain, that some cope extraordinarily poorly with pain, and that others maintain pain entirely by psychologic factors. These are the "problem patients" who demand and consume inordinate amounts of pain medications and medical resources, yet leave everyone dissatisfied with the outcome. Little is truly understood about such patients, and our frustrations with them are generally projected upon the patients themselves. Yet it would be both unwise and unfair to label as psychopathology all the deviations from normal emo-

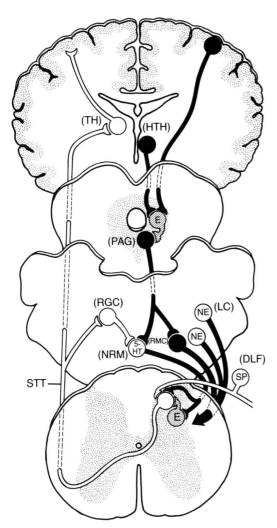

FIGURE 3–5. Endogenous analgesic mechanisms are shown. The ascending nociceptive output of the spinothalamic tract (STT) is modulated by connections in the dorsal horn via descending pathways in the dorsolateral funiculus (DLF). Cerebral inputs from the cortex, amygdala, thalamus (TH), and hypothalamus (HTH) converge on the periaqueductal grey (PAG), where endorphinergic neurons play a major role. The PAG projects to the rostral ventral medulla from which serotonin-containing cells of the nucleus raphe magnus (NRM) and the nucleus reticularis magnocellularis (RMC) project via the DLF to the dorsal horn. The STT supplies ascending pain signals to the nucleus reticularis gigantocellularis (RGC), which feeds into the descending system of the PAG and rostral ventral medulla. Noradrenergic neurons of the locus ceruleus (LC) and adjacent nuclei also contribute to descending pain modulation via the DLF. (E = endorphin; NE = norepinephrine; SP = substance P; 5-HT = serotonin.)

tional behavior that are seen in patients with pain. Although it is likely that chronic pain brings out latent psychopathology, it is also true that pain invariably involves both cognitive and emotional aspects.

Much evidence from careful reports of human studies, as well as knowledge of nociceptive physiology, indicates that the affective-motivational aspects of pain can be distinguished from its sensory intensity. For example, the unpleasantness of a dental procedure may respond to diazepam, whereas the sensory intensity responds to fentanyl. Nowhere is this distinction more clear than in anticipatory distress, which in certain cases may be disabling.

In the acute phase following injury, the experience of pain as well as the recognition of damage gives rise to emotional distress. Generally, the greater the anxiety the greater is the perceived pain; but, which is cause and which effect may be difficult to say.[39] A patient with a history of anxiety may complain more of pain following a procedure but may not experience more intense pain than a patient who is more characteristically calm.

The emotional accompaniments of chronic pain include anxiety but tend more toward depression and anger. The incidence of depression in chronic pain is hard to estimate, because many of the indicators of depression, such as vegetative signs, are consequences of pain itself. Furthermore, evidence exists that patients with chronic pain tend to somatize their conflicts rather than experience their affect. Whether this indicates "masked depression" is debatable. Certainly, the destructive impact of chronic pain on determinants of well-being would be expected to cause depression. Not only are there loss of autonomy, reduction in pleasurable activities, social isolation, and a host of frustrating and defeating confrontations with one's environment, but there is also the constant grinding assault of pain itself. What is remarkable is the ability of some patients with chronic pain to avoid emotional deterioration.[40]

Some chronic pain sufferers display anger and become demanding and manipulative. Indeed, their unrewarding, sometimes punitive experiences within the health care system may encourage these traits. The clinician should avoid the conclusion that such patients' pain complaints are less likely to be valid.

Large scale studies utilizing instruments such as the MMPI indicate that chronic pain patients rate high on scales of not only "depression" but also "hypochondriasis" and "hysteria." Hypochondriasis indicates a fascinated absorption with bodily symptoms and the conviction of disease associated with a phobic attitude. Hysteria indicates the conversion of fears into somatic symptoms—in the present instance, pain. Other elements of somatization related to pain include loss of function (paralysis) and loss of sensation other than pain (numbness). Evidence suggests that with increasing chronicity these abnormalities grow. Whether they exist as latent traits in persons destined to develop pain, whether they perpetuate the pain, or whether they represent maladaptations to the stress of a chronic illness remains to be seen.

Psychodynamic models of pain are interesting but currently beyond proof. They draw our attention to the interpretation of pain as punishment, its relationship to guilt and shame, and its role in satisfying masochistic needs. On the one hand, pain is a threat to the autonomy of the ego and brings out dependency. On the other hand, pain legitimizes behaviors that may have considerable secondary gains. In psychopathic individuals, complaints or demonstrations of pain may simply be malingering. No one can doubt the relevance of psychodynamic mechanisms in pain, and appreciation of their role is essential in the management of patients in pain.

A more general model of the impact of emotions on pain is that of stress, acting to enhance and perpetuate pain. Stress as a general concept refers to the magnitude of adaptive reactions brought into play by life changes or demands. Stress increases affective responses and the physiologic arousal accompanying them. This model is often applied to explain the numerous disorders implicating a cycle of muscle contraction (tension-pain-anxiety), in which stress appears to turn up the gain in the circuit. As attractive and straightforward as this model seems, it is not so easily proved.[41]

Cognitive theories of pain focus on the concepts of stress and coping. In these models, the patient's cognitive appraisal of the situation depends on his or her perception of the consequences of a painful event, its personal meaning, and the available resources for coping. Belief systems are critical to each of these areas. Maladaptive responses are likely to have resulted from previous failed attempts to cope. So the therapeutic approach is to re-educate the pain patient to recognize previous errors in attribution, to appreciate and enhance the realm of control, and to practice strategies for managing the pain.[42] These stategies include relaxation techniques, diversion of attention, reinterpretation of stimuli, and positive self-reinforcement.

One approach to the overwhelming psychologic complexity of pain is the application of behaviorism. Rather than speculating on unobservable psychologic mechanisms, behavioral theories are confined to the observable: behavior is governed by its consequences. Pain behavior, for example, may be elicited at first by a noxious stimulus, but later it may persist despite the disappearance of the stimulus if environmental reinforcers are sufficiently strong. Strength of a reinforcer in operant conditioning depends on individual circumstance. As an example, food is a powerful reinforcer if one is hungry, not if one is full.

The object of behavioral therapy is to alter pain behavior. Examples of such behavior include quantifiables such as "number of blocks walked," "time sitting still," "number of references to pain in an hour," and even grimaces and vocalizations. Once the behaviors and their consequences are delineated for the patient, effective reinforcers are found to modify them, and these are systematically applied. Extinction of maladaptive behaviors and establishment of healthy behaviors are objectively monitored, irrespective of the issues concerning pain itself. The evidence suggests that behavioral therapy is effective in reducing disability due to pain. If pain has fewer negative consequences, something valuable has been accomplished.

PAIN DUE TO NERVE INJURY

Nerve injury represents a special case of tissue damage, and the characteristics of pain arising from injured nerves are distinctive in many ways. Whereas it is usual for pain to subside when damaged tissues heal and inflammation abates, injured nerves may never heal completely and the pain arising from them is independent of inflammation. Acute trauma to a nerve trunk causes an immediate shock-like pain projected to the site of sensory innervation (e.g., hitting the "funny bone"), followed by an aching pain at the site of the injury. The first represents mechanically induced axonal discharge, and the second represents an example of regular nociception in the nerve sheath by the nervi nervorum.

Following the acute phase, there are three different mechanisms by which neuritic pain is generated.[44] First, dysesthesias, or distorted sensations, occur when an abnormal pattern of impulses reaches the central nervous system. This pattern may be an altered ratio of inputs from various receptors (selective damage), excessive or repetitive firing of fibers when stimulated, leakage of signals between adjacent fibers (ephaptic transmission or cross talk), mismatching of central and peripheral processes (aberrant regeneration), or disturbed central processing due to cell injury. Painful dysesthesias may be shock-like, burning, jabbing, or lancinating. Innocuous stimuli may become noxious (allodynia). Thresholds may be changed, so that warmth becomes burning or light pressure, crushing (hypersensitivity, hyperpathia).

Second, paresthesias, or spontaneous sensations, arise from activity of damaged nerves in the absence of peripheral stimulation. The most common experience of paresthesias is the "pins and needles" after prolonged pressure on a nerve. Shortly after injury, during the process of regeneration, and in the presence of nerve scarring, spontaneous discharges are frequent. Usually they are not painful, but they can be shock-like, burning, jabbing, cramping, or crushing.

Third, reflex sympathetic dystrophy, or causalgia, was originally described following injuries to major nerve trunks in the limbs, although it is now recognized to occur in the absence of overt nerve involvement. The precise mechanism of this pain remains unknown, but it clearly involves the sympathetic nervous system. The pain is characterized by intense burning and throbbing with an incredible degree of hypersensitivity, so that in extreme cases, a draft of air or the vibration of a door being closed nearby is sufficient to trigger the pain. The involved limb swells; it alternates between dusky cold and red hot. The skin, hair, nails, and joints undergo pathologic changes; the sufferer is intensely affected. Speculations on the origin of reflex sympathetic dystrophy include abnormal connections between the peripheral somatic and autonomic nerves and distortions of the central processing in the dorsal horn of the spinal cord.[45]

The keys to recognition of neuritic pains are the existence of disturbed sensory discrimination in the affected zone, the correspondence of the pain projection sites to known nerve distributions, the occurrence of shock-like or bizarre sensory qualities to the pain, and the transformation of innocuous into painful stimuli, although the last may occur as well when there is inflammation.

Sciatica is perhaps the best known example of neuritic pain. This pain arises from irritation or damage to any of the nerve roots or major constituents of the sciatic nerve. In the typical situation, a herniated disc or bone spur presses on the exiting nerve root, causing an ache in the low back in the region of injury and a shooting pain down the leg following the distribution of the nerve to the skin, muscle, and other tissues (dermatomal, myotomal, sclerotomal). Reflexive paraspinal muscle spasm; mechanical sensitivity to motion of the lower spine and to nerve traction; and sensory, motor, or reflex dysfunction in the corresponding distribution occur. The equivalent condition affecting the upper cervical nerves may refer pain to the head.

Trigeminal neuralgia is characterized by sudden shock-like jabbing pains on the face, most often near the corner of the mouth but occurring anywhere in the territory of the trigeminal nerve. During a susceptible phase, innocuous stimuli in the trigger zone are capable of causing an excruciating siege of pain, so that affected persons may avoid talking or exposure to drafts of air. In idiopathic cases, no interim sensory deficits occur, but careful examination may disclose exaggerated sensory summation or prolonged after sensation. In cases of trigeminal neuralgia due to recognized disease, such as multiple sclerosis, sensory deficits are frequently present. Many patients respond well to anticonvulsant medications; others respond to minor lesions of the appropriate root of the sensory ganglion.

Postherpetic neuralgia is a residual, sometimes permanent pain in the territory of nerve damage resulting from an attack of herpes zoster. When the acute herpetic attack subsides, an intensely disturbing dysesthetic pain commences in the same area. Sometimes there are shock-like bouts, sometimes burning, and sometimes indescribable qualities. Often, contact with clothes is unbearable. Always, there are sensory deficits. Spontaneous pricking may come from a region where cutaneous stimulation is barely felt. Currently, no therapy is available for postherpetic neuralgia that is generally successful, although some patients may gain a modicum of relief from certain antidepressant medications.

When a nerve is severed and scarring prevents sprouts from the regenerating proximal portion from re-establishing connections, a neuroma may be formed. This ball of tangled nerve sprouts possesses exquisite mechanical and chemical sensitivity so that the mere pulsation of nearby arterial blood or the local sympathetic release of norepinephrine may exite paroxysms of pain in severe cases.[46] Surgical resection of the neuroma may be effective, but the same problem is likely to be repeated at the new cut end. In fact, all cut nerves form neuromas at least at the microscopic level, although not all of them present pain problems. The signature of a neuroma is an exquisitely sensitive spot proximal to an area of sensory deficit signifying the cut proximal end of a nerve.

PAIN DUE TO TISSUE INJURY

The prototype of acute pain is that arising in the immediate setting of tissue injury—traumatic, surgical, or related to an active disease process, such as cancer or infection. As such, the local response to injury is an essential aspect of the pain. Sensitization by substances released during the inflammatory response is the primary mechanism of the hyperalgesia that characterizes clinical pain. In addition, changes in the patterns of central processing at the spinal cord may also be responsible for hyperalgesia. It is the shift of effective mechanical thresholds to pain that determines loss of function, and it is the generation of ongoing peripheral discharge and central transmission that produces the continual background of discomfort. Such is the degree of sensitization that the repeated shock of normal arterial pulsations can be a source of agonizing throbbing pain.

Examples of pain due to tissue injury are all too numerous and familiar. Of pains referred to the region of the face and oral cavity, examples include abscessed teeth, trauma to the temporomandibular joint, infection of the perinasal sinuses, cancer of the jaw, and extraction of a tooth. Each instance has its characteristic signature, composed of its spatial and temporal profiles, responses to specific mechanical stimuli, and mixture of sensory qualities related to the proportional excitation of the constituent nerves. Many times our perception of these distinctions is poor, but much depends diagnostically on such nuances; therefore, efforts to read various pain signatures are worth the trouble.

Migraine is an example of acute pain associated with reactive changes in tissues but not resulting from tissue injury as such. In a certain respect, migraine represents a local inflammatory response in the larger intracranial arteries, which alternately constrict and dilate, thereby exciting sensitized nociceptors in their walls. The injurious nature of the inciting stimulus is far from obvious (e.g., a glass of wine, an argument) and the evidence for tissue injury is subtle, but no one doubts the pain of a migraine attack. This is attributable to the common experience of the condition and the recognition of its underlying pathophysiology, both of which socially and medically validate the pain.

Frequently, the inciting event for pain or the cause of its perpetuation is not overt injury in the usual sense but rather dysfunction. Careful analysis will usually disclose ongoing injury, perhaps only on the microscopic level. Most often this injury is occurring in muscles or connective tissues, such as ligaments, tendons, or fascia. "Myofibrositis," "myofascial pain," "tension myalgia," and "fibromyalgia" are some of the terms used to describe these disorders.[47] A lack of consensus exists as to whether these disorders are disease entities, whether they are all in fact the same, or whether they are merely epiphenomena. The hallmark of these conditions is the existence of tender spots in the affected tissues. Sometimes it can be demonstrated that these represent trigger zones, because blocking them with an injection of local anesthetic abolishes the pain over a much wider or distant area. Because the existence of tender spots is associated with spasm in the affected muscles, it is postulated that the condition is maintained by a cycle of pain-inducing spasm through local nociceptor reflexes, which in turn induces pain and sensitivity through microscopic injury by tissue ischemia or other means. Initial trauma, such as a sprain or bruise, may start the cycle, while emotional and behavioral factors, by facilitating muscle tension and reactivity, establish the chronic state. Situations are known in which no initial injury is required, such as tension headaches (also known as muscle contraction headaches). Additionally, situations occur in which a continuation of an abnormal contraction during normal use results in dysfunctional use and consequent pain, as is postulated in many cases of chronic low back pain.

PAIN APPARENTLY UNRELATED TO PERIPHERAL NOCICEPTION

Far more problematic are those conditions in which the relationship of pain to injury is remote and the evidence for ongoing inflammation or other recognized pathophysiology is missing. Doubtless, there are conditions that are just as real as migraine but remain unrecognized because they are more rare and lack validation because they are not understood. How are these to be differentiated from disorders that bear no relationship to nociception in the periphery? At present, this question is unanswerable in the general sense.

Current prejudice maintains that patients without recognizable disorders may not have "real pain." The approach of modern investigators is to accept that the complaint of pain is truly pain and to proceed with an understanding of the mechanisms involved, which in many cases may not have anything to do with excitation of peripheral nociceptors.

Conditions arise analogous to those that arise from damage to peripheral nerves in which pain is a consequence of damage to central sensory mechanisms. The best recognized example of this is "thalamic pain" following a stroke or other pathology affecting the sensory thalamus. Patients describe extremely disagreeable spontaneous and induced sensations from the affected contralateral body, concurrent with impairment of sensory discrimination. Less often, a similar occurrence results from lesions in the somatosensory cortex or sensory projection pathways in the brain stem or spinal cord. No reason exists to consider these pains as less real than others that result from peripheral damage to the nervous system. If there are cases in which the central pathology is obvious, then cases may exist in which the central pathology is subtle. No lesion may be seen on the macroscopic level, but, perhaps, a derangement of the functional connections in central pain pathways occurs. At the present time, the delineation of such states is beyond our ability to distinguish, but the theoretic possibility exists.

"Chronic pain" is usually employed as a generic term for all pains that persist over 6 months, irrespective of pathology. That such a generic concept is at all viable reflects the communality of mechanisms brought into play by pain over time. The emphasis shifts from primary nociceptive events to affective, cognitive, and behavioral patterns. In all cases of chronic pain, a thorough search must be made for an underlying nociceptive source, followed, of course, by specific means to remedy it. Many times the source is not found, or if found, there is no remedy. More often, the source seems insufficient to cause the degree of pain expressed, but since no truly objective criteria exist, the estimation relies on the judgment of the examiner. In the end, however, the function of the clinician is not to legitimize chronic pain, but to help the patient live and function with it to the extent that it cannot be eliminated. No neurophysiologic model of chronic pain exists at the present time. Therefore, available models are limited to psychodynamic and behavioral descriptions, and therapies are designed to match. This practice, born of necessity, should not constitute a prejudice concerning the "reality" of the pain.

Temporomandibular disorders probably reflect the full gamut from pain entirely dependent upon injury, to pain arising from continued dysfunctional use after injury, to pain caused entirely by emotionally triggered contraction. With the passage of time, distinctions among these types may fade, so that correction of the problem may require addressing both the mechanical and behavioral aspects, irrespective of the mode of onset. The entity of chronic pain is only a theoretic pole toward which a given patient's syndrome tends to approach with time. Intervention is always better sooner than later, and a physiologic analysis of the problem is appropriate at every point.

REFERENCES

1. Merskey, H.: Pain terms: a list with definitions and notes on usage. Pain 6:249–252, 1979.
2. Beecher, H.K.: *Measurement of Subjective Responses.* Oxford University Press, New York, 1959.
3. Melzack, R., Wall, P.D., and Tye, T.C.: Acute pain in an emergency clinic: latency of onset and descriptor patterns related to different injuries. Pain 14:33–43, 1982.
4. Wall, P.D.: On the relation of injury to pain: The John J. Bonica lecture. Pain 6:253–264, 1979.
5. Hardy, J.D., Wolff, H.G., and Goodell, H.: *Pain Sensation and Reactions.* Williams & Wilkins, Baltimore, 1952.
6. Torebjork, H.E.: Sensory correlates of somatic afferent fibre activation. Human Neurobiol. 3:15–20, 1984.
7. Wolff, B.B.: Factor analysis of human pain responses: pain endurance as a specific pain factor. J. Abnorm. Psychol. 78:292–298, 1971.
8. Gracely, R.H.: Psychophysical assessment of human pain. In *Advances in Pain Research and Therapy,* vol. 3. J.J. Bonica, J.C. Liebeskind, and D.G. Albe-Fessard (eds.). Raven Press, New York, 1979.
9. Melzack, R.: The McGill pain questionnaire: major properties and scoring methods. Pain 1:275–299, 1975.
10. Sherrington, C.S.: *The Integrative Action of the Nervous System.* Scribner, New York, 1906.
11. Bessou, P. and Perl, E.R.: Response of cutaneous sensory units with unmyelinated fibers to noxious stimuli. J. Neurophysiol. 32:1025–1043, 1969.
12. Campbell, J.N. and Meyer, R.A.: Primary afferents and hyperalgesia. In *Spinal Afferent Processing.* T.L. Yaksh (ed.). Plenum Press, New York, 1986.
13. LaMotte, R.H. and Campbell, J.N.: Comparison of responses of warm and nociceptive C-fiber afferent in monkey with human judgments of thermal pain. J. Neurophysiol. 41:509–528, 1978.
14. Torebjork, H.E. and Hallin, R.G.: Perceptual changes accompanying controlled preferential blocking of A- and C-fiber responses in intact human skin nerves. Exp. Brain Res. 16:321–332, 1973.
15. Meyer, R.A. and Campbell, J.N.: Myelinated nociceptive afferents account for the hyperalgesia that follows a burn to the hand. Science 213:1527–1529, 1981.
16. Campbell, J.N. and LaMotte, R.H.: Latency to detection of first pain. Brain Res. 266:203–208, 1983.
17. Van Hess, J. and Gybels, J.M.: C-nociceptor activity in human nerve during painful and nonpainful skin stimulation. J. Neurol. Neurosurg. Psychiatry 44:600–607, 1981.
18. Raja, S.N., Campbell, J.N., and Meyer, R.A.: Evidence for different mechanisms of primary and secondary hyperalgesia following heat injury to the glabrous skin. Brain 107:1179–1188, 1984.
19. Torebjork, H.E., Ochoa, L.J., and Schady, W.: Referred pain from intraneural stimulation of muscle fascicles in the median nerve. Pain 18:145–156, 1984.
20. Heppelman, B., Schaible, H.G., and Schmidt, R.F.: Effects of prostaglandins E1 and E2 on the mechanosensitivity of group III afferents from normal and inflamed cat knee joints. In *Advances in Pain Research and Therapy,* vol. 9. H.L. Fields, R. Dubner, and F. Cervero (eds.). Raven Press, New York, 1985.
21. Dubner, R.: Neurophysiology of pain. Dent. Clin. North Am. 22:11–30, 1978.
22. Rethelyi, M.: Geometry of the dorsal horn. In *Spinal Cord Sensation.* A.G. Brown and M. Rethelyi (eds.). Scottish Academic Press, Edinburgh, 1981.
23. Darian-Smith, I.: The trigeminal system. In *Handbook of Sensory Physiology,* vol. 2. A. Iggo (ed.). Springer Verlag, Berlin, 1973.
24. Marfurt, C.F. and Turner D.F.: The central projections of tooth pulp afferent neurons in the rat as determined by the transganglionic transport of horseradish peroxidase. J. Comp. Neurol. 223:535–547, 1984.
25. Jessell, T.M. and Dodd, J.: Neurotransmitters and differentiation antigens in subsets of sensory neurons projecting to the spinal dorsal horn. In *Neuropeptides in Neurologic and Psychiatric Disease.* J.B. Martin and J.D. Barches (eds.). Raven Press, New York, 1986.
26. Melzack, R. and Wall, P.D.: Pain mechanisms: a new theory. Science 150:971–979, 1965.
27. Wall, P.D.: The dorsal horn. In *Textbook of Pain.* P.D. Wall and R. Melzack (eds.). Churchill Livingstone, New York, 1989.
28. Price, D.D. and Dubner, R.: Neurons that subserve the sensory-discriminative aspect of pain. Pain 3:307–338, 1977.
29. Willis, W.D.: The pain system. The neural basis of nociceptive transmission in the mammalian nervous system. Karger, Basel, 1985.
30. Denny-Brown, D. and Yanagisawa, N.: The functions of the descending root of the fifth nerve. Brain 96:783–814, 1973.
31. Kenshalo, D.R., Jr., Giesler, G.J., Leonard, R.B., and Willis, W.D.: Responses of neurons in primate ventral posterior lateral nucleus to noxious stimuli. J. Neurophysiol. 43:1594–1614, 1980.

32. Penfield, W. and Rasmussen, T.: *The Cerebral Cortex of Man.* The Macmillan Company, New York, 1950.
33. Anderson, S.A., Keller, O., Roos, A., and Rydenhag, B.: Cortical projection of tooth pulp afferents in the cat. In *Pain in the Trigeminal Region.* D.J. Andersson and B. Matthews (eds.). Elsevier-North Holland Publishing Co., Amsterdam, 1977.
34. Kenshalo, D.R., Jr. and Isensee, O.: Responses of primate SI cortical neurons to noxious stimuli. J. Neurophysiol. 50:1479–1496, 1983.
35. Mayer, D.J. and Liebeskind, J.C.: Pain reduction by focal electrical stimulation of the brain: an anatomical and behavioral analysis. Brain Res. 68:73–93, 1974.
36. Fields, H.L.: An endorphin-mediated analgesia system: experimental and clinical observations. In *Neurosecretion and Brain Peptides: Implications for Brain Function and Neurologic Disease.* J.B. Martin, S. Reichlin, and K.L. Bick (eds.). Raven Press, New York, 1981.
37. Duggan, A.W., Hall, J.G., and Headly, P.M.: Morphine, encephalin and the substantia gelantinosa. Nature 264:456–458, 1976.
38. Lewis, J.W., Cannon, J.T., and Liebeskind, J.C.: Opioid and nonopioid mechanisms of stress analgesia. Science 208:623–625, 1980.
39. Sternbach, R.A.: Clinical aspects of pain. In *The Psychology of Pain,* 2nd ed. R.A. Sternback (ed.). Raven Press, New York, 1986.
40. Sternbach, R.A.: *Pain Patients: Traits and Treatment.* Academic Press, New York, 1974.
41. Dolce, J.J. and Raczynski, J.M.: Neuromuscular activity and electromyography in painful backs: psychological and biomechanical models in assessment and treatment. Psychol. Bull. 97:502–520, 1985.
42. Turk, D.C., Miechenbaum, D., and Genest, M.: *Pain and Behavioral Medicine: A Cognitive-Behavioral Perspective.* Guilford Press, New York, 1983.
43. Fordyce, W.E.: *Behavioral Methods for Chronic Pain and Illness.* C.V. Mosby Co., St. Louis, 1976.
44. Ochoa, L.J., Torebjork, E., Marchettini, P., and Sivak, M.: Mechanisms of neuropathic pain: cumulative observations, new experiments, and further speculation. In *Advances in Pain Research and Therapy,* vol. 9. H.L. Fields, R. Dubner, and F. Cervero (eds.). Raven Press, New York, 1985.
45. Bonica, J.J.: Causalgia and other reflex sympathetic dystrophies. In *Advances in Pain Research and Therapy,* vol. 3. J.J. Bonica, J.C. Liebeskind, and D.G. Albe-Fessard (eds.). Raven Press, New York, 1979.
46. Wall, P. and Gutnick, M.: Ongoing activity in peripheral nerves: the physiology and pharmacology of impulses originating from a neuroma. Exp. Neurol. 43:580–593, 1974.
47. Travell, J.: Myofascial trigger points: clinical view. In *Advances in Pain Research and Therapy,* vol. 1. J.J. Bonica and D. Albe-Fessard (eds.). Raven Press, New York, 1976.

Rebecca Castaneda

CHAPTER 4

Occlusion

The etiology of temporomandibular disorders (TMDs) has been the subject of much controversy. Basic and clinical research, however, has brought about a better understanding of the causative factors and a recognition of the presence of multiple, often coexisting, causative factors.

McNeill and coworkers[1] have described three etiologic factors in TMDs as follows: (1) predisposing factors, (2) precipitating or triggering factors, and (3) perpetuating or sustaining factors.

Predisposing factors include the structural, neurologic, vascular, hormonal, and metabolic features of an individual. A factor that can increase joint loading and predispose a patient to a TMD is loss of posterior teeth. Psoriasis may predispose a patient to systemic arthritic changes, including the temporomandibular joint (TMJ). Hypothyroidism may predispose a patient to muscular pain.

Precipitating factors generally fall into the following four categories: (1) overt, extrinsic trauma to the head, neck or jaw; (2) repeated, low-grade extrinsic trauma, such as nail biting, chewing on pencils, and violin playing; (3) repeated low-grade intrinsic trauma, such as clenching or bruxism; and (4) stress that passes a certain threshold, which is individual for each patient.

Perpetuating or contributing factors are those that aid in the continuation of symptoms and often go unrecognized by the clinician.[1] Examples include underlying systemic disease and chronic cervical spine pathology.

Considerable overlap occurs in these categories, and what may be a predisposing factor in one patient may be a perpetuating or precipitating factor in another. It is unclear in which category occlusal disturbances belong. Clinicians make strong arguments for occlusion acting both as a predisposing factor and as a perpetuating factor despite the lack of scientific evidence.

The role of occlusion in TMDs is muddled in disagreement. Little evidence supports the theory that occlusion is a primary etiologic factor, although a secondary or contributing role is probable. Cacchiotti[2] has reviewed the literature on this subject and observed that variations in research methodology make it difficult to derive definite conclusions. Ingervall and associates,[3] on the one hand, found significant statistical association between the presence of nonworking side interferences and signs of TMDs. On the other hand, Butler and coworkers[4] found no such correlation.

Ingervall's group found that the presence of a discrepancy between centric relation and maximum intercuspal position (CR-IP) was significantly associated with signs of TMDs. In contrast, both Pullinger[5] and Solberg's groups[6] could find no such relationship. Butler and associates[4] concluded that Angle's occlusal classification had no correlation with patient and nonpatient populations, whereas Pullinger and coworkers,[5] Castaneda and coworkers,[7] and Perry[8] have shown a statistically higher incidence of signs of TMDs in class II, division 2 patients (Fig. 4–1). Loss of molar support has been reported to be associated with signs and symptoms of TMDs by Mejersjo and Hollender,[9] Castaneda and associates,[10] and Oberg and associates[11] (Fig. 4–2).

McNeill[12] theorized that a broader array of biomechanical factors contributes to the development of TMDs rather than occlusal factors alone and suggests that research should broaden its focus from local occlusal factors to all of the biomechanical components of the stomatognathic system. A study by McNeill and previous work by Agerberg and Eckerdal[13] suggested that occlusal interferences can cause a shift in the condylar position within the fossa. Resulting increases in distractive or compressive forces may in turn be responsible for the development of regressive changes in the TMJ. Loss of molar support, as mentioned, is believed to increase or at least change the direction of joint loading, initiating remodeling and osteoarthrotic changes.[14] Lack of molar support is thought to cause a fulcrum in a more anterior position, resulting in greater joint loading.

Distractive forces due to second or third molar fulcruming may also result in biomechanical deviation and can cause joint instabil-

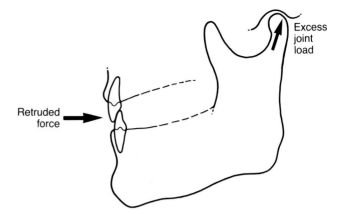

FIGURE 4–1. Class II, division 2 occlusion. Distal thrust may result in posterior compression of the temporomandibular joint.

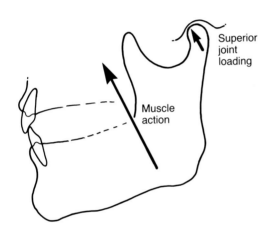

FIGURE 4–2. Loss of molar support. The anterior teeth serve as an anterior fulcrum resulting in increased temporomandibular joint loading.

ity (Fig. 4–3).[15] These distractive forces are also believed to increase neuromuscular activity necessary for joint stabilization.[16]

Many studies attempting to show a relationship between occlusion and TMDs have been criticized because of a failure to include specific diagnostic groups. Instead, symptoms were used as the criteria for identifying a particular group of patients. Other studies failed to utilize control groups. In addressing these issues, Seligman and Pullinger[32] conducted a study of 196 patients and 222 controls. They divided the patients into the following five separate well-defined diagnostic groups: (1) disc displacement with reduction; (2) disc diplacement without reduction; (3) osteoarthrosis with a history of prior derangement; (4) osteoarthrosis with no history of prior derangement; and (5) masticatory myalgia only.

They found the following results:

1. Large symmetric and asymmetric retruded contact position-intercuspal position (RCP-ICP) (greater than 1 mm) slides were more common in patients diagnosed as having

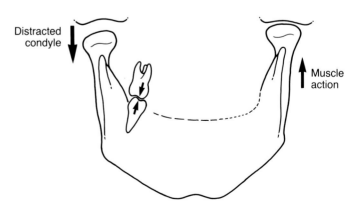

FIGURE 4–3. The second or third molar fulcrum motion may result in distraction of the temporomandibular joint on the same side.

osteoarthrosis, with or without histories of prior derangements, than in controls. Patients diagnosed as having masticatory myalgia were also more likely to have a large RCP-ICP slide.

2. Asymmetric RCP-ICP slides were more common in patients with a diagnosis of disc displacement with reduction and in patients with osteoarthrosis with or without histories of prior derangements.

3. A combination of unilateral RCP contacts and a lack of RCP-ICP slide was more common among females with disc diplacement with reduction.

4. Anterior open bite was more common in patients with osteoarthrosis with or without prior derangements and patients with myalgia only.

5. Cross bite and class II, division 2 patients showed no correlation with any diagnostic group.

These investigators, in this well-designed study, caution that their results do not prove a definite etiologic role of occlusion in causing TMDs. The relationships observed may have been a consequence of TMD; some may be predisposing factors, and others may be protective.

The role that occlusion plays in the development of functional disturbances of the masticatory system may be controversial, but its potential effects on the biomechanics of the craniofacial complex cannot be ignored. Occlusion as a single entity is probably not enough to precipitate mandibular dysfunction. However, occlusal pathology coexisting with other behavioral, psychologic, or somatic systemic factors appears to be significant. The multifactorial nature of TMDs together with the wide range of adaptive capacity among individuals continues to complicate the assessment of the specific role of occlusion in causing mandibular dysfunction.

STUDY OF OCCLUSION

The study of occlusion is an integral part of any dental curriculum. Historically, the emphasis has been on mechanical approaches, which led to the development of technically elaborate, precision instrumentation and conceptual engineering applications. Attention was paid strictly to the teeth and how they meet while ignoring other parts of the masticatory system.

Mohl,[28] in *A Textbook of Occlusion*, presented a biologic approach, calling for the ap-plication of the scientific method to test the clinical impressions and empirical judgments that the dental profession has employed in formulating treatment philosophies and principles. In the biologic approach, occlusion must not be limited to the study of how teeth come together but must encompass the functional and structural components of the entire masticatory system. Occlusion has been defined by many experts and has evolved to reflect physiologic principles. In 1899, Angle defined occlusal relationships in terms of static tooth contacts.[17]

In contrast, Jablonski[18] defined occlusion as follows:

The relationship between all the components of the masticatory system in normal function, dysfunction, and parafunction, including the morphological and functional features of contacting surfaces of opposing teeth and restorations, occlusal trauma and dysfunction, neuromuscular physiology, temporomandibular joint and muscle function, swallowing and mastication, psychophysiological status, and the diagnosis, prevention, and treatment of functional disorders of the masticatory system.

For the purposes of this discussion, occlusion can be classified into three groups: ideal, physiologic, and nonphysiologic. The clinical distinction of these three groups must be understood before pathologic changes can be diagnosed and properly treated.

IDEAL OCCLUSION

Occlusion is often described as being anatomically "ideal" if it follows a classic cusp-fossa, tooth-to-tooth pattern (Fig. 4–4). But to do so is to promulgate the outdated tooth-oriented concepts ignoring the other elements of

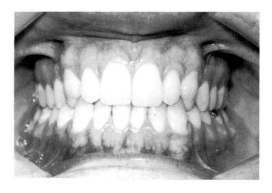

FIGURE 4–4. "Ideal" occlusion shown with an "ideal" tooth-to-tooth relationship.

the masticatory system. A description of a truly ideal occlusion must incorporate the other anatomic structures of the masticatory system in their respective ideal states and must also incorporate their functional interrelationships.

An ideal occlusion allows for the TMJs to be in their optimal functional position while the teeth are in maximal intercuspation. McNeill[19] has described the optimal condylar position as being "The structural or anatomical position (in a healthy joint) of the condyle with its biconcave disk braced against the eminence in an anterior superior direction . . . (and) with optimum integrated muscle activity as well as with maximal occlusal stability. . . . The muscle action with ligamentous support or restriction determines the optimum position of the condyle." The muscle pull across the TMJ determines the most stable condylar position—a statement that holds true for all joints.

The *Glossary of Prosthodontic Terms*[20] defines centric relation (CR) as follows:

A maxillary-mandibular relationship in which the condyles articulate with the thinnest vascular portion of their respective discs with the complex in the anterior-posterior position against the slopes of the articular eminence. This position is independent of tooth contact. This position is clinically discernible when the mandible is directed superiorly and anteriorly and restricted to purely rotary movements about a transverse horizontal axis (Fig. 4–5).

Centric occlusion (CO) is defined as "The occlusion of opposing teeth when the mandible is in centric relation. This may or may not coincide with the maximal intercuspal position."[20] In an ideal occlusion, centric occlusion coincides with maximal intercuspation. An ideal occlusion should also be stable, and there should be no evidence of change in tooth position or in the periodontium. The teeth should be aligned in the dental arches so that the masticatory forces are directed as much as possible

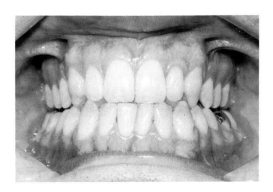

FIGURE 4–6. Anterior guidance illustrated in protrusive movement.

along their long axes without torquing lateral movement. This alignment of the dentition is the result of forces from the surrounding musculature that act on the dentition from all directions and position the teeth in the "neutral zone."[21]

In CO, the holding contacts are on the posterior teeth. The anterior teeth guide the mandible in functional movements when the teeth are in contact. In protrusive and laterotrusive movements, the posterior teeth are separated by the anterior teeth (Figs. 4–6 and 4–7).

The lingual cusps of maxillary posterior teeth, the buccal cusps of the mandibular posterior teeth, and the supporting cusps are responsible for maintaining a constant vertical dimension of occlusion (VDO). They also function in breaking down food in mastication. The buccal cusps of the maxillary posterior teeth, the lingual cusps of the mandibular posterior teeth, and the nonsupporting cusps help to maintain a bolus of food on the occlusal table. The posterior teeth are aligned so that they can adequately support the powerful ver-

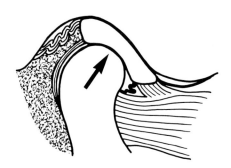

FIGURE 4–5. The optimal centric relation position of the condyle interposed with the meniscus.

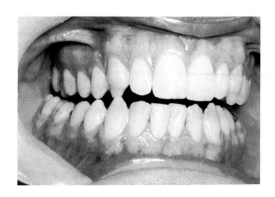

FIGURE 4–7. Anterior guidance illustrated in laterotrusive movement.

tical forces of mastication. In contrast the anterior teeth are labially inclined and cannot adequately support vertical forces. For this reason, the posterior teeth protect the anterior teeth from the extreme vertical forces of mastication while the anterior teeth maintain only slight CO contacts.[22]

The anterior teeth guide the mandible in protrusive and laterotrusive movements. In protrusive movement, the incisors should come into contact disoccluding the posterior teeth (incisal guidance). In laterotrusive movements, the canines disocclude all other teeth (canine guidance). Canine and incisal guidance are collectively termed anterior guidance. Because the anterior teeth are farther from the elevator muscles than the posterior teeth, less force is applied to the anterior teeth. Consequently, the anterior teeth are best suited for absorbing the horizontal forces of eccentric mandibular movements, which can be destructive to the posterior teeth.[23] In particular, the canine has the best suited bony architecture and crown-to-root ratio to tolerate horizontal forces. Williamson and Lundquist[24] have shown how masticatory muscle activity decreases when the posterior teeth disocclude in protrusive and laterotrusive movements. Rugh and colleagues[33] have shown that this can also occur with molar guidance as well. It seems that a single tooth contact as opposed to multiple tooth contacts is advantageous as a guide for lateral movement.

An ideal occlusion therefore provides for "mutual protection" of anterior and posterior teeth. There should be even, bilateral, simultaneous contact of all posterior teeth and only slight contact of the anterior teeth in CO. This relationship gives maximal stability to the TMJs and minimizes occlusal forces on each individual tooth. In eccentric contacts, the anterior teeth guide the mandible and protect the posterior teeth from horizontal forces.

In addition, an ideal occlusion should maintain the low postural tonicity of the masticatory muscles. Such an occlusion is void of local or peripheral stimuli, such as nonworking side interferences that together with extrinsic factors elevate the activity of these muscles.

Another requirement of an ideal occlusion is optimal function. The masticatory system is involved in speech, mastication, and swallowing. The position of the dentition is critical in these functions. For instance, the ideal position of the maxillary incisors allows for contact of the incisal edges with the wet-dry line of the lower lip for a clear and distinct "f" or "v"

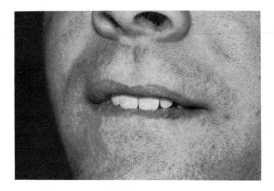

FIGURE 4–8. Patient producing "f" or "v" sound. Note the position of the maxillary incisal edges at the wet-dry line of the lower lip.

sound (Fig. 4–8). The maxillary and mandibular incisors must come to an edge-to-edge relationship for the proper incision of food. Opposing posterior teeth should be oriented along their long axes for efficient grinding of food to occur. The ideal occlusion must also be comfortable and aesthetically pleasing to the patient.

Even if all of the previously described requirements are present, occlusion can be considered pathologic if there is painful function, discomfort, or aesthetic displeasure. Occlusal factors not considered pathologic in one individual may, in combination with other stimuli, be pathologic in another. Adaptive capacity plays a role in each individual's tolerance to occlusal factors, whether ideal by definition or not ideal.

PHYSIOLOGIC AND FUNCTIONAL OCCLUSION

Few individuals actually have ideal occlusions,[5] yet most who have "malocclusions" function well. The adaptive capacity in most people is high enough that a significant deviation from the ideal occlusion may be very "normal," stable, and harmonious. Pullinger and associates[5] found that in a nonpatient population of 120 males and 102 females with a mean age of 29, ICP and RCP were coincident in only 29% of the sample. Of this sample, 60% were found to have unilateral molar contact in RCP. No statistically significant association was found between those with ICP-RCP slides and those with TMJ clicking or tenderness. Likewise, no relationship was found between unilateral molar contact in RCP and TMJ clicking or tenderness.

Studies on mandibular dysfunction patients have failed to date to identify which occlusal variables predispose these patients to TMDs. Thomson[26] compared 100 patients who had signs and symptoms of TMJ pain and dysfunction with 100 controls. No statistically significant differences in the prevalence of displaced path of closure, lack of posterior tooth support, wear facets, or clenching habits were found between these two groups.

As Carlsson[27] observed, "One individual's occlusion may have marked deviations from 'normal' orthodontic standards but provide excellent function, while another subject may have an occlusion with optimal morphologic relationships yet be suffering mandibular dysfunction. This is the background for the controversy regarding the consequences of occlusal interferences." He goes on to say that "The dentition's lack of distinct influence on mandibular and TMJ dysfunction that is pointed out (by research) may be explained by the wide range of adaptability in individuals' masticatory systems and by the multifactorial etiology of dysfunction."

Mohl[28] has described the prerequisites for a physiologic occlusion as follows:

It could very well be a malocclusion, but it is a malocclusion in a state of health. It is an occlusion that has adapted well to its environment, is aesthetically satisfactory to the patient, has no pathological manifestations or dysfunctional problems, is in a state of harmony and requires no therapeutic intervention.

As with an ideal occlusion, a physiologic occlusion is also stable. There should be no drifting or extrusion of teeth, nor should there be any changes in tooth mobility, periodontal ligament thickness, or wear on teeth or increased dental sensitivity. Signs of change in the masticatory system may be indicative of parafunction which unlike normal function is damaging.

Mandibular function should be comfortable and painless. There should be no complaints regarding ease of mandibular movement. A complaint of an inability to chew for whatever reason is nonphysiologic for that patient. A patient may complain of a lack of sufficient teeth on one or both sides, muscle fatigue, or TMJ pain while chewing. Any recurring pain or discomfort during function is a sign of dysfunction.

A physiologic occlusion should be aesthetically pleasing to the patient. What may be an unsightly tooth arrangement to the dentist may be satisfactory or even pleasant to the patient.

Provided the other criteria for a physiologic occlusion are met, it is irresponsible and unnecessary to impose corrective treatment for a patient who has no complaint in this regard.

NONPHYSIOLOGIC OCCLUSION IDENTIFICATION AND THERAPIES

Most people have occlusions that deviate from the ideal. Most, however, have the adaptive potential to tolerate this deviation and function without signs or symptoms of dysfunction. A segment of the population does suffer from signs and symptoms of mandibular dysfunction—some of whom deviate from the ideal but others who don't. Pullinger and coworkers[5] showed that in a population of healthy individuals, the incidence of TMJ clicking was greatest in subjects with no ICP-RCP slide and in subjects with unilateral as opposed to bilateral molar contact in RCP.

In the same way that the masticatory muscles and the TMJs exhibit signs and symptoms of mandibular dysfunction, so can the dentition and its supporting structures. Signs of dysfunction at the tooth level include mobility, occlusal wear, tooth fractures, hypersensitive or painful teeth, and drifting of teeth. The presence of these signs may reflect a functional disturbance that has exceeded the adaptive capacity of the dentition and its supporting structures.

Mohl[28] explains that "Such signs and symptoms may be the result of how the individual uses the occlusion and not a result of its structural features. Thus, the term nonphysiologic occlusion does not imply cause and effect. It merely suggests that a problem already exists or that a physiologic outcome is doubtful and that treatment may be indicated."

Mohl, when talking about "how the individual uses the occlusion," was likely referring to bruxism and clenching—parafunctional habits, common in the general population. Helkimo[29] reported the frequency in two nonpatient populations to be 42%. Solberg and colleagues[6] reported that signs and symptoms of bruxism were observed in 80 to 90% of a study population.

Parafunctional behavior does not necessarily lead to a TMD or to a nonphysiologic occlusion. Parafunction is a central nervous system phenomenon and thus the occlusion is a secondary consideration. The pattern, frequency, and nature of the behavior, as well as the adaptive capacity of the individual, will determine if the outcome will be destructive. The effect of parafunction may be short-lived, i.e., temporary jaw fatigue, or it may be chronically destructive and eventually debilitating. The most prominent feature of parafunctional behavior is excessive loading. Whether intermittent or constant, the increased loading may damage the teeth, joints, and muscles.

Parafunctional behaviors differ from normal function in that they are often subconscious (Table 4–1). It is common for patients to deny that they have such habits. Forces applied during nocturnal bruxism can exceed three times that of normal function. The forces generated in normal function, such as eating and swallowing, are better tolerated because these forces are directed along the long axes of the teeth. In comparison, parafunctional activities frequently have horizontal components.

Most functional activities occur close to the maximal intercuspal position, distributing forces over a maximum number of teeth. Parafunctional activities occur in eccentric positions and apply forces to a fewer number of teeth and often in an unstable joint position. The likelihood of damage to the teeth and the TMJs is increased. Furthermore, parafunctional isometric activity inhibits the normal blood flow necessary for tissue oxygenation and by-product elimination, resulting in muscle pain and fatigue. Protective reflexes that control functional activities are less responsive or absent during parafunctional activities.[22]

Because of the close association between parafunction and tissue damage and the prevalence of parafunctional behavior, it is critical for the dentist to identify and manage any oral parafunctional habits.

A telltale sign of parafunction is increased tooth mobility in a patient with a healthy periodontium. The mobility is due to occlusal overload. Radiographically, the width of the

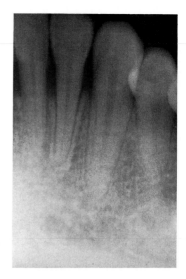

FIGURE 4–9. Increased periodontal ligament space from primary occlusal trauma often caused by parafunction.

periodontal ligament space may be increased (Fig. 4–9). In the absence of periodontal inflammation, the effects of occlusal trauma are believed to be reversible after the management and elimination of excessive loading. In the presence of periodontal inflammation, however, occlusal trauma can contribute to the rapid and irreversible destruction of bony support.[30]

Tooth wear and fracture are often destructive signs of parafunction (Fig. 4–10). Wear facets are simply identified as noncontiguous anatomy on occlusal or incisal tooth surfaces. If an abrasive diet is not a factor, such wear will usually be due to nonfunctional activities. Examination of wear patterns or "facets" often reveals that bruxism occurs in eccentric mandibular positions, beyond the normal functional range and in contrast to the normal

TABLE 4–1. Comparison of Functional and Parafunctional Activities Using Five Common Factors

FACTOR	FUNCTIONAL ACTIVITY	PARAFUNCTIONAL ACTIVITY
Forces of tooth contacts	17,200 lb-sec/day	57,600 lb-sec/day (possibly more)
Direction of applied forces to teeth	Vertical (well-tolerated)	Horizontal (not well-tolerated)
Mandibular position	Centric occlusion (relatively stable)	Eccentric movements (relatively unstable)
Type of muscle contraction	Isotonic (physiologic)	Isometric (nonphysiologic)
Influence of protective reflexes	Present	Absent
Pathologic effects	Unlikely	Very likely

Reprinted with permission from Okesson, J.: *Fundamentals of Occlusion and TMD*, 2nd ed. C.V. Mosby Co., St. Louis, 1989.

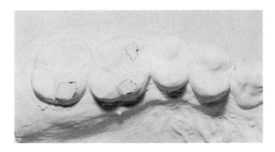

FIGURE 4–10. Study model showing wear facets resulting from parafunctional activity.

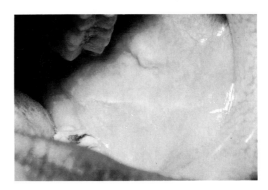

FIGURE 4–12. A linea alba indicative of cheek biting.

physiologic wear of aging seen in the functional range (Fig. 4–11).

Tooth fractures are often the result of horizontal loads placed on cusp inclines. Another symptom sometimes associated with parafunction is tooth hypersensitivity or pulpitis. A complaint of hypersensitivity or pain to heat or cold may be only the beginning of a pulpal necrosis. Although decay is the most common cause of this condition, the clinician often sees a patient with tooth pain and no sign of clinical or radiographic pathology. Occlusal parafunction should be considered as part of the differential diagnosis.

Soft tissue changes indicating parafunction include the presence of a linea alba from cheek biting (Fig. 4–12), a scalloped tongue (Fig. 4–13), and muscle hypertrophy. The coexistence of these signs with the presence of wear facets helps determine if bruxism or clenching is a current or past behavior.

A nonphysiologic occlusion is not necessarily the result of parafunction. Loss of teeth, for instance, can cause drifting and supereruption

of teeth (Fig. 4–14), resulting in working and nonworking interferences. The loss of teeth may cause unilateral function and overload of the remaining teeth and TMJs. Excessive load on the tissues of the TMJ may lead to remodeling.[7] Lack of posterior support, particularly in the presence of a compromised periodontium, often leads to maxillary anterior tooth flaring, creating spaces between teeth and overclosing the vertical dimension of occlusion further loading the TMJs.

MALOCCLUSION RESULTING FROM A TEMPOROMANDIBULAR DISORDER

Most clinicians and researchers focus their discussions on the ability of malocclusions to cause TMDs. Malocclusion, however, may be the direct effect of a TMD—the *result* of articular or neuromuscular pathology. For instance, a patient with osteoarthrosis may develop an anterior open bite or a unilateral posterior oc-

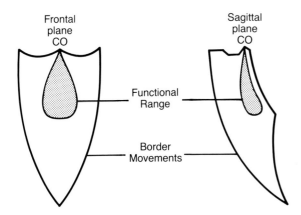

FIGURE 4–11. Parafunction often occurs beyond the normal functional range. (CO = centric occlusion.)

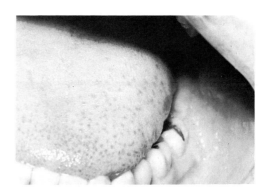

FIGURE 4–13. A scalloped tongue indicative of tongue biting.

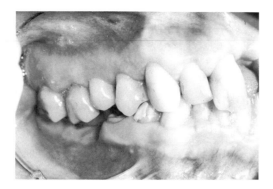

FIGURE 4–14. Loss of teeth may result in severe drifting and supereruption of teeth.

clusion secondary to condylar shortening associated with this disease process (Figs. 4–15 and 4–16). Schellhas[31] has described how joint inflammation and avascular necrosis can lead to transient and permanent severe occlusal dis-

turbances (see Chapter 16). Developmental anomalies, neoplastic lesions, and maxillary and mandibular fractures are other examples of pathologies that can lead to malocclusion. These occlusal changes can be so severe that their correction requires a combination of prosthodontic, orthodontic, and surgical treatment.

A malocclusion can also be the result of asymmetric muscle hyperactivity. The term "acute malocclusion" describes a transient malocclusion due to muscle spasm and is characterized by premature contacts on the contralateral side and no contact on the ipsilateral side.[22]

SUMMARY

Occlusion is a part of the masticatory system. The entire system functions as a unit and is influenced not only by the teeth but by all the

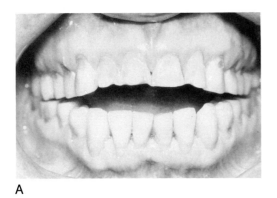

A

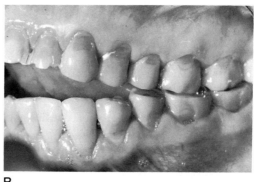

B

FIGURE 4–15. A and B, Anterior open bite in a patient suffering from osteoarthrosis.

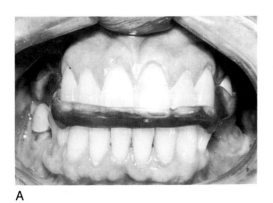

A

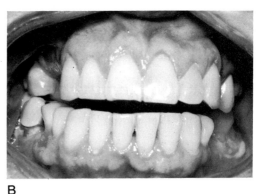

B

FIGURE 4–16. Unilateral posterior open bite in a patient with osteoarthrosis. A, With a stabilization appliance. B, Without a stabilization appliance.

components. The clinical must recognize that the individual's physical and psychologic makeup and adaptive capacity can have dramatic effects on this system. The weak correlation between occlusal disturbance and mandibular dysfunction shown in the current research points to the importance of the multifactorial etiology of TMDs.

REFERENCES

1. McNeill, C., Danzig, W.M., Farrar, W.B., et al: Craniomandibular (TMJ) disorders—the state-of-the-art. J. Prosthet. Dent. 44:434–437, 1980.
2. Cacchiotti, D.: Etiologic factors associated with TMJ dysfunction. U.C.S.F. Dental Explorer 2:9–12, 1988.
3. Ingervall, B., Mogin, B., and Thylander, B.: Prevalence of symptoms of functional disturbances of the masticatory system in Swedish men. J. Oral Rehab. 7:185–197, 1980.
4. Butler, J.H., Folke, L.E.A., and Bandt, C.L.: A descriptive survey of signs and symptoms associated with the myofascial pain-dysfunction syndrome. J. Am. Dent. Assoc. 90:635–639, 1975.
5. Pullinger, A.G., Seligman, D.A., and Solberg, W.K.: Temporomandibular disorders. Part II. Occlusal factors associated with temporomandibular joint tenderness and dysfunction. J. Prosthet. Dent. 59:363–367, 1988.
6. Solberg, W.K., Woo, M.W., and Houston, J.B.: Prevalence of mandibular dysfunction in young adults. J. Am. Dent. Assoc. 98:25–34, 1979.
7. Castaneda, R., McNeill, C., and Guerrero, A.: Biomechanics in TMJ osteoarthritis. Part II. J. Dent. Res. 68:43, 1989.
8. Perry, H.T.: Relation of occlusion to TMJ dysfunction: the orthodontic viewpoint. J. Am. Dent. Assoc. 79:137–141, 1969.
9. Mejersjo, C. and Hollender, L.: TMJ pain and dysfunction: relation between clinical and radiographic findings in the short- and long-term. Scand. J. Dent. Res. 92:241–248, 1984.
10. Castaneda, R.C., McNeill, C., and Noble, W.: Biomechanical factors in TMJ osteoarthritis. J. Dent. Res. 67:87, 1988.
11. Obserg, T., Carlsson, G.E., and Fajers, C.M.: The temporomandibular joint: a morphologic study of a human autopsy material. Acta Odontol. Scand. 29:349–384, 1971.
12. McNeill, C.: Mandibular position indicator. J. Dent. Res. 68:43, 1989.
13. Agerberg, G. and Eckerdal O.: Occlusal and temporomandibular joint relations: a comparative study. J. Craniomandib. Pract. 5:3, 234–239, 1987.
14. Smith, D.M., McLachian, D.R., and McCall, W.D., Jr.: A numerical model of TM joint loading. J. Dent. Res. 65(8):1046–1052, 1986.
15. Roth, R.H.: TM joint pain-dysfunction and occlusal relationships. Angle Orthod. 43:136–153, 1973.
16. Hylander, W.L.: Functional anatomy. In *The TMJ*, 3rd ed. B.G. Sarnett and D.M. Laskin (eds.). Springfield, Charles C Thomas, 85–113, 1979.
17. Angle, E.H. Classification of malocclusion. Dent. Cosmos. 41:248, 1899.
18. Jablonski, S.: *Illustrated Dictionary of Dentistry.* W.B. Saunders Co., Philadelphia, 1982.
19. McNeill, C.: The optimal TMJ condylar position in clinical practice. Int. J. Periodont. Rest. Dent. 6:53–76, 1985.
20. *Glossary of Prosthodontic Terms.* J. Prosthet. Dent. 58:6, 715–762, 1987.
21. Dawson, P.E.: *Evaluation, Diagnosis and Treatment of Occlusal Problems,* 2nd ed. C.V. Mosby Co., St. Louis, 1989.
22. Okeson, J.P.: *Fundamentals of Occlusion and Temporomandibular Disorders.* C.V. Mosby Co., St. Louis, 1985.
23. Lee, R.L.: Anterior guidance. In *Advances in Occlusion.* H. Lundeen and C.H. Gibbs (eds.). John Wright PSG Inc., Boston, 1982.
24. Williamson, E.H. and Lundquist, D.O.: Anterior guidance: its effect on electromyographic activity of the temporal and masseter muscles. J. Prosthet. Dent. 49:816–821, 1983.
25. Manns, A., Chan, C., and Miralles, R.: Influence of group function and canine guidance on electromyographic activity of elevator muscles. J. Prosthet. Dent. 57:494–500, 1987.
26. Thomson, H.: Mandibular dysfunction syndrome. Br. Dent. J. 130:187–193, 1971.
27. Carlsson, G.E.: Consequences of occlusal interferences. In *Prosthodontic Treatment in Partially Edentulous Patients.* G.A. Zarb et al (eds.). C. V. Mosby Co., St. Louis, 1978.
28. Mohl, N.D.: Diagnostic rationale: an overview. In *A Textbook of Occlusion.* N.G. Mohl, G.A. Zarb, G. Carlsson, and J. Rugh (eds.). Quintessence Books, Chicago, 1988.
29. Helkimo, M.: Studies on function and dysfunction of the masticatory system. II. Index for anamnestic and clinical dysfunction and occlusal state. Swed. Dent. J. 67f:101–108, 1974.
30. Glickman, I.: Inflammation and trauma from occlusion: codestructive factors in chronic periodontal disease. J. Periodontol. 34:5, 1963.
31. Schellhas, K.P.: Unstable occlusion and TMJ disease. J. Clin. Orthodont. 22:5, 332–337, 1989.
32. Seligman, D. and Pullinger, A.: Association of occlusal variables among defined TM patient diagnostic groups. J. Craniomandib. Dis. 3:227–236, 1989.
33. Rugh, J., Graham, G., Smith, J., and Ohrbach, R.: Effects of canine versus molar occlusal splint guidance on nocturnal bruxism and craniomandibular symptomatology. J. of Craniomandib. Dis. 3:4, 203–210, 1989.

Jeffrey S. Mannheimer
John Dunn

CHAPTER 5

Cervical Spine

Evaluation and Relation to Temporomandibular Disorders

Many patients with craniofacial pain do not present with obvious dysfunction of the temporomandibular joints (TMJs). A significant number of patients who present with TMJ pain or dysfunction may have no history of direct trauma or known intrinsic etiology. These patients, however, are seen often at facial and TMJ pain clinics. Prior to their visit to these specialty clinics, many of these patients have previously seen family practitioners, chiropractors, neurologists, otolaryngologists, dentists, and psychiatrists. The patient also has often gone through great expense, frustration, and despair.

A working knowledge of extrinsic etiology that can produce temporomandibular disorders (TMDs) is imperative. Perhaps the most common extrinsic factor is dysfunction of the cervical spine. The cervical spine is intimately related to the cranium and masticatory system via specific joint articulations, muscle attachments, and neural and vascular innervations. Postural abnormalities that alter the normal relationship between the head and the neck frequently lead to TMDs that are often overlooked by the dentist as well as the physician.

Abnormal posture can result in compression of the suboccipital region and produce pain referred to the temporomandibular region as well as alter the normal resting position of the mandible. The net effect can change normal TMJ arthrokinematics, increase compression forces, and produce intrinsic derangements either by acute or cumulative macrotrauma or microtrauma.

Therapeutic procedures that focus on the pain or dysfunction, or both, of the TMJ may have very little relation to the true etiology. The patient becomes dependent on medications or other pain control techniques, and long-term splint usage is common. Sometimes, misdirected surgical interventions are used. Many patients thus develop chronic pain syndromes and are frequently given a diagnosis of myofascial pain dysfunction (MPD) or chronic facial pain.

It is the purpose of this chapter to highlight the relationship of the head and neck while presenting the procedures by which a dentist can perform a screening of the cervical spine as part of the temporomandibular evaluation. A working knowledge of cervical spine anatomy, including joint, muscle, vascular, and neural relationships, is thus imperative along with an understanding of pain and dysfunction mechanisms, prior to performing the evaluation and determining the need to refer the patient.

ANATOMY OF THE CERVICAL SPINE

The cervical spine is the prime component of what is known as the upper quarter. The upper quarter, however, also consists of the cranium, mandible, TMJs, dentition, upper or suboccipital and midlower cervical spine, hyoid bone, cervicothoracic junction, upper thoracic spine, first and second ribs, sternum, clavicle, shoulder girdle, and upper extremity. The relationship among all of the upper quarter components is so intertwined that abnormalities of any one structure can frequently cause or contribute to pain and dysfunction of an adjacent structure. The entire upper quarter is therefore considered to represent a functional unit, because the position or movement of one component part can easily influence another.

Skeletal Relationships

The cervical spine is composed of seven vertebrae. These can be further subdivided into the upper cervical spine, consisting of occiput, atlas (C1) and axis (C2), and the C3-C7 vertebrae, comprising the midlower cervical spine. The upper cervical spine, also known as the suboccipital spine and craniovertebral region, is structurally different from the remainder of the cervical region. Support of the head is a prime function of the atlas and axis, which differ structurally from the other cervical vertebrae (Fig. 5–1). The atlas does not have a vertebral body but an anterior and a posterior arch with palpable transverse processes, without a palpable spinous process. Superior facets on the lateral masses of the anterior surface articulate with those of the occipital condyles to form the occipital atlantoid joint (OA). Inferior facets articulate with the superior facets of the axis forming the atlantoaxial (AA) joint. The axis is also structurally different from the atlas and remaining cervical vertebrae. Its transverse processes are short and not palpable, whereas its spinous process is the largest of all cervical vertebrae and is bifid, making it simple to palpate. The vertebral body is minimal and contains the odontoid process or dens, which has an anterior facet that articulates with the atlas at its anterior arch. The anterior arch also possesses an articulating facet to the odontoid process of the axis located behind the anterior tubercle. Figure 5–2 illustrates the occiput-atlas-axis complex from a variety of views.

The remainder of the cervical vertebrae possess significant anterior vertebral bodies, superior and inferior articulating facets, plus small transverse and posterior spinous processes. Unlike the spinous process of the axis, which is directed posteriorly, those of C3-C7 also have an inferior inclination (Fig. 5–3).

Intervertebral discs are absent between occiput and atlas as well as between atlas and axis. However, the vertebral bodies of all other cervical vertebrae are separated by discs. The discs help to promote a normal cervical lordosis in comparison with the suboccipital region, which is oriented into a slight kyphosis. These curvatures are altered by active movements of the head and neck as well as by abnormal postures.

The first and most superior cervical joint where movement can occur is the OA joint between the occiput and atlas. This is a saddle-shaped joint in which the articular surfaces are oriented to promote a sliding movement of the

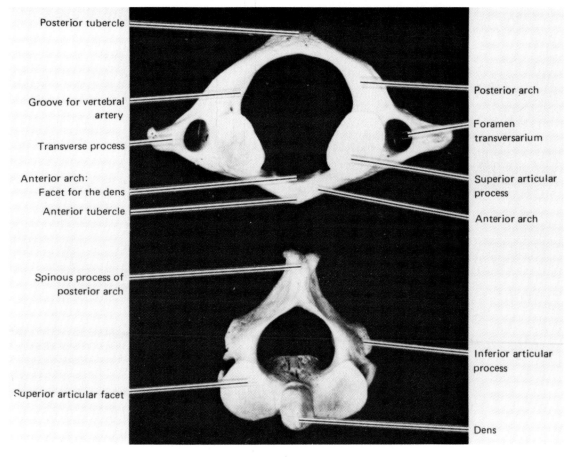

FIGURE 5–1. Superior view of atlas (top). Superior view of axis (bottom). (Reprinted with permission from Hiatt, J.L. and Gartner, L.P.: *Textbook of Head and Neck Anatomy,* 2nd ed. Williams & Wilkins, Baltimore, 1987.)

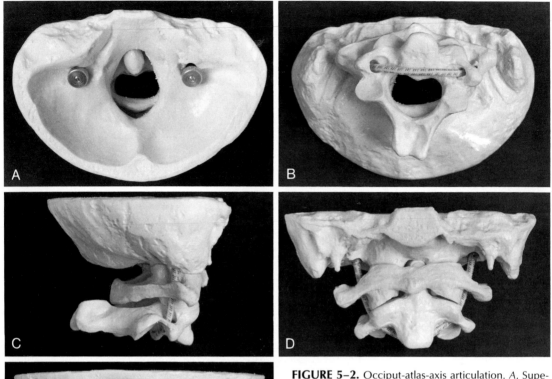

FIGURE 5–2. Occiput-atlas-axis articulation. *A,* Superior view. *B,* Inferior view. *C,* Lateral view. *D,* Anterior view. *E,* Posterior view.

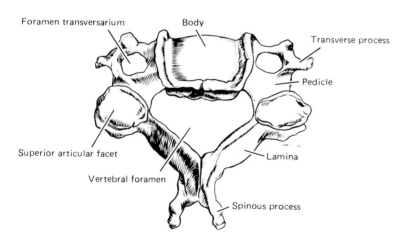

FIGURE 5–3. Typical midcervical vertebra. (Reprinted with permission from Hiatt, J.L. and Gartner, L.P.: *Textbook of Head and Neck Anatomy,* 2nd ed. Williams & Wilkins, Baltimore, 1987.)

convex cranium (occiput) forward and backward on the concave atlas. This motion is more appropriately termed nodding or anterior and posterior cranial rotation and occurs within a range of 15 to 20 degrees from neutral.[1,2] A greater degree of anterior cranial rotation (ACR) occurs at AA in comparison to OA. However, twice as much posterior cranial rotation (PCR) takes place at OA than AA (Fig. 5–4).[1,3]

Sidebending and rotation in the suboccipital area, known as axial rotation, occur independently of one another, whereas in the mid to lower cervical spine these motions occur together.[2] Motion in this area has been reviewed in a three-dimensional analysis: sidebending occurs in the same direction as rotation at segments below the C3-C4 level and in the opposite direction of rotation above the C2-C3 level (OA and AA).[4] This finding represents a natural coupling motion of the craniovertebral complex. An equal amount (5 to 10 degrees) of sidebending takes place at OA and AA. The greatest degree of craniovertebral rotation takes place at AA and is considered to be 50 to 70% of the entire cervical region, which represents about 105 degrees to either side from the neutral position. A minimal degree of pure rotation occurs at OA that ranges from 0 to 5 degrees. Each segment below AA demonstrates only 4 to 8 degrees of rotation.[4]

The majority of cervical motion occurs between C2-C7. Flexion and extension also known as forward and backward bending, respectively, are greatest at C5-C6, with the C4-C5 and C6-C7 segments a close second. The facet joints at these levels are oriented to promote forward and backward bending while inhibiting rotation and sidebending from occurring separately. Thus, whenever sidebending is performed, in the midlower cervical spine, rotation also occurs simultaneously to the same side.[3] Forward bending occurs with rotation below the C5-C6 level and backward bending with rotation above the C4-C5 level. The net result is that whenever cervical spine rotation occurs the greatest degree of weight bearing is on the anterior edge of the vertebral bodies below the C5-C6 segments and the posterior edge above C4-C5.[4] This factor presents strong implications to the site of the degenerative joint disease known as spondylosis.

The facet joints also known as zygopophyseal joints consist of a superior and inferior articular process from adjacent vertebrae that move in a gliding motion, which is most pronounced in forward bending. There are 14 facet joints from the occiput to the first thoracic vertebrae. These are all of the synovial variety and are highly innervated. The cervical spine is also unique in that from C3-T1 there are additional saddle-shaped articulations known as uncovertebral joints of Luschka. These are situated at the superior aspect of the vertebral body and serve to inhibit sidebending, as they are most pronounced posterolaterally.[5] There are ten uncovertebral joints that can develop synovial and arthritic degenerative changes.

Range of motion at the midlower cervical spine is much greater than that of the craniovertebral region in forward and backward bending as well as sidebending and is explained further in the chapter. The importance of test-

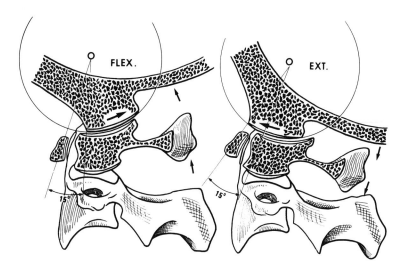

FIGURE 5–4. Forward and backward nodding of the occipital-atlantal complex. (Reprinted with permission from Kapandji, I.A.: *The Physiology of the Joints, vol. 3. The Trunk and Vertebral Column.* Churchill Livingstone, New York, 1974.)

ing upper and midlower cervical components separately is a prime consideration when dealing with craniofacial pain, occlusal alterations, or both that may originate from the craniovertebral complex.[6-8]

The cervical thoracic junction consists of the last cervical vertebrae and the first two thoracic vertebrae. Also present at this region is the beginning of the rib cage, and ribs 1 and 2 thus are considered part of the upper quarter. Joint articulations between the ribs and vertebral bodies are known as the costovertebral joints.

Soft tissue connections between upper quarter skeletal structures consist of the ligaments, fascia, and muscle. In the suboccipital region, strong ligamental arrangements are the most important and provide for stability and coordinated movements of the OA and AA joints. The transverse ligament of the atlas stabilizes the odontoid process against the anterior arch of the atlas, as it courses across the posterior aspect of the odontoid shaft.

The function of the alar ligaments is to maintain the odontoid process between the lateral mass of the atlas. Additional posterior ligamental bands course between the superolateral odontoid region to the medial aspect of each occipital condyle.[9]

The importance of this region in the examination, as it relates to the neck, is to assess the integrity of the alar-odontoid complex prior to performing any active or passive movements. This assessment may necessitate specific radiologic or manual evaluation to rule out fractures or displacement of the atlas or axis. Subluxations can commonly occur from automobile accidents as well as from rheumatoid arthritis (RA) and Down's syndrome. In RA, subluxation is due to inflammation of the soft tissues at the AA joint, including the synovium and transverse ligament producing a rupture. The process may even extend to the occipital condyles and lateral mass of the atlas causing erosion and osteolysis.[10-12]

Arthrokinetics of the OA region results in an anterior glide of the atlas upon forward nodding of the head on the neck and a posterior glide with backward nodding (see Fig. 5–4). Any joint restriction in this region could be observed by the chin's deviating to the affected side upon nodding. When sidebending occurs, the atlas will normally glide to the same side as the occiput. Discussion of the entire arthrokinematic sequence in the suboccipital area is beyond the scope of this chapter. However, the dentist should observe for head tilt, assess range of motion (ROM), order a radiologic ex-

amination, or refer the patient for a medical consult whenever blurred vision, tinnitus, dizziness syncope, concentration difficulties, vertigo, or nausea is reported. This practice is especially important following acute trauma, such as a whiplash injury, or in a chronic condition, such as RA, that can lead to subluxation. This symptomatology may be indicative of an odontoid fracture and any passive head positioning should be avoided.[10-13]

The course of the vertebral artery from the posterosuperior aspect of the subclavian and behind the anterior scalene muscle and transverse process of C7 extends through the transverse foramina of C1-C6. This artery is in close contact with the uncovertebral joints. The vertebral artery then enters the suboccipital area and courses into the foramen magnum. This distribution makes it a prime suspect in the aforementioned symptomatology. The artery lies along a groove on the superior surface of the atlas before coursing through the transverse foramina into the foramen magnum and may easily be impinged by abnormal suboccipital posture.[14,15]

Other ligamental structures that join the cranium to the suboccipital spine include the posterior longitudinal ligament, the posterior and anterior atlanto-occipital membranes, the ligamentum nuchae, and the apical ligament. The ligamentum nuchae is important because it is composed of fibroelastic tissue and provides a septum for the attachment of other regional musculature. Its distribution is from the external occipital protuberance to the spine of C7. The ligamentum nuchae is continuous with the supraspinous and interspinous ligaments. Connections between the occipital base and foramen magnum to the atlas and axis are most significant.[9]

Ligamental support of the spine consists primarily of the anterior and posterior longitudinal ligaments, which course along the front and back of the cervical vertebral bodies, respectively. In addition, the supraspinous and interspinous ligaments exist between the spinous processes of C7 to the sacrum. The prevention of excessive motion and stabilization are prime functions of these structures. Intertransverse ligaments joining adjacent transverse processes are underdeveloped in the cervical region and thus offer minimal stability.

Intervertebral Discs

The first intervertebral disc lies between the axis and the third cervical vertebra. Intervertebral discs have vertebral end plates, which articulate with the adjacent vertebral bodies. The posterior portion of the discs lies anterior to the intervertebral foramina, which contain the spinal nerve roots. The discs are composed of an external cartilaginous annulus fibrosis and internal cottage cheese–like nucleus pulposus. The posterolateral outer third of the annulus has nociceptive innervation, whereas the nucleus does not. Because of their location and function, intervertebral disc degeneration can commonly lead to encroachment upon the nerve roots, dysfunction, and pain. Degeneration usually begins with increased compression forces resulting in an attempt by the body to stabilize via the laying down of calcium. Vertebral lipping and spurring are thus promoted, giving rise to spondylosis or degenerative arthritis. Involvement of the facet joints is quite common.[16]

NEUROMUSCULAR RELATIONSHIPS

Support and stabilization of the spine relative to upper quarter posture also involve contractile elements. The interplay between temporomandibular and craniocervical musculature is quite complex and even more so when one considers the neural interplay that exists between the two.

The major muscles that need to be evaluated are those that connect the occiput to the upper cervical spine, first and second ribs, clavicle, and scapula. Thus, hyperactivity or shortening (contracture or spasm) of a muscle that spans more than one upper quarter structure can be understood to contribute to postural abnormalities as well as pain and dysfunction at local and distal sites. A detailed analysis of anatomic and kinesiologic properties of each muscle is beyond the scope of this chapter. The dentist, however, needs to be aware of their general location, function, and innervation in order to realistically perform a screening evaluation of the cervical spine.

Suboccipital Fossa

The depression between the spinal column and mastoid process of the temporal bone is the suboccipital fossa or triangle. Bordered superiorly by the occiput and distally by the axis, small suboccipital muscles course between the occiput and axis, thus influencing head and neck posture and function.

The obliquus capitis superior and inferior, rectus capitis posterior major, and rectus capitis posterior minor are the deepest and smallest of the suboccipital muscles. They are actively involved in extension, rotation, and sidebending of the head. They are all innervated by the C1 spinal nerve root but cannot be palpated individually or as a group, as they lie underneath the more superficial and longer semispinalis and splenius capitis (Fig. 5–5).[17]

The semispinalis capitis originates from the transverse processes of T6-C7 and articular processes of C4-C6 to insert at the occipital bone between the superior and inferior nuchal lines. The splenius capitis originates from the

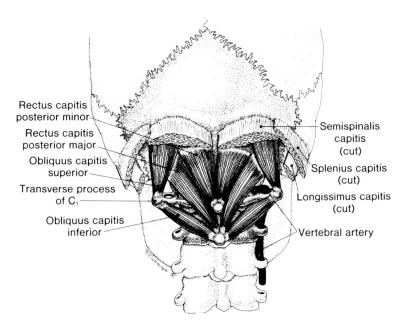

FIGURE 5–5. The muscles of the suboccipital fossa. (Reprinted with permission from Travell, J.A. and Simons, D.A.: *Myofascial Pain and Dysfunction, The Trigger Point Manual.* Williams & Wilkins, Baltimore, 1983.)

Rectus capitis posterior minor

Rectus capitis posterior major

Obliquus capitis superior

Transverse process of C$_1$

Obliquus capitis inferior

Semispinalis capitis (cut)

Splenius capitis (cut)

Longissimus capitis (cut)

Vertebral artery

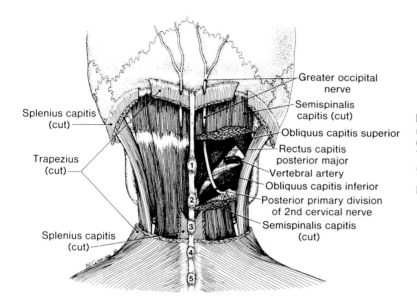

Greater occipital
nerve

Semispinalis
capitis (cut)

Obliquus capitis superior

Rectus capitis
posterior major

Vertebral artery

Obliquus capitis inferior

Posterior primary division
of 2nd cervical nerve

Semispinalis capitis
(cut)

Splenius capitis
(cut)

Trapezius
(cut)

Splenius capitis
(cut)

FIGURE 5–6. Occipital attachments of the upper trapezius. (Reprinted with permission from Travell, J.A. and Simons, D.A.: *Myofascial Pain and Dysfunction, The Trigger Point Manual.* Williams & Wilkins, Baltimore, 1983.)

nuchal ligament and spinous processes of T4-C7 to insert on the mastoid process of the temporal bone and lateral aspect of the superior nuchal line of the occiput. The action of these muscles is also to extend, rotate, and sidebend the head. They are innervated by the C1-C6 spinal nerves, and palpatory assessment in this region is primarily limited to these larger muscles in conjunction with the occipital attachment of the upper trapezius and the mastoid attachment of the sternocleidomastoid (SCM) (Figs. 5–5 to 5–7).

Laterally, the longissimus capitis and SCM muscles insert upon the posterior aspect of the mastoid process and the lateral half of the superior nuchal line of the occiput, respectively. The upper trapezius (UT) and SCM are two of the most important upper quarter muscles. The trapezius runs from the superior nuchal line and external occipital protuberance to the ligamentum nuchae and spinous processes of the thoracic vertebrae and C7. The upper division inserts upon the clavicle, acromion, and scapular spine. When contraction of one UT occurs it results in backward bending, ipsilateral sidebending, and contralateral rotation similar to that of the SCM. Bilateral UT contraction produces backward bending of the head and an increase in cervical lordosis. The SCM has both a sternal and clavicular head to the manubrium of the sternum and medial third of the clavicle, respectively (see Fig. 5–7). These two muscles share common innervation via the C3 nerve root and spinal accessory nerve with C2 and C4, also providing inner-

vation to the SCM and UT, respectively.[18,19] A branch of the accessory nerve also joins the vagus and hypoglossal nerves with an additional anastomosis upon nerve fibers at the

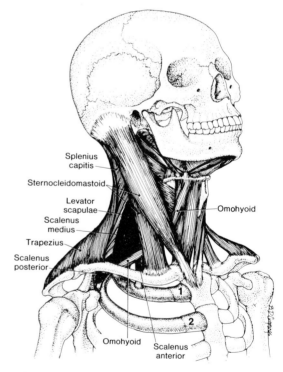

Splenius
capitis

Sternocleidomastoid

Levator
scapulae

Scalenus
medius

Trapezius

Scalenus
posterior

Omohyoid

Omohyoid

Scalenus
anterior

FIGURE 5–7. Anterolateral view of the significant muscular attachments between the craniomandibular region and shoulder girdle. (Reprinted with permission from Travell, J.A. and Simons, D.A.: *Myofascial Pain and Dysfunction, The Trigger Point Manual.* Williams & Wilkins, Baltimore, 1983.)

TABLE 5–1. Accessory Nerve

CRANIAL AND SPINAL (CRANIAL NERVE 11)

Somatic Efferent

Intimately related to hypoglossal and vagus (communicates with superior ganglion)
Intimately related to dorsolateral section of ventral horn C2-6—foramen
Magnum—dura mater

Jugular foramen—anterior to TP of atlas → SCM $\underset{\text{(cranial portion)}}{\text{pierces}}$ →
Post △ of neck → midpart of posterior aspect → trapezius

Anastamoses

Fibers of C2-C4 segments   Cranial (occipital section of upper trapezius)
Fibers of C5-C6   With vagus and hypoglossal
                   (dorsolateral) aspect of ventral horn

Lesions

May affect vagus and hypoglossal   Occipital FX
                                     Cervical lymph node
                                     Inflammation
                                     Tumor, abscess

∴ Majority of fibers cross midline

TP = transverse process; SCM = sternocleidomastoid; Post △ = posterior triangle; FX = fracture.

dorsolateral aspect of the ventral horn of C5-C6 (Table 5–1).[20]

A synergistic action of the SCM and its homolateral UT takes place in sidebending of the head. The SCM also has a more specific action on the head in that it sidebends ipsilaterally but rotates contralaterally. Thus, the left SCM will sidebend the head to the left but rotate it to the right simultaneously. This characteristic has strong implications in the patient who presents with a sidebent or rotated head. Bilaterally both SCMs produce forward inclination of the head and posterior rotation.[19]

Other important muscles that should be assessed in this region are the scalenes and levator scapulae, which along with the upper trapezius, inferior belly of the omohyoid, platysma, and splenius capitis, constitute what is known as the posterior triangle of the neck.[17–19]

The anterior and middle scalenes originate from the transverse processes of the C3-C6 and C2-C7 vertebrae, respectively, to insert upon the first rib. The posterior scalene originates from the transverse processes of the C4-C6 vertebrae to insert on the second rib. Composite innervation consists of the C3-C8 spinal nerves. The scalenes are also accessory muscles of respiration, as they can elevate the rib cage. They can also produce sidebending of the head or forward bending of the cervical spine, when acting unilaterally or bilaterally (Fig. 5–8).

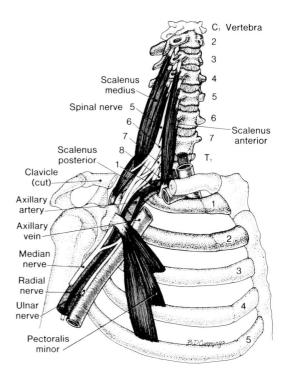

FIGURE 5–8. Thoracic inlet region illustrates the location of the scalenes, pectoralis minor, brachial plexus, and blood vessels. (Reprinted with permission from Travell, J.A. and Simons, D.A.: *Myofascial Pain and Dysfunction, The Trigger Point Manual.* Williams & Wilkins, Baltimore, 1983.)

The levator scapula runs from the superior medial angle of the scapula to the transverse processes of C1-C4. Its main function is scapula elevation. However, if the scapula is fixed contraction of this muscle can backward bend and side tilt the head ipsilaterally. Innervation is via the C3-C5 levels (Fig. 5–9).[17–20]

The rhomboids consist of a minor and major division. The former arises from the ligamentum nuchae and spinous processes of C7 and T1 to insert into the root of the scapular spine. The major division may be attached to the minor and courses just below it from the spinous processes of T1-T5 and the related supraspinous ligaments to insert into the vertebral border of the scapula from the spine to inferior angle. Innervation is via the C3-C5 spinal nerves. The main action of these muscles is to adduct or retract the scapulae.

Other significant muscles of the anterior cervical region include the longus colli, supra hyoids and infra hyoids, and pectorals. Bound close to the anterior aspect of the vertebral bod-

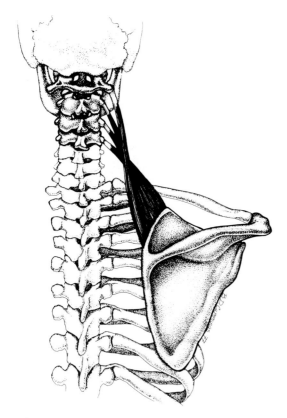

FIGURE 5–9. The levator scapulae. (Reprinted with permission from Travell, J.A. and Simons, D.A.: *Myofascial Pain and Dysfunction, The Trigger Point Manual.* Williams & Wilkins, Baltimore, 1983.)

ies and transverse processes of C1-T3, the longus colli thus functions as a flexor of the head and neck. The longus capitis, rectus capitis, anterior and rectus capitis lateralis lie anterior to the longus colli, and thus any palpation in this region really includes the status of all of these muscles. Innervation is via the C1-C3 spinal roots for the most superficial muscles and C2-C7 for the longus colli. When contracting bilaterally, the normal lordosis is lost and a straight cervical spine may result. Palpation of the longus colli region necessitates gentle finger placement between the SCM and trachea.[17–20]

The supraclavicular sulcus is the natural depression that exists between the clavicle, UT, and SCM overlying the first rib. The most superficial muscle of the anterior cervical region, however, is the platysma. This muscle is extremely thin and cannot be differentiated from the skin and superficial fascia that overlie it. Its extensive distribution includes the inferior border of the mandible, skin, and hypodermis of the face to the deltoid and pectoral fascia. The platysma thus covers the entire submandibular, hyoid, and anterior cervical region. This region has great significance in postural abnormalities that can result in mandibular repositioning and concomitant TMJ pain and dysfunction, which is discussed subsequently. The depth of the supraclavicular sulcus can increase dependent on the degree of activity or spasm of the SCM, scalenes, and levator scapulae—all of which can produce elevation of the shoulder girdle. However, the sulcus may also decrease in the presence of edema following a fracture of the clavicle or first rib, the presence of swollen glands, or a cervical rib.[17–19]

Inferior to the clavicle lies the pectoral musculature on the anterior chest wall. The pectoralis major spans the region from the sternal half of the clavicle, upper anterior surface of the sternum and the upper rib cage to the outer bicipital ridge of the humerus. The pectoralis minor lies under the major and runs from ribs 3 to 5 to the coronoid process of the scapula (see Fig. 5–8). Both of these muscles can easily become shortened in the presence of postural abnormalities. Their actions are upon the upper extremity and shoulder girdle, driving it into the thoracic region and internally rotating the shoulder. Innervation is via C5-T1 and C8-T1 spinal nerves for the major and minor, respectively.

The remaining musculature that needs a brief anatomic description is that of the shoulder itself. The muscles are the deltoid, supraspinatus, and infraspinatus plus the teres minor. The deltoid is a triangular-shaped muscle, surrounding the shoulder joint in front, back, and laterally. Periosteal connections include the clavicle, acromion, and scapular spine to the midshaft of the humerus. The deltoid's function is to elevate, extend, and abduct the arm. Innervation is via the C5-C6 spinal nerves.

The SIT muscles of the shoulder consist of the *s*upraspinatus, *i*nfraspinatus, and *t*eres. The most superior is the supraspinatus located within the supraspinous fossa of the scapula above its spine. This muscle can be palpated directly behind and below the upper trapezius superior to the spine of the scapula. The infraspinatus occupies the superior position below the scapular spine. The teres minor lies just inferior to the infraspinatus. These muscles compose the soft tissue overlying the posterior aspect of the scapula (Fig. 5–10). They all insert in descending order upon the posterior aspect of the greater tuberosity of the humerus. Other muscles in the shoulder girdle area, such as the teres major and latissimus dorsi, are more inferior. The subscapularis and the serratus anterior are anterior to the scapula and not essential to a dental screening examination. They may, however, become a source of pain; adversely affect shoulder girdle function; or produce postural abnormalities, such as scapular winging. The definitive evaluation of the shoulder girdle area is out of the realm of dentistry, and appropriate referral is warranted. Specific illustrations of the musculature not shown in this chapter can be found in anatomy texts.

The composite innervation of all the shoulder girdle and upper extremity musculature is via the C2-T1 distribution. Therefore, any major functional disturbance should be observed as part of this screening examination.

Peripheral Neuroanatomy

Knowledge of the segmental relationship of the spinal cord is essential in order to explain the innervation of skin, muscle, and bone. A total of 31 pairs of spinal nerves exit from the vertebral column segmentally at intervertebral foramina except for those of C1 and C2.[16] The intervertebral foramina are bordered anteriorly by the intervertebral discs except at OA and AA, posterior longitudinal ligament, and adjacent portions of the vertebral bodies. The articular process of the facet joints and their capsules constitute the posterior border with the lateral edge of the ligamentum flavum.[20-23]

Spinal nerves are typically mixed, thus containing motor, sensory, and sympathetic components. Nerve fibers from the dorsal (posterior) and ventral (anterior) horns of each spinal cord segment form the sensory (afferent) and motor (efferent) roots, respectively. The dorsal and ventral roots converge and exit the foramen as a mixed spinal nerve.[20-23]

Nerve roots must perforate the dura mater and pass through dural sleeves within the intervertebral foramen that are continuous with the epineurium of the nerves. The dura mater is composed of tough fibrous connective tissue and runs from the interior of the cranium, through the foramen magnum, and surrounds the spinal cord throughout its distribution. The dura mater is uninterrupted from the cranium to the coccyx at the second sacral level (S2). It is also attached to the posterior surfaces of C2 and C3.[20-23] Thus, postural abnormalities or suboccipital joint dysfunction may be a source of dural irritation.

Nerve roots further subdivide into anterior and posterior primary rami. The anterior primary ramus (APR) innervates the skin (dermatome), muscles (myotome), and bone (sclerotome) of the extremities, anterolateral trunk, and neck via its lateral and anterior

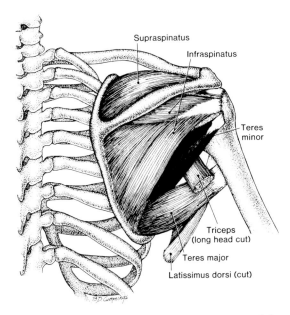

FIGURE 5–10. Muscles of the posterior aspect of the shoulder girdle. (Reprinted with permission from Travell, J.A. and Simons, D.A.: *Myofascial Pain and Dysfunction, The Trigger Point Manual.* Williams & Wilkins, Baltimore, 1983.)

Supraspinatus
Infraspinatus
Teres minor
Triceps (long head cut)
Teres major
Latissimus dorsi (cut)

branches. Innervation of the skin, muscle, and bone plus the fibrous septa of the scalp, neck, and trunk is via the posterior primary rami (PPR). Lateral branches innervate ligaments and muscles lateral to the facet joints. Medial branches innervate the posterior aspect of the facet joints and capsule. Another branch arises from the anterior aspect of the spinal nerve exits 2 to 3 mm from the intervertebral foramen, receives a sympathetic component and then re-enters the foramen. This is known as the sinuvertebral or recurrent meningeal nerve which innervates the posterior longitudinal ligament, vertebral body, outer third of the annular fibers of the intervertebral discs, anterior aspect of the dura mater, and epidural blood vessel walls.[16,20–24] Although there are no intervertebral discs at the OA and AA segments, a sinuvertebral nerve (SNV) still exists. The SNVs of C1 and C2, however, join with that of C3 to further innervate the cruciate ligaments, tentorial membrane, and dura of the posterior cranial fossa (Table 5–2).[16,22,24,25] Peripheral nerves originate from limb plexuses, which are formed by the ventral rami of spinal nerves. Peripheral nerves that emerge from a plexus are supplied by fibers from two or more spinal cord segments resulting in an overlap of innervation to each dermatome and myotome. The cervical plexus is composed of ventral and dorsal rami from C1-C4 and communicates with cranial nerves 11 and 12 (Table 5–3).[21,22,27] The dorsal and ventral rami of C5-T1 compose the brachial plexus. Thus, overlap occurs from C4 to both plexuses.

The last neural structure of significance is the primary sympathetic chain of ganglia extending from T2-L3 anterolaterally along the spinal column. An important consideration is that three additional ganglia exist above T2, namely the superior, middle, and inferior cervical sympathetic ganglia: these communicate with the inferior, middle, and superior cardiac nerves from the vagus, which can account for cardiac referral to the face and neck.[20,24] In the cervical

TABLE 5–2. Sinovertebral Nerve of C3

INNERVATES
Outer third of annulus fibrosis, PLL, anterior DM, epidural blood vessel walls
Ligaments of AA, paramedian dura of postcranial fossa
SVN of C1 and C2 join C3-cruciate ligaments, tentorial membrane and dura of postcranial fossa

PLL = posterior longitudinal ligament; DM = dura mater; AA = atlantoaxial joints; SVN = sinuvertebral nerves.

TABLE 5–3. Cervical Plexus*

Ventral Rami of C1-C4	Innervates skin, ligaments, and joints of anterior neck, shoulders, upper chest, plus motor to neck musculature and phrenic nerve
Dorsal Rami of C1-C4	Muscles, ligaments and joints of posterior head and neck, skin from vertex and lower mandibular region to the spine of the scapula

*Communicates with the hypoglossal and spinal accessory

region, sympathetic ganglia are situated in front of the transverse processes. Vasomotor, pilomotor, glandular, and visceral innervation is provided via the autonomic nervous system (ANS).

The cervical portion of the sympathetic chain also innervates the walls of the internal and external carotid arteries, the dura mater, and the cervical spinal nerves. Nerves arising from the cervical sympathetic chain anastomose with those from the cervical nerve roots around the vertebral artery as a source of innervation.[20–25]

A segmental relationship of visceral innervation also exists. Visceral afferents that convey nociceptive input enter the spinal cord and synapse in the same segment as the preganglionic fibers of the efferent (motor) distribution. Preganglionic fibers course from the APR to the sympathetic chain via the white rami communicantes (WRC). Postganglionic fibers course back to the APR from the sympathetic chain via the grey rami communicantes (GRC). Descending input from the hypothalamus synapses with the preganglionic fibers to provide a facilitatory or inhibitory effect upon the ANS.[20,22,24,26,27]

Other than the cervical portion of the sympathetic chain, visceral innervation is primarily limited to the thoracolumbar distribution. Blood vessels, however, are also considered to be viscera. Visceral motor and sensory nerves innervate blood vessel walls, hair, and glands and most importantly accompany the trigeminal, facial, glossopharyngeal, and vagus nerves.[20,24,28] However, afferent input from the lower esophagus, central tendon of the diaphragm, portions of the pericardium and the biliary tract, mediated by the phrenic nerve, can represent a visceral mechanism of referred pain to the shoulder.[20,26,28,29] Associated hyperalgesia, hyperesthesia, sweating, piloerection, and muscular rigidity can occur.

In addition, the gallbladder can refer pain to the inferior angle of the right scapula. The dermatomal innervation of this region is the T7-T9 segments, which also give rise to the visceral afferent innervation of the gallbladder. The gallbladder, located in the right thoracic region, is thus innervated from the right side of the spinal cord. A viscerosomatic reflex results in acute discomfort described as an ache. Eating greasy, fatty, or fried foods can precipitate gallbladder pain.[29] This type of pain is unchanged by rest, movement, or position—which is not the case with somatic pain. Active, passive, and resistive movement testing are thus required as evaluative tools because visceral problems may also be precipitated by vagal irritation at the suboccipital region as discussed further.

The chronology of visceral pain is opposite to that of somatic pain. Acute somatic pain is characteristically sharp, superficial, and not difficult to localize whereas acute visceral pain is dull or vague, deep, achy, and difficult to localize. In addition, viscera are sparsely innervated and acute damage or irritation to a small localized area usually does not result in a perceptible stimulus. A long-lasting or chronic, strong stimulus or one that excites visceral afferents over a large region is thus necessary for the perception of chronic visceral pain that has the quality of acute somatic pain. This pain may occur from obstruction, distention, inflammation, ischemia, and hyperacidity as well as traction or compression forces upon mesentery and associated blood vessels.[28-30]

The anatomic relationship of the spinal cord and its segments to each related spinous process, intervertebral foramen, and nerve root is nonuniform. This is most pronounced at the lumbosacral levels and most uniform or segmental at the thoracic (T3-T12) levels. In the cervical region, spinal segments give rise to nerve roots that exit above their corresponding vertebral bodies. The first cervical root exits between atlas and axis. There are, however, eight cervical nerve roots but only seven cervical vertebrae; therefore, the C8 root exits between the seventh cervical and first thoracic vertebrae.[23]

For the purpose of evaluation, the cervical spinous processes correspond with the spinal cord segment one greater than itself. Thus, the spinous process of C5 provides the landmark for the sixth cervical segment giving rise to the C6 nerve root exiting from the foramen at C5-C6. The C7 spinous process is level with the eighth cervical segment giving rise to the C8 nerve root exiting from the C7-T1 foramen. The spinous process will usually correspond to the inferior articular process of the facet joint of the same vertebral body, unless a malalignment or structural fault is present.[23]

If spinous processes are to be used as landmarks in the evaluation procedure accuracy necessitates that the patient stand with the arms alongside the trunk. Palpation that begins from the occipital protuberance will descend into a depression between the occiput and the first palpable spinous process of C2. The atlas does not possess an easily palpable spinous process, but its posterior arch lies within the depression between occiput and axis (see Fig. 5–2).

The posterior direction of the remainder of the cervical spinous processes produces a degree of overlap and makes isolation difficult. However, because the spinous process of C7 is very prominent, but sometimes difficult to distinguish from that of C6 or T1, the index finger can be placed on what is thought to be the C7 spinous process and the middle finger on the one above (C6), while the patient's head is gently bent backward. If finger placement is correct the spinous process of C6 becomes less prominent, as it moves anteriorly establishing the one below as C7. This test is most demonstrative at the C6-C7 vertebrae.[23] The spinous processes of T3 and T7 are other important landmarks, as they correspond to the level of the scapular spine and its inferior angle, respectively.

Dermatome, Myotome, and Sclerotome

A knowledge of the differences between the dermatome, myotome, and sclerotome of the upper quarter region is imperative in order to understand the phenomenon of referred pain. A dermatome is considered to represent the cutaneous region innervated by one spinal nerve through both of its rami.[27] This factor accounts for the existence of both anterior and posterior dermatomes innervated by the same segment. However, cervical dermatomes are not as segmental as they appear on various anatomic charts.[23,26,27]

Hilton's law specifies that the neural innervation of the myotome acting upon a given joint is the same as that of the joint (sclerotome) and the overlying cutaneous region.[31] This finding is not apparent at the head and pectoral and scapular regions of the upper quarter. A uniform segmental relationship only exists among the dermatome, myotome, and sclerotome in the T3-T12 region.

The cutaneous innervation of the head is via the trigeminal nerve. However, the occiput (up to and including the vertex of the head and the inferior to submandibular region) is supplied by the occipital nerves originating from the C1-C3 segment (Fig. 5–11A and 5–11B). Irritation of the C1 root has been shown to provide some sensory innervation to the anterior half of the head. Experimental stimulation of C1 rootlets has caused orbital, frontal, and vertex pain, although it is not considered to have a cutaneous distribution.[16,31,33] The area from midcervical to the acromion laterally and distally to the spine of the scapula primarily consists of the C3-C4 dermatome and myotome. Cutaneous and underlying muscle innervation is segmental, including that of the deeper skeletal structures. Nerve roots from C5-T2 provide the remainder of the upper-quarter innervation, which consists of the entire upper extremity as well as the scapular and interscapular region below its spine. Therefore, involvement of the C5-T2 nerve roots can produce referred pain to the inferior angle of the scapula as well as the finger tips as illustrated in Figure 5–11C to 5–11H.

The T3-T7 dermatome, however, extends from the spine of the scapula to its inferior angle, whereas the underlying myotome is purely of cervical origin providing a nonuniform arrangement. Cutaneous (skin) pain is

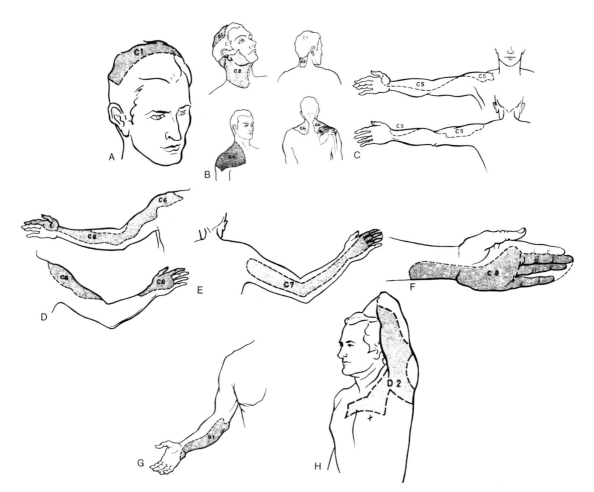

FIGURE 5–11. *A*, The C1 dermatome. *B*, The C2–C4 dermatomes. *C*, The C5 dermatome. *D*, The C6 dermatome. *E*, The C7 dermatome. *F*, The C8 dermatome. *G*, The T1 dermatome. Thoracic and dorsal (D) are used interchangeably. *H*, The T2 dermatome. Thoracic and dorsal (D) are used interchangeably. (Reprinted with permission from Hernandez C.S. and Argote, M.L.: *A Visual Aid to the Examination of Nerve Roots.* Bailliere Tindall, London, 1976.)

commonly perceived as superficial itching, burning, pricking, or a pins-and-needles (paresthesia) sensation.[16,22,26,33] Muscle pain is classically described as dull, deep, and achy.[23] Therefore, pain arising from the cervical spine that is perceived solely in the thoracic dermatome of the interscapular region is deep, dull, and achy and commonly gives rise to myalgic or trigger points in the scapular musculature innervated by the cervical spine. The location of the pain may mislead the clinician into suspecting a pathology of thoracic origin, but delineation via manual compression/distraction tests of the cervical spine and pain quality helps to determine the true origin.

A general awareness of the distribution of the cervical and upper thoracic dermatomes and myotomes is a necessity for the dentist. The T1 and T2 dermatomes are located not on the thorax but along the ulnar border of the arm. The cutaneous innervation of the fourth and fifth fingers plus the region alongside the ulnar area of the forearm to the elbow is primarily innervated by the T1 root. The region extending from the elbow into the axilla is supplied by the T2 root. The remainder of the upper extremity is innervated by the C5-C8 nerve roots. Thus, both a dermatomal and myotomal distribution to the upper extremity occur. This can account for pain sensations indicative of the pins and needles called paresthesia and the muscular aching known as myalgia. Both sensations may exist simultaneously in similar regions or separately in different areas. A classic example is that of a muscular ache in the posterolateral arm above the elbow (deltoid and triceps dis-

tribution) in association with paresthesia in the thumb and index finger. Nerve root irritation possibly from spondylosis or a posterolateral disc herniation at the C5-C6 level may be implicated as the etiologic factor.

TRIGEMINOCERVICAL COMPLEX

In the suboccipital region, a dense neural interplay exists between specific cranial and spinal nerves that makes anatomic differentiation virtually impossible. Connections thus exist among the trigeminal, facial, glossopharyngeal, and vagus, with those of the upper C1-C4 cervical spinal nerves. The nucleus caudalis of the trigeminal nerve contains a substantia gelatinosa region that is continuous with that of the dorsal horn of the spinal cord.[34–37] Furthermore, the spinal accessory nerve communicates with the superior ganglion of the vagus, anastamoses with fibers from the C2-C4 spinal segments, and is considered to be an efferent portion of the pharyngeal plexus and vagus.[24,34] A majority of accessory nerve fibers cross the midline, which has implications for referred pain from the SCM (see Table 5–1). The hypoglossal nerve communicates with the inferior ganglion of the vagus, and both are bound together by dense connective tissue at OA. It also joins the pharyngeal plexus and spinal nerves of C1 to form the ansa cervicalis (Table 5–4). Hypoglossal efferents additionally innervate the hyoid and tongue musculature.[24,34] The vagus nerve provides both efferent and afferent innervation to the viscera. In addition, various branches innervate the dura of the pos-

TABLE 5–4. Ansa Hypoglossi (Cervicalis)

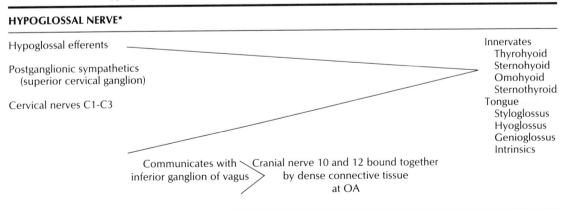

HYPOGLOSSAL NERVE*

Hypoglossal efferents

Postganglionic sympathetics (superior cervical ganglion)

Cervical nerves C1-C3

Communicates with inferior ganglion of vagus

Cranial nerve 10 and 12 bound together by dense connective tissue at OA

Innervates
Thyrohyoid
Sternohyoid
Omohyoid
Sternothyroid
Tongue
Styloglossus
Hyoglossus
Genioglossus
Intrinsics

*Courses below belly of posterior digastric
OA = occipital atlantoid.

terior cranial fossa as well as the dorsal wall of the external auditory meatus and concha, thus possibly mimicking TMJ pain. A superior laryngeal branch provides motor and sensory input to the larynx, vocal cords, soft palate, lateral pharynx, posterior part of the tongue, and superior surface of the epiglottis (Table 5–5).[24,34] Thus, the trigeminocervical complex actually represents cranial nerves 5, 7, 9, 10, 11, and 12, plus spinal nerves C1-C4.

The vertebral artery also courses through the suboccipital region, and any compression along its distribution may lead to intracranial vasoconstriction and the possibility of widespread symptomatology. Innervation of the vertebral artery is via nerves from the cervical sympathetic chain and upper cervical roots.[9,14,16,22] The facet joints, capsules, and ligaments of the atlas and axis have dense mechanoreceptor innervation.[38] Proprioceptive input from this region thus plays a significant role in the control of equilibrium.[22,38] The innervation of the facet joints, capsules, and ligaments of the atlas, axis, and to a lesser degree the third cervical vertebra is quite dense and is provided by cervical nerves C1-C3 (Table 5–6).[16,18,31,38,39,40] Normal, non-nociceptive input from this area to the central nervous system is essential for and contributes to the control of balance and equilibrium. Visual plus vestibular input combines with proprioception to stabilize gaze during natural movements of the head.[40] The interaction between all of this afferent signaling takes place at the vestibular nucleus. Right rotation of the head sufficient to

TABLE 5–5. Vagus Nerve*

VISCERAL EFFERENTS AND AFFERENTS
Also innervates dorsal wall of EAM and concha

Branches

Meningeal ramus	Jugular foramen to dura mater of postcranial fossa
Superior laryngeal nerve	Lateral pharynx and larynx and vocal cords (motor and sensory)
Anastomose with	5,7,9,11,12 and C2-C4
Pharyngeal plexus	(vagus plus glossopharyngeal and cervical sympathetics)
Motor to	Pharyngeal constrictors Soft palate (levator palatini) Palatal arches
Sensory to	Mucous membranes of pharynx Posterior part of tongue Superior surface of epiglottis

*Passes through diaphragm.
EAM = external auditory meatus.

TABLE 5–6. Cervical Nerves 1 to 3

INNERVATE
Ligaments and joints of C1-C3
Anterior/posterior musculature
SCM, trapezius
Posterior cranial dura mater (tentorium and falx cerebelli)
Vertebral artery
Ventral ramus of C2-meningeal branches to hypoglossal and vagus (lateral walls of posterior cranial fossa)

SCM = sternocleidomastoid.

stretch the C1-C3 joint capsules thus excites neurons in the right vestibular nucleus, which in turn facilitates neurons in the left abducens and right oculomotor nucleus to maintain proper orientation. Any imbalance of such afferent input in favor of nociception, stemming from suboccipital dysfunction, can cause nystagmus or vertigo.[40] When vertigo exists, sudden movements of the head can result in imbalance.[39,40]

The SCM is the prime muscular source of proprioceptive input relative to orientation of the head in space. Trigger points of the clavicular head of the SCM due to shortening and hyperactivity have been stated to contribute to spatial disorientation, dizziness, and vertigo (Table 5–7).[41] Unilateral hyperactivity may also result in ipsilateral suboccipital compression.

Postural abnormalities resulting from various acute or chronic etiologies that produce suboccipital compression can therefore be responsible for craniofacial pain anywhere in the head. In addition, pharyngeal, laryngeal, aural, visual, and abdominal symptoms may also occur separate from or in conjunction with dizziness, vertigo, or nystagmus based upon the anatomic relationships that have previously been presented (Table 5–8).

Postural Considerations

The upper-quarter postural analysis is the most important part of the cervical evaluation.

TABLE 5–7. Suboccipital Spine

DISRUPTION OF NORMAL PROPRIOCEPTIVE INPUT
Nystagmus—involuntary repetitive movement of eyes
Dizziness—sensation of altered spatial orientation
Vertigo—sensation of head floating, swimming, or rotating.

TABLE 5–8. Dysfunction of Trigeminocervical Complex*

Craniofacial pain
Occipital neuralgia
Pharyngeal, laryngeal, aural, abdominal, and visual symptoms
Dizziness, vertigo, and nystagmus

*Can mimic or contribute to craniomandibular pain and dysfunction.

The dentist should be able to identify abnormalities and understand how abnormal posture can cause facial pain and TMJD.

Diagnosis of postural abnormalities first requires an awareness of what is normal. Three planes of reference (pupilar, otic, and occlusal) should be assessed and found parallel to one another. Ramus height should be equal bilaterally. In normal erect posture, a gravitational plumb line can be used as a standard. The center of gravity of the skull exists at the bisection of the vestibular apparatus (otic plane) of the inner ear.[42] Normally, the plumb line should fall just behind the apex of the coronal suture through the external auditory meatus, odontoid process, and just posterior to the cervical vertebral bodies. The line would continue to descend through the glenohumeral joint, lumbar vertebral bodies, and sacral promontory. Distally, it would fall slightly posterior to the center of the hip joint, just anterior to the center of the knee joint, through the calcaneocuboid joint, and end just anterior to the lateral malleolus.[2,3,19]

An analysis of the lower quarter is not necessary for the dentist to perform, but there should be an awareness of major abnormalities that can alter the craniovertebral relationship. Lower-quarter abnormalities, such as asymmetries of the medial plantar arch, leg length, and iliac crests, are well-known causes of asymmetry of shoulder height and head tilt. Leg length discrepancies have been shown to cause electromyographic abnormalities of the masticatory muscles, which may lead to malocclusion.[43] Curvature of the lumbar spine with a loss of the normal lumbar curve or lordosis is commonly associated with the development of a forward head posture (FHP). The normal lordosis is lost when one assumes a slouched sitting position. Cumulative factors weigh heavily in the development of a flat lumbar spine, and occupations that require prolonged standing or sitting have been implicated.[44]

Normal Upper-Quarter Posture

Normal upper-quarter posture exists when the shoulders are slightly retracted from the line of gravity with the clavicles just posterior to the first rib. The clavicles should be horizontal, and their articulation with the shoulder (acromioclavicular joint) and sternum (sternoclavicular joint) should not demonstrate prominence or asymmetry. Scapular spines should also be relatively horizontal and symmetric without significant prominence of one vertebral border in comparison to the other (winging). The depth of each supraclavicular sulcus should be the same, and shoulder elevation must be equal.[44]

The upper thoracic spine should possess a normal degree of kyphosis without the development of a dowager's hump. The mid to lower cervical spine should demonstrate a 30- to 35-degree lordosis. The SCMs, from origin to insertion, should have a 45- to 60-degree angulation. The horizontal distance from a vertical plumb line posterior to the apex of the thoracic spine to the midcervical region can be measured. Normally, this should fall within 6 to 8 cm.[7,44–48]

In the suboccipital area, a slight kyphosis should exist between the cranium and C1-C2. The mid-low cervical lordosis and slight kyphosis of the upper cervical region allow for simultaneous forward and backward bending of the head independent of the rest of the cervical spine.[45–48]

The hyoid bone should be situated just anterior and inferior to the vertebral body of C3. Its posterior horn should be level with the C2-C3 disc. Alterations in its position can occur with abnormal craniovertebral posture as a result of length-tension changes in the hyoid musculature. The normal mandibular resting position, in the presence of normal upper quarter posture, should have a freeway space of 2 to 4 mm.[8]

Abnormal Upper-Quarter Posture

The most common abnormality in the cervical spine with direct impact upon the craniofacial area is the FHP. Any increase in the SCM angulation or distance from the thoracic apex to midcervical region manifested by forward inclination of the head and neck constitutes an FHP. This is considered to be minimal at 60 degrees, moderate at 60 to 75 degrees, and maximal at 75 to 90 degrees. There will usually be an associated decrease in the cervical lordosis approaching a straight cervical spine. This is most common following acute trauma, such as a hyperextension injury, when reflex guarding of the longus colli, SCMs, and scalenes occurs.[49,50] Cumulative microtrauma resulting from improper home, work, and driving postures can also eventually lead to development of an FHP.[44] Continued increases in forward inclination may lead to inversion of the cervical lordosis and, therefore, cause kyphosis. This postural abnormality can even result in ACR when correction of the line of sight is not possible.[44]

An FHP may exist with or without posterior cranial rotation (PCR). Identification of PCR requires a lateral view of the patient when standing. In the presence of PCR, the distance between occiput and atlas decreases resulting in greater suboccipital compression Rocabado[7] recommends measuring this distance on a cervical radiograph and considers normal to be 4 to 9 mm.

A hyperflexion/hyperextension injury or whiplash will acutely cause reflex guarding of the small suboccipital extensors, SCMs, and upper trapezius and levator scapulae, resulting in an FHP with PCR. Over time, a habitual slumped posture can cause posterior cranial rotation in order to maintain proper eye level for work and play.

In the presence of a prolonged FHP with PCR, pain at the cervicothoracic junction and shoulder girdle can occur. The shoulder girdle cannot remain in its normal position in the presence of muscular forces that result from a prolonged FHP: increased tension results, and postural changes occur. The occiput will approximate the posterior shoulder girdle causing shortening of the upper trapezius and levator scapulae. Significant pain may occur in this region manifested by a palpable band or knot. This has been termed the crossed-shoulder syndrome and usually is most prominent on the side of the dominant arm.[18] The middle and lower trapezius and the rhomboids are stretched or lengthened in the presence of scapular abduction and protraction. Forward migration of the shoulder girdle results and eventually is compounded by shortening of the pectorals.

Postural forces upon the shoulder girdle also produce forward migration and internal rotation of the glenohumeral joint, resulting in round shoulders (RS), scapula abduction, alar scapulae, and winging. An associated upper

TABLE 5–9. Forward Head Posture

CONTRIBUTES TO

Alteration of proprioceptive input
Compression of occiput on upper cervical spine
Degenerative disc disease
Occlusal alteration
Increased posterior tooth contact } Mandibular repositioning
Increased TMJ compression
Upper thoracic kyphosis
Shoulder impingement
Shortening of anterior cervical musculature
Thoracic inlet compression and neurovascular compression syndromes
Dural irritation

---

thoracic kyphosis may exist. The combination of PCR and RS will eventually lead to glenohumeral instability.

Clavicular angulation and compression of the sternoclavicular and acromioclavicular joints hinder normal posterior rotation of the clavicle that accompanies any elevation of the shoulder. Impingement and entrapment forces leading to tendinitis, bursitis, and rotator cuff tears at the shoulder can occur on the dominant side.[44] Entrapment of the suprascapular nerve and traction on the C5-C6 roots of the brachial plexus may lead to increased shoulder girdle and upper extremity pain (Table 5–9). The brachial plexus tension test explained subsequently in this chapter may be very helpful in diagnosis. Weakness and atrophy can develop secondary to nerve compression and should be evaluated by an orthopedist or neurologist.

Neurovascular Compression

A longstanding FHP may eventually lead to compression at the supraclavicular region. The thoracic inlet lies deep to this region and is bordered by the first thoracic vertebrae posteriorly, the superior border of the manubrium of the sternum anteriorly, and the first rib laterally. The subclavian artery and vein and the lower trunk of the brachial plexus are situated here and may be compressed by FHP or the existence of a cervical rib.[44]

Symptoms known generally as thoracic inlet syndrome (TIS) need more specific evaluation by a physician or physical therapist to determine specific etiology. Symptoms include irritation of a peripheral nerve, distal paresthesia, tenderness of innervated musculature, possible hyperesthesia, and burning pain. In addition, vascular symptoms may occur when the entrapment includes blood vessels. Neurovascular compression in the thoracic inlet area is most common in females between the ages of 20 and 40.[51] This is also a common age group with TMJ complaints. Shortening of the scalenus anterior, scalenus medius, and pectoralis minor muscles can cause entrapment of neurovascular structures at the thoracic inlet region as illustrated in Figure 5–8.

Referred pain into the upper extremity resulting from thoracic inlet compression is generally perceived in the C8-T1 dermatomal distribution as paresthesia and the myotomal distribution as muscular ache and tenderness. The dermatomal and myotomal distribution correlates with the segmental origin of the ulnar nerve. The more distal the symptomatology, the greater the degree of involvement. Progression to heaviness, weakness, and sensory loss within the ulnar distribution is a sign of increased neurovascular compression. In the hand, symptoms can involve the fourth and fifth finger and may even lead to trophic changes and peripheral vascular insufficiency. This occurrence, however, is much more common in the lower extremity.[44]

Hyperactivity and shortening of the levator scapulae give rise to a related but different syndrome of referred pain. The symptom complex includes unilateral suboccipital pain with referral across the spine of the scapula to the anterolateral fourth and fifth intercostal region and distally into the posterolateral arm and the dorsal surface of the forearm and fourth and fifth fingers. This is known as the scapulocostal syndrome.[52] Specifically, discomfort is within the dorsal surface of the forearm and ulnar side of the fingers. This is distinct from TIS referral on the volar (palm) surface in addition to the ulnar side. Thus, evaluation has to be quite specific and include objective assessment as well as the patient's subjective report.

Patients with TIS are frequently awakened at night by pain. Nocturnal paresthesia occurs when the lower trunk of the brachial plexus is lifted off the first rib in the supine position. While sleeping, compression is thus decreased and pain impulses can travel beyond the lesion to the supraspinal appreciation centers. When upright, in positions of abnormal posture (e.g., FHP), compression occurs and pain decreases. Vascular signs, such as paresthesia and numbness, may thus become more pronounced during the day.

It is difficult to differentiate one specific neurovascular compression syndrome in the tho-

racic inlet region from another solely by pain quality and distribution. Specific diagnosis becomes even more difficult when considering the possibility of referral from cervical nerve root irritation or compression. Posture and pain distribution should, however, be noted by the dentist. All of these syndromes may be characterized by an FHP, but if the syndrome is unilateral the involved side may demonstrate shoulder elevation, deeper supraclavicular sulcus, or greater clavicular angulation. Pain distribution from scalene involvement will affect the anterior (pectoral) region of the arm, whereas in the presence of levator scapulae involvement posterior (scapular) and rib cage discomfort will exist along with upper extremity referral.

Palpation for tenderness constitutes part of the evaluation. The location and function of the related muscles have been discussed and should become a general part of the cervical evaluation.

Headaches and Craniofacial Pain

Many headaches of muscle contraction origin and some vascular headaches are precipitated by postural and degenerative changes of the upper cervical spine. Guarding of the splenius and semispinalis capitis muscles gives rise to pain referral in the suboccipital, occiput, and vertex regions. The greater occipital nerve courses through the semispinalis capitis and possibly the occipital attachment of the upper trapezius.[16,22,31–33,41] An FHP with associated PCR may thus represent the somatic etiology of posterior and vertex headache (Table 5–10).

The upper trapezius refers pain to the temporal and retro-orbital area. Reflex activation of the ipsilateral SCM has been shown to precipitate associated dizziness or vertigo.[41] Persis-

TABLE 5–10. Forward Head Posture with Posterior Cranial Rotation

INCREASES
Suboccipital compression forces upon the trigeminocervical complex and vertebral artery
Increased craniofacial pain
Alteration of proprioceptive input
Increases tension on suprahyoids and promotes greater mandibular repositioning
May contribute to abnormal tongue position, tongue thrust, and anterior open bite
Hyperactivity of masticatory muscles

tent pain in the temporalis muscle, producing spasm, stemming from upper trapezius referral, can result in secondary referral to the ipsilateral maxillary teeth.[41] This may also give rise to mandibular hypomobility due to elevation and retrussive force. The entire process may be perpetuated by upper trapezius pressure in buxom women who wear bras with thin and tight straps, especially those with associated FHP.[44]

Compression of the vertebral artery occurs with postural dysfunction and compression of the suboccipital complex. Compression of the posterior cervical sympathetic network can result in widespread cranial nerve symptomatology due to compromised circulation. The syndrome of Barré-Liéou thus includes tinnitus, vestibular problems, blurred vision, hoarseness, rhinorrhea, lacrimation, hot flashes, and sweating along with a throbbing headache.[53] Such symptomatology is not unlike that caused by TMDs. The etiology may be craniovertebral, temporomandibular, or a combination of the two, underscoring the need for thorough evaluation of both regions.

Innervation of the cranial dura by the first three cervical nerves, the hypoglossal, and the vagus may represent a source of tractional headache. The dura mater is extremely sensitive at the cranial base. Stimulation of the tentorium cerebelli and falx cerebri has been shown to cause referred pain to the forehead.[15]

Postural dysfunction that irritates or compresses the trigeminocervical complex also can be an extrinsic source of intraoral pain. A burning or stabbing paroxysmal pain at the base of the tongue and soft palate may implicate involvement of the glossopharyngeal nerve.[24,54] Vagal involvement can also be perceived at the base of the tongue and glottis along with upper thoracic referral indicative of superior laryngeal neuralgia.[24,54] Ipsilateral numbness of the tongue along with a homolateral occipital headache and postauricular pain can occur by sudden rotation of the head stretching the AA capsule, which is termed the cervicolingual syndrome.[39,55,56]

Cranial nerves 5, 7, 9, and 10 also innervate the ear.[24,27] Many other overlapping innervation patterns exist, but a complete review is beyond the scope of this chapter. The primary cervical source of craniofacial pain is thus the trigeminocervical complex. Sensory and motor innervation to both the temporomandibular and craniovertebral region stems from this complex. Table 5–11 summarizes the neuroanatomic causes of craniofacial pain. When postural dysfunction causes an impact directly upon the TMJ, pain referral from hyperactive masticatory muscles occurs, further com-

TABLE 5–11. Trigeminocervical Complex

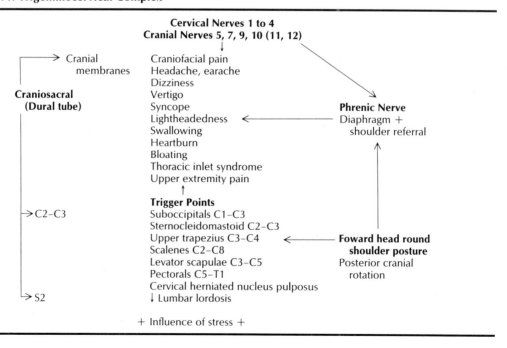

pounding the symptoms and leading the clinician to assume that the etiology is solely TMJ related and craniovertebral dysfunction is not considered.

TEMPOROMANDIBULAR PAIN AND DYSFUNCTION

Many factors can influence the resting position of the mandible and affect occlusion, respiration, masticatory muscle activity, and TMJ compression forces. The cumulative effects of FHP produce adaptive changes in the anterior and posterior cervical musculature. The posterior extensors shorten, and the anterior flexors lengthen. A similar effect occurs upon the hyoid musculature. The suprahyoids shorten, and the infrahyoids lengthen, resulting in hyoid bone elevation, especially in the presence of PCR. The degree of elevation increases proportionately to the decline of cervical lordosis and increases even more so when kyphosis or inverted lordosis occurs.[7,8,44,46–48]

Shortening of the suprahyoids leads to hyperactivity and an associated hyoid elevation and a depressive force on the mandible. A retrussive force will also occur in part because of the contraction of the digastrics when the hyoid bone is anchored.[57] Retrusion will be more pronounced when the mandible is fixed in the presence of clenching. An opposite action occurs upon the condyles as they are forced up into the glenoid fossa and translated forward as the body of the mandible is depressed and retruded.[44] This action may load the retrodiscal tissue and predispose a patient to internal derangement. The amount of condylar elevation and translation increases as the amount of PCR increases.

Mouth breathing can increase mandibular depression. Daly and associates,[58] Vig and Showfety,[59] and Hellsing and associates[60] have studied the effects of anterior open bite, nasal obstruction, and head position. They showed that head extension (e.g., PCR) can be induced by creating an anterior open bite or obstructing the nasal airway. An increase in suprahyoid activity promoted mandibular depression with an associated increase in freeway space.[57–60] However, when the head is forward flexed on the upper cervical spine the mandible is forced up and forward, decreasing freeway space.

Some have theorized that a prolonged FHP when present early in life may be a significant factor in the later development of micrognathia and retrognathia.[61] Forward head posture has also been shown to be associated with a large hyocervical distance.[62]

Head extension produces an increase in the electromyographic activity of the infrahyoids and suprahyoids. The passive stretch on the suprahyoids that results from PCR produces superior displacement of the hyoid bone. The infrahyoids contract at the same time to maintain stability.[63] Increased extension of the head has been found to be associated with a progressive decrease in posterior cervical muscle activity, because the center of gravity is altered in favor of extension.[63] An increase in masseter activity has been demonstrated to occur at 10 and 20 degrees of PCR without a rise in anterior temporalis activity. Other studies have also shown a related increase in temporalis activity.

The effect of postural changes at the craniovertebral region on masticatory muscle activity has been studied. Boyd and coworkers[64] found increased activity in PCR in the anterior temporalis but decreased activity in the masseter and anterior digastrics. In flexion, a decrease in anterior temporalis activity was seen with an increase in masseter and anterior digastric activity.[64]

However, Hellsing and associates[60] found reduced anterior temporalis activity in 28 of 30 normal adults under the experimental influence of nasal obstruction. These investigators observed increased suprahyoid activity allowing for mandibular depression and stabilization of the hyoid bone to maintain an open airway.

Chewing and the resting position of the tongue are also affected by an elevation of the hyoid bone. The tongue can begin to rest on the floor of the mouth, and a tongue thrust pattern can develop. In the presence of FHP with PCR, the support-suspension mechanism of the tongue is altered. The styloid process moves anteriorly and the mandible posteriorly, decreasing the sling-like tension system. Hyoid elevation results in slackening of the inferior extrinsic muscular attachments.

Genioglossus activity is elevated in the presence of PCR. This, together with tongue positioning on the floor of the mouth, promotes a thrusting activity and an anterior open bite.[65,66] Furthermore, a tongue thrust swallow produces greater posterior intercuspation, which is normally minimal. The assistive action of the tongue in moving a bolus of food posteriorly is affected. Greater intercuspation may lead to masticatory hyperactivity, ultimately leading to greater loading of the TMJ.[6,46,65,66]

Shoulder girdle, cervical, and temporomandibular hyperactivity resulting from postural stress and strain are thought to be prime etiologic factors in the development of the myofascial pain dysfunction syndrome. Muscle hyperactivity leads to activation of trigger point mechanisms that easily mimic other pain syndromes in the upper quarter.[41,44]

Continued loss of normal muscle rest length and associated joint hypomobility lead to continued muscular spasm, trigger point tenderness, poor waste-product liberation, and localized ischemia of adjacent muscle and nerve fibers.

Ongoing nociceptive input from muscle, joint, and ligamentous mechanoreceptors into the segmentally related dorsal horn leads to facilitation. The net result is sympathetic excitation producing greater secretory activity, reduced skin impedance, and lowered pain threshold to gentle palpation and joint oscillation.[43,67] This may be the reason for the constant muscular tenderness that is apparent in myofascial pain dysfunction.

An anterior repositioning splint in a patient with FHP can cause increased craniofacial pain, tinnitus, and fullness of the ear. Muscular forces causing mandibular retrussion are already in play, and an anterior repositioning appliance will be attempting to counteract this force. The result is greater muscle activity promoting trigger point mechanisms. A few weeks of manual soft tissue release techniques, joint mobilization, and postural corrective exercises are thus recommended prior to splint therapy.[68-70] If unloading the TMJ is necessary in the acute stage then a flat plane splint should be used, which will not hinder mandibular positioning changes resulting from correction of upper-quarter posture.[68,70] Specific therapeutic interventions have been described elsewhere.[44,68-71]

In conclusion, the incidence of an abnormal craniovertebral relationship is common among patients with craniofacial pain. The dentist should be aware of the anatomic, neuromuscular, neural, and circulatory mechanisms and should be able to at least generally screen the cervical region during the initial evaluation.

EVALUATION OF THE CERVICAL SPINE

The evaluation of the cervical spine is necessary to rule out its potential as a source of pain. Once the true source of pain has been identified, the treatment becomes systematic and logical.

History

Besides gathering information, taking a history is an opportunity to establish rapport with a patient who may be anxious and uncertain about his or her prognosis.

The chief complaint, history of the present illness, and pertinent past medical and dental history are taken. When taking the history, the physical therapist or dentist may elicit patient complaints not within the area of expertise. At the outset, it is important that the practitioner refer the patient to the appropriate professional for a more comprehensive evaluation.

Subjective Examination

The cervical spine is the most flexible region of the vertebral column and falls prey to the cumulative effects of microtrauma caused by faulty posture. This leads to changes in structure and function frequently producing pain in both the temporomandibular and craniocervical regions. The close interrelationship must always be kept in mind—the upper quarter must always be considered as one functional unit.

Several areas of the cervical spine give rise to symptoms often seen in patients with craniocervical and temporomandibular pains. As previously discussed, the upper cervical spine may refer pain that spreads just below the occiput; the origin of the pain may be the C1-C2 or C2-C3 apophyseal joints.[74] If pain is located in the occipital area it is likely coming from the OA joint. Findings of cervical spine pain are often seen in patients referred for TMJ evaluations.[32,39,75,76,83]

Upper cervical spine pathology may cause dizziness, lightheadedness, nausea, visual disturbances, and tinnitus.[39,83] Irritation of the sympathetic plexus surrounding the vertebral artery by osteoarthritic processes may cause decreased blood flow producing vertebrovascular insufficiency.[84]

Other areas to which cervical pain can be referred include the spine, the pectoral region, the scapula and its medial border, and the entire upper extremity.[74]

Characteristics of Symptoms

Patients may experience many sensations with musculoskeletal dysfunctions. Most frequently they describe pain, stiffness, aching, fatigue, and weakness.

Pain is usually the cause for patients' seeking help. Pain has various qualities that may give insight into its nature. It might be described as a "deep aching pain," which may implicate an intervertebral disc. Pain that is superficial and localized may implicate a zygapophyseal joint. Chronic nerve root pain is often described as nagging and annoying, whereas acute root pain is severe, shooting, burning, and unrelenting.[85] Patients will complain that they are unable to get relief even if they are lying down.

The severity of the pain helps guide examination and management. Testing may be limited on the first visit if pain is severe.

Behavior of Symptoms

The behavior of symptoms over a 24-hour period assists the clinician in formulating a diagnosis and its effect on the activities of daily living (ADL). A patient who works all day as a waiter and at 10:00 P.M. experiences discomfort in the cervical spine, is able to sleep through the night, and wake in the morning without pain or discomfort has a slight problem. This patient requires movement testing to provoke the pain. This patient can be contrasted with the patient who rises in the morning, walks ten steps, and is in severe unrelenting pain. The cervical spine screening form, specifically adapted for the dentist, allows the recording of these data (Table 5–12).

The irritability of a disorder is determined by the degree of activity necessary to provoke a symptom response. The severity of the symptoms and the time before the symptoms subside provide important information regarding possible pathology.[73]

Pain experienced during ADL, such as backing up a car or reading or writing at a desk, provides information on the effects of rotation and flexion of the cervical spine. This activity-position relationship can later help guide manual therapy techniques, which may be indicated.

Therefore, specific questions regarding activities and postures of a sustained nature should be asked and may include questions about sitting, driving, and sleeping. Pain in the cervical spine produced by sitting, especially in FHP is frequently observed especially in typists, keypunch operators, office clerks, and assembly plant workers.[86-88]

Rest generally will ease pain of a mechanical nature. If rotation to the right in the cervical spine produces pain, and movement away from right rotation eases the pain, it is likely of a mechanical nature. Symptoms that remain the same with many positional changes or after rest may be of a nonmechanical origin, often inflammatory or systemic. Mechanical disorders do not follow this rule and are aggravated by specific reclining positions. Typically, patients can sleep but may wake up in pain. The pain eases as the patient starts moving through the day.

Postural Assessment

The purpose of postural assessment is to observe static and dynamic deviations, position abnormalities, protective deformities, asymmetry, and general muscle tone.

Posture is generally observed from frontal, lateral, and posterior views. During evaluation, the patient should stand on a level surface without shoes and in his or her normal relaxed posture.

From the frontal view, the clinician should observe sidebending and rotation of the head on the neck. The SCM and scalenes should be observed, and their effect on the supraclavicular sulcus and angulation of the clavicle noted. Figures 5–12 A and B show a patient with hyperactivity of the left SCM. Prime symptoms were fullness of the left ear, occipital headache, pain around the orbit of the left eye, and pain of the left face. Upper trapezius discomfort was also present. Internal and external rotation and depression or elevation of the shoulder girdle may elicit a painful response. Symmetry of the soft tissues and osseous structures of the face with attention to the orbital ridge, zygoma, maxilla, and mandible should be checked. Figure 5–13 is a relatively normal frontal view and can be compared with Figure 5–12.

Lateral observation is particularly useful for identification of patients with FHP.[44,78,89] Forward head posture moves the cranium anterior to the anatomic plumb line causing shortening of the cervical extensors and elongation of the flexors. This effect causes PCR and the lower cervical spine to be maintained in flexion, leading to a loss in cervical lordosis. An increase in the angulation of the SCM will be seen from a normal of 45 to 60 degrees to 90 degrees. Figure 5–14 shows a normal standing posture as compared with Figure 5–15, which shows FHP with PCR. Internal rotation of the glenohumeral joint and protraction and elevation of the shoulder girdle may also be observed.

Date _____/_____/_____ Age _____ Sex _____   Occupation _____

Name _____

SITES OF PAIN AND PARAESTHESIAE

ACTIVE ROM

IMMEDIATE HISTORY

Forward Head Posture	☐ Mild	☐ Mod.	☐ Sev.
Forward Shoulders	☐ Mild	☐ Mod.	☐ Sev.
Head Tilt	☐ R	☐ L	
Shoulder High	☐ R	☐ L	
Iliac Crest High	☐ R	☐ L	

PAIN

Degree
Nature
Constant   Periodic   Occasional
Increasing   Static   Decreasing
Night Pain
Sleep Position
A.M. Pain
AGGRAVATES
Cough/Sneeze   Deep Breath
EASES

SOFT TISSUE PALPATION

	L	R
–Supraclavicular Sulcus	_____	_____
–Suboccipital Fossa	_____	_____
–Longus Colli	_____	_____
–Sternocleidomastoid	_____	_____
–Scaleni	_____	_____
–Trapezius	_____	_____
–Levator Scapulae	_____	_____
–Rhomboids	_____	_____
–Pectorals	_____	_____
–Supraspinatus	_____	_____
–Infraspinatus	_____	_____
–Deltoid	_____	_____
–Teres	_____	_____
Compression _____ Distraction _____		
Vertebral Artery L _____ R _____		

Myotome Scan _____ Dermatome Scan _____

Shoulder Girdle Restriction   R   L   ☐ Mild   ☐ Mod.   ☐ Sev.

TABLE 5–12. Cervical Spine Screening Form

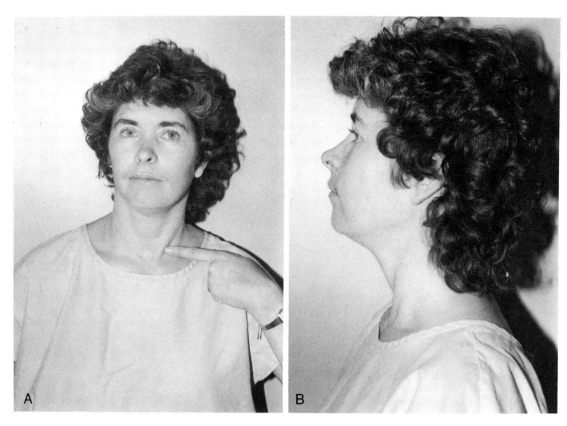

FIGURE 5-12. *A*, Hyperactivity of the left sternocleidomastoid (SCM). Note the prominence of both the sternal and clavicular attachments. *B*, Hyperactivity of the left SCM. Note the prominence of the sternal and clavicular heads as well as the presence of forward head posture (FHP) with posterior cranial rotation (PCR).

The posterior view confirms what was seen on the first two views and provides additional postural information. The scapulae may be protracted, retracted, elevated, or winged. This is assessed by observing the relationship of the medial border and the superior and inferior angles of the scapulae with the cranium and the cervical and thoracic spine. Deviations indicate a structural or muscular imbalance (Fig. 5–16).

If there are pathomechanical findings in the upper quarter, further investigation lower down the kinetic chain may be warranted. Iliac crest heights and hip, knee, and ankle dysfunctions may cause or perpetuate upper-quarter dysfunctions. Proper evaluation may necessitate referral.

Active Movement Tests

Active movement of the cervical spine helps the clinician to evaluate the available range of motion, the patient's willingness to move, and the pain or stiffness at the end of the range. Limitation may be caused by pathology in the muscle, ligament, capsule, and facet joints. If movement is limited during active range but does not produce pain, gentle overpressure can be applied by the clinician. Provocation with overpressure may produce pain, providing important information as to location and severity of the pathology. A movement is considered normal when it is full and pain free with sustained overpressure. In the presence of an FHP, the atlas is pushed posteriorly, inhibiting forward nodding of the head on the neck.

In active movement testing, the last motion assessed should be the most painful. Pure forward bending is first observed and should be 80 to 90 degrees with the chin to the chest (Fig. 5–17). Next, full rotation is examined—normal being when the chin is almost over the acromion (70 to 90 degrees) as shown in Figure 5–18. It is important that patients perform pure rotation and do not bend backward during this

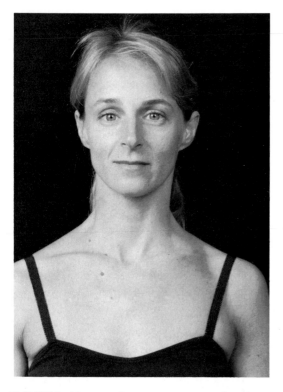

FIGURE 5–13. Normal anterior view. Note the relative equivalent prominence of sternocleidomastoid (SCM) tendons.

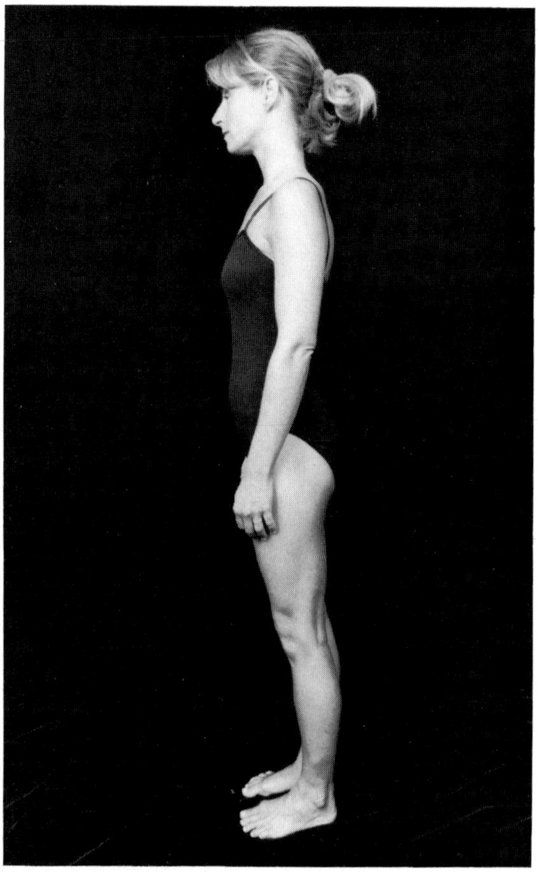

FIGURE 5–14. Normal standing posture.

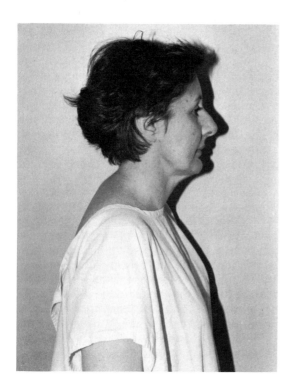

FIGURE 5–15. Abnormal upper quarter posture. Note the presence of forward head, posterior cranial rotation, "dowager's hump," and internal rotation of the shoulders.

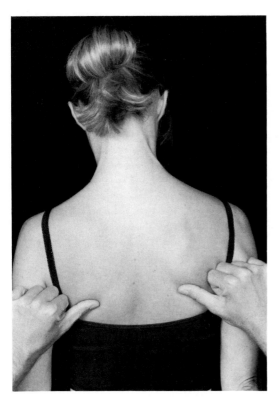

FIGURE 5–16. Posterior view demonstrating assessment of scapular position.

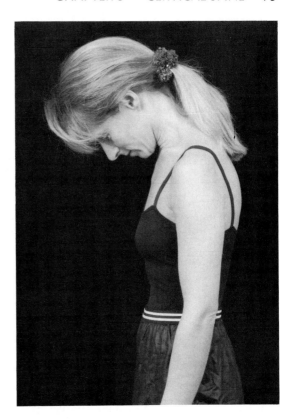

FIGURE 5–17. Active forward bending of the cervical spine. A distance of no more than two fingerbreadths between the chin and sternum is considered to be within normal limits.

procedure. Normal sidebending produces 20 to 45 degrees of motion, bringing the ear toward the shoulder. The curve of the lateral cervical spine away from the side of motion is observed for flexibility or straightness (Fig. 5–19). Side-to-side comparisons in sidebending and rotation are helpful. Backward bending is best viewed from the anterior position. Restrictions will cause cranial deviation to the right or left side. Muscle symmetry and tone are also noted. In Figure 5–20, the patient has increased tone in the left scalenes and SCM. Figure 5–21 shows a side view of backward bending, which demonstrates a normal vertical plane of the face being parallel with the ceiling. It is helpful to first have the patient perform backward bending from a normal standing position and then from the corrected position. In the presence of FHP, backward bending is diminished and can result in an increase in suboccipital compression.

Combined active movement tests can be employed for quick identification of local restriction. The OA joint can be grossly tested by asking the patient to fully rotate the cervical spine

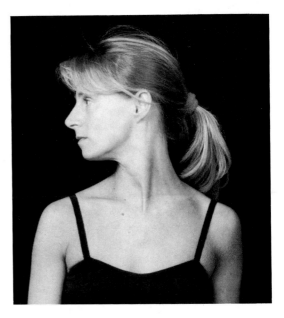

FIGURE 5–18. Active rotation of the cervical spine.

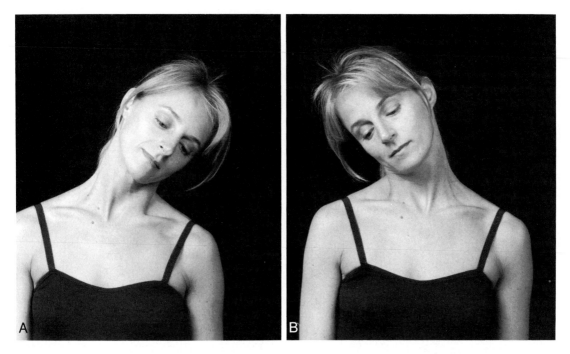

FIGURE 5–19. *A,* Active left side bending. *B,* Active right side bending.

and then nod the chin. Movement of the right and left sides are compared. Figure 5–22 illustrates this motion also called the scalene cramp test position as described by Travell.[41] Pain referred to the ipsilateral arm is considered a positive sign.

The AA joint may also be grossly tested by having the patient sidebend maximally and then rotate the head to the opposite side. Figure 5–23 shows a decreased ability to sidebend, but rotation appears adequate. The integrity of the alar ligament can be assessed by palpating each side of the spinous process of C2 while

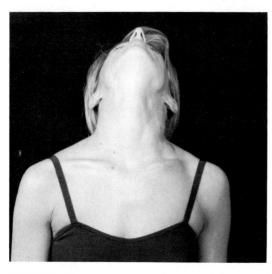

FIGURE 5–20. Active backward bending of the cervical spine. Note the small degree of deviation to the left.

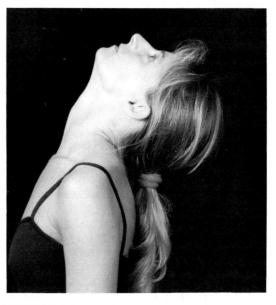

FIGURE 5–21. Active backward bending of the cervical spine as viewed laterally.

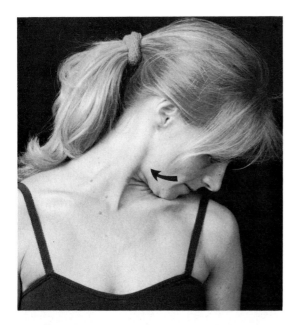

FIGURE 5–22. Active rotation with nodding. Normal movement should allow for the chin to be positioned near or within the supraclavicular fossa.

passively sidebending the OA joints. The spinous process of C2 should move immediately to the opposite side if the alar ligament is intact. These tests provide general impressions of possible dysfunction. In the presence of positive findings, further mobility testing is needed to isolate the exact joint and its degree of restriction so that appropriate therapy can be initiated.

Passive Range of Motion

Cervical movement may be further evaluated by passive movement testing. The available range, the quality of movement, and most importantly the joint "end feel" are determined during passive testing. Comparisons of adjacent segments and their hypermobility or hypomobility are assessed.

Gentle passive provoking movements are applied by the clinician to assess "joint play" in flexion, extension, lateral flexion, and rotation. It is sometimes necessary to combine mo-

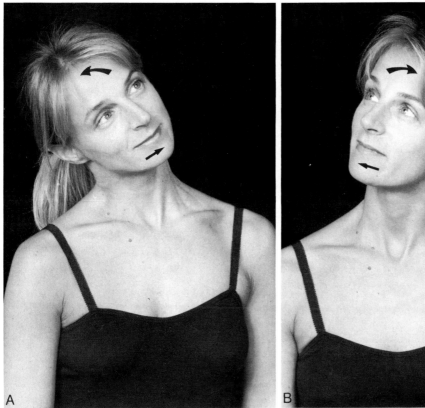

FIGURE 5–23. *A*, Active right side bending and left rotation of the upper cervical spine. *B*, Active left side bending and right rotation of the upper cervical spine.

tions during testing to reproduce painful movement, to increase range, or to relieve joint pain. Passive range of motion (ROM) for testing the cervical spine is common practice for knowledgeable physical therapists, but beyond the training of most dentists.

The passive testing of right sidebending is demonstrated at the C3-C4 segment (Fig. 5–24). This technique is first applied segmentally to one side of the cervical spine and then to the other. Upper cervical spine extension (Fig. 5–25) and lower cervical spine extension (Fig. 5–26) are tested in a standing position. Chin nodding in upper cervical flexion is demonstrated in Figure 5–27. Passive provocation of FHP with PCR may recreate cervical pain and suboccipital headache when this position is maximized. This test position may also provoke TMJ pain because of the compression forces on the TMJ that occur in this position. Onset of symptoms will generally occur within 30 seconds and will be similar to those of FHP maintained for long periods of time (Fig. 5–28). Overpressure can be applied to any joint to provoke symptoms but should not be greater than the maximal pathologic position assumed by the patient during the day.

The physical therapist also performs specific oscillations and vertebral pressures in the sub-

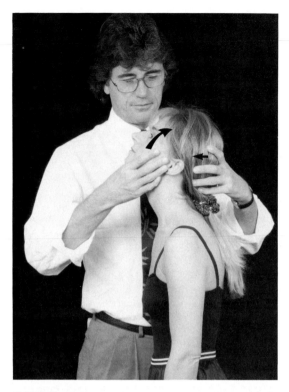

FIGURE 5–25. Passive extension of the upper cervical spine. Note that this extension imparts significant suboccipital compression.

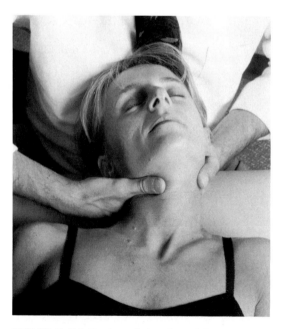

FIGURE 5–24. Passive side bending of the C3–C4 segments. The therapist's right hand is the fulcrum, and the left hand provides the passive motion.

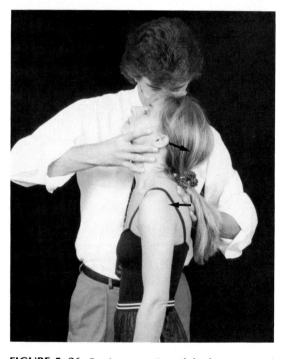

FIGURE 5–26. Passive extension of the lower cervical spine.

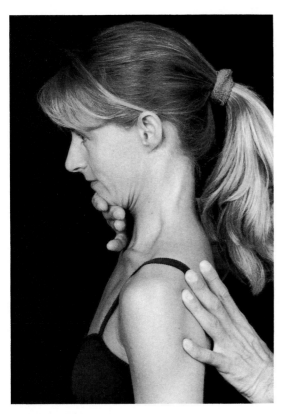

FIGURE 5–27. Passive nodding that imparts flexion at the upper cervical region and stretch of the suboccipital extensors.

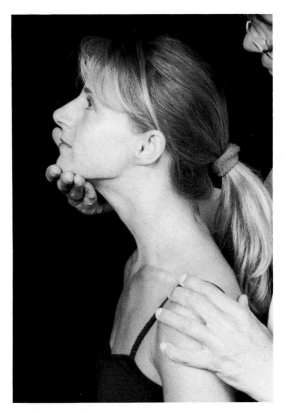

FIGURE 5–28. Passive postural provocation into the forward head position (FHP) with posterior cranial rotation (PCR).

occipital area, especially when headache or craniofacial pain exists. Gentle posterior to anterior glides of the atlas and axis in central and unilateral directions can be applied to the posterior arch of the atlas and the spinous process or lamina of the axis. Transverse pressures can be applied to the spinous process of the axis. These techniques are performed while the patient is in the prone position, with additional techniques to the anterior vertebral body, in the supine position. Assessment of the degree of hypomobility and pain and of the relief of pain is helpful in diagnosis.[15,36,72–74] These tests provide important information relative to the direction of movement to be performed by the physical therapist during treatment.

Resisted Range of Motion

The musculature of the cervical spine can be a source of pain and dysfunction and can be independent or dependent on underlying structural pathology.

Isometric testing of cervical musculature without the compression of underlying joints and neural structures is virtually impossible. Differentiation of muscle and joint dysfunction is assessed after assembling all historical and physical examination information and after trial treatment of a structure is judged for symptomatic relief.

In the presence of cervical spine dysfunction frequent alteration of muscle length and tone occurs. This is significant because muscle influence in one area tends to lead to imbalance in other areas,[18] often leading to alteration of joint mechanics as well. Thus, both muscle and joint dysfunctions may exist together and require simultaneous treatment. The muscles should be assessed as to length, bulk, fiber texture, and strength and should be included in routine evaluation of cervical and shoulder girdle pain. If the patient is having referred symptoms to the upper extremities, this finding becomes particularly important.

Isometric myotomal testing of involved segmental muscle groups may reveal weakness

TABLE 5–13. Myotome Scan: Isometric Test Bilaterally

IN NEUTRAL POSITION
1. C1-C2   Neck flexion
2. C3   Neck sidebending
3. C4   Shoulder shrugs
4. C5   Shoulder abduction
5. C6   Elbow flexion/wrist extension
6. C7   Elbow extension/wrist flexion
7. C8   Thumb extension
8. T1   5th finger abduction/index finger abduction

when comparing left and right extremities. If weakness is noted, it must be differentiated from neurologic deficits and disuse atrophy.

Isometric muscle testing, as listed in Table 5–13, are reliable only if the patient is instructed to contract with equal force on each side. Patients in severe pain should not be tested, as it may lead to increased discomfort.

Peripheral Joint Scan

Sometimes, symptoms that appear to originate in the cervical spine and refer to the upper extremity may actually originate elsewhere. Symptoms may also originate from one or more pathologic peripheral joints coexisting with cervical dysfunction.

Shoulder girdle pathology often coexists with FHP, particularly when a result of a traumatic incident. A cervical hyperextension injury in which the automobile was hit from behind while the patient held the steering wheel can disrupt the integrity of the shoulder girdle.[49]

Patients with pain in the scapular region require examination of the cervical spine and the glenohumeral and scapulothoracic joints. Patients with headaches and lateral facial pains require examinations of the upper cervical spines and TMJs.[85]

Evaluation of the shoulder joint may commence with Apley's flexion and extension tests (Fig. 5–29). These two tests cover most joint motions and will provoke the appropriate joint structures. If shoulder pain cannot be provoked, other movements are needed to create maximal stress on the rotator cuff, bursa, coracoacromial arch, and glenoid labrum. Pain located over the apex of the shoulder may require examination of the acromioclavicular and sternoclavicular joints. Comprehensive assessment of the shoulder complex is beyond the dental evaluation but should be included in the physical therapy evaluation. Painful and stiff shoulder joints must be considered as possible causes of shoulder and arm pain, and the isolated glenohumeral joint should be tested. Locking tests can be performed by passive abduction, extension, and slight medial rotation. An anterior force can be applied, and the production of pain implicates the glenohumeral joint. More distal pain referred over the elbow, wrist, and hand would require testing of all joint motions through physiologic ranges with overpressure.

If two joints are implicated, for instance, the cervical spine and shoulder girdle, and there is difficulty with differentiation, only one joint should be initially treated. The patient should be re-evaluated before proceeding to treatment of the other joint.

Specific Tests

A group of specific tests help differentiate tissue involvement, particularly in the cervical, thoracic, and shoulder girdle region.

Evaluation of referred pain from the cervical spine requires combined movement tests that compress articular surfaces and constrict intervertebral foramina. These tests are often useful to reproduce referred symptoms.[90–92] The Cervical Spine Compression Test (Fig. 5–30) is performed with the patient sitting with the head in slight flexion. Force is directed downward and equally so as not to affect one side more than the other. The test finding is positive if articular or neural signs are provoked. The more distal the experienced pain in the upper extremity, the more positive the test result. This test can be modified to introduce unilateral compression to either side of the cervical spine by sidebending and rotating to the same side followed by extending the head (Spurling's test). Foraminal encroachment will cause the symptoms to be more distal, as the force of these three motions is increased.

The Cervical Distraction Test is performed by lifting the head at the mastoid region while maintaining the neutral position (Fig. 5–31). This test is designed to alleviate pressure from the suspected implicated tissues. The test finding is positive when symptoms are decreased. A positive distraction test result may be a strong indicator that cervical traction may be helpful.[91] Cervical traction with TMDs should be performed suboccipitally to avoid the TMJ compression commonly produced by mandibular halters.[44]

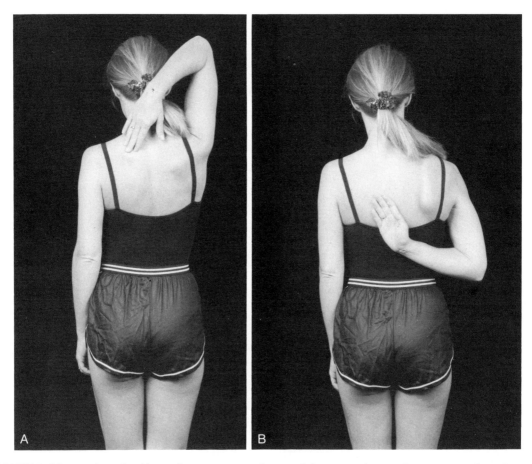

FIGURE 5–29. *A,* Apley's shoulder girdle test imparting flexion, abduction, and external rotation. *B,* Apley's shoulder girdle test imparting extension, adduction, and internal rotation.

Vertebral Artery

The vertebral artery is one of the major sources of blood supply to the brain stem. This artery may fall prey to stretching or compressive forces throughout its length. Occlusion can occur from the C6 segment to the suboccipital region.[14] Extremes of motion during rotation of the cranium can cause a decrease in blood flow in the contralateral vertebral artery at the AA and OA joints.[93] Compromise of the artery has also been reported in extension.[94] Figure 5–5 illustrates the vertebral artery.

Clinically, symptoms experienced with vertebral artery insufficiency include dizziness, nausea, tinnitus, and visual disturbances. Patients with temporomandibular and craniocervical disorders often present with these symptoms. These patients most often have soft tissue and joint impingements restricting the suboccipital regions.

Clinical testing of the vertebral artery is indicated when such symptoms are present. The Vertebral Artery Test is performed both in weightbearing and nonweightbearing positions.[14,90] In the weightbearing position, the patient is seated with the head in a neutral position. The patient is first instructed to rotate the head to both sides. If symptoms are not produced, the head is placed in extension and active rotation to either side is performed. If symptoms still do not develop, the clinician passively moves the head through all motions to full range and asks the patient to report any change in symptoms (Fig. 5–32). It is important that the head be moved through the full available range for the test to be valid. Patients with restricted motion may not allow valid testing.

The nonweightbearing Vertebral Artery Test is performed with the patient in the supine po-

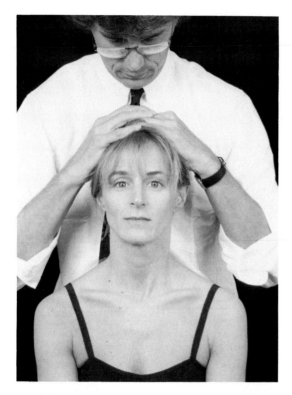

FIGURE 5–30. Manual cervical spine compression.

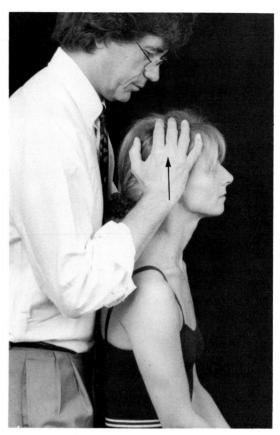

FIGURE 5–31. Manual cervical spine distraction.

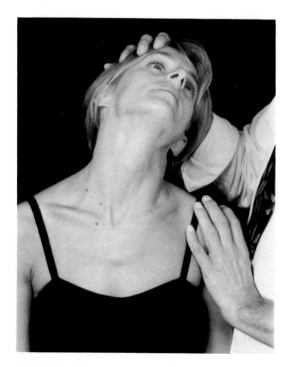

FIGURE 5–32. Passive testing of the left vertebral artery in the seated position.

sition (Fig. 5–33). The patient's head is fully extended and rotated to either side and held for approximately 15 seconds. During this test, the clinician observes for pupillary asymmetries and the patient reports any dizziness, light-headedness, or visual disturbance. A patient may also experience giddiness, nausea, or tinnitus.[14,72,93] Another means of assessment is to have the supine patient maximally extend the head on a pillow and hold that position for 15 to 30 seconds. This method may compromise both vertebral arteries. It is important to note that osseous or myofascial restriction may hamper tests of the vertebral artery—there may not be adequate ROM to compromise the artery sufficiently. However, if symptoms arise the test is discontinued, especially in the elderly patient in whom RA and osteoarthritic and atherosclerotic pathology may be involved. This test must always be performed before any subcranial treatment is started.

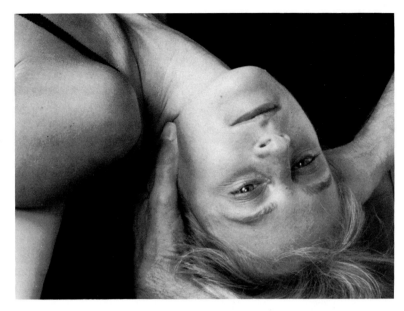

FIGURE 5–33. Passive testing of the left vertebral artery in the supine position.

Brachial Plexus Tension Tests

Combinations of movement in the upper extremities may produce symptoms in the cervical spine.

Elvey[92] demonstrated that movements of the upper extremity in various planes could produce tension in the cervical nerve roots, surrounding sheaths, and dura. The movements of horizontal abduction and external rotation of the glenohumeral joint, coupled with elbow and wrist extension, shoulder depression, and sidebending of the cervical spine to the opposite side produced the greatest tension in the C5, C6, and C7 nerve roots. This test is performed with the patient in the supine position and may be helpful in the identification of a source of vague shoulder and upper arm pain. Positive findings suggest a tensional component of the neural tissues. The severity is determined by observing the amount of full extension of the elbow available on the affected side compared with the unaffected side.

A tension test for the neuromeningial tissues of the entire spinal cord is the slump test (Fig. 5–34). The therapist applies a full longitudinal stretch on the neuromeningial structures (dura mater), placing the spine in maximum flexion combined with hip flexion, knee extension, and ankle dorsi flexion.[85] Symptoms of pain, paresthesia, or both produced in the cervical and thoracic spine by this general test support the need for additional testing.

Neurovascular Compression Tests

Thoracic inlet syndromes produce compression of the lower trunk of the brachial plexus and the subclavian artery and vein. It is generally thought that the compression is located in the supraclavicular fossa between the anterior and medial scalene musculature and first rib (Fig. 5–35). Forward head posture, direct trauma, and anatomic variations can produce impingement of these neurovascular structures.[95–97]

Symptoms include poorly localized pain and aching in the supraclavicular fossa, anterior shoulder, and arm. Paresthesia classically affects the eighth cervical and first thoracic dermatomes.[95] Patients frequently describe heaviness, clumsiness, and subjective weakness of the upper extremity.

Vascular symptoms and signs will be evident if the subclavian artery is impinged. Ischemic pain of the arms and forearms may occur with mild exercise. The patient may complain of "coldness," "whiteness," and "blueness." Vascular symptoms can become worse in cold weather. Impaired venous drainage may cause swelling of the arms and stiff fingers. Examination of the supraclavicular fossa may also disclose fullness from contracted muscles, tenderness to palpation, or impaired circulatory and lymphatic flow (Fig. 5–35).

Many tests have been described to provoke the tissues of the thoracic inlet. The reliability

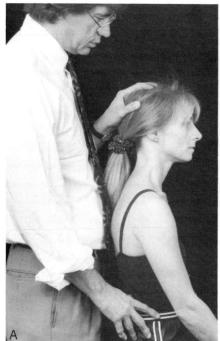

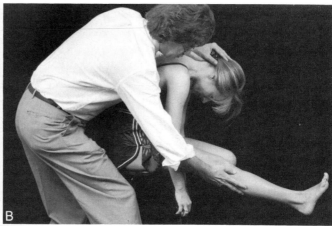

FIGURE 5–34. *A*, Starting position for the slump test. *B*, End position for the slump test.

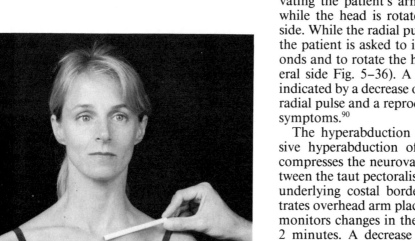

FIGURE 5–35. Location of the supraclavicular fossa.

of these tests is questionable. Reproduction or exacerbation of subjective complaints seems to be a more useful indicator.

The Adson's test evaluates compression of the subclavian artery by pressure exerted by the anterior scalene. This test is performed by elevating the patient's arm parallel to the floor, while the head is rotated to the contralateral side. While the radial pulse is being monitored, the patient is asked to inhale for 10 to 15 seconds and to rotate the head toward the ipsilateral side Fig. 5–36). A positive test finding is indicated by a decrease or an obliteration of the radial pulse and a reproduction of the patient's symptoms.[90]

The hyperabduction maneuver causes passive hyperabduction of the shoulder, which compresses the neurovascular components between the taut pectoralis minor tendon and the underlying costal borders. Figure 5–37 illustrates overhead arm placement, as the clinician monitors changes in the radial pulse for up to 2 minutes. A decrease or obliteration of the pulse and a reproduction of the symptoms constitute positive test results.

The Costoclavicular Test or Exaggerated Military Position is done by bringing the shoulder girdle into retraction and depression for up to 2 minutes while the clinician monitors the radial pulse. This position may compress the subclavian vessels and brachial plexus during approximation of the first rib and clavicle (Fig. 5–38.[95]

The Three-Minute Elevated Arm Exercise or Overhead Stress Test is performed with the

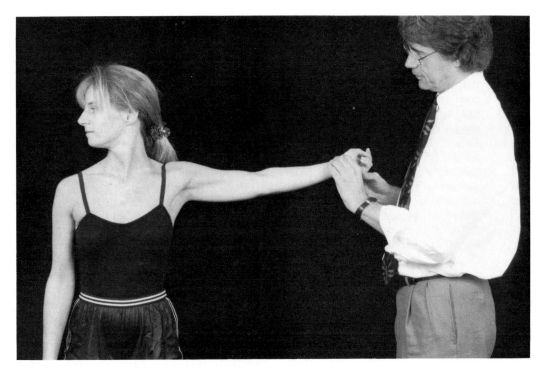

FIGURE 5–36. Adson's test for neurovascular compression.

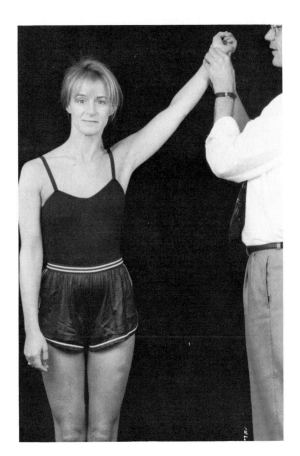

FIGURE 5–37. Hyperabduction test for neurovascular compression.

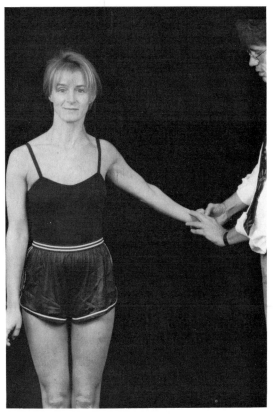

FIGURE 5–38. Costoclavicular test for neurovascular compression.

arms elevated to 90 degrees and the shoulder girdle slightly retracted. The patient is asked to open and close the fist slowly and steadily for 3 minutes. A positive test finding is noted if the patient is unable to complete the test or reproduction of symptoms occur (Fig. 5–39).[90]

The test for scapulocostal involvement (levator scapula) is performed by palpating the superior medial angle of the scapula while the examiner pulls the arm into hyperextension, depression, and internal rotation. A tender trigger point at the superior medial angle is quite common along with elevation of the scapula and reproduction or exacerbation of pain as previously described.

Tinel's test reproduces radiating pain or paresthesia by tapping on the scalenes in the supraclavicular fossa.

Dizziness Testing

Dizziness related to rapid head movement and not to head posture requires additional testing. Dizziness provoked by quick rotary or flexion-extension movements can arise from the vestibular apparatus. This is tested by having the patient stand, and while the head is stabilized the trunk is rotated to the left and right. Figure 5–40 shows the head held in a sustained rotary hold position for a minimum of 10 seconds, as the trunk is rotated. If nystagmus occurs for a few seconds, it will be due to distortion of the cervical spine proprioceptive input. If nystagmus lasts longer, is latent, and increases with prolonged testing a vascular origin is suspected.[93]

Palpation Examination

Palpation will verify and supplement the information gained from the preceding test findings. A thickening, swelling, or painful response to palpation over a facet or joint capsule should correlate with areas of decreased movement, primary painful areas, and referred pain patterns. Muscles are palpated from origin to insertion. The clinician should palpate for texture and tightness and search for fibrous bands and nodules. Trigger points and their referral patterns should be carefully assessed.[41]

Elevated or lowered temperature and dryness and tension of the skin may indicate chronic underlying pathology. Altered tissue can be compared from one side with the other.

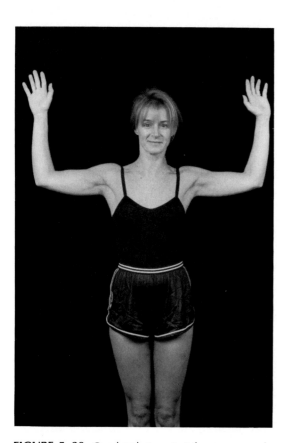

FIGURE 5–39. Overhead stress test for neurovascular compression.

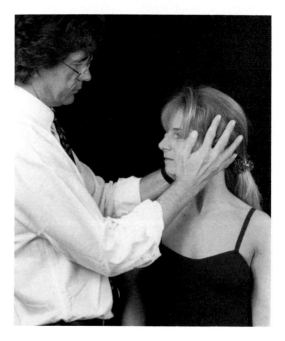

FIGURE 5–40. Dizziness testing of the vestibular apparatus.

A thorough knowledge of three-dimensional structure and function is necessary for the clinician to make a proper diagnosis. The pressure, direction, and force of palpation must be consistent to gain valid information comparing left and right sides.

Soft Tissue Palpation

Soft tissue palpation is divided into superficial and deep intersegmental muscles, ligaments, and apophyseal joints.

Palpation of the occiput down to C3 and from C3 to the lateral mass of the atlas and back to the occiput constitutes examination of the suboccipital triangle. The deep suboccipital muscles provide stability and attach the occiput, atlas, and axis. The splenius capitis is best palpated within the upper part of the muscular triangle formed by the trapezius behind, SCM in front, and levator scapula below. Isolation of the semispinalis capitis requires slight flexion of the head with the patient seated, side lying or prone with the head cupped in the hands.[41] Figures 5–5 and 5–6 illustrate the anatomic locations of these muscles. Palpation of the interlaminar spaces and the capsules of occiput-C1, C1-C2, and C3 is also valuable.

The interlaminar space, joint casules, and supraspinous ligaments should be palpated from C3-C7. C7-T1 is a common area of soft tissue alteration, which can give rise to symptoms.

The mandible, hyoid bone, cervical spine, and shoulder girdle function as a unit.[7,98] Thus, complete palpation should include all of the suprahyoid and infrahyoid musculature. The longus colli may be particularly tender in patients with hyperextension injuries and can be responsible for straightening of the cervical lordosis.[49] The scalenes should be scrutinized carefully. The anterior scalene is the most commonly involved followed by the middle and posterior.[41] The anterior scalene is best palpated under the posterior border of the clavicular division of the SCM. Finger pressure just above the clavicle may occlude the jugular vein with the anterior scalene alongside (Fig. 5–41).[41]

The middle scalene can be palpated deep and anterior to the upper trapezius alongside the cervical transverse processes. It is difficult to palpate the posterior scalene because it is obscured by the levator scapula. If the levator scapula is pushed aside where it emerges from under the upper trapezius, isolated palpation

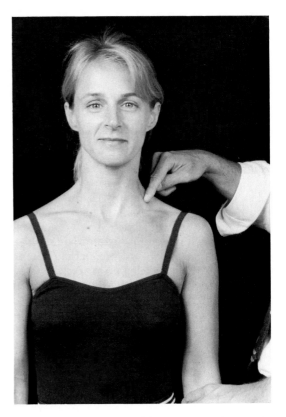

FIGURE 5–41. Location of the anterior scalene in the supraclavicular fossa.

may be possible. Scalene and SCM spasms may produce neurovascular entrapment indicative of TIS.[99]

The SCM is best palpated with the patient seated or supine. The head should be bent to the palpating side and slightly rotated to the opposite side. Each belly should be lifted and palpated between the thumb and index fingers.[41] Figure 5–12A illustrates moderate hyperactivity of the left SCM with prominence of the sternal and clavicular heads.

The C5, C6, and C7 nerves of the brachial plexus may be palpated as they exit the foraminal gutter by sliding the finger tip laterally along the articular pillars and then moving anteriorly. Pain with radiation in the upper extremity may be produced.

The SCM, upper trapezius, and levator scapula must be palpated superficially. The levator scapulae, scalenes, upper trapezius, and SCMs should be palpated with the patient in a side-bent or rotated head posture. In the sitting position with elbow support the upper trapezius and levator scapula slacken. The upper trapezius can be pushed posteriorly and the levator scapula can be isolated when the head is rotated to the opposite side. This maneuver produces tightening of the levator and lifts it against the palpating fingers.[41]

The middle trapezius and rhomboids can be palpated along the vertebral border of the scapula. The supraspinatus, infraspinatus, and teres minor muscles are palpated in descending fashion over the supraspinous and infraspinous fossa and inferior angle of the scapula (see Fig. 5–10).

Pectoralis major palpation is illustrated in Figure 5–42. The palpating fingers should move lower to assess the sternal and costal sections. The pectoralis minor is more difficult to palpate. It is best done with the patient supine and the arm elevated slightly to slacken the pectoralis major. One or two fingers are then placed at the apex of the axilla and begin to slide along the chest wall under the pectoralis major. Palpation continues toward the midline to the pectoralis minor muscle. Pain referral from the pectoralis minor is difficult to distinguish from that of scalene entrapment.[14]

Osseous Palpation

Changes palpated on vertebral body structures provide evidence of dysfunctional intervertebral mechanics. Generally, the spinous and transverse processes are assessed for position. Position changes may cause abnormal forces to be applied on ligamentous and muscular tissues throughout the kinetic chain. Muscle and vetebral body imbalances feed the soft tissue and osseous receptors, which result in pain and dysfunction. Of particular importance is the position of the lateral mass of the atlas. When the atlas is rotated or laterally deviated in relation to the occiput and axis, it may be palpated as an asymmetry in depth and position in relation to the mastoid bone.

The spinous processes of the cervical spine C2, C6, and C7 are located without difficulty because of their size and position, whereas those of C3-C5 are generally shorter and deeper. A test for specific delineation has been previously described.

The hyoid bone joins the mandible to the shoulder girdle through the suprahyoid and infrahyoid musculature. This bone is also indirectly united with the cervical spine by the posterior digastric and stylohyoid connection to the cranium. The omohyoid joins the hyoid with the upper scapula. Pain in these structures

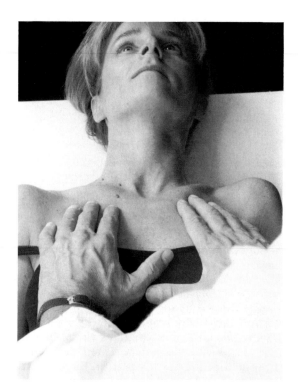

FIGURE 5–42. Palpation of the upper anterior rib cage and pectoralis muscle.

may be elicited on swallowing or passive movement testing. The glenohyoid, sternohyoid, and omohyoid are innervated from the C1 nerve roots and the hypoglossal nerve. A patient with suboccipital impingement or FHP may have possible nerve root irritation leading to hypertonicity of this musculature.[100] Any pain on palpation suggests dysfunction. Symptoms may relate to myalgia of the tongue, masticatory musculature, or both. Patients often describe fullness and tightness of the floor of the mouth or anterior neck, indicating muscular involvement in this region.

Cervical spine posture can influence the position of the mandible; FHP often changes its rest position.[66,68–70,101,102] Any change in mandibular position will influence the submandibular musculature and its relationship to the hyoid. In FHP, the net effect is to increase submandibular muscle tone and retrognathia.[46,102]

The first two ribs are important osseous anchors for the scalene musculature. The first rib is the shortest and is normally positioned in an oblique downward direction toward the sternum. The anterior and middle scalenes insert on the most lateral aspect of this rib. The second rib is twice as long and anchors the posterior scalene. Rib dysfunction may occur in the upper costovertebral joints, referring pain to the posterior cervicothoracic region.[90] This may be caused by rotary fixation of a thoracic vertebra restricting motion of the costovertebral joints on inhalation and exhalation. Restriction may be tested by assessing the pump handle motion of the ribs as illustrated in Figure 5–42. Asymmetry of rib motion would indicate rib dysfunction. Limited motion is evident on the dysfunctional side when a deep inspiration is taken. Further assessment of thoracic vertebral motion is then necessary. Vertebra and rib dysfunctions may occur independently because of soft tissue adaptations. Palpation of a bulge at the level of the clavicle between the anterior and middle scalenes may represent a cervical rib, which may also cause thoracic inlet syndrome; this finding should be confirmed with radiographs.[41]

Soft tissue examination of the supraclavicular fossa may disclose a fullness brought about by tension of the scalene group. This fullness can often be visualized, and palpation of the fossa for elevated and anteriorly displaced first and second ribs will confirm the observation. Thoracic inlet symptoms may be present with restricted sidebending and rotational movements of the cervical and thoracic joints. As the ribs elevate and move anteriorly, the brachial plexus and its associated vessels become impinged. This is often seen in FHP as well as in trauma, obesity, and occupational stress.[95–97,103]

SIGNS AND SYMPTOMS INDICATING PHYSICAL THERAPY REFERRAL

Patients may present with a myriad of signs and symptoms. Clinicians dealing with craniovertebral and temporomandibular pathology must be alert to specific problems arising from the cervical spine.

A history of gradual onset of symptoms after minor or prolonged physical activity may be indicative of mechanical derangement.[72] Activity can include long duration driving, bicycling on a racer, or repeated microtrauma of holding a telephone with one shoulder to the ear. Patients may experience craniocervical pain with referral patterns. These patterns have been explored by many investigators, such as Kellgren[104] and Cloward.[105] They found typical pain referral patterns with cervical disk involvement. Pain usually started in the cervical spine and was referred to the scapula, shoulders, or as far distally as the forearm and hand. The compression and distraction tests previously described are generally used to separate nerve root pathology from facet joint or other tissue involvement. Differentiation of the specific tissue at fault is often elusive.

When nerve root involvement occurs, pain and paresthesia may be more distinct. A patient's pathology may be judged as worsening when the pain refers more distally into the upper extremity. Such signs of nerve root irritation are usually accompanied by hyperactive reflexes, muscular ache, dermatomal paresthesia, or all three.[72] As nerve root compression increases, there may be diminished or absent deep tendon reflexes as well as weakness. When testing the tendon reflex, the tendon should be tapped six times to ascertain if a fading reflex response is present, which is indicative of a developing root sign.[106]

Weakness in muscle strength is confirmed by testing one muscle of a representative cord segment. Muscle weakness that is not due solely to pain is a strong indicator of a neurologic deficit.[106]

Sensory testing is appropriately performed with the patient's eyes closed while tactile stimulation is applied to various dermatomes. Complete patterns of anesthesia should be further tested with pin pricks.

Severe nerve root pain has a prominent quality of deep aching.[72] The patient is often holding the extremity and describes a heaviness, especially after movement. Burning and shooting pain may be present. The extremity may be cold and swollen, indicating neurovascular involvement.

If a cervical disk is bulging or extruded, the spinal cord may become compressed. Thus, examination may disclose spasticity, a positive plantar response, or clonus, each of which is a myelopathic sign.[107] Other signs of root or cord compression may include muscle wasting and trophic skin changes. Patients with these signs are often surgical candidates.

Patients with constant pain despite bed rest, anti-inflammatory medications, and muscle relaxants may have severe nerve root entrapments, inflammatory processes, or malignancies. A red flag should go up if the patient has recently had an unplanned weight loss. The possibility of malignancy should weigh heavily in the examiner's mind. Pancoast's tumor may refer pain into the upper extremity and cervical

Name _____   Occupation _____

Age _____   Sex _____   Date _____   Referred by Dr: _____

Recent History:

A/A   W/C   C/M   Other: _____

_____

_____

_____

Previous History: Treatment/Surgery & Results

_____

_____

Medical Background: RA   OA   Other Illness: _____

_____

Medication: _____

_____

Sites of Pain & Paresthesia

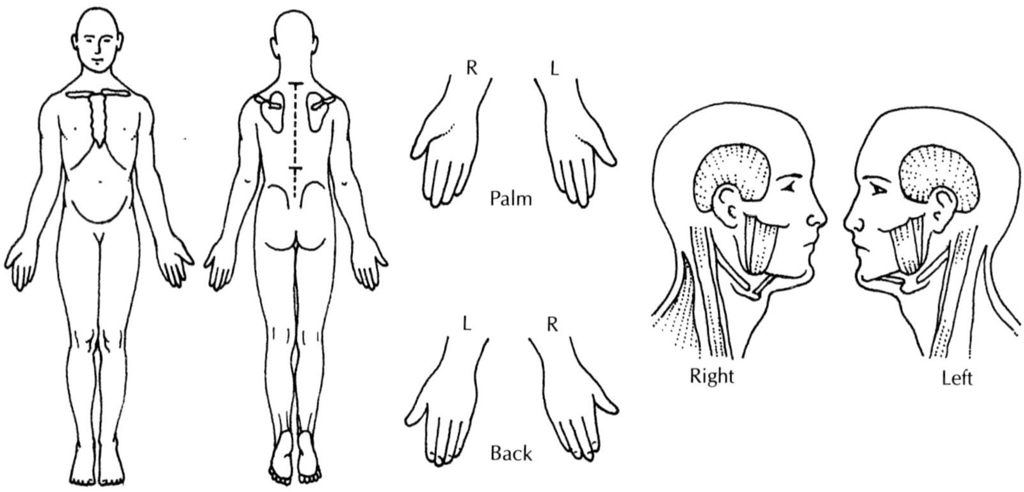

Pain Characteristics

Degree	0 -------------------------- 10	
Nature		
Constant	Periodic	Occasional
Increasing	Static	Decreasing
Night Pain		
Sleeping position	Supine	Prone
	SDLY	L/R
Read/TV in bed	_____	
Best time	AM	PM

Aggravates

Standing	Walking	Driving
Sitting	Rising from	Computer
Sustained flexion	Sustained ext.	Reading
Cough/sneeze	Deep breath	

Eases

Postion	Movement

Associated S/S:

Dizziness, vertigo, nausea, lightheaded, blurred vision

TABLE 5–14. Assessment Form for the Upper Quarter.

Static Posture & Muscle Guarding

Palpation Findings

O Sore/Tender	**x** Hypomobile segment	**V** Prominent
P Pain	**B** Boggy	**R** Rotated
∿∿ Hypermobile	**S** Elicited Spasm	⬜ Step

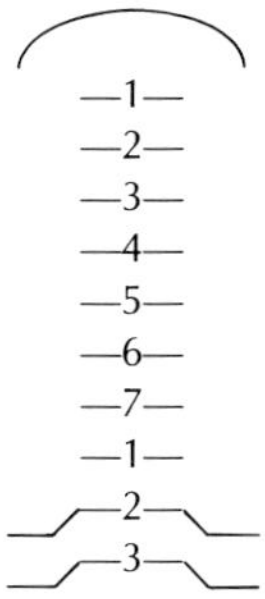

—1—
—2—
—3—
—4—
—5—
—6—
—7—
—1—
—2—
—3—

Postural Provocation Testing

Passive / **Active**

		Pain		FB
Side glide	WNL	Hypomobile		
Ant. glide	WNL	Hypomobile	LSB	RSB
Post. glide	WNL	Hypomobile		
Rotation OA	WNL	Hypomobile	RL	RR
Central P.A.				BB
Vert. Pressure	WNL	Hypomobile		
Unilat. P.A.			P = Pain active	
Vert. Pressure	WNL	Hypomobile	OP = Pain on overpressure	
Transverse				
Vert. Pressure	WNL	Hypomobile		

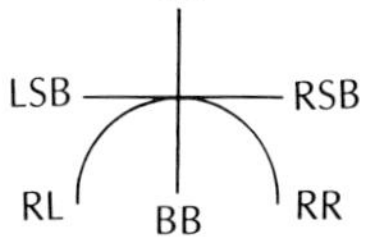

MUSCLES

	L	R
Supraclavicular region	___	___
Suboccipital region	___	___
Longus Colli	___	___
Sternocleidomastoid	___	___
Scaleni	___	___
Upper trapezius	___	___
Mid trapezius	___	___
Levator scap.	___	___
Rhomboids	___	___
Pectorals	___	___
Supraspinatus	___	___
Infraspinatus	___	___
Deltoid	___	___
Teres	___	___
Cervical facet tenderness	___	___

Peripheral Joint Scan:
T/M
A/C
S/C
Shoulder
Elbow
Wrist
Hand

Specific Tests
Compression _____
Distraction _____
Scalene Cramp _____
Spurlings _____
Quadrant Comp. _____
Vertebral Artery   L   R
TIS _____

Isometric Testing

X-ray (date)

Neurological Screen
Neck F (Dural)
Weakness
Atrophy
Reflexes
Sensation

CONCLUSION   Posture   Trauma   Dysfunction   Derangement   Spondylosis

Suggest Craniomandibular Evaluation _____

Goals _____

Initial Treatment _____

TABLE 5–14. Assessment Form for the Upper Quarter *Continued*

spine.[108] Often, brachial plexus tension testing will recreate the patient's pain in this clinical situation.

Other pathologies, such as traumatic fractures of the cervical spine, collagen disease with longstanding steroid use, and osteoporotic changes, especially in elderly women, must be considered by the alert clinician in dealing with the complete medical picture.

CERVICAL SPINE SCREENING FOR THE DENTIST

The cervical spine screening examination form provides the dentist with the information for a precise and rapid scan of the upper quarter (see Table 5–12). The purpose of this form is to assess structure and function such that an appropriate referral for physical therapy can be made. It is only necessary that the dentist perform a brief upper-quarter screening examination. The extensive assessment techniques normally performed by a knowledgeable orthopedist, neurologist, or physical therapist are not necessary. Table 5–14 shows a more comprehensive assessment form for the upper quarter appropriate for a physical therapist.

It is hoped that the dentist will recognize postural and functional abnormalities of the upper quarter and the effects upon the temporomandibular and craniocervical system. The specific diagnostic implications and the necessity to evaluate, refer, and involve others, such as the physical therapist, in the comprehensive management process should be evident.

REFERENCES

1. Worth, D.R. and Seluik, G.: Movements of the craniovertebral joints. In *Modern Manual Therapy.* G. Grieve (ed.). Churchill Livingstone, New York, 1986.
2. Kapandji, I.A.: *The Physiology of the Joints, vol. III. The Trunk and Vertebral Column.* Churchill Livingstone, Edinburgh, 1974.
3. Panjabi, M., Dvorak, J., Duranceau, J., et al: Three-dimensional movements of the upper cervical spine. Spine 13:726–730, 1988.
4. Miniura, M., Moriya, H., Watanabe, T., et al: Three-dimensional motion analysis of the cervical spine with special reference to the axial rotation. Spine 14:1135–1139, 1989.
5. Willis, T.A.: Luschka's joints. Clin. Orthop. Relat. Res. 46:121, 1966.
6. Makofsky, H.W.: The effect of head posture on muscle contact position: The sliding cranium theory. J. Craniomandib. Pract. 7:286–292, 1989.
7. Rocabado, M.: Biomechanical relationship of the cranial, cervical and hyoid regions. J. Craniomand. Pract. 1:61–66, 1983.
8. Kraus, S.L.: Cervical spine influence on the craniomandibular region. In *TMJ Disorders: Management of the Craniomandibular Complex.* S.L. Kraus (ed.). Churchill Livingstone, New York, 1988.
9. Buckworth, J.: Anatomy of the suboccipital region. In *Upper Cervical Syndrome.* H. Vernon (ed.). Williams & Wilkins, Baltimore, 1988.
10. Rana, N.: Natural history of atlanto-axial subluxation in rheumatoid arthritis. Spine 14:1054–1056, 1989.
11. Kawaida, H., Sakou, T., Morizono, Y., et al: Magnetic resonance imaging of upper cervical disorders in rheumatoid arthritis. Spine 14:1144–1148, 1989.
12. Ohsawa, T., Izawa, T., Kvroki, Y., et al: Follow-up study of atlanto-axial instability in Down's syndrome without separate odontoid process. Spine 14:1149–1153, 1989.
13. Esmark, H. and Kalen, R.: Injuries of the atlas and axis. A follow-up study of 85 axis and 10 atlas fractures. Clin. Orthop. 217:257–260, 1987.
14. Aspinall, W.: Clinical testing for cervical mechanical disorders which produce ischemic vertigo. Orthop. Sports Phys. Ther. 11:176–182, 1989.
15. Steiger, H,: The anatomy of headache. Man. Med. 3:37–40, 1987.
16. Bogduk, N.: Innervation and pain patterns of the cervical spine. In *Physical Therapy of the Cervical and Thoracic Spine.* R. Grant (ed.). Churchill Livingstone, New York, 1988.
17. Hiatt, J.L. and Gartner, L.P.: *Textbook of Head and Neck Anatomy.* Williams & Wilkins, Baltimore, 1987.
18. Janda, V.: Muscles and cervicogenic pain syndromes. In *Physical Therapy of the Cervical and Thoracic Spine.* R. Grant (ed.). Churchill Livingstone, New York, 1988.
19. Kendall, F. and McCreary, E.: *Muscles: Testing and Function.* Williams & Wilkins, Baltimore, 1983.
20. Warwick, R. and Williams, P.L.: *Gray's Anatomy,* 35th ed. W.B. Saunders Co., Philadelphia, 1973.
21. Sunderland, S.: Anatomical perivertebral influences on the intervertebral foramen. In *The Research Status of Spinal Manipulative Therapy.* M. Goldstein (ed.). HEW Publication No. (NIH) 76-998, Bethesda, 1975.
22. Bogduk, N.: The clinical anatomy of the cervical dorsal rami. Spine 7:319–330, 1982.
23. Mannheimer, J.S. and Lampe, G.N.: Electrode placement sites and their relationship. In *Clinical Transcutaneous Electrical Nerve Stimulation.* J.S. Mannheimer and Lampe G.N. (eds.). F.A. Davis, Philadelphia, 1984.
24. Brodal, A.: *The Cranial Nerves. Anatomy and Anatomicoclinical Correlations.* Blackwell Scientific Publications, Oxford, 1965.
25. Kramer, J.: *Intervertebral Disc Diseases.* Yearbook Medical Publishers, Chicago, 1981.
26. Chusid, J.G.: *Correlative Neuroanatomy and Functional Neurology,* 16th ed. Lange Medical Publications, Los Altos, 1976.
27. Haymaker, W. and Woodhall, B.: *Peripheral Nerve Injuries,* 2nd ed. W.B. Saunders Co., Philadelphia, 1953.
28. Sweet, W.: *Autonomic Contributions to Pain Syndromes.* W.B. Saunders Co., Philadelphia, 1969.
29. Doran, F.: The sites to which pain is referred from the common bile duct in man and its implications for the theory of referred pain. Br. J. Surg. 54:599–606, 1967.

30. Spiro, H.: Acute pancreatitis. Chest pain: Probl. Diff. Diagn. 3:1, 1978.

31. Wyke, B.: The neurology of joints. Ann. R. Coll. Surg. 41:25, 1977.

32. Dugal, A. and Ansemon, N.: The entrapped greater occipital nerve and internal derangement of the TMJ. J. Craniomand. Pract. 2:51–54, 1983.

33. Cyriax, J.: *Textbook of Orthopaedic Medicine,* vol. 1. *Diagnosis of Soft Tissue Injuries.* Bailliere Tindall, London, 1982.

34. Gray, H.: *Gray's Anatomy,* 29th ed. C. Goss (ed.). Lea & Febiger, Philadelphia, 1973.

35. Hassler, R. and Walker, A.E.: *Trigeminal Neuralgia.* W.B. Saunders Co., Philadelphia, 1970.

36. Edmeads, J.: Headaches and head pains associated with diseases of the cervical spine. Med. Clin. North Am. 62:533, 1978.

37. Elvidge, A.R. and Li, C.: Central protrusion of cervical intervertebral disc involving descending trigeminal tract. Arch. Neurol. Psych. 63:455, 1950.

38. Driscoll, D.: Anatomical and biomechanical characteristics of upper cervical ligamentous structures. A review. J. Manipulative Physiol. Ther. 10:107–112, 1987.

39. Jull, G.A.: Headaches associated with the cervical spine. In *Modern Manual Therapy.* A. Grieve (ed.). Churchill Livingstone, Edinburgh, 1986.

40. Baloh, R.W.: *The Essentials of Neurotology.* F.A. Davis, Philadelphia, 1984.

41. Travell, J.G. and Simons, D.G.: *Myofascial Pain and Dysfunction: The Trigger Point Manual.* Williams & Wilkins, Baltimore, 1983.

42. Seemann, D.C.: Center of gravity of the skull: A review of theories and a pilot study to determine location. J. Manipulative Physiol. Ther. 4:15–18, 1981.

43. Robinson, M.F.: The influence of head position on temporomandibular joint dysfunction. J. Prosth. Dent. 16:169, 1966.

44. Mannheimer, J.S.: Prevention and restoration of abnormal upper quarter posture. In *Postural Considerations in the Diagnosis and Treatment of Cranio-Cervical-Mandibular and Related Chronic Pain Disorders.* H. Gelb and M. Gelb (eds.). Ishiyaku Euro-American. (In press.)

45. Pal, G.P. and Sherk, H.H.: The vertebral stability of the cervical spine. Spine 13:447–449, 1988.

46. Kraus, S.L.: Cervical spine influences on the craniomandibular region. In *TMJ Disorders: Management of the Craniomandibular Complex.* S.L. Kraus (ed.). Churchill Livingstone, New York, 1988.

47. Rocabado, M.: Course notes: Heak, neck and TMJ joint dysfunction. Rocabado Institute for Craniomandibular and Vertebral Therapeutics, Southfield, Michigan, 1979.

48. Rocabado, M.: Course notes: Advanced upper quarter. Rocabado Institute for Craniomandibular and Vertebral Therapeutics, Southfield, Michigan, 1980.

49. Mannheimer, J.S., Attanasio, R., Cinotti, W.R., et al: Cervical strain and mandibular whiplash: Effects upon the craniomandibular apparatus. Clin. Prev. Dent. 11:29–32, 1989.

50. McCall, J.: Electromyography of muscles of posture: Posterior vertebral muscles in man. J. Physiol. (London) 157:33, 1961.

51. Calliet, R.: *Shoulder Pain.* F.A. Davis, Philadelphia, 1966.

52. Tarsy, J.: *Pain Syndromes and Their Treatment.* Charles C Thomas, Springfield, 1953.

53. Gayral, L. and Neuwirth, E. Oto-neuro-ophthalmologic manifestations of cervical origin: Posterior cervical syndrome of Barré-Liéou. N.Y. State J. Med. 54:1920–1926, 1954.

54. Pawl, R.P.: *Chronic Pain Primer.* Yearbook Medical Publishers, Chicago, 1979.

55. Bogduk, N.: Cervical Causes of Headache and Dizziness. In *Modern Manual Therapy.* G. Grieve (ed.). Churchill Livingstone, Edinburgh, 1986.

56. Lous, I.: The cervicolingual syndrome. Man. Med. 3:63–65, 1987.

57. Solow, B. and Krieberg, S.: Soft tissue stretching: A possible control factor in craniofacial morphogenesis. Scand. J. Dent. Res. 85:505, 1976.

58. Daly, P., Preston, C.B. Evans, W.A.: Positional response of the head to bite opening in adult males. Am. J. Orthod. 82:157, 1982.

59. Vig, P.S. and Showfety, K.J.: Experimental manipulation of head posture. Am. J. Orthod. 77:258, 1980.

60. Hellsing, E., Gorsberg, C.M. Linder-Aronson, S.: Changes in postural EMG activity in the neck and masticatory muscles following obstruction of the nasal airways. Eur. J. Orthod. 9:247, 1986.

61. Solow, B. and Tallgren, A.: Head posture and craniofacial morphology. Am. J. Phys. Anthropol. 44:412, 1976.

62. Tallgren, A. and Solow, B.: Hyoid bone position, facial morphology and head posture in adults. Eur. J. Orthod. 9:1, 1987.

63. Forshey, C.M., Hellsing, E., Linder-Aronson, S., et al: EMG activity in neck and masticatory muscles in relation to extension and flexion of the head. Eur. J. Orthod. 7:177, 1985.

64. Boyd, C.H., Sloyle, W.F., MacBoyd, C., et al: The effect of head position on electromyographic evaluation of representative mandibular positioning muscle groups. J. Craniomand. Pract. 5:50–54, 1987.

65. Lowe, A. and Johnston, W.: Tongue and jaw muscle activity in response to mandibular rotations in a sample of normal and anterior open bite subjects. Am. J. Orthod. 76:565, 1979.

66. Kraus, S.L.: Physical therapy management of TMJ dysfunction. In *TMJ Disorders: Management of the Craniomandibular Complex.* S.L. Kraus (ed.). Churchill Livingstone, New York, 1988.

67. Korr, I.: Sustained sympathicotonia as a factor in disease. In *The Neurobiologic Mechanisms in Manipulative Therapy.* I. Korr (ed.). Plenum Press, New York, 1978.

68. Kraus, S.L.: Second Annual Meeting of the International College of Craniofacial and Vertebral Therapeutics, Atlanta, Georgia, 1989.

69. Darling, D., Kraus, S., Glasheen-Wray, M.,: Relationship of head posture and the rest position of the mandible. J. Prosthet. Dent. 52:11–115, 1984.

70. Goldstein, D., Kraus, S., Williams, W., et al: Influence of cervical posture on mandibular movement. J. Prosthet. Dent. 52:421, 1984.

71. Dunn, J.: Physical therapy. In A. Kaplan (ed.). *Temporomandibular Disorders: Diagnosis and Treatment.* W.B. Saunders Co., Philadelphia, 1991.

72. Maitland, G.D.: *Vertebral Manipulation,* 5th ed. Butterworth, London, 1986.

73. Magarey, M.E.: Examination and assessment in spinal joint dysfunction. In *Modern Manual Therapy of the Vertebral Column.* G.P. Grieve (ed.). Churchill Livingstone, Edinburgh, 1986.

74. Magarey, M.E.: Examination of the cervical spine. In *Modern Manual Therapy of the Vertebral Column.*

G.P. Grieve (ed.). Churchill Livingstone, Edinburgh, 1986.

75. Lader, E.: Cervical trauma as a factor in the development of TMJ dysfunction and facial pain. J. Craniomand. Pract. 1:86, 1983.

76. Trott, P.H.: Passive movements and allied techniques in the management of dental patients. In G.P. Grieve (ed.). *Modern Manual Therapy of the Vertebral Column.* Churchill Livingstone, Edinburgh, 1986.

77. Rocobado, M.: Course notes: Diagnosis and treatment of abnormal craniocervical and craniomandibular mechanics. Rocobado Institute for Craniomandibular and Vertebral Therapeutics, Southfield, Michigan, 1981.

78. Clark, G.T.: Examination of temporomandibular disorder patients for craniocervical dysfunction. J. Craniomand. Pract. 2:56, 1983.

79. Kemper, J.T. and Okeson, J.P.: Craniomandibular disorders and headaches. J. Craniomand. Pract. 49:702, 1983.

80. Kreisberg, M.K.: Headache as a symptom of craniomandibular disorders. II. Management. J. Craniomand. Pract. 4:219, 1986.

81. Shan Kland, W.E.: Differential diagnosis of headaches. J. Craniomand. Pract. 4:47, 1986.

82. Alanen, P.J. and Kirves Kari, P.K.: Occupational cervicobrachial disorder and temporomandibular joint dysfunction. J. Craniomand. Pract. 3:69, 1985.

83. Edeling, J.S.: The true cervical headache. South Afr. Med. J. 62:531, 1982.

84. Braaf, M.M. and Rossner, S.: Trauma of the cervical spine as a cause of chronic headache. J. Trauma 15:441, 1975.

85. Magarey, M.E.: Examination of the cervical and thoracic spine. In *Physical Therapy of the Cervical and Thoracic Spine.* R. Grant (ed.). Churchill Livingstone, New York, 1988.

86. Maeda, K.: Occupational cervicobrachial disorder in assembly plant. Kurume Med. J. 22:231–239, 1975.

87. Waris, P.: Occupational cervicobrachial Syndromes. Scand. J. Work Environ. Health 6:3–14, 1980.

88. Valtonen, E.: The tension neck syndrome: Its etiology, clinical features and results of physical treatment. Ann. Med. Int. Fenn. 57:139–142, 1968.

89. Sahrman, S.A.: Adult posturing. In *TMJ Disorders: Mangement of the Craniomandibular Complex.* S. Kraus (ed.). Churchill Livingstone, New York, 1988.

90. Stratton, S.A. and Bryan, J.M.: Dysfunction, evaluation, and treatment of the cervical spine and thoracic inlet. In *Orthopaedic Physical Therapy.* R. Donatelli and M.J. Wooden (eds.). Churchill Livingstone, New York, 1988.

91. Kaput, M.: Orthopedic Physical Therapy. In *Physical Therapy of the Cervical and Thoracic Spine.* R. Grant (ed.). Churchill Livingston, New York, 1988.

92. Elvey, R.H.: The investigation of arm pain. In *Modern Manual Therapy of the Vertebral Column.* G. Grieve (ed.). Churchill Livingstone, Edinburgh, 1988.

93. Grant, R.: Dizziness testing and manipulation of the cervical spine. In *Physical Therapy of the Cervical and Thoracic Spine.* R. Grant (ed.). Churchill Livingstone, New York, 1988.

94. Okawara, S. and Nibbelink, D.: Vertebral artery occlusion following extension and rotation of the head. Stroke 5:640, 1974.

95. Phillips, H. and Grieve, G.P.: The thoracic outlet syndrome. In *Modern Manual Therapy of the Vertebral Column.* G. Grieve (ed.). Churchill Livingstone, New York, 1989.

96. Greenfield, B.: Upper quarter evaluation: Structural relationships and interdependence. In R. Donatelli and M. Wooden (eds.). *Orthopaedic Physical Therapy.* Churchill Livingstone, New York, 1989.

97. Darnell, M.: A proposed chronology of events for forward head posture. J. Craniomand. Pract. 2:50, 1983.

98. Brodie, A G · Anatomy and physiology of head and neck musculature. Am. J. Orthod. 36:831, 1950.

99. Campbell, J.K.: Post-traumatic headaches. J. Cranio. Dis. 1:75–77, 1987.

100. Upledger, J.: *Craniosacral Therapy. II. Beyond the Dura.* Eastland Press, Seattle, 1987.

101. Kraus, S.: Influences of the cervical spine on the stomatognathic system. In *Orthopedic Physical Therapy.* R. Donatelli and M. Wooden (eds.). Churchill Livingstone, New York, 1989.

102. Mohl, N.D.: Head posture and its role of occlusion. N.Y. State Dent. J. 42:17–23, 1984.

103. Howell, J.W.: Evaluation and Management of the thoracic outlet syndrome. In R. Donatelli (ed.). *Physical Therapy of the Shoulder.* Churchill Livingstone, New York, 1987.

104. Kellgren, J.: Observation of referred pain arising from skeletal structures. Clin. Sci. 3:175–190, 1938.

105. Cloward, R.B.: The clinical significance of the sinovertebral nerve. J. Neurosurg. Psychiatr. 23:321–326, 1960.

106. Grieve, G.: *Mobilization of the Spine,* 3rd ed. Churchill Livingstone, London, 1979.

107. Brian, L. and Wilkinson, M.: *Cervical Spondylosis and Other Disorders of the Cervical Spine.* W.B. Saunders Co., Philadelphia, 1967.

108. Hannington-Kiff, J.: *Pain Relief.* J.B. Lippincott Co., Philadelphia, 1974.

Ronald Burakoff

CHAPTER 6

Epidemiology

Over the last 57 years, the entity first described in the literature as Costen's syndrome[1] has been renamed, redefined, and re-examined by several generations of dentists and other health practitioners. This chapter reviews the contributions of epidemiology to our knowledge and understanding of such temporomandibular disorders (TMDs). A brief overview of some of the principles and tools of epidemiology are presented. The reader is advised to consult an epidemiology textbook for a more detailed description of the concepts introduced in this chapter. Information gleaned from population-based studies that have been published concerning TMDs is summarized.

Epidemiology is the study of the distribution and determinants of disease and injuries in the population.[2,3] Epidemiology is clearly in its early developmental stage in relation to the study of TMDs. However, despite its youth, epidemiology shows a great deal of potential to help clinicians develop effective treatment plans for their patients. The epidemiologist is concerned with the maintenance of health and the prevention of disease. The epidemiologist's major responsibility is to identify those individuals in the population that have the highest and lowest rates of the particular disease under investigation.

Common characteristics of the different groups are identified. Hypotheses are developed as to the causes of one group being diseased and the other being free from disease. Because TMDs generally include a number of separate entities and because many of these disorders are of multiple etiology, the epidemiologist's task is formidable.[4] Compounding the epidemiologist's problem is the fact that many TMDs are chronic in nature, and the line separating diseased individuals from "not diseased" individuals is often arbitrary. Tempo-romandibular disorders are believed to be progressive in nature, and many persist for several years. Unfortunately, the natural history of TMDs has not been fully documented.[5]

In determining the extent of disease in a population, the epidemiologist studies rates: incidence and prevalence. Incidence rates measure the number of new cases of disease in a specified time period. Prevalence rates are a measure of the total number of cases of a particular disease in a specified population at a particular time.

In testing hypotheses about the etiology of disease, there are two approaches: experimental and observational. In the experimental approach, one studies the impact of varying factors he or she controls. Although the experimental model is practical for animal studies, it is often not practical for human population studies. It is usually impossible or unethical to conduct human experimental hypothesis testing studies. The epidemiologist mainly employs observational studies to add validity to a hypothesized cause and effect relationship between a postulated risk factor and disease. In observational studies the differences between groups are observed and analyzed—they are not experimentally created by the investigator. The major difficulty with observational studies is that the investigator does not have the ability to isolate the variables under study. It is virtually impossible to control for all possible competing causative factors for a disease in study groups. Nonetheless, observational studies have contributed a great deal to our understanding of many diseases.

Observational studies can be divided into descriptive and analytic. Descriptive studies are concerned with the occurrence of the disease under investigation and employ prevalence rates to qualify and quantify the extent of the disease in the population. Cross-sectional studies determine the prevalence of a particular disease in a population or sample at a given time. Cross-sectional studies are performed once and tend to be fact-finding in nature. The population group is selected without prior knowledge of the health status under investigation. Analytic studies are employed to test hypotheses about etiology. They can be either retrospective or prospective.

In retrospective studies, individuals are diagnosed as having a particular disease and are compared with those not having the disease (controls). The aim of the study is to identify what determinant causes the difference between the groups. These studies are also referred to as case controls. The study is retrospective because the population has previously been influenced by the determinant under study.

Prospective studies or cohort studies begin with individuals who are disease-free and are followed longitudinally over time. The individuals in prospective studies are divided into groups depending on their exposure to a suspected causative factor. Incidence rates of the two groups are then analyzed and with statistical methodology inferences can be made about the validity of the initial hypothesis. Epidemiologic studies are applicable to populations, and results can only add support to a particular etiologic hypothesis, but not absolute proof. However, the epidemiologist can build a convincing case for an etiologic hypothesis with repeated sampling studies, which have a cumulative effect on the probability of the hypothesis being correct.[2]

SIGNS AND SYMPTOMS

Laskin[6] contended that the most unfortunate consequence of grouping conditions under a term such as "TMJ syndrome" is the creation of a one disease/one treatment philosophy merely because the symptoms are similar. This is inappropriate because the underlying diseases are unique. Epidemiologic studies tend to focus on prevalence of signs and symptoms of diseases. Symptoms according to Gross and associates[7] should be defined as " . . . those factors bothering the patient," and thus they are generally subjective in nature.

Symptoms are determined by the clinician through interviews, questionnaires, or both. Signs are objective, and it is up to the clinician to identify the presence or absence of signs from the physical examination or the analysis of laboratory data. Gross has appropriately pointed out that "Clinical signs are important, but symptoms are perhaps more important in that they lead to treatment seeking behavior." With TMDs, signs and symptoms are often interchangeable. For example, joint sounds are often reported by the patient as a symptom and by the clinician as a sign of the disease. Also, there is considerable overlap of signs and symptoms, e.g., tenderness to palpation of masticatory muscles is not an entirely objective finding but a highly subjective one.

Greene and Marbach[8] presented some doubts about the inferential value of most epidemiologic TMD studies. They suggest "The criteria used in recent epidemiologic studies to determine how many people in the population have mandibular dysfunction do not correspond directly to the incidence of clinical disorders of facial pain related to TMJ disease or masticatory muscle dysfunction." This dilemma is a result of disease definition. When a definition is too broad, a situation may result in so many individuals being labeled as diseased that one might infer an epidemic has occurred. Conversely, when the disease definition is too narrow, individuals with pathology of the same etiology are inappropriately excluded. Eversole and Machado[9] presented a classification for internal derangements of the temporomandibular joint. They suggested that previous epidemiologic studies aggregated individuals with internal derangements and myofascial dysfunctions. They further suggest that in future studies these individuals should be treated as having separate disease entities. A growing consensus exists that a TMD should not be looked upon as a single entity or considered from a single point of view.[10]

Despite the problems in defining TMDs, a growing consensus has been building as to the signs and symptoms that should be evaluated. These include the following: limitation of range of mandibular movement, masticatory muscle pain, TMJ pain, joint sounds, pain on jaw opening, pain on jaw movement, and recurrent headache and ear pain and associated stuffiness. In addition, some studies have incorporated the following signs and symptoms in their investigations: tooth wear, bruxism, clenching, occlusal stability, and centric relation discrepancies.[6,11–17] Unfortunately, most investigators have chosen to aggregate a different constellation of signs and symptoms, which has made it difficult to compare results of studies. The dental literature, which has paid a great deal of attention to joint sounds, has one common feature, according to Wabke and co-workers:[18] " . . . a pronounced lack of clarity." They underscore the difficulty of comparing published studies and state that "Little can be distilled about which complete agreement exists," concerning the importance of joint sounds.

Indices are used to allow comparisons of the health status between populations and of the same population over time. Dentistry has effectively utilized indices to measure the severity and extent of dental caries and periodontal disease for many years (e.g., decayed, missing, filled teeth rates and various measures of periodontal health). Helkimo[11,19,20] presented an index for measuring dysfunction of the masticatory system. The Helkimo index has three components: (1) clinical dysfunction index (Di), (2) anamnestic dysfunction index (Ai), and (3) occlusal state index (Oi). The Di is comprised of the following determinants: impaired range of mandibular motion, impaired function of the temporomandibular joint, pain on movement of the mandible, muscle pain, and temporomandibular joint pain. For each determinant a numeric score of 1 to 5 is awarded based on written criteria. The higher the numeric score, the more severe the dysfunction. Similarly, the Ai and Oi result in numeric scores that can be used for statistical manipulation. The Helkimo index grades the severity of dysfunction—it is not a diagnostically sensitive instrument as far as subgroups of TMDs are concerned. Because of this lack of diagnostic sensitivity, it cannot be utilized to list etiologic hypotheses. It is helpful in characterizing the extent of general dysfunction in a given population.

Additional attempts have been made to create indices that will measure the severity of TMDs.[21] At the present time, no particular index developed has gained wide acceptance among the research community. Because TMDs include many disease entities, it is not surprising that a powerful index has not been created (Table 6–1).

STUDIES ON INFANTS, CHILDREN, AND ADOLESCENTS

Razook and colleagues[22] have reviewed the literature on the prevalence of TMDs and found that virtually nothing has been reported and little is known or understood about the entity in children under 1 year of age. They presented three cases of joint sounds in infants and described possible anatomic factors and mechanical explanations for the signs observed clinically. They concluded that there may be no significance to these early signs and the development of TMJ dysfunction later in life. Bernal and Tsamtsouris[23] questioned the parents and examined 136 children, 3, 4, and 5 years old, in Cambridge, Massachusetts. According to the parent's reports, 17% of the children ground their teeth and 7% suffered from occasional headaches. Examination revealed 5% of the children demonstrated clicking of the TMJ and 20% had irregular movements of the

condyles. The mean maximal mandibular opening was 42 mm, and 11% exhibited deviation of the mandible during opening. These investigators found no relationship among age and sex and the variables under study except that dental wear correlated with age. Symptoms exceeded signs in the population, but the symptoms recorded were those perceived by the parents not articulated by the children.[23]

For older children, Williamson[24] reported that 35% of pretreatment orthodontic patients, ages 6 to 16, had symptoms that included muscle pain, clicking of the TMJ, or both. Nilner and Lassing[25] examined 440 Swedish children, 7 to 14 years old, and found 36% with symptoms, 19% with recurrent headaches or pain in the temporal region, 13% with reported clicking sounds from the TMJ, and 14% with history of trauma to the face. Upon examination, 64% of the children reported tenderness on palpation of the masticatory muscles. Temporomandibular joint sounds were recorded in 8% of the children, and 32% exhibited irregular jaw movements. Nilner and Lassing concluded that mandibular dysfunction is prevalent in children.

Egermark-Eriksson and associates[26] studied three groups of Swedish children ages 7, 11, and 15. These investigators reported that joint sounds were found in more girls than boys. There were no sex or age differences for reduced movement capacity, deviation in opening, locking or luxation of the mandible, pain on movement, or TMJ tenderness. Joint sounds and muscle tenderness were two symptoms that increased with age. These workers stated that although the prevalence of symptoms was high (39%, 67%, and 74%) for each age group respectively, the severity was judged to be slight. Grosfeld and colleagues[27] reported on two groups of 400 Polish people age 15 to 18 and 19 to 22. In this study, although both age groups had similar prevalence of disorders (68.25% and 67%, respectively), females had higher rates in both age groups. The clinical signs of mandibular deviation were found to be more prevalent to the left. This finding, although unexplained, was also reported in other studies.[25,28,29] Nilner[30] reported on findings from two groups of Swedish school children that she had earlier reported individually. The first group consisted of 440 children age 7 to 14, and the second group, age 15 to 18. The older group had a higher prevalence of symptoms (41% to 36%) and clicking (17% to 13%). Both groups reported recurrent headaches at nearly

TABLE 6–1. Prevalence of Signs and Symptoms in Selected Epidemiologic Studies

STUDY	METHOD	N	POPULATION	AGE	SEX MALE/ FEMALE	AT LEAST ONE SYMPTOM	AT LEAST ONE SIGN	AT LEAST ONE SYMPTOM OR SIGN
1. Agerberg[46]	Q	1106	Urban Swedes	15–74	531/575	57	41	
2. Helkimo[20]	Q,E	321	Finnish Lapps	15–65	156/165	57	88	
3. Hanson[45]	E,I	1069	Swedish shipbuilders	17–73	987/82			79
4. Swanljung[44]	E,I	583	Finnish workers	18–64	256/341	58	41	
5. Ingervall[47]	Q,E	389	Swedish men	21–54 $\bar{x} = 32$	389/0	15	60	
6. Osterberg[41]	Q,E	384	Swedish retirees	70	186/198	59	86	
7. Agerberg[42]	E,I	194	Swedish retirees	70	85/109	23	74	
8. Molin[50]	Q,E	253	Swedish conscripts	18–25 $\bar{x} = 19$	253/0	12	28	
9. Heloe[37]	I	246	Norwegian adults	25	110/136	31*		
10. Wanman[32]	E,Q	285	Swedish adolescents†	17	146/139	20	56	62
11. Wanman[34]	E	258	Swedish adolescents†	17–19			76	
12. Grosfeld[27]	I,E	800	Polish teens	15–18	197/203			68
			Polish adults	19–22	208/192			67
13. Szentpetery[48]	Q,E	600	Hungarian urbanites	12–85 $\bar{x} = 40$	285/315	20	80	
14. Nilner[29]	E,I	309	Swedish school children	15–18	147/162	41	77	
15. Nilner[25]	E,I	440	Swedish school children	7–14	222/218	36	72	
16. Egermark-Eriksson[26]	Q,E	402	Swedish children	7	62/74	39		
				11	70/61	67		
				15	76/59	74		
17. Magnusson[36]	Q,E	121	Swedish adolescents†	15–20	65/56	70	62	
18. Pullinger[38]	Q,E	222	U.S. dental and dental hygiene students	$\bar{x} = 23.9$	120/102	39		
19. Bernal[23]	Q,E	149	U.S. Head Start children	3–5	79/70	38	21	
20. Solberg[28]	Q,E	739	U.S. college students	19–25	369/370	26	76	
21. Gross[7]	Q	1109	Non-TMJ patients from a general dental practice	3–89 $\bar{x} = 39.8$	468/641	21*		
22. Droukas[40]	E,Q	48	Swedish dental students	20–38 $\bar{x} = 25$	25/23	31	65	
23. Williamson[24]	I,E	304	pretreatment orthodontic U.S. patients	6–16 $\bar{x} = 12.9$	129/175	35		
24. de Laat[39]	I,E	121	Belgian dental students	22–28	71/50	40	72	
25. De Boever[25]	Q,E	75	Flemish children	8–11	33/42		68	

*Joint sounds only
†Longitudinal study
Q = questionnaire; E = examination; I = interview.

the same rate (14% for the younger, 16% for the older). Clinically, sounds were heard in both the younger and older groups, 8% and 14%, respectively. In this study, there was no significant difference in symptoms between boys and girls.

LONGITUDINAL STUDIES ON ADOLESCENTS

Wanman and Agerberg[31–34] have reported on the results of a 2-year longitudinal study that began with 285 adolescents, 17 years old,

living in Skellerftea, Sweden. These workers assessed temporomandibular sounds and signs of mandibular dysfunction. Each participant was administered a questionnaire and examined during the month of their birthday at ages 17, 18, and 19. Clicking sounds as reported by questionnaire increased from a prevalence of 13% at age 17 to 16.3% at age 19. The study showed statistically significant differences in TMJ sounds for girls over time and in the group at 19 years old. The incidence in the first year of the study was 5.7% and 13.3% for the 2-year period. A 24% period prevalence was reported for the entire population. Only 5.8%

consistently reported TMJ clicking sounds. Nearly one third of those reporting clicking at age 17 reported no sounds at age 18. This was also true for the reports at 18 and 19 years.

Clinically, the prevalence of sounds was recorded at nearly 20% for all three study intervals. Girls had significantly higher prevalence at 18 and 19. Similar to the findings of the questionnaire, TMJ sounds fluctuated with time, and nearly 50% of those with sounds were free of them the following year. The incidence during the first year was 8.3% and 17.5% during the 2-year period. For the total sample, the 2-year period prevalence was 36%; 9.3% recorded sounds at all three examinations. These investigators found a high correlation between those reporting TMJ sounds and clinical findings. No subjects were clinically judged to have crepitation. In this study, no consistent patterning relationship occurred between reported and recorded sounds and single factors explored in the questionnaire (pain in face, jaws, or during jaw movement; difficulties in opening wide or chewing; fatigue in jaws; locking or luxation of the TMJ; recurrent headaches; grinding; clenching; nail biting; trauma to jaw; orthodontia; and tinnitus). Wanman and Agerberg concluded that "In view of the natural longitudinal fluctuations of clicking, most only need to be supervised and treatment can seldom be advocated."[34] Using the Helkimo clinical dysfunction index (Di) to measure the prevalence of signs of mandibular dysfunction, 56%, 48%, and 50% of the population at the three observation intervals had at least one mild sign. The period prevalence for those individuals reporting at least one sign was 76%. Girls had significantly higher values at all examinations. As with TMJ sounds, the longitudinal pattern showed almost 60% of the individuals showing no change over time and the remainder improved or became impaired equally often.

De Boever and van den Berghe[35] reported on the results of a 5-year longitudinal study that began with 510 Flemish 3- to 7-year-old children who were symptom-free at the start of the study. These workers reported " . . . a tremendous increase in the frequency of signs and symptoms of mandibular dysfunction" at the 5-year interval when the children were 8 to 11 years old. A total of 60% had demonstrated deviation on opening, 2% had restricted opening (less than 30 mm), 29% had TMJ sounds on the right, and 24% had TMJ sounds on the left. Of this population, 68% recorded at least one

sign of dysfunction; however, most had only mild to moderate symptoms.

Magnusson and associates[36] re-examined 119 Swedish 15-year-olds who participated in an earlier study by Egermark-Eriksson and associates.[26] The participants were given the same questionnaire and examined clinically. The TMJ sounds increased between the ages of 15 and 20 with females reporting more sounds than males. Nearly 70% of the population reported at least one of the following symptoms at ages 15 and 20: TMJ sounds, tiredness in jaws, difficulty in mouth opening, and pain or tiredness in the jaw or face during chewing. When the last symptom (tiredness in the jaw) was disaggregated from the study, a significant increase (p<0.01) occurred from 27% to 39% between the 15-year-olds and 20-year-olds. Headaches (more than one a month) were reported by 44% of the 20-year-olds compared with 35% of the 15-year-olds. Of the 20-year-olds, 62% had one or more signs of dysfunction " . . . but signs of severe dysfunction were rare."[36] In 48% of the participants, no change occurred in the clinical dysfunction index and the rate of improvement and impairment was equal in the rest of the study population. Of the three subjects who had the most severe signs of dysfunction at the initial examination, they had no or mild dysfunction 5 years later.

Although a frequent finding at both examinations, TMJ sounds exhibited the same longitudinal variability as described by Wanman and Agerberg. Nearly half of those with clicking at age 15 had no clicking at age 20, and those with recorded clicking at 20 had negative findings 5 years earlier.

STUDIES ON YOUNG ADULTS

Nonpatient studies on young adults consist of two basic types: those performed on the general population and those on university students. Heloe and Heloe[37] reported on 246 25-year-old individuals living in Norway and compared them to a study whose sample was drawn from the general adult populations of Norway. These investigators pointed out that there is difficulty in comparing two studies because "unequal methods and criteria" are often used. However, they believed that they controlled many variables to make the following inference: symptoms tended to decrease with age and "Women more than men stated having some symptoms" (i.e., mandibular dysfunction). Of the 25-year-olds, 31% reported that they had experienced clicking and crepitation from their mandibles. Molin[50] studied 19-year-old Swedish conscripts and found 14% were aware of clicking of the TMJ. Clinical investigation revealed 28% of the sample had signs of dysfunction, which predominantly consisted of tenderness to palpation of the TMJ and the muscles of mastication and irregular movements of the mandible. Frequent headaches (greater than one per week) were reported by 11% of the group. The relatively low rates of dysfunction were more consistent with studies of adolescents than with the general population.

Several studies included young adults who also were dental, dental hygiene, or university students.[28,38-40] Pullinger's group found in their study of 253 dental and dental hygiene students the following: masticatory, cervical, and headache pain, 14%; restricted range of mandibular movement, <1%; joint sounds, 29%; crepitus, 3%; muscles tender to palpation, 48%; and symptom-free on Helkimo Di, 45%. Only 1% of the study group had clinical signs of dysfunction that were considered severe. Women were found to have statistically significant more headaches, TMJ clicking, TMJ tenderness on palpation, and masticatory muscle tenderness on palpation. These findings were comparable with previous studies of this age group.[38] Solberg's[28] examination of 739 university students with an average age of 22.5 years supported the assertion that women had higher incidences of positive findings than men. In this university population, 76% had clinical signs of dysfunction, but only 26% reported symptoms. Little sex difference was noted for awareness of symptoms except for headaches: women greater than men. Men were twice as likely to be free of both signs and symptoms as compared with women.[28] De Laat and van Steenberghe[39] looked at 121 Belgian dental students and found similar findings to other studies of older adolescents. Droukas and colleagues[40] examined 48 Swedish dental students and found " . . . relatively frequent but mainly mild signs and symptoms of mandibular dysfunction."

STUDIES ON OLDER INDIVIDUALS

Osterberg and Carlsson[41] examined 384 residents of Gothenburg, Sweden, all age 70. The participants were administered a questionnaire and examined clinically. A modified Helkimo Di and Ai were used to rate the severity of dys-

function. Of the population, 41% reported no symptoms, and 46% were judged to have seven dysfunctions according to the Ai. Signs of clinical dysfunction were found to be present in 84% of the sample. Temporomandibular joint sounds were diagnosed in 37%. Tenderness to palpation near the TMJ was rare, but more than 50% of participants had masticatory muscles that were tender to palpation. Statistical analysis of reported symptoms of men and women showed no significant differences. Severe clinical signs were more prevalent in women than in men; however, only tenderness of the TMJ and masseter muscles produced significant differences. Persons with natural teeth reported less impaired chewing ability, but answers to other questions about function or clinical examination revealed no significant differences between the groups. These investigators concluded that "The frequency of signs and symptoms of mandibular dysfunction in men and women was remarkably similar."[42]

Agerberg and Osterberg[42] examined and interviewed 194 men and women and found 74% with clinical signs of dysfunction. These signs included TMJ sounds and deviation or tenderness to palpation of the masticatory muscles and TMJs. When the subjects were questioned, 23% " . . . remembered that they had earlier symptoms." Men had larger mean maximal openings, but there were insignificant differences for the horizontal movements.

Choy and Smith[43] looked at 160 persons who were complete denture wearers and who attended a university dental clinic in the United States. They found 15% to have TMJ disturbances. The disturbances consisted of muscle tenderness, joint sounds, and restricted movements. Tenderness associated with the lateral pterygoid was the most common site of muscle involvement. These investigators concluded that the use of a questionnaire was " . . . not very reliable as a primary method of identifying TMJ patients." Swanljung and Rantanen[44] reported that complete denture wearers had more symptoms than younger individuals with natural dentitions.

STUDIES ON GENERAL NONPATIENT POPULATIONS

Helkimo used a population of 321 Finnish-Lapps, aged 15 to 65, as the basis for material that produced several descriptive and analytic reports, which became the foundation for the indices bearing his name. The subjects were representative of ethnic Finnish-Lapps who lived in a geographic district of Finland in 1969–1970. Each participant was administered a questionnaire and examined clinically by a dentist. Of these, 29% reported a feeling of fatigue in the jaws, 15% reported facial pain, and 43% reported some symptoms related to movement of the mandible. Temporomandibular joint sounds were reported by 35% of the participants. A total of 21% reported experiencing headaches at least twice a week or more. Clinical examination revealed a mean maximal opening of the mouth of 46 mm and maximal horizontal movements of 8 to 9 mm. Of the subjects, 63% exhibited deviations or irregularities on opening of the jaw, or both, and about 33% reported pain on maximal opening. Positive palpatory findings were found at the region of the TMJ in 45% and of the masticatory muscles in 66% of subjects.[11,19]

Of the individuals who reported no subjective symptoms, 82% were judged to have some clinical signs. Of those with clinical signs, more than half had only mild clinical symptoms. Of those individuals who were clinically symptom-free, 65% were also subjectively symptom-free. Helkimo[20] concluded there was " . . . relatively good agreement between dysfunction reported by the patient and found at examination." There was little sex and age difference of reported symptoms. Clinical findings were higher among individuals over 35 years of age and those with dentures.

Hanson and Nilner[45] examined 1069 Swedish people in a shipyard in 1964. Clicking of the TMJ was the most common symptom (65%), followed by palpatory findings in the muscles of mastication (37%), and tenderness of TMJ (10%).

Agerberg and Carlsson[46] questioned every 35th individual age 15 to 74 residing in Ulmae, Sweden, in 1971 for a total sample of 1106. Facial pain and headache were reported by 24%, pain on maximal opening was reported by 12%, and 7% reported impaired mandibular movement. Females reported more joint sounds (44% vs. 34%), impaired movement of mandible (6% vs. 3%), and previous treatment for mandibular functional disorders than males (9% vs. 7%). The investigators concluded that although sex differences were noted in their study, the differences were much less than those reported in previous studies. The study also reported that pain and symptoms of dysfunction of the masticatory system were common. All ages had the same symptoms except

that pain on movement of the mandible was more common among younger individuals.

Ingervall and associates[47] reported on the results of a study of 389 Swedish soldiers between the ages of 21 and 54 years. The study participants were in active military service and presumably free of serious illness. Difficulty with mouth opening was reported by 9.9%, and 3.4% had TMJ or muscle pain. The prevalence of headaches was less than in other studies (5% reported more than one per week). Of the population, 15% reported at least one symptom of dysfunction, and 60% had at least one sign of dysfunction. The most frequent signs of dysfunction were locking or luxation of the mandible (23%), reduced movement (18%), deviation on opening (19%), muscle tenderness (17%), and clicking (16%).

Swanljung and Rantanen[44] looked at a random sample of 593 Finnish workers. Of the sample, 58% reported at least one symptom, and 41% were clinically judged to have signs of functional disorders of the masticatory system. No sex differences were reported, and individuals over 38 had more symptoms than those who were younger.

Szentpetery and coworkers[48] studied 600 randomly selected individuals from an urban community in Hungary, using the Helkimo anamnestic and clinical dysfunction indices. The population age ranged from 12 to 85 years—285 males and 315 females. Females reported statistically significant differences in the following: fatigue or stiffness in the masticatory muscles; pain in the face, neck, and around the ears; headaches; tooth clenching; and tooth grinding. Clinical signs were found in 80% of the population. However, the majority of signs were mild; less than 1% had severe signs. The most common signs were TMJ sounds and mastication muscle palpation pain (lateral pterygoid most frequent). A gender preference for females was reported.

Dworken and associates[49] have reported on the preliminary findings of the first large population-based epidemiologic study on a United States population. They are examining a representative study sample of 320,000 enrollees in a prepaid health plan located in Puget Sound, Washington. Their research objectives are directed at the shortcomings of existing studies. Namely, there are no studies that " . . . have used identical study methods to compare the following groups of subjects: (1) those who are both symptomatic and seeking treatment, (2) those from the same community who are asymptomatic, and (3) those who are symptomatic but either are not currently seeking treatment or have never sought treatment." The clinical examination included an assessment of range of motion, joint sounds, palpation of muscles and joints, classification of occlusion, and dental and oral health status. Preliminary findings indicate that "TMD cases are distinguishable from controls in the range of vertical jaw opening possible, with or without assistance." Other variables, such as range of excursive movement, joint sounds, and classification of occlusion, did not distinguish TMD cases from controls. Individuals who had symptoms, but were not patients, scored between the true patients and controls on the variables assessed.

CONCLUSIONS

Epidemiology's contribution to our knowledge and understanding of TMDs faces many barriers. First among them is the development of a standardized case definition and diagnostic subgroups. A classification system must be established that will aid, not obscure, the diagnosis. Secondly, uniform criteria to measure the severity of the disease must be developed along with reliable and reproducible examination methodologies. For example, should joint sounds be recorded by Doppler ultrasound, the ear, the stethoscope, or some other method? How does one control for examiner variability when using digital pressure to measure tenderness to palpation of the TMJ or muscles of mastication? Once the first two criteria are met, several long-term, population-based studies need to be done to determine the incidence, natural history, and etiology of the various entities that make up TMDs.

REFERENCES

1. Costen, J.: A syndrome of ear and sinus symptoms dependent upon disturbed function of the temporomandibular joint. Ann. Otol. Rhinol. Laryngol. 43:1–5, 1934.
2. Mausner, J.S. and Kramer, S.: *Mausner and Bahn Epidemiology—An Introductory Text,* 2nd ed. W.B. Saunders Co., Philadelphia, 1985.
3. Last, J.: Epidemiology and health information. In *Public Health and Preventive Medicine,* 12th ed. J. Last (ed.). Appleton-Century-Crofts, Norwalk, Connecticut, 1986.
4. Rugh, J. and Solberg, W.: Oral health status in United States: Temporomandibular disorders. J. Dent. Educ. 49:398–405, 1985.
5. Solberg W.: Epidemiology, incidence and prevalence of temporomandibular disorders. In *The President's Conference on the Examination, Diagnosis and Management of Temporomandibular Disorders.* D. Laskin, W. Greenfield, W. Gale, et al (eds.). American Dental Association, Chicago, 1983.
6. Laskin, D.: Etiology of the pain-dysfunction syndrome. J. Am. Dent. Assoc. 79:147–153, 1969.
7. Gross, A., Rivera-Morales, W., and Gale, E.: A prevalence study of symptoms associated with TM disorders. J. Craniomand. Disorders/Facial Oral Pain 2:191–195, 1988.
8. Greene, C. and Marbach, J.: Epidemiologic studies of mandibular dysfunction: A critical review. J. Pros. Dent. 48:184–190, 1982.
9. Eversole, L. and Machado, L.: Temporomandibular joint internal derangements and associated neuromuscular disorders. J. Am. Dent. Assoc. 110:69–78, 1985.
10. Morawa, A., Loos, P., and Easton, J.: Temporomandibular joint dysfunction in children and adolescents: Incidence, diagnosis, and treatment. Quintessence International 11:771–777, 1985.
11. Helkimo, M.: Studies on function and dysfunction of the masticatory system. II. Index for anamnestic and clinical dysfunction and occlusal state. Swed. Dent. J. 67:101–121, 1974.
12. De Boever, J.: Functional disturbances of the temporomandibular joint. In *Temporomandibular Joint.* A. Zarb, et al (eds.). C.V. Mosby Co., St. Louis, 1979.
13. Isaacsson, G., Linde, C., and Isberg, A.: Subjective symptoms in patients with temporomandibular joint disk displacement versus patients with myogenic craniomandibular disorders. J. Prost. Dent. 61:70–77, 1989.
14. Schwartz, L.: Pain associated with the temporomandibular joint. J. Am. Dent. Assoc. 51:394–403, 1955.
15. McNeil, C., Danzig, W., Farrar, W., et al: Craniomandibular (TMJ) disorders. The state of the art. J. Prost. Dent. 44:434–437, 1980.
16. Rugh, J.D. and Solberg, W.K.: Psychological implications in temporomandibular pain and dysfunction. In *Temporomandibular Joint—Function and Dysfunction.* G.A. Zarb and G.E. Carlsson (eds.). Munksgaard, Copenhagen, 1979.
17. Solberg, W.K.: Neuromuscular problems in the orofacial region: Diagnosis classification, signs and symptoms. Int. Dent. J. 31:206–215, 1981.
18. Wabke, K., Hansson, T., Hoogstraten, J., and van der Kuy, P.: Temporomandibular joint clicking: A literature review. J. Craniomand. Dis./Facial Oral Pain 3:163–173, 1979.
19. Helkimo, M.: Studies on function and dysfunction of the masticatory system. I. An epidemiological investigation of symptoms of dysfunction in Lapps in North Finland. Proc. Finn. Dent. Soc. 70:37–49, 1974.
20. Helkimo, M.: Studies on function and dysfunction of the masticatory system. III. Analyses of anamnestic and clinical recordings of dysfunction with the aid of indices. Swed. Dent. J. 67:165–182, 1974.
21. Friction, J. and Schiffman, E.: Reliability of a craniomandibular Index. J. Dent. Res. 65:1359–1364, 1980.
22. Razook, J., Gotcher, J., and Bays, R.: Temporomandibular joint noises in infants: Review of the literature and report of cases. Oral Surg. Oral Med. Oral Pathol. 67:658–663, 1989.
23. Bernal, M. and Tsamtsouris, A.: Signs and symptoms of temporomandibular joint dysfunction in 3 to 5-year-old children. J. Pedo. 10:127–140, 1986.
24. Williamson, E.: Temporomandibular dysfunction in pretreatment adolescent patients. Am. J. Orthod. 72:429–433, 1977.

25. Nilner, M. and Lassing, M.: Prevalence of functional disturbances and diseases of the stomatognathic system in 7—14 year olds. Swed. Dent. J. 5:173–187, 1981.
26. Egermark-Eriksson, I., Carlsson, G., and Ingervall, B.: Prevalence of mandibular dysfunction and orofacial parafunction in 7, 11, and 15 year old Swedish children. Eur. J. Orthod. 3:163–172, 1981.
27. Grosfeld, O., Jackowska, M., and Czarnecka, B.: Results of epidemiological examinations of the temporomandibular joint in adolescents and young adults. J. Oral Rehab. 12:95–105, 1985.
28. Solberg, W.K., Woo, M., and Houston, J.: Prevalence of mandibular dysfunction in young adults. J. Am. Dent. Assoc. 98:25–33, 1979.
29. Nilner, M.: Prevalence of functional disturbances and diseases of the stomatognathic system in 15—18 year olds. Swed. Dent. J. 5:189–197, 1981.
30. Nilner, M.: Functional disturbances and diseases in the stomatognathic system among 7 to 18 year olds. J. Craniomand. Pract. 3:358–367, 1985.
31. Wanman, A. and Agerberg, G.: Mandibular dysfunction in adolescents. I. Prevalence of symptoms. Acta Odontol. Scand. 44:47–54, 1986.
32. Wanman, A. and Agerberg, G.: Two-year longitudinal study of signs of mandibular dysfunction in adolescents. Acta Odontol. Scand. 44:333–342, 1986.
33. Wanman, A. and Agerberg, G.: Relationship between signs and symptoms of mandibular dysfunction in adolescents. Commun. Dent. Oral Epidemiol. 14:225–230, 1986.
34. Wanman, A. and Agerberg, G.: Temporomandibular joint sounds in adolescents: A longitudinal study. Oral Surg. Oral Med. Oral Pathol. 69:2–9, 1990.
35. De Boever, J.A. and van den Berghe, L.: Longitudinal study of functional conditions in the masticatory system of Flemish children. Commun. Dent. Oral Epidemiol. 15:100–103, 1987.
36. Magnusson, T., Egermark-Eriksson, I., and Carlsson G.: Five-year longitudinal study of signs and symptoms of mandibular dysfunction in adolescents. J. Craniomand. Pract. 4:338–344, 1986.
37. Heloe, B. and Heloe, L.: Frequency and distribution of myofascial pain-dysfunction syndrome in a population of 25 year olds. Commun. Dent. Oral Epidemiol. 7:357–360, 1979.
38. Pullinger, A., Seligman, D., and Solberg, K.: Temporomandibular disorders. Part I. Functional status, dentomorphic features, and sex differences in a nonpatient population. J. Prosthet. Dent. 52:228–235, 1985.
39. de Laat A. and van Steenberghe D.: Occlusal relationships and temporomandibular joint dysfunction. Part I. Epidemiologic findings. J. Prosthet. Dent. 54:835–842, 1985.
40. Droukas, B., Lindee, C., and Carlsson, G.: Relationship between occlusal factors and signs and symptoms of mandibular dysfunction. Acta Odontol. Scand. 42:277–283, 1984.
41. Osterberg, T. and Carlsson, G.: Symptoms and signs of mandibular dysfunction in 70-year-old men and women in Gothenburg, Sweden. Commun. Dent. Oral Epidemiol. 7:315–321, 1979.
42. Agerberg, G. and Osterberg, T.: Maximal mandibular movements and symptoms of mandibular dysfunction in 70-year-old men and women. Swed. Dent. J. 67:147–164, 1974.
43. Choy, E. and Smith, D.: The prevalence of temporomandibular joint disturbances in complete denture patients. J. Oral Rehab. 7:331–332, 1980.
44. Swanljung, O. and Rantanen, T.: Functional disorders of the masticatory systems in Southwest Finland. Commun. Dent. Oral Epidemiol. 7:177–182, 1979.
45. Hanson, T. and Nilner, M.: A study of the occurrence of symptoms of diseases of the temporomandibular joint masticatory musculature and related structures. J. Oral Rehab. 2:313–324, 1975.
46. Agerberg, G. and Carlsson, G.: Functional disorders of the masticatory system. I. Distribution of symptoms according to age and sex as judged from investigation by questionnaire. Acta Odont. Scand. 30:597–613, 1972.
47. Ingervall, B., Mohlin, B., and Thilander, B.: Prevalence of symptoms of functional disturbances of the masticatory system in Swedish men. J. Oral Rehab. 7:185–197, 1980.
48. Szentpetery, A., Hohn, E., and Fazekas, A.: Prevalence of mandibular dysfunction in an urban population in Hungary. Commun. Dent. Oral Epidemiol. 14:177–180, 1986.
49. Dworkin, S., Von Korff, M., LeResche, L., and Truelove, E.: Epidemiology of temporomandibular disorders. I. Initial clinical and self-report findings. In *Proceedings of the 5th World Congress on Pain*. R. Dubwer, G. Gelbhart, and M. Bonds (eds.). Elsevier Science Publishers, New York, 1988.
50. Molin, C., Carlsson, G.E., Friling, B., and Hedegard, B.: Frequency of symptoms of mandibular dysfunction in young Swedish men. J. Oral Rehab. 3:9–18, 1976.

SECTION II

PATHOLOGY

Andrew S. Kaplan

CHAPTER 7

Classification

Among the controversial aspects of temporomandibular disorders (TMDs), the one that adds the most confusion is the lack of uniform diagnostic terminology. Starting in the 1920s, the existence of TMDs was recognized by Goodfriend[1] and Wright.[2] Costen[3] later described a syndrome consisting of impaired hearing, jaw stiffness, tinnitus, vertigo, and headache. He grouped these symptoms into a syndrome that became known as Costen's syndrome. Although his anatomic description of the mechanism of this disorder was proved to be invalid, he nevertheless recognized a group of signs and symptoms causing facial pain

In 1959, Schore[4] described a similar group of symptoms, which he called the "TMJ dysfunction syndrome." Schwartz,[5] that same year, coined the term "temporomandibular pain syndrome." In 1962, Ramfjord and Ash,[6] in their textbook on occlusion, classified temporomandibular joint (TMJ) disorders into two subgroups: (1) acute traumatic TMJ arthritis/ muscle spasm and (2) chronic TMJ arthritis/ recurrent muscle spasms. The first subgroup was described as starting with a sharp pain of the TMJ leading to a dull ache. Trismus and deviation on opening were often seen. The second group had a characteristic gradual onset, with unilateral dull pain and restricted movement. Deviation toward the affected side, clicking, and crepitus were often seen. According to Okesson,[7] Gerber[8] described a similar group of signs and symptoms, which he termed "occlusomandibular disturbance." Graber[9] used the term "myoarthropathy of the TMJ" and Voss,[10] the term "pain dysfunction syndrome."

In 1969, Laskin[11] delineated specific criteria for the diagnosis of a disorder that he described mainly as muscular in origin. Laskin called the disorder the "myofacial pain dysfunction syndrome" (MPDS). He specified that at least three of five criteria had to be present for this diagnosis to be made. The five criteria were facial pain, generally unilateral; pain on palpation of the masticatory muscles; clicking of the TMJ during function; limited or deviated opening; and absence of positive findings on radiography. Laskin's description and a series of papers that followed led to the popularization of this term. Unfortunately, MPDS was used by many clinicians as a catchall phrase for any pain and dysfunction affecting the masticatory system.

Later, in the 1970s, several papers were published by Farrar.[12-14] These led to an interest in "internal derangement" or displacement of the disc, causing clicking and, at least in some patients, locking in the TMJ. As occurred with the popularization of the MPDS diagnosis, an era of internal derangement diagnoses began. Many practitioners began attributing all pain in and around the TMJ to disc displacement.

It is not difficult to see how the diversity of terms used to describe a rather heterogeneous group of symptoms led to confusion. Clinicians who discuss a patient with a diagnosis of MPDS have no way of knowing how their treatment results compare with those in a patient with the same treatment but a diagnosis of TMJ dysfunction syndrome. Likewise, comparative analysis of much of the TMJ literature is impossible because of the different diagnostic terminology and the lack of specific diagnostic criteria.

Moffet[15] believed that diagnostic terminology should be considered a "clinical instrument" that must be employed carefully, because the use of the wrong words to identify an illness can lead to wrong thinking and possibly wrong treatment. Fricton and associates[16] stated that misdiagnosis is the most common reason for treatment failure. Diagnostic terms should ideally relate to a specific pathologic process of a particular tissue. Diagnostic terminology should not always be based on pain in a particular structure, because pathologic processes are not necessarily painful.

Diagnostic terms describing TMDs as syndromes have the possible pitfall of collecting heterogeneous groups with different diagnoses with overlapping symptoms into one group. The danger is that the same treatment modality will not necessarily be appropriate for all those in the group. Butterworth and Deardorff[17] pointed out the need for diagnostic homogeneity. They also pointed out the vast differences in frequencies of specific diagnoses from various TMJ clinics. These workers also noted the unlikelihood that patients' disorders differ significantly from clinic to clinic. They theorized that the differences exist because of variation of terminology, theoretic orientation of etiology, and treatment rationales of the individual clinics.

The first attempt to classify TMDs into specific subgroups was undertaken by Bell,[18] in 1960. He divided the disorders into three groups: (1) intracapsular conditions, (2) capsular conditions, and (3) extracapsular conditions.

In 1980, the American Academy of Craniomandibular Disorders developed a classification system (Table 7–1).[19] The system tended to be complex, and some of the subgroups seemed to reflect theoretic bias and overlapped. Bell[20] criticized the attempt as not being based on symptoms and as such not practical.

In 1982, Bell[21] refined his classification. Disorders were divided into five subcategories: masticatory muscle disorders, disc-interference disorders, inflammatory disorders, chronic hypomobilities, and growth disorders. Each disorder was described in terms of four symptoms: masticatory muscle pain, restriction in movement, interference, and acute malocclusion.

At the President's Conference on the Examination, Diagnosis, and Management of TMJ Disorders in 1982, the adopted classification system was heavily based on Bell's but was, in part, based on etiology rather than symptoms.[22] Because etiology is often multifactorial and often proves to be elusive, the scheme was not ideal.

In 1986, Bell[23] further refined his diagnostic categories (Table 7–2). His classification system is utilized today by many practitioners, and its elements are found in most classification schemes proposed by others.[24–26] The classification system used in this book is no exception.

Stegenga and colleagues[31] proposed a classification system for TMDs based on synovial joint pathology. Emphasizing the similarities of the TMJ with other synovial joints in the body rather than the differences, they developed a rather complex system. These workers separated TMDs into articular and nonarticular disorders and inflammatory and noninflammatory disorders into a "two-by-two" grid (Table 7–3). This scheme was adapted from a classification system developed by the American Rheumatism Association.[32] A later proposal for establishing a generally accepted classification system has been undertaken by the American Academy of Craniomandibular Disorders.[26] Disorders of the TMJ have been reclassified to "fit" into the existing headache classification system of the International Headache Society.[30] The inclusion of TMDs into this larger medical classification has at least three advantages:

1. The presence of TMDs in a well-accepted medical classification will allow the practitioner to put these problems into perspective with other diagnoses that affect the head and neck. The need for a true differential diagnosis will be more apparent.

2. The presence of TMDs in this larger classification may help treatment be more readily accepted by third party carriers.

3. The classification scheme, and specific diagnostic criteria, if generally adopted, will create uniformity in the terminology. Diagnostic terms will eventually be standardized.

In this system, the disorders that specifically affect the TMJ and the muscles of mastication fall under three existing categories: (1) cranial bones, (2) masticatory muscle disorders, and (3) TMJ disorders (see also Table 7–4).

Although most attention is given to disorders specific to the TMJ and the masticatory system, the practitioner must be generally familiar with a much broader spectrum of disease and consider other diagnoses that can cause problems throughout the head and neck. The possibility of systemic disease has to be suspected as well. Fricton and coworkers[24] emphasize this point by recommending the exclusion of intracranial and extracranial pathology before entertaining the possibility of TMD. The presence of systemic disease must be ruled out as well. This practice will decrease the possibility that a life threatening disease will remain untreated while the patient is treated for a TMD.[27–29]

CLASSIFICATION SYSTEMS

Classification systems have been based on signs and symptoms, tissues of origin,[24] etiology, structural and functional disorders,[22] frequency,[32] and medical classification.[26,31,32] Currently, no one ideal or accepted system for classification is used. One ideal system, for use by all practitioners in the near future, is unlikely. The particular system adopted by a particular practitioner will reflect his or her theo-

TABLE 7–1. Classification of TMJ Disorders (A)

I. Craniomandibular disorders of organic origin
    A. Articular disturbances
        1. Disc derangements
            a. Disc dysfunction
            b. Disc displacement
            c. Disc dyscrasias
        2. Condylar displacement
        3. Inflammatory conditions
            a. Synovitis
            b. Discitis
            c. Capsulitis
            d. Contusion
            e. Rupture
        4. Arthritides
            a. Osteoarthritis (arthrosis)
            b. Rheumatoid arthritis
            c. Polyarthritis (gout, lupus, Reiter's syndrome)
            d. Rheumatoid variants (psoriatic, juvenile)
            e. Infectious arthritis
        5. Ankylosis
            a. Fibrous
            b. Osseous
        6. Fractures
        7. Neoplasias
            a. Chondroma
            b. Osteoma
         8. Developmental abnormalities
            a. Hyperplasia
            b. Hypoplasia
            c. Agenesis
    B. Nonarticular disturbances
        1. Neuromuscular conditions
            a. Myofascitis (muscle tenderness)
            b. Contracture (mechanical shortening)
            c. Trismus/spasm (reflex splinting)
            d. Dyskinesia (weakness and incoordination)
        2. Dental occlusal conditions
            a. Unstable occlusion (structural imbalance)
            b. Premature posterior tooth contacts (posterior fulcruming)
            c. Lack of posterior occlusal support
            d. Distal thrust to mandible
        3. Disturbances involving referral of secondary symptoms
            a. Latent myofascial tenderness
            b. Active myofascial trigger points
II. Craniomandibular disorders of nonorganic (functional) origin
    A. Myofascial pain-dysfunction (MPD) syndrome
    B. Phantom pains
    C. Positive occlusal sense
    D. Conversion hysteria
III. Craniomandibular disorders of nonorganic origin combined with secondary organic tissue changes
    A. Articular
    B. Nonarticular
        1. Neuromuscular
        2. Oral
            a. Teeth
            b. Periodontium
            c. Soft Tissues

Reprinted with permission from McNeil, C., Danzig, D., Farrar, W., et al: J. Prosthet. Dent. 44:434, 1980.

TABLE 7–2. Classification of TMJ Disorders (B)

I. Masticatory muscle disorders
    1. Protective muscle splinting
    2. Muscle spasm activity
        a. Elevator muscle spasm
        b. Inferior lateral pterygoid muscle spasm
        c. Superior lateral pterygoid muscle spasm
    3. Muscle inflammation
II. Disc-interference disorders
    1. Class I interference (during maximum intercuspation)
    2. Class II interference (following maximum intercuspation)
    3. Class III interference (during *normal* translatory cycle)
        a. Due to excessive passive interarticular pressure
        b. Due to structural incompatibility between the sliding surfaces
        c. Due to impaired disc-condyle complex
            1. Adhesions between disc and condyle
            2. Damaged articular disc
            3. *Functional* displacement/dislocation of the disc
            4. Dysfunctional superior retrodiscal lamina
    4. Class IV interference (joint hypermobility)
    5. Class V interference (*spontaneous* dislocation)
III. Inflammatory disorders of the joint
    1. Synovitis and capsulitis
    2. Retrodiscitis
    3. Inflammatory arthritis
        a. Traumatic arthritis
        b. Degenerative arthritis
        c. Infectious arthritis
        d. Rheumatoid arthritis
        e. Hyperuricemia
IV. Chronic mandibular hypomobilities
    1. Contracture of elevator muscles
        a. Myostatic contracture
        b. Myofibrotic contracture
    2. Capsular fibrosis
    3. Ankylosis
        a. Fibrous
        b. Osseous
V. Growth disorders of the joint
    1. Aberration of development
    2. Acquired change in joint structure
    3. Neoplasia
        a. Benign
        b. Malignant

Reprinted with permission from Bell, W.: *Temporomandibular Disorders*, 2nd ed. Year Book Medical Publishers, Chicago, 1986.

retic bias or specialty orientation. For example, diagnoses made by proponents of condylar displacement theories will discuss "posterior or anterior condylar displacement" (see Chapters 18 and 23). Oral and maxillofacial surgeons who use arthroscopy use diagnostic terms such as "adhesions" and "synovial chondromatosis" (see Chapter 31).

Although it is less important that a particular system be adopted by all practitioners, it is important that the definitions of specific diagnoses become uniform. This will be useful, starting at the dental school level as an aid in teaching and decreasing confusion when comparing studies found in the literature and throughout TMD and facial pain centers across the country. The uniformity of terminology will allow clinicians from around the world to know when they are reliably talking about the same disease process. When discussing, for instance, internal derangement of the TMJ, there should be consistent agreement as to what the term means. The definition of each diagnostic group as proposed by the American Academy of Craniomandibular Disorders is reproduced in Table 7–4. The general acceptance of these definitions is encouraged and will go a long way toward eliminating the confusion that al-

Text continued on page 115

TABLE 7–3. Classification of Temporomandibular Disorders (C)

	NONINFLAMMATORY	INFLAMMATORY	
		Primary	Secondary

Articular*	Osteoarthrosis (OA):
	a. primary
	  not associated with TMJ derangements (e.g., generalized OA)
	  associated with TMJ internal derangements
	    a. initial OA
	    b. reducible anterior disc displacement (1. early; 2. late)
	    c. semipermanent disc displacement
	    d. permanent disc displacement
	    e. OA terminal stage
	b. secondary (e.g., trauma, hypermobility syndrome)
	Mechanical TMJ derangements (other than internal derangements associated with OA)
	a. related to articular disc movement
	  acute anterior disc displacement
	  posterior disc displacement†
	b. related to condylar movement
	  subluxation (possibly related to hypermobility syndrome)
	  luxation
	c. traumatic (e.g., fracture of condylar head/neck)
	d. ankylosis† (fibrous, osseous)
	Congenital and developmental disorders† (e.g., condylar agenesis, dysplasia, hypoplasia, hyperplasia)
	Neoplasia†
	a. benign (chondroma, synovial chondromatosis)
	b. malignant (primary, metastatic)
		Diffuse connective tissue disturbances†:
		†Rheumatoid arthritis
		†Juvenile chronic arthritis (Still's disease)
		Other forms of arthritis†
		†ankylosing spondylitis (M. Bechterew)
		†psoriatic arthritis
		†infectious arthritis
		†Reiter's syndrome
			TMJ synovitis
			acute (contusion)
			secondary to (mechanical) irritation
			Capsulitis, secondary to ligamentous sprains
			Crystal-induced arthropathy
			hyperuricemia (gout)
			calciumpyrophosphate dihydrate deposition
			hydroxyapatite deposition
			
			Drug/allergen induced rheumatic syndromes†

Nonarticular	Bruxism gnashing clenching Fibromyalgia (myofascial pain syndrome) Others†: muscular contracture Eagle's syndrome Coronoid hypertrophy (impingement) orofacial dyskinesia biochemical connective tissue disorders	Diffuse connective tissue diseases†: a. polymyalgia rheumatica b. arteritis temporalis c. scleroderma d. others (incl. polymyositis/dermatomyositis, systemic lupus erythematosus, Sjögren syndrome)	Tenomyositis of masticatory muscles

*Extra-articular symptoms not classified separately. These include (a) muscular: hyperfunction (e.g., protective muscle splinting) with/without contribution to dysfunction, weakness, myalgia, atrophy/hypertrophy, spasm (rare) and (b) changes in occlusion due to joint and/or muscle dysfunction.
†Uncommon in TMJ.
Reprinted with permission from Stegenga, B., de Bont, L., and Boering, G.J.: Craniomandib. Pract. 7:107–117, 1989.

TABLE 7–4. Proposed Definition of Each Diagnostic Group

11. Headache or facial pain associated with disorder of cranium, eyes, ears, nose, sinuses, teeth, mouth, or other facial or cranial structures

11.1 Cranial bones including mandible

Comment: Most disorders of the skull and mandible (e.g., congenital abnormalities, aplasia, hypoplasia, osteolysis, hyperplasia, neoplasia, fracture) are not accompanied by facial pain. Important exceptions are osteomyelitis, pain associated with altered function, multiple myeloma, and Paget's disease.

11.1.1 Congenital or developmental disorders

11.1.1.1 Aplasia (agenesis) (ICD #524.8)

Condylar aplasia is a failure in development of the cranial bones or mandible. The most common development defect is the absence of the condyle, usually resulting from failure of appearance of the primordium of the condyle in embryonic development. In this case there is no articular fossa; the eminence is rudimentary or absent. The auditory apparatus is frequently affected.

11.1.1.2 Hypoplasia (ICD #526.89)

Incomplete development or underdevelopment of cranial bones or mandibular condyle that is congenital or acquired. It is less severe than aplasia. Condylar hypoplasia can be associated with fibrous ankylosis.

11.1.1.3 Condylolysis (ICD #524.9)

Mandibular condylolysis is related to a lytic event. The condyle becomes progressively smaller and may disappear. It is distinguished from aplasia by not being associated with facial anomalies. Normal development proceeds until a lytic event occurs. It is not usually associated with ankylosis or erosive changes in the fossae. Serologic tests are negative.

11.1.1.4 Hyperplasia (ICD #526.89)

Overdevelopment of the cranial bones or mandible that is congenital or acquired. A non-neoplastic increase in the number of normal cells. It can occur as a localized enlargement (i.e., condylar hyperplasia or coronoid hyperplasia) or as an overdevelopment of the entire mandible or side of the face.

11.1.1.5 Neoplasm (ICD #213.1 and 170.1)

A neoplasm is a new, abnormal, uncontrolled growth of the cranial bones or mandible. Benign tumors are most commonly found in the TMJ (e.g., osteoma, chondroma, and chondromatosis). Malignant tumors (e.g., osteosarcomas, chondrosarcomas) are exceedingly rare.

11.7 Temporomandibular joint disorders

11.7.1 Deviation in form (ICD #719.68)

(Previously used term: dyscrasia.) Irregularities of intracapsular soft and hard articular tissues.

Diagnostic criteria:
(1) Pain not present
(2) Repetitive, nonvariable joint noise, if present, occurs at the same condylar position on opening and closing of the mandible

11.7.2 Articular disc displacement

11.7.2.1 Disc displacement with reduction (ICD #718.38)

(Previously used terms: internal derangement, anterior disc displacement, reciprocal click.) Alteration, usually abrupt, of the disc-condyle structural relationship during mandibular translation; usually characterized by reciprocal clicking.

Diagnostic criteria:
(1) Pain, when present, precipitated by joint movement and caused by inflammation
(2) Reproducible joint noise at different positions during opening and closing mandibular movements; closing noise (click) usually located close to intercuspal position
(3) Soft tissue imaging reveals displaced disc that reduces, usually on opening

Table continued on following page

TABLE 7–4. Proposed Definition of Each Diagnostic Group *Continued*

(4) No coarse crepitus
(5) Range of motion usually normal

11.7.2.2 Disc displacement without reduction (ICD #718.28)
(Previously used terms: nonreducing disc, "closed lock.") Altered disc-condyle structural relationship that is maintained during translation; can be acute or chronic.
Diagnostic criteria (acute):
(1) Pain, usually extreme, precipitated by function and caused by inflammation
(2) Marked limited mandibular opening
(3) No joint noise
(4) Straight line deviation to the affected side on opening
(5) Marked limited laterotrusion to the contralateral side
(6) Soft tissue imaging reveals displaced disc without reduction
Diagnostic criteria (chronic):
(1) Usually not painful, or pain markedly decreased from acute stage
(2) History of joint noise and/or limitation of mandibular opening
(3) No joint noise other than possible crepitus
(4) Slight limited mandibular opening
(5) Slight limited laterotrusion to the contralateral side
(6) Soft tissue imaging reveals displaced disc without reduction

11.7.3 Temporomandibular joint hypermobility (ICD #728.5)
(Previously used terms: subluxation, hypertranslation, hyperextension, ligament laxity.) Excessive disc and/or condylar translation, usually well beyond the eminence.
Diagnostic criteria:
(1) Excess range of motion
(2) Clicking, when present, may not be reproducible and can usually be eliminated by superior support or loading of the mandible; the noise can be present with rapid mandibular movement but may disappear with routine function
(3) Usually not associated with pain
(4) Soft tissue imaging usually negative

11.7.4 Dislocation (ICD #718.38)
(Previously used terms: "open lock," subluxation, luxation.)
A condition in which the condyle is positioned anterior to the articular eminence and/or disc and is unable to return to a closed position.
Diagnostic criteria:
(1) Excessive range of motion
(2) Inability to close mandible
(3) Pain, if present, occurs at time of dislocation with residual pain after the episode
(4) If true dislocation, patient cannot reduce the dislocated mandible without help from a clinician; the condition is termed "subluxation" if the patient can reduce the condyle, usually in a brief period of time

11.7.5 Inflammatory conditions

11.7.5.1 Synovitis (ICD #727.09)
(Previously used terms: capsulitis, discitis, retrodiscitis, arthritis.)
An inflammation in the synovial lining of the TMJ.
Diagnostic criteria:
(1) Localized pain exacerbated by function, especially with superior and/or posterior joint loading
(2) Limited range of motion secondary to pain
(3) Possibly characterized by fluctuating swelling caused by effusion, preventing occlusion of ipsilateral posterior teeth
(4) No radiographic evidence of structural changes unless accompanied by arthrosis

11.7.5.2 Capsulitis (ICD #716.98)
(Previously used terms: retrodiscitis, arthritis, arthralgia, contusion.)
Inflammation of the joint capsule; usually includes an inflammation of the synovium.

TABLE 7–4. Proposed Definition of Each Diagnostic Group *Continued*

Diagnostic criteria:
(1) Point tenderness on palpation of TMJ
(2) Pain at rest and exacerbated by function, especially with stretching of capsule
(3) Range of motion limited by pain
(4) No radiographic evidence of structural bony change
Comment: This problem may be secondary to trauma of the TMJ. However, the differences between synovitis and capsulitis are almost impossible to detect clinically.

11.7.6 Arthritides

11.7.6.1 Osteoarthrosis (ICD #715.38)
(Previously used terms: osteoarthritis, arthritis, degenerative joint disease, arthrosis deformans.)
Osteoarthrosis is a degenerative noninflammatory condition of the joint characterized by structural changes of the joint surfaces.
Diagnostic criteria:
(1) No pain present
(2) No point tenderness on palpation
(3) Crepitus
(4) If range of motion is limited, it is secondary to degeneration
(5) If range of motion is limited, deviation to the affected side on opening
(6) Radiographic evidence of structural bony change

11.7.6.2 Osteoarthritis (ICD #716.98)
(Previously used terms: arthritis, osteoarthrosis, degenerative joint disease.)
Osteoarthritis is a degenerative condition accompanied by secondary inflammation (synovitis) of the TMJ.
Diagnostic criteria:
(1) Pain caused by synovitis
(2) Usually point tenderness on palpation
(3) Crepitus or multiple joint noises
(4) Range of motion limited, with deviation to the affected side on opening; limitation is secondary to pain or degeneration
(5) Radiographic evidence of structural bony change

11.7.6.3 Polyarthritides (ICD #714.9)
Arthritis caused by a generalized systemic polyarthritic condition. Temporomandibular joint polyarthritides include rheumatoid arthritis, juvenile rheumatoid arthritis (Still's disease), spondyloarthropathies (ankylosing spondylitis), crystal-induced diseases (gout, hyperuricemia), and Reiter's syndrome. This group of arthritides includes multiple diagnostic categories best diagnosed with serologic tests and managed by rheumatologists. Dental management relates to secondary complaints and craniomandibular disorder (CMD) contributing factors.
Diagnostic criteria:
(1) Pain during acute and subacute stages
(2) Point tenderness on palpation may be present
(3) Crepitus may be present
(4) Radiographic evidence of structural bony change
(5) Range of motion limited, secondary to pain and/or degeneration
(6) Abnormal serologic findings usually present
(7) Anterior open bite may be present

11.7.7 Ankylosis
(Previously used term: arthrokleisis.)
Ankylosis is restricted mandibular movement with deviation to the affected side on opening.

11.7.7.1 Fibrous ankylosis (ICD #718.58)
Fibrous ankylosis is produced by adhesions within the TMJ.
Diagnostic criteria:
(1) Not usually associated with pain
(2) Limited range of motion on opening
(3) Deviation to the affected side

Table continued on following page

TABLE 7–4. Proposed Definition of Each Diagnostic Group *Continued*

        (4) Limited laterotrusion to the contralateral side
        (5) No radiographic findings other than absence of ipsilateral condylar translation on opening

11.7.7.2 Bony ankylosis (ICD #718.58)
    The union of the bones of the TMJ by proliferation of bone cells, resulting in complete immobility of that joint.
Diagnostic criteria:
(1) Not associated with pain
(2) Limited range of motion on opening
(3) Marked deviation to the affected side
(4) Marked limited laterotrusion to the contralateral side
(5) Radiographic evidence of bone proliferation

11.8 Masticatory muscle disorders

11.8.1 Myofascial pain (ICD #729.1)
    (Previously used terms: myofascial pain dysfunction [MPD] syndrome, fibromyalgia, myalgia, trigger point pain, muscle contraction headache, tension headache.)
Myofascial pain is a regional aching pain associated with localized tenderness in firm bands of muscle and tendons (also termed trigger points).
Diagnostic criteria:
(1) Continuous pain, usually dull, in one or more muscles
(2) Localized tenderness in firm bands of muscle
(3) Can have reproducible alteration of pain complaints with palpation of specific tender areas termed "active" trigger points of pain referral
(4) May be associated with parafunction, postural hypertonicity, or secondary to trauma

11.8.2 Myositis (ICD #728.81)
    (Previously used term: tendomyositis.)
Myositis is a painful generalized inflammation usually of the entire muscle; may occur in tendinous attachments of muscle as well.
Diagnostic criteria:
(1) Pain, usually acute, in a muscle
(2) Tenderness over entire region of the muscle
(3) Possible swelling of the muscle
(4) Range of motion limited because of pain and swelling
(5) Associated with trauma or infection of the muscle
Comment: When muscle tissue ossifies, condition is termed "myositis ossificans."

11.8.2.1 Tendomyositis (ICD #727.8)

11.8.2.2 Tendonitis (ICD #727.8)

11.8.3 Spasm (ICD #728.85)
    (Previously used terms: acute trismus, myospasm, cramp.)
Muscle spasm is a sudden, involuntary contraction of a muscle.
Diagnostic criteria:
(1) Acute pain is present
(2) Marked, limited range of motion
(3) Continuous muscle contraction (fasciculation)
(4) Increased electromyogram activity even at rest
(5) Usually caused by overstretching or acute overuse of a muscle

11.8.4 Reflex splinting (ICD #728.89)
    (Previously used terms: protective splinting, muscle guarding, trismus.)
Reflex rigidity of a muscle occurring as a means of avoiding pain caused by movement of the parts.
Diagnostic criteria:
(1) Pain usually present
(2) Muscle tenderness on palpation
(3) Limited range of motion
(4) Rigidity of jaw upon manipulation

TABLE 7–4. Proposed Definition of Each Diagnostic Group *Continued*

11.8.5 Muscle contracture (ICD #728.9)
(Previously used terms: chronic trismus, muscle fibrosis, muscle scarring.)
Muscle contracture is chronic resistance of a muscle to passive stretch, as a result of fibrosis.
Diagnostic criteria:
(1) Usually not painful
(2) Limited range of motion, not caused by joint disorder
(3) Unyielding firmness on passive stretch

11.8.6 Hypertrophy (ICD #728.9)
Muscle hypertrophy is a generalized abnormal enlargement of muscle tissue.
Diagnostic criteria:
(1) Usually not painful
(2) Grossly enlarged muscle
(3) Range of motion may be limited, but not usually

11.8.7 Neoplasm
Craniofacial muscle neoplasia is a new, abnormal, and uncontrolled growth of muscle tissue (e.g., myxoma, myxosarcoma, rhabdomyosarcoma).

11.8.7.1 Malignant (ICD #171.0)

11.8.7.2 Benign (ICD #215.0)

Reprinted with permission from American Academy of Craniomandibular Disorders, Guidelines for Evaluation, Diagnosis, and Management. Quintessence Publishing Co., Lombard, IL, 1990.

ready exists. The International Classification of Disease (ICD) number accompanies each diagnostic category.

The classification system in this text is not unique, original, or presented to supplant other classification systems. Like all the others, it will have its proponents and its critics. This classification system is meant to be used as an organizational framework from which to orient the clinician to the various possibilities of differential diagnosis and includes the categories defined in Table 7–4.

All classifications have their limitations. Recognition of this fact may well be the strength of classification systems, in general. It allows the clinician to see what falls under the heading of TMDs. As important, by setting specific criteria for diagnosis, the classification system, by virtue of exclusion, defines what is *not* a TMD. This helps guide the clinician as to when and who to refer patients. Unfortunately, the overdiagnosis of TMD has become all too common. Because patients are suffering with pain in the head or neck does not mean they have TMDs. Treatment may not necessarily fall within the realm of a dentist.

Some patients can have multiple diagnoses. It is common for a patient to have internal derangement coexisting with myofascial pain and dysfunction. There is no rule stating "one pa-

tient, one disease." It is also unwise to assume that each patient's disorder will fit into a specific classification of disease of any system. Clearly, some patients cannot be categorized utilizing any one specific diagnosis.

The classification system in this text is based on similar systems published by Fricton,[16] Bell,[23] and others. It divides TMDs into two major categories, disorders that affect the musculature and disorders that affect the joint. Each of these groups are further divided into subcategories. The muscle disorder group is delineated into eleven diagnostic categories. The joint disorder group is subdivided into eight different categories, several of which are further subdivided. Each subgroup is based on a pathologic process or a particular stage of a pathologic process.

Chapters 9 through 15 are devoted to detailed discussions of each of these areas. There are chapters devoted to muscular disorders, internal derangement, arthritides, developmental disease, and neoplastic disease. Each of these chapters specifically describes the particular pathologies falling under its subheading. In addition, the subject of trauma, although an etiology, is discussed in detail in two chapters—one devoted to soft tissue changes and the other to osseous damage. A thorough discussion of related cervical spine disorders is found in chapter 2 and should not be overlooked as an important part of the differential diagnosis.

CLASSIFICATION OF TEMPOROMANDIBULAR DISORDERS

I. Muscular Disorders
  A. Muscle tension (hyperactivity)
  B. Muscle spasm (sustained)
  C. Muscle inflammation (myositis)
  D. Myofascial pain and dysfunction (trigger points)
  E. Fibrosis and contracture
  F. Atrophy
  G. Hypertrophy
  H. Muscle tears/lacerations
  I. Protective splinting/trismus
  J. Fibromyalgia
  K. Neoplasia

II. Temporomandibular Joint Disorders (Arthrogenous disorders)
  A. Internal derangement
    1. Deviation in form
      a. Frictional disc incoordination
      b. Articular surface defects
      c. Disc thinning and perforation
    2. Disc displacement
      a. Partial (anteromedial) disc displacement
      b. (Anteromedial) disc displacement with reduction
        (1) Partial displacement
        (2) Complete displacement
    3. (Anteromedial) disc displacement with intermittent locking
    4. (Anteromedial) disc displacement without reduction
      a. Acute
      b. Chronic
    5. (Anteromedial) disc displacement with perforation of the retrodiscal tissue
    6. Adhesive disc hypomobility
    7. Displacement of the disc/condyle complex
      a. Subluxation
      b. Dislocation
  B. Arthritis of the TMJ
    1. Noninflammatory arthritis (osteoarthrosis)
    2. Inflammatory arthritis
      a. Rheumatoid arthritis
      b. Juvenile rheumatoid arthritis
      c. Psoriatic arthritis
      d. Ankylosing spondylitis
      e. Lupus erythematosus
    3. Infectious arthritis
      a. Direct extension
      b. Systemic infection
    4. Metabolic disease
      a. Gout arthritis
      b. Chondrocalcinosis
  C. Capsulitis/synovitis
  D. Retrodiscitis
  E. Fractures of the TMJ
  F. Ankylosis
    1. Fibrous
    2. Bony
  G. Developmental disturbances of the TMJ
    1. Condylar hyperplasia
    2. Condylar hypoplasia
    3. Condylar aplasia
  H. Neoplasia

REFERENCES

1. Goodfriend, D.: Symptomatology and treatment of abnormalities of the mandibular articulation. Dent. Cosmos. 75:844, 1933.
2. Wright, W.: Deafness as influenced by malposition of the jaws. Nat. Dent. A. J. 7:979, 1920.
3. Costen, J.: Classification and treatment of temporomandibular joint problems. Ann. Otol. Rhinol. Laryngol. 65:35, 1956.
4. Shore, N.: *Occlusal Equilibration and Temporomandibular Joint Dysfunction.* J.P. Lippincott Co., Philadelphia, 1959.
5. Schwartz, L.: A temporomandibular joint pain dysfunction syndrome. J. Chron. Dis. 3:284, 1956.
6. Ramfjord, S. and Ash, M.: *Occlusion.* W.B. Saunders Co., Philadelphia, 1966.
7. Okesson, J.: *Management of TMJ Disorders and Occlusion.* C.V. Mosby Co., St. Louis, 1989.
8. Gerber, A.: Kiefergelenk und Zahnokklusion. Dtsch Zahnaerztl Z. 26:119, 1971.
9. Graber, G.: Neurologische und Psychosomatische aspekte der Myoarthropathien des Kauorgans. Z.W.R. 80:997, 1971.
10. Voss, R.: Die Behandlung von Beschwerden des Kiefergelenkes mit Aufbisplatten. Dtsch Zahnaerzil Z. 19:545, 1964.
11. Laskin, D.: Etiology of the pain dysfunction syndrome. J. Am. Dent. Assoc. 79:147, 1969.
12. Farrar, W.: Diagnosis and treatment of painful temporomandibular joints. J. Prosthet. Dent. 28:629–636, 1972.
13. Farrar, W.: Diagnosis and treatment of anterior dislocation of the articular disc. N.J. Dent. J. 41:348–351, 1971.
14. Farrar, W.: Differentiation of the temporomandibular joint dysfunction to simplify treatment. J. Prosthet. Dent. 28:629, 1972.
15. Moffet, B.: *Diagnosis of Internal Derangements of the Temporomandibular Joint,* vol. I. University of Wash-

ington Continuing Dental Education, Seattle, Washington, 1984.

16. Fricton, J., Kroening, R., and Hathaway, K.: *TMJ and Craniofacial Pain.* Ishiyaku EuroAmerica Inc., St. Louis, 1989.

17. Butterworth, W. and Deardorff, J.: Psychometric profiles of craniomandibular pain patients. Part II. A multidisciplinary case report. J. Craniomandib. Pract. 5:367, 1987.

18. Bell, W.: *Temporomandibular Joint Disease.* Egan Co., Dallas, 1960. [See Press Conference Book.]

19. McNeil, C., Danzig, D., Farrar, W. et al: Craniomandibular (TMJ) disorders—The state of the art. J. Prosthet. Dent. 44:434, 1980.

20. Bell, W.: *Temporomandibular Disorders,* 2nd ed. Year Book Medical Publishers, Chicago, 1986.

21. Bell, W.: Classification of TM disorders. In The President's Conference on the Examination, Diagnosis and Management of Temporomandibular Disorders. D. Laskin, et al (eds.). Am. Dent. Assoc. 1982.

22. Laskin, D., et al (eds.): The President's Conference on the Examination, Diagnosis and Management of Temporomandibular disorders. Am. Dent. Assoc. 1982.

23. Bell, W.: *Temporomandibular Disorders,* 2nd ed. Year Book Medical Publishers, Chicago, 1986.

24. Fricton, J., Kroening, R., and Hathaway, K.: *TMJ and Craniofacial Pain.* Ishiyaku EuroAmerica Inc., St. Louis, 1989.

25. Clark, G.: Three principles of treatment for managing temporomandibular disorders. In *Perspectives in Temporomandibular Disorders.* Clark, G. and Solberg, K. (eds.). Quintessence Publishing Co., Lombard, IL, 1987.

26. American Academy of Craniomandibular Disorders (ed.): *Craniomandibular Disorders, Guidelines for Evaluation, Diagnosis and Management.* Quintessence Publishing Co., Lombard, IL, 1990.

27. Kaplan, A., Lawson, W., and Som, P.: Coexistence of myofacial pain dysfunction syndrome and mucoepidermoid carcinoma of the parotid gland. J. Am. Dent. Assoc. 112:495–496, 1986.

28. Roistacher, S. and Tannenbaum, D.: Myofacial pain associated with oropharyngeal cancer. Oral Surg. Oral Med. Oral Path. 61:459–462, 1986.

29. Grace, E. and North, A.: TMJ dysfunction and orofacial pain caused by parotid gland malignancy. J. Am. Dent. Assoc. 116:348, 1988.

30. International Headache Society: Classification and diagnostic criteria of headache disorders, cranial neuralgias and facial pain. Cephalgia 8:Suppl. 7, 1988.

31. Stegenga, B., deBont, L., and Boering, G.: A proposed classification of TMD based on synovial joint pathology. J. Craniomandib. Pract. 7:107–117, 1989.

32. McCarty, D.: Differential diagnosis of arthritis: analysis of signs and symptoms. In *Arthritis and Allied Conditions.* D. McCarty (ed.). Lea & Febiger, Philadelphia, 1985.

Noshir Mehta

C H A P T E R   8

Muscular Disorders

Symptoms of temporomandibular disorders (TMDs) include pain and dysfunction in the head, neck, face, and jaw areas.[1] [1] The symptoms are often multiple and varied,[5-8] and they are primarily related to the musculoskeletal system. The system can be divided into three main areas termed the "triad of dysfunction,"[9] which accounts for the majority of patient complaints:

1. *Myofascial pain and dysfunction* relates to pain and dysfunction of the skeletal muscles of the body. It has often been confused with myofacial pain, a term used to denote *masticatory* muscle dysfunction. Myofascial pain and dysfunction may affect any skeletal muscle singly or in combination and does not limit itself to the face and jaws.
2. *Internal derangement of the temporomandibular joint (TMJ)* relates to problems within the TMJs themselves. Symptoms range from noise on movement to pain and locking and can be followed by osteoarthritic changes in the joints over time. The muscles are often secondarily affected, and the patient may present with muscle pain.
3. *Cervical spine dysfunction* relates to disorders of the spinal column, the vertebrae, and the ligaments. The muscles that support, move, and protect the cervical spine are often symptomatic in patients with TMDs, and patients with cervical spine pathology often complain of facial pain.

In each of these areas is a common denominator. Whether primary or secondary, the muscular system is involved. An understanding of muscle function and dysfunction is essential to be able to properly evaluate and treat the patient with TMD.

The purpose of this chapter is to familiarize the reader with the most common muscle dysfunctions and their association with TMDs.

MUSCLE FUNCTION

To understand muscle dysfunction, a brief description of muscle function is important. For more detail, perusal of a physiology text is recommended.

Muscles of the skeletal system are striated and are divided into two groups. One group provides for rapid or phasic movement; these muscles are pale in color, have a fast rate of contraction, and fatigue quickly.[10] The second group is characterized by a dark red color. These muscles provide for tonic or postural activities and are more resistant to fatigue.

Each striated muscle has an origin (fixed end) and an insertion. Muscles promote movement by contraction. They cannot push but only pull. Muscle function requires that antagonist muscles act in harmony for physiologic skeletal movement. The contraction of a muscle relies on groups of fibers to contract while other groups in the same muscle rest. These groups alternate in their contracting and resting phases. Group interchange allows a muscle to function without fatigue.

Force generation through muscle function relies on several factors—the frequency and number of motor units activated by the contraction; the original length and the velocity at which the muscles shorten; and the rate of fatigability.

Fatigability of muscles will vary depending on fiber type. According to Eriksson and Thornell,[12] masticatory muscles contain a predominance of low threshold fatigue resistant motor units. Muscles of the extremities, in contrast, have an equal distribution of low threshold fatigue resistant type I motor units, high threshold fatigue sensitive type IIA motor units, and high threshold fatigue resistant type IIB motor units.[13]

Muscle fatigue and pain can be predicted on the basis of contraction time. Muscles that have the fastest contraction time have a quicker onset of fatigue. The muscles of mastication, for example, have the fastest contraction times of any skeletal muscles other than the external ocular muscles. Therefore, it is common for parafunctional movement of the jaws to produce fatigue and pain.[14]

CLASSIFICATION OF MUSCLE DYSFUNCTION

Many classifications of muscular disorders have been proposed. Bell[15,16] has described myogenous pains that emanate from the orofacial structures. He classified them as being musculoskeletal pains of the deep somatic type and categorized them as (1) protective muscle splinting, (2) myofascial trigger point pain, (3) muscle spasm pain, and (4) muscle inflammation pain.

Travell and Rinzler[17] introduced the myofascial genesis of pain in 1952 to the dental profession, and the term myofascial pain dysfunction syndrome was used by Laskin[18] to designate a muscular variation of the term "TMJ syndrome."[19,20]

The concept espoused by Travell and Rinzler identifies the trigger point as the primary source of myofascial pain, and they differentiate this from (1) myalgia (diffuse), (2) muscle spasm, and (3) contracture.

Kraus[21] classified muscle pain into four groups: (1) muscle spasm, (2) muscle tension, (3) muscle deficiency, and (4) trigger points.

The International Headache Society's[22] classification for headache disorders, cranial neuralgias, and facial pain addressed the issue of muscle pain under the following headings: (1) myalgia due to trauma, (2) myalgia secondary to parafunction, (3) myalgia secondary to postural hypertonicity, (4) myofascial pain, (5) reflex splinting/trismus, (6) spasm (sustained), (7) myositis, and (8) contracture (fibrosis).

A great deal of overlap occurs in these classifications. A consensus seems to exist that muscles spasm, develop trigger points, or become inflamed thus causing pain. Treatment may vary depending on the location and function of the muscle and whether the muscle is the site of the primary pathology or is activated secondarily as a response to pathology in another structure. For example, if a patient presents with a masseter spasm, the diagnostician must differentiate between trauma-related spasm of the muscle itself and protective splinting related to an injured TMJ.

A classification should clearly identify the primary or secondary nature of a muscular problem, its anatomic location, and if possible its etiology. These determinations facilitate communication with the patient and other health-care professionals and help guide treatment. The following classification based on the triad of dysfunctions concept has been proposed:[9]

ETIOLOGIC AND STRUCTURAL CLASSIFICATION OF MUSCULAR DISORDERS

  I. *Primary myofascial and muscle pain dysfunction*
   A. Myalgia due to localized acute muscular injury
    1. Muscle tear/laceration
    2. Muscle inflammation (myositis)
    3. Muscle spasm/splinting
    4. Myofascial pain and trigger points
   B. Myalgia due to chronic sustaining parafunctional activity
    1. Muscle tension (hyperactivity)
    2. Muscle spasm sustained
    3. Muscle inflammation (myositis)
    4. Myofascial pain and trigger points
    5. Fibrosis/contracture
    6. Atrophy
   C. Myalgia due to chronic sustaining postural factors
    1. Muscle tension
    2. Muscle spasm sustained
    3. Muscle inflammation (myositis)
    4. Myofascial pain and trigger points
    5. Fibrosis/contracture
    6. Atrophy
 II. *Secondary to internal derangement of the TMJ*
   A. Muscle tension
   B. Muscle spasm/protective splinting
   C. Muscle inflammation (myositis)
   D. Myofascial pain and trigger points
   E. Fibrosis/contracture
   F. Atrophy
III. *Secondary to cervical spinal dysfunction*
   A. Muscle tension
   B. Muscle spasm/protective splinting
   C. Muscle inflammation (myositis)
   D. Myofascial pain and trigger points
   E. Fibrosis/contracture
   F. Atrophy

DEFINITIONS OF TERMINOLOGY

MYALGIA. Myalgia is defined as pain in a muscle or muscles[23] and was first introduced into the literature in 1938 by Gutstein.[24] Later, writing under the name of Good,[25] he described trigger points as myalgic spots. Since then, the term has been used synonymously with myositis, localized trigger points,[25] myofascial syndrome,[17] and myofascitis.[26,27] This usage has resulted in confusion, and "myalgia" is often employed as a broad general term under which other more specific diagnoses exist.

MYOSITIS. Myositis is defined as inflammation in a muscle resulting in localized muscle soreness. This inflammation can occur from acute strain with unaccustomed use, abuse, external trauma, and infection.[28] Muscle inflammation can also occur following muscle tear and laceration as a normal stage of healing.

MUSCLE SPASM. Muscle spasm is defined as a painful contraction of striated muscle caused by chronic or acute trauma, excessive tension, or organic disorders.[79]

MUSCLE SPLINTING. Muscle splinting, also referred to as muscle guarding and protective muscle splinting,[30] is a reflex protective mechanism. Skeletal muscles contract into a hypertonic and painful state as a means of stabilizing an injured part.[31] It is nature's way of preventing further injury.

MYOFASCIAL TRIGGER POINT. According to Travell and Simons,[32] a myofascial trigger point is defined as "a hyperirritable spot, usually within a taut band of skeletal muscle or in the muscle's fascia, that is painful on compression and that can give rise to characteristic referred pain, tenderness, and autonomic phenomena." Trigger points may be active or latent and can be classified as primary, associated, satellite, and secondary.

MYOFASCIAL PAIN. Myofascial pain is defined as pain arising from myofascial trigger points.

MYOFASCIAL PAIN DYSFUNCTION SYNDROME. This syndrome was defined by Laskin[18] as facial pain characterized by myofascial trigger points, muscle tenderness, joint dysfunction, and difficulty in jaw movement.

MUSCLE FATIGUE. As previously noted, muscles function by group interchange. Muscle fatigue results when the contractile activity exceeds the capability of muscle fiber group interchange.[30] A muscle that is in chronic spasm or overworked will ultimately become fatigued and painful.

FIBROSITIS. Fibrositis is a term introduced by Bowers[33] in 1904 to denote muscular rheumatism. It is generally described as inflammation of the fibrous tissues and can occur in any skeletal muscle in the body. The word fibrositis is used interchangeably with several different diagnoses, including myofibrositis,[34] fibromyalgia,[35] muscular fibrositis,[32] and interstitial myofibrositis.[36]

MYOTATIC CONTRACTURE. When a muscle is not allowed to function within its full range of motion, it eventually loses its stretch reflex capability, and shortening or contracture occurs. The specific cause is usually an inhibitory influence due to muscle splinting or immobilization of the part for an extended period of time. Myotatic contracture is usually reversible with appropriate therapy.[15]

MYOFIBROTIC CONTRACTURE. This occurs as a response to an inflammatory process or from an untreated myostatic contracture, ultimately resulting in fibrosis of the muscle or its sheath. This contracture is not reversible.[15]

Primary Myofascial and Muscle Pain Dysfunction

Primary myofascial and muscle pain dysfunction is the most common cause of pain and discomfort of all TMDs and originates from the muscles of the head and neck. Recognition of primary muscle pain is important for successful treatment of patients with acute and chronic pain. Frequently, patients diagnosed as having pain related to internal derangement are actually suffering from muscle pain. Treatment aimed at orthopedic correction may lead to ongoing pain and dysfunction.

Muscle pain may originate from the muscle body, the tendon attachments, or the fascia as a result of macrotrauma, stretching, forceful contraction, ischemia, hyperemia, or microtrauma. General characteristics of muscle pain have been described by Bell[16] as being of the deep somatic category, having the following characteristics:

1. The pain is usually of a dull and deep quality.
2. The pain is of a diffuse nature.
3. The incidence and severity of the pain vary with the stimulus.
4. Associated restriction in movement may be present.

Myalgia Due to Localized Acute Injury

Tissue injury initiates an inflammatory reaction that induces pain.[37] The exact nature of the pain depends on the location, severity, and type of injury. Injury in a muscle that does not have constant use allows for resolution of the inflammatory process. A muscle subject to constant movement, parafunction, or both will have delayed healing.

In the inflammatory process, prostaglandins and bradykinins act in conjunction to increase capillary permeability by local vasodilation, lowering the pain threshold.[38,39] The affected area is more sensitized to a wider variety of stimuli, and as a result spontaneous pain and hyperalgesia take place. Injury to a muscle will also result in myositis and cellulitis.

Damage to a muscle can occur from acute muscle strain or from direct trauma. Soft tissue injury can result in bleeding, inflammation, and swelling causing the muscle to respond with myalgia, muscle spasm, muscle splinting, or myositis. Myofascial trigger points occur in various combinations within the muscle and are considered by Travell[40] to be the primary source of muscular pain.

Injury results in a deep sharp ache on contraction of the muscle. Depending on the area of injury, the pain may emanate from the tendon attachments (tendonitis), the fascial component (myofascitis), or the body of the muscle (myospasm and myositis).

Myositis

Injury due to a direct blow to a muscle can trigger a localized inflammatory response accompanied by swelling, pain, and immobilization of the part. In the case of the masticatory system, there is restriction in jaw movement with a possible lateral shift of the mandible. This will evidence itself by a change in the patient's perception of occlusion.

Injury to the head and neck muscles will result in an accompanying reduction in neck movement and changes in shoulder height and head posture as a means of protecting against further trauma.[41] The pain may be perceived by the patient as a headache.[42] An accompanying feeling of weakness in the neck will be experienced. Other inflammatory myogenous pains may be related to the tendons, fascia, and bursae.[43] Immobilization of a muscle due to inflammation and pain may progress to contracture and atrophy. Other factors giving rise to myositis may be localized infections, surgical procedures, and diseases.

Diagnosis

A diagnosis of myositis can be made using the following criteria:

History. Patients generally have the ability to point to a single cause, often trauma, abuse, infection, or surgery.

Symptoms. Patients complain of localized soreness, swelling, and pain along with weakness and immobilization of the affected part. Pain is described generally as dull, deep, boring, and constant. There may be episodes of sharp pain related to movement of the affected area.

Patients with myositis of the masticatory musculature may complain of a change in the bite with inability to chew, swallow, and speak comfortably. In cervical muscle injury, headaches, neck pain, reduction in movement of the head along with weakness of the head and neck muscles would be reported.[44]

Clinical Signs. Depending on the extent of the injury, the area may appear swollen and discolored because of extravasation of inflammatory products. An inflamed muscle on palpation will appear as a soft painful mass. Pain will be associated with active as well as passive movement of the affected part. The skin surface may be warmer to the touch. The patient may present with low-grade fever if there is secondary infection involved. Electromyographic evaluation will show a low resting tension and an inability of the muscle to function fully due to protective splinting,[45] evidenced by low electromyographic readings (Fig. 8–1).

Pressure threshold measurements, utilizing a threshold meter,[46] show a reduction from the baseline threshold of force that induces discomfort (Fig. 8–2). Thermography demon-

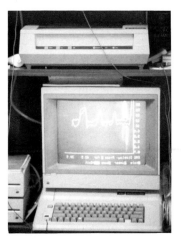

FIGURE 8–1. Electromyographic readout using bilateral electrodes for comparison of left and right side muscles. The level readings are at rest with the mouth open; the spikes are full bites. (Davicon, Boston.)

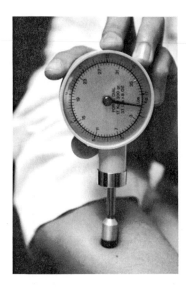

FIGURE 8–2. Pressure threshold meter.

strates increased temperature over the site of injury. Proximal to the injury, there may be a cold spot showing vasoconstriction, which may affect healing of the injured areas.[46]

Clinical Course. This depends on the severity of the injury and the ability of the part to remain immobilized during the initial phase of healing. Protective splinting of the injured muscle must be treated in a timely manner to prevent contracture and atrophy.

Treatment

Initial therapy of the acute symptoms of myositis includes the following:

1. Ice is applied to the affected part to reduce swelling if the patient is seen immediately after the injury. This can be followed by heat, as acute symptoms subside.

2. The patient should be restricted to painless limits of movement.

3. No injections, ultrasound, or massage should be used at the time of acute injury.

4. Anti-inflammatory medication can be prescribed.

5. Antibiotic therapy is necessary if infection is present.

After the acute symptoms have subsided treatment includes (1) increased heat and mobilization of the affected area, (2) institution of an exercise program to regain full range of motion, and (3) institution of muscle-strengthening exercises.

Muscle Splinting

Muscle splinting is a reflex mechanism by which skeletal muscles stabilize an injured area and protect it from further injury. The involved muscles become hypertonic and painful. An associated feeling of weakness may be alarming to the patient. This is a normal body defense to reduce function of the affected part.

Muscle splinting often occurs as a sequel to muscle injury and follows myositis. If splinting remains over a protracted period, muscle spasm may follow with or without trigger points leading to a chronic cycle of myofascial pain and dysfunction.[47]

Diagnosis

History. Because this is a protective mechanism, the history should indicate an injury to a muscle or internal derangement.

Symptoms. Pain will be experienced when the involved muscle is contracted. A feeling of stiffness and muscular weakness is experienced. The patient may report restriction of movement due to pain.

In the masticatory system, splinting of the elevator muscles may affect occlusal contact patterns. Because of the accompanying weakness, occlusal forces and chewing are affected. Pain limits jaw activity, mimicking trismus or an anteriorly displaced disc without reduction (closed lock).

Injury to the cervical muscles would cause protective splinting and decrease mobility of the head and neck. The accompanying weakness is frightening to patients who report that they cannot keep their head upright for any appreciable period of time. Pain in the cervical muscles will be present with movement of the head and neck.

Patients may report numerous secondary symptoms related to the protective adaptation that takes place. These may include, but are not limited to, vertigo, headaches, eye pain, neck and arm pain, and face and jaw pain. Protracted splinting of the cervical area may further cause mild low back symptoms, as the body goes through an adaptive process in an attempt to help the injured area.

Clinical Signs. A muscle in protective splinting elicits pain on palpation and stretching. Muscle tightness and muscle weakness may be noticed during evaluation of range of motion and muscle palpation. Electromyographic changes are not seen during rest. Electromyographic activity of the masticatory muscles will be normal as activity is increased until pain is experienced, at which point the activity is decreased in response to the splinting action. Pressure threshold measurements may or may not show the reduced tolerance to pain. Thermography will not show any change unless myositis is present.

Treatment

Initially, therapy should consist of restriction of movement of the affected area. In the masticatory system, if there is a noticeable shift of the mandible, the patient may complain of difficulty in keeping the mandible in a relaxed position. A stabilization splint during this acute phase will allow for occlusal stability. Care must be taken to reduce the time the appliance is worn, as healing takes place so as to permit the occlusion to return to normal.

If the patient is in pain due to an inability of the muscles to maintain a stable head posture, a cervical collar with the smaller width positioned under the chin may be prescribed until initial healing occurs. Once the muscles are capable of control, the collar should not be worn.

Injections generally are not indicated. Stretching, ultrasound, or massage can be used in the initial stages. Rest and relaxation form the basis of acute therapy.

Once the muscles have started to heal, splinting will decrease. At this stage, muscle therapy can begin. The aim is to regain mobility. Mobilization techniques, gentle stretching, and range of motion exercises are required to prevent myospasm, contracture, and atrophy.

Muscle Spasm

Muscle spasm is defined as the painful contraction of a striated muscle caused by trauma, tension, or disease.[21] The spasm manifests as pain and interference in function. Contraction occurs in response to increased excitability of alpha motoneurons. Once it occurs, the pain and spasm tend to perpetuate each other and become cyclic.

The maintenance of muscle spasm is thought to be due to the ischemia induced in a skeletal muscle by its continued contraction. The muscle fatigues and lactic acid builds up leading to the release of bradykinin, causing pain.

Muscle spasm may occur spontaneously, followed by myositis or protective splinting. It may also present itself in response to the central excitatory effect of deep pain located elsewhere.[30] True muscle spasm is to be differentiated from myofascial trigger points. In true muscle spasm, motor unit activity contracts the whole muscle, overriding group exchange and resulting in shortening. The symptoms of myofascial pain dysfunction syndrome (MPDS), as described by Laskin,[18] have sometimes been attributed to muscle spasm.[31,47] Pa-

tients with MPDS have been observed to have tense and shortened muscles and increased resting electromyographic levels.[47] Travell and coworkers,[26] as far back as 1942, proposed the pain-spasm-pain theory for cyclic muscle spasm; however, their concept does not hold true in all cases of muscle shortening.

Motor activity is evident in a muscle that contains trigger points when it is stretched to a point of pain. This is a protective response to limit stretching and to bring the muscle back to resting level. Currently, it is thought that spasm may occur in muscles that have trigger points. The actual spasm is distinguished from trigger points by muscular rigidity and shortening accompanied with pain and dysfunction of the structure the muscle attaches to.[31]

In the masticatory musculature, a spasm of the masseter or temporalis muscle results in limited range of motion, which in turn causes a deflection to the ipsilateral side on opening. If a spasm is isometric, the muscle will be rigid and resistant to stretch. Although the exact nature of the attachment to the disc is controversial, most workers concede that the lateral pterygoid muscle influences disc function and that spasm of the inferior lateral pterygoid can cause malocclusion. Condylar position can be affected in true spasm of the elevator muscles and may predispose a patient to internal derangement.[49]

In the cervical area, a muscle spasm can create a host of problems[50] including severe pain and rigidity of the neck, secondary vertebral shifts and locking, entrapment of nerves with pain radiating to the innervated area, and forced adaptation to a new postural position.[51] Eventually, this spasm can affect the middle and low back muscles.[52] In addition to severe headaches and dysfunction, a change may occur in the maxillomandibular relationship, resulting in a malocclusion.[54] As with all chronic pain, the severe pain and inability to function can bring about psychosocial problems.[55]

Diagnosis

History. There will be a history of trauma, although there may be a time lag between the injury and the spasm. This interval is due to the development of spasm followed by myositis and protective splinting that went untreated.

Symptoms. The onset of symptoms is usually sudden and is related to an acute contraction of the muscle and an increase in pain, as the muscle is moved or stretched. An associated reduction in movement of the affected structure occurs. The pain is of the somatic type and is described as deep, boring, and constant. Depending on the area of spasm, secondary symptoms may be reported and may be related to nerve entrapment, vertebral restriction, postural adaptive syndromes, and trigger points.

Clinical Signs. Acute muscle spasm of the masticatory system can cause a noticeable shift in the occlusion. Subtle changes in the face may be seen and reported along with a noticeable shift in occlusal contact patterns.

Spasm of the cervical muscles may be more dramatic as seen in patients presenting with acute torticollis. Such spasm can cause tremendous pain and dysfunction on any jarring or change in head position.

Spastic muscles must be differentiated by palpation from the painful soft muscle of myositis, relatively normal albeit painful muscle splinting, and localized taut bands and areas of myofascial trigger points. In contrast, a muscle in spasm has a stiff hard surface that is painfully resistant to stretch.

Electromyographic recordings show a high degree of standing tension. The muscle will not show an appreciable increase in activity on function but will show a decrease in electromyographic activity in contrast to the contralateral side.

Pressure threshold meters and tissue compliance measurements may be useful for identification of the particular muscles in spasm. Thermography is also being investigated for routine diagnostic use.[46,56]

Treatment

Initial treatment should be directed toward eliminating the cycling spasm.

The patient should be restricted to movement within painless limits, but all function should not be eliminated. Function is necessary to regain a normal stretch reflex, which helps relax the muscle.

A stabilization (flat plane) appliance can be used to disengage the teeth for spasm in the masticatory muscles. Splints are thought to work by shutting off proprioceptive input from the teeth, which may play a role in the maintenance of spastic activity.

Muscle relaxants administered judiciously can help reduce dysfunction and spasm and can act as adjuncts to other therapy.[56]

Injection of spastic muscles,[21,32] spray and stretch techniques using vaporcoolants (ethyl chloride or fluoromethane spray),[32] and massage and accupressure techniques[58] are of help in reducing spastic activity.[57]

As the muscle starts to respond to treatment, stretching and range of motion exercises can be instituted to prevent contractures and to bring the muscle into full function.[29]

Structural factors should be corrected only after the muscle is pain-free and fully functional.

Myofascial Pain and Trigger Points

As mentioned, in 1952 Travell and Rinzler[17] introduced the myofascial pain and trigger point concept to the medical and dental professions. A myofascial trigger point is a hyperirritable locus within a taut band of skeletal muscle that is located in muscular tissue or in its associated fascia or tendon. The spot is painful on compression and can evoke characteristic referred pain and autonomic phenomena.[30]

Trigger points may be active or latent. Active trigger points may cause pain spontaneously or during movement. Latent trigger points are not painful but create weakness and restriction of movement in a muscle. These trigger points are activated by sudden overloading contraction, viral infection, cold temperature, and fatigue. Increased emotional stress can also activate a latent trigger point.

Latent trigger points afflict nearly half of the population by early adulthood.[59] Sola and Williams[60] in a study of 100 male and 100 female 19-year-old recruits, reported evidence of latent trigger points in shoulder muscles. Focal tenderness was found in 45% of the men and 54% of the women, and satellite trigger points were found in 5% of these subjects. The evidence supporting the presence of myofascial pain in acute and chronic pain is convincing.[61-63]

Because of the complex nature of the myofascial trigger points and their common presence in acute and chronic muscle dysfunction, an understanding of their clinical features is necessary. According to Travell and Simons,[32] there are seven clinical features: (1) local tenderness over the trigger point; (2) referred pain, tenderness, and autonomic phenomena; (3) palpable taut band associated with the trigger points; (4) a local twitch response of a trigger point is usually present in a palpable taut band; (5) perpetuation of trigger points; (6) a therapeutic effect when stretching a muscle with trigger points; and (7) weakness and fatigability of muscles afflicted with trigger points.

Local Tenderness of the Trigger Point

Simons[59] believes that the exquisite local tenderness is well explained by sensitization of the nerve endings of group III and group IV muscle receptors. He based this opinion on the work of Mense[64] and the fact that they are also responsible for tenderness and pain in tissue injury and inflammation.[65] Potassium and bradykinin prostaglandins, histamine, serotonin, substance-P, and leukotrienes have all been implicated in tissue sensitization. Of these, group III and group IV muscle receptors are most affected by bradykinin[66] and by prostaglandins.[67]

Referred Pain, Tenderness, and Autonomic Phenomena

These are explained by Simons[59] by four physiologic mechanisms.

Convergence projection is a mechanism in which a single cell in the spinal cord receives pain input from an internal organ and from a muscle or skin source. Because the brain has no way to distinguish the source, the pain may be interpreted as originating from the skin or muscles rather than from the internal organ.

Convergence facilitation takes place when information from a sensory nerve responding to a stimulus from the reference zone on the ascending (spinothalmic tract) neuron is facilitated by augmented activity from a trigger point or visceral source.

Axon branching of primary afferent nociceptors or peripheral branching of a sensory nerve to different parts of the body can create confusion within the brain as to the source of the pain.

Activity of sympathetic nerves may mediate referred pain from trigger points by releasing substances that sensitize primary afferent endings in the area of the referred pain.

All of these mechanisms are thought to influence referred pain phenomena. The reported location of the clinical pain from a trigger point is often not the source of the pain.

Palpable Taut Bands Associated with Trigger Points

These are characteristic of myofascial trigger points and are explained by a shortening of the muscle fiber sarcomeres within a taut band.[68] A local twitch response (LTR) is characteristic of a taut band and diagnostic of myofascial trigger points. A palpable taut band has a nodular or ropy feeling on palpation.[68]

Normal muscle function depends on an equal length of all sarcomeres throughout the muscle fiber. When a sarcomere shortens in the region of a trigger point, those distant from the trigger point have to compensate by becoming longer, affecting function.

Taut bands exhibit an *absence* of electrical activity, a quality differentiating them from muscle spasm. A muscle in a shortened position for prolonged periods may activate a latent trigger point. Attempts to stretch a muscle with a taut band to its full length produces unbearable pain.

Shortened sarcomeres are associated with depletion of ATP in the sarcoplasmic reticulum, disrupting the calcium pump causing loss of calcium uptake.[69] This effect causes temporary contraction of the muscle fiber. Rupture of the sarcoplasmic reticulum due to stressful overload may release the calcium. With an impaired or absent recovery mechanism, an uncontrolled localized contraction will be initiated. This contraction produces ischemia preventing restoration of the ATP to the sarcoplasmic reticulum, utilizing large amounts of energy with the ultimate result of muscular fatigue. This occurrence may also explain why muscles shortened for a prolonged period as in sleep may demonstrate a change from latent to acute trigger points.[68]

Local Twitch Response of a Trigger Point in a Palpable Taut Band

This is a characteristic transient contraction or "twitch" of muscle fibers in a taut band. The twitch can be stimulated by palpation and can be seen as a dimpling near the musculotendinous attachment. It is also demonstrable on an electromyogram.[70]

Perpetuation of Trigger Points

A trigger point is a region of metabolic distress due to local generation of sensitizing agents and compromise of the muscle's physiologic systems.[68] This compromise can be perpetuated by continued stress on the involved muscle. Some workers believe that nutritional factors, such as vitamin inadequacy, may play a role. Hormonal factors, hypothyroidism being the most common, can also perpetuate trigger points.

Therapeutic Effect of Stretching the Muscle with Trigger Points

The stretching of affected sarcomeres helps release contractile tension and returns the muscle to normal metabolic function with an equalization in the length of individual sarcomeres.[68] This effect is the rationale for stretching muscles before and after exercise and following physical therapy with range of motion exercises.

Weakness and Fatigability of Muscle Afflicted with Trigger Points

Muscle weakness and fatigability are often seen in patients with trigger points due to reduced circulation and hypoxia in the affected muscles.[70]

Diagnosis

History. In acute trauma, such as an automobile accident, the patient is usually specific as to the onset. If trauma was not a cause, identification of any event that may have initiated the pain and the position the patient was in at the time can give valuable information as to the etiology.

Symptoms. The pain is usually a dull or intense ache that varies daily. The pain is strongly related to posture and muscle activity. The pain can usually be localized by the patient and can be indicated on a diagramatic representation of the body. The muscles of posture and mastication are commonly affected by trigger points. The pain may occur in the same dermatome, myotome, or sclerotome. Satellite trigger points may occur within the pain reference zone. Travell and Simons[32] have delineated the pain referral zones as illustrated in Figures 8–3 to 8–20.

Clinical Signs. There will be a restricted movement with pain on passive stretching, and strong contraction will dramatically increase pain.[72] Resistive testing reveals weakness due to protective splinting.

Trigger points are palpated by rubbing the finger tip lightly along the long axis of the muscle. If present, a taut band will first be located and then the more sensitive trigger point. Applying pressure on a trigger point elicits a grimace or an involuntary sound from the patient called the "jump sign."[32] Snapping palpation of the taut band will produce an LTR confirming the presence of the trigger point. Final confirmation comes on reproduction of the patient's pain by digital pressure.

Pressure algometers quantify the amount of pressure applied to a trigger point.[46] This measurement allows the patient to visualize and

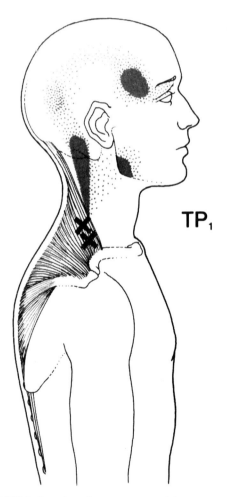

FIGURE 8–3. Referred pain pattern and location (Xs) of trigger point one in the upper trapezius muscle. Solid areas show the essential referred pain zone. Stippling maps the spillover zone. (Reprinted with permission from Travell, J. and Simons, D.: *Myofascial Pain and Dysfunction: The Trigger Point Manual.* Williams & Wilkins, Baltimore, 1983.)

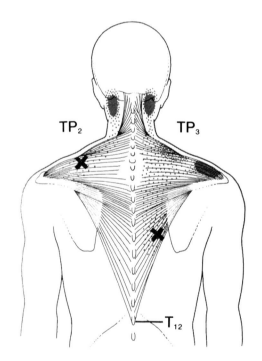

FIGURE 8–4. Referred pain patterns and locations (Xs) of trigger point two in the left upper trapezius and of trigger point three in the right lower trapezius. (Conventions are as in Figure 8–3.) (Reprinted with permission from Travell, J. and Simons, D.: *Myofascial Pain and Dysfunction: The Trigger Point Manual.* Williams & Wilkins, Baltimore, 1983.)

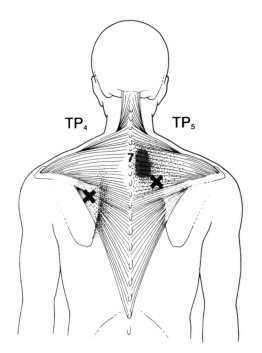

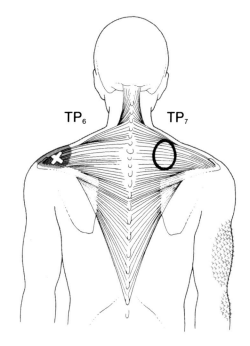

FIGURE 8–5. Referred pain patterns and locations (Xs) of trigger point four in the left lower trapezius and of trigger point five in the right middle trapezius. (Conventions are as in Figure 8–3.) (Reprinted with permission from Travell, J. and Simons, D.: *Myofascial Pain and Dysfunction: The Trigger Point Manual.* Williams & Wilkins, Baltimore, 1983.)

FIGURE 8–6. Referred pain pattern and location of trigger point six (X) in the left middle trapezius. (Conventions are as in Figure 8–3.) Trigger point seven on the right lies within the *encircled area* of the middle trapezius. The zone to which it refers pilomotor activity, or "gooseflesh," is identified on the right upper extremity by ">" symbols. (Reprinted with permission from Travell, J. and Simons, D.: *Myofascial Pain and Dysfunction: The Trigger Point Manual.* Williams & Wilkins, Baltimore, 1983.)

the clinician to document the severity of the trigger point. It may also be used to objectively record the efficacy of treatment.[73,74]

Thermography may help visualize "hot spots" that are 5 to 10 cm in diameter. Confusion exists, however, as to the thermographic presentation of the trigger point itself or the zone of referred pain. Different researchers have found the referred pain zone to be hot[75] and cold.[32] Therefore, at this time, thermogra-

phy has little application in differentiating a trigger point from a referred pain zone.

Magnetic resonance imaging (MRI) is being considered as a method of detecting active trigger points by looking for changes in the phosphorus concentration and thus the levels of ATP.[68]

Text continued on page 132

FIGURE 8–7. Referred pain patterns (*solid* shows essential zones and *stippling* shows the spillover areas) with location of corresponding trigger points (Xs) in the right sternocleidomastoid muscle. *A,* The sternal (superficial) division. *B,* The clavicular (deep) division. (Reprinted with permission from Travell, J. and Simons, D.: *Myofascial Pain and Dysfunction: The Trigger Point Manual.* Williams & Wilkins, Baltimore, 1983.)

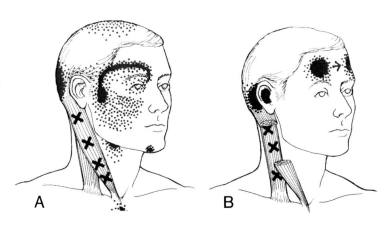

A   B

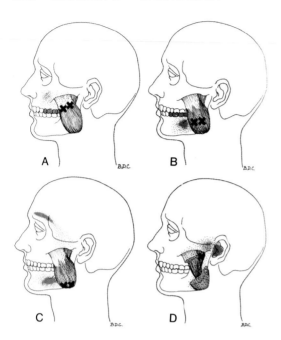

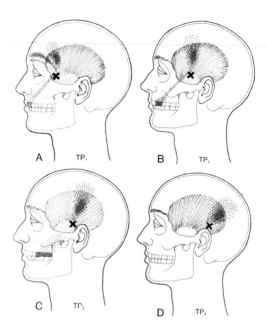

FIGURE 8–8. The Xs locate trigger points in various parts of the masseter muscle. *Solid areas* show essential referred pain zones, and *stippled areas* are spillover pain zones. *A,* Superficial layers, upper portion. *B,* Superficial layer, midbelly. *C,* Superficial layers, lower portion. *D,* Deep layer, upper part—just below the temporomandibular joint. (Reprinted with permission from Travell, J. and Simons, D.: *Myofascial Pain and Dysfunction: The Trigger Point Manual.* Williams & Wilkins, Baltimore, 1983.)

FIGURE 8–9. Referred pain patterns from trigger points (Xs) in the left temporalis muscle (essential zone *solid,* spillover zone *stippled*). *A,* Anterior "spokes" of pain arising from the anterior fibers (trigger point one region). *B* and *C,* Middle spokes (trigger point two and trigger point three regions). *D,* Posterior supra-auricular spoke (trigger point four region). (Reprinted with permission from Travell, J. and Simons, D.: *Myofascial Pain and Dysfunction: The Trigger Point Manual.* Williams & Wilkins, Baltimore, 1983.)

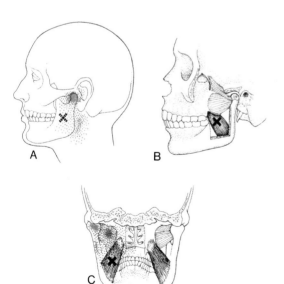

FIGURE 8–10. Referred pain pattern *(solid)* and location of the responsible trigger point (X) in the left medial pterygoid muscle. *A,* External areas of pain to which the patient can point. *B,* Anatomical cutaway to show the location of the trigger point area in the muscle, which lies on the inner side of the mandible. *C,* Coronal section of the head through the temporomandibular joint, looking forward, showing internal areas of pain. (Reprinted with permission from Travell, J. and Simons, D.: *Myofascial Pain and Dysfunction: The Trigger Point Manual.* Williams & Wilkins, Baltimore, 1983.)

FIGURE 8–11. The referred pain pattern *(stippled area)* of trigger points (Xs) in the left lateral pterygoid muscle (right). (Reprinted with permission from Travell, J. and Simons, D.: *Myofascial Pain and Dysfunction: The Trigger Point Manual.* Williams & Wilkins, Baltimore, 1983.)

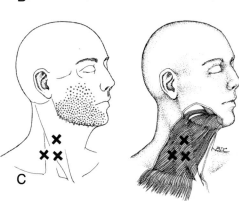

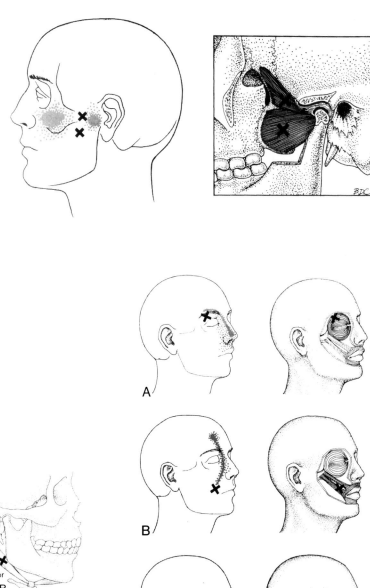

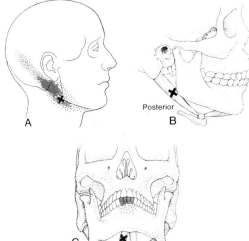

FIGURE 8–12. Referred pain pattern (essential portion, *solid area;* spillover portion, *stippled area*) of trigger points (Xs) in the right digastric muscle. *A* and *B,* Posterior belly, side view. *C,* Anterior belly, front view. (Reprinted with permission from Travell, J. and Simons, D.: *Myofascial Pain and Dysfunction: The Trigger Point Manual.* Williams & Wilkins, Baltimore, 1983.)

FIGURE 8–13. Pain patterns *(stippled areas)* and the trigger points (Xs) from which the pain is referred. *A,* Orbital portion of the right orbicularis oculi muscle. *B,* Right zygomaticus major muscle. *C,* Right platysma muscle. (Reprinted with permission from Travell, J. and Simons, D.: *Myofascial Pain and Dysfunction: The Trigger Point Manual.* Williams & Wilkins, Baltimore, 1983.)

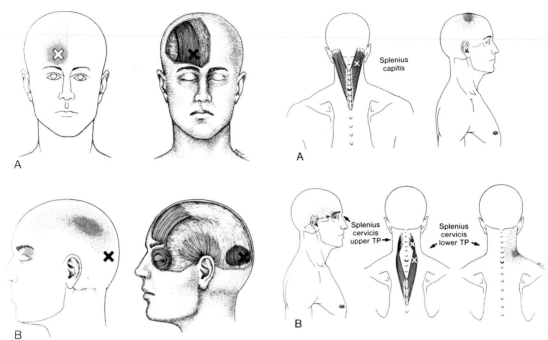

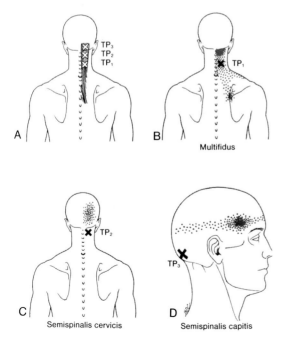

FIGURE 8–14. Pain patterns *(stippled areas)* referred from trigger points (Xs) in the occipitofrontalis muscle. *A,* Right from talis belly. *B,* Left occipitalis belly. (Reprinted with permission from Travell, J. and Simons, D.: *Myofascial Pain and Dysfunction: The Trigger Point Manual.* Williams & Wilkins, Baltimore, 1983.)

FIGURE 8–15. Trigger points (Xs) and referred pain patterns *(stippled areas)* for the right splenius capitis and splenius cervicis muscles. *A,* The splenius capitis trigger point, which overlies the occipital triangle. *B,* The upper splenius cervicis trigger point (figure on the *left*) refers pain to the orbit. The *dash line* and *arrow* indicate that the pain seems to shoot through the inside of the head to the back of the eye. The lower splenius cervicis trigger point (figure on the *right*) refers pain to the angle of the neck. The *middle* figure shows upper and lower splenius cervicis trigger points. (Reprinted with permission from Travell, J. and Simons, D.: *Myofascial Pain and Dysfunction: The Trigger Point Manual.* Williams & Wilkins, Baltimore, 1983.)

FIGURE 8–16. Referred pain patterns and their trigger points (Xs) in the medial posterior cervical muscles. *A,* Three major trigger point (TP) locations. *B,* TP_1 lies deep at the C_4 or C_5 level in the multifidi or rotatores. It is the posterior cervical trigger point most commonly found and often leads to entrapment of the greater occipital nerve. *C,* TP_2 in the third-layer semispinalis cervicis. *D,* The uppermost TP_3 in the semispinalis capitis. (Reprinted with permission from Travell, J. and Simons, D.: *Myofascial Pain and Dysfunction: The Trigger Point Manual.* Williams & Wilkins, Baltimore, 1983.)

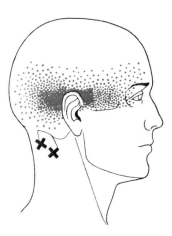
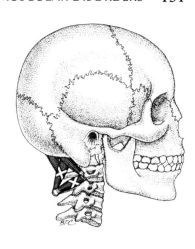

FIGURE 8–17. Referred pain pattern *(stippled area, left)* of trigger points (Xs) in the right suboccipital muscles *(right)*. (Reprinted with permission from Travell, J. and Simons, D.: *Myofascial Pain and Dysfunction: The Trigger Point Manual.* Williams & Wilkins, Baltimore, 1983.)

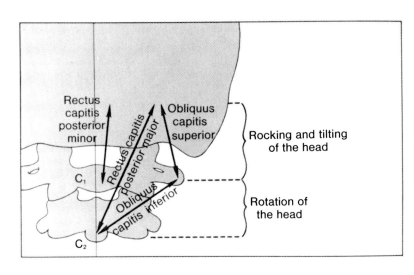

FIGURE 8–18. Graphic summary of the actions of the right suboccipital muscles. (Reprinted with permission from Travell, J. and Simons, D.: *Myofascial Pain and Dysfunction: The Trigger Point Manual.* Williams & Wilkins, Baltimore, 1983.)

FIGURE 8–19. Consolidated referred pain pattern of the two trigger point locations (Xs) for the right levator scapulae muscle. The essential pain pattern is *solid,* and the spillover pattern is *stippled.* (Reprinted with permission from Travell, J. and Simons, D.: *Myofascial Pain and Dysfunction: The Trigger Point Manual.* Williams & Wilkins, Baltimore, 1983.)

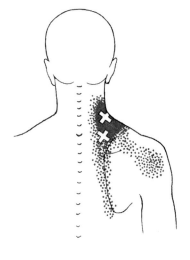
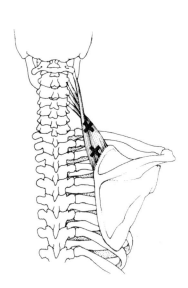

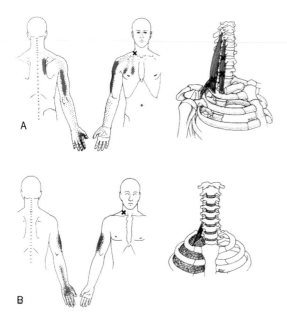

FIGURE 8–20. Composite pain pattern (*solid areas* are the essential and *stipples areas* are the spillover pain reference zones) with location of trigger points (Xs) in the right scalene muscles. *A,* Scalenus anterior, medius, and posterior. Some trigger points may have only one essential reference zone. *B,* Scalenus minimus. (Reprinted with permission from Travell, J. and Simons, D.: *Myofascial Pain and Dysfunction: The Trigger Point Manual.* Williams & Wilkins, Baltimore, 1983.)

Treatment of myofascial trigger points includes the following:

1. Spraying the involved muscle with ethyl chloride or fluoromethane followed by stretching.[76]
2. Hot compresses and range of motion exercises.
3. Trigger point injections of procaine (0.5% solution in saline) or lidocaine (2% *without* epinephrine).[68]
4. Ischemic compression for 30 to 60 seconds.[68]
5. Accupressure.[58]
6. Pharmacologic therapy, including analgesics, muscle relaxants, antidepressants, and nonsteroidal anti-inflammatory medication.[56,77]
7. Correction of posture.[41,53]
8. Stress management.[78]
9. Sleep management.
10. Stabilization of nutritional and metabolic factors.[32]
11. Exercise.[21]
12. Occlusal appliances and correction of occlusion for masticatory muscle involvement.

Fibrositis and Fibromyalgia

The term fibrositis was introduced in 1904 by Bowers[33] to describe muscular rheumatism. Fibrositis has been synonymous with myofascial trigger points,[32] myofibrositis,[34] and fibromyalgia and describes a chronic generalized aching in muscles accompanied by fatigue and disturbed sleep. This condition is a form of nonarticular rheumatism[80] and is considered a connective tissue disorder.

Fibrositis and fibromyalgia can be confused with myofascial trigger points and the myofascial pain syndrome.[81] It has a predilection for females,[82] an unknown etiology, and tends to be of a systemic nature.[82] The more generalized symptoms may be the only distinguishing factor from myofascial trigger points.

Diagnosis
Symptoms. The symptoms include widespread aching lasting more than 3 months,[83] accompanied by disturbed sleep, stiffness, and fatigue. An increase in symptoms may occur on exposure to cold and sudden changes in temperature. Anxiety and depression often accompany the symptoms.

Signs. The patient will complain of tender sites in muscles but no trigger points or taut bands will be detected. Other signs include

- Skin roll tenderness over the upper scapular region
- Normal joint and muscle strength
- Muscle spasm accompanied by tender, fibrotic nodules and erythema at the palpated site
- No significant electromyographic change (muscle functions)
- Reduced tolerance compared with normal tissue in pressure and pain threshold meters.

Treatment
Currently, no therapy other than supportive therapy is available for fibrositis. Nonsteroidal anti-inflammatory agents, antidepressants, and muscle relaxants can be provided for muscle pain. Psychologic support for anxiety and depression may be necessary. Physical therapy and stretching exercises for maintaining muscular range of motion and other exercises to build up muscle strength are sometimes helpful.

Fibrosis and Contracture

Myotatic contracture occurs in muscles that are not allowed to function within their full range of motion. The muscle will tend to lose its stretch reflex capabilities, and a gradual shortening of the muscle occurs. Pain or immobilization of a part for a prolonged period leads to myotatic contracture.[15]

In the masticatory musculature this problem can occur owing to the unwillingness or inability of patients to open their mouths fully. Patients frequently report avoiding opening wide for fear of hearing clicking or crepitus; others may not open wide because of past or present pain. Over time, this practice leads to the development of a habituated protective pattern causing myotatic contracture. Likewise, restricted movement of the cervical region results in myotatic contracture. This condition is alleviated with treatment.

Myofibrotic contracture often occurs as a result of an inflammatory process leading to fibrous changes in the muscle or its sheath. Trauma to a muscle and the resultant inflammation and muscle splinting may lead to fibrosis—an irreversible condition.[15] Radiation therapy, incision through a muscle with fibrotic healing, and disuse for long periods (more than 6 weeks) also can result in myofibrotic contracture.

Diagnosis

Symptoms. In patients with masticatory muscle involvement, myotatic or myofibrotic contracture will appear with limited interincisal opening. If the elevator muscles are involved, there will be deviation on opening but not on protrusion. Lateral movement will be normal.

Pain will not be present without sudden and forceful stretching or biting. Usually, a history of injury or long-term immobility of the mandible exists. Acute or chronic malocclusion will not occur as a result of contracture.

Signs. Palpation will generally not elicit pain, especially with a myofibrotic type of contracture.

Tests. Decreased electromyographic activity will be seen when the muscle is contracted. Pressure and pain tolerance meters show lower thresholds. Plain radiography, computerized tomographic (CT) scan, arthrography, or MRI scan of the TMJ can be done to rule out internal derangement.

Treatment

The treatment for myotatic contracture is gradual stretching of the involved muscle. Ultrasound, with 5 to 10% hydrocortisone cream, can be used as adjunct therapy. Massage and myofascial release along with daily stretching

and exercise will bring the muscle slowly back to function.

Myofibrotic contracture is irreversible and requires surgical intervention for a patient whose function is severely impaired.

Myalgia Due to Chronic Sustaining Parafunctional Activity

Oral parafunction includes bruxism,[84,85] clenching, lip biting, thumb sucking, and any other oral habit not associated with mastication, deglutition, and speech.[86,87] Bruxism and clenching are the most common of the parafunctional activities with a prevalence of up to 90% in the general population.[88,89]

In most patients, parafunction occurs in a milder intermittent form and does not require treatment. If moderate or severe, bruxism and clenching can create havoc on the oral structures causing wear of the teeth, breakdown of the periodontium in the presence of inflammation, and internal derangement and muscular dysfunction.[90]

Studies on bruxism and clenching have reported excessive force occurring for extended periods,[91] whereas normal tooth contact during a 24-hour period is about 20 minutes, occurring during chewing and swallowing.[87] Parafunctional forces exceed normal masticatory forces, and the resultant force vector is primarily horizontal. Under such conditions, damage is likely to occur to the teeth and periodontium. Ironically, most treatments are designed to protect the occlusion in function rather than in parafunction.

It appears that damage occurs based on the "weakest link" theory.[93] If one considers the teeth, periodontium, TMJs, and muscles as "links in a chain" working together for proper function, the detrimental effects of parafunction cause breakdown in the weakest of these structures. The other structures remain relatively healthy or become secondarily affected. For example, an individual may initially show parafunctional wear of the canines, leading to a shift of forces to the other teeth. If these teeth are strong enough to withstand the excessive force, the pathology may shift to the TMJ. The patient can, therefore, present with both tooth and joint pathology.

Bruxism and clenching have been explained historically by theories of occlusion,[94] but to date have yet to be substantiated by research. Theories relating bruxism as a nervous system disorder have also been proposed.[95] Nocturnal bruxism is currently classified as a sleep disorder, the duration and intensity of which varies nightly based on the emotional stress and pre-sleep activities of the individual.[84] Sleep studies have shown that bruxism occurs during body movement [95] and changes in heart rate and respiration.[91] Bruxism occurs during the rapid eye movment (REM) stage of sleep and during the transition from a deeper to a lighter stage of sleep.[84]

Numerous studies have been done on the personality characteristics of "bruxers."[95,97] People who clench and grind their teeth have been shown to exhibit higher degrees of anxiety, aggressiveness, and hostility.[95,98] The conclusions of these and other studies have confirmed an emotional etiology of diurnal (daytime) parafunction.[99,100] Diurnal parafunctions include lip biting, nail biting, thumb sucking, clenching, and habitual bruxism. The pathologic effects are the same as those for nocturnal parafunction.

Myalgia Secondary to Chronic Sustaining Parafunctional Activity

Excessive tension in the masticatory muscles due to nocturnal or diurnal parafunction can lead to muscle dysfunction. Headache, neck pain, and facial pain are common sequelae.[100] Chronic parafunction may lead to hypertrophy, spasm, tears, and development of myofascial trigger points.[32,90]

Diagnosis

Symptoms. Hypertrophy of the masseter can secondarily obstruct the opening of the parotid gland (Stensen's duct), causing a back-up of saliva with associated swelling, pain,[101] and occasional xerostomia. Depending on the muscles involved, the patient may complain of pain in the affected areas or, when trigger points are activated, in the referral zones.

Associated internal derangement can occur in the presence of myalgia of the elevator or lateral pterygoid muscles. Excessive contraction of the elevator muscles will load the TMJs if posterior tooth support has been compromised. Chronic contraction of the lateral pterygoid muscle from parafunction may predispose a patient to internal derangement.

Excessive muscle tension generated during sleep may cause muscle tears and myositis with swelling.[90] Patients may present with pain in the cervical muscles due to chronic bruxism and clenching. Electromyographic studies have shown an interrelationship of cervical muscle activity and occlusal contact (Fig. 8–21).[102] The patient may report restless sleep, waking up with limited mandibular range of motion and headache, facial pain, and neck pain. The pain and stiffness usually improve as the day progresses.

If a patient complains of stiffness and pain increasing as the day progresses, diurnal activity should be suspected. The patient may report high levels of stress and depression. Palpable muscle soreness will primarily affect the elevators and the lateral pterygoid. Increased pain will be noted if the patient is asked to clench on the wear facets by moving the mandible laterally—this is called a provocation test.

A testing device known as a Bruxscore has been used as a means of quantifying nocturnal activity (Fig. 8–22).[103,104] A portable electromyographic biofeedback instrument has also been utilized to monitor bruxism.[98] A tape recorder can monitor bruxing noises but is not very reliable because clenching does not produce significant noise.

Repeated monitoring on different nights at a sleep laboratory will give the most accurate monitoring; however, this is rarely necessary. Electromyographic analysis may show a higher resting tension level than normal but is dependent on the specific type of muscle disorder and the specific muscle being analyzed.

Treatment

The treatment of parafunctional activity must attend to three areas:

Therapeutic modalities for stress leading to parafunctional activity include biofeedback,

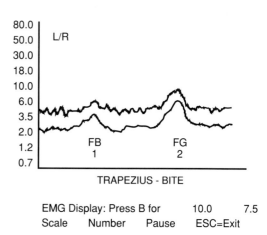

FIGURE 8–21. Bilateral electromyographic activity of the trapezius muscles showing the response of the muscles to occlusal full bites (FB).

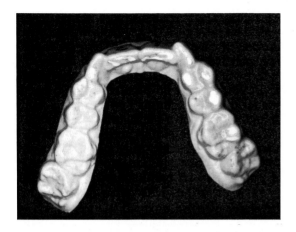

FIGURE 8–22. Bruxscore device to evaluate parafunction. The device is constructed of four laminated colored plastic sheets approximately $\frac{1}{200}$-inch in total thickness, with 14,400 microdots/inch^2 on the surface. The material can be vacuformed on the patient's model. Scoring is done by counting the surface microdots missing and multiplying by the level of color 1–4. (Courtesy of Dr. Forgione, Tufts University School of Dental Medicine, Boston.)

stress management,[105] medication,[106] and psychologic counselling.[105] The goal is to decrease parafunction to within the adaptive capacity of the individual.

Protective treatment of the oral structures is best accomplished with occlusal appliances worn at night, during the day, or both, which reduce loading on the TMJ, stress on the dentition and periodontium, and muscle activity.

Treatment of the muscles themselves includes oral medication, trigger point injection, and physical therapy. The individual's muscular problems should be diagnosed and treated. Specific treatments have been previously discussed.

Myalgia Secondary to Posture

The stability and function of the cervical region depends on the position of the head on the shoulders. The position is affected by gravity and the functional adaptation of the individual.[107]

A healthy craniocervical complex maintains a stable head position through a series of learned complex antagonistic muscle interactions. An infant cannot keep the head up on the shoulders because coordinated neuromuscular control has not yet been learned. Once control develops, low-grade postural tension is constant, maintaining a normal curve.[108,109]

Studies on different head postures have shown that forward head posture (FHP) leads to shortening and greater tension of the posterior cervical muscles.[107,110] The trapezius, sternocleidomastoid, and deeper muscles contract to prevent the head from tipping forward, leading to muscle hyperactivity and chronic tension.

Often, the patient develops a level of tension that leads to pain. A common example is the general muscle aches that plague the sedentary office worker.[111,112] Over time, shortened muscles tend to develop trigger points and the accompanying symptoms. Chronic postural inactivity may lead to fibromyalgia. The cervical spine is forced to adapt to the forces applied by strong cervical muscles, and this may result in a loss of normal cervical lordosis.[53]

The body adapts to FHP by rounding of the shoulders, leading to chronic shortening of the pectoral muscles, which further maintains FHP. Pectoral muscle tension along with FHP leads to upper thoracic breathing and tighter intercostal muscles.[113] The anterior and middle scalenes may entrap the brachial plexus at the thoracic outlet, or the first rib can be pulled up to the clavicle resulting in costoclavicular entrapment.[9]

Mehta and Forgione[113] have discussed the effect of chronic FHP and the relative position of the occiput, atlas, and axis with respect to each other and the craniomuscular complex. Forward head posture and cervical muscle tension can lead to changes in occlusal contacts.[102,114] Analyzing occlusal contact in maximum intercuspation with the patient in a supine position will not allow an accurate evaluation of occlusion in function. Likewise, posture and stability of the cervical region should be considered before definitive occlusal therapy is instituted.

Sleep Posture

Proper positioning during sleep is important for resting the postural muscles. A patient who habitually sleeps on his or her stomach and twists the neck at 90 degrees to the body experiences the same effects as the individual who keeps the head turned to one side all day long. People who sleep on their sides with the arms outstretched under the pillow and head may have a tendency to entrap the brachial plexus at the costoclavicular level. This side position can be abusive to the cervical muscles and can result in acute torticollis of the sternocleidomastoid muscle. Neck stiffness and trigger points are observed in patients with sleep habits that involve strained head positions.[115]

Standing posture may be affected by leg length discrepancies, hip rotation, and flat feet.[113] Individuals who work over machinery in a leaning position are likely to suffer from cervical and low back symptoms. Shoes that are unevenly worn or that have extremely high heels affect balance and tend to cause a secondary protective adjustment of the postural muscles.[79] This adjustment may result in chronic muscular shortening, trigger points, and spasm. Shifts in body posture and compensatory cervical changes affect mandibular position and tooth contact patterns (Fig. 8–23).

Diagnosis

Symptoms

1. Pain and stiffness related to the patient's sleep or daily activity
2. Chronic aching in the postural cervical muscles especially evident in the trapezius and sternocleidomastoids
3. A feeling of the head being too heavy on the neck
4. Forward head position
5. Pain and burning at the root of the neck
6. Pain and restriction on full range of motion of the head

Signs

1. Pain on palpation with symptoms ranging from TPs to acute spasm
2. Limited active range of motion with pain
3. Plumb line evaluation from the ear showing extent of FHP
4. Having the patient stand against a wall and measuring the distance to the neck, head, and midback will give an indication of the degree of postural problems (see chapter 5).

5. Cervical and spinal plain films, CT or MRI scans may be needed to evaluate spinal curvature and to rule out other pathology.
6. Having the patient demonstrate positions they occupy during the day and inquiring about sleep positions will help determine etiology.

Treatment

Treatment of the affected muscle groups and correction of the posture includes the following:

1. Short-term exercise to increase range of motion and improve postural position
2. Muscle re-education to strengthen the muscles in the therapeutic postural position
3. Maintenance of muscle flexibility with a home exercise program to maintain the therapeutic postural position.

Muscle Disorders Secondary to Internal Derangement

In the presence of acute or chronic internal derangement, the muscles that support and move the joints can be secondarily affected. Protective muscle splinting helps to prevent further injury to the joint. Immobilization of the injured joint is frequently seen with anterior disc displacement without reduction (closed lock). Splinting of the masticatory elevatory muscles is maintained until the joint is healed.

The clinical finding of elevator spasm often causes the physician or dentist who is unfamiliar with TMD to prescribe muscle relaxants. These override the body's defense mechanisms

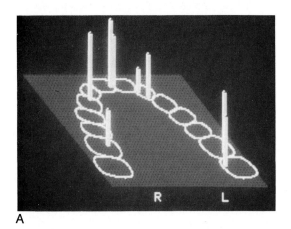
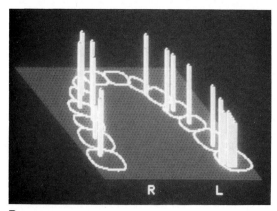

A   B

FIGURE 8–23. Computerized readout of occlusal contact patterns before (A) and after (B) ultrasound treatment of the trapezius muscle.

and proper treatment of the internal derangement would result in cessation of the muscle splinting.

If the internal derangement is not adequately treated, the muscles remain chronically shortened and may eventually undergo contracture.[15] A patient with acute closed lock often presents with a history of clicking. The patient may or may not be able to pinpoint an eliciting event. Sometimes, the patient wakes up in the morning with the jaw locked. Other times, it can occur during chewing. The patient will often have loss of posterior support through tooth wear, tooth breakdown, or missing or poorly restored posterior teeth.[116]

Closed lock may be accompanied by a change in occlusion resulting from disc displacement, accompanying spasm of the lateral pterygoid, or both. There may be a shift of the occlusion to the contralateral side with a corresponding posterior open bite developing on the ipsilateral side. The patient may attempt to position the posterior teeth into contact but is hampered by the joint pain and by the lateral pterygoid, pulling the mandible in the opposite side.

In acute trauma, the occlusion settles back to its preinjured state once the TMJ inflammation has subsided. If, however, the patient has a parafunctional habit or a lost vertical dimension,[116] the joint will continue to be loaded and healing will be delayed. In such instances, the joint may become chronically inflamed and the muscles of mastication may continue to be in a state of protective splinting, spasm, or both.

If a patient has a combination of acute trauma, loss of posterior teeth, and moderate to severe parafunction, it is likely to bring about an anterior disc displacement with intermittent locking of the TMJ. Patients will often report histories of trauma that are followed by a variable period of clicking, progressively increasing in frequency, culminating in an abrupt disappearance and an inability to open the mouth. Differential diagnosis of a patient who has limited opening must include internal derangement as well as muscle trismus.

Muscle Disorders Secondary to Cervical Spinal Dysfunction

Muscle disorders may occur secondarily to rotations, fixations, fusions, or injury or locking of the facets of the cervical, thoracic, lumbar, and sacral vertebrae. The history, physical examination, and radiographic evaluation, often done in conjunction with a physiatrist or orthopedist, will reflect the acuteness and severity of the vertebral problem.[117]

Disc herniations can secondarily affect the cervical muscles through protective splinting, which can eventually lead to chronic postural changes. Nerve impingement and nerve root injuries can also affect muscle function. Commonly seen cervical problems in relation to TMDs occur at the following cervical levels.

Occiput/Atlas

A reduction in the space between the posterior spine of the atlas and the base of the occiput as reported by Rocabado[53] (Fig. 8–24) may cause pain by compression of the suboccipital tissues. The pain will be perceived as a headache starting from the back of the head.

Acute or long-standing trauma can cause a shift in the occiput/atlas relationship and may lead to chronic tension in the suboccipital muscles with resulting fixation and nerve irritation of the C1 and C2 nerves. The pain will be referred from the back of the head to the eye, along the side of the head, along the skin over the TMJ, and down along the angle of the mandible, radiating into the neck.[118]

Rotation of the atlas is commonly seen in patients with TMDs and may be linked to changes in occlusal contact patterns and insta-

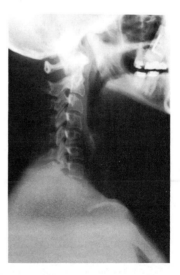

FIGURE 8–24. Cervical radiograph of patient with whiplash injury. Note the loss of normal curve, especially at C_4–C_6; also note the reduction of the suboccipital space between occiput and atlas.

bility of mandibular position.[113] Osteoarthritic degeneration and ligament and muscle injury also occur at this level in acceleration/deceleration injuries.

Atlas/Axis Level

Trauma to this level may cause a disruption of the transverse ligament holding the odontoid process of the axis against the anterior arch of the atlas.[118] This can allow for a forward subluxation or dislocation of the atlas on the axis.

A disruption of the C1-C2 articulation also may result in excessive stretching or kinking of the vertebral artery due to hypermobility. This may lead to temporary vertebrobasilar syndrome with symptoms of vertigo, nausea, tinnitus, and visual disturbances.[119]

A reduction in cervical rotation will be seen because 40 to 50% of rotation occurs around the atlas/axis articulation.[118] Pain also limits movement. Fractures are always to be considered in trauma to the atlas/axis region.

C4, C5, and C6

The level of greatest instability against acceleration/deceleration forces appears to be the C5-C6 region,[120] with C4-C5 being primarily affected in hyperextension and C5-C6 in hyperflexion.[121] Trauma can be to the ligaments, discs, and vertebral bodies dependent on the direction and magnitude of the force.

The cervical curve can be affected (see Fig. 8–24), and the patient will often have a compensatory FHP further perpetuating the problem. Nerve root injuries or spinal cord impingement may occur in cervical trauma and must be evaluated (Fig. 8–25).

Other cervical, thoracic, lumbar, and sacral

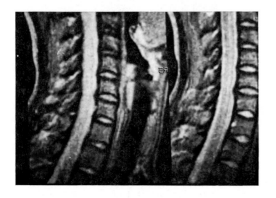

FIGURE 8–25. Magnetic resonance imaging of patient showing constriction of spinal cord at C_5–C_6.

areas may also be affected as discussed elsewhere in this text.

Diagnosis

The patient will have a history of direct or indirect injury to the head and neck.

The symptoms range from headaches, nausea, visual disturbances, neck weakness, pain, and stiffness accompanied by noises on rotation, flexion, and extension of the head.[119] Depending on the level of the initial injury, branches of the cervical and brachial plexus and the areas they supply can also be affected. Secondary muscles affected can cause superimposed acute or chronic pain; therefore, a specific cervical evaluation must be done.

Testing for cervical damage requires full orthopedic and neurologic evaluation.[122] Plain radiography and CT or MRI imaging are useful for visualizing hard and soft tissue damage of the vertebral area. Electromyography, nerve conduction, thermography, and pressure algometry testing are helpful in evaluating nerve and muscle function.

Treatment

Treatment may require initial immobilization if there is structural damage. This initial phase should last only as long as it takes to allow healing.

Next, the patient should receive soft tissue mobilization to regain lost range of motion (see chapter 24).

Depending on the effect of the cervical problem on the masticatory system or vice versa, occlusal appliances may be worn to reduce muscle tension.[79]

Pain management includes muscle relaxants, nonsteroidal anti-inflammatory agents, and antidepressants.

Specific muscle therapy depends on the nature of the muscular problem. Generally, techniques of spray and stretch, trigger point injections, heat and ultrasound, electrogalvanic stimulation, transcutaneous electrical nerve stimulator (TENS) accupressure, and acupuncture are acceptable for reducing muscle symptoms.

Chronic pain brings about anxiety and depression, which may require psychologic management. Sleep is often disturbed and antidepressant medication may be required until the pain subsides.[105,106]

After the pain and dysfunction are controlled, range of motion exercises are started to regain full movement. This is imperative to prevent chronic myotatic or myofibrotic contractures.[15]

The patient should follow a muscle rehabilitation program, including slow controlled muscle strengthening to prevent ongoing muscle dysfunction.

The patient's nutritional needs and general health need to be considered.

REFERENCES

1. Scheman, P.: The differential diagnosis of so-called temporomandibular joint disease. N.Y. Dent. J. 4:46, 1980.
2. Arlen, H.: The otomandibular syndrome. In *Clinical Management of Head, Neck and TMJ Pain and Dysfunction*, 2nd ed. H. Gelb (ed.). W.B. Saunders Co., Philadelphia, 1985.
3. Graham, G.: Differential diagnosis of temporomandibular disorders. Gen. Dent. 31:474, 1983.
4. Clark, G.: Examining temporomandibular disorder patients for craniocervical dysfunction. J. Craniomand. Pract. 2:55–63, 1983.
5. Malkin, D.P.: The role of TMJ dysfunction in the etiology of middle ear disease. Ind. J. Orthodont. 25:20, 1987.
6. Gelb, H. and Gelb, M. Taking the mystique out of the diagnosis and treatment of craniomandibular (TMJ) disorders. Intern. Dent. J. 39:129, 1989.
7. Bezuur, J.N., Hansson, T., and Wilkinson, T.M.: The recognition of craniomandibular disorders. An evaluation of the most reliable signs and symptoms when screening for CMD. J. Oral Rehabil. 16:367, 1989.
8. Schellhas, K.P., Wilkes, C.H., and Baker, C.C.: Facial pain, headache and temporomandibular joint inflammation. Headache 29:228, 1989.
9. Mehta, N.R., Forgione, A.G., Rosenbaum, R., and Holmberg, R.: "TMJ" triad of dysfunctions: A biological basis of diagnosis and treatment. J. Mass. Dent. Soc. 4:173, 1984.
10. Bishop, B.: *Basic Neurophysiology*. Medical Examination Publication Co., Garden City, NY, 1982.
11. Eriksson, P.O., Eriksson, A., Ringquist, M., and Thornell, L.E.: Special histochemical muscle fibre characteristics of the human lateral pterygoid muscle. Arch. Oral Biol. 26:495–507, 1981.
12. Eriksson, P.O. and Thornell, L.E.: Histochemical and morphological muscle fibre characteristics of the human masseter, the medial pterygoid and the temporal muscles. Arch. Oral Biol. 28:781–795, 1983.
13. McCall, W.D., Jr.: The musculature. In *A Textbook of Occlusion*. N. Mohl, G. Zarb, G. Carlson, and J. Rugh (eds.). Quintessence Publishing Co., Lombard, IL, pp. 97–108, 1988.
14. Christensen, L.V.: Jaw muscle fatigue and pains induced by experimental tooth clenching. A review. J. Oral Rehabil. 8:27–36, 1981.
15. Bell, W.: *Clinical Management of Temporomandibular Disorders*. Year Book Medical Publishing, Chicago, 1982.
16. Bell, W.: *Orofacial Pains. Classification, Diagnosis and Management*, 4th ed. Year Book Medical Publishing, Chicago, 1989.
17. Travell, J. and Rinzler, S.H.: The myofascial genesis of pain. Postgrad. Med. 11:425–434, 1952.
18. Laskin, D.M.: Etiology of the pain-dysfunction syndrome. J. Am. Dent. Assoc. 79:147–153, 1969.
19. Bell, W.E.: Clinical diagnosis of the pain-dysfunction syndrome. J. Am. Dent. Assoc. 79:154–160, 1969.
20. Hansson, T.: Temporomandibular joint changes related to dental occlusion. In *Temporomandibular Joint Problems*. W.K. Solberg and G.T. Clark (eds.). Quintessence Publishing Co., Lombard, IL, 1980.
21. Kraus, H.: *Diagnosis and Treatment of Muscle Pain*. Quintessence Publishing Co., Lombard, IL, 1988.
22. Headache Classification Committee of the International Headache Society: Classification diagnostic criteria for headache disorders, cranial neuralgias and facial pain. Cephalgia 8(Suppl 7):1–96, 1988.
23. *Dorland's Illustrated Medical Dictionary*, 27th ed. W.B. Saunders Co., Philadelphia, 1988.
24. Gutstein, M.: Diagnosis and treatment of muscular rheumatism. Br. J. Phys. Med. 1:301–321, 1938.
25. Good, M.G.: Rheumatic myalgias. Practioner 146:167–174, 1941.
26. Travell, J., Rinzler, S., and Herman, M.: Pain and disability of the shoulder and arm: Treatment by intramuscular infiltration with procaine hydrochloride. J.A.M.A. 120:417–422, 1942.
27. Gillette, H.E.: Office management of musculoskeletal pain. Texas State J. Med. 62:47–53, 1966.
28. Alling, C.C. II and Mahan, P.C.: *Facial Pain*, 2nd ed. Lea & Febiger. Philadelphia, 1977.
29. Bell, W.E.: *Orofacial Pains*, 4th ed. Yearbook Medical Publishers, Chicago, 1989.
30. Kraus, H.: *Muscle Spasm in Diagnosis and Treatment of Muscle Pain*. Quintessence Publishing Co., Lombard, IL, 1988.
31. Bell, W.E.: Masticatory muscle function. In *Clinical Management of Temporomandibular Disorders*. Year Book Medical Publishers, Chicago, 1982.
32. Travell, J.G. and Simons, D.G.: *Myofascial Pain and Dysfunction: Trigger Point Manual*. Williams & Wilkins, Baltimore, 1983.
33. Bowers, W.R.: Lumbago. Its lessons and analogies. Br. Med. J. 1:117–121, 1904.
34. Llewellyn, L.J. and Jones, A.B.: *Fibrositis*. Rebman, New York, 1915.
35. Hench, P.K.: Nonarticular rheumatism. In *Rheumatic Diseases: Diagnosis and Management*. W.A. Katz (ed.). J.B. Lippincott, Philadelphia, 1977.
36. Awad, E.A.: Interstitial myofibrositis. Hypothesis of the mechanism. Arch. Phys. Med. 54:440–453, 1973.
37. Wolff, H.G. and Wolf, S.: *Pain*, 2nd ed. Charles C Thomas, Springfield, IL, 1958.
38. Lim, R.J.S.: Pain Ann. Rev. Physiol. 32:269–270, 1970.
39. Handwerker, H.O.: Influences of algogenic substances and prostaglandins on the discharges of unmyelinated cutaneous nerve fibers identified as nociceptors. In *Advances in Pain Research and Therapy*. J.J. Bonica and D.G. Albe-Fessard (eds.). Raven Press, NY, 1976.
40. Travell, J.: Referred pain from skeletal muscle; pectoris major syndrome of breast pain and soreness and sternomastoid syndrome of headache and dizziness. N.Y. State J. Med. 55:331–340, 1955.
41. Rocabado, M., Johnson B.E., Jr., and Blakney, M.: Physical therapy and dentistry: An overview. J. Craniomand. Pract. 1:46–49, 1983.
42. Gordon, E.J.: Diagnosis and treatment of common neck disorders. Med. Trial Tech. 26:162–194, 1980.
43. Bland, J.H.: Cervical spine syndromes. J. Musculoskel. Med. 23–41, Nov. 1986.

44. Blumenthal, L.S.: Injury to the cervical spine as a cause of headache. Postgrad. Med. 56:147–153, 1974.
45. Forgione, A.: Personal communication, 1989.
46. Fischer, A.A.: Documentation of muscle pain and soft tissue pathology. In *Diagnosis and Treatment of Muscle Pain.* H. Kraus (ed.). Quintessence Publishing Co., Lombard, IL, 1988.
47. Frost, H.M.: Musculoskeletal pain. In *Facial Pain,* 2nd ed. C.C. Alling and P.E. Mahan (eds.). Lea & Febiger, Philadelphia, 1977.
48. Zseisengreen, H. and Elliott, H.W.: Electromyography in patients with orofacial pain. J. Am. Dent. Assoc. 67:798, 1963.
49. Mehta, N.: Personal communication, 1989.
50. Gelb, H. and Tarte, J.: A two-year clinical dental evaluation of 200 cases of chronic headache. The craniocervical mandibular syndrome. J. Am. Dent. Assoc. 91:1230–1236, 1975.
51. Valtonen, E.: The tension neck syndrome: its etiology, clinical features and results of physical treatment. Ann. Med. Int. Tenn. 57:139–142, 1968.
52. Waris, P.: Occupational cervicobrachial syndromes. Scand. J. Work Environ. Health 6(Suppl 3):3–14, 1980.
53. Rocabado, M.: Biomechanical relationship of the cranial cervical and hyoid regions. J. Craniomand. Pract. 7:61–65, 1983.
54. Schokker, R.P., Hansson, T.L., and Ansink, J.J.: Craniomandibular disorders in headache patients. J. Craniomand. Dis. Facial Oral Pain 3:71–74, 1989.
55. Lee, Y.O. and Lee, S.W.: A study of the emotional characteristics of temporomandibular disorder patients using SCL-90-R. J. Craniomand. Dis. Facial Oral Pain 3:25–34, 1989.
56. Pogrel, M.A., Erbez, G., Taylor R.C., and Dodson, T.B.: Liquid crystal thermography as a diagnostic aid and objective monitor for TMJ dysfunction and myogenic facial pain. J. Craniomand. Dis. Facial Pain 3:65–70, 1989.
57. Bell, W.E.: Orofacial pains. In *Management of Patients in Pain,* 4th ed. Year Book Medical Publishers, Chicago, 1989.
58. Forgione, A.: Personal communication, 1990.
59. Simons, D.G.: Myofascial pain syndrome due to trigger points. Intern. Rehab. Med. Assoc. IRMA Monograph Series No. 1., Nov. 1987.
60. Sola, A. E. and Williams, R.C.: Myofascial pain syndromes. Neurology 6:91–95, 1956.
61. Fishbain, D.A., Goldberg, M., Meagner, B.R., et al: Male and female chronic pain patients characterized by DSM III psychiatric and diagnostic criteria. Pain 26:181–197, 1986.
62. Simons, D.G. and Travell, J.G.: Myofascial origins of low back pain: Principles of diagnosis and treatment. Postgrad. Med. 73:66–77, 1983.
63. Fricton, J.R., Kroening, R., Haley, D., and Siegart, R.: Myofascial pain syndrome of the head and neck: A review of clinical characteristics of 164 patients. Oral Surg. 60:615–623, 1985.
64. Mense, S.: Nervous outflow from skeletal muscle following chemical noxious stimulation. J. Physiol. 267:75–88, 1987.
65. Perl, E.R.: Unraveling the story of pain. In *Advances in Pain Research and Therapy,* vol. 9. H. L. Fields, et al (eds.). Raven Press, New York, 1985.
66. Franz, M. and Mense, S.: Muscle receptors with group IV afferent fibres responding to application of bradykinin. Brain Res. 92:369–383, 1975.
67. Frost A.: Diclofenac vs. lidocaine as injection therapy in myofascial pain. Scand. J. Rheumatol. 15:153–165, 1986.
68. Simons, D.G. and Travell, J.G.: Myofascial trigger points: a possible explanation. Pain 10:106–109, 1981.
69. Rowland, L.P., Araki, S., and Carmel, P.: Contracture in McArdle's disease. Arch. Neurol. 13:541–544, 1965.
70. Fricton, J.R., Auvinen, M.D., Dykstra, D., and Schiffrman, E.: Myofascial pain syndrome: Electromyographic changes associated with local twitch response. Arch. Phys. Med. Rehabil. 66:314–317, 1985.
71. Lund, N., Bengtsson, A., and Thorborg, P.: Muscle tissue oxygen pressure in primary fibromyalgia. Scand. J. Rheumatol. 15:165–173, 1986.
72. McDonald, A.J.R.: Abnormally tender muscle regions and associated painful movements. Pain 8:197–205, 1980.
73. List, T., Helkimo, M., and Falk, G.: Reliability and validity of a pressure threshold meter in recording tenderness in the masseter muscle and the anterior temporalis muscle. J. Craniomand. Pract. 7:223–229, 1989.
74. Reeves, J.L., Jaeger, B., and Graff-Radford, S.B.: Reliability of the pressure algometer as a measure of myofascial trigger point sensitivity. Pain 24:313–321, 1986.
75. Fischer, A.A.: Correlation between site of pain and "hot spots" on thermogram in lower body. Academy of Neuromuscular Thermography: Clinical Proceedings. Postgrad. Med. (Custom communications) March, 1986.
76. Simons, D.G.: Myofascial pain syndromes due to trigger points. 2. Treatment and single-muscle syndromes. Manual Med. 1:72–77, 1985.
77. Gessel, A.H.: Electromyographic biofeedback and tricyclic antidepressents in myofascial pain dysfunction syndrome. Psychological predictors of outcome. J. Am. Dent. Assoc. 92:1048–1052, 1975.
78. Carlsson, S.G., Gale, E.N., and Ohman, A.: Treatment of temporomandibular joint syndrome with biofeedback training. J. Am. Dent. Assoc. 91:602–605, 1975.
79. Gelb, H.: Craniocervical mandibular disorders. In *Diagnosis and Treatment of Muscle Pain.* H. Kraus (ed.). Quintessence Publishing Co., Lombard, IL, 1988.
80. Kaplan, H.: Psychogenic rheumatism. Ariz. Med. 32:280–281, 1975.
81. Bennet, R.M.: The fibrositis fibromyalgia syndrome: Current issues and prospectives. Am. J. Med. 81(Suppl 3a):8–15, 1986.
82. Wolfe, F.: The clinical syndrome of fibrositis. Am. J. Med. 81(Suppl 3a):7–14, 1986.
83. Smythe, H.A.: Fibrositis and other diffuse musculoskeletal syndromes. In *Textbook of Rheumatology,* vol. 1. W.N. Kelly, et al (eds.). W.B. Saunders Co., Philadelphia, 1989.
84. Wruble, M.K., Lumley, M.A., and McGlunn, F.D.: Sleep-related bruxism and sleep variables: A critical review. J. Crandiomand. Disord. Facial Oral Pain 3:152–158, 1989.
85. Nadler, S.C.: Bruxism: A critical review. Psych. Bull. 84:767–781, 1972.
86. Scharer, P.: Bruxism. In *Frontiers of Oral Physiology, Physiology of Mastication,* vol. 1. Y. Kawamura (ed.). Basel, Switzerland, S. Karger, 1974.

87. Graf, H.: Bruxism. Dent. Clini. North Am. 13:659, 1969.
88. Reding, G.R., Rubright, W.C., and Zimmerman, S.O.: Incidence of bruxism. J. Dent. Res. 45:1198–1204, 1966.
89. Solberg, W.K., Woo, M.W., and Houston, J.B.: Prevalence of mandibular dysfunction in young adults. J. Am. Dent. Assoc. 98:25–34, 1979.
90. Rugh, J.D. and Orbach, R.: Occlusal parafunction. In *A Textbook of Occlusion.* N. Mohn, G. Zarb, G. Carlsson, and J. Rugh (eds.). Quintessence Publishers, Lombard, IL, 1988.
91. Reding, G.R., Zepelin, H., Robinson, J.E., Jr., et al: Nocturnal teeth grinding: All night psychologic studies. J. Dent. Res. 42:786–797, 1968.
92. Mehta, N.R., Glickman, I., Haddad, A.W., and Roeber, F.W.: Portable electronic system for studying tooth contact patterns in bruxism. Int. Assoc. Dent. Res. Abstract no. 993, 1972.
93. Mehta, N.R.: Bruxism and its interrelationship to the oral structures—The weak link theory. In preparation, 1990.
94. Ramfjord, S.P.: Bruxism, a clinical and electromyographic study. J. Am Dent. Assoc. 62:36–58, 1961.
95. Olkinuora, M.: A psychosomatic study of bruxism with emphasis on mental strain and familiar predisposition factors. Proc. Finn. Dent. Soc. 68:110–123, 1972.
96. Ware, J.C. and Rugh, J.D.: Destructive bruxism: Sleep stage relationship. Sleep, 11:172–181, 1988.
97. Glaros, A.G. and Rao, S.M.: Bruxism: A critical review. Psych. Bull. 84:767–781, 1977.
98. Vernallis, F.E.: Teeth-grinding: Some relationships to anxiety, hostility and hyperactivity. J. Clin. Psychol. 11:389–391, 1955.
99. Christensen, L.V.: Experimental teeth clenching in man. Swed. Dent. J. Suppl. 60, 1989.
100. Villarosa, G.A. and Moss, R.A.: Oral behavioral patterns as factors contributing to the development of head and facial pain. J. Prosthet. Dent. 54:427–430, 1985.
101. Ahlgren, J., Omnell, K.A., Sonesson, B., and Toremalm, N.G.: Bruxism and muscle hypertrophy of the masseter muscle. Pract. Otorhinolaryngol. 31:22–29, 1969.
102. Mehta, N.R.: Evaluation of a possible cervical/occlusal interrelationship. Presented at the Annual Meeting of the American Equilibration Society. Chicago, Feb. 15–16, 1989.
103. Forgione, A.: A simple but effective method quantifying bruxism behavior. J. Dent. Res. 53(Special issue): Abstract No. 292, P127, 1975.
104. Mejias, J. and Mehta, N.R.: Subjective and objective evaluation of bruxing patients undergoing short-term splint therapy. J. Oral Rehab. 9:279–289, 1982.
105. Rugh, J.: Behavioral therapy. In *A Textbook of Occlusion.* N. Mohl, G. Zarb, G. Carlsson, and J. Rugh (eds.). Quintessence Publishing Co., Lombard, IL,1988.
106. Greg, J.M. and Rugh, J.: Pharmacological therapy. In *A Textbook of Occlusion.* N. Mohn, G. Zarb, G. Carlsson, and J. Rugh (eds.). Quintessence Publishing Co., Lombard, IL, 1988.
107. Duncan, J. and Feguson, D.: Keyboard operating posture and symptoms. Operating Ergonomics 17:651–662, 1974.
108. Brodie, A.G.: Anatomy and physiology of head and neck musculature. Am. J. Orthod. 11:831–834, 1950.
109. Last, R.J.: The muscles of the head and neck. A review. Int. Dent. J. 5:338–354, 1955.
110. Alanen, P.J. and Kirveskari, P.K.: Occupational cervicobrachial disorder and temporomandibular joint dysfunction. J. Craniomandib. Pract. 3:70–72, 1985.
111. Onishi, N., Nomura, H., Sakai, K., et al: Shoulder muscle tenderness and physical features of female industrial workers. J Hum. Ergol. 5:87–102, 1976.
112. Waris, P.: Occupational cervicobrachial syndromes. Scand. J. Work Environ. Health 6(Suppl. 3): 3–14, 1980.
113. Mehta, N. and Forgione, A.: Postural effects on occlusal contacts. In press, 1990.
114. Goldstein, D.F., Kraus, S.L., Williams, W.B., and Glasheen-Wray, M.: Influence of cervical posture on mandibular movement. J. Prosthet. Dent. 52:421–424, 1984.
115. Travell, J. and Simons, D.: Scalene muscles. *Myofascial Pain and Dysfunction: The Trigger Point Manual.* Williams & Wilkins, Baltimore, 1983.
116. Kipp, S. and Carlsson, G.: The temporomandibular joint: Problems related to occlusal function. In *A Textbook of Occlusion.* N. Mohl, G. Zarb, G. Carlsson, and J. Rugh (eds.). Quintessence Publishing Co., Lombard, IL, 1988.
117. Fitz-Ritson, D.E.: Neuroanatomy and neurophysiology of the upper cervical spine. In *Upper Cervical Spine.* H. Vernon (ed.). Williams & Wilkins, Baltimore, 1988.
118. Grice, A.S.: Pathomechanics of the upper cervical spine. In *Upper Cervical Syndrome.* H. Vernon (ed.). Williams & Wilkins, Baltimore, 1988.
119. Croft, A.C.: Soft tissue injury long and short term effects. In *Whiplash Injuries.* S. Foreman and A.C. Croft (eds.). Williams & Wilkins, Baltimore, 1988.
120. McKenzie, J.A. and Williams, J.F.: The dynamic behavior of the head and cervical spine during whiplash. J. Biomech. 4:477–490, 1971.
121. Jackson, R.: Anatomy. In *The Cervical Syndrome.* R. Jackson (ed.). Charles C Thomas, Sprinfield, IL, 1977.
122. Hoppenfeld, S.: *Orthopedic Neurology.* J.B. Lippincott, Co., Philadelphia, 1977.
123. Conley, T.E.: A neurologist's view of myofascial pain. In *Diagnosis and Treatment of Muscle Pain.* H. Kraus (ed.). Quintessence Publishing Co., Lombard, IL, 1988.
124. Sonkin, L.S.: Myofascial pain in metabolic disorders. In *Diagnosis and Treatment of Muscle Pain.* H. Kraus (ed.). Quintessence Publishing Co., Lombard, IL, 1988.

Richard A. Pertes
Ronald Attanasio

CHAPTER 9

Internal Derangements

With the advent of sophisticated diagnostic and imaging techniques and the development of arthroscopy, a great deal of information concerning craniomandibular disorders (CMD) has emerged. What formerly was anecdotal evidence has now been confirmed by many researchers and clinicians.

Various researchers have reported that the frequency of signs of dysfunction in a general population may vary from 25 to 50%, depending on the particular study. The most frequently reported sign was a clicking sound in the temporomandibular joint (TMJ) that was evenly distributed among all age groups and sexes.[1-3] Clicking is considered to be characteristic of an internal derangement (ID) of the TMJ.

Probably the most often quoted definition of ID of the TMJ has been provided by Dolwick[4] who defined it as "an abnormal relationship of the articular disc to the mandibular condyle, fossa, and articular eminence."

Although not specifically stated, the term ID implies that there is a mechanical disturbance of normal function. Clinically, internal derangements are characterized by interference of restriction of joint function during mandibular movement. Joint noise, especially clicking, is a common finding. Whether any dysfunction is accompanied by pain depends on the adaptive capacity of the patient, because each individual reacts to the same noxious input at different levels of suffering.

In addition to ID, degenerative joint disease is another common intracapsular disorder involving the TMJ. In the past, these terms had been used interchangeably. As defined by Moffett,[5] however, degenerative joint disease is "the pathologic final common pathway for all diseases, injuries, and derangements that affect a joint during its life cycle." A cause and effect relationship appears to exist between these two entities, and in many patients an untreated ID may progress through a series of gradual changes to degenerative joint disease or arthrosis.[6,7] Both ID and degenerative joint disease are noninflammatory disorders. Continuation of the degenerative process may result in true inflammatory degenerative arthritis (see chapter 10).

Many members of the general population with the characteristic click of an ID do not develop pain, experience significant dysfunction, or progress to a more serious disorder.[8] Therefore, questions concerning clinical management arise. Should asymptomatic patients with clicking be treated or should any derangement be allowed to progress to a chronic disease state? Is repositioning the mandible through appliance therapy to reduce a displaced disc a valid objective of treatment? And, if repositioning is successful, is permanent stabilization of the joint through occlusal changes necessary to prevent a recurrence of any symptoms?

Thus, even in the light of new and abundant findings, there are conflicting viewpoints regarding treatment of a patient with an ID. This chapter attempts to provide some insight into a most perplexing problem.

HISTORICAL PERSPECTIVE

Interest in intracapsular disorders of the TMJ is not of recent origin. The first descriptions of the structural characteristics of internal derangements of the TMJ were published by Annandale,[9] in 1887, and Pringle,[10] in 1918. Wakely,[11] in 1929, discussed the causal relationship of trauma to the posterior attachment of the disc and to disc displacement. Correlation of clinical symptoms to structural dysfunction was also reported by Goodfriend,[12] in 1932.

It was not until 1934, when Costen,[13] an otolaryngologist, described a group of apparently unrelated clinical symptoms about the ear, sinus, and head areas related to a derangement in the TMJ that the problem received serious attention. In attributing these symptoms to mandibular overclosure due to "the lack of molar teeth or badly fitting dental plates permitting overbite," Costen made "TMJ" a dental problem. He reasoned that trauma to the meniscus as a result of the condyles being shoved upward and backward probably caused perforation of the meniscus, compression of the eustachian tubes, and pressure and irritation to various nerves in the area.

Costen's theory, however, was unable to account for those symptoms that were initially related to the masticatory musculature and fell into disrepute. In the 1950s, Schwartz[14] advanced the new view that many of the symptoms were caused by spasm within the masticatory muscles as a result of muscle tension due to stress. Laskin,[15] in the 1960s, further refined Schwartz's concepts and proposed the psychophysiologic theory that also implicated emotional factors. The various symptoms were gathered into one syndrome that he called the "myofascial pain dysfunction syndrome (MPDS)." A shift in thinking occurred that emphasized the neuromuscular system rather than occlusion and the structures of the joint.

Nevertheless, investigation into the mechanics of the joint continued. Ireland,[16] in 1951, described how a disc displacement of the TMJ could create clicking sounds and progress to locking of the joint. Documentation of his observations was provided through tomograms. With the development of arthrography, Norgaard[17] was able to provide visualization of disc displacements. Wilkes further advanced the use of this technique by adding fluoroscopy.[18,19] It was not until Farrar[20-22] published several articles on internal derangements in the 1970s and challenged the muscle spasm concepts that the emphasis shifted back to the articular structures of the joint.

The 1980s have seen the development of computerized tomographic (CT) scanning and magnetic resonance imaging (MRI) to both diagnose internal derangements and assess treatment results. Arthroscopic surgery, once utilized primarily for knees, is now an acceptable technique both as a diagnostic tool and in the management of some intracapsular disorders. Although the emphasis is now on the joint, almost all clinicians agree that an unbiased approach to diagnosis and treatment must be used without regard to any particular "camp" or technique.

BIOMECHANICS OF THE TEMPOROMANDIBULAR JOINT

In order to understand abnormal joint function, the clinician must have a working knowledge of normal TMJ function. The TMJ is unique in the respect that the joint of one side cannot function without movement in the op-

posite joint, thereby creating a bilateral articulation between the mandible and the cranium—the craniomandibular articulation. It is also the only joint in the human body with a rigid end point of closure, which is provided by the teeth.[23] This relationship between the teeth and the joint structures places the management of craniomandibular disorders in the field of clinical dentistry.

The true key to normal joint function lies in understanding the active role of the articular disc in maintaining joint stability throughout all movements of the mandible. By dividing the joint cavity into two distinct cavities each with a different function, the articular disc creates a double joint, one above the other. The condyle articulates with the disc to form the lower joint, the disc-condyle complex, where only hinge or rotational movement occurs in a healthy joint. An upper joint is formed by the articulation of the disc-condyle complex with the posterior slope of the articular eminence. Normally, only translatory movement takes place in the upper joint.[24-26]

During the translatory cycle, a combination of rotation in the disc-condyle complex occurs in conjunction with sliding movement in the upper joint. As the disc-condyle complex moves forward on the articular eminence in the opening phase, the condyle rotates anteriorly in the inferior concavity of the disc while, at the same time, the disc rotates posteriorly on the condyle. This mechanism provides stability in the joint during movement by having the condyle function against the thin, intermediate zone of the disc, which is avascular and non-innervated.[24,25]

It has been assumed until lately that fibers of the superior belly of the lateral pterygoid acted to protract the disc. New anatomic studies, however, have revealed that most of the fibers of the superior lateral pterygoid attach to the neck of the condyle with very few, if any, going directly to the disc.[27-29] The question of whether a protractor of the disc exists is now the subject of considerable debate.

Posterior rotation of the disc is accomplished by the superior retrodiscal lamina that is part of the posterior attachment. This structure, which is attached to the posterior border of the disc, is composed of connective tissue giving it the property of elasticity. During rest and in the closed joint position, the superior retrodiscal lamina is relaxed and does not influence disc position. Only during the forward phase of the translatory cycle does the superior retrodis-

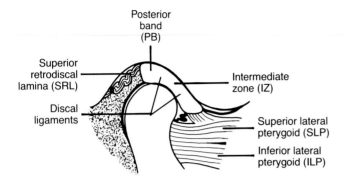

FIGURE 9–1. Lateral view of the normal disc-condyle relationship in the closed-joint position. Superior retrodiscal lamina (SRL), posterior band (PB), intermediate zone (IZ), discal ligaments, superior lateral pterygoid (SLP), and inferior lateral pterygoid (ILP). Note the self-seating capacity of the disc due to its biconcave shape. (Modified from Okeson, J.P.: *Management of Temporomandibular Disorders and Occlusion,* 2nd ed. C.V. Mosby Co., St. Louis, 1989.)

cal lamina become active and retract the disc posteriorly on the condyle.

Normal joints do not exhibit any sliding movement between the condyle and disc primarily because of the firm attachment of the disc to the condyle at the medial and lateral poles by discal ligaments. Similar to all ligaments, they are nonelastic and cause the disc to move passively with the condyle in an anterior and posterior direction.[30] Another factor preventing translation between the condyle and disc is the self-seating capacity of the disc. This is due to the biconcave shape of the disc created by a thin central or intermediate zone connecting a thick posterior and slightly less thick anterior band.[31] When viewed sagittally, the posterior band ends at the apex of the condyle in the 12-o'clock position when the teeth are in maximum intercuspation (Figs. 9–1 and 9–2).[16]

All movements of the TMJ should be friction-free, noise-free, and pain-free. Any damage to joint structures can interfere with normal function, possibly leading to pain, dysfunction, or both.

ETIOLOGY OF INTERNAL DERANGEMENTS

Most internal derangements appear to be related to either acute or chronic insult to the TMJ complex. In general, causes of internal derangements can be classified under the broad headings of acute macrotrauma, chronic microtrauma, or developmental and acquired defects.

Acute Macrotrauma

Macrotrauma involves an external source of injury to the TMJ, such as a blow to the mandible, mandibular whiplash, and mandibular hyperextension. Katzberg and coworkers[32] reported that one fourth of patients who had IDs that were confirmed by arthrography revealed a histories of injury to the mandible just before the onset of symptoms. In another study, 43% of patients presenting with symptoms related to a TMJ disorder had a previous history of injury to the head or neck.[33]

With trauma to the mandible, the extent of

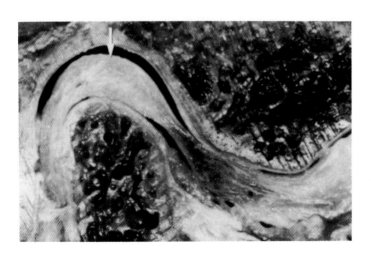

FIGURE 9–2. Sagittal section of a temporomandibular joint autopsy specimen with the biconcave disc in the normal (superior) position. Arrow indicates posterior band superior to the condyle. (Reproduced with permission from Rohlin, M., Westesson, P.L., and Eriksson, L.: J. Oral Maxillofac. Surg. 43:194, 1985.)

damage is dependent on the magnitude and direction of the force of impact. If a direct blow to the chin from a face-on direction is involved, a condyle may fracture or both condyles may be driven into the retrodiscal structures. An inflammatory response in these highly vascularized and innervated tissues is likely to occur as well as damage to the temporomandibular ligament. Should the blow be offset to one side of the mandibular symphysis, the contralateral condyle may sustain more damage than the ipsilateral joint.

Various studies have shown that mandibular whiplash can occur concurrently with cervical whiplash.[34–37,94] In such an event, it has been hypothesized that the extreme hypertranslation of the condyle from the glenoid fossa may stretch and possibly tear the posterior attachment as well as the medial and lateral discal ligaments. This action could predispose the patient to disc displacement.

There have been reported cases of patients associating the onset of TMJ-related symptoms to oral surgical procedures or intubations for general anesthesia.[23] The mechanism appears to be similar to that encountered with mandibular whiplash and involves excessive condylar hypertranslation for a prolonged period of time.

Cervical traction with a chin strap may provide an excessive loading force on the TMJ.[38] This may precipitate symptoms in patients who already have compromised TMJ structures because of a previous injury or a lack of posterior dental support as a result of missing teeth. The presence of posterior teeth allows forces from cervical traction to be distributed over a wider area including the maxilla rather than concentrating them in the joint area. A pre-existing disc displacement may also be exacerbated by cervical traction. Fortunately, newer cervical traction units have been modified to eliminate this potential problem. Macrotrauma is discussed in detail in chapters 11 and 12.

Chronic Microtrauma

Microtrauma involves a source of low-grade trauma to the TMJ over a long period of time. Included in this category are forces that overload the joint complex or disturb the normal relationship of the condyle, disc, and eminence.

Bruxism, and clenching in particular, can have a destructive effect on the TMJ through excessive overloading. Normal TMJ biomechanics may be altered, as synovial fluid is expressed. Any extended compressive forces on these tissues may cause deformation by altering the delicate balance between form and function.[31] Articular remodeling, which is the normal adaptive response of healthy tissue to mechanical forces acting on the joint, can be replaced by degenerative changes. In the TMJ, the articular disc is more vulnerable to degeneration and deformation than are the articular surfaces of the condyle and eminence. This likely occurs because the disc does not appear to have the capacity for cellular remodeling due to a lack of blood vessels.[5]

Loss of posterior support of the dental arches may contribute to overloading of the joint structures. In fact, any deficiency in molar support may permit the condyle to impact against the disc, causing deformation or deterioration.[30] Whether the result is a deepening of the central bearing area of the disc or a change in the borders of the disc depends on disc location at the time of overloading. Articular surfaces may be roughened by abrasive movement, setting the stage for a true disc displacement in the future.

Although bruxism appears to be the primary activating agent involved in any excessive pressure produced on the joint structures, the role of emotional tension must also be considered.[15,40] Sustained emotional stress increases muscle tonus in the elevator muscles and interarticular pressure within the joint. These can activate any pre-existing condition and precipitate an ID.

Role of Occlusion

The role of occlusal factors, such as prematurities and interferences in the etiology of internal derangements, is muddled in controversy.[41,42] To date, no conclusive studies have yet demonstrated a positive correlation between occlusal factors and internal derangements, although a relationship has been shown to exist between masticatory muscle function and occlusal factors. The nature of occlusion as an etiologic factor in internal derangements, therefore, may well be an indirect one related to chronic microtrauma. Perhaps Bell's statements that "Occlusal interference serves primarily as a predisposing factor that requires activating before it becomes etiologically important" and that "Emotional tension and bruxism are the important activating factors" are most appropriate.[24]

Confusion also abounds with respect to malocclusion as an etiologic factor in the development of ID. Clinical studies that have attempted to establish a relationship have been equivocal. Pullinger and associates[43] found that among dental students, TMJ tenderness was more frequent in class II division 2 subjects than in class I. However, these investigators were not able to associate clicking with a specific Angle class.

What may be of more significance than either occlusal factors or malocclusions may be the orthopedic relationship of the mandible to the maxilla. This relationship, of course, is determined by the inclined planes of the teeth meeting in maximum intercuspation. Proponents are of the opinion that malrelationship of the mandible to the maxilla may cause the various components of the disc-condyle complex to be malpositioned with respect to optimum function. In particular, they have focused on abnormal condylar position in the fossa as a prime factor in the etiology of internal derangements.[44-47] This focus has led to therapeutic procedures designed to place the condyle into a more "normal" position in the fossa. Unfortunately, various studies in this area have not been in agreement and the link between abnormal condylar position and internal derangements is still not clear.

Developmental and Acquired Defects

Numerous developmental, growth, and acquired defects can alter the structural integrity of the TMJ components. Developmental anomalies include hypoplastic and hyperplastic condyles and various skeletal facial asymmetries.[48] Various endocrine and nutritional disturbances as well as tumors can involve the TMJ, leading to a disruption in function.[49]

TREATMENT PHILOSOPHY

Most patients who present for treatment related to a TMJ disorder have pain or dysfunction as the chief complaint. Other patients present with minimal symptoms and are concerned about preventing a future problem. And, unfortunately, there are those TMJ patients who have been suffering for many years possibly as a result of misdiagnosis and mistreatment. Some of these individuals might be categorized as chronic pain patients, especially if they have signs of depression and they exhibit patterns of pain behavior. Chronic pain may accompany any organic pathology of the joint. Effective therapy involves more than a mechanistic approach. Treatment should focus on the psychologic component of pain as well.

The clinician treating a patient with an ID is often asked "Can the condition be cured?" In our opinion, it is unrealistic to expect a "cure." At best, we are only managing signs and symptoms to the best of our ability within the framework of the patient's ability to cope with the disorder.

Patients who have internal derangements commonly have accompanying masticatory muscle tenderness, hyperactivity, or both.[50] In some cases, the muscle hyperactivity is the cause of the ID, whereas, in others, it is secondary to the derangement. In one study, Isberg and coworkers[51] reported that masticatory muscle activity was provoked by disc displacement and disappeared when disc position was normalized on mouth opening. Proper management, therefore, must also include the neuromuscular system for treatment to be successful.

In addition, a significant number of patients with ID may also have signs and symptoms in the cervical spine and upper back.[52] Therefore, an evaluation of the cervical spine should be part of the clinical examination.[53] Patients with positive findings should be referred for additional consultation with the appropriate health practitioner.

As part of an overall management program, those etiologic factors that initiated the disorder should be identified and their influence be reduced or eliminated. Other contributing factors can have a direct or indirect bearing on successful treatment. For example, a patient may have sustained trauma to a previously asymptomatic joint in a motor-vehicle accident that precipitated the onset of symptoms. With the stress of living with pain and disability, the patient may have also developed a persistent clenching habit. This parafunctional activity could serve as a perpetuating factor in the continuation of symptoms by overloading the joint and causing the development of masticatory muscle spasm. Failure to address the perpetuating factor in this case by not including behavior modification in the form of stress reduction or psychologic therapy would probably compromise treatment.

Temporomandibular joint therapy itself is usually divided into two phases: phase I is designed to reduce the degree of the patient's chief complaints and to encourage repair and regeneration of damaged tissues, thereby improving joint function. Treatment modalities in phase I are essentially reversible. Phase II has as its primary goal stabilization of joint structures after signs and symptoms have been significantly reduced. It involves irreversible procedures and incorporates various dental therapies, such as orthodontics, prosthetic rehabilitation, and equilibration.[54,55] Phase II is discussed elsewhere in this text.

From a long-term viewpoint, therapy for internal derangements has two main objectives: (1) the restoration of relatively normal joint function without pain and (2) the elimination of contributing factors to enable the patient to be independent of professional health care.

Management, therefore, usually involves a regimen of conservative or nonsurgical therapy over a period of several months. If conservative therapy does not significantly improve the condition within 3 to 4 months, the diagnosis should be reviewed and therapy re-evaluated. At that point, a surgical consultation may be in order. Before the advent of arthroscopy, a great deal of prolonged nonsurgical treatment took place because of the morbidity associated with open joint surgery. Arthroscopy, although a surgical procedure, is far less invasive and is often employed as an adjunct to conservative therapy both from a therapeutic as well as a diagnostic viewpoint.[56,57]

If either the conservative or the surgical approach is to be successful, consideration must be given to all aspects of patient care. Successful management, therefore, involves an understanding of the patient.

PHASE I TREATMENT

Internal derangement is essentially a biomechanical problem. Probably the most popular approach to treatment is a mechanical one, involving intraoral occlusal appliances or splints. Splint therapy cannot be used in a vacuum and must be combined with other treatment modalities to be successful.

Appliance Therapy

For many years, intraoral occlusal appliances, or splints, have been employed in conjunction with other treatment methods to manage signs and symptoms of craniomandib-

ular disorders, including IDs. Traditionally, a flat plane or stabilization splint was applied to reduce pressure on joint structures and to neutralize any harmful effect of occlusal discrepancies. Most appliances were placed in the maxillary arch and adjusted to achieve maximum contact with the opposing arch in centric relation. For the most part, no effort was made to eliminate joint noise which, on occasion, disappeared while the splint was worn.

Not until Farrar's era did the concept of repositioning the mandible anteriorly to recapture a displaced disc gain popularity. The use of anterior repositioning splints for internal derangements became widespread, and several different appliance designs evolved.

The goal of repositioning therapy is to maintain a normal relationship of the disc to the condyle when the appliance is worn. This is achieved through inclines on the splint that encourage a forward mandibular posture. Lundh and Westesson and colleagues[62] compared an anterior repositioning splint with a flat occlusal splint in the treatment of anteromedial disc displacement (ADD) with reduction. They reported that the anterior repositioning splint decreased joint pain during rest, chewing, and protrusion while eliminating the characteristic reciprocal clicking. Palpatory tenderness of the joint and masticatory muscles was also reduced. With the flat plane occlusal splint, joint tenderness was reduced but reciprocal clicking or muscle tenderness was not affected. They concluded that these cases can be successfully treated by means of positioning the mandible anteriorly.

At this point, the term "success" should be defined. The long-term effect of repositioning therapy has been questioned along with the possibility of iatrogenically introducing irreversible changes in the occlusion. Is it necessary to have both relief of pain and an absence of clicking when appliances are removed? In separate studies, Okeson[64] and Moloney and Howard[65] reported that although pain symptoms were essentially eliminated with discontinuation of the appliances, clicking returned in most cases. If these criteria apply, the success rate for repositioning therapy is low. If the clinician is willing to accept the perseverance of nonpainful joint sounds and catching during mandibular movements along with a significant reduction in pain, however, the success rate is encouraging. For those patients who have pain when splint therapy is stopped, either nighttime wearing of an appliance may be indicated or a second phase of treatment may be necessary.

Two types of appliances are frequently utilized for treating internal derangements.[66] One is a stabilization splint that is made in the patient's habitual arc of closure. The splint's primary purpose is to reduce pressure on joint structures, although the splint has been shown to reduce parafunctional activity as well. This appliance can be made for either dental arch. The appliance maintains full contact with the opposing teeth in centric occlusion and allows for movement in all directions.

The other appliance is a repositioning appliance that has as its main objective the recapture of the disc.[60] Usually, a combination of an upper and a lower appliance insures the patient's compliance. The upper appliance is worn at night and frequently has a repositioning ramp behind the maxillary incisors to prevent the mandible from retruding when the patient is reclining. A lower appliance with occlusal indents to guide the mandible into a protrusive position is worn during the day.[54] All appliances need constant monitoring and adjustment to insure that they are effective.

No "cookbook" approach is available to using occlusal splints in the treatment of internal derangements. This treatment should be based on a thorough knowledge of TMJ biomechanics. Each patient must be evaluated individually with respect to specific treatment objectives.

Pharmacologic Therapy

To control pain initially, nonsteroidal antiinflammatory agents are recommended. They should be administered in combination with rest and a mechanically soft diet, along with heat and cold applications where indicated. If chronic pain is a factor and is accompanied by a sleep disturbance, antidepressants are often effective. Muscle relaxants can be prescribed if acute muscle spasm is complicating the joint problem.[67]

Physical Medicine

Physical therapy is a necessary adjunct in many cases to control pain and restore function. Electromodalities, such as TENS, ultrasound, and iontophoresis, are particularly helpful in controlling pain. Mobilization of joint structures along with myofascial release

techniques has also been reported to be effective. An exercise program is essential, not only for its specific therapeutic benefit, but also because it involves the patient in the therapy.[68,69]

Behavior Modification

Behavior modification can be extremely valuable to reduce parafunctional activity and emotional tension. Long-standing stress has been implicated in musculoskeletal pain and dysfunction and must be considered in any management program.[70]

Medical Consultations

Frequently, a medical problem may be both a predisposing and a complicating factor. Outside referrals to various medical specialists are indicated in these cases. All treatment should be preceded by an in-depth patient education program to show the interrelationship between causative factors and various contributing factors, which may be present. Only through knowledge and awareness can the patient actively participate in recovery.

DIFFERENTIAL DIAGNOSIS OF INTERNAL DERANGEMENTS

The first step in successful management is to reach a working diagnosis in order to formulate appropriate objectives so that therapy will be effective.

Internal derangement is an intracapsular disorder. However, some signs and symptoms commonly associated with IDs may also be encountered with MPDS, which is an extracapsular disorder related to the muscles of mastication.[71,72]

Unilateral muscle tenderness, preauricular pain, headaches, and limitation of jaw function are common to both disorders. A clicking or popping noise in the TMJ has been listed by Laskin[73] as another common symptom of MPDS. Its origin is thought to be muscular incoordination of the two heads of the lateral pterygoid as opposed to the clicking in IDs, which is due to disc displacement. A simple test to differentiate between these two types of clicks is to have the patient move the mandible to the opposite side. If the click persists, it is more likely to be due to a disc displacement. Pain emanating from either source can display similar clinical characteristics that are strongly related to functional demands. Manual palpation of the muscles or functional manipulation of the TMJ will increase pain in a graduated manner.[74] Usually, joint pain is reported to be less upon awakening because it decreases with rest. However, pain related to MPDS should be expected to be worse in the morning, because it may be related to parafunctional activity, such as nocturnal bruxism.[75]

A limited opening may also be encountered with other extracapsular and intracapsular problems, including coronoid impingement, elevator muscle spasm, trismus, intracapsular adhesions, ankylosis, and even hysterical conversion reaction.[76]

In addition, the possibility of encountering an ID in both joints must be considered. Sanchez-Woodworth and associates[77] evaluated 211 patients with signs and symptoms of ID using MRI. Their results suggested that because both TMJs are interrelated, a mechanical dysfunction on one side can potentially affect the opposite joint. They also emphasized the complexity of treatment by noting that some patients may have a different stage of ID occurring in each joint.

A TMJ examination for a suspected ID should include an extensive history, a thorough clinical examination, study casts of the teeth, and screening radiographs of the TMJ. The most common radiograph for this purpose is a panoramic or lateral oblique transcranial view. Roberts and coworkers[78] reported that clinical findings alone or in conjunction with plain radiographs of the TMJ were not accurate enough to assess the specific stage of ID. They recommended an image modality that depicted the condition of the soft tissue structures. This would include arthrography or MRI with surface coils.[79,80] Direct visualization of the joint employing an arthroscope also has diagnostic merit, although it has been employed more for its therapeutic value. Diagnostic anesthetic blocks to locate the source of pain are often valuable in the differential diagnostic process.

CLASSIFICATION OF INTERNAL DERANGEMENTS

Dolwick's definition of ID as "an abnormal relationship of the articular disc to the mandibular condyle, fossa, and articular eminence" is rather restrictive in that it is limited to disc displacement. Change in disc morphology is recognized as an important feature of IDs and

may, in fact, contribute to functional impairment of the TMJ.[81] Therefore, in our expanded definition of ID, we have included disc deformations as well as dislocations of the disc-condyle complex in addition to true disc displacements. These categories are clinically related and imply an anatomic disturbance in the normal mechanics of the joint.

Medical disease classification strives for complete consistency with mutually exclusive categories. It is essentially a pragmatic affair and is designed to aid in treatment. But nature does not operate in the same manner, and several disease processes may be occurring within the TMJ at the same time, either independently or as a cause and effect relationship. Each is capable of interfering with normal function and may be a source of pain. For example, Westesson and coworkers[82,83] found a high frequency of disc deformation and articular surface irregularities associated with disc displacement.

Some categories have been deliberately omitted because of the infrequency of occurrence. These would include posterior and lateral disc displacements. It is possible that, in the future, with increased diagnostic capabilities, more cases will be reported, which would warrant their inclusion in a classification system.

Within these limits, the following classification is proposed for internal derangements of the TMJ:

I. Deviation in form
  A. Frictional disc incoordination
  B. Articular surface defects
  C. Disc thinning and perforation
II. Disc displacements
  A. Partial anteromedial disc displacement
  B. Anteromedial disc displacement with reduction
    1. Partial
    2. Complete
  C. Anteromedial disc displacement with intermittent locking
  D. Anteromedial disc displacement without reduction
    1. Acute
    2. Chronic
  E. Anteromedial disc displacement with perforation of retrodiscal tissue
III. Adhesive disc hypomobility
IV. Displacement of disc-condyle complex
  A. Subluxation
  B. Dislocation

Deviation in Form

Frictional Disc Incoordination

Optimum joint function indicates that the disc must be free to rotate on the condyle and translate against the eminence. Excessive pressure may exhaust the lubrication on the articular surface of the eminence or disc and cause roughness on the superior surface of the disc or physical adhesions between the disc and eminence.[84] According to Bell,[24] this condition may result from occlusal disharmony that displaces the disc-condyle assembly during clenching. Bruxism, excessive biting force, and trauma with the teeth together are other causes. Frictional disc incoordination usually occurs after a prolonged period of inactivity. Thus, when the translatory cycle begins, the disc may stick to the eminence and be immobile. By straining the discal ligaments, frictional disc incoordination predisposes the patient to a true disc displacement of the joint.

Clinical Signs and Symptoms. A discrete opening click may be discerned, as the inertia of the disc is overcome and it snaps back onto the condyle. Momentary discomfort may accompany the click, but the remainder of the translatory cycle is accomplished without difficulty.[84,85]

Treatment. The primary goal of treatment should be the elimination of the occlusal disharmony, which is the main etiologic factor involved. Obviously, abusive use and clenching should also be reduced. Some healing may occur if the disc-condyle complex can be prevented from returning to the closed position. This is best accomplished by applying a stabilization splint on a full-time basis for a few months. The splint should be fabricated without any repositioning component and should be balanced for both day and night wear. When symptoms have been reduced, the patient should be weaned off the splint during the day and eventually, night. At that point, occlusal equilibration should be done to eliminate the occlusal disharmony.

Articular Surface Defects

A structural defect located on the articulating surface of the eminence, the superior surface of the disc, or both may cause an impediment to normal translatory movement of the disc. The defect may be caused by trauma to the mandible when the teeth are apart, abusive use, and developmental and growth anomalies.[24]

Clinical Signs and Symptoms. Because the interference occurs at the same point in the translatory cycle, a reciprocal click can be detected at that point both during opening and closing movements. Frequently, a deviation of the incisal path occurs on opening, as the patient attempts to avert the interference. Although the condition itself is painless, it can be worsened by any increase in interarticular pressure.[24,25,85]

Treatment. Habit training to develop a path of mandibular movement that avoids the interference may allow resolution at the affected site. This should be accompanied by a conscious effort to reduce the force of chewing and eliminate abusive habits. Chewing on the affected side, by decreasing the interarticular pressure, may also be helpful. A stabilization splint may serve to reduce pressure on the joint structures.[24,25]

Disc Thinning and Perforation

As previously stated, excessive pressure on the TMJ can cause deformation in joint structures. If overloading occurs while teeth are together, thinning of the central part of the disc may result. Continuous pressure may eventually cause perforation, which usually appears as a circular hole with fragmented borders in the midbody of the disc. Fracture of the disc, leading to degenerative changes in articular surfaces of the joint, has also been reported.[31]

Clinical Signs and Symptoms. Symptoms depend on the extent of damage to the disc. From a theoretic viewpoint, thinning of the central part of the disc should not result in pain because that part of the disc is noninnervated. Practically, however, any activity that deepens the central bearing area of the disc undoubtedly will exert harmful effects on other joint structures and associated musculature. Variable joint tenderness and muscle pain should be expected.

If the disc should perforate, grating sounds or crepitus during the translatory cycle is likely because of damage of the articular surfaces.[39,86] Pain is usually a concomitant feature, which conversely may diminish as the extent of damage increases. Fracture of the disc can manifest itself clinically as an alteration in occlusion when the teeth are in maximum intercuspation. A suspected diagnosis of disc perforation should be confirmed by imaging, preferably arthrography.[79,87]

Treatment. A stabilization splint should be utilized in cases of disc thinning to prevent a perforation. If perforation has occurred, surgical intervention may be indicated because the disc lacks the capacity for regeneration. This course of treatment should be considered only in the case in which the patient can no longer tolerate the symptoms.

Disc Displacement

Because the only physiologic movement permitted between the disc and condyle is rotation, any sliding movement between the disc and condyle is abnormal. Tight discal ligaments and self-seating wedges provided by thick anterior and posterior borders of the disc preclude sliding movements. In order for the disc to slide on the condyle, a deformation of the borders of the disc must occur along with sufficient damage to the discal ligaments. The posterior margin of the disc has been thinned in most internal derangements, allowing the disc to be displaced in an anteromedial direction.[24,25] Because of joint anatomy, the lateral discal ligament is usually compromised before the medial ligament, accounting for the medial component of the displacement. Both medial and lateral ligaments may be involved in rare cases resulting in medial displacement.[87] In any of the disc displacements, the posterior attachment elongates to a varying degree, resulting in compromised function.

Disc displacements are usually viewed as a series of progressively worsening clinical entities. A study on the life history of TMJ dysfunction by Rasmussen[88] concluded that there were three phases. Phase one was characterized by clicking and lasted from 3 to 6 years. Painful locking and limited range of mandibular motion were the main features of phase two, which lasted approximately 1 year followed by crepitation and arthrosis in phase three. Other studies were not able to duplicate the findings of Rasmussen. In their study, Lundh and colleagues[89] found that only 9% of patients with reciprocal clicking (ADD with reduction) developed locking. Patients initially had more pain, joint tenderness, dental abrasion on the affected side, and increased frequency of missing molar support than patients who did not progress to locking. In another study, Pullinger and Seligman[90] concluded that "... not all closed-lock patients are the result of a dysfunction progression beginning with disk derangement." Therefore, although this classification is presented as a continuum, caution is advised before reaching any definite conclusions regarding interceptive treatment.

As previously stated, the clinical signs and symptoms of ID are nonspecific for each stage and are not consistently reliable in determining the status of the disc-condyle relationship. Kozeniauskas and Ralph[91] reported that even asymptomatic joints may have an ID as revealed by arthrography. Therefore, it may be necessary to use MRI, arthrography, or arthroscopy to confirm the clinical impression.

Partial Anteromedial Disc Displacement

In a healthy joint, the center of the posterior band of the disc is in the 12-o'clock position on the condyle when the teeth are occluded. With partial anterior disc displacement, the end of the posterior band of the disc terminates anteriorly to this position on the condyle in the closed-joint position. This effect occurs primarily because of some thinning of the posterior band in combination with minimal elongation of the discal ligaments permitting the disc to slide anteriorly on the condyle. Elongation of the disc itself is a common finding, and some stretching of the posterior attachment undoubtedly occurs (Fig. 9–3).[85]

Clinical Signs and Symptoms. Because the degree of disc displacement is not sufficient to cause a collapse of disc space, signs of clicking are usually absent. Although no gross interference with function occurs, a slight early deviation to the affected side on opening may occur. Discomfort in the joint area after prolonged clenching as well as tenderness on joint palpation may be reported by the patient. The inclusion of partial anterior disc displacement as a diagnostic category, however, is not because of its significance as a clinical entity but rather because of its role as a precursor to more damaging disc displacements.[85]

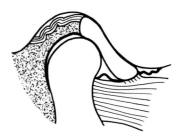

FIGURE 9–3. Partial anteromedial disc displacement in resting, closed-joint position. Because no collapse of disc space has occurred, minimum interference with joint function is encountered. (Modified from Okeson, J.P.: *Management of Temporomandibular Disorders and Occlusion,* 2nd ed. C.V. Mosby Co., St. Louis, 1989.)

Treatment. Because signs and symptoms are usually minimal, treatment is directed at preventing any worsening of the disc displacement. Intraoral appliances in combination with stress reduction are the therapies of choice. Theoretically, at least, it would appear that some degree of mandibular repositioning would be indicated to keep the condyle in proper relationship with the disc. Clinically, even a stabilization appliance appears to be helpful and it has the added advantage of minimizing the possibility of phase II therapy.

Anteromedial Disc Displacement with Reduction

Increased elongation of discal ligaments and posterior attachment can allow the disc to be displaced even farther anteromedially, creating an obstruction to normal condylar translation (Figs. 9–4 and 9–5). At the same time, deformation may be occurring in that part of the disc that is anteriorly positioned. In an autopsy study, Westesson and colleagues[83] were able to "... demonstrate a high frequency of disk deformation and irregularities of the articular surfaces associated with internal derangement." Thickening and enlargement of the posterior band was the most frequent type of disc deformation, but the most pronounced deformations included the entire disc and were often associated with a perforation of the posterior attachment. These investigators concluded that disc deformation appeared to be preceded by anterior disc displacement and was closely associated with disturbed joint function.

Although a high degree of variability of condylar position exists in patient subgroups with ID, Ronquillo and associates,[92] using arthrography, reported "... A tendency for posterior condylar position was found in patients with meniscal displacement with reduction but not in symptomatic normals or patients with meniscus displacement without reduction."

By using electromyography, Isberg and coworkers[51] were able to demonstrate an increase in elevator muscle activity with disc displacement during closing, which ceased when disc position was normalized on opening. They concluded that this finding was most likely due to an arthokinetic reflex similar to a protective mechanism seen in other joints. This activity could prevent the condyle from passing over the posterior band of the condyle to achieve reduction of the disc and could account for some of the pain associated with disc displacement. Roberts and colleagues,[93] in a study comparing arthrographic findings of the TMJ with muscle palpation, found that some muscles were tender to palpation, but they cautioned against relying on muscle palpation alone as an indicator for specific treatment of an ID.

Clinical Signs and Symptoms. Patients with ADD with reduction usually have the classic "reciprocal clicking" so well described by Farrar and McCarty.[94,95] Upon closing, a click may be detected that represents displacement of the disc anteromedially. Condylar movement recordings of patients with ID, done by Mauderli and colleagues,[96] found that a figure eight–shaped pattern was usually associated with reciprocal clicking joint sounds. An opening click representing reduction of the displaced disc coincided with the sharp upward deflection of the condyle. A soft closing click that represented displacement of the disc occurred during the deflection just proceeding full closure. These deflections in the condylar path were caused by the thick posterior band of the disc, passing between the condylar and articu-

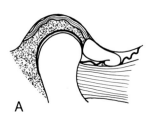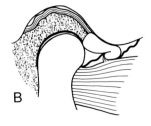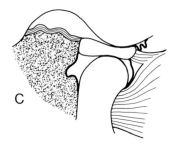

FIGURE 9–4. Anteromedial disc displacement with reduction. *A,* Resting, closed-joint position. *B,* Early stage of translation. *C,* Reduction of disc that is usually accompanied by an opening click. If reduction occurs late in the translatory cycle, the prognosis for permanent stabilization of the disc on the condyle is poor. (Modified from Okeson, J.P.: *Management of Temporomandibular Disorders and Occlusion,* 2nd ed. C.V. Mosby Co., St. Louis, 1989.)

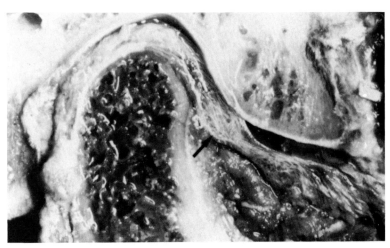

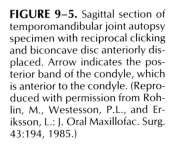

FIGURE 9–5. Sagittal section of temporomandibular joint autopsy specimen with reciprocal clicking and biconcave disc anteriorly displaced. Arrow indicates the posterior band of the condyle, which is anterior to the condyle. (Reproduced with permission from Rohlin, M., Westesson, P.L., and Eriksson, L.: J. Oral Maxillofac. Surg. 43:194, 1985.)

lar eminence. According to Oster and coworkers,[97] these opening and closing clicking sounds differed from the opening and closing sounds that were observed in patients with disc displacement without reduction and from the crepitation observed in patients with degenerative arthritis.

In a study correlating mandibular range of motion with arthrographic findings in patients with ID, Roberts and associates[98] found that patients with ADD with reduction tended to exhibit slight hypermobility in the affected joint and had a maximum opening within, or slightly greater than, the normal range. During early opening, deviation of the mandible to the affected side may be noted. When the disc is reduced, the mandible deviates away from the involved joint and returns to the midline and may even go past the midline.

A word of caution regarding occlusal interferences should be noted. With ADD, the disc space often narrows and the condyle is often found to be displaced in a posterior and superior position, resulting in occlusal interferences on the affected side. In these cases, permanent occlusal changes should not be contemplated until disc position has been normalized.[51]

Although some studies have attempted to show the progression of patients through the various stages of disc displacement to disc deformation to articular surface changes, the subject is still controversial. Why some patients remain in the category of anterior disc displacement with reduction for years while others proceed to intermittent locking and anterior disc displacement without reduction within a matter of months is still not clear. It has been hypothesized that the answer may lie

in differentiating between partial and complete ADD with reduction.[99,100]

Partial. The displacement involves only the lateral pole, and the disc rotates around the medial pole. Thus, the medial part of the disc maintains the vertical distance between the condyle and eminence. This condition may become chronic and not progress to the stage of locking.

Complete. If the entire disc is displaced anteromedially involving both the lateral and medial poles, the vertical distance between the condyle and eminence may not be maintained. The posterior band of the disc is likely to become thickened, preventing reduction and increasing the likelihood of progression to disc displacement without reduction.

Treatment. In both partial and complete ADD with reduction, mandibular repositioning appliances that stabilize a protrusive position to keep the disc in a more optimal relationship with the condyle have been advocated.[60,62,64] These appliances may also reduce pain by decreasing adverse loading in the joint. Because the long-term success for maintaining the disc in its most physiologic position is questionable, the primary purpose of protrusive splint therapy may be to allow repair and regeneration to occur in the retrodiscal tissue and possibly in the discal ligaments.[25,63] Anterior repositioning splints apparently have little effect on the condylar movement pattern.[96]

Although treatment appears to be simple from a conceptual viewpoint, several problems may be encountered. Often, the elimination of both clicking and mandibular deviation on opening and closing along with pain reduction are the guidelines to determine the effectiveness of splint therapy. However, Manzione and colleagues,[101] utilizing lower space single contrast arthrography, found that in about 50% of clinically successful cases they had, in fact, failed to recapture the disc.[101]

Another potential problem with protrusive splint therapy is that the amount of mandibular anterior repositioning needed to prevent disc displacement may be too great to stabilize through phase II occlusal changes. This factor may necessitate a compromise in terms of disc recapture, and a stabilization appliance may be indicated. Irreversible changes in occlusion (i.e., posterior open bite), as a result of protrusive splint therapy, have been reported. In spite of these drawbacks, repositioning appliance therapy appears to be a useful way of nonsurgically managing ADD with reduction, but this therapy must be employed with an awareness of potential problems in carefully selected patients.

Anteromedial Disc Displacement with Intermittent Locking

If the disc remains displaced for longer periods of time, the shape of the disc may slowly change from biconcave to biconvex, making passage of the condyle under the disc more difficult. To recapture the disc, the patient must learn to move the mandible to the opposite side in order to activate the superior retrodiscal lamina. Unfortunately, at this point, the retrodiscal tissue has thinned considerably and lost much of its elasticity, making disc reduction difficult to achieve. If untreated, this condition invariably progresses to the stage of anterior disc displacement without reduction.[4,94]

Clinical Signs and Symptoms. Intermittent locking may occur at any time, but it most often occurs in the morning upon awakening, especially after a prolonged period of clenching. Eating may also precipitate the intermittent lock, particularly if the patient chews on the affected side. Often, the patient relates a previous history of jaw clicking on opening except when trauma is involved. More pain may be reported when the TMJ is locked. By relaxing the muscles through medication, physical means, moving the mandible to the opposite side, or their combination, many patients learn to reduce displaced discs. Of critical importance in terms of prognosis are the frequency and duration of the intermittent locking.[4,94]

Treatment. Mandibular repositioning appliance therapy to keep the disc in proper alignment with the condyle is the first step in treatment. The appliance sequence is modified by having the patient wear a maxillary appliance with a small ramp full time for one week. A lower appliance is then placed for daytime use and the maxillary appliance is worn only at night. Finally, the ramp on the maxillary appliance is extended to insure that the mandible does not retrude at night.[54]

Anteromedial Disc Displacement Without Reduction

As a result of continued disc deformation along with elongation of discal ligaments and loss of tension in the posterior attachment, the disc may remain anteromedially displaced creating a "closed lock." Contact is lost between condyle, disc, and articular eminence and the articular disc space collapses trapping the disc in front of the condyle—preventing translation (Figs. 9–6 and 9–7). Except for cases involving trauma, there is usually a history of clicking followed by limitation of opening.[95,100,102]

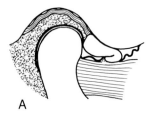 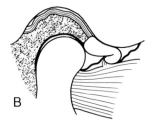 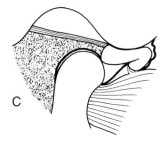

A   B   C

FIGURE 9–6. Anteromedial disc displacement without reduction. *A,* Resting, closed-joint position. *B,* Early stage of reduction showing the condyle pushing the disc forward. *C,* Late stage of translation showing the changes in the disc shape and jamming of the disc in front of the condyle preventing normal translatory movement. A normal range of vertical opening may be achieved with time. (Modified from Okeson, J.P.: *Management of Temporomandibular Disorders and Occlusion,* 2nd ed. C.V. Mosby Co., St. Louis, 1989.)

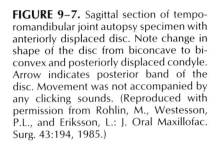

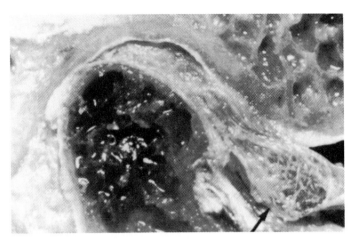

FIGURE 9–7. Sagittal section of temporomandibular joint autopsy specimen with anteriorly displaced disc. Note change in shape of the disc from biconcave to biconvex and posteriorly displaced condyle. Arrow indicates posterior band of the disc. Movement was not accompanied by any clicking sounds. (Reproduced with permission from Rohlin, M., Westesson, P.L., and Eriksson, L.: J. Oral Maxillofac. Surg. 43:194, 1985.)

Eriksson and Westesson[103] found that patients placed in the category of ADD without reduction had more pain than patients with ADD with reduction. These workers also reported that crepitation, lateral tenderness of the TMJ, and joint pain were frequently found in patients with ADD without reduction and seldom found in patients with ADD with reduction.

Disc deformation has been reported to be a common occurrence in patients with a nonreducing disc. Therefore, for the purpose of treatment planning as well as overall prognosis, this stage should be subdivided into an acute and a chronic substage depending on the duration of the displacement. In general, if the disc has been displaced for 6 months or less, the condition may be labeled acute. The chronic substage can best be determined by taking an accurate history from the patient.

Acute

A restricted maximum opening of 20 to 25 mm is the most obvious clinical sign of acute ADD without reduction. In addition, the mandibular midline is sharply deflected to the affected side at the end of opening. The term deflection must be differentiated from deviation (Figs. 9–8 and 9–9). Deviation is a discursive movement of the mandible that ends in the centered position and is indicative of interference during movement. It is characteristic of anterior disc displacement with reduction.[24,25]

Limited opening due to ADD without reduction must be differentiated from limited opening due to elevator muscle spasm or capsular restraint. By inducing a passive stretch to the joint after the patient has actively opened to the full extent, the "end-feel" can be determined. If a displaced disc is responsible for limited opening, there will be a hard end-feel with little or no play. In contrast, a gummy end-feel is present when muscle spasm or capsular connective tissue is preventing full opening.[104] With elevator muscle spasm, only vertical movement is restricted and protrusive and lateral excursions are normal. Cases of ADD without reduction, however, exhibit restricted movement in both protrusive and contralateral excursions. Movement to the side of the involved joint is usually not mechanically restricted because the main movement occurring in the joint is rotation. Pain restriction may be due to impingement upon inflamed retrodiscal tissues, particularly when a history of trauma is present.[94] Secondary muscle spasm of the ele-

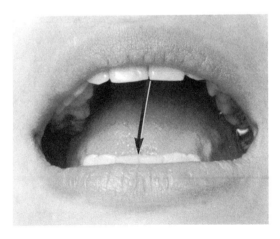

FIGURE 9–8. Deflection of the mandibular incisal path. On opening, the mandibular midline is continuously displaced to the affected side and does not return to the centered position. This is a sign of restricted mandibular movement and is characteristic of acute anteromedial disc displacement without reduction or unilateral elevator muscle spasm.

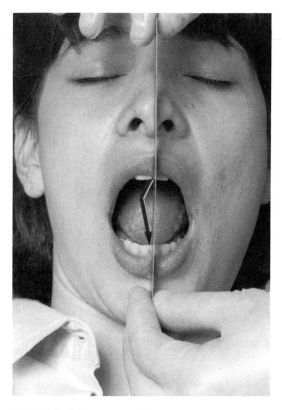

FIGURE 9-9. Deviation of the mandibular incisal path. On opening, the mandibular midline shifts to the side of interference but returns to the centered position at maximum opening. Deviation is characteristic of anteromedial disc displacement with reduction.

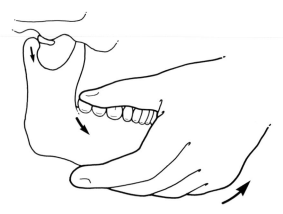

FIGURE 9-10. Reductive mobilization of the temporomandibular joint. This procedure is used to distract the condyle in an effort to manually reduce a displaced disc. Downward pressure is exerted on the posterior teeth while pulling upward on the patient's chin.

vator muscles may add to the restricted opening as well as capsular involvement.

In the acute stage, joint noise is usually absent. However, if ADD without reduction represents the next stage in a continuum, crepitation may be detected as the displacement becomes chronic and changes occur in the articular surfaces.

In general, the more acute the condition, the greater the chances for successful reduction of the disc through reductive mobilization and appliance therapy.

Treatment

Initial therapy should have as its primary objective reduction of the displaced disc through mobilization of the joint[105] (Fig. 9-10). This procedure attempts to recreate the space between the condyle and eminence in order to allow retraction of the disc by the superior retrodiscal lamina. Success is contingent upon the presence of a functional retrodiscal lamina to retract the disc as well as minimal deformation of the displaced disc. Some patients are able to reduce the displaced disc without assistance from the clinician. This involves having the patient open as wide as possible without discomfort and then moving the mandible toward the opposite joint. If unsuccessful, the clinician may then attempt to reduce the disc manually through downward pressure on the last molar on the involved side.[25] Success in reducing the disc can usually be clinically determined by comparing the amount of vertical opening and contralateral movement after mobilization with the amount of movement before mobilization. This difference should be verified through imaging, for clinical criteria alone may not be accurate.

Because secondary elevator muscle spasm is usually present as well as some inflammation of joint structures, it may be of benefit to provide a skeletal muscle relaxant and a nonsteroidal anti-inflammatory agent prior to the procedure. In some cases, changes in the connective tissue capsule may be contributing factors. Stretching of the vertical fibers of the capsule through the use of a pivot appliance or exercise may be indicated. Blocking the auriculotemporal nerve may be necessary if the patient experiences considerable discomfort during mobilization. Immediately after successful mobilization, appliances must be placed to prevent the condyle from returning to a closed-joint position.[25,100]

We recommend a maxillary appliance with a protrusive guide ramp on a full-time basis for a minimum of 10 days. The appliance must be worn during eating, and a bite prop should be given to the patient to use when they remove the appliance for toothbrushing. A soft diet is recommended along with chewing on the opposite side. After 10 days, if the disc remains reduced, a mandibular repositioning appliance can be placed for day wear alternating with a maxillary appliance for night. Biweekly visits to evaluate progress, monitor appliances, and treat soft tissues are necessary.

Chronic

In chronic cases, the disc is permanently deformed and the posterior attachment dysfunctional, making reduction of the disc all but impossible. Early in this stage, there may be some deflection to the affected side on opening and limited opening. Over time, a normal range of opening is achieved, owing to elongation of the posterior attachment and continued stretching and tearing of the discal ligaments.[85,103] Radiologic evidence of a displaced disc may be necessary to confirm the diagnosis. Crepitation is usually present, which may represent degenerative changes in the articular surfaces.

Treatment. If the closed lock is borderline with respect to duration, an attempt should still be made to reduce the disc through mobilization. If successful, it may be treated as an acute closed lock, although the prognosis is poor for permanent stabilization of the disc. Unsuccessful reduction necessitates a decision regarding surgical intervention or treating the patient "off the disc." This decision should be based on the degree of pain and dysfunction that may be present. Many patients function with little discomfort, although the disc is permanently displaced. In these patients, the posterior attachment has apparently fibrosed creating a "pseudo disc." Other patients with the same disorder may experience significant pain and dysfunction. In part, this finding may be due to the presence of hyperplastic connective tissue in the posterior part of the fossa.[106] Pain occurs when the condyle compresses this tissue when the mouth is closed. In general, an attempt should be made to decompress the joint, employing intraoral appliances to encourage pseudo disc formation and to reduce pressure against retrodiscal tissue. If pain persists, a surgical procedure may be indicated.[75]

Anteromedial Disc Displacement with Perforation of Retrodiscal Tissue

According to Farrar and McCarty,[95] if the disc is displaced anteromedially when the patient closes in habitual centric occlusion, the condyle is usually displaced posteriorly and superiorly. Therefore, the anterior part of the posterior attachment may be subjected to abnormal compressive loading. Invariably, this leads to structural changes in the posterior attachment. Initially, this may appear as an elongation of the inferior retrodiscal lamina when viewed arthrographically. In some cases, this elongation may progress to herniation of the posterior attachment (Figs. 9–11 and 9–12). In other cases, however, compressive forces on the tissues of the posterior attachment may lead to remodeling.

In separate studies, Scapino[107] and Blaustein and Scapino[108] studied the pathologic morphology of the disc and posterior attachment in cases of anteromedial disc displacement without reduction. They found that the collagen fibers of the anterior part of the posterior attachment took on a fibrotic character. A compact mass of fibers was present that contained fewer of the small vessels that were normally present. They concluded that the fibrosis represented a remodeling process brought on by compressive loading of the posterior attachment.

Why some patients were able to adapt to these abnormal forces through remodeling and others underwent the pathologic process is a subject of great conjecture.[109] Perhaps systemic factors are involved in addition to local factors. In any event, the treatment implications are obvious and are discussed under appliance therapy.

For those patients in whom a perforation has occurred, there is usually a history of previous clicking and locking, pain, and perhaps crepitus. The exception to this is when trauma is the initiating event.

Clinical Signs and Symptoms. Pain may be variable depending on patient tolerance and

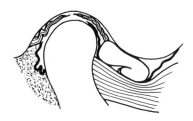

FIGURE 9–11. Anteromedial disc displacement with perforation of retrodiscal tissue. With the loss of elasticity in the superior retrodiscal lamina, the disc displacement is permanent. (Modified from Okeson, J.P.: *Management of Temporomandibular Disorders and Occlusion*, 2nd ed. C.V. Mosby Co., St. Louis, 1989.)

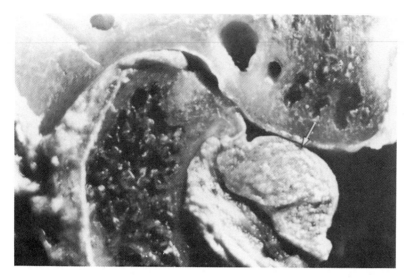

FIGURE 9–12. Sagittal section of temporomandibular joint autopsy specimen with anteriorly displaced and deformed disc indicated by the arrow. A large perforation is present, and the condyle articulates directly against the temporal bone. Movement was accompanied by crepitation. (Reproduced with permission from Rohlin, M., Westesson P.L., and Eriksson, L.: J. Oral Maxillofac. Surg. 43:194, 1985.)

pressure against the area. Joint tenderness and crepitus, which is indicative of degenerative articular surface changes, are usually present. Any limitation of movement may be caused by associated muscle involvement and the restriction imposed by pain. Diagnosis of a perforation is best accomplished through arthrography or arthroscopy. Magnetic resonance imaging, which is ideal for disc displacement, may not be as accurate for a perforation.[110]

Treatment. The only definitive treatment for a perforation of the posterior attachment is surgery.[75] Whether appliance therapy to decompress the area to allow for remodeling will be effective at this stage is doubtful. As with any surgical procedure, the patient's ability to tolerate the condition is a major determinant.

Adhesive Disc Hypomobility

Most documented cases of intracapsular restriction of mandibular movement or closed lock are due to ADD without reduction. With the emergence of arthroscopy has come more of an awareness that intracapsular adhesions occurring in the superior joint cavity between the disc and eminence may also cause closed lock.[11] Trauma is frequently implicated as a causative factor. If the trauma is slight, only mild surface damage to the disc may occur, resulting in frictional disc incoordination or a surface defect in form. A more severe incident could cause intracapsular bleeding and effusion, leading to disc fibrillation and eventually, adhesions. The disc is fixed to the eminence, preventing normal translation (Fig. 9–13). Adhesions may also occur in the inferior joint cavity between the disc and condyle but are more difficult to document.

Clinical Signs and Symptoms. Clinically, adhesive disc hypomobility is indistinguishable from acute ADD without reduction. Because translation does not occur, opening is limited. If pain is present, it is variable and may be due

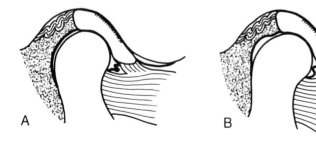

A   B

FIGURE 9–13. Adhesive disc hypomobility. *A,* Closed. *B,* Open. An adhesion occurring between the disc and fossa may prevent normal translatory movement creating a "closed-lock" with a vertical opening of 25 to 30 mm. No collapse of the articular disc space occurs, and the disc is not anteriorly displaced. (Modified from Okeson, J.P.: *Management of Temporomandibular Disorders and Occlusion,* 2nd ed. C.V. Mosby Co., St. Louis, 1989.)

to stretching of the discal ligaments, as forced opening is attempted. If the disc is permanently fixed to the eminence, continued opening may force the condyle against the anterior border of the disc, causing thinning and stretching of discal ligaments. Eventually, posterior displacement of the disc may occur.[25] In order to differentiate closed lock due to disc displacement and limited opening due to adhesions, imaging studies are required.

Inferior joint adhesions would not inhibit the amount of translation and opening would be normal. However, rotational movement in the disc-condyle complex would be eliminated and rough, irregular, noisy movements would be encountered.[24]

Treatment. Surgical arthroscopic procedures with lysis and lavage have been reported to be successful in elminating adhesions and freeing the disc.[56,57,111] Any splints employed for either nonsurgical or postoperative treatment should only decompress the joint and not attempt to reposition the mandible anteriorly.

Displacement of the Disc-Condyle Complex

Subluxation:

During normal opening, the disc rotates posteriorly on the condyle as the disc-condyle complex translates on the eminence. As a result of excessive opening, the condyle and the disc may be forced anteriorly beyond the normal limits of the translatory cycle. If the disc cannot rotate any farther posteriorly and the condyle continues to translate, a partial dislocation or subluxation can occur between the disc and articular eminence. Usually, the patient will have a history of jaw popping with opening the mouth wide when yawning or eating or during a dental procedure. Both subluxation and its sequel, complete dislocation, appear to have a common predisposing factor— an articular eminence with a short steep posterior slope.[24,25] This structural feature seems to be more common in skeletal deep bite facial types in which the associated occlusion is characterized by a deep overbite.

Clinical Signs and Symptoms. During wide opening, a momentary pause occurs after which the condyle jumps forward into maximum opening creating a void behind the condyle. This movement is rough and irregular and is often characterized by joint noise described as a click or a "thud."[25,84] Usually, pain

does not accompany subluxation unless it becomes habitual. Diagnostically, for treatment purposes, this wide opening click must be differentiated from a click that signifies reduction of a displaced disc. A subluxation type of click occurs only on wide opening and not on protrusive movement or lateral excursion. The click associated with reduction of a displaced disc, however, can occur during both protrusive and contralateral excursion.

Treatment. Habit training to voluntarily limit mouth opening within normal limits is the most conservative approach. This should be accompanied by exercises that strengthen the elevator muscles. Occasionally, injection of a sclerosing solution to reduce the laxity of the capsule may be tried. If these efforts fail, an eminectomy to flatten the articular eminence in order to reduce the amount of posterior rotation of the disc on the condyle is the definitive treatment of choice.[24]

Dislocation

As opposed to subluxation, which is a partial loss of contact between the disc and eminence, dislocation involves a collapse of the articular disc space. The disc is trapped anteriorly to the condyle that is now in direct contact with the eminence. This condition is caused by additional rotation of the condyle beyond its biomechanical limit. Because of the collapsed disc space, the superior retrodiscal lamina cannot retract the prolapsed disc. Adding to the problem is the elevator muscle spasm that frequently accompanies dislocation and preserves the decrease in articular disc space (Fig. 9–14).[25]

Clinical Signs and Symptoms. After opening wide, there is an inability to close the mandible that is locked open in a prognathic position and cannot be moved vertically. Depressions may be noted in the preauricular area formerly occupied by the condyles. An acute malocclusion is present with an anterior open bite and contact between only the most posterior teeth. Pain may be variable, which increases as the patient attempts to close, thus straining the inferior retrodiscal lamina and the collateral discal ligaments. Myospasm of the elevator muscles may add to the discomfort.[25]

Treatment. The main objective of treatment is to widen the articular disc space to allow the superior retrodiscal lamina to retract the disc. Forcefully closing the mandible should be avoided because it may add to elevator muscle

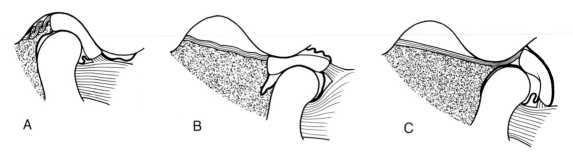

FIGURE 9–14. Dislocation of the condyle-disc complex. *A,* Resting, closed-joint position. *B,* Full, forward position of disc-condyle complex. *C,* Dislocation due to movement beyond the biomechanical limit. The disc is prolapsed anteriorly in front of the condyle. The articular space is collapsed, and the condyle is in contact with the eminence. (Modified from Okeson, J.P.: *Management of Temporomandibular Disorders and Occlusion,* 2nd ed. C.V. Mosby Co., St. Louis, 1989.)

spasm and aggravate dislocation. Reduction of the displaced mandible is best accomplished by having the patient yawn as widely as possible while the clinician exerts slight posterior pressure on the chin. If reduction is not achieved, placement of thumbs behind the molars and pressing down while the patient yawns may yield the necessary additional articular space. Should these digital manipulations fail, stimulation of the gag reflex by touching a mouth mirror to the soft palate may inhibit elevator muscle activity, thus increasing the articular disc space. If dislocation is chronic, the patient should be taught how to self-reduce the mandible. Habit training similar to that employed for subluxation should be instituted. Surgical intervention in the form of an eminectomy may be necessary if the condition becomes intolerable.[24,25]

CONCLUSIONS

At the beginning of this chapter, questions concerning clinical management of ID were raised. Perhaps the most significant question concerns treatment of the patient with a non-symptomatic click. Because all clicks are not alike and may represent different clinicial entities, a differential diagnosis is necessary. Some clicks may respond to simple exercises or to habit training. "To treat or not to treat" usually concerns painless reciprocal clicking associated with ADD with reduction, and this has been a controversial topic for years.

Many factors should enter into the clinician's decision. Two important factors are the age of the patient and the circumstances surrounding the onset. Patients who have had painless reciprocal clicking for many years do not warrant treatment for they have adapted to

their dysfunction. Conversely, the emergence of a click in a mature patient who has missing teeth on the affected side along with evidence of bruxism may herald the beginning of a serious problem. Any tenderness to palpation in the joint should be noted and the patient placed on periodic visits to monitor the condition.

The presence of painless reciprocal clicking in a teenager must be carefully assessed. If the patient's history reveals that the clicking is occurring with increasing frequency and clinical examination demonstrates joint and muscle tenderness to palpation, we would be inclined to recommend treatment. This would consist of appliance therapy and behavior modification, if indicated. However, if there is some masticatory muscle tenderness without any joint involvement, a stress reduction program alone might suffice. Of course, periodic monitoring of the patient's signs and symptoms is mandatory. All patients, regardless of age, should be educated with respect to their condition and warned of possible sequelae.

Repositioning therapy is another controversial area. When first presented by Farrar in the late 1970s, the concept was enthusiastically received and adopted. However, its long-term effect on joint structures has been questioned, particularly after appliances have been discontinued. In our opinion, mandibular repositioning therapy still has considerable merit in the treatment of some stages of internal derangements. In the event that symptoms had been significantly reduced in phase I therapy but returned after the patient was weaned off appliances, there appears to be some alternatives. One is to have the patient wear a stabilization appliance at night and monitor the symptoms periodically. If symptoms still persist, the patient should be placed back on a stabilization day appliance as well. Should symptoms still remain, resumption of full-time repositioning appliances would seem to be indicated. At that point, a decision on phase II stabilization therapy to restore the patient to a therapeutically derived position should be made. Any contributing factor that might be perpetuating the symptoms should be eliminated, if possible. Arthroscopic intervention as an adjunct to conservative therapy should also be explored prior to irreversibly altering the occlusion.

It is obvious that much confusion is still present with respect to management of a patient with an ID.[112] Equally apparent is the observation that we are still in the process of gathering information and learning about this disorder. It is hoped that the 1990s will shed more light on the subject and lead to a consensus among clinicians and researchers.

REFERENCES

1. Solberg, W.K.: Temporomandibular disorders: background and the clinical problems. Br. Dent. J. 160:157, 1986.
2. Vincent, S.D. and Lilly, G.E.: Incidence and characterization of temporomandibular joint sounds in adults. J.A.D.A. 116:203, 1988.
3. Rieder, C.E., Martinoff, J.T., and Wilcox, S.A.: The prevalence of mandibular dysfunction. Part I. Sex and age distribution of related signs and symptoms. J. Prosthet. Dent. 50:81, 1983.
4. Dolwick, M.F.: Diagnosis and etiology. In *Internal Derangements of the Temporomandibular Joint.* C.A. Helms, R.W. Katzberg, and M.F. Dolwick (eds.). University of California Press, San Francisco, 1983.
5. Moffett, B.C.: Definitions of temporomandibular joint derangements. In *Diagnosis of Internal Derangements of the Temporomandibular Joint.* vol. 1. B.C. Moffett (ed.). University of Washington, Seattle, 1984.
6. Dolwick, M.F., Katzberg, R.W., and Helms, C.A.: Internal derangements of the temporomandibular joint: Fact or fiction? J. Prosthet. Dent. 49:415, 1983.
7. Brand, J.W., Whinery, J.G., Anderson, Q.N., and Keenan, K.M.: The effects of temporomandibular joint internal derangement and degenerative joint disease on tomographic and arthrotomographic images. Oral Surg. Oral Med. Oral Pathol. 67:220, 1989.
8. Greene, C.S. and Laskin, D.M.: Long-term status of TMJ clicking in patients with myofascial pain and dysfunction. J.A.D.A. 117:461, 1988.
9. Annandale, T.: Displacement of the interarticular cartilage of the lower jaw and its treatment by operation. Lancet 1:411, 1887.
10. Pringle, J.H.: Displacement of the mandibular meniscus and its treatment. Br. J. Surg. 6:385, 1918.
11. Wakely, C.P.G.: The causation and treatment of displaced mandibular cartilage. Lancet 217:543, 1929.
12. Goodfriend, D.J.: Dysarthrosis and subarthrosis of the mandibular articulation. Dent. Cosmos. 74:523, 1932.
13. Costen, J.B.: Syndrome of ear and sinus symptoms dependent upon disturbed function of the temporomandibular joint. Ann. Otol. Rhinol. Laryngol. 43:1, 1934.
14. Schwartz, L.L.: Disorders of the temporomandibular joint. W.B. Saunders Co., Philadelphia, 1959.
15. Laskin, D.M.: Etiology of the pain-dysfunction syndrome. J.A.D.A. 79:147, 1969.
16. Ireland, V.E.: The problem of "the clicking jaw." Proc. R. Soc. Med. 44:363, 1951.
17. Norgaard, F.: Arthrography of the mandibular joint. Acta Radiol. 25:679, 1944.
18. Wilkes, C.H.: Arthrography of the temporomandibular joint in patients with the TMJ-pain dysfunction syndrome. Minn. Med. 61:645, 1978.
19. Wilkes, C.H.: Structural and functional alterations of the temporomandibular joint. Northwest Dent. 57:287, 1978.
20. Farrar, W.B.: Diagnosis and treatment of anterior dislocation of the articular disc. N.Y. State Dent. J. 41:348, 1971.
21. Farrar, W.B.: Characteristics of the condylar path in internal derangements of the temporomandibular joint. J. Prosthet. Dent. 39:319, 1978.
22. Farrar, W.B. and McCarty, W.L.: The TMJ dilemma. J. Ala. Dent. Assoc. 63:19, 1979.
23. Mohl, N.D.: Functional anatomy of the temporomandibular joint. In *The President's Conference on the Examination, Diagnosis and Management of Temporomandibular Disorders.* D.M. Laskin, et al (eds.). American Dental Association, Chicago, 1983.
24. Bell, W.E.: *Temporomandibular Disorders: Classification, Diagnosis, and Management,* 2nd ed. Chicago, Year Book Medical Publishers, 1986.
25. Okeson, J.P.: *Fundamentals of Occlusion and Temporomandibular Disorders.* C.V. Mosby Co., St. Louis, 1985.
26. DeBrul, E.L.: The craniomandibular articulation. In *Sicher's Oral Anatomy,* 7th ed. C.V. Mosby Co., St. Louis, 1980.
27. Mahan, P.E., Wilkinson, T.M., Gibbs, C.H., et al: Superior and inferior bellies of the lateral pterygoid muscle EMG activity at basic jaw positions. J. Prosthet. Dent. 50:710, 1983.
28. Wilkinson, T.M.: The relationship between the disk and the lateral pterygoid muscle in the human temporomandibular joint. J. Prosthet. Dent. 60:715, 1988.
29. Carpentier, P., Yung, J.P., Marguelles-Bonnet, R., and Meunissier, M.: Insertions of the lateral pterygoid muscle: An anatomic study of the human temporomandibular joint. J. Oral Maxillofac. Surg. 46:477, 1988.
30. Mahan, P.E.: The temporomandibular joint in function and pathofunction. In *Temporomandibular Joint Problems.* W.K. Solberg and G.T. Clark (eds.). Quintessence Publishing Co., Lombard, IL, 1980.
31. Moffett, B.C.: Histological aspects of temporomandibular joint derangements. In *Diagnosis of Internal Derangements of the Temporomandibular Joint,* vol. 1. B.C. Moffett (ed.). University of Washington, Seattle, 1984.
32. Katzberg, R.W., Dolwick, M.F., Helms, C.A., et al: Arthrotomography of the temporomandibular joint. Am. J. Roentgenol. 134:995, 1980.
33. Harkins, S.J. and Marteney, J.L.: Extrinsic trauma: A significant precipitating factor in temporomandibular dysfunction. J. Prosthet. Dent. 54:271, 1985.

34. Mannheimer, J., Attanasio, R., Cinotti, W.R., and Pertes, R.A.: Cervical strain and mandibular whiplash: Effects upon the craniomandibular apparatus. Clin. Prev. Dent. 11:29, 1989.

35. Weinberg, S. and LaPointe, H.: Cervical extension-flexion injury (whiplash) and internal derangement of the temporomandibular joint. J. Oral Maxillofac. Surg. 45:653, 1987.

36. Roydhouse, R.H.: Whiplash and temporomandibular dysfunction. Lancet 1:1395, 1973.

37. Leder, E.: Cervical trauma as a factor in the development of TMJ dysfunction and facial pain. J. Craniomand. Pract. 1:85, 1983.

38. Shore, N.A., Shaefer, M.G., and Hoppenfeld, S.: Iatrogenic TMJ difficulty: Cervical traction may be the etiology. J. Prosthet. Dent. 41:541, 1979.

39. Stegenga, B., de Bont, L.G.M., and Boering, G.: Osteoarthrosis as the cause of craniomandibular pain and dysfunction: A unifying concept. J. Oral Maxillofac. Surg. 47:249, 1989.

40. Rugh, J.D.: Psychological factors in the etiology of masticatory pain and dysfunction. In *The President's Conference on the Examination, Diagnosis and Management of Temporomandibular Disorders.* D.M. Laskin, et al (eds.). American Dental Association, Chicago, 1983.

41. Carlsson, G.E. and Droukas, B.C.H.: Dental occlusion and the health of the masticatory system. J. Craniomand. Pract. 2:141, 1984.

42. Roberts, C.A., Tallents, R.H., Katzberg, R.W., et al: Comparison of internal derangements of the TMJ with occlusal findings. Oral Surg. Oral Med. Oral Pathol. 63:645, 1987.

43. Pullinger, A.G., Seligman, D.A., and Solberg, W.K.: Temporomandibular disorders. Part II. Occlusal factors associated with temporomandibular tenderness and dysfunction. J. Prosthet. Dent. 59:363, 1988.

44. Levy, P.H.: Clinical implications of mandibular repositioning and the concept of an alterable centric relation. Dent. Clin. North Am. 19:543, 1975.

45. Gelb, H.: Effective management and treatment of the craniomandibular syndrome. In *Clinical Management of Head, Neck and TMJ Pain and Dysfunction,* 2nd ed. H. Gelb (ed.). W.B. Saunders Co., Philadelphia, 1985.

46. Weinberg, L.A.: Role of condylar position in TMJ dysfunction-pain syndrome. J. Prosthet. Dent. 41:636, 1979.

47. Katzberg, R.W., Keith, D.A., Ten Eick, W.R., and Guralnick, W.C.: Internal derangements of the temporomandibular joint: An assessment of condylar position in centric occlusion. J. Prosthet. Dent. 49:250, 1983.

48. Habets, L.L., Bezuur, J.N. van Ooij, C.P., and Hansson, T.L.: The orthopantomogram. An aid in diagnosis of temporomandibular joint problems. I. The factor of vertical magnification. J. Oral Rehab. 14:475, 1987.

49. Keith, D.A.: Etiology and diagnosis of temporomandibular pain and dysfunction: Organic pathology (other than arthritis). In *The President's Conference on the Examination, Diagnosis and Management of Temporomandibular Disorders.* D.M. Laskin, et al (eds.). American Dental Association, Chicago. 1983.

50. Isacsson, G., Linde, C., and Isberg, A.: Subjective symptoms in patients with temporomandibular disk displacement versus patients with myogenic craniomandibular disorders. J. Prosthet. Dent. 61:70, 1989.

51. Isberg, A., Widmaim, S.E., and Ivarsson, R.: Clinical,

radiographic, and electromyographic study of patients with internal derangement of the temporomandibular joint. Am. J. Orthod. 88:453, 1985.

52. Rocabado, M., Johnston, B.E., and Blakney, M.G.: Physical therapy and dentistry: An overview. J. Craniomand. Pract. 1:745, 1982–3.

53. Clark, G.T.: Examining temporomandibular disorder patients for cranio-cervical dysfunction. J. Craniomand. Pract. 2:56, 1983–4.

54. Pertes, R.A., Attanasio, R., Cinotti, W.R., and Balbo, M.: Use of occlusal splint therapy in the treatment of MPD and internal derangements of the TMJ. J. Clin. Prev. Dent. 11:26, 1989.

55. Lundh, H. and Westesson, P.L.: Long-term follow-up after occlusal treatment to correct abnormal temporomandibular joint disk position. Oral Surg. Oral Med. Oral Pathol. 67:2, 1989.

56. Sanders, B. and Buoncristiana, R.: Diagnostic and surgical arthroscopy of the TMJ: Clinical experience with 137 procedures over a two-year period. J. Craniomand. Disord. Facial Oral Pain 1:202, 1987.

57. Moses, J.J., Sartoris, D., Glass, R., et al: The effect of arthroscopic surgical lysis and lavage of the superior joint space on TMJ disc position and mobility. J. Oral Maxillofac. Surg. 47:674, 1989.

58. Farrar, W.B.: Differentiation of temporomandibular joint dysfunction to simplify treatment. J. Prosthet. Dent. 28:629, 1972.

59. Pertes, R.A.: Updating the mandibular orthopedic repositioning appliance (MORA). J. Craniomand. Pract. 5:351, 1987.

60. Clark, G.T.: The TMJ repositioning appliance: A technique for construction, insertion, and adjustment. J. Craniomand. Pract. 4:38, 1986.

61. Fox, C.W., Abrams, B.L., Williams, B, and Doukoudakis, A.: Protrusive positioners. J. Prosthet. Dent. 54:258, 1985.

62. Lundh, H., Westesson, P.L., Kopp, S., and Tillstrom, B.: Anterior repositioning splint in the treatment of temporomandibular joints with reciprocal clicking: Comparison with a flat occlusal splint and an untreated control group. J. Oral Surg. Oral Med. Oral Path. 60:131, 1985.

63. Lundh, H.: Correction of temporomandibular joint disk displacement by occlusal therapy. Swed. Dent. J. Suppl 51:1987.

64. Okeson, J.P.: Long-term treatment of disk-interference disorders of the temporomandibular joint with anterior repositioning occlusal splints. J. Prosthet. Dent. 60:611, 1988.

65. Moloney, F. and Howard, J.A.: Internal derangements of the temporomandibular joint. III. Anterior repositioning splint therapy. Aust. Dent. J. 31:30, 1986.

66. Clark, G.T., Lanham, F., and Flack, V.F.: Treatment outcome results for consecutive TMJ clinic patients. J. Craniomand. Disord. Facial Oral Pain 2:87, 1988.

67. Clark, G.T.: Diagnosis and treatment of painful temporomandibular disorders. Dent. Clin. N Am. 31:645, 1987.

68. Kirk, W.S. and Calabrese, D.K.: Clinical evaluation of physical therapy in the management of internal derangement of the temporomandibular joint. J. Oral Maxillofac. Surg. 47:113, 1989.

69. Mannheimer, J.S.: Physical therapy concepts in evaluation and treatment of the upper quarter. In *TMJ Disorders: Management of the Craniomandibular Complex.* S.L. Kraus (ed.). Churchill Livingstone, New York, 1988.

70. Gale, E.N.: Behavioral management of MPD. In *The President's Conference on the Examination, Diagnosis and Management of Temporomandibular Disorders*. D.M. Laskin, et al (eds.). American Dental Association, Chicago, 1983.
71. Gross, A. and Gale, E.N.: A prevalence study of the clinical signs associated with mandibular dysfunction. J.A.D.A. 107:932, 1983.
72. Eversole, L.R. and Machado, L.: Temporomandibular joints internal derangements and associated neuromuscular disorders. J.A.D.A. 110:69, 1985.
73. Laskin, D.M.: Myofascial pain-dysfunction syndrome: Etiology. In *The Temporomandibular Joint*, 3rd ed. B.G. Sarnat and D.M. Laskin (eds.). Charles C Thomas, Springfield, 1980.
74. Solberg, W.K.: Temporomandibular disorders: Physical tests in diagnosis. Br. Dent. J. 160:273, 1986.
75. Kryshtalskyj, B. and Weinberg, S.: Surgical correction of internal derangements of the TMJ. Oral Health 78:19, 1988.
76. Howard, J.: Differential diagnosis of mandibular hypomobility. In *Diagnosis of Internal Derangements of the Temporomandibular Joint*, vol. 1. B.C. Moffett (ed.). University of Washington, Seattle, 1984.
77. Sanchez-Woodworth, R.E., Tallents, R.H., Katzberg, R.W., and Guay, J.A.: Bilateral internal derangements of temporomandibular joint: Evaluation by magnetic resonance imaging. Oral Surg. Oral Med. Oral Pathol. 65:281-285, 1988.
78. Roberts, C.A., Katzberg, R.W., Tallents, R.H., et al: Correlation of clinical parameters to the arthrographic depiction of temporomandibular joint internal derangements. Oral Surg. Oral Med. Oral Pathol. 66:32, 1988.
79. Westesson, P.L.: Arthrography of the temporomandibular joint. J. Prosthet. Dent. 51:535, 1984.
80. Helms, C.A., Doyle, G.W., Orwig, D., et al: Staging of internal derangements of the TMJ with magnetic imaging: Preliminary observations. J. Craniomand. Disord. Facial Oral Pain 3:93, 1989.
81. Heffez, L. and Jordan, S.: A classification of temporomandibular disk morphology. Oral Surg. Oral Med. Oral Pathol. 67:11, 1989.
82. Westesson, P.L.: Structural hard-tissue changes in temporomandibular joints with internal derangements. Oral Surg. Oral Med. Oral Pathol. 59:220, 1985.
83. Westesson, P.L., Bronstein, S.L., and Liedberg, J.: Internal derangement of the temporomandibular joint: Morphologic description with correlation to joint function. Oral Surg. Oral Med. Oral Pathol. 59:323, 1985.
84. Mahan, P.E.: *Seminar on TMJ Disorders and Facial Pain*. Northeast Dental Seminars, Boston, Dec. 11–12, 1985.
85. Ross, J.B.: Diagnostic criteria and nomenclature for TMJ arthrography in sagittal section. Part I. Derangements. J. Craniomand. Disord. Facial Oral Pain 1:185, 1987.
86. Rohlin, M., Westesson, P.L., and Eriksson, L.: The correlation of temporomandibular joint sounds with joint morphology in fifty-five autopsy specimens. J. Oral Maxillofac. Surg. 43:194, 1985.
87. Katzberg, R.W.: Temporomandibular joint imaging. Radiology 170:297, 1989.
88. Rasmussen, O.C.: Description of population and progress of symptoms in a longitudinal study of temporomandibular arthropathy. Scand. J. Dent. Res. 89:196, 1981.
89. Lundh, H., Westesson, P.L., and Kopp, S.: A three-year follow-up of patients with reciprocal temporomandibular joint clicking. Oral Surg. Oral Med. Oral Pathol. 63:530, 1987.
90. Pullinger, A.C. and Seligman, D.A.: TMJ osteoarthrosis: A differentiation of diagnostic subgroups by symptom history and demographics. J. Craniomand. Disord. Facial Oral Pain 1:251, 1987.
91. Kozeniauskas, J.J. and Ralph, W.J.: Bilateral arthrographic evaluation of unilateral temporomandibular joint pain and dysfunction. J. Prosthet. Dent. 60:98, 1988.
92. Ronquillo, H.I., Guay, J., Tallents, R.H., et al: Tomographic analysis of mandibular condyle position as compared to arthrographic findings of the temporomanidbular joint. J Craniomand. Disord. Facial Oral Pain 2:59, 1988.
93. Roberts, C.A., Tallents, R.H., Katzberg, R.W., et al: Comparison of arthrographic findings of the temporomandibular joint with palpation of the muscles of mastication. Oral Surg. Oral Med. Oral Pathol. 64:275, 1987.
94. Farrar, W.B. and McCarty, W.L.: *A Clinical Outline of Temporomandibular Joint Diagnosis and Treatment. Normandie Study Group for TMJ Dysfunction.* Normandie Publications, Montgomery, 1982.
95. Farrar W.B. and McCarty, W.L.: Inferior joint space arthrography and characteristics of the condylar path in internal derangements of the TMJ. J. Prosthet. Dent. 41:548, 1979.
96. Mauderli, A.P., Lundeen, H.C., and Loughner, B.: Condylar movement recordings for analyzing TMJ derangements. J. Craniomand. Disord. Facial Oral Pain 2:119, 1988.
97. Oster, C., Katzberg, R.W., Tallents, R.H., et al: Characterization of temporomandibular joint sounds. Oral Surg. Oral Med. Oral Pathol. 58:10, 1984.
98. Roberts, C.A., Tallents, R.H., Espeland, M.A., et al: Mandibular range of motion versus arthrographic diagnosis of the temporomandibular joint. Oral Surg. Oral Med. Oral Pathol. 60:244, 1985.
99. Kerstens, H.C.J., Golding, R.P., Valk, F.R.C.R., and van der Kwast, W.A.M.: Magnetic resonance imaging of partial temporomandibular joint disc displacement. J Oral Maxillofac. Surg. 42:25, 1989.
100. Westesson, P.L.: Clinical and arthrographic findings in patients with TMJ disorders. In *Diagnosis of Internal Derangements of the Temporomandibular Joint*, vol. 1. B.C. Moffett (ed.). University of Washington, Seattle, 1984.
101. Manzione, J.V., Tallents, R., Katzberg, R.W., et al: Arthrographically guided splint therapy for recapturing the temporomandibular joint meniscus. Oral Surg. 57:235, 1984.
102. Schwartz, H.C. and Kendrick, R.W.: Internal derangements of the temporomandibular joint: Description of clinical syndromes. Oral Surg. Oral Med. Oral Pathol. 58:24, 1984.
103. Eriksson, L. and Westesson, P.L.: Clinical and radiological study of patients with anterior disc displacement of the temporomandibular joint. Swed. Dent. J. 7:55, 1983.
104. Rocabado, M.: Arthrokinematics of the temporomandibular joint. In *Clinical Management of Head, Neck and TMJ Pain and Dysfunction*, 2nd ed. H. Gelb (ed.). W.B. Saunders Co., Philadelphia, 1985.
105. Howard, J.: Reductive mobilization of the acute closed lock in the temporomandibular joint. In *Diagnosis of Internal Derangements of the Temporo-*

mandibular Joint, vol 1. B.C. Moffett (ed.). University of Washington, Seattle, 1984.

106. Isberg, A., Isacsson, G., Johansson, A., and Larson, O.: Hyperplastic soft-tissue formation in the temporomandibular joint associated with internal derangement. Oral Surg. Oral Med. Oral Pathol. 61:32, 1986.
107. Scapino, R.P.: Histopathology associated with malposition of the human temporomandibular joint disc. Oral Surg. 55:382, 1983.
108. Blaustein, D.I. and Scapino, R.P.: Remodeling of the temporomandibular joint disk and posterior attachment in disk displacement specimens in relation to glycosaminoglycan content. Plast. Reconstruct. Surg. 78:756, 1986.
109. Hall, M.B., Brown, R.W., and Baughman, R.A.: His-
tologic appearance of the bilaminar zone in internal derangement of the temporomandibular joint. Oral Surg. 58:375, 1984.
110. Schelhas, K.P., Wilkes, C.H., Fritts, H.M., et al: Temporomandibular joint: MR imaging of internal derangements and postoperative changes. Am. J. Neuroradiol. 8:1093, 1987.
111. Sanders, B.: Arthroscopic surgery of the temporomandibular joint: Treatment of internal derangement with persistent closed lock. Oral Surg. Oral Med. Oral Pathol. 62:361, 1986.
112. Wabeke, K.B., Hansson, T.L., Hoogstraten, J., and van der Kuy, P.: Temporomandibular joint clicking: A literature overview. J. Craniomand. Disord. Facial Oral Pain 3:163, 1989.

Andrew S. Kaplan
Daniel Buchbinder

CHAPTER 10

Arthritis

Rheumatologic diseases of the temporomandibular joint (TMJ) present the dentist with diagnostic challenges. Many of these diseases affect similar populations and have similar clinical characteristics. The astute clinician has to be familiar with these disorders and their differential diagnoses. Distinguishing between these disease entities is important, as the clinical course, long-term prognosis, therapy, and need for referral will vary.

Different classifications of rheumatologic diseases affecting the TMJ have appeared in several sources.[1-4] We believe that the most straightforward classification is that of Kreutziger and Mahan.[1] They divide the arthritides into four categories:

1. Noninflammatory arthritis
2. Inflammatory arthritis
3. Infectious arthritis
4. Metabolic disease

Noninflammatory arthritis or osteoarthrosis has as its hallmark the initial involvement of the cartilaginous and subchondral layers of the joint. The synovium is secondarily involved. Inflammation, when present, is a secondary finding. The inflammatory arthritides include rheumatoid arthritis, ankylosing spondylitis, psoriatic arthritis, juvenile rheumatoid arthritis, lupus erythematosus, and Reiter's syndrome. The initial involvement in this group is the synovium with secondary effects on the articulating surfaces.

The infectious arthritides are divided into two subgroups. The first subgroup includes arthritic changes due to direct extension of odontogenic or soft tissue infection as well as those due to secondary infection, such as after surgery or traumatic injury. The second subgroup is infection due to systemic disease. Such diseases as gonorrhea, syphilis, tuberculosis, actinomycosis, and Lyme disease are reported to have occasional involvement with the TMJ.

Arthritis related to metabolic disease includes gout and synovial chondromatosis. Each of these diseases is reviewed with respect to epidemiology, etiology, pathology, clinical and radiographic presentations, laboratory findings, and treatment.

OSTEOARTHROSIS

Osteoarthrosis is the most common form of arthritis affecting the human body.[5-7] Its high frequency accounts for one of the major causes of loss of time at work. This disease is also commonly referred to as degenerative joint disease and osteoarthritis. The different names used to identify this condition reflect the ongoing controversy as to the existence of an inflammatory component. Most research indicates that this disorder is noninflammatory in nature. Inflammatory infiltrate, sometimes found in the synovial fluid of an affected joint, represents a secondary change due to the disease process and is not a cause of it.

Osteoarthrosis is divided into two major classifications: primary and secondary.[23] Primary osteoarthrosis includes those cases in which the disease is of an unknown origin or stems from a genetic cause. Most cases of osteoarthrosis fall into this category. Secondary osteoarthrosis are those cases in which the cause can be better identified. Causes can include trauma; underlying disease state, causing a deviation in form within the joint; and occupational stress, among others. Because so little is known about the causes of osteoarthrosis, these subgroups are somewhat artificial and greatly overlap. As more is learned, the primary subgroups of this disease will likely change.

Epidemiology of osteoarthrosis has been a subject of much research over many years.[6] Osteoarthrosis shows a higher frequency with increased age, arthritic changes being evident in as much as 80% of the general population by the sixth decade of life. Only 5% show evidence of degenerative changes below the age of 25. Early onset of osteoarthrosis is commonly related to mechanical joint problems and to stress induced by occupation. Osteoarthrosis affects men and women with approximately the same frequency but is more common in men younger than the age of 45. Above the age of 45, women are affected more frequently.[6]

Research has failed to show a significant relationship with ethnic group, geographic location, or genetic predisposition, with two exceptions discussed further in this chapter.

Studies on the bilaterality of osteoarthrosis in the various joints of the human body show a frequency of approximately 85%.[5] The dominant side usually shows greater severity. The joints most commonly affected include those of the knees, hands, feet, and hips.[6]

The areas of the spine most commonly involved are the lumbar and cervical regions.[6] With the high frequency of TMJ patients complaining of pain in the cervical region, this fact cannot be ignored. The cervical spine is more commonly affected in females and the lumbar region in males.

Osteoarthrosis is the most common form of arthritis of the TMJ.[2] The reported frequency varies widely probably because of methodologic reasons. Blackwood[8] studied 400 TMJs histopathologically and reported a frequency of 40%. Macalister,[9] in a study of 69 cadavers, reported a frequency of 69%.

Clinical studies using different criteria show much lower frequencies. Toller[10] reported an incidence of about 8% in data collected from 1573 TMJ patients. Mejersjo[11] reported the clinical incidence to be as high as 16%. With radiographic change as a criterion, frequencies as low as 14% and as high as 44% have been reported.[12,13]

As is the case with osteoarthrosis in the rest of the human body, there seems to be an increasing frequency with advancing age. The peak, however, is in the fourth and fifth decades.[14] Osteoarthrotic changes can occur in a significant number of 20 and 30 year olds. Stewart and Standish[15] reported on six patients younger than the age of 19. Radiographic changes are sometimes seen in younger children as well.

As with most temporomandibular disorders (TMDs), osteoarthrosis shows a strong predilection for females, with as much as a 6:1 ratio.[14] Clinically, the disease tends to be predominantly unilateral, although bilateral disease does occur.[16] Ackerman and coworkers[27] have shown in an autopsy study, however, that there often is correlation of degenerative change between right and left sides.

Etiology

The understanding of the etiology of osteoarthrosis is far from complete. As previously mentioned, age appears to be a factor. Osteoar-

throsis is also associated with obesity.[5] One might postulate that the increased loading of the weight bearing joints provides a simple cause-and-effect relationship. This reasoning, however, is an oversimplification because this finding holds true for some of the nonweight bearing joints, such as the distal interphalangeal joints, but not in the ankle, a weight bearing joint.

It is well-known that individuals engaging in certain physical activities on a repeated basis have higher incidences of osteoarthrosis. Often cited as examples are basketball players (knees), football players (talar joints), miners (spines and knees), and pneumatic drill operators (wrists). These findings are likely due to repeated loading on the involved joints, which overcomes adaptive capacity. This subject is discussed subsequently in relationship to the TMJ.

Genetic factors have not been shown to have a strong link with osteoarthrosis with two exceptions, ochronosis and congenital dislocation of the hip.[5] The latter is related to systemic joint laxity, whereas the former is due to a missing systemic enzyme resulting in deposition of homogentisic acid in cartilage causing degenerative changes. A familial disposition seems to exist in the development of Heberden's nodules,[7] bony enlargements of distal interphalangeal joints affected by osteoarthrosis, but the relationship is controversial.

Hormonal and dietary factors have not been shown to be primary ones in the etiology of osteoarthrosis. Mechanical factors that affect the functional contours of a joint can lead to osteoarthrosis. These can include postural and bony abnormalities and prior trauma.[5] Traumatic injury often is used as an experimental animal model in the study of osteoarthrosis.

Etiologic factors with respect to the TMJ have been studied. It seems that local factors play the major role, but much is not understood. The most often implicated local factor is repetitive overloading of the joint.[17] Parafunctional habits (bruxism and clenching) are probably the most common causes. Clinicians most often have implicated occlusal interferences[17] and malocclusion. Evidence exists that missing teeth can lead to osteoarthrosis.[26]

It is widely believed that the presence of a displaced meniscus precedes the onset of arthritic changes. Pullinger and Seligman[18] analyzed a group of 122 patients with internal derangement and osteoarthrosis. They were able to identify distinct groups of patients, one of which showed evidence of progressing through the stages of internal derangement with reduction to internal derangement without reduction to osteoarthrosis. Another group of patients with osteoarthrosis had no history of locking or clicking. These patients in general tended to be older and were more likely to be males. The group with a history of internal derangement tended to be younger and female. These researchers postulate that systemic joint laxity may be part of the cause.

Many clinicians believe that internal derangement can lead to osteoarthrosis of the TMJ in some patients, but osteoarthrosis can be primary and lead to disc derangement (Fig. 10–1).

Macrotrauma can cause osteoarthrosis. Macrotrauma can include such incidents as a motor vehicle accident, a fight with impact to the mandible, and a fall with impact to the mandible. This subject is discussed in detail in chapters 11 and 12.

Intracapsular fractures can result in deviations in form enough to cause regressive remodeling of the TMJ, leading to osteoarthrosis. Likewise, any of the systemic arthritides, developmental disturbances, and neoplastic diseases leaving altered joint surfaces can result in the final common pathway of osteoarthrosis.

Pathology

All joints go through a constant process of adaptation or remodeling, in response to functional demands and local conditions. Histologically, as seen in Figure 10–2, the structures of the condyle and articular eminence can be divided into five distinct zones. The functional area is a layer of fibrous connective tissue. Below this area is a transitional layer or proliferative zone. This zone is made up of undifferentiated mesenchyme, a tissue that is pluripotential. This tissue allows for the remodeling capacity of the joint and serves as the major protective factor to increased demand. Next is a layer of fibrous cartilage. Finally, there is a calcified cartilage layer, which is compact and spongy bone.

The thickness of the cartilaginous and fibrous layers will vary according to functional demand.[17,19] The functional area of the condyle is the anteriosuperior slope. Not surprisingly, this tends to be the area with the greatest thickness. On the articular eminence, the posterior inferior slope is the functional area (Fig. 10–3).

As functional demands are increased, but are

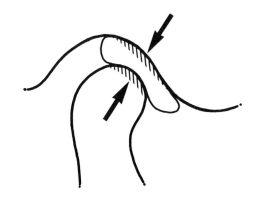

FIGURE 10–3. The functional surfaces of the temporomandibular joint.

within the physiologic capacity of the joint, progressive remodeling takes place. As described by Kreutziger and Mahan,[1] the peripheral and weight bearing areas of the condyle and temporal component show the most change. Cartilage forms within the proliferative zone. At the same time or subsequently, the cartilage in contact with the subchondral bone mineralizes. This process is followed by resorption and replacement with haversian systems. It is thought that the articular surface of the condyle and the temporal component react passively to these changes.[19] The meniscus, assuming it is in proper position, also adapts passively to changes in contour and may eventually become pathologic in nature.

Hansson[17] has studied progressive remodeling and notes that the changes often create a deviation in form. These changes can be seen on gross specimens as flattenings and elevations of both the condyle and temporal component and occur with a high frequency. Hansson and coworkers[20] noted these changes in 26 of 30 cadavers ranging in age from 17 to 37 at the time of death.

When the reparative capacity of a joint is exceeded, degenerative changes begin. As this process unfolds, a decrease in the cellular element of the proliferative zone is seen. The elastic capacity of the cartilaginous layers is decreased. A lack of cohesion occurs between the collagen bundles within the cartilage allowing the accumulation of fluid. This accumulation weakens the structure of the functional surface enough to cause cracks, which eventually deepen, and cartilage breaks away. This process is known as "fibrillation."[10]

Reactive bone forms beneath the fibrocartilage layer. Resorption of the articular bone then occurs or can occur after the bone is denuded. Channels into the medullary bone can form, and they eventually form subarticular cysts, also known as "Eli's cysts" (Fig. 10–4). If the cyst wall collapses it can cause severe changes in the shape of the condyle. The spongy bone reacts by mounting a reparative process—the proliferation of vascular mesenchyme, which forms granulation tissue. Occasionally, this tissue proliferates through surface defects and can mature into a dense fibrous connective tissue on the functional surface. The process may stop at this point and give sufficient function to the joint.[1]

The bone eventually becomes denuded and can exhibit pitting and severe changes in contour (Figs. 10–5 and 10–6). The condylar bone in the functional area also thickens, a process known as eburnation. If the meniscus was not previously affected its damage is likely at this time. Toller[10] has emphasized the importance of an intact meniscus for the best chance at repair.

Completing the picture is the proliferation of bone at the margins of the condylar head, resulting in lipping (Fig. 10–7). These bony growths are often referred to as osteophytes. If a bony fragment breaks free and is present in the synovial fluid it is referred to as a "loose body" and also by some as "joint mice."

Cartilaginous debris and occasional loose bodies are sometimes found in the synovial fluid and may give rise to an inflammatory reaction in the synovial tissues. This reaction is a secondary rather than a primary finding of osteoarthrosis. Hence, its classification as noninflammatory arthritis.

One can gain insight into the biochemical processes occurring in osteoarthrotic cartilage breakdown by referring to the medical literature.[5–7] Cartilage is mainly made up of chondrocytes, fibrocytes, collagen fibrils, proteoglycan molecules, and water. The collagen forms a woven network in which the proteoglycan molecules reside. The proteoglycan molecule is manufactured within the cartilage chondrocytes.

The proteoglycan aggregate is made up of a stem of hyaluronic acid from which the proteoglycans are suspended as side chains (Fig. 10–8). These molecules are hydrophilic. One of the characteristics of cartilage is that it absorbs shock well. At least in part, cartilage is protective of the joint structures. The other greater shock absorber is the bone itself because of its greater mass. The ability of cartilage to absorb and express water as function dictates is thought to give it this quality, known as "weeping lubrication."

As described by Moll,[5] one of the first changes in osteoarthrosis is a disruption of the proteoglycan structures. These side chains apparently shorten and allow a greater accumulation of fluids, lowering the capacity to absorb stress. This disruption allows for proteolysis and eventual degradation.

Progressive remodeling is more likely to occur on the condylar head, whereas osteoarthrotic changes are more likely on the temporal component.[21] This finding is probably due to the relatively better capacity of the condyle to adapt to changes in function as evidenced by a thicker soft tissue covering.[17]

Clinical Features

Osteoarthrosis usually has a gradual onset, but acute onset is occasionally seen. Progression of the disease can last months or years.

The disease tends to have acute and chronic stages. During the acute stage, pain may be present and likely corresponds to the period of regressive remodeling. The pain may be due to the presence of inflammation of the synovium. The patient may complain of pain over the TMJ and may exhibit point tenderness to palpation in this area. Many patients exhibit pain on palpation of one or more muscles of mastication because of muscle guarding in an attempt not to move the painful joint. Curiously, many patients progress through the acute stage without an awareness of any pain at all. Some

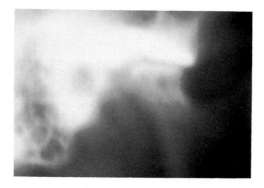

FIGURE 10–4. Tomogram demonstrating the presence of an "Eli's cyst" in the subchondral portion of the condylar head.

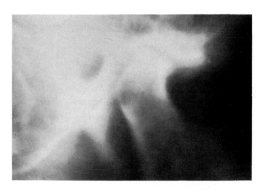

FIGURE 10–7. Tomogram demonstrating an anterior anvil-shaped deformity and lipping of the head of the condyle.

patients present without any clinical signs other than crepitus.

Irby and Zetz[14] and Mejersjo[11] estimate that the acute painful stage lasts about 9 months. The exact duration will vary from patient to patient, depending on local and systemic factors. The disease process tends to "burn out," and the joint is often left with characteristic osseous changes and surprisingly good function.

The patient may exhibit limited opening and pain throughout the range of mandibular motion. The cause of loss of range of motion may

be due to muscle guarding, capsular contracture, severe incongruity of joint structures, or mechanical blockage due to fibrosis or disc displacement.[5] The pain will often be unilateral and when involving the TMJ is often not evident in other joints throughout the body. Morning stiffness generally is not a feature of osteoarthrosis but can be present. It usually lasts no more than 30 minutes.[6] The clinician must be careful not to confuse stiffness, which is secondary to habitual clenching, with osteoarthrosis.

The joint noise associated with osteoarthrosis is crepitation[24]—a grating sound usually heard during both opening and closing. Crepitation is likely to be a late finding of the disease. If it is not present, one cannot rule out a diagnosis of osteoarthrosis, as osseous changes in the early stages may not be sufficient to cause crepitation.

Radiographic Features

The radiographic presentation of advanced osteoarthrosis can be dramatic. Changes include condyle flattening, osteophytes, eburnation, and decreased joint space. Flattening in combination with the formation of bone on the anterior joint margin gives the condyle a characteristic appearance sometimes referred to as an anvil-shaped deformity. Radiopaque loose bodies may be seen. There may be small radiolucent areas or Eli's cysts visible within the condylar head (see Figs. 10–5 and 10–10). Decreased range of motion may or may not be evident in the open views.

These changes are best demonstrated on computerized tomography (CT) or tomogram.[25,28] Only changes on the lateral portion of the condyle can be seen on a transcranial film. The temporal component and condylar head are more easily visualized, and the joint space better evaluated on a tomogram. Several examples of transcranial, panoramic, and tomographic films with osteoarthrotic changes are seen in Figures 10–9 through 10–14.

Osteoarthrosis may *not* show any radiographic evidence, particularly in the early stages. Conversely, it is not unusual to see striking changes on a radiograph with the patient complaining of no pain or pain from the contralateral side. It is impossible to determine the activity of the osteoarthrotic process from a radiograph alone. Some clinicians advocate bone scanning for this purpose (see chapter 18).[22]

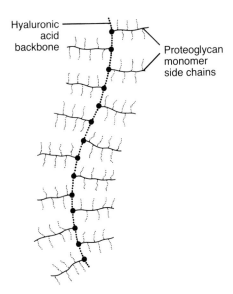

Hyaluronic acid backbone

Proteoglycan monomer side chains

FIGURE 10–8. The molecular structure of a proteoglycan molecule.

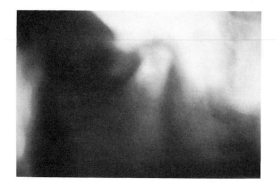

FIGURE 10–9. Severe osteoarthrotic changes 2 years after severe trauma was sustained to the chin.

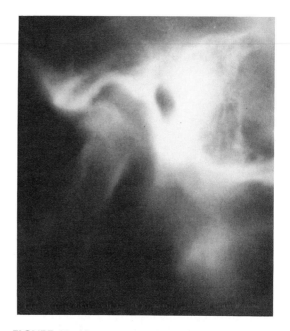

FIGURE 10–10. Severe osteoarthrotic changes 5 years after the patient suffered a severe fall and struck his chin.

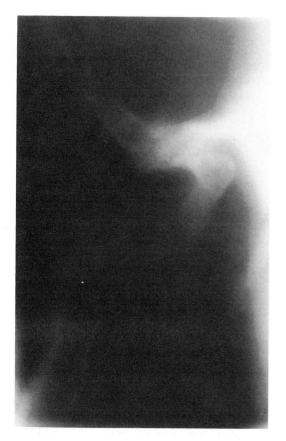

FIGURE 10–11. Tomogram demonstrating ''beaking'' of the condylar head commonly seen in late osteoarthrosis.

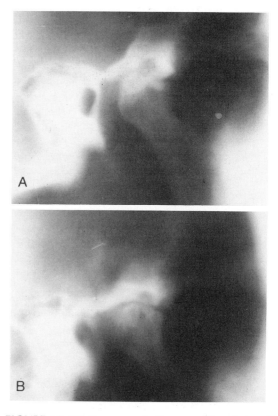

FIGURE 10–12. Tomogram in the open (*A*) and closed (*B*) positions demonstrating flattening, sclerosis, and ''Eli's cysts'' in both the condyle and temporal component.

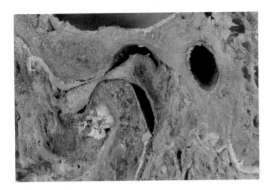

FIGURE 10–1. Sagittal section of a human temporomandibular joint showing degenerative changes of the condylar head without disc displacement. Note the thin midportion of the disc.

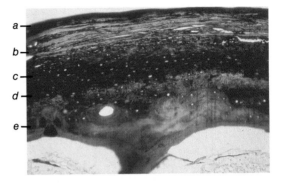

FIGURE 10–2. Photomicrograph of an adult condyle demonstrating the five layers of the articular surface. *a,* Articular surface; *b,* proliferative zone; *c,* fibrocartilage; *d,* calcified cartilage, and *e,* compact bone.

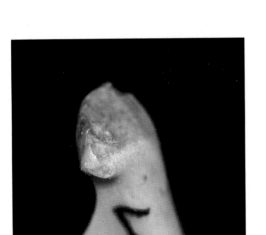

FIGURE 10–5. Dry condylar specimen demonstrating degenerative changes of the articular surface of the condyle.

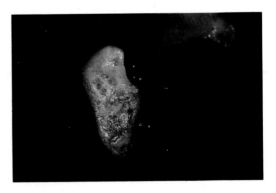

FIGURE 10–6. A second dry condylar specimen as in Figure 10–5.

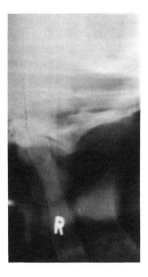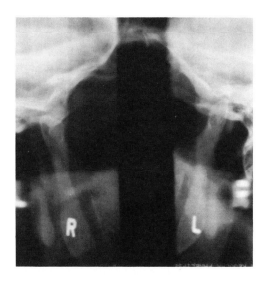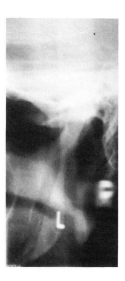

FIGURE 10–13. Panoramic film demonstrating osteoarthrotic changes of the right temporomandibular joint.

Laboratory Findings

The dentist will rarely have need to send a patient for laboratory testing. The diagnosis of osteoarthrosis is generally made from the history, TMJ examination, and radiographs. Laboratory findings, in contrast with some of the other arthritides, are unremarkable.[5,6,10] The erythrocyte sedimentation rates and rheumatoid factor findings are normal. Serum calcium, phosphate, and alkaline phosphatase levels are also normal. Antinuclear factor, urate, protein, and urine analyses would be within normal limits as well.

Synovial fluid content in osteoarthrotic joints has been studied.[5] Good viscosity and normal mucin clot formation are observed. Cartilage debris may be present, and a mildly elevated white blood cell count may be present with mostly mononuclear cells.

Treatment

To date no treatment exists that can reverse the anatomic and biochemical alterations of osteoarthrosis. The treatment approach has to be aimed at restoring function and managing pain through the acute phase of the disease. Little has been written comparing different techniques of treatment, specific to the osteoarthrotic TMJ. Indeed, it has yet to be shown that any of the treatment modalities shorten the course of the disease. Much of what is presented in the ensuing discussion is based on clinical experience.

The first step in treatment is to provide the patient with an explanation of the problem along with reassurance. The patient should be told about the acute painful stage and the "burn out" phase of the disease. The practitioner should not detail a particular time frame but should indicate that the clinical course is usually self-limiting. A description of the changes that the joint will go through, in terms the patient can understand, should be given, and a clear description of the proposed treatment plan with any alternatives should also be given. The patient will be more accepting of treatment if a clear rationale is provided. Reassurance is the only treatment for the patient who is asymptomatic except for crepitus associated with mandibular movement.

Treatments provided include one or more of the following: (1) medication, (2) physical therapy, (3) splint therapy, and only rarely (4) surgery. Because each of these areas is covered in detail elsewhere in this text, only a brief discussion is included here.

The most frequently used medications in the treatment of osteoarthrosis are the nonsteroidal anti-inflammatory drugs (NSAIDs). Aspirin is the most frequently given, and according to Lipstate and Ball,[6] it still is the preferred medication. Aspirin's long-term safety record, low cost, and good analgesic and anti-inflammatory properties are the reasons.

Many other NSAIDs are available. Common examples include naproxen (Naprosyn), sulindac (Clinoril), tolmetin sodium (Tolectin), and choline magnesium trisalicylate (Trilisate). The

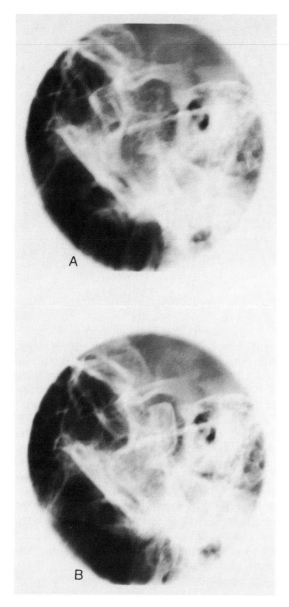

FIGURE 10–14. Transcranial film in the open (A) and closed (B) positions demonstrating flattening due to osteoarthrosis.

scribing. It is most important that the medication be taken as frequently as prescribed and for the recommended length of time. Patients who take these medications "only when it hurts" may not allow for sufficient blood levels for the anti-inflammatory effects.

Some practitioners advocate intra-articular steroids. This kind of treatment is the subject of much controversy because of reports of detected deterioration of joints.[30–32] Toller suggests that if a problem exists it is probably a function of the *frequency* of injection.[29]

Toller's clinical study indicates that *single* injections may be helpful for patients over 30 years old but are not indicated for younger patients. He cautions that other nonsurgical avenues of treatment should be exhausted first. Friedman and Moore[33] have questioned the efficacy of steroid injections. Their work showed that the beneficial effects are transient after 4 weeks. In our clinical experience, steroid injections for treatment of osteoarthrosis are rarely needed.

Muscle relaxant medications, antianxiety agents, or both are occasionally helpful in the treatment of this problem. They are particularly useful in the acute stages for those who are severe bruxers or clenchers. These drugs, in combination with NSAIDs, are also very effective. Examples of these medications include diazepam (Valium), methocarbamol (Robaxin), orphenadrine citrate (Norgesic Forte), and chlorzoxazone (Parafon Forte). Pharmacologic treatment of TMDs is discussed in detail in chapter 25.

Splint therapy is commonly applied in the treatment of osteoarthrosis. We recommend a flat plane splint to be worn all the time for the initial 2 weeks and then at night only. The splint should be of the full coverage type and provide full and simultaneous contact around the arch, with freedom of movement in all directions.

Unless the presence of an easily reducible internal derangement can be demonstrated, long-term repositioning therapy is not indicated for the patient with osteoarthrosis. Because the disease is self-limiting and the clinical course is benign, it makes little sense to reposition the mandible, necessitating expensive and time-consuming prosthetic and orthodontic therapy. Splint therapy is discussed in detail in chapter 23.

Physical therapy modalities can be successfully prescribed to reduce pain and increase or maintain range of motion. Hot packs can help

advantages of these medications when compared with aspirin include increased gastric tolerance with some and lower dosage frequency. These increase the probability of patient compliance. Curiously, one of these medications may prove to be very effective for one patient and not help another patient at all. The clinician may have to "shop around" before an effective medication is found. As with all medications, the practitioner should be familiar with the potential complications before prein relaxing involved muscles and decreasing pain in the muscles and joints themselves. Some patients find that ice compresses are superior. Patients need to be cautioned that ice compresses should be applied for no more than 20 minutes in any hour, or skin damage may result.

Physical therapists can make use of ultrasound, high voltage electrogalvanic stimulation, and massage techniques to help increase mandibular range of motion and decrease pain. In addition, gentle mobilization can be tried. The patient can be instructed to perform mild exercises at home.

Surgical approaches have been advocated for the osteoarthrotic TMJ but are rarely necessary.[10,32] The approaches include both arthroscopy and open joint surgery. Chapters 31 and 32 discuss these procedures in detail.

RHEUMATOID ARTHRITIS

Rheumatoid arthritis is a chronic systemic disorder of unknown etiology. This debilitating disease affects people of all ages.[34] The characteristic feature of rheumatoid arthritis is persistent inflammatory synovitis, usually involving peripheral joints in a symmetric distribution.[35] This disorder often results in destruction of articular cartilage, bony erosion, and disruption of physiologic form and function of the involved joint. The clinical course may vary from mild joint discomfort of short duration to chronic polyarthritis, pain, and gross deformity. The systemic nature of this disease may affect skin, blood vessels, eyes, pleura, lungs, peripheral nerves, and exocrine glands.

About 50% of patients with rheumatoid arthritis will present with TMJ complaints.[36] In the adult, these can vary from mild joint stiffness to total joint disruption and occlusal-facial deformity.[35] During childhood, rheumatoid arthritis can have a devastating effect on skeletofacial development[36,37] and can in some cases even cause ankylosis of the joint.[38]

Epidemiology and Etiology

A total of 7 million Americans are afflicted with rheumatoid arthritis.[39] There is a 3:1 female predilection and an increased incidence and decreased predilection for females with age. The peak age of onset is between 35 and 45 years.[35] There is no known etiology; however, strong genetic, autoimmune, and postinfectious factors are associated with the inci-

dence of rheumatoid arthritis. It is seen four times as often in first-degree relatives of patients with seropositive disease.[34] Rheumatoid arthritis has also been associated with the class II major histocompatibility gene complex antigen HLA-DR4, which may play a role in pathogenesis.[39] This antigen may leave these patients more susceptible to environmental factors. It is generally thought that an autoimmune reaction against antigen from a systemic infection[37] or an infection-altered IgG initiates the inflammatory response in the affected joints. The Epstein-Barr virus has been associated with rheumatoid arthritis in some etiologic manner.[35] Of patients with rheumatoid arthritis, 80% are seropositive for rheumatoid factor (RF) (antibodies against the patients' own IgG).[35] Even though the presence of RF is not conclusive for rheumatoid arthritis, it remains a useful diagnostic "marker" for the disease.[35]

Histologic and Pathophysiologic Features

Joints affected by rheumatoid arthritis show destructive and degenerative changes. These changes are first seen at the periphery of the joints. A nonspecific inflammatory response occurs in the synovial lining. An intense infiltration of macrophages, granulocytes, and plasma cells into the synovium is associated with a fibrin exudate.[40] The synovium becomes hypertrophic and is then referred to as a pannus. The pannus enlarges and extends into the joint space, forming villous folds (Fig. 10–15).[39] The pannus takes on a granulomatous[37] and edematous nature, which interferes with joint function and stretches the soft tissues, causing pain.[39] Lysosomal enzymes are released from macrophages and granulocytes in the synovium. These enzymes cause breakdown and erosion of the articular cartilage condylar head and temporal bone.[36] These degenerative changes may progress to impaired joint function, collapse, fibrous and bony ankylosis,[37,41] occlusal-facial deformity, and occlusal discrepancies.[42]

The synovial fluid of rheumatoid arthritic joints possesses characteristic pathologic changes. The fluid is usually sterile[36] and often turbid. Reduced viscosity, showing the mucus-string sign; decreased mucin clot complement[36] and glucose levels; and increased protein content are observed. The white blood cell count is usually above 20,000/mm³, with a predomi-

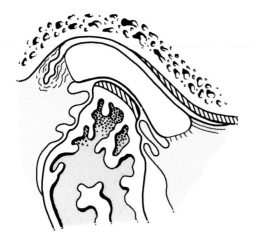

FIGURE 10–15. Schematic representation of a pannus eroding the temporomandibular joint in rheumatoid arthritis.

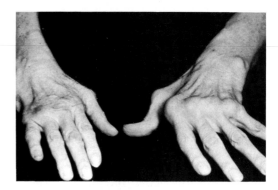

FIGURE 10–16. Rheumatoid arthritis. Ulnar drift. (Reproduced with permission from the American College of Rheumatology. *The Revised Clinical Slide Collection on the Rheumatic Diseases,* 1981.)

nance of polymorphonuclear leukocytes. Ragocytes or phagocytes with cytoplasmic inclusion bodies are often seen.[36,43]

General Clinical Course

Rheumatoid arthritis has both articular and systemic involvement. The joints of the hands, wrists, feet, elbows, shoulders, hips, knees, ankles, and TMJs may be involved symmetrically.[35,36] The first presentation of rheumatoid arthritis may be systemic: weight loss, fever, and fatigue.[39] The articular symptoms may include joint pain, morning stiffness of greater than 30 minutes (gelling),[36] joint swelling and loss of function,[34,44] rupture of tendons, and surrounding muscle ache. Continued degenerative changes may produce characteristic joint deformities, e.g., ulnar drift and swan-neck deformity of the fingers (Figs. 10–16 to 10–18).[36,45] About 15% of rheumatoid arthritis patients possess disabling deformities of the larger joints.[39] Subluxation of the first cervical vertebra on the second cervical vertebra from weakening of the transverse ligament may be present but asymptomatic. External trauma, however, may cause dislocation.[36] Rheumatoid nodules are present in 20% of rheumatoid arthritis patients; these nodules are most often found on frictional areas (Fig. 10–19).[39] Rheumatoid granulomas may also involve the myocardium, lung parenchyma, and sclera. These may be associated with cardiac arrhythmias, pericarditis, pulmonary fibrosis, pleuritis, epi-

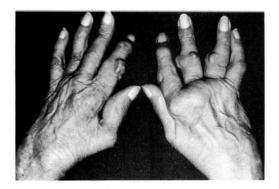

FIGURE 10–17. Rheumatoid arthritis. Finger deformity. (Reproduced with permission from the American College of Rheumatology. *The Revised Clinical Slide Collection on the Rheumatic Diseases,* 1981.)

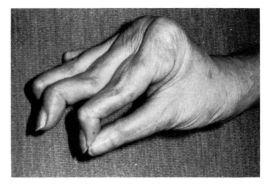

FIGURE 10–18. Rheumatoid arthritis. Swan-neck deformity.

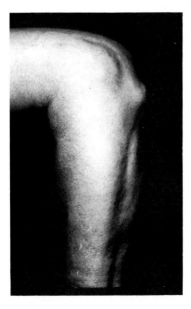

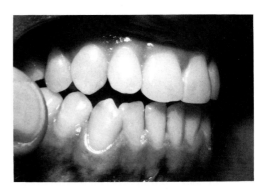

FIGURE 10-20. Class II anterior open bite in a patient with rheumatoid arthritis.

FIGURE 10-19. Rheumatoid arthritis. Subcutaneous nodules. (Reproduced with permission from the American College of Rheumatology. *The Revised Clinical Slide Collection on the Rheumatic Diseases,* 1981.)

scleritis, iritis, keratoconjunctivitis, and vasculitis leading to skin ulcerations and osteoporosis.[36] Of rheumatoid arthritis patients, 80% enter a prolonged period of remission.[35,39] Rheumatoid arthritis, hypersplenism, anemia, thrombocytopenia,[39] and neutropenia are seen in combination in Felty's syndrome.[36] Of rheumatoid arthritis patients, 5% suffer from Sjögren's syndrome. These patients are more susceptible to lymphoid malignancies.[36]

Clinical Course— Temporomandibular Joint

Reported incidence of bilateral involvement of the TMJ in patients with rheumatoid arthritis (RA) varies from 34 to 75%.[36,37,46] The most common clinical complaints are deep dull preauricular pain during function[36,47,48]; joints that are tender to palpation; morning joint stiffness, usually of greater than 30-minutes duration; clicking[49]; crepitus[36,47]; and decreased bite force.[50] Subsequent degeneration of joint architecture can lead to further functional loss, decreased mobility, and occlusal-facial deformity. The most common deformity is a class II anterior open bite (Fig. 10-20).[36] Fibrous and bony ankylosis is infrequently seen.[36,38,47]

Radiographic Findings

Radiographic changes are seen in 60% of patients with rheumatoid arthritis.[36] These changes are not usually visualized early in the disease. Irregular erosion or deossification of the condylar head, at the anterior and medial surfaces, is commonly the first radiographic change. Early changes are poorly visualized with panoramic imaging.[36] Complete erosion of the condylar head has been reported (Fig. 10-21).[36] Condylar destruction may lead to narrowing of the joint space and anterior positioning of the condylar head.[36] Flattening of the articular eminence and erosion of the roof of the glenoid fossa can be seen.[51] Marginal proliferation and flattening of the condyle may be associated with a remittent phase.[36] Joints

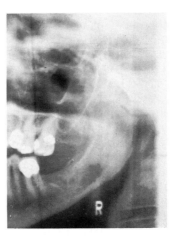

FIGURE 10-21. Panoramic film showing changes in the mandibular condyle in a patient with rheumatoid arthritis.

with advanced disease may display a spiked condylar appearance.[36] Deepened antigonial notching, posterior premature occlusion, shortened posterior ramus length,[52] osteoporotic bony trabecular pattern,[36] lipping,[36] and osteophyte formation[36] have also been described.

Laboratory Findings

Rheumatoid arthritis is often accompanied by characteristic but not pathognomonic laboratory findings. Patients with rheumatoid arthritis usually have seropositive findings for RF. An RF titer of greater than 1:1280 is highly suggestive of rheumatoid arthritis[36] and is associated with a poor prognosis. However, 20% of people who do not have rheumatoid arthritis are seropositive for RF. The latex fixation test for RF is useful, but the results must be interpreted with caution. They can be positive in patients with other diseases and negative in 20% of patients with rheumatoid arthritis.[39] About 50% of rheumatoid arthritis patients have seropositive findings for antinuclear antibodies.[36] Mild anemia and increased platelet count are often associated with active disease.[39] Leukocytosis and leukopenia, with a normal white blood cell count, are often seen. The Westergren erythrocyte sedimentation rate is usually elevated above 20 mm/hour during active disease.

Treatment Alternatives

The systemic nature of rheumatoid arthritis dictates that the treatment involve the patient's internist or rheumatologist. As mentioned, the TMJ involvement often parallels that of the general disease. The TMJ often becomes asymptomatic with improvement of the systemic disorder.[37] The approach includes nonsurgical, medical, and dental treatment (palliative and remittent) and surgical procedures. Treatment is combined physiotherapy,[53] splint therapy, and joint rest.[44] Occlusal adjustment can alleviate anterior open bites of small magnitudes.

Palliative therapy includes analgesics, NSAIDs, and injectable steroids. Although intra-articular corticosteroids can be effective in reducing pain, they may bring about additional degenerative changes, leading to fibrous ankylosis.[36,54]

The anti-inflammatory effect of NSAIDs is mediated by inhibition of prostaglandin cyclooxygenase and inhibition of leukocyte migration.[39,55] Very often, palliative therapy is very effective in managing the rheumatoid arthritic patient. Remittent therapy includes antimalarial drugs, e.g., hydrochloroquine; gold compounds; and D-penicillamines.[44] Low-dose corticosteroids, when used, are usually used temporarily. Immunosuppressive drugs, plasmaphoresis, and total lymph node irradiation have been used experimentally.[39]

Surgical Treatment

Surgical therapy is indicated when pain is unresponsive to other modes of therapy and to improve function and to correct a secondary occlusal-facial deformity.[36] A preoperative workup should include consultation with the patient's physician to fully understand the overall condition. Results of the Westergren erythrocyte sedimentation rate, complete blood workup, and RF titers should be known. Surgery is most successful when the disease is nonactive.[36]

In patients with early rheumatoid disease, the goals of surgery are to " . . .improve function, maintain vertical height, and reduce pain."[36] Kent and associates[37] suggest achieving these through conservative condylar shave and placement of an allogenic implant, with or without meniscectomy. Long-term success of this procedure, however, has been questioned. Fragmentation of the implant and the resultant severe foreign-body reaction have led to the abandonment of the use of these implants. At present, autogenous interpositional materials are used.

Surgical treatment of the patient with advanced TMJ rheumatoid disease, who presents with occlusal-facial deformities, may require total joint replacement to alleviate pain and to restore form, function, and facial aesthetics. The chance for recurrent deformity is thereby minimized. Arthroplasty and interpositional implants would not be adequate to correct the deformity. The patient may present with erosion of the condyle, vertical loss, convex facial appearance, mandibular deficiency, class II occlusal relationship, anterior open bite, and joint hypomobility. Cephalometric analysis may reveal the shortening of the mandibular rami, high mandibular plane angle, and retrognathic deformity. Radiographic imaging, including tomography, can demonstrate a spiked condylar remnant and erosion of the glenoid fossa.[36] Cephalometric analysis and model surgery are essential to determine the true nature of the deformity and the possible need for other corrective procedures (maxillary or chin augmentation procedures).

Kent and associates[37] recommend the Vitek-Kent fossa and condylar prosthesis for TMJ reconstruction. The length of the condyle analog and the size of the fossa replacement are established with the radiographs. Retromandibular and preauricular approaches are made. Coronoidectomy and suprahyoid myotomy may be necessary to rotate the mandible into the original occlusion. Because the vertical height has been lost, condylar bone is seldom removed. After modification, the fossa replacement is fixated to the zygomatic arch. Following preparation of the lateral ramus, the condylar prosthesis is secured with two self-tapping screws and one self-tapping bolt. Once beyond the healing stages, the patient usually enjoys normal joint function except lateral and protrusive movements and correction of the deformity.

Alternatively, some surgeons reconstruct the TMJ employing costochondral grafts.

Patients who already suffer from rheumatoid arthritis–induced deformity, but who at present are free of active disease, are functioning well, and are free of pain, may be managed utilizing orthognathic surgical techniques. Cephalometric predictions, model analysis, and model surgery are used in the workups of these patients. Corrective surgery may include maxillary, mandibular, or bimaxillary osteotomies. Chin and angle of mandible augmentation procedures may further enhance facial aesthetics.[36]

ANKYLOSING SPONDYLITIS

Ankylosing spondylitis is an arthropathy characterized by inflammation of the ligamentous insertion of the muscles on the bone. Spondylitis, sacroiliitis, ocular changes, and asymmetric oligarthritis of the large joints are associated with the presence of HLA-B27.[58]

This arthropathy afflicts 1% of whites and 0.25% of blacks. Females are affected three times as often as males by spondylitis but are equally affected by sacroiliitis. The onset of symptoms usually occurs in the second and third decades of life. A strong familial incidence is noted among first-degree family members.

Clinical Course

The presenting symptoms of ankylosing spondylitis often begin with mid to low back pain and stiffness, often after prolonged rest. Exercise and mobility often alleviate these symptoms. The pain may radiate into the buttocks and posterior areas of the legs. The central cartilaginous joints of the thoracic cage and the manubriosternal and sternoclavicular joints may be involved and cause pleuritic pain upon respiration. Dactylitis, Achilles tendonitis, plantar fasciitis, and iliac crest involvement may cause enthesopathic pain. Polyarthritis and polyarthralgia are common in the large and small distal joints. Early morning stiffness and joint swelling are often noted and are often asymmetric.

Ocular changes consist of anterior uveitis. Approximately a fourth of patients with ankylosing spondylitis experience this. Intermittent pain, redness, and photophobia may be either unilateral or bilateral. Patients with ankylosing spondylitis show decreased spinal mobility, loss of lumbar lordosis, and increased thoracic and cervical kyphosis. Reduced respiratory excursions, stooped posture, fixation of the spine with head inflection, and shuffling gait are latent findings.

In ankylosing spondylitis, the axial skeleton is affected by chronic inflammatory arthritis. This induces a fibrotic response that later calcifies, creating ossified ligaments, bony bridging between vertebrae, and skeletal immobility. Temporomandibular joint involvement can be as high as 50%,[59] and it is often accompanied by pain, stiffness, and decreased range of motion of the jaw including ankylosis. These findings are most common in older patients with more advanced stages of disease.[60]

Radiographic Findings

The radiographic changes seen in ankylosing spondylitis include pseudowidening of the sacroiliac joints due to destruction of cartilage and subchondral erosion. Osteoblastic response causes sclerosis of the bony margins; osteoid tissue ingrowth and calcification cause bridging of the joint spaces. Juxta-articular osteopenia is seen later. Flattening of the normal concave surface of the vertebral bodies gives a square appearance to the vertebrae. These are often the first radiographic changes seen in ankylosing spondylitis. The syndesmophytes that bridge the vertebrae immobilize the spine and give it a bamboo-like appearance (Fig. 10–22). Radiographic findings in the TMJ include bony erosion, subchondral sclerosis, and usually narrow joint space.[61]

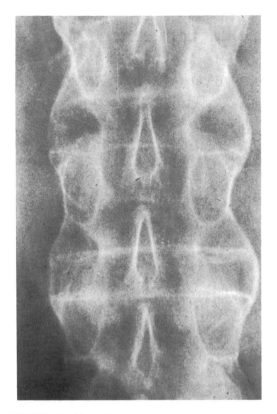

FIGURE 10–22. Ankylosing spondylitis, radiograph of the spine. Note the calcified joint spaces. (Reproduced with permission from the American College of Rheumatology. *The Revised Clinical Slide Collection on the Rheumatic Diseases,* 1981.)

Laboratory Findings

No specific laboratory test exists for ankylosing spondylitis. Early elevation of the erythrocyte sedimentation rate is consistent with the inflammatory process. Alkaline phosphatase levels may be elevated during the osteitis phase. Approximately 90% of white and 50% of black patients with ankylosing spondylitis harbor HLA-B27.[58]

Treatment Alternatives

The treatment of ankylosing spondylitis relies mostly on physical therapy and NSAID therapy. The NSAIDs help promote exercise and function, inhibiting calcification and axial immobility and thereby promoting maximal motion and function. "Spondylitic" jackets have been used to maintain posture and alleviate vertebral pain. Treatment of TMJ symptoms also involves NSAID and aggressive phys-

ical therapy. Intra-articular steroid injections have been advocated as an effective means of reducing the symptoms, but this remains controversial. In cases of ankylosis of the TMJ, surgical correction, including total joint reconstruction, may be necessary.

PSORIATIC ARTHRITIS

Psoriatic arthritis is an inflammatory process that affects approximately 6% of patients with psoriasis. Psoriasis occurs in approximately 1.2% of the population.[62] The onset of the disease is usually between the ages of 35 and 45 years. Psoriatic arthritis is characterized by the following triad: (1) psoriasis, (2) erosive polyarthritis, and (3) negative rheumatoid factor findings. Unlike rheumatoid arthritis, psoriatic arthritis affects men more frequently than women (1:1.4)[62] and has a predilection for the distal rather than the proximal interphalangeal joints. It is, therefore, a distinct pathologic entity from rheumatoid arthritis.

Clinical Course

Psoriatic arthritis is diagnosed through the clinical symptoms and findings on examination. Patients often present with fatigability, morning stiffness of the affected joints, joint swelling, limitation of motion, joint pain, myalgia, weight loss, fever, and malaise. The clinical aggressiveness of psoriasis does not necessarily parallel that of rheumatoid arthritis. The clinical features, however, are similar. Therefore, the history of psoriasis is necessary to confirm the diagnosis. The absence of RF and subcutaneous nodules usually present in the patient with rheumatoid arthritis will also aid in the diagnosis. Improvement of the arthritis generally follows improvement in the skin lesions. Remission of joint symptoms tends to be more frequent and complete in psoriatic arthritis than in rheumatoid arthritis. The finding of synovitis often alludes to the onset of psoriatic arthritis.

Patients are divided into three groups. Group I patients present with asymmetric articular synovitis, often of the distal interphalangeal or the proximal interphalangeal joints of the hands and feet. Clinically, the fingers may appear as "sausage digits" (Fig. 10–23). This appearance is due to the attendant flexor tendon sheath effusion. These patients often experience a less aggressive and disabling course.

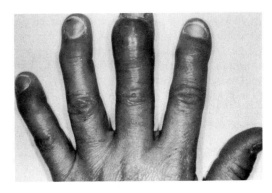

FIGURE 10–23. "Sausage" digits in a patient with psoriatic arthritis. (Reproduced with permission from the American College of Rheumatology. *The Revised Clinical Slide Collection on the Rheumatic Diseases,* 1981.)

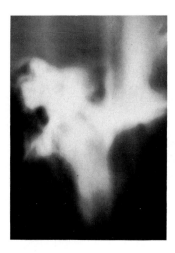

FIGURE 10–24. Tomogram of a patient with psoriatic arthritis showing severe degeneration and ankylosis of the temporomandibular joint.

Group II patients present with symmetric involvement of the joints. Approximately 50% of these patients may experience erratic, destructive, deforming, disabling, and aggressive courses.

Group III patients, or psoriatic spondyloarthritic patients, present with sacroiliitis or ankylosing spondylitis with psoriasis. These patients have clinical complaints similar to those of patients with idiopathic ankylosing spondylitis.

Arthritis mutilans is a complication of psoriatic arthritis, occurring equally among the three groups of PsA patients. Arthritis mutilans is characterized by a severe destructive arthritis with a very aggressive course affecting the small joints of the hands and feet. Osteolysis, bone absorption, ankylosis, and osteoporosis of the metacarpals, metatarsals, and phalanges are often seen radiographically.

Temporomandibular joint involvement is characterized by episodic, unilateral, painful joints and restricted motion.[63] A history of sudden onset and spontaneous remission is typical. Symptoms may last for many months. In severe cases, ankylosis of the joint has been reported (Fig. 10–24).[64,65]

Laboratory Findings

No specific laboratory findings exist for psoriatic arthritis. Because it is a seronegative disease, the diagnosis is based on clinical and radiographic findings consistent with psoriatic arthritis. Owing to widespread inflammation, the erythrocyte sedimentation rate and the C-reactive protein level are often elevated. These cases are associated with the presence of HLA antigens B17, Bw38, Bw39, and DRw4.[62]

Radiographic Findings

The radiographic findings consistent with psoriatic arthritis include soft tissue swelling of the peripheral joints, loss of cartilage space, demineralization, erosions, bony ankylosis, subluxation, and subchondral cysts. Arthritis mutilans often occurs with "whittling, pencil-in-cup, opera-glass hand, and telescope-finger" deformities on radiographic studies (Fig. 10–25). In such patients, there is often evidence of coexisting osteoporosis, osteolysis, and ankylosis. Radiographs of the TMJ often appear normal, but erosive and osteoporotic changes have been observed.[66]

Treatment Alternatives

Acute psoriatic arthritis is treated with bed rest, physical therapy, orthotics, and NSAIDs including aspirin. Corticosteroids may be given to treat patients who do not respond to conservative therapy. In severe cases, a remittent agent, such as gold salts, 6-mercaptopurine, and methotrexate, may be used. Treatment of the TMJ symptoms is usually limited to NSAIDs and physical therapy to maximize joint mobility during exacerbation of symptoms. In cases of true bony ankylosis, condylectomy and interpositional gap arthroplasty have been advocated by Stimson and Leban[64] and by Kudryk and coworkers.[65]

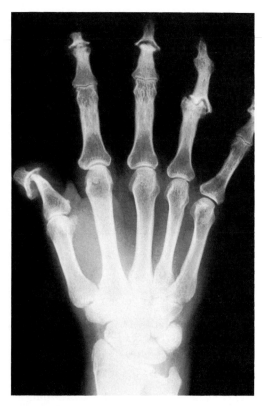

FIGURE 10–25. Radiograph of the hand of a patient with psoriatic arthritis. (Reproduced with permission from the American College of Rheumatology. *The Revised Clinical Slide Collection on the Rheumatic Diseases,* 1981.)

JUVENILE RHEUMATOID ARTHRITIS

Juvenile rheumatoid arthritis, or Still's disease, is a chronic disease characterized by synovitis. Extra-articular findings are variable. It is seen in children younger than 16 years. These patients often present with fever, myalgia, arthralgia, sore throat, rash, lymphadenopathy, and leukocytosis.[67] Usually, no history of rheumatoid arthritis has been recorded in the family. The diagnosis is made clinically, once all other possibilities are ruled out.

Juvenile rheumatoid arthritis is a chronic disease. Often, a recent history of systemic infection, trauma, or psychologic stress is reported. The proposed pathophysiology is similar to that of the adult form of rheumatoid arthritis. These cases are associated with HLA-DR5,DR8.

Clinical Course

Juvenile rheumatoid arthritis is divided into five subgroups according to clinical presentation.[67] The first group is polyarticular (RF positive) juvenile rheumatoid arthritis. Approximately 10% of children with juvenile rheumatoid arthritis experience this form of the disease. They are seropositive for RF. A female predilection and a symmetric involvement of the joints are noted. Symptoms often appear late in childhood.

These children present with swelling of the joints of the fingers, neck pain, limited motion, and subluxation of the atlantoaxial joint. The systemic nature of this disease is defined by fever, weight loss, anemia, and growth retardation. Morning stiffness and rheumatoid nodules are also seen.

The TMJ may be involved in this patient group and may be unilateral or bilateral. Patients often experience preauricular pain, ear pain during during mandibular function, and decreased range of motion of the mandible. Micrognathia and ankylosis are often seen in these children (Fig. 10–26).[68,69] These cases have positive findings for rheumatoid factor, and 75% have antinuclear antibodies. Treatment of this condition requires surgical intervention not only to restore joint mobility (release of the ankylosis) but also to correct the resulting malocclusion and dentofacial deformity.

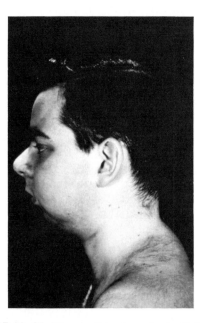

FIGURE 10–26. Micrognathia of a patient with juvenile rheumatoid arthritis. (Reproduced with permission from the American College of Rheumatology. *The Revised Clinical Slide Collection on the Rheumatic Diseases,* 1981.)

Polyarticular (RF negative) juvenile rheumatoid arthritis makes up 30% of diagnosed juvenile rheumatoid arthritis cases. This disease differs from polyarticular (RF positive) disease in that patients are seropositive for RF, prognoses are more favorable, and rheumatoid vasculitis does not occur. Onset can occur at any age. About 5% are seropositive for antinuclear antibodies. Temporomandibular joint involvement is also common in this group.

Polyarticular juvenile rheumatoid arthritis, type I, affects females four times that of males. Onset is usually in early childhood. This form of juvenile rheumatoid arthritis is associated with acute iridocyclitis. The large joints are usually involved, but less than four joints during the first 6 months of the disease. Temporomandibular joint involvement is possible. Patients rarely experience severe arthritis.

Periarticular juvenile rheumatoid arthritis, type II, affects males more often than females. Onset is usually in late childhood. The patients lack rheumatoid factor and antinuclear antibodies. The disease usually progresses to Reiter's syndrome or ankylosing spondylitis. Sacroiliitis and acute iridocyclitis are seen.

Systemic-onset juvenile rheumatoid arthritis, or febrile Still's disease, constitutes 20% of juvenile rheumatoid arthritis cases. This form usually occurs before the age of 5 years. A slight male predilection is noted. These children usually present with a high fever and a pink rash on the trunk and upper arms. Lymphadenopathy and hepatosplenomegaly can be present. Pleuritis, pericarditis, arthralgia, muscle spasm, and morning stiffness are also observed. Patients lack rheumatoid factor and antinuclear antibodies in the serum. Late in the course, only arthritis remains.

SYSTEMIC LUPUS ERYTHEMATOSUS

Systemic lupus erythematosus (SLE) is classified as a connective tissue or, more appropriately, a collagen and vascular disorder of unknown etiology. Its frequency among the inflammatory arthritides is second to that of rheumatoid arthritis. This disorder results from the formation of antinuclear antibodies that form immune complexes that deposit within vessel walls, causing widespread multisystemic disturbances.

Systemic lupus erythematosus occurs primarily in women (90 to 95%),[70] usually between 20 and 40 years of age. The problems associated with SLE can be subdivided into vasculitis and polyserositis. Small vessel vasculitis leads to renal, central nervous system, and cutaneous involvement. Polyserositis leads to synovial, pleural, pericardial, and peritoneal involvement. The major causes of SLE-related deaths are renal failure, central nervous system disease, hemorrhage, and infection.

Clinical Course

Diagnosis of SLE is often difficult. Patients present with vague symptoms including joint pain, butterfly skin rash on the face (Fig. 10–27), weakness, malaise, and fever. Joint involvement is very common. The disorder typically appears as a migratory polyarthralgia or as an asymmetric polyarthritis, without obvious joint deformity. Aseptic necrosis of the femoral head can be seen, especially in the patient who is receiving corticosteroid therapy.[70]

Temporomandibular joint involvement is relatively common. Jonsson and colleagues[71] reported that two thirds of the SLE patients they evaluated reported having had temporomandibular symptoms in the past, with 59% having had severe symptoms. The most frequent clinical manifestations of the disease include reduced mobility of the mandible, locking or dislocation, tenderness to palpation, and pain on movement of the TMJs. Tuggle[72] re-

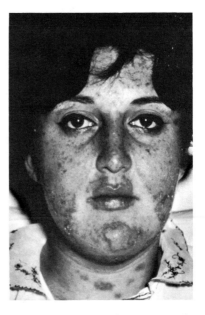

FIGURE 10–27. Skin rash of a patient with systemic lupus erythematosus. (Reproduced with permission from the American College of Rheumatology. *The Revised Clinical Slide Collection on the Rheumatic Diseases,* 1981.)

ported a case in which TMJ symptoms were the only arthritis-related complaints of a patient who was later diagnosed with SLE.

Radiographic Findings

The most common radiographic finding in the affected condyle is the flattening of its head. Erosions, osteophytes, and sclerosis can also be seen.[73,74]

Treatment

Treatment of this condition is geared toward management of the underlying systemic condition. Temporomandibular symptoms are treated palliatively, using a combination of analgesic and anti-inflammatory medications with physical therapy to improve the range of motion.

REITER'S SYNDROME

Reiter's syndrome has been classically described as a triad of arthritis, conjunctivitis, and urethritis.[75] Today, the findings of seronegative oligoarticular asymmetric arthritis and urethritis are sufficient to make the diagnosis of Reiter's syndrome (Figs. 10–28 through 10–30).

Reiter's syndrome is the most common cause of arthritis in young males.[75] There are two forms of the disease: postvenereal and postdysenteric. Females are less affected by the postvenereal type. There seems to be an equal sex predilection of the postdysenteric type.

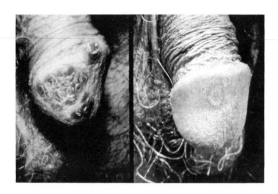

FIGURE 10–29. Reiter's syndrome. Urethritis. (Reproduced with permission from the American College of Rheumatology. *The Revised Clinical Slide Collection on the Rheumatic Diseases,* 1981.)

The exact pathogenesis of this disease is unknown. The HLA-B27 alloantigen occurs with high frequency in the diseased population.[76] Up to 90% of Reiter's syndrome cases are found to be HLA-B27 seropositive. An infectious process of the urogenital tract or gut coupled with a specific genetic background seems to predispose the patient to develop Reiter's syndrome. Reports of TMJ involvement are rare. Bomalsky and Jiminez[77] reported a patient with arthritic symptoms of TMJ, and they believe that this finding may be grossly under-

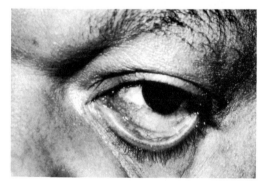

FIGURE 10–28. Reiter's syndrome. Uveitis. (Reproduced with permission from the American College of Rheumatology. *The Revised Clinical Slide Collection on the Rheumatic Diseases,* 1981.)

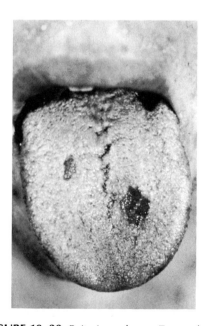

FIGURE 10–30. Reiter's syndrome. Tongue lesion.

reported in the literature.[77] This syndrome lacks a specific histopathologic lesion.

Clinical Course

The first manifestation of the disease is urethritis. This is usually followed by the development of conjunctivitis and finally arthritis. The urethral discharge can be asymptomatic with a moderate amount of serous discharge. However, it may also be accompanied by a profuse purulent and blood-stained discharge. This can sometimes lead to urologic complications, which may include prostatitis, internal strictures, seminal vasculitis, cystitis, and urethral stenosis. The conjunctivitis is frequently minimal and of short duration. Symptomatic conjunctivitis has also been described in rare instances.[76] When this is the case, the patient will present with burning, itching "red eyes" accompanied by profuse purulent discharge. Rare ocular complications include nongranulomatous anterior uveitis, superficial keratitis, posterior uveitis, and optic neuritis.

A rheumatologic manifestation of Reiter's syndrome includes an acute onset of an asymmetric oligarticular arthritis, predominantly affecting the joints of the lower extremities. Fever and malaise will often accompany the arthritic symptoms. Examination of the affected joints will reveal warm erythematous joints, painful to palpation.

Other clinical features often associated with Reiter's syndrome are mucocutaneous lesions that can be found in the mouth, the palms and soles, and the glans penis. Furthermore, 30% of the patients afflicted with Reiter's syndrome of the postvenereal type will have a skin lesion termed keratoderma blennorrhagicum.[75] This lesion consists of crusted, scaly papules distributed on the palms, soles, and glans penis. Occasionally, the skin of the scalp, trunk limbs, and scrotum can also be affected.

Rare manifestations of Reiter's syndrome include pleuropericarditis, aortic regurgitation, neurologic findings, and secondary amyloidosis.

Laboratory Findings

There are no specific diagnostic tests for Reiter's syndrome. Some of the common laboratory findings include mild anemia of chronic disease, leukocytosis, and elevated erythrocyte sedimentation rates and C-reactive protein levels. Findings of rheumatoid factor and antinuclear antibodies are negative.

Radiographic Findings

Radiographically, the acute phase of the disease is not accompanied by bony changes but may reveal soft tissue edema over the affected joint. In the chronic phase, radiographic findings include bony erosion and narrowing of the joint space. Periosteal bony apposition along the shaft adjacent to the involved joint can also be seen. This finding can be suggestive of Reiter's syndrome. Temporomandibular joint findings include erosive changes of the condylar head and narrowing of the joint space.[77]

Treatment

Treatment of Reiter's syndrome is often empirical and palliative in nature. The acute arthritis is treated with analgesics and NSAIDS.[75] The conjunctivitis and oral lesions rarely require treatment. The uveitis, however, is treated with corticosteroids administered topically, periocularly, or systemically, depending on the severity of the symptoms. The administration of systemic corticosteroids can exacerbate the mucocutaneous eruptions.

INFECTIOUS ARTHRITIDES

Septic or infectious arthritides of the TMJ are extremely rare. The mechanism of inoculation of the causative microorganism is usually a penetrating wound from an injection into the joint or a direct extension from an adjacent structure, such as the middle ear or parotid gland. Sometimes, the infectious organism can gain access to the joint from a distant site in the body via hematogenous dissemination. Generally, the patient who would be most susceptible to this type of arthritis is the patient with diabetes mellitus, SLE, rheumatoid arthritis, and other immunosuppressive diseases. Rheumatoid arthritis patients are at risk because of the presence of a decreased immune response as well as damaged joint structures. Trimble and associates[78] reported a case of septic arthritis of the TMJ in a rheumatoid arthritis patient.

Various microorganisms have been implicated in the pathogenesis of septic arthritis of the TMJ. Although *Neisseria gonorrhoeae,*

Staphylococcus aureus, and streptococci account for 95% of the acute pyogenic arthritis in adults, *Haemophilus influenzae* has been implicated as an etiologic factor in children.[79]

Malignant otitis externa, a rare and severe form of otitis externa caused by *Pseudomonas aeruginosa* and seen in the elderly diabetic patient, can spread to involve the TMJ.

Clinical Course

Clinical findings are variable. Preauricular swelling and pain and limitation in jaw opening are all signs of the disease.[80] The cardinal signs of the infectious process (redness, heat, and swelling) may be masked because most of these patients are debilitated and immunosuppressed. In addition, the presence of fascial attachments around the joint will limit the extension of the process to the surface where it would be more apparent clinically.

Radiographic Findings

Radiographic findings are seen late in the disease progression, usually in the form of destruction of the articular cartilage. Changes may be best observed utilizing CT imaging.[80]

Laboratory Findings

Laboratory findings include elevated erythrocyte sedimentation rates and leukocytosis. Aspiration with examination of joint fluid is the best diagnostic test that can be performed when one suspects a septic joint. The sample can be analyzed microscopically for the presence of microorganisms and cultured. A total leukocyte count and a fasting synovial glucose sample can also be obtained. The fasting synovial glucose level is decreased by 50% in the presence of bacterial infections. If a disseminated source is suspected blood culture results can be obtained to confirm the diagnosis.

Treatment

Treatment of septic arthritis of the TMJ is generally surgical management. The administration of parenteral antibiotics has limited success because of the difficulty in penetrating the affected area. Treatment ranges from repeated aspiration, incision, and drainage, to arthrotomy and debridement of the joint.[80]

LYME DISEASE

Lyme disease is a spirochetal infection transmitted by the tick *Ixodes dammini*.[81] The patients exposed to this infection present with fever, headache, neck stiffness, myalgia, arthralgia, and erythema chronicum migrans.[82] Erythema chronicum migrans often begins as a red macule or papule (Fig. 10–31). The surrounding erythematous tissues may cover a diameter of 15 cm. The center of these lesions may become clear, indurated, vesicular, or necrotic. Several red rings may be seen at the

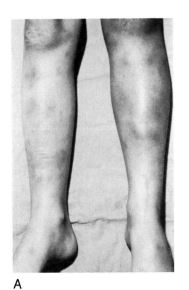
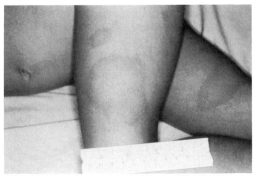

A   B

FIGURE 10–31A and B. Lyme disease. Macular rash.

outer border of these lesions. Secondary lesions may also be observed. These lesions are warm but nontender. Regional lymphadenopathy is common. The cutaneous lesions usually fade within a month.

Of all infected patients, 15% develop neurologic involvement weeks after the onset of symptoms. This often includes meningoencephalitis, cranial nerve involvement, and peripheral radiculoneuropathy. The cerebrospinal fluid of these patients contains 100 lymphocytes/μL. Many patients show signs of cardiac involvement, including atrioventricular block, myopericarditis, and cardiomegaly. Early in the course of this disease, arthralgia and myalgia may be severe. Late in the disease, arthritis develops. Patients present with joint swelling but little pain. Usually, only one or two large joints, often the knee, are affected.[81] This arthritis may recur for years following the disease. About 10% of patients develop chronic arthritis. The TMJ may be involved in as many as a third of the patients.[83] In a number of cases, TMJ involvement can be the initial sign. Some patients will complain of preauricular pain and limited mouth opening.

Diagnosis is confirmed by the presence of IgM antibody to the spirochete. The neurologic, cardiac, and joint involvement parallels the IgM level. Synovial fluid contains approximately 25,000 cells/μL, mostly neutrophils. The serum glutamic-oxaloacetic transaminase level is elevated.

Treatment Alternatives

Once the disease is diagnosed, the antibiotic regimen most commonly employed is doxycycline 100 mg twice a day for 14 to 21 days. Alternatively, amoxicillin 500 mg four times a day in combination with probenecid (Benemid) 500 mg twice a day for 21 days can be used. For those patients who fail to respond to the oral regimen, intravenous ceftriaxone for 2 weeks may be given. This disease should be managed in close cooperation with a rheumatologist.

METABOLIC ARTHRITIDES
Gout and Pseudogout

Gout is a disease entity that manifests itself by one or many of the following:

- Increase in the serum urate concentration

- Recurrent attacks of a characteristic acute arthritis
- Tophi (deposits of monosodium urate monohydrate) in and around the ear and joints of the extremities (Fig. 10–32)
- Renal disease
- Uric acid nephrolithiasis.

The prevalence of gout in the western world ranges from 0.13 to 0.37% of the general population. Gout is primarily a disease of adult men, with a peak incidence in the fifth decade. Women account for only 5% of the cases.[84]

The identification of several specific factors associated with the development of gout indicates the disorder is most likely a clinical manifestation of a group of diseases. Genetic as well as environmental factors that will tend to increase the serum urate concentration seem to be involved in the pathogenesis of gout. Gout is inherited as an autosomal dominant trait, but more commonly genetic studies suggest multifactorial inheritance.[84] Two specific enzymatic causes of gout are hypoxanthine guanine phosphoribosyltransferase deficiency and 5-phosphoribosyl-1-pyrophosphate synthetase overactivity.

Clinical Course

The clinical course of gout may be subdivided into four stages: asymptomatic hyperuricemia, acute gouty arthritis, intercritical gout,

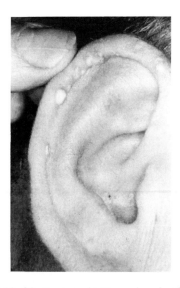

FIGURE 10–32. Gouty tophi. (Reproduced with permission from the American College of Rheumatology. *The Revised Clinical Slide Collection on the Rheumatic Diseases*, 1981.)

and chronic tophaceous gout. Nephrolithiasis may occur in stages two through four.

Stage I: Asymptomatic Hyperuricemia. During this stage, the serum urate level is raised, but arthritic symptoms, tophi, and uric acid deposits are not present. The tendency toward acute gouty arthritis will increase as a function of the hyperuricemia level and duration. The risk of nephrolithiasis also correlates with these findings. The first stage of gout usually ends with the first attack of gouty arthritis or nephrolithiasis.

Stage II: Acute Gouty Arthritis. Acute gouty arthritis is exquisitely painful. It is initially manifested as a monoarticular arthritis with no systemic symptoms, rapidly progressing to a polyarticular form with an accompanying fever.

Acute gouty arthritis is predominantly a disease of the distal extremities. The more distal the site of involvement the more typical the attacks. Approximately 90% of affected patients experience acute attacks that involve the great toe (podagra).[85] Following the great toe, the sites of initial involvement are the insteps, ankles, heels, knees, fingers, and elbows. In patients with severe disease other joints may also be involved including the hips, shoulders, spine, sacroiliac, sternoclavicular, and temporomandibular. A few cases have been reported with TMJ symptoms of pain and limitation of movement.[86–88]

Usually, the first attack is sudden and explosive in nature, often at night. Trigger factors include alcohol ingestion, certain drugs, dietary excess, trauma, and surgery. The painful arthritis is often accompanied by a febrile state. Laboratory findings usually include leukocytosis and elevated sedimentation rate.

Stage III: Intercritical Gout. This is an asymptomatic phase beginning at the time the symptoms of the acute gouty arthritis subside. The patient is completely symptom-free. Of affected patients, 60% will experience a relapse within the first year; 7% will never have a relapse.[84]

The intercritical phase may last up to 10 years. Should a second attack occur, the succeeding attacks will occur more frequently and will usually be polyarticular, more severe, prolonged, and associated with fever.

Stage IV: Chronic Tophaceous Gout. This stage is characterized by the formation of tophaceous deposits. The degree and duration of the hyperuricemia and the severity of the renal disease will determine the amount of tophaceous deposits. The classic location for the deposits is the helix and antihelix of the ear. They can also be found along the ulnar surface of the forearm, the olecranon bursae, and the Achilles tendon. Tophi rarely become infected. They may ulcerate and exude a material high in monosodium urate crystals.

Up to 90% of patients afflicted with gout exhibit some degree of renal dysfunction. Prior to the advent of long-term hemodialysis renal failure accounted for 17 to 25% of the fatal outcomes of gout.[84]

Radiographic Findings

Radiographic features of gouty arthritis, when present, may include erosive changes in the condylar head. Degenerative changes of the articular surface of the condyle will be associated with the presence of tophi within the joint.[89]

Laboratory Findings

Hyperuricemia is a hallmark in gout. Leukocytosis and an increased erythrocyte sedimentation rate, which are nonspecific, are usually associated with gouty arthritis. The aspiration of a tophus and the examination of the aspirate under a polarizing microscope will reveal the presence of monosodium urate crystals and will obviously confirm the presence of a tophus.[90]

Treatment

The treatment of gout is aimed at terminating the acute attack as promptly as possible. In addition, preventing relapses; preventing systemic complications of the disease, such as nephropathy; preventing or reversing contributing factors, such as obesity, hypertriglyceridemia, and hypertension; and preventing nephrolithiasis are the other objectives.

Anti-inflammatory medications are usually used, and the drug of choice is colchicine. Standard therapy for acute gout involves the administration of 0.6 mg qh or 1.0 mg q2h orally, until one of the following occurs: symptoms improve, gastrointestinal side effects develop, or a maximum of 6 mg is taken without any signs of relief. Most patients show signs of relief within the first 12 hours of treatment. However, almost 80% of all patients will not be able to tolerate an optimal dose of colchicine because of gastrointestinal side effects. In these cases, indomethacin is given. It is generally better tolerated than colchicine and may therefore be the drug of choice for the patient afflicted with acute gouty arthritis.[84]

Calcium pyrophosphate dihydrate crystal deposition disease, a syndrome that clinically mimicks gout, is also a metabolic arthritis. This disease is often referred to as pseudogout. The absence of urate crystal deposition and the lack of acute attacks have led to the more appropriate name of pyrophosphate arthropathy.

Pyrophosphate arthropathy occurs in approximately 5% of the adult population. Two types of meniscal calcifications (chondrocalcinosis) are seen in these patients. The primary form, usually seen in the elderly, is associated with the presence of diffuse calcium salt deposits in the menisci of the hip, shoulder, and sternoclavicular and temporomandibular joints. A secondary form of the disease is observed in the younger patient. A history of trauma to the affected joint can be elicited. A 1.5:1 male predominance occurs in the primary form of the disease. Trauma or joint surgery is often associated with chondrocalcinosis. The definitive diagnosis is based on the presence of calcium pyrophosphate dihydrate crystals.

Radiographic Findings

Radiographic findings include punctate and linear radiolucent lesions of the fibrocartilaginous joint structures. Even though large joints are usually affected, TMJ involvement has been reported by several workers.[91–93] Subchondral bone cysts and osteoarthrosis are often associated with pyrophosphate arthropathy. Fibrocartilaginous structures are most dramatically involved; hence, the frequency of TMJ involvement. During an acute attack, the synovium becomes infiltrated with polymorphonuclear lymphocytes. With the resolution of the acute phase, these become replaced by mononuclear cells and fibroblasts. Microscopic evidence of crystalline deposition in the superficial synovium is evident.

Treatment

Acute attacks of "pseudogout" are treated with repeated aspiration of joint fluids to extract the crystals and intra-articular corticosteroid injections. In cases with severe degenerative changes, arthroplasty and meniscectomy are advocated.[86] Nonsurgical management with anti-inflammatory and analgesic medica-

tions is usually sufficient, as it is a self-limiting disease process that will resolve spontaneously.

REFERENCES

1. Kreutziger, K. and Mahan, P.: Temporomandibular degenerative joint disease. Oral Surg. Oral Med. Oral Path. 40:165–182, 1975.
2. Jarrerr, M. and Schmid, F.: Rheumatic disorders of the TMJ. In *The President's Conference of the Examination, Diagnosis and Management of TMJ Disorders.* D. Laskin, et al (eds.). Am. Dent. Assoc., Chicago, 1982.
3. Lundeen, T., Levitt, S., and McKinney, M.: Evaluation of TMJ disorders by clinician ratings. J. Prosthet. Dent. 59:202–211, 1988.
4. Tanaka, T.: A rational approach to the differential diagnosis of arthritic disorders. J. Prosthet. Dent. 56:727–731, 1986.
5. Moll, J.: Osteoarthritis. In *Rheumatology in Clinical Practice.* J. Moll (ed.). Blackwell Publishers, Boston, 1987.
6. Lipstate, J. and Ball, G.: Osteoarthritis. In *Clinical Rheumatology.* G. Ball and W. Koopman (eds.). W.B. Saunders Co., Philadelphia, 1986.
7. Bole, G.: Osteoarthritis. In *Rheumatology and Immunology,* 2nd ed. A. Cohen and J. Bennett (eds.). Grune & Stratton, New York, 1986.
8. Blackwood, H.: Arthritis of the mandibular joint. Br. Dent. J. 115:317–326, 1963.
9. Macalister, A.: A microscopic study of the human temporomandibular joint. N.Z. Dent. J. 50:161–172, 1954.
10. Toller, P.: Temporomandibular arthropathy. Proc. R. Soc. Med. 67:153–159, 1974.
11. Mejersjo, C.: Therapeutic and prognostic considerations in TMJ osteoartrosis: A literature review and a long-term study in 11 subjects. J. Craniomandib. Pract. 5:70–78, 1987.
12. Kellgren, J. and Moore, R.: Generalized osteoarthritis and Heberden's nodes. Br. Med. J. 1:181–187, 1952.
13. Madsen, B.: Normal variations in anatomy, condylar movements and arthrosis frequency of the TMJs. Acta Radiol. 4:273–288, 1966.
14. Irby, W. and Zetz, M.: Osteoarthritis and rheumatoid arthritis affecting the TMJ. In *The President's Conference on the Examination, Diagnosis and Management of TMJ Disorders.* D. Laskin, et al (eds.). Am. Dent. Assoc., Chicago, 1982.
15. Stewart, C. and Standish, S.: Osteoarthritis of the TMJ in teenaged females: report of cases. J. Am. Dent. Assoc. 106:638–640, 1983.
16. Gray, R.: Pain dysfunction syndrome and osteoarthrosis related to unilateral and bilateral TMJ symptoms. J. Dent. 14:156–159, 1986.
17. Hansson, T.: TMJ changes related to dental occlusion. In *Temporomandibular Joint Problems.* W. Solberg and G. Clark (eds.). Quintessence Publishing Co., Lombard, IL, 1980.
18. Pullinger, A. and Seligman, D.: TMJ osteoarthrosis: A differentiation of diagnostic subgroups by symptom history and demographics. J. Craniomandib. Disorders 1:251–256, 1987.
19. Solberg, W.: TMJ disorders: clinical significance of TMJ changes. Br. Dent. J. 160:231–236, 1986.
20. Hansson, T., Oberg, T., Solberg, W., and Penn, M.:

Anatomic study of the TMJs of young adults: A pilot investigation. J. Prosthet. Dent. 41:556–560, 1979.

21. Solberg, W., Hansson, T., and Nordstrom, B.: The TMJ in young adults at autopsy: a morphologic classification and evaluation. J. Oral Rehab. 12:303–321, 1985.

22. Gates, G.: Radionuclide diagnosis. In *Oral and Maxillofacial Surgery,* vol. 1. D. Laskin (ed.). C.V. Mosby Co., St. Louis, 1980.

23. Liberman, D.: Osteoarthritis. In *Internal Medicine for Dentistry.* L. Rose and D. Kaye (eds.). C.V. Mosby Co., St. Louis, 1983.

24. Rohlin, M., Westesson, P., and Eriksson, L.: The correlation of TMJ sounds with joint morphology in fifty-five autopsy specimens. J. Oral Maxillofac. Surg. 43:194–200, 1985.

25. Bean, L., Omnell, K., Oberg, T.: Comparison between radiologic observations and macroscopic tissue changes in TMJs. Dentomaxillofac. Radiol. 6:90–106, 1977.

26. Christensen, L. and Ziebert, G.: Effects of experimental loss of teeth on the TMJ. J. Oral Rehab. 13:587–598, 1986.

27. Ackerman, S., Rohlin, M., and Kopp, S.: Bilateral degenerative changes and deviation in form of TMJs. Acta Odontol. Scand. 42:45–53, 1984.

28. Hansson, L., Hansson, T., and Peterson, A.: A comparison between clinical and radiologic findings in 259 TMJ patients. J. Prosthet. Dent. 50:89–94, 1983.

29. Toller, P.: Use and misuse of intra-articular corticosteroids in treatment of TMJ pain. Proc. Soc. Med. 70:461–463, 1977.

30. Slater, R., Gross, A., and Hall, J.: Hydrocortisone arthropathy—an experimental investigation. Canad. Med. Assoc. J. 97:374–377, 1967.

31. Moskowitz, R., Davis, W., Sammareo, J., et al: Experimentally induced corticosteroid arthropathy. Arthritis Rheum. 13:236–243, 1970.

32. Poswillo, D.: Experimental investigation of the effects of intra-articular hydrocortisone and high condylectomy on the mandibular condyle. Oral Surg. Oral Med. Oral Path. 30:161–173, 1970.

33. Friedman, D. and Moore, M.: The efficacy of intra-articular steroids in osteoarthritis: a double-blind study. J. Rheumatol. 7:850–856, 1980.

34. Germain, B., Vasey, F., and Espinoza, L.: Early recognition of rheumatoid arthritis. Compr. Ther. 5:16, 1979.

35. Braunwald, E., Isselbacher, K.J., Petersdorf, R.G., et al: *Harrison's Principles of Internal Medicine,* 11th. ed. McGraw-Hill, New York, 1987.

36. Tabeling, H.G. and Dolwick, M.F.: Rheumatoid arthritis: Diagnosis and treatment. Fla. Dent. J. 56:1, 1985.

37. Kent, J.N., Carlton, D.M., and Zide, M.F.: Rheumatoid disease and related arthropathies: Surgical rehabilitation of the temporomandibular joint. Oral Surg. Oral Med. Oral Path. 40:584, 1975.

38. Irby, W. and Zetz, R.: Osteoarthritis and rheumatoid arthritis affecting the temporomandibular joint. In *The President's Conference on the Examination, Diagnosis and Management of TMJ Disorders.* D. Laskin, et al (eds.). Am. Dent. Assoc., Chicago, 1982.

39. Seymour, R., Crouse, V., and Irby, W.: Temporomandibular ankylosis secondary to rheumatoid arthritis. Oral Surg. Oral Med. Oral Path. 40:584, 1985.

40. Zide, M.F., Carlton, D.M., and Kent, J.N.: Rheumatoid disease and related arthropathies. Oral Surg. Oral Med. Oral Path. 61:119, 1986.

41. Trenwith, J. and Beale, G.: Rheumatoid arthritis in the temporomandibular joint. N.Z. Dent. J. 73:195, 1977.

42. Ogus, H.: Degenerative disease of the temporomandibular joint in young persons. Br. J. Oral Surg. 17:17, 1979.

43. Larheim, T.A., Storhaug, K., and Tveito, L.: Temporomandibular joint involvement and dental occlusion in a group of adults with rheumatoid arthritis. Acta Odontol. Scand. 41:301, 1983.

44. Harvey, A., Johns, R., Owens, A., and Ross, R.: *Principles and Practice of Medicine,* 19th ed. Appleton-Century-Crofts, New York, 1976.

45. Fries, J.: The approach to the rheumatic disease patient. Compr. Ther. 5:8, 1979.

46. Bennett, R.: Management of rheumatoid arthritis. Compr. Ther. 5:23, 1979.

47. Syrjanen, S.M.: The temporomandibular joint in rheumatoid arthritis. Acta Radiologica Diagnosis Fasc., 1985.

48. Tegelberg, A. and Kopp, S.: Clinical findings in the stomatognathic system of individuals with rheumatoid arthritis and osteoarthritis. Acta Odontol. Scand. 45:65, 1987.

49. Fileni, A., Amato, L., and Brizi, M.G.: Radiologic findings related to the TMJ in cases of rheumatoid arthritis. RAYS (Rome) 11:49, 1986.

50. Etalla-Ylitalo, U.M., Syrjanen, S., and Halonen, P.: Functional disturbances of the masticatory system related to temporomandibular joint involvement by rheumatoid arthritis. J. Oral Rehab. 14:415, 1987.

51. Larheim, T.A. and Floyfstrand, F.: Temporomandibular joint abnormalities and bite force in a group of adults with rheumatoid arthritis. J. Oral. Rehab. 12:477, 1985.

52. Chalmers, I.M. and Blair, G.S.: Rheumatoid arthritis of the temporomandibular joint. A clinical and radiological study using circular tomography. Quart. J. Med. 42:369, 1973.

53. Redlund-Johnell, I.: Severe rheumatoid arthritis of the temporomandibular joints and its coincidence with severe rheumatoid arthritis of the cervical spine. Scand. J. Rheumatol. 16:347, 1987.

54. Hollingsworth, J. and Saykalay, R.: Systemic complications of rheumatoid arthritis. Symposium on rheumatic disease. Med. Clin. North Am. 61:271, 1977.

55. Tegelberg, A. and Kopp, S.: Short-term effect of physical training on temporomandibular joint disorder in individuals with rheumatoid arthritis and ankylosing spondylitis. Acta Odontol. Scand. 46:49, 1988.

56. Poswillo, D.: Experimental investigation of the effects of intra-articular hydrocortisone and high condylectomy on the mandibular condyle. Oral Surg. Oral Med. Oral Path. 30:161, 1970.

57. Goodwin, J.S.: Mechanism of action of nonsteroidal anti-inflammatory agents. Am. J. Med. 77:57, 1984.

58. Calin, R.: In *Arthritis and Allied Conditions,* 10th ed. D.J. McCarty (ed.). Lea & Febiger, Philadelphia, 1985.

59. Wenneberg, B.: Inflammatory involvement of the temporomandibular joint of individuals with ankylosing spondylitis. Swed. Dent. J. Suppl 20, 1983.

60. Davidson, C., Wojtulewsky, J.A., Bacon, P.A., and Winstock, D.: Temporomandibular joint disease in ankylosing spondylitis. Ann. Rheum. Dis.: 34:87, 1975.

61. Wenneberg, B., Hollender, L., and Kopp, S.: Radio-

graphic changes in the temporomandibular joint in ankylosing spondylitis. Dentomaxillofac. Radiol. 12:25, 1983.

62. McCarty, D.J.: In *Arthritis and Allied Conditions,* 10th ed. Lea & Febiger, Philadelphia, 1985.

63. Kononen, M.: Subjective symptoms from the stomatognathic system in patients with psoriatic arthritis. Acta Odontol. Scand. 44:337, 1986.

64. Stimson, C.W. and Leban, S.G.: Recurrent ankylosis of the temporomandibular joint in a patient with chronic psoriasis. J. Oral Maxillofac. Surg. 40:678, 1982.

65. Kudryk, W.H., Baker, G.L., and Percy, J.S.: Ankylosis of the temporomandibular joint from psoriatic arthritis. J. Otolaryngol. 14:336, 1985.

66. Kononen, M.: Radiographic changes in the condyle of the temporomandibular joint in psoriatic arthritis. Acta Radiol. [Diagn.] 27:185, 1987.

67. McCarty, D.: *Arthritis and Allied Conditions.* D. McCarty (ed.), Lea & Febiger, Philadelphia, 1985.

68. Larheim, T.A, Hoyeraal, H.M., Starbrun, A.E., and Haanaes, H.R.: The temporomandibular joint in juvenile rheumatoid arthritis. Scand. J. Rheumatol. 11:5, 1982.

69. Larheim, T.A. and Haannaes, H.R.: Micrognathia, temporomandibular changes and dental occlusion in juvenile rheumatoid arthritis of adolescents and adults. Scand. J. Dent. Res. 89:329, 1981.

70. Dubois, E.L.: *Lupus Erythematosus,* 2nd ed. University of Southern California Press, Los Angeles, 1976.

71. Jonsson, R., Lindvall, A.M., and Nyberg, G.: Temporomandibular joint involvement in lupus erythematosus. Arthritis Rheum. 26:1506, 1983.

72. Tuggle, J.W.: Systemic lupus erythematosus involvement of temporomandibular joint: A case report. Texas Dent. J. December, 1985.

73. Leibling, M.R. and Gold, R.H.: Erosions of the temporomandibular joint in systemic lupus erythematosus. Arthritis Rheum. 24:848, 1981.

74. Gerbacht, D. and Shapiro, L.: Temporomandibular joint erosion in systemic lupus erythematosus. Arthritis Rheum. 25:597, 1982.

75. Wilson, J., Braunwald, E., Isselbacher, K., et al: *Principles of Internal Medicine,* 12th ed. McGraw-Hill, New York, 1991.

76. Weiberg, H.W., Ropes, M.W., Kulka, J.P., et al: Reiter's syndrome—clinical and pathologic observations. Medicine 41:35, 1962.

77. Bomalsky, J.S. and Jiminez, S.A.: Erosive arthritis of the temporomandibular joint in Reiter's syndrome. J. Rheumatol. 11:400, 1984.

78. Trimble, D.L., Shoenaers, J.A.H., and Steolinga, P.J.W.: Acute suppurative arthritis of the temporomandibular joint in a patient with rheumatoid arthritis. J. Maxillofac. Surg. 11:92, 1983.

79. Schmidt, F.R.: Bacterial arthritis In *Arthritis and Allied Conditions,* 10th ed. D.J. McCarty (ed.). Lea & Febiger, Philadelphia, 1985.

80. Bounds, G.A., Hopkins, R., and Shugar, A.: Septic arthritis of the temporomandibular joint. A problematic diagnosis. Br. J. Oral Maxillofac. Surg. 25:61, 1987.

81. Steere, A.C. and Malawista, S.E.: Cases of Lyme disease in the United States: Locations correlated with distribution of *Ixodes dammini.* Ann. Int. Med. 93:1, 1980.

82. Steere, A.C. and Malawista, S.E.: Erythema chronicum migrans and Lyme arthritis: The enlarging clinical spectrum. Ann. Int. Med. 86:685, 1977.

83. Harris, R.: Lyme disease involving the temporomandibular joint. J. Oral Maxillofac. Surg. 46:78, 1988.

84. Braunwald, E., Isselbacher, K., Petersdorf, R., et al (eds.): *Harrison's Principles of Internal Medicine,* 11th ed. McGraw-Hill, New York, 1987.

85. Holmes, E.W.: Clinical gout and the pathogenesis of hyperuricemia. In *Arthritis and Allied Conditions,* 10th ed. D. J. McCarty (ed.). Lea & Febiger, Philadelphia, 1985.

86. Gross, B.D., Williams, R.B., DiCosimo, D.J., and Williams, S.V.: Gout and pseudogout of the temporomandibular joint. Oral Med. Oral Surg. Oral Path. 63:551, 1987.

87. Kleinman, H.Z. and Ewbank, R.L.: Gout of the temporomandibular joint: Report of 3 cases. Oral Surg. 27:281, 1969.

88. Flour, E., Haverling, M., and Molin, C.: Gout in the temporomandibular joint: Report of a case. J. Otorhinolaryngol. Relat. Spec. 36:16, 1974.

89. Kleinman, H.Z. and Ewbank, R.L.: Gout in the temporomandibular joint: Report of 3 cases. Oral Surg. 27:281, 1969.

90. Bullough, P.G. and Vigorita, J.: *Atlas of Orthopaedic Pathology.* Gower Medical Publishing Ltd., New York, 1984.

91. Hutton, C.W., Doherty, M., and Dieppe, P.A.: Acute pseudogout of the temporomandibular joint: A report of three cases and a review of the literature. Br. J. Rheumatol. 26:51, 1987.

92. DeVos, R.A.I., Brants, J., Kusen, G.J., and Becker, A.E.: Calcium pyrophosphate dihydrate arthropathy of the temporomandibular joint. J. Oral Surg. 51:497, 1981.

93. Good, A.E. and Upton, L.G.: Acute temporomandibular joint arthritis in a patient with bruxism and calcium pyrophosphate deposition disease. Arthritis Rheum. 25:353, 1982.

94. Axhausen, G.: Pathologie und Therapie des Keifergleukes. Fortschr Zahnheilk 9:171, 1933.

95. Spujt, H.J., Dorfman, H.D., and Fechner, R.E.: *Tumors of Bone and Cartilage, Atlas of Tumor Pathology,* 2nd series, fascicle 5. Armed Forces Institute of Pathology, Washington, 1971.

Jay R. Goldman

CHAPTER 11

Soft Tissue Trauma

Trauma is a major etiologic factor in practically all types of temporomandibular disorders (TMD).[1-6] Interestingly, it is usually the first or second etiology on most lists of TM disorders. Many types of trauma not normally associated with TM disorders are notable and deserve attention. Bruxism and a direct blow to the jaw are examples of microtrauma and macrotrauma, respectively. Nail biting, violin playing, scuba diving, whiplash, and a "banana-peel" fall are not universally recognized as causing damage to the TMJs. But some believe they can do just that. Yet, which structure of the joint is damaged? Which structure or structures in the joint, around the joint, or a substantial distance from the joint are causing the pain? What is primarily traumatized? What injury was secondary? What is the actual pathogenesis of the injury? These questions encouraged the writing of this chapter, the purpose of which is threefold: first, establishing trauma as a major etiologic factor of TM disorders; second, describing the mechanism of different traumatic events in causing them; and third, identifying and describing intracapsular and extracapsular structural damage.

Because no significant differences may be evident in the signs, symptoms, and treatment outcomes of TM disorders from varying etiologies,[7] a traumatic event eliciting pain or dysfunction becomes most significant in making a proper diagnosis. This factor is especially true because most TMDs clinically mimic other pathologies and injuries of the head and neck.[8]

We live in a litigious society; consequently, some emphasis is placed on the ramifications of TMJ trauma as it relates to the law and to insurance regulations.

Trauma causes a TMD when normal protective processes become decompensated or when they are abruptly altered.[9] Microtrauma or macrotrauma can result in osseous remodeling[9-11]; disc displacement[12-15]; alteration of normal morphology, capsulitis, and discitis[11,16,17]; alteration of condylar position; and degenerative changes.[14,15,18-21]

A forced inappropriate motion to a joint[22] or body part will result in swelling and pain. The TMJ and its associated parts are all vulnerable to trauma. Pullinger and Monteiro[23] reported that trauma was the most significant factor characterizing patients with TM disorders. Harris and coworkers[24] reported that trauma is a fairly common cause of clinical symptoms of the TMJ and masticatory muscles. Morgan and associates[25] studied more than 1000 patients over a 15-year period and concluded that all components of the joint can be damaged by trauma. The magnitude, duration, and direction of the insult determines the type of injury sustained.[26] Minor trauma strains the capsule and ligaments. Severe trauma will result in synovial membrane damage. Extremely severe trauma, short of fracture, can damage the articular surfaces, subchondral bone, or both and eventually leads to degenerative joint disease.[27,28]

Trauma is becoming increasingly recognized in its etiologic role in TM disorders. In the study by Pullinger and Monteiro,[23] a TMJ patient population was compared with a group of control subjects. Trauma was the most common etiologic factor.

Trauma should take on a more important role in treatment planning and prognosticating than it has in the past. Brooke and Stenn[29] showed that a less favorable outcome is associated with postinjury TM disorders. Observers agree that the demand for treatment is on the rise because of the increases in traumatic events from sports participation and motor vehicle accidents.[30-32]

The specifics of the traumatic event must be understood; they can reveal the structures primarily injured and those secondarily injured. This understanding is fundamental to the successful management of the injury. For example, masticatory muscle pain, TM arthropathy, musculotendinous pathology, and synovial tissue damage seemingly lead to similar symptomology. Consequently, misdirected approaches aimed at the incorrect pathology may be taken. Laskin[33] stated that understanding the etiology is as important as the diagnosis in establishing a rational treatment plan. The conglomeration of symptoms into a "syndrome" establishes undesirable results. Treatment is directed at a malady with diverse etiology. Because there are many paths of entry in TM disorders, the extraneous must be identified. Terms such as extrinsic, extracapsular, and macrotrauma and microtrauma are not diagnostically useful. These terms are acceptable for general discriptions and epidemiologic study but misleading and vague for clinical application. It is necessary to abandon the syndrome concept with regard to etiology just as it is with regard to diagnosis and classification. Moffet's[34] view is that the syndrome concept is inappropriate because it fails to focus a diagnostic label on the problem of the individual patient. Dentistry no longer considers malocclusion as the primary etiologic factor in TM disorders but recognizes other etiologic factors as well.[35] It follows that as specific anatomic parts are identified as being injured, appropriate therapy can be directed to the individual patient rather than providing the same therapy to all patients. Any successful treatment must be based on an undersatnding of the pathogenesis of the disease.[36] The condition in which the anatomic components of the joint exists at a particular time, therefore, deserves consideration.

In the emergency room, internal derangement, traumatically induced synovitis, and other traumatically induced conditions of the TMJs are not of the highest priority. However, after treating the life-threatening injuries, a diagnosis relative to the TMJs aids in future treatment.[37] This practice has special significance because a TM disorder can devastate its victim. Solberg[38] stated that the soft tissue alterations can have "crippling" effects. A TM disorder, although not being life threatening, is certainly life altering.

HISTORICAL PERSPECTIVE AND STUDIES

Traumatic events are being recognized as precipitating factors with increasing frequency.[39–41] Silver and colleagues[41] reported that in 32% of their patients who had surgical repairs the causative events were traced to trauma. Stringert and Worms[42] stated that trauma (both indirect and direct) was a major cause of TMJ damage or TMJ-related pathology. Christiansen and colleagues[43] examined and treated 43 patients who had sustained direct blows to their jaws, faces, or deep facial structures. At least 37% had documented articular disc derangements, and 74% had degenerative joint changes. The injuries sustained resulted from motor vehicle accidents (42%), falls (19%), battery (14%), industrial accidents (4%), and a variety of other types of trauma (21%).

Trauma to the joint can induce deleterious changes that range from articular surface damage to fracture and dislocations[44] to minor muscular aches, major muscle pathology, and psychologic problems such as anxiety and depression.[1,45] In a group of 165 patients studied with TM disorders, trauma was implicated as the causative factor. Some 38% with histologically proven osteoarthritis reported a history of trauma. In these patients, 62.6% of recurrent mandibular dislocations and 62.5% of mandibular ankylosis were caused by trauma. Norman[19] further postulated that mandibular trauma may precipitate other disorders of the TMJ.

Epidemiologic research has shown that 50 to 88% of the general population have or have had signs and symptoms of TM disorders.[46–48] As much as 25% of this population suffers from severe symptoms. Of the 175 patients studied by Norman who had pain dysfunction syndromes, 12% had undisputed trauma. This investigator further concluded, after operating on over 200 joints, that trauma was of singular importance in the etiology of a number of nonfracture disorders of the TMJ.[19]

Rasmussen's[49] longitudinal study of the three stages of TM arthropathy indicated that the first stage, consisting of clicking and intermittent locking, is often by-passed with the eliciting event of trauma. The patients often enter directly into stage 2 or closed lock. In other cases, stage 1 merely predisposed the individual. Trauma, as the eliciting event, drew the patient into stage 2. This finding was true in 20% of the patients surveyed. Any kind of trauma can trigger a TM disorder. Muggings, sports injuries, weight lifting, scuba diving, motor vehicle accidents, and childbirth are adequate events to trigger TMJ pain and pathology. Silver and Simon[50] reported that over 50% of the cases they studied were induced by macrotrauma or microtrauma. Pullinger and Monteiro[23] studied a student population and identified orthodontic treatment, molar surgery, and trauma as etiologic factors. With regard to the last, 30.1% of the TM disorder patients had histories of notable trauma and 12.1% mild trauma, compared with the asymptomatic control group who reported 1.7% notable trauma and 8.7% mild trauma.

The significance of this study was that prior trauma was the strongest link to symptomatic status in the groups studied. Traumatic effects could also be insidious and cumulative, thereby adding to the difficulty of reporting an accurate and a precise history. Hohmann and coworkers[51] reported that two thirds of their TMD patients had histories of trauma causally related to arthrosis. They also related intra-articular hemorrhage to trauma. Kopp[52] showed traumatic arthritis as a sequelae to TMJ trauma. Meyer[53] reported disc displacement as the result of trauma. Harkins and Marteney[54] studied a large heterogeneous, symptomatic population in order to evaluate the roll of extrinsic trauma as a precipitating factor in TM disorders. Of 661 patients displaying objective signs and symptoms, 555 (84%) experienced some form of significant trauma to the body. A total of 284 patients reported that extrinsic trauma to the head or neck was the precipitating factor in the onset of dysfunctional symptoms. Only 14 (2%) who suffered head or neck trauma reported no relationship of trauma to pain and dysfunction. Some 128 patients (19%) reported whiplash injury as the precipitating factor of the TM disorder. A single blow to the head or neck was reported by 144 (22%) as the causative factor of the TM disorder. Of 348 patients studied by Takada and associates,[55] 28.7% cases were attributable to some form of trauma.

Acute extrinsic trauma is a major precipitating factor in the onset of TM disorders. Numerous workers have cited this factor but failed to expand on the mechanism of pathogenesis.[56] Two exceptions are the descriptions of cervical sprain (whiplash) by Lader[57] and Rocabado[58] who proposed a sequence of events leading to the development of TMJ arthropathy and muscular pathosis. Minor injury or apparently harmless trauma may be enough to produce symptoms.[59,60] Moses[61] reported that a whiplash injury could be sustained in a rear end collision at a speed of just 5 mph.

None of the studies presented tell us anything about the patient's pretrauma status. Investigation into disease-producing trauma must include pre-existing conditions, such as parafunction and stress disorders. It must also take into account the high frequency of individuals with asymptomatic internal derangements and other TM signs without symptoms.[1] The interaction of pre-existing components and trauma has been extensively discussed elsewhere.[46–48,62] In one theory, the role of trauma has been entwined with occlusal disharmony. A traumatic event may sprain one or both TMJs, and the injury is prevented from resolving because of pre-existing occlusal factors, which act to perpetuate the injury. Muscle involvement now plays a secondary role, in that splinting of the injured joint takes place. Muscles of mastication, of the cervical area, and of the shoulders and arms can be involved.[63]

TRAUMATIC ARTHRITIS

Traumatic arthritis describes a diverse group of pathologies that develop from single or repeated episodes of trauma.[22] Historically, many poorly understood disorders were attributed to trauma. Rheumatoid arthritis, tuberculous arthritis, gout, and other maladies that altered the structural integrity of the joints and predisposed them to inflammation were among the pathologies "swept" into the etiologic trauma "basket."[64] However, with better understanding of pathologic mechanisms, even osteoarthritis, which was considered a traumatically induced disorder in the early literature, is being explained as an altered cartilage metabolism not necessarily related to trauma. Solberg[9] states that onset is the result of inadequate articular remodeling response and not the result of spontaneous events. The emphasis on the etiologic role of multiple microtrauma in osteoarthritis is diminishing,[22] although some still maintain that joint degeneration follows trauma. Some consider traumatic arthritis synonymous with osteoarthritis.[22] Others make a distinction between the two based on the presence of degenerative change with or without inflammation.[65,66]

Bora and Miller[67] implicated trauma as a cause of osteoarthritis and proposed two possible mechanisms. First, in the absence of a meniscus, such as in an internal derangement or perforation, the synovial lining and subchondral bone are subject to inflammatory changes from microtrauma. The reparative properties are compromised and increase the potential of traumatic arthritis. Second, because the periarticular tissues and surrounding musculature offer resistance against joint overloading, any compromise of these structures increases the potential of developing traumatic arthritis. Clark[18] reported that repetitive behavior patterns, such as grinding, clenching, and chronic gum chewing, traumatize and injure muscle and synovial lining causing osteoarthritis. Bollet[20] suggested that physical stress brought to bear on cartilage is important but minor compared with muscle pull, which generates much more physical stress on cartilage. In view of the parafunctional habits involving the mandible and the frequent microtrauma that the TMJ sustains, Bollet's findings may apply to the TMJ—local stress may rupture lysosomes in cartilage cells, activating proteolytic enzymes,[20] and it may be responsible for the initiation of osteoarthritis. It is likely that no single event is responsible for the onset of osteoarthritis.

Hohmann and coworkers[68] reported that TMJ osteoarthritis secondary to acute or chronic trauma is a frequent occurrence in the spectrum of TMDs. They divided degenerative osteoarthritis into two groups. The *primary* type of osteoarthritis is more commonly seen in an older patient population, with deterioration of the articular cartilage surfaces and fibrocartilage meniscus. Radiographic findings may be marked with lipping, spurring, or flattening of the condyle, whereas symptoms of trismus pain and crepitation are usually mild. The *second* type, degenerative arthritis, is usually seen in the young or middle-aged patient, preceded by a traumatic event to the teeth, joint, or mandible. Radiographic findings are less impressive, but symptoms may be severe locking, profound myospasm, head and neck pain, and hypomobility, and otologic symptoms.[68,69]

Ricketts[70] proposed that a single traumatic episode may cause degenerative changes and that a continuous reinjury may occur from the mechanical traumatic effects of occlusal interferences.

Mayne and Hatch[71] defined traumatic arthritis as joint lesions produced by acute direct trauma. The amount of trauma sustained by the TMJ depends on magnitude, duration, and direction of the insult. Minor trauma may cause strain of the ligaments or capsule with subsequent edema, but healing is usually rapid and complete because of a rich blood supply.[72] Severe injuries can traumatize the synovium, which may heal or persist depending on the presence of perpetuating factors. Very severe trauma may damage articular surfaces, subchondral bone, or both. Traumatic arthritis may develop, and an irregular joint surface results. Katzberg and colleagues[15] suggested that direct trauma displacing the meniscus stimu-

lates osteoclastic activity of the articular fibrocartilage. Histopathologic analysis of 25 patients who underwent surgical corrections demonstrated degenerative arthritis in 13 (52%) and remodeling in all 25. Vertical and horizontal splitting of the articular fibrocartilage to complete loss of the fibrous surface and exposure of the bone were observed. The pathologic features are dependent on the severity of the injury. Inflammation of the synovium, intra-articular and extra-articular hemorrhage, compression or rupture of the meniscus, and compression or fracture of the articular surface of the condyle may occur.[46]

In order to diagnose traumatic arthritis, guidelines have been suggested. Hanlon and Estes[73] listed the following criteria:

1. The arthritic changes must be severe enough to produce synovitis with pain, swelling, effusion, and dysfunction.
2. The traumatized joint must be the only one with such inflammation.
3. Normal articular function must have been present before the injury.
4. Progressive articular changes may occur, which in time can be demonstrated by radiographs.

Pinals[22] accepted a traumatic episode as the etiology of osteoarthritis with the following criteria:

1. The joint was normal before injury.
2. Effusion or structural damage shortly after the injury was documented.
3. Similar disease has not occurred in nontraumatized joints.

Traumatic arthritis or osteoarthritis may develop in joints that are repeatedly traumatized as a result of occupational or sports activities.[22] Positive radiographic findings, such as joint narrowing and osteophytes, were common in groups studied,[22] but the subjects were largely asymptomatic. Farrar and McCarty[74] have reported positive radiographic findings of degenerative joint disease in asymptomatic populations. These changes occur in the hands and wrist of boxers and workers who use pneumatic hammers, in the ankles of soccer players, in the first metatarsophalangeal joint of ballet dancers, and in the elbows of foundry workers. These injuries are commonly termed repetitive articular trauma.[22] Certainly, many investigators[75,76] have implicated parafunctional habits, such as bruxism, as an etiology of traumatic arthritis. Bora and Miller[67] suggested that excessive stress on the articular cartilage may be the initiating factor. Less emphasis has been placed on aging and the wear-and-tear theories because chondrocytes would be expected to show signs of degeneration and decreased synthetic activity. The synthesis of all matrix components, however, is markedly higher in osteoarthritis.[67]

Clark[18] suggested that osteoarthrotic changes may occur in young people and that macrotrauma and microtrauma are thought to be common contributing factors.

Several pathways exist in the development of traumatic arthritis. Radin and associates[77] have shown that excessive stress leads to traumatic arthritis and joint degeneration. Guralnick and coworkers[78] reported that these may occur as a result of a dislocation or a single traumatic experience, such as biting an extremely hard substance or excessive opening over a prolonged time. Effusion may develop, and fluid may be aspirated from the joint. Provided infectious arthritis is first ruled out, steroids may be injected into the superior joint space with dramatic amelioration of symptoms. Long-standing traumatic arthritis may alter the occlusion, resulting in an open bite. This too responds favorably with the local administration of steroids.

Mayne and Hatch[6] believe that the term traumatic arthritis should be reserved for those joint lesions that are produced by acute direct trauma and not for joint lesions that are produced by microtrauma caused by mechanical stresses. They prefer the term "osteoarthritis secondary to repeated trauma" for the last type of joint pathology. Their criteria for diagnosing traumatic arthritis from acute direct trauma is the presence of primary synovitis.

The nature of traumatic arthritis is best evaluated by history and physical examination. Hemorrhage may be found in the joint with an increase of protein content in the joint's fluid. Mucin content and mucin clot test findings are normal. Clinically, localized tenderness, pain, and swelling over the joint will be present. Treatment consists of heat application, splint therapy, rest, analgesics, and if necessary aspiration of joint fluid.[6] It is generally agreed that, if severe enough, and if healing does not occur uneventfully as it should in most cases, traumatic arthritis may develop into osteoarthritis.[18,22,67,73,78,79] In this instance, the articular surfaces are no longer protected, and the underlying innervated and vascular osseous tissues become inflamed. This effect may be the source of persistent arthralgia that is intensified as movement causes the inflamed surfaces to press and rub against each other. If long lasting, symptoms of capsulitis ensue,[80] with palpable tenderness over the joint, formation of inflammatory exudate, and occasionally acute malocclusion.

Healing of the articular surface in traumatic arthritis appears dependent, in part, on the synovial lining. The degree to which traumatic arthritis may heal or progress is influenced by metabolic and physical determinants. Experiments by Izumi[81] demonstrated no articular cartilage repair occurred when "lacerating microtrauma" was applied to the articular surface of monkey TMJs. However, when the induced microtrauma was not confined to the cartilage but included the peripheral synovial lining, the wound demonstrated healing. Immature mesenchymal cells began to invade along the bottom of the incisive cleavage from the synovial lining to the wound. Details of osteoarthritis (degenerative joint disease) are discussed in chapter 10.

Acute or chronic intermittent injury may result in soft tissue lesions with effusion into the joint space, arthritic and osteoarthritic changes, and even intracapsular fractures that may go undetected on radiographs.[24] Small cracks, linear fractures, and early degenerative changes are not easily detected on radiographs. Furthermore, 30 to 50% of diseased bone must be resorbed or destroyed in order to be visualized on a radiograph.[82]

Early detection of traumatic intracapsular change is necessary in order to pre-empt the irreversible changes that may occur, such as interference with joint movement and, in children, growth inhibition.[70,83] Traumatic influence on growth factor is discussed subsequently in this chapter. Harris and colleagues[24] studied post-traumatic changes in the TMJs with scintigraphy. They showed that following TMJ trauma, a bone scan may reveal early changes particularly in the absence of radiologic evidence.[24] These workers concluded that the greater uptake of radiopharmaceutic agents in the TMJ may be due to the following:

1. Metabolic and biochemical changes resulting from contusion in the joint's bony surfaces.
2. Intracapsular fracture
3. Remodeling of the articular surface after the impact of the condyle—this process of repair and remodeling may take months, even

years, before it becomes metabolically quiescent.

4. Secondary osteoarthrotic changes.

A similar study on patients with TMJ pain and osteoarthrosis revealed a better correlation between scintigraphic changes and clinical and histologic findings than between radiographic changes and clinical and histologic findings.[84] In this study, Harris noted that morphologic changes on radiographs did not always correspond with symptoms and histology. He suggested that old structural changes may be viewed radiographically with little or no biochemical activity. In addition, symptomless joints showed increased uptakes of radiopharmaceutic agents, which may be caused by the sensitivity of the scintigram in showing early metabolic changes before the onset of symptoms. This finding could also be caused by false positive results.[84] In view of the fact that arthritic changes from indirect and direct trauma are being reported with greater frequency and, in view of the fact that early detection is required for efficacious treatment, scintigraphy as a diagnostic tool may be of benefit.

Computerized tomography (CT) may be used in the early diagnosis and detection of traumatic injuries. The advantages of conventional and tomographic radiographs have been described in chapter 18. Their disadvantages lie in their inability to demonstrate soft tissue damage and, according to Christiansen and associates,[43] osseous trauma to the craniofacial region may not be depicted. Even magnetic resonance imaging (MRI) is not indicated during the first 24 hours after trauma because of its inability to distinguish between blood and edema until the formation of methemoglobin, which facilitates this differentiation.[85]

The advantages of CT over other imaging techniques were demonstrated in patients with fractures who continued to have unexplained symptoms and in patients without fractures who continued to have post-traumatic TMJ pain and dysfunction.[43] As an imaging modality, CT is recommended to detect damaged tissue early.

In summary, it appears osteoarthritis has no one specific cause. If a traumatic event was causally related, the term traumatic arthritis is appropriate. If the traumatic arthritis progresses, the term osteoarthritis or osteoarthrosis can be used. The pathogenesis of osteoarthritis is described in chapter 10. A traumatic insult causes the release of proteolytic and collagen-olytic enzymes from chondrocytes capable of degrading the cartilage matrix. Attempts at repair fail to keep pace with degradative activity, and cartilage breakdown continues. Trauma and a host of nonmechanical factors accentuate the process.[86] Undiagnosed microfractures and crush damage to the head of the condyle may have a role in the etiology of osteoarthritis.[19]

CHONDROMALACIA

Chondromalacia is the softening of the articular cartilage due to matrix (collagen fibrils and proteoglycans) decomposition.[87] This breakdown is thought to be caused by microtrauma—repetitive loading—and macrotrauma—sudden, violent impact causing contusion of the articular surface.[88] Loss of local nutrition and normal physical stimulation often resulting from immobilization are the other causes of chondromalacia.[88,89] This traumatically induced, generally irreversible disorder is a degenerative process and is thought to be a precursor to osteoarthritis in the knee.[90-92] However, no such opinion can be found in the literature regarding the TMJ.

The four stages of chondromalacia are based on arthroscopic findings:

Stage 1:   Softening caused by loss of vertical collagen fibers and altered cartilage metabolism.

Stage 2:   Blister formation caused by a separation and then a filling in of collagen fibers with a resultant bulge, having the consistency of a cutaneous blister.

Stage 3:   Ulceration and fragmentation of the blister results in the articular surface having a crab meat–like appearance.

Stage 4:   Progression leads to complete loss of cartilage and exposed subchondral bone surrounded by a rim of cartilage. This crater-like appearance is followed by a rubbing or polishing of the sclerotic bone, further resulting in a glistening, ivory-like appearance. This is the process of eburnation.[93,94]

CAPSULITIS

The capsule is composed of an outer and inner lining.[95,96] The outer lining is a vascularized, innervated fibrous layer. The inner layer is lined with synovial membrane. Inflammation of the outer layer is termed capsulitis, whereas inflammation of the inner layer (synovium) is termed synovitis. Clinically, these two entities are indistinguishable[97] and are manifested by the following:

1. Masticatory pain and restricted movement
2. Swelling due to effusion into the joint cavity
3. Malocclusion if the effusion and inflammation are severe enough.

Synovitis and capsulitis are secondary to inflammatory arthritis, periarticular conditions, or pre-existing capsular fibrosis; if these are not the etiologic factors, trauma is usually the factor.[98] A blow to the mandible is a common type of capsular trauma. This macrotrauma results in pain, joint effusion, and reflex muscle guarding, all of which end clinically as immobilization,[99] which is discussed subsequently in this chapter. During the healing process, the capsule may adhere to adjacent tissue (ankylosis) and even heal in a shortened state. Microtrauma to the capsule may occur via a malocclusion of the teeth resulting in a change in the maxillomandibular relationship and joint position. Capsular stress due to habits is also a major etiologic factor. Chewing gum, biting finger nails, and leaning the jaw on the hands are all examples of intrinsic microtrauma.

Capsulitis or inflammation of the outer capsular layer is usually caused by local trauma, abusive use, or infection. Strain and injury are caused by forced excessive condylar movement with the resultant inflammation readily involving the collateral discal or TMJ ligaments or both. Capsular pain is characterized by palpable tenderness directly over the joint and by pain if condylar movement stretches the capsule. Pain is increased with maximum intercuspation. The pain is decreased if the patient bites on a tongue depressor. Dysfunction due to capsulitis ranges from minor restriction to total immobilization.

CAPSULAR FIBROSIS

Persistent capsular inflammation predisposes a patient to capsular fibrosis. This is a fibrotic contracture of the capsular ligament usually due to trauma, including the trauma from surgery.[100] Capsular fibrosis may result from joint damage, such as a blow directly over the joint or to the mandible, which may readily sprain (tear or stretch) the capsule. Scarring of the capsule (fibrosis) results in capsular restraint, which is due to the reduction in size and flexibility of the capsule. Bruising or lacerating the articular surfaces, ligaments, or retrodiscal tissue, or their combination, with or without hemarthrosis, can result in capsular fibrosis. Restrained movement from capsulitis is almost always in the outer ranges, effecting extreme translatory movement in opening and protrusive and lateral excursion. Capsular fibrosis alone is a nonpainful condition, but one of two situations can induce pain: first, if the inflammation is in conjunction with the fibrotic capsule and, second, if a forced opening or traumatic event in the presence of capsular fibrosis produces inflammation. In either case, capsular fibrosis should be treated as capsulitis. Restriction in movement is almost always due to pain and not to the actual fibrosis or physical restraint.

SYNOVITIS

Inflammation of the synovial membrane (inner lining of the capsule) due to local trauma or abusive use (macrotrauma or microtrauma) is termed traumatic synovitis. Intracapsular infection may also result in synovitis. Both cause fluctuating swelling due to effusion, discomfort in mandibular movements or palpation, and alteration of synovial fluid. Localized synovitis of the posterior aspect of the joint occurs with edema in the posterior joint space. This is referred to, in dental literature, as posterior capsulitis or retrodiscitis.[101]

Chase and coworkers[102] suggested that synovitis is associated with chronic trauma of the TMJs.

As described by Mahan,[103] the synovial membrane extends anteriorly and posteriorly from the capsule itself without a fibrous backing and is bound by loose areolar connective tissue. As such, it makes up the anterior and posterior boundaries of the joint capsule. Just beyond these structures lie the innervated vascular, bilaminar zone, posteriorly, and the vulnerable lateral pterygoid muscle, anteriorly. A direct blow to the jaw or the hyperflexion stage of whiplash results in retrusion of the condyle into the posterior joint space. The hyperextension stage of whiplash injures the anterior aspect of the TMJ and the lateral pterygoid muscle. Hence, Mahan applied the term "the Achilles tendon" of the TMJ.[103] Pain, mostly at the outer border positions, and repositioning of the mandible may ultimately develop. This repositioning is due to either intracapsular edema or *avoidance phenomenon,* which is initiated by nociceptive input into the central nervous system that alters muscular function.[104]

A long-standing synovitis may also result in gelation or chronic stiffness of the joint.[96]

The patient with osteoarthritis may be predisposed to synovitis,[105] making the joint especially vulnerable even to minor trauma.

Acute forms of retrodiscitis or synovitis may develop immediately from trauma. This diagnosis should be suspected with or without fracture.

Whether the traumatic synovitis or capsulitis is chronic or acute it may be treated by injection of corticosteroid if the eliciting trauma is not likely to be repeated. If the inflamed capsule is caused by another underlying condition treatment must be based on the primary condition.

In some instances, synovitis may result in deformation of the articular cartilage as has been demonstrated using an animal model.[106] This finding has not been demonstrated with TMJ articular cartilage. Increased deformability may alter force transmission to the underlying bone and its vascular structures. Following synovitis, care should be exercised to prevent the application of inappropriate loading to the deformable joint cartilage so as not to produce permanent change in form.[106]

SYNOVIAL HEMANGIOMA

Although this is an unusual soft tissue lesion of the TMJ, it should be included in the differential diagnosis, especially because one hypothesis concerning its pathogenesis is posttraumatic degeneration of the TMJ soft tissue elements.[107] Enzinger and Weiss[108] and Thomas and Evarts[109] suggested that trauma may be a possible initiating factor in the formation of this lesion. Moon's review[110] of 134 patients with synovial hemangiomas of the knees revealed over 26% had significant trauma prior to developing symptoms. There is a female predilection, and synovial hemangioma usually occurs in children and young adults. Clinically, intermittent preauricular pain, restriction of motion, and jaw deviation on opening are experienced. Radiographically, a radiolucency may be seen posterior to the condyle, widening the joint space. Laboratory test results are within normal limits. Excisional biopsy is the conclusive diagnostic test and treatment of choice.[107]

SYNOVIAL ADHESION

Inflammation from trauma and its effect on the synovial lining have been observed arthroscopically.[111] If this inflammatory process is severe enough necrosis and fibrin deposition on the synovial surfaces occur. This deposition serves as the scaffolding onto which adhesions may form, even without further trauma.

The amount of connective tissue proliferation in the synovial lining is dependent on the degree of inflammation and can be caused by trauma. If severe enough, obliteration of the anterior synovial pouch may occur. Kaminishi[112] observed fibrotic restrictions in the superior compartment. He described simple fibrous adhesions progressing to bands of fibrous tissue that are so large they actually reduced joint space. These falsely appear to be the outer boundary of the synovium and are thus termed *fibrosynovial pseudowalls.* If extensive they may totally ankylose the joint. Arthroscopic diagnosis and treatment are discussed in greater detail in chapter 31.

DISCAL ATTACHMENT INJURY

The clinical symptoms of a disc derangement are clicking, popping, and discoordination. Symptoms are due to the loosening or tearing of the lateral disc and capsular attachments.[14,113] This occurs when the hinge movement, restricted and governed by the discal ligaments, is exceeded or violated,[114] which may result in inflammation in the early stages, progressing into capsulitis. In later stages it can result in detachment. Trauma from motor vehicle and sports accidents can result in elongation of the collateral ligaments, producing instability of the disc with subsequent subluxation or total dislocation.[115]

This pathologic change should be considered a separate entity from internal derangement into which it may develop. Pain from disc interference emanates from the disc attachment tissue where nociception takes place and not from the disc itself, which lacks nociception.[114]

Initially, disc attachment injury can occur from trauma with no clinical signs or symptoms. It may develop its own pain pattern and clinical features. At first, slight pain is experienced during function and slight tenderness is noted upon palpation of the lateral aspect of the joint. Discomfort is intermittent and may accompany a low-grade click. This click should be distinguished from a loud click that becomes indistinct over time. The last is a sign of disease progression and not the mild intermittent click of an early discal attachment injury. Bell[116] termed this type of injury *discitis,* which implies the discal attachment and not the disc proper is injured or inflamed. This injury results from intrinsic trauma, such as occlusal disharmony, or from external violence or extrinsic trauma. Discitis may be considered an early stage in the pathogenesis of an internal disc derangement. Extreme or persistent trauma will determine its course of progression, if any, into this derangement.

RETRODISCITIS (POSTERIOR CAPSULITIS)

The most common type of TMJ synovitis is the insidious chronic form due to chronic trauma[102] or, more specifically, to condyles that load the synovial membranes by continuously encroaching on the highly vascularized retrodiscal tissues. Loss of molar support, excessive tooth wear and occlusal habits, and prematurities are examples of intrinsic trauma that result in retrodiscal synovitis not involving the lateral wall of the capsule.[117] Long-term retrodiscal impingement can result in metaplasia of the loose connective tissue into a denser fibrotic tissue, altering synovial fluid metabolism[118,119] and adding insult to the already existing functional displacement.

Acute trauma to the mandible can induce an immediate inflammatory response in the retrodiscal tissues.[17,97] A forceful retrusion of the condyle into the vascular, innervated posterior joint space is marked by swelling, pain, extravasation of inflammatory fluid into the synovial sacs, and if severe acute malocclusion. It has also been called "retrosynovitis."[108] Macrotrauma is usually an obvious causative factor with resultant pain and dysfunction. Acute retrodiscitis, in contrast to the insidious chronic form, can be accompanied by hemarthrosis, which can lead to adhesion between the disc and temporal fossa or the disc and condyle.[97] (See chapter 12.)

Retrodiscitis attributed to microtrauma or intrinsic trauma is a greater diagnostic challenge. Although experimental evidence is lacking, abusive habits[115] and disharmony between occlusion and surrounding musculature[120] may cause chronic retrodiscitis but requires an accurate and a thorough history to diagnose. Firmly occluding the teeth together or pressing the jaw posteriorly, as in a provocation test (see chapter 17), will elicit immediate pain in retrodiscitis. The differential diagnosis of retrodiscitis, lateral pterygoid muscle spasm, capsulitis, and discal attachment injury is essential because treatment for each varies.[17] Selective loading and unloading, as described by Widmer[121] and Friedman[122] will help distinguish these disorders from each other.

Trauma to the retrodiscal tissue may result in clicking. Clicking that occurs at the extreme limits of opening indicates greater damage to the posterior discal attachments and is the most difficult to treat.[122]

Retrodiscitis from reptitive microtrauma or insidious injury may be preceded by posterior condylar displacement but only after considerable deterioration of the disc and discal ligaments and elongation of the posterior, inner, and horizontal portions of the temporomandibular ligament.[123] Pain emanating from the retrodiscal tissue has been termed nonarthritic temporomandibular arthralgia[97] and typically elicits no proprioceptive response in the chronic form but may result in secondary myospastic activity in the acute traumatic form.[96]

TEMPOROMANDIBULAR JOINT EFFUSION AND THE SYNOVIUM

Effusion is defined as the escape of fluid from the blood vessels or lymphatics into a tissue or cavity.[91] In the case of the TMJ, the "cavity" or capsule is fully lined with synovial membrane except over the articular cartilage surface. The lining is two to three cells thick with its deeper tissue consisting of fibrous tissue, fat, or loose connective tissue[103,124] and is equipped for support, filtration, phagocytosis, and motility. Synovial lining is extremely vascular and well-suited for rapid exchange of fluid and solutes from joint space to vessels and vice versa.[125] Synovial fluid is a clear, viscous fluid, relatively acellular (<1000 cells/mm^3). It functions to lubricate and provide nutrition for the avascular cartilage.

Trauma to the joints can produce cartilage damage, meniscal damage, or both with resultant joint noises and locking. Joint swelling may occur, however, without internal derangement.[125] Aspiration and analysis of joint fluid can help identify this kind of injury. Bloody fluid suggests traumatic injury. With bloody fluid, bone marrow spicules, fat, or immature red blood cells may suggest small fractures. Harris and associates[24] reported that many intracapsular fractures remain undiagnosed, thereby emphasizing the importance of joint fluid analysis, especially in patients with persisting symptoms and negative radiographic findings. Magnetic resonance imaging (MRI) can effectively demonstrate joint effusion but only 24 hours after the initial trauma.[85] A T2-weighted image is required to effectively demonstrate joint fluid.[126] Blood within the joint fluid may not appear until several days after hemarthrosis owing to rapid phagocytic action in the synovial fluid.[125]

Cloudy fluid aspirated from the joint can suggest a variety of disease entities so it is not specific for traumatic effusion. Totally clear fluid may be considered uncomplicated traumatic joint effusion[125] and may exist without much warmth, erythema, or tenderness. A yellow tinge is characteristic of traumatic arthritis. White and coworkers[124] reported a post-traumatic chylous (fatty) effusion in the knee following blunt trauma without evidence of hemarthrosis or fracture. They further suggested that disruption of the synovial lining, allowing fat leakage into the joint is a possible mechanism in traumatic arthritis of the knee. Weinberger and Schumacher,[127] using the knee joints of dogs, demonstrated that blunt trauma produces a clear, nonbloody effusion containing fat. This fat released from either the bone marrow or synovial membrane may be responsible for the altered vascular permeability. Fat in traumatized joints has been studied by others. Pinals[128] reported that fracture into the joint space produced effusion containing fat. Gregg and colleagues[129] documented fat in traumatic effusions with no evidence of fracture. Schmid and MacNair[130] reported the presence of a substantial amount of cholesterol and lipoproteins in the synovial fluid of a patient with traumatic arthritis. More studies are needed to clarify the diagnostic role of joint fluid analysis in the TMJ.

Treatment recommendations for joint effusions are sparse in the medical literature and almost nonexistent for TMJs; however, the application of cold and rest have been shown experimentally to decrease synovial blood flow, thereby reducing acute effusion.[92]

Clinically, acute malocclusion may result from inflammatory effusion within the TMJ.[78]

This effect may occur from macrotrauma or microtrauma; a sensation of disocclusion of the ipsilateral posterior teeth and premature contact of the contralateral anterior teeth may result.[123] In addition, a "gummy" end feel may be detected on examination in the presence of joint effusion because of the capsular tightness due to distention of the joint capsule.[131] Normally, the capsule allows a certain range of motion, but because of the loss of laxity, restriction and deviation occur on opening.

OTHER PAIN SYNDROMES

Even with a history of trauma, establishing a diagnosis for head, face, jaw, and neck disorders is a challenge for both medical and dental clinicians. The literature is full of cases in which the TMJ refers pain to other structures, but little attention is paid to disorders that may refer pain to the TMJ.[132] A "TMD patient" may not present with pain in the TMJ itself but in other areas.[8] The clinician must discover the origin of the painful condition and render treatment or make the appropriate referral. Pain to the temple, ear, throat, and neck has been reported as a common finding of some TM disorders.[74,133] Consequently, pain syndromes involving those anatomic parts should be ruled out. Additionally, it has been reported in the literature that myofascial pain dysfunction (MPD) syndrome may result from trauma[29,134,135] and that this syndrome and hyoid bone and styloid process syndromes can be confused.[136] It is necessary to describe these conditions so that proper differential diagnostic procedures can be incorporated into standard examination procedures. Sicher[137] reported that in certain types of MPD syndromes, temporal pain may originate in the temporal muscle; pain in the neck and jaws may originate in the masseter muscle; and pain in the throat may originate in the pterygoid muscles. Earache is common to these syndromes.

HYOID BONE SYNDROME

The hyoid bone syndrome is a symptom complex of chronic or recurrent facial pain. It was described in 1954 by Brown[138] as a symptom complex of neck and throat pain, which was referred to the ear. Brown demonstrated that bidigital movement of the hyoid bond from side to side reproduced the pain. Kopstein,[139] in 1975, redefined this syndrome as being caused by the hyoid apparatus consisting of the styloid process, stylohyoid ligament, thyroid cartilage, and hyoid bone. In 1982, Lim[136] reported treating 18 patients with head and neck pain by excising the greater horn of the hyoid bone, which relieved the pain permanently. Originating at the tip of the greater horn of the hyoid bone in the carotid area, the pain radiates to the ipsilateral ear, temporal area, sternocleidomastoid muscle, posterior pharyngeal wall, or supraclavicular area.[136] Of the 50 patients treated and reported by Lim, ten had excruciating temporal headaches and were treated previously for migraines. Four had bilateral carotid pain radiating to the ears, supraclavicular areas, and sternocleidomastoid muscles. All the patients had been taking various analgesics, tranquilizers, and antibiotics and had been managed by various clinicians including psychiatrists.

The pain is usually initiated and aggravated by swallowing or by bowing the head toward the affected side. Essential hypertension may be present, and physical findings may reveal enlargement of the carotid sinus with tenderness.

When hyoid bone syndrome is suspected, bidigital motion from side to side, as described by Brown,[138] is necessary along with intraoral palpation and local anesthetic diagnostic block. Treatment consists of anti-inflammatory medication and, if ineffective, surgical excision.

STYLOID AND ERNEST'S SYNDROMES

Styloid syndrome, also known as Eagle's syndrome, is caused by mineralization of the stylohyoid ligament and elongation of the styloid process.[140] This condition causes facial pain; earache; temporal headache; vertigo; and pain on swallowing, turning the head, and opening the mouth.[141] Styloid syndrome may cause carotid arteritis by encroaching on the carotid artery.[79]

In contrast to Eagle's syndrome, injury and inflammation of the stylomandibular ligament at its mandibular insertion have been reported and termed Ernest's syndrome.[132,142] Shankland[142] studied 68 patients who fulfilled the following three criteria: (1) pain reported at the ligament insertion, (2) pain palpated at this insertion, and (3) pain relieved after diagnostic anesthetic injection into the ligamentous insertion. Motor vehicle accident was reported as

the causative factor in 32% of the cases. Blow to the mandible was reported in 16% of the patients. Other traumatic episodes were reported for 41%. In five patients, prolonged dental treatment, traction, and intubation were the causative factors.

The symptoms of Ernest's syndrome include TMJ and temporal pain, earache, pain at the angle of the mandible, posterior toothache, and eye and throat pain. Its pathogenesis, however, has not been clearly elucidated. Burch[143] and Spalteholz-Spanner[144] classified the stylomandibular ligament as an accessory ligament that becomes slack with jaw opening and tight with full protrusion or overclosing of the mandible beyond its normal vertical relation. The contralateral ligament tightens during lateral jaw border movement. A tearing Ernest's syndrome may occur during the hyperflexion phase of whiplash. Individuals lacking posterior support are thought to be predisposed to this type of injury. Patients with parafunctional habits placing the mandible in extreme border positions may also be predisposed to this condition.

In summary, styloid pain syndromes may mimic craniofacial and TMJ pain patterns. The diagnosis of "insertion tendonitis" as described by Shenoi[145] and Steinmann[146] may challenge the most astute clinician. Therefore, the differential diagnosis of TMD must include stylohyoid and stylomandibular attachment disorders.[147]

INFECTIOUS ARTHRITIS

Septic or infectious arthritis of the TMJs is rare[148,149] but nonetheless reported in the literature.[78,150] Mayne and Hatch[6] observed that any pathogenic bacteria may cause infectious arthritis, which can progress to mild synovitis, destructive joint lesions, and even death. Early diagnosis and vigorous and prolonged antibiotic treatment are strongly recommended[151] because of the unusually high incidence of mortality.[152,153]

The organisms most commonly involved in a septic joint are *Neisseria gonorrhoea, Staphylococcus aureus,* and streptococci. Children are most often afflicted with this disease, and in 10% of the cases, *Haemophilus influenzae* is the pathogen.[150] Even a tentative impression of sepsis warrants culturing the joint fluid.[6]

Organisms may enter the joint via a penetrating wound; a ruptured capsule; an invasion from adjacent infection, such as otitis media; or a hematogeneous spread from a distant site. Individuals with impaired immune responses or pre-existing joint damage, such as the patient with rheumatoid arthritis, are at particular risk in developing infectious arthritis.[148]

Infectious arthritis must be distinguished from rheumatoid arthritis, gout, pseudogout, rheumatic fever, and traumatic arthritis because its clinical features are similar. These are extreme pain; a hot, red, swollen joint; tenderness on palpation with slight fluctuation; and limitation of movement. Systemic evidence is fever, leukocytosis, and septicemia.[6]

Bony changes can take place within several weeks. Joint space may change as well owing to the accumulation of pus and exudate and the destruction of the meniscus.

Phagocytic action is critical for rapid healing but can be impaired with administration of steroidal or nonsteroidal drugs.[149]

DIZZINESS, VERTIGO, AND OTHER OTOLOGIC SYSTEMS

Dizziness and vertigo are common symptoms in post-traumatic syndrome.[154] These symptoms are controlled by the central nervous system that obtains its information from three different sensory inputs: eyes, vestibular apparatus, and proprioceptive system. The proprioceptive system receives its input from the mechanoreceptors in joints, ligaments, and muscles. Morgan and coworkers[155] cited the traumatic malrelationships of the TMJ with the adjacent structures of the ear as causes of vertigo. Weeks and Travell[156] reported that trigger areas in the sternocleidomastoid muscle are responsible for *postural vertigo.*

Libin[157] reported that masticatory muscle spasm may affect all the muscles innervated by the mandibular division of the trigeminal nerve, especially the tensor tympani and tensor veli palatini muscles. These muscles are sensitive to the contractions of the pterygoids and temporalis muscles, which may result in their own contraction.[158] Arlen[159] and Malkin[160] described this as *reflex hypertonia* and associated otologic symptoms with spasm of the lateral pterygoid muscle.

Fullness in the ear, a common symptom in whiplash victims, may be due to spasm of the tensor veli palatini muscle, which is due to

spasm of one of the pterygoids. Loss of hearing, another common post-traumatic symptom, has been theorized to result from increased tension on the tympanic membrane, which may be caused by contraction of the tensor tympani muscle.[157]

Tinnitus, another otologic symptom commonly present in post-trauma patients, is reported to be associated with spasm in the stapedius muscle. This muscle responds via reflex hypertonia in the presence of spasm in other muscles innervated by the facial nerve. This effect was demonstrated by Watanabe and colleagues[161] who severed the stapedial tendon, which was followed by the immediate cessation of the tinnitus.

MACROTRAUMA

An acute single episode that disturbs, impairs, restricts, or otherwise causes swelling, tenderness, pain, or their combination to the TMJs is termed macrotrauma. If the eliciting event comes from an external source it is termed extrinsic. If the trauma is generated from within the stomatognathic system it is termed intrinsic. An example of intrinsic macrotrauma is the act of unexpectedly biting down on an extremely hard substance while chewing soft food, e.g., contacting a pit while eating cherry pie. If this causes a sudden, painful stimulus, the masticatory muscles automatically react to withdrawal from the noxious source.[162] This is a nociceptive reflex and accounts for the jaw-opening reflex, which is a protective mechanism.[163]

Whiplash; a blow to the chin during an altercation; a fall from a bicycle; a nonimpact jolting of the mandible, such as a "banana-peel" fall; and iatrogenic (medical and dental) procedures described later in this chapter, are examples of extrinsic macrotrauma.[23,24,31,50,54,164]

YAWNING AND EPILEPTIC SEIZURE

Yawning has been implicated as an etiologic event in developing a TM disorder. An overzealous yawn can stretch the discal attachments and can result in discitis, synovitis, subluxation or total dislocation of the meniscus, or myospasm of the anterior digastric muscle.[165–168] Dislocation of the condyles has also been reported as a consequence of yawing.[78,169,170] An epileptic seizure can also induce TMJ injury owing to the abrupt jaw movements with resultant injury similar to that of yawning.[171,172]

WHIPLASH

Whiplash, also called extension-flexion injury, is the most common cervical insult associated with motor vehicle acceleration/deceleration accidents.[173]

In 1948, Wakeley described anterior-medial displacement of the articular disc as a result of trauma.[174] He believed that this type of injury was particularly significant if the trauma occurred when the mouth was open and the posterior attachment was already stretched. This is precisely the mandibular position during the hyperextension phase of whiplash. Gay and Abbott,[175] in 1953, described the role of muscle spasm in the pathophysiology of whiplash syndrome. In 1968, Rowe and Killey[2] discussed the effects of sheer stress on the discal attachment, resulting in loss of synchronization of the disc and condyle, leading to disc derangement, clicking, and pain. Rocabado,[176] followed by Lader,[57] believed pathofunction in the cervical musculature can play an important etiologic role in the development of TM disorders and craniomandibular and cervicomandibular pain syndromes.

Weinberg and La Pointe[173] studied 28 whiplash patients. Of these, 18 were involved in rear end collisions, six in front end, and four in side impacts. These patients were examined, on the average, 126 days from the date of the motor vehicle accident. All stated that there were no pre-existing TMJ symptoms. Limited mouth opening was reported by nine patients, whereas TMJ clicking and numbness were reported by four patients. Six patients reported immediate onset of symptoms, ten experienced symptoms by the first day, five patients by the second day, four patients between the third and sixth day, and three developed symptoms after 1 week. Arthrograms revealed 12 anterior meniscus dislocations with reduction, eight meniscus dislocations without reduction, one meniscus dislocation without reduction with perforation, and one meniscus dislocation with reduction and perforation. There were three normal joints arthrographically, but the patients were diagnosed with MPD syndrome. Weinberg and La Pointe concluded that there was a relationship between acceleration/deceleration accidents and internal derangements.

MECHANISM OF INTERNAL DERANGEMENT IN WHIPLASH

Structural alteration of the TMJ occurs in a rear end collision. Initially, there is *acceleration* of the victim's car and torso, but because of their own inertia, the head and neck move rotatively backward in a direction opposite that of the impact (Fig. 11–1) This *hyperextension phase* takes place around a fulcrum at some point in the cervical spine. Simultaneously, two mechanisms provide for the sudden, wide opening of the mouth. First, the mandible, because of its own inertia, moves much slower than the cranium (Fig. 11–2A), resulting in jaw opening. Secondly, the suprahyoid muscles fail to elongate quickly enough to accommodate the hyperextended head.[103] The net result is the anchoring of the mandible aided by a stabilized hyoid bone (Fig. 11–2B). Therefore, during the initial impact, snapping back of the head and neck, extensive opening of the mouth, and hypertranslation of the condyle and disc assembly occur (Figs. 11–2C and 11–2D). Dunn[177] stated that mandibular whiplash, causing hyperextension of the cervical spine, may result in signif-

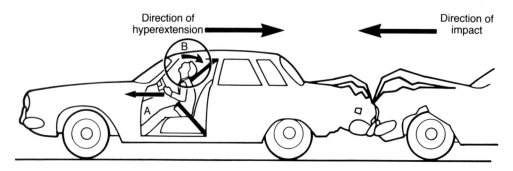

FIGURE 11–1. Car and torso move forward (*A*), while head and neck hyperextend backward (*B*).

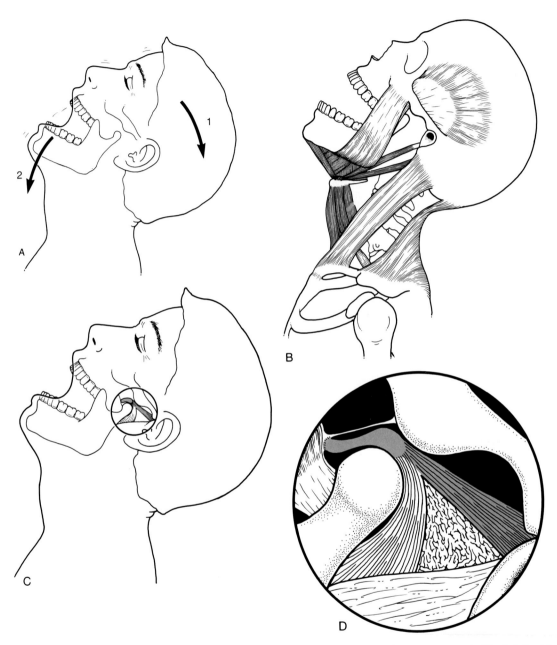

FIGURE 11-2. *A,* The mandible lags behind the hyperextending head because of its own inertia. B, The infrahyoid and suprahyoid muscles anchor the mandible downward, as the head hyperextends, effecting a sudden, wide opening of the jaw. *C* and *D,* The condyle hypertranslates, forcing the disc assembly forward, stretching and possibly tearing the superior lamina of the posterior attachment.

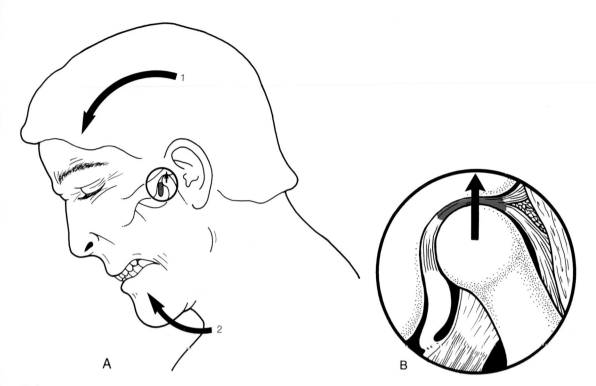

FIGURE 11–3. *A and B*, During the deceleration phase, the head is hyperflexed abruptly (arrow 1), closing the mouth (arrow 2). Note the retrusion of the condyle and the anteriorly displaced meniscus.

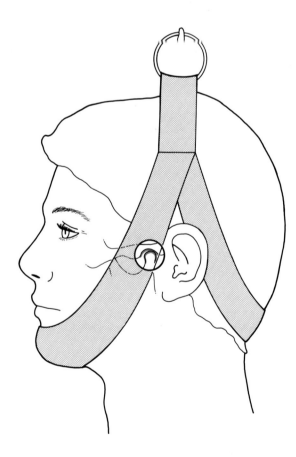

FIGURE 11–10. Although cervical traction ameliorates neck symptoms, it results in intrusion of the condyle into the glenoid fossa.

icant damage to the supramandibular and submandibular musculature. This damage results in excessive opening of the mouth, leading to stretching of the retrodiscal tissue and possibly the superior belly of the lateral pterygoid muscle. The probability of internal derangement increases proportionally with severity of the hyperextension injury.

Injury to the joint during hypertranslation is likely because of the joint's "Achilles tendon." The medial half of the anterior aspect of the TMJ is not bounded by a true capsule. The synovial membrane lining the superior joint cavity at this junction is supported by loose areolar connective tissue.[103,178] Likewise, the lateral half of the anterior aspect is also loose areolar connective tissue not a thick sheet of collagen fibers. This weak, loosely bound tissue cannot limit joint movement and probably accounts for the high incidence of damage to the synovial tissue and lateral pterygoid muscle. The posterior deep temporal nerves are easily traumatized by the hypertranslating condyles, which rub on the temporal bone at the anterior portion of the eminence.[103] Other investigators[164] have also identified the hyperextension phase as causing anterior meniscus displacement and myalgia.

Next, the *deceleration phase* occurs, as the vehicle brakes to a sudden stop or hits a vehicle or object in front. This propels the head and torso forward until the head hits the windshield, steering wheel, or dashboard or is halted abruptly by the seat/torso restraint (shoulder seat belt).[179] The flexing of the head forward abruptly closes the mouth. As the mouth closes, the condyle moves up and back into the glenoid fossa, crushing the stretched out posterior attachment owing to the inability of the disc to translate backward as quickly as the condyle (Figs. 11–3A and 11–3B). This leaves the disc dislocated anterior to the condylar head. The net result during the *hyperflexion* or *deceleration phase* is damaged retrodiscal tissue and internal derangement. The posterior attachment may be stretched, crushed, torn, or perforated.[173] Additional injury such as discitis, synovitis, effusion, hemarthrosis, and capsulitis may also occur. Muscle splinting, discussed in chapter 8, further insults the displaced disc by shortening of the lateral pterygoid muscle. The arthropathy and pain increase muscle tension that is, in and of itself, guarding against the bobbing about of the head. Ernest reported a case of whiplash injury inducing the pain-spasm-pain cycle.[133]

INDIRECT MECHANISM OF WHIPLASH

The indirect effect of cervical trauma or whiplash via reflex postural alterations of the craniovertebral and craniomandibular relationship can ultimately result in a TM disorder. The sequence begins with an acceleration/deceleration accident. Cervical myospasm and cervical sprain stimulate neuroreceptors to reflexly compensate for the cervical postural alteration.[57,61,176,180] The suprahyoid musculature responds with increased hypertonicity, altering mandibular position with respect to the maxilla resulting in malocclusion. This effect is defined as an alteration in the normal interrelationship of the cusps and fossa of the occlusal system.[57,181] Neuroreceptors in the periodontal ligament and joint capsule provide afferent central nervous system input, resulting in muscle bracing or splinting in addition to the guarding that already developed from direct trauma.

The development of TM disorders from cervical trauma has been discussed in the literature[177,182–184] and the interrelationship between internal derangement and mandibular muscular disorders seems plausible.[101,185] However, the actual compilation of statistics by the National Highway Traffic Safety Administration (NHTSA) is lacking in this field. No raw data have been ever compiled by the National Accident Sampling System (NASS) of the NHTSA. Because TMDs are categorized as *minor* trauma, there is little to no support for its placement on the agenda for study by federal agencies.[179] It is impossible to calculate the actual number of TMD victims in motor vehicle accidents. However, years of studies have shown vast numbers of cervical trauma victims from motor vehicle accidents.[32,186–190] Because cervical trauma may result in TM disorders, it can be logically deduced that motor vehicle accidents are causative events for a multitude of TM disorders. Having established a cause and effect relationship between neck trauma and onset of TM disorders, some of the statistics and some of the features of motor vehicle accidents that presumably have a distinct connection with TM problems are reviewed.

Assuming hyperextension/hyperflexion accidents are major etiologic factors in the development of TMDs, the statistics published by the United States Department of Transportation concerning head and neck injuries become most relevant. Almost 17 million people and more than 11 million motor vehicles were involved in almost 6.5 million crashes reported by police in 1986. Another 11 million crashes were reported to sources other than police.

The number of neck injuries due to motor vehicle accidents is quite impressive. There are well over 500,000 police reports of whiplash (nondirect impact) accidents and an additional 750,000 injuries due to direct impact of the neck.[187] The true number is probably twice that because all whiplash accidents are not reported to the police but rather to someone else, e.g., insurance company representatives, service station attendants, and lawyers.

The enactment of "mandatory restraint use" laws in many states has resulted in a nationwide increase in safety belt use from about 15% in 1974 to 40% in 1986 for front seat passengers of automobiles.[32]

The use of seat belts has had a profound yet paradoxical effect on head and neck injuries. First, lap restraints have reduced severe injuries when compared with no restraints at all. Lap and shoulder or torso restraints reduced *serious* injury to the head and neck dramatically compared with lap restraints only. Interestingly, the incidence of *minor* neck injury rose with the use of lap and torso systems. In one study,[187] 3.6% of unrestrained occupants and 2.6% of lap belt–restrained occupants suffered whiplash injury compared with 4.8% of lap and torso belt–restrained occupants. Partyka[187] described the mechanism responsible for this increase in whiplash symptoms. Without a torso restraint there would be head contact, which dissipates some of the energy of hyperflexion. With a torso restraint there would be more neck movement. As a consequence, distinctly fewer disfiguring facial injuries and life-threatening head injuries occur, but more minor neck injuries. Benham[191] formulated a mathematic model that described head, neck, and torso movement in a head on or rear end crash that propelled the car until it stopped suddenly against another vehicle or object. He demonstrated that the energy transferred to the head and neck is greater with a torso and lap restraint system. This increases the inertial forces during hyperflexion, as compared with the decreased energy transferred to the head and neck when the unrestrained torso is permitted to move forward during hyperflexion. More energy is absorbed by the moving torso—with a lap restraint only—and, therefore, the head and neck are hyperflexing with less force (Figs. 11–4A and 11–4B).

Eppinger[179] supported the findings of Partyka[187] and Benham[191] and, in another comparative study of neck injury mechanisms in frontal collisions, Ommaya and coworkers[186] reported that restrained occupants show a higher proportion of neck injuries. To further illustrate the effect of energy transfer to the head and neck, they observed that shorter occupants have a risk of neck injury of about 40% less than taller occupants. This finding is also noted in Benham's model (Fig. 11–5A). The cause and effect relationship between motor vehicle accidents, torso restraints, and TM disorders has not been established employing scientific methods. However, the pathogenesis of cervical injury and TM disorders juxtaposed with statistics presented by the NHTSA and NASS is highly suggestive of such a causal relationship. Evidence compiled through careful research and controlled studies is needed to validate these relationships.

Cervical trauma can occur with no TMJ sequelae, but there are many cases of undiagnosed TMDs in which the etiologic event is a motor vehicle accident *without* a direct blow to the jaw. Recognition of this fact is essential if victims are to receive timely treatment instead of suffering needlessly, often for years.

ENDOTRACHEAL INTUBATION

Joint subluxation or condylar dislocation is an occasional complication after general anesthesia.[192–195] Intubation procedures, along with prolonged bronchofiberoscopy,[196] may cause pathologic changes in TMJs. Lipp and colleagues,[197] in a double-blind study of 140 patients, concluded that the mandibular range of motion was reduced in the patient group receiving routine oral intubation compared with two other groups receiving nasal intubation and face mask anesthesia. Temporomandibular joint hematoma with intra-articular adhesion may occur because of damage to the highly vascular retrodiscal tissue. Disc displacement can occur as well.[198]

A forward and sometimes vigorous jaw thrust is part of the routine procedure in general anesthesia.[199,200] It is also recommended that a patient's mouth be maximally opened for endotracheal intubation.[201,202] (Fig. 11–6) A mouth gag[199] or prop is also sometimes employed.[168] These maneuvers may induce a meniscus dislocation or worsen a pre-existing condition. Because the prevalence of internal derangements is estimated to be as high as 25

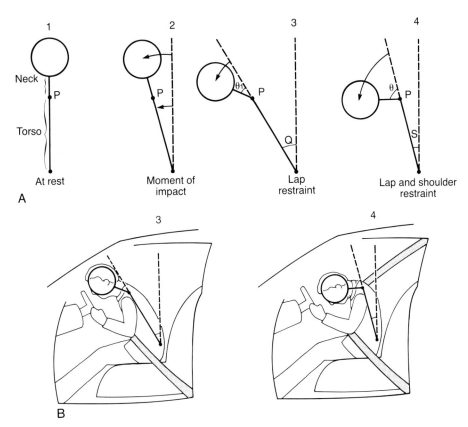

FIGURE 11–4. *A,* Benham demonstrated that after the moment of impact, the head and torso start moving forward (*2*); with a lap restraint, the torso moves forward and the head and neck hyperflex (*3*); with a shoulder restraint, movement of the torso is limited and more energy is transferred to the head and neck, resulting in greater hyperflexion (*4*). Because damage to the temporomandibular joint (TMJ) is proportional to the magnitude of hyperflexion and hyperextension, the lap and shoulder restraint may be directly responsible for increased insult to the TMJ. *B,* Benham's demonstrations superimposed on the victim.

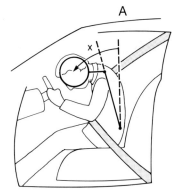

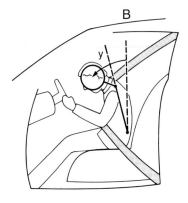

FIGURE 11–5. Because of the greater inertia of the taller victim's head (*A*) compared with the shorter victim (*B*), increased hyperflexion occurs.

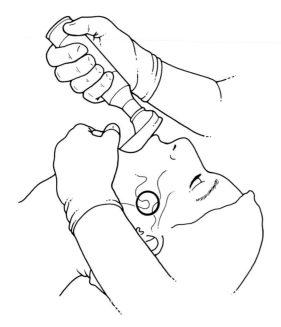

FIGURE 11-6. Although different techniques of orotracheal intubation may be employed, the head must be extended and the mouth maximally opened. This maneuver may result in the injury described, especially in a patient with pre-existing intracapsular damage.

to 50% of the general population,[200] it is advisable that the anesthesiologist determine the status of the TMJs prior to the intubation procedure. This determination is especially significant because the TMJ is frequently taken for granted and is considered of little consequence during tracheal intubation.[202]

EARLY TEMPOROMANDIBULAR JOINT TRAUMA—FORCEPS AND BREECH PRESENTATION DELIVERIES

Although difficult to verify, *forceps* and *breech presentation deliveries* have been identified as etiologic factors in traumatically induced TMDs. A preliminary study by Clayman and Goldberg[203] demonstrated a correlation between forceps deliveries and subsequent problems with the TMJ. Proper placement of forceps applies pressure directly over the TMJ. Garry[204] reported that the meniscus may be damaged if the forceps compress the preauricular area. Fortunately, the injured tissues of an infant regenerate rapidly and often heal uneventfully. Because forceps delivery is on the decline, it will be necessary to compare the frequency of early TM disorders in future years

with that of past years and examine the correlation with forceps delivery.

Grosfeld and associates,[205] investigated 156 children—83 born by vaginal breech presentation and 73 born spontaneously by vertex presentation. Almost 60% of these children showed signs of TM injuries, with slightly over two thirds of them breech deliveries. These numbers were statistically significant, particularly when observing severe TM disorders. It was concluded, therefore, that many early injuries to the TMJ that were considered congenital were probably caused by vaginal breech delivery. Obstetricians should consider that possibility when choosing a delivery technique (breech vs. surgical). In addition, early dental consultations with frequent followups are highly recommended.

DIRECT BLOW

Many patients have difficulty describing accurately the onset of TM disorders. Direct blow to the jaw is the exception, providing the symptoms are immediate. Delayed onset of symptoms is discussed in the section *Latency.* Direct blow most commonly occurs from an altercation, a forward fall off a bicycle,[70] a sports injury, or a secondary impact in a motor vehicle accident (i.e., the body being thrust into a structure inside the vehicle after the vehicle sustains the primary impact).[187]

MENISCUS INJURY FROM DIRECT BLOW

Depending on the degree of trauma, the meniscus may sustain varied damage—some temporary, e.g., inflammation in the posterior retrodiscal tissue, and some permanent, e.g., complete tearing from its capsular attachments. Because a direct blow may be from more than one direction, different parts of the joint may be structurally damaged. A blow that violently directs the jaw backward can detach the retrodiscal tissue and discal ligaments, or it can thin out or perforate the retrodiscal tissue, leading to detachment. If the meniscus remains attached to the anterior capsule and lateral pterygoid muscle, the meniscus anteriorly dislocates. If the mouth is opened and the condyle has translated forward during impact, the anterior capsule may be injured, thereby detaching the meniscus. Similar injury may occur if the individual is anticipating the blow and profoundly contracting the masticatory muscles in a protective, guarded manner. When the impact is delivered, the mandible thrusts backward more quickly than the contracted upper head of the lateral pterygoid muscle can relax.[206] The result is a tearing of the muscle fibers from the anterior wall of the capsule and a detaching of the meniscus from its anterior boundary.

The severity of a direct blow varies and therefore may cause differences in types and degrees of injury. An acute inflammatory episode may result. Capsulitis or synovitis may develop as well. Collateral discal attachment stretching and weakening may occur. Articular surfaces, ligaments, and retrodiscal tissues may be bruised. Naturally, a combination of any of the aforementioned is indeed possible. In addition, inflammatory muscle injury may result in myofibrotic contracture, in which case the muscle resting length is shortened and hypomobility and pain ensue.[207]

The mouth guard worn by professional boxers protects the osseous structures; meniscus; and attachment tissues, particularly the posterior attachment, by virtue of restricting backward movement of the condyle and creating joint space by distracting the condyle inferiorly.[208]

CHILDBIRTH

During labor and delivery, women sometimes clench the teeth and induce severe TMJ symptoms. Often these symptoms are blamed on the pressures of having a new baby and certainly that may be a related cause. But the clinician must recognize the potential of traumatizing both muscle and intracapsular structures with the profoundly heavy clenching induced during childbirth. In addition to muscular overuse and joint overloading, the postural position of a woman during delivery is often with the head and neck flexed forward while she is in a supine position (Fig. 11–7). According to Kraus,[209] this postural position exceeds the physiologic adaptive range of the cervical spine causing adverse effects to develop on the craniomandibular region. Add this factor to the clenching from emotional and physical stress and another common form of macrotrauma becomes apparent.

TEMPOROMANDIBULAR JOINT TRAUMA AFFECTING GROWTH

Traumatically induced growth disturbances have been reported in the literature[70,210–214] and often are due to fractures of the condylar head and neck. In many cases, these childhood fractures remain undiagnosed until interference with growth and development becomes apparent.[210] Macrotrauma, without fracture, and microtrauma can cause growth inhibition. Ricketts[70] claimed that a blow to the jaw is sufficient to alter mandibular growth. The most com-

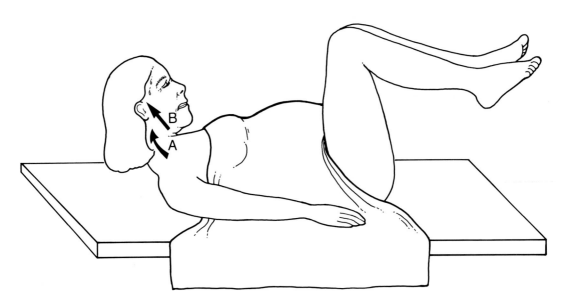

FIGURE 11–7. A flexed head and neck and clenched mandible may easily traumatize the temporomandibular joints, especially in combination with tremendous physical and emotional strain, as in childbirth.

mon macrotrauma in children is falling, face forward, off a bicycle and may be related to the high incidence of condylar undergrowth.

Ricketts also reported on a young individual with a history of continued use of a neck collar. Retrognathia resulted because of the resorption of condyles bilaterally, slight resorption of the chin, and obvious growth inhibition. In a second case, he theorized that microtrauma resulted in traumatic arthritis. The timing of this arthropathy coincided with a growth period, and condylar undergrowth resulted.

I have treated an 18-year-old woman who presented with signs and symptoms of "whiplash" injury. A motor vehicle accident occurred 3 months prior to her presentation for treatment. She had headaches, restricted range of motion, bilateral clicking, muscle tenderness, and a host of craniocervicomandibular symptoms indicating acceleration/deceleration injury. Magnetic resonance image findings revealed hypoplastic condyles, bilaterally (Fig. 11-8). Further questioning revealed a traumatic forceps delivery at birth. The patient had a retrognathic profile. Her dentist of record denied any pre-existing signs or symptoms prior

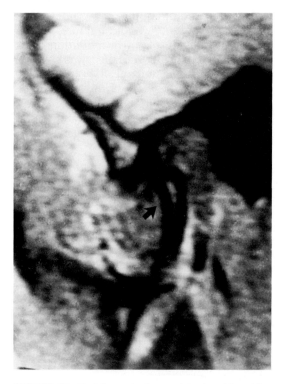

FIGURE 11-8. A hypoplastic condylar head is evident and is apparently due to a traumatic delivery, based on history and hospital records.

to the motor vehicle accident, as did the patient and her mother. The TM disorder was refractory to nonsurgical treatment except for substantial, but not total, amelioration of headaches.

Of course, one can only speculate as to what the whiplash effect would have been had there been normal morphologically formed TMJs. It seems reasonable to speculate that the undersized condyles and incongruous joint structures were responsible for treatment failure. This finding is in view of the fact that all other skeletal parts were morphologically sound, that all other organ systems functioned normally, and that no other trauma was ever reported.

Berger and Stewart[215] reported a similar case in which a traumatic forceps delivery and compression of the mother's uterus from a motor vehicle accident 5 days before delivery were part of the history. Facial asymmetry was noted 4.5 months later. Radiographically, the infant had a shallow sigmoid notch, a short condylar process, and a hypoplastic condyle with a shorted ramus.

The condylar neck and head are particularly vulnerable to trauma. The growth center is directly beneath the condylar head. Normally, balanced bilateral growth occurs in a downward and forward direction. Trauma in children can damage this growth center and can result in disfigurement and disability.[2] The key factors in traumatically induced growth disturbances are the severity of the injury; the precise anatomic location; and, perhaps most influential, the timing of the trauma with regard to normal growth and development.

"BANANA-PEEL" FALL

Falling onto the lower back and injuring the coccyx is a common occurrence and has been widely reported in the orthopedic literature.[216,217] The "banana-peel" fall occurs when the legs and feet slip out from under the torso as seen in Figure 11-9. The body falls abruptly to the ground with a profound impact on the victim's back—notably the coccyx. Two mechanisms are responsible for developing TMJ pain and dysfunction. First, the inertia of the head and neck propels these structures backward after the body jolts to a sudden stop. This head and neck hyperextension is similar to the hyperextension of whiplash. Secondly, a reflex protective mechanism, *muscle splinting*,[218] is activated to stabilize the threatened parts and protect them from further injury. The cervi-

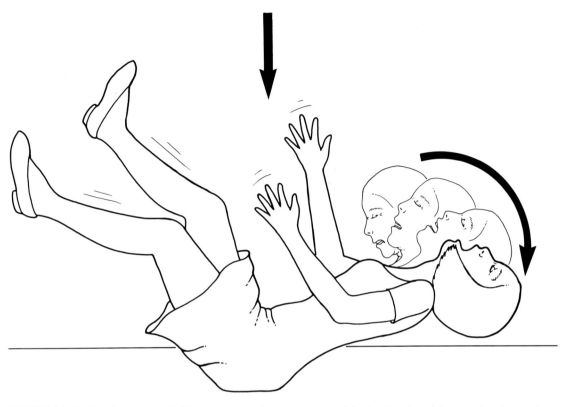

FIGURE 11–9. The "banana-peel" fall may result in hyperextension of the head and neck besides the obvious back injury. Cervical strain and temporomandibular joint insult occur.

comandibular musculature becomes hypertonic and painful, especially if splinting is protracted. Two case histories illustrate this kind of trauma:

A 20-year-old female patient presented for biyearly prophylaxis. In updating the medical history, she reported bilateral earache and occipital-frontal headache 6 to 8 weeks prior to the examination. Careful questioning revealed that she had slipped on a wet surface in an ice cream parlor 3 months earlier with immediate onset of lower back pain. Three weeks later, earaches commenced; three weeks later, headaches. Medical examination findings were negative, but a TMJ examination revealed discitis, traumatic synovitis, and myositis/myospasm of several masticatory and cervical muscles. Prior to this traumatic event, there were no signs or symptoms of any TM disorders. Treatment commenced immediately, and amelioration of symptoms soon followed.

A 50-year-old obese female was referred for injuries sustained from an unusual fall. She reported stepping onto a shuffleboard disk and slipping. With her feet up in the air, she fell squarely onto her back. Upon presentation for examination, she had a 23-mm maximum opening and a host of other signs of a TM disorder. Her dentist of 15 years reported that

the patient had had a full range of motion, no joint noise, and no history of chronic headaches or masticatory pain prior to the fall. Treatment yielded satisfactory results. A stabilization splint was inserted, and physical therapy was initiated. Although range of motion increased to 38 mm, intermittent pain persisted. The MRI revealed a chronic locked condition.

MICROTRAUMA

Microtrauma is a repetitive, low-grade trauma that continuously places a body part into a position of stress or abuse. Injury results when the body part can no longer adapt to the prolonged stress. Normal protective mechanisms, e.g., muscle guarding and avoidance phenomena, prevent damage because microtrauma generally occurs without the individual's awareness.[209]

Frequent gum chewing, nail biting, resting of the jaw on one's hand, lip biting, bruxism, and clenching are examples of microtrauma. These are classified as *intrinsic* microtrauma because they arise from within the stomatognathic system. *Extrinsic* microtrauma originates from outside the system but similarly affects the craniomandibular complex. Examples include postural or occupational microtrauma, such as violin playing or scuba diving, excessive unprotected cervical traction, and prolonged use of a cervical collar. Other common abusive habits are biting on a pipe stem, pencil, or other object between the teeth; use of toothpicks; and habitual mannerisms, such as protrusive and lateral movements of the mandible. All of these examples can result in disc interference disorders; intracapsular adhesions; structural alterations in the condylar head, eminence morphology, or both; disc thinning; discal ligament damage; traumatic synovitis; and degenerative joint disease.[219,220]

The pre-existing condition of the TMJ will influence the nature of the resulting pathology. For example, a steep eminence increases the force of impact loading and causes a greater burden on the disc-condyle assembly.[220] Pre-existing posterior condylar position can weaken the posterior and lateral discal attachments resulting in posterior synovitis, discitis, and disc displacement.

CERVICAL TRACTION AND CERVICAL COLLARS

Whiplash victims often wear immobilizing collars to support and protect the head and neck and relax the soft structures.[61] A cervical collar may aggravate a primary TMJ arthropathy or initiate a secondary one,[57,221] by pushing the lower jaw up and backward resulting in joint loading. Some cervical traction devices can have the same effects (Fig. 11–10).[43,61,166,222] Although these modalities are effective for cervical problems, retrusion of the mandible can cause impingement on the retrodiscal tissue, which may result in traumatic synovitis, crushed and severed posterior attachment, disc displacement or vascular engorgement, and lateral pterygoid muscle spasm. In addition, retrusion of the mandible with respect to the maxilla establishes a temporary malocclusion with premature contacts, which may induce TMJ and muscle pain and dysfunction.[223] In some cases, cervical traction may induce painful symptoms rather quickly. Frankel and colleagues[222] reported the occurrence of TMJ symptoms 2 days after cervical traction. Along with others,[57,224] this group has advocated the use of a stabilization splint to prevent distali-

zation and vertical displacement of the mandible. Patients with cervical injuries with missing posterior teeth and those with predispositions to postural irregularities should be especially careful.[61] The clinician should consider a neck-traction device, which eliminates the upward and backward pull on the patient's mandible.

OVERLOADING

Repetitive microtrauma or a single traumatic episode can overload the TMJ beyond its functional capacity. The osseous-supported articulating surfaces can remodel and adjust to compressive forces, provided they do not exceed physiologic limits.[225] The articular disc cannot remodel[226] but deforms and deteriorates under compressive forces.[227,228] *Static overloading* initiated by the microtraumatic effects of bruxism[229] can thin out the central bearing area of the disc, presdisposing the patient to disc perforation and degenerative joint disease.

IMPACT LOADING

Impact loading is caused by posterior overclosure and bruxism, which apply excessive forces on the TMJ. This loading results in loss of contour of the disc, and the patient is predisposed to traumatic arthritis and internal derangement of the joint.[230] The traumatic effects of impact loading on the TMJ have been the subject of research. This may give some insight into the pathogenesis of traumatically induced arthropathy. Traumatic arthritis and degenerative joint disease are thought to be initiated or at least perpetuated by continued mechanical damage.[231]

Repetitive loading experiments mimicking naturally occurring microtrauma were first conducted by Radin and Paul.[227] They studied the progression of the disease by oscillating bovine joints under high constant loads, intermittently subjecting them to impact dynamic loading. Their observations resulted in two possible explanations for the dramatic wear of the articular cartilage. One is that repeated impact loading squeezes out cartilaginous interstitial fluid, increasing shear or friction that induces wear. The other is that high compressive stress damages the integrity of the cartilage, increasing its vulnerability to shear stress. In these experiments, the impact loads were introduced, interrupted, and then applied again.

The friction was almost double compared with static loading. This model may mimick loading in clenching, bruxism, or other parafunctional habits. Mahan[103] cited the Radin study demonstrating that impact loading, rather than sliding and gliding movements, results in degenerative arthritic changes. Mahan further suggested that clenching the jaw with a loss of posterior teeth tends to impact load the TMJs. The mandibular elevator muscles, working collectively with the premolars acting as the fulcrum, load the lever arm producing a driving force between the condyle and fossa articular eminence. Mahan suggests this effect may be related to the degenerative changes in the TMJ.[103] The rounded head of the condyle being thrust onto the posterior slope of the eminence during traumatic repetitive impact loading may account for degeneration occurring in the center of articular surfaces and progressing outward toward the joint periphery.

The response of joints to impact loading is consistent in all experimental studies: stiffening of the underlying subchondral bone along with trabecular microfracture. This causes the cartilaginous articular surface to lose its underlying resilient shock-absorbing[77] capacity, and then degenerative arthritis ensues.[232] Bollet[233] concluded that greater physical stress is probably responsible for initiating the enzymatic processes that actually destroy the cartilage.

Experiments by others have shown the formation of primary and secondary fissures that ultimately coalesce to produce cartilage fragments in the subchondral bone.[234,235] Zimmerman and colleagues[231] found that the amount of load was more significant than the number of cycles to which the joint was subjected. In fact, this experimental model failed to produce cartilage disruption after 120,000 cycles, but doubling the load caused fissure formation after only 500 cycles.

A disruption in normal biomechanics seems to be a critical factor in producing cartilage lesions. Fengler and Franz[236] suggested that a one time trauma above a certain level of severity can produce serious cartilage lesions with loss of proteoglycans, flaking, and collagen fibril exposure.

Mongini[10] investigated impact loading and subsequent remodeling of the condyle. Others have suggested that occlusal discrepancies may be significant in adversely loading the TM joints.[237] Bruxism, "collapsed bite," and cervical spine influences have also been implicated in the pathogenesis of osteorarthritis.

IMMOBILIZATION

When one thinks of TMJ trauma, repetitive loading and macrotrauma, such as a fracture or a blow to the jaw, immediately come to mind. *Immobilization* is another type of trauma and has a different form and mode of action.

Immobilization can occur because of an intermaxillary fixation, a prolonged illness or injury with joint effusion, a reflex muscle guarding,[238] or a self-imposed protective mechanism due to fear or pain. The last is most commonly found in young patients.[239] Immobilization can result in ankylosis, particularly following trauma with hemarthrosis. Other effects of immobilization of the TMJs are osteoarthritis, joint stiffness, capsular tightness, increased vulnerability to traumatic arthritis, and myopathy.

Immobilization results in thinning of articular cartilage[240,241]; decreased diffusion of nutrients into the articular cartilage[240]; egress of catabolites from the articular cartilage[240]; decreased proteoglycan synthesis, which has been demonstrated experimentally in the knees of dogs[67,242] and TMJs of monkeys[241]; and increased water content, which may then contact and combine with either collagen or proteoglycan, resulting in gel formation.[67] Water content is significantly higher in osteoarthritis and may be responsible for the biomechanical disruption of the tissue.[240]

Immobilization causes two distinct alterations to take place in the capsule. Biochemically, there is a reduction in the content of water and glycosaminoglycan. This effect diminishes the lubrication between the collagen fibers of the outer capsule and results in decreased capsular extensibility. This *capsular stiffness* is due to the loss of freely gliding collagen fibers.[243]

Painful muscle spasm and muscle atrophy are also results of immobilization. Immobility can build up muscle tension and activate latent trigger points.[244]

The effects of immobilization on the joint cartilage, capsule, and mandibular musculature increase the vulnerability of the TMJs to traumatic arthritis. The coexistence of immobilization with parafunctional habits may also result in more rapid development of pathology.

POSTURAL MICROTRAUMA

Scuba diving has been implicated in the etiology of TM disorders. Although no studies have been reported, some have cited this sport as a definite trigger for TMJ pain and dysfunction. Many divers have chronic daily headaches and disc interference disorders and blame the headaches on the depths of the dives or length of time under water.[12] Divers are susceptible to MPD syndrome because the biting down on the regulator or mouthpiece causes the jaw to be in a forward posture. This position is maintained throughout the dive and is an example of intrinsic microtrauma, especially in commercial divers. In a series of 23 commercial divers evaluated and treated by me, cervical and TM disorders were observed in the form of disc-interference disorders, myospasm, synovitis, and tendonomyositis. No other eliciting event could be identified, and exacerbation of symptoms coincided with each dive.

In addition to clenching down hard on the breathing apparatus, two other contributing factors are proposed. First, abnormal head and neck posture has been reported to initiate TM disorders.[61,182,245] Secondly, Kraus[209] reported that cervical extension causes the mandible to retrude. This retrusion causes the condyles to impinge on retrodiscal tissue and stretch the lateral pterygoid muscle.

If one observes the head and neck of a scuba diver as he or she swims forward (Fig. 11–11A), the strained position is quite apparent. In order to look forward in an unstrained position, the diver must right the body somewhat (Fig. 11–11B). Playing the violin and some other musical instruments can have similar effects. A series of 18 violinists with signs and symptoms of TMD were evaluated. In order to hold the instrument, the musician presses the jaw down while the head and neck are in the forward head posture (FHP) (Fig. 11–12A). Kraus proposed that FHP effects and elevation and retrusion of the mandible lead to altered occlusal contacts.[209] In addition, the violin player generally keeps the mouth tightly closed and, as is seen in Figure 11–12B, the head and neck are tilted to the instrument's side. Travell observed that the lateral pterygoid muscle activity is increased when maintaining mandibular side pressure in fixed protrusion, while holding a violin in the playing position.[246] Activities thought to cause TM disorders are swimming,[247] weight lifting,[31] and nail biting.[62,248] When swimming the crawl stroke, the head turns repeatedly and the mandible moves anteriorly and laterally to facilitate breathing. Racing with vigorous movement, or slower repetitive lap swimming, may cause the joint structures or the lateral pterygoid muscle, or both, to be overstressed and injured. Some weight lifters demonstrate profound clenching during their events, overload the joints, induce sustained contraction in the masseters, and eventually

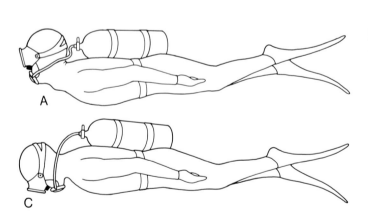
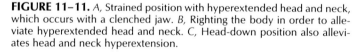
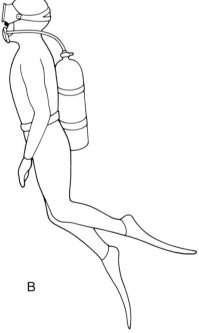

FIGURE 11–11. *A,* Strained position with hyperextended head and neck, which occurs with a clenched jaw. *B,* Righting the body in order to alleviate hyperextended head and neck. *C,* Head-down position also alleviates head and neck hyperextension.

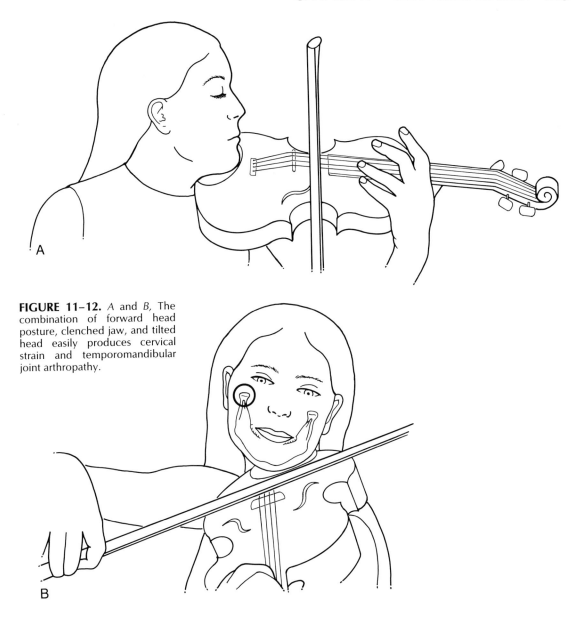

FIGURE 11–12. *A* and *B,* The combination of forward head posture, clenched jaw, and tilted head easily produces cervical strain and temporomandibular joint arthropathy.

develop TM disorders. Nail biting, in addition to elevating the load on joint tissues, increases activity in the lateral pterygoid muscle.[249–251] This common oral habit frequently accompanies bruxism.[62,252]

LATENCY

Temporomandibular joint pain may develop weeks or months after initial trauma for several reasons. Mannheimer[183] suggested that FHP, which develops from cervical trauma, eventually gives rise to muscle imbalance. This can lead to a TM disorder with the passage of

time—1 week, several months, or even a few years. Friedman and Weisberg[253] stated that clicking may *eventually* lead to a complete anterior dislocation of the meniscus. Rasmussen[49] observed that patients usually seek treatment at the onset of pain, which can be 2 years after the actual incident.

Hansson[36] suggested that symptoms caused by overloading are not manifested until several years after a precipitating event. Leonard and Anderson[254] reported on two cases, the first in which disc perforation, condylar degeneration, and aseptic necrosis occurred several years after the patient sustained a jaw fracture. In the second case, a fistfight led to the development of a closed lock with extensive meniscus and condylar head destruction 1 year later.

Meyer[167] suggested that over a period of time the abnormal positioning of a displaced meniscus and the contracture of associated ligaments and muscles lead to myofascial pain and degenerative changes. He reported a case in which a blow to the chin, displacing the meniscus, initally caused no pain. A study of 28 patients with histories of trauma revealed only six whose TMD symptoms developed immediately and 22 whose symptoms developed subsequently.[173]

The key word in understanding latency is *development*—the time needed for joint adhesions to develop on the synovial membrane, for sustained muscle contraction to develop into fibrotic contracture, for loosened discal ligaments to develop into an internal derangement, or for poor head and neck posture to eventually develop into muscular disharmony. Rocabado's description[176] of the progression from a whiplash injury to a TM disorder illustrates the concept of latency as being a function of the time needed for pain and dysfunction to develop. Figure 11–13 illustrates the pathways in the development of TM disorders.

MOVEMENT DISTURBANCES

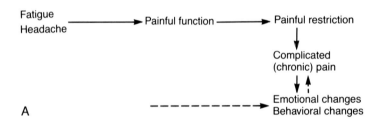

DISCOMFORT

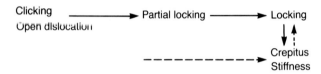

A

FIGURE 11–13. *A,* Progression of temporomandibular disorders. (Reprinted with permission from Solberg, W. K.: Current concepts on the development of TMJ dysfunction. In *Developmental Aspects of Temporomandibular Disorders.* D. Carlson, J.A. McNamara Jr., and K.A. Ribbens (eds.). University of Michigan, Ann Arbor, 1985.) *B,* Etiologic pathways of temporomandibular disorders according to the multifactorial concept. Temporomandibular disorders result from adverse loading of the jaw system, differentially generated by repetitive loadings due to stress, postural loading due to biomechanical factors, and macrotrauma. (Reprinted with permission from Solberg, W.K. and Seligman, D.A.: Temporomandibular orthopedics. In *New Vistas in Orthodontics.* L.E. Johnston (ed.). Lea & Febiger, Philadelphia, 1985.)

Etiology of temporomandibular (TMJ) disorders

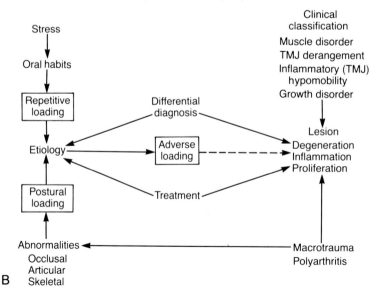

B

Psychologic variables play a role in latency, owing, in part, to the sequential relationship of anxiety, muscular tension, pain, and dysfunction, as described by Rugh and Solberg.[45] Additionally, a non-TMJ injury may secondarily cause TMJ symptoms. For example, tension myositis syndrome of the lower back can result in anxiety and depression.[255] These psychologic factors could maintain a coexisting TM disorder.[256] Latent TMD symptoms confuse patients and clinicians, especially in the absence of specific findings during the examination in the emergency room or after radiographic evaluation.

A traumatized patient may not seek immediate care[36] or may not be immediately referred to a dentist for treatment,[8,257] which is reflected as a delay from onset to treatment. A thorough history is necessary to help make the distinction from true latency.

PSYCHOLOGIC ASPECTS

The psychologic aspects of TMJ trauma cannot be overstated. The worst problems occur in the patient whose pain remains undiagnosed. Tanaka[258] reported that the average TM disorder patient has been seen by at least seven physicians, dentists, psychologists, or other health professionals. Of these patients, 7 out of 10 have been incompletely diagnosed or misdiagnosed because of the lack of understanding of the differential diagnosis or the disease processes involved.

In microtrauma or macrotrauma with latent symptoms, the patient may be unable to identify the precipitating traumatic incident. The patient experiences symptom progression with increasing severity and secondary physical and autonomic effects.[259] The pain-spasm-pain cycle is activated,[260] and disability ensues. Eating, sexual activity, sleep, speech, and sporting activities may be disturbed.[1] These problems impair the patient's emotional state,[261] which is further aggravated if the dentist or physician dismisses the problem because radiographic findings are lacking. Speculand and Goss[256] reported that most patients have no radiographically detectable pathology.

Chronicity leads to anxiety and depression.[1] The persistence of pain is the greatest factor in producing psychologic effects. Chronic pain is the most threatening and debilitating factor in the TMD patient.[262] Sarno[255] reported that pain causes fear of physical deterioration, of further injury, and of potential disability, and fear of

pain itself. Rugh and Solberg[262] reported that chronic pain (lasting more than 6 months) becomes as clinically important as the disease state with which it is associated and that the amount of pain can have little to do with the amount of damaged tissue.[263] Therefore, treatment must be directed not only at the injured structure but at the patient's mental state as well.

LITIGATION AND INSURANCE

Many trauma patients are involved in litigation. The legal process is lengthy and adds more stress to an already painful and stressful condition. This situation can prolong and intensify the injurious effects and can result in a more difficult management problem.[264]

Patients in litigation often undergo insurance examinations, examination before trial, courtroom appearances, negotiations of possible settlement, and innuendos of malingering. The emotional state of the injured patient is sensitized. The psychologic stress becomes a perpetuating factor.[265]

In some cases, the end of litigation marks the end or reduction of chronic symptoms. This effect has been explained as malingering for secondary gain during the legal action.[45] Two other possibilities should be considered. First, in the absence of *chronic factitious illness,*[266] it is possible that the end of the legal proceedings substantially reduces emotional stress, thereby eliminating a perpetuating factor. Second, a reduction in symptoms often takes place in the chronic phase of osteoarthritis.[49] This phase could coincide with the 3- to 4-year duration of the average personal injury case.[267]

The opposite can happen—the pain and dysfunction continue or even worsen. This scenario has been observed in studies involving chronic back injury. One study revealed that litigants are not "cured by a verdict."[268] Two other studies failed to demonstrate exaggerated psychologic effects of litigation and failed to support the contention that patients involved in litigation develop an "accident" or "compensation neurosis."[269,270] In yet another study, patients were divided into three categories; "litigation pending," "litigation settled," and "no litigation." There was no significant difference in the prevalence of symptoms 6 to 26 months after the injury.[271]

The belief that litigants, claiming financial reward because of industrial or traffic accidents, improve and return to work a short time after finalization of their claims, irrespective of outcome, was largely supported by Miller[272] and others.[273-276] Several studies, however, not only failed to support their contention, but strongly suggested the opposite. Thompson[277] studied 500 patients with post-traumatic psychoneurosis and reported that "The effects of financial settlement on the course of the illness had negligible benefit." Balla and Moraitis[278] found that in 31 of 82 patients injuries worsened after litigation was concluded. Mendelson[279] reviewed 101 patients, all working at the time of their injury; 67% did not return to work for at least 16 months after finalization of legal proceedings. Macnab[280] studied 145 whiplash victims 2 years or more after the conclusion of litigation and reported that 121 still had symptoms.

The view that patients invariably become symptom-free and resume work within months of the end of litigation appears to be untrue.

Because TM disorders can occur from acute extrinsic trauma[55] and because there is a surge in public and professional awareness, personal injury claims abound.[56] The monetary awards have dramatically escalated. More controlled studies are needed regarding TMJ injuries, including the psychologic and physical effects on the individual during and after litigation. In an analysis of 900 traumatically induced TM disorder patients by Goldman,[281] there was little difference regarding treatment outcome between those in or not in litigation. In a survey of 171 patients, no significant difference was observed in residual signs and symptoms between these groups (Table 11–1).

Many TMJ trauma victims lose benefits because of the denial of payment by some insurance examiners. The basis of denial is the opinion that no causal relationship to the traumatic

event exists or that the TM disorder was pre-existing and unrelated to the accident. In order to substantiate a claim, communication must be established with the patient's dentist and physician to establish the preaccident status. A clear distinction between "predisposing" and "pre-existing" conditions must be made and understood by the insurance companies and their consultants. Clinical knowledge of the traumatized TMJ must be part of the emergency room physician's understanding when initially treating the accident victim. In this way, early diagnosis and treatment may be rendered. In the case of a developing TM disorder that surfaces clinically weeks or months later, appropriate care should be offered and appropriate insurance benefits distributed.

MALINGERING

Dorland's Illustrated Medical Dictionary defines malingering as "the willful, deliberate, and fraudulent feigning or exaggeration of symptoms of illness or injury, done for the purpose of a consciously desired end."[282] Malingering seems to be a form of *abnormal illness behavior* or "patients who behave in a manner inappropriate for the degree of somatic injury observed."[256] Bell[283] stated that malingering is commonplace in today's socioeconomic world and that this compensation pain serves the purpose of secondary gain—financial, behavioral, or both. This type of behavior presents serious problems in pain management and is difficult to detect because treatment failures also occur in the nonmalingering patient population. The tragedy lies with the patient who legitimately was injured but has an unsuccessful treatment outcome. The patient may be mislabeled a "a psychiatric case,"[256] a malingerer, or a "litigant

TABLE 11–1. Persistence of Symptoms in Patients Pending Litigation, After Litigation, and No Litigation

	TRAUMATICALLY INDUCED TMD* (NO. OF PATIENTS)	POST-TREATMENT: NO TMD SYMPTOMS (NO. OF PATIENTS)	POST-TREATMENT: REMAINING TMD SYMPTOMS (NO. OF PATIENTS)	REMAINING TMD SYMPTOMS 2 YRS. AFTER ACCIDENT (APPROXIMATE % OF PATIENTS)
Pending litigation	21	14	7	33%
After litigation	118	80	38	32%
No litigation	32	23	9	28%
Total	171	117	54	

*Temporomandibular disorders.

personality." This inappropriate attitude may damage the relationship between clinician and patient, possibly worsening the symptoms.

Patients with latent symptoms may often be labeled as malingerers. An example of this is the patient injured in a motor vehicle accident who had negative radiologic findings, no objective findings during the emergency room examination, and onset of TMJ pain that developed secondarily as a result of wearing a prescribed cervical collar[284] or traction device.[221] Some clinicians may mislabel these patients.

REFERENCES

1. Solberg, W.: Temporomandibular disorders: Background and the clinical problems. Br. Dent. J. 160:157–161, 1986.
2. Rowe, N.L. and Killey, H.C.: *Fractures of the Facial Skeleton,* 2nd ed. Livingstone, Edinburgh, 1968.
3. Sanders, B.: Presentation on TMJ Internal Derangement and Arthrosis. AAOMS Clinical Congress, Philadelphia, 1982.
4. Meyenburg, K., Kubik, S., and Palla, S.: Relationships of the muscles of mastication to the articular disc of the temporomandibular joint. Helv. Odont. Acta 30:1, 1986.
5. Carlsson, G.E., Kopp, S., and Öberg, T.: Arthritis and allied disease of the temporomandibular joint. In *Temporomandibular Joint Function and Dysfunction.* G.A. Zarb and G.E. Carlsson (eds.). C.V. Mosby Co., St. Louis, 1979.
6. Mayne, J.G. and Hatch, G.S.: Arthritis of the temporomandibular joint. J.A.D.A. 79:125–130, 1969.
7. Truelove, E., Burgess, J., Dworkin, S., et al; Abstract #1482, University of Washington, Seattle, 1989.
8. Morgan, D.H.: The great imposter, J.A.M.A. 35:22, 1976.
9. Solberg, W.K.: Temporomandibular disorders: Clinical significance of TMJ changes. Br. Dent. J. 160:233, 1986.
10. Mongini, F.: Remodeling of the mandibular condyle in the adult and its relationship to the condition of the dental arches. Acta Anat. 82:437, 1972.
11. Sokoloff, L.: The remodeling of articular cartilage. Rheumatology 7:11–18, 1982.
12. Okeson, J.P.: *Fundamentals of Occlusion and Temporomandibular Disorders.* C.V. Mosby, St. Louis, 1985.
13. Leopard, P.J.: Anterior dislocation of the temporomandibular disc. Br. J. Oral and Maxillofac. Surg. 22:9–17, 1984.
14. Dolwick, M.F. and Sanders, B.: Pathology. In *TMJ Internal Derangement and Arthrosis.* C.V. Mosby, St. Louis, 1985.
15. Katzberg, R.W., Keith, D., Guralnick, W., et al: Internal derangements and arthritis of the temporomandibular joint. Radiology 146:107–112, 1983.
16. Benson, F.: TMJ disorders. In *TMJ Disorders—Management of the Craniomandibular Complex.* S.L. Kraus (ed.). Churchill Livingstone, New York, 1988.
17. Bell, W.E.: *Orofacial Pains: Classification, Diagnosis, Management,* 3rd ed. Year Book Medical Publishers, Chicago, 1985.
18. Clark, G.: Diagnosis and treatment of painful TM disorders. Dent. Clin. North Am. 31:4, 1987.
19. Norman, J.E. de Burgh: Post-traumatic disorders of the jaw joint. Ann. R. Coll. Surg. 64:27–36, 1982.
20. Bollet, A.J.: An essay on the biology of osteoarthritis. Arthritis Rheum. 12:2, 1969.
21. Clement, R., Hanlon, M., Willis, E., Jr.: Osteoarthritis aggravated by trauma. Am. J. Surg. Nov.:556–569, 1949.
22. Pinals, R.S.: Traumatic arthritis and allied conditions. In *Arthritis and Allied Conditions—A Textbook of Rheumatology,* 10th ed. D.J. McCarty (ed.). Lea & Febiger, Philadelphia, 1985.
23. Pullinger, A.G., and Monteiro, A.A.: History factors associated with symptoms of temporomandibular disorders. J. Oral Rehab. 16:117–124, 1988.
24. Harris, S., Rood, J.P., and Testa, H.J.: Post-traumatic changes of the temporomandibular joint by bone scintigraphy. Int. J. Oral Maxillofac. Surg. 17:173–176, 1988.
25. Morgan, D., House, L., Hall, W., and Vamvas, S.: Surgery of the TMJ. In *Diseases of the Temporomandibular Apparatus.* D. Morgan, L. House, W. Hall, and S. Vamvas (eds.). C.V. Mosby, St. Louis, 1982.
26. Benson, F.: TMJ disorders. In *TMJ Disorders—Management of the Craniomandibular Complex.* S.L. Kraus (ed.). Churchill Livingstone, New York, 1988.
27. Freyberg, R.: The joints. In *Pathologic Physiology: Mechanisms of Disease.* W. Sodeman, and W. Sodeman, Jr. (eds.). W.B. Saunders Co., Philadelphia, 1967.
28. Nuelle, D.G., Alpern, M.C., and Ufema, J.W.: Arthroscopic surgery of the temporomandibular joint. Ang. Orthod. 56:118–142, 1986.
29. Brooke, R. and Stenn, P.G.: Post injury myofascial pain dysfunction sysndrome: Its etiology and prognosis. Oral Surg. 45:846–850, 1978.
30. Benson, F.: TMJ disorders. In *TMJ Disorders—Management of the Craniomandibular Complex.* S.L. Kraus (ed.). Churchill Livingstone, New York, 1988.
31. Irby, W.B. and Baldwin, H.K.: *Emergencies and Urgent Complications in Dentistry.* C.V. Mosby Co., St. Louis, 1965.
32. National Accident Sampling System: A report on traffic crashes and injuries in the United States. U.S. Department of Transportation, National Highway Traffic Safety Administration, 1986.
33. Laskin, D.M.: Etiology of the pain-dysfunction syndrome. J.A.D.A. 79:147–153, 1969.
34. Moffet, B.C.: Classification and diagnoses of temporomandibular joint disturbances. In *Temporomandibular Joint Problems.* W.K. Solberg and G.T. Clark (eds.). Quintessence Publishing Co., Lombard, IL, 1980.
35. McLaughlin, R.P.: Malocclusion and the temporomandibular joint—an historical perspective. Ang. Orthod. 58:186–190, 1988.
36. Hansson, L.: Current concepts about the TM joint. J. Prosth. Dent. 55:3, 1986.
37. Marciani, R.D. and Ziegler, R.C.: Temporomandibular joint surgery: A review of 51 operations. Oral Surg. 56:472, 1983.
38. Solberg, W.K.: Temporomandibular disorders: Functional and radiological considerations. Br. Dent. J. 160:195, 1986.

39. McNeill, C., et al: Craniomandibular (TMJ) disorders—The state of the art. J. Prosth. Dent. 44:434, 1980.

40. McNeill, C.: Craniomandibular (TMJ) disorders—The state of the art. Part II. Accepted diagnostic and treatment modalities. J. Prosth. Dent. 49:393–397, 1983.

41. Silver, C., Simon, S., and Savastano, A.: Meniscus injuries of the temporomandibular joint. J. Bone Joint Surg. 38A:3, 1956.

42. Stringert, H.G. and Worms, F.W.: Variations in skeletal and dental patterns in patients with structural and functional alterations of the temporomandibular joint: A preliminary report. Am. J. Orthod. 89:293, 1986.

43. Chrisiansen, E.L., Thompson, J.R., and Hasso, A.N.: CT evaluation of trauma to the TM joint. J. Oral Maxillofac. Surg. 45:920–923, 1987.

44. Hellsing, G., L'Estrange, P., and Holmlund, A.: Temporomandibular joint disorders: A diagnostic challenge. J. Prosthet. Dent. 56:600–604, 1986.

45. Rugh, J.D. and Solberg, W.K.: Psychological implications in temporomandibular joint function and dysfunction. In *Temporomandibular Joint Function and Dysfunction.* G. Zarb and G.E. Carlsson (eds.). Munksgaard, Copenhagen, 1979.

46. Gerschman, J.A. and Reade, P.C.: Disorders of the TM joint and related structures. Aust. Fam. Physician, 17:4, 1988.

47. Helkimo, M.: Epidemiological surveys of dysfunction of the masticatory system. In *Temporomandibular Joint Function and Dysfunction.* G.A. Zarb and G.E. Carlsson (eds.). Copenhagen, Munksgaard, 1979.

48. Clark, G.T., Solberg, W.K., and Monteiro, A.A.: TM disorders: New challenges in clinical management, research, and teaching. In *Perspectives in TM Disorders.* G.T. Clark and W.K. Solberg (eds.). Quintessence Publishing Co., Lombard, IL, 1987.

49. Rasmussen, O.C.: Description of population and progress of symptoms in a longitudinal study of temporomandibular arthropathy. Scand. J. Dent. Res. 89:196–203, 1981.

50. Silver, C.M. and Simon, S.D.,: Meniscus injuries of the temporomandibular joint: Further experiences. J. Bone Joint Surg. 45:1, 1958.

51. Hohmann, A., Wilson, K., and Nelms R.C.: Surgical treatment in temporomandibular trauma. Symposium on trauma to the head and neck. Otolaryngol. Clin. North Am. 16:549, 1983.

52. Kopp, S.: Pain and functional disturbances of the masticatory system—A review of etiology and principles of treatment. Swed. Dent. J. 6:49, 1982.

53. Meyer, R.A.: Clicking sounds owing to temporomandibular injury. J.A.D.A. 346:38, 1982.

54. Harkins, S.J. and Marteney, J.L.: Extrinsic trauma: A significant precipitating factor in temporomandibular dysfunction. J. Prosthet. Dent. 54:271–272, 1985.

55. Takada, K. Yoshimura, Y., Endoh, N., et al: Clinical study of the temporomandibular joint disturbances, statistical observation of patients with temporomandibular arthrosis. J. Osaka Univ. Dent. Sch. II:7–16, 1971.

56. Harkins, S.J.: Extrinsic trauma and TM dysfunction. J. Craniomand. Pract. 4:1, 1986.

57. Lader, E.: Cervical trauma as a factor in the development of TMJ dysfunction and facial pain. Craniomand. Pract. 1:86–90, 1983.

58. Rocabado, M.: Arthrokinematics of the temporomandibular joint. Dent. Clin. North Am. 27:581–584, 1983.

59. Dolwick, F.M.: Diagnosis and etiology. In C.A. Helms, R.W. Katzberg, and M.F. Dolwick (eds.). *Internal Derangements of the Temporomandibular Joint.* Radiology Research and Education Foundation, San Francisco, 1983.

60. Speck, J.E. and Zarb, G.A.: Temporomandibular pain-dysfunction: A suggested classification and treatment. J. Canad. Dent. Assoc. 6:305–310, 1976.

61. Moses, A.: Cervical whiplash and TMJ. Similarities in symptoms. Trial, 61–63, March, 1986.

62. Helkimo, E. and Westling, L.: History, clinical findings, and outcome of treatment of patients with anterior disk displacement. J. Craniomand. Pract. 5:3, 1987.

63. Reade, P.C.: An approach to the managment of TMJ pain dysfunction syndrome. J. Prosthet. Dent. 51:91–96, 1984.

64. Thomas, H.O.: *Diseases of the Hip, Knee, and Ankle Joints, with their Deformities, Treated by New and Effective Methods,* 3rd ed. H. K. Lewis, London, 1878.

65. Benson, F.: TMJ disorders. In *TMJ Disorders—Management of the Craniomandibular Complex.* S.L. Kraus (ed.). Churchill Livingston, New York, 1988.

66. Bourbon, B.: Anatomy and biomechanics of the TMJ. In *TMJ Disorders—Management of the Craniomandibular Complex.* S.L. Kraus (ed.). Churchill Livingstone, New York, 1988.

67. Bora, W. and Miller, G.: Joint physiology, cartilage metabolism, and the etiology of osteoarthritis. Hand Clin. 3:325–334, 1987.

68. Hohmann, A., Wilson, K., and Nelms, C.R., Jr.: Surgical treatment in temporomandibular joint trauma. Otolaryngol. Clin. North Am. 16:549–573, 1983.

69. Myrtaugh, H.: The incidence of ear symptoms in cases of malocclusion and temporomandibular joint dysfunction. Br. J. Oral Surg. 2:28–32, 1984.

70. Ricketts, R.M.: Clinical implication of the temporomandibular joint. Am. J. Orthod. 52:416–438, 1966.

71. Mayne, J. and Hatch, G.: Arthritis of the temporomandibular joint. J.A.D.A. 79:125,1969.

72. Freyberg, R.: The joints. In *Pathologic Physiology: Mechanisms of Disease.* W. Sodeman and W. Sodeman, Jr. (eds.). W.B. Saunders Co., Philadelphia, 1967.

73. Hanlon, C. and Estes, W.: Osteoarthritis aggravated by trauma. Am. J. Surg. 78:555, 1949.

74. Farrar, W.B. and McCarty, W., Jr.: *Clinical Outline of Temporomandibular Joint Diagnosis and Treatment, Funt-Stack Index,* 7th ed. Normandie Publications, Montgomery, Alabama, 1983.

75. Rugh, J.D. and Ohrback, R.: Occlusal parafunction. In *A Textbook of Occlusion.* N.D. Mohl, G.A. Zarb, G.E. Carlsson, and J.D. Rugh (eds.). Quintessence Publishing Co., Lombard, IL, 1988.

76. Juniper, R.P.: The superior pterygoid muscle? Br. J. Oral Surg. 19:121, 1981.

77. Radin, E.L., Paul, I.L., and Rose, R.M.: Role of mechanical factors in pathogenesis of primary osteoarthritis. Lancet i: 519, 1972.

78. Guralnick, W., Kaban, L.B., and Merrill, R.: TMJ afflictions. N. Engl. J. Med. 299:3, 1978.

79. Bell, W.: *Orofacial Pains: Classification, Diagnosis, Management,* 4th ed. Year Book Medical Publishers, Chicago, 1989.

80. Bell, W.: *Orofacial Pains: Classification, Diagnosis,*

Management, 4th ed. Year Book Medical Publishers, Chicago, 1989.

81. Izumi, Y.: The effects of immobilization on the healing process of experimental microtrauma of the articular disc on the temporomandibular joint of monkeys. J. Stomatolog. Soc. 50:378–417, 1983.

82. Borak, J.: Relationship between the clinical and roentgenological findings in bone metastases. Surg. Gynecol. Obstet. 75:599–604, 1942.

83. Carlsson, G.E., Kopp, S., and Oberg, I.: Arthritis and allied diseases of the temporomandibular joint. In *Temporomandibular Joint Function and Dysfunction.* G. Zarb and G.E. Carlsson (eds.). Munksgaard, Copenhagen, 1979.

84. Harris, S.A.: An investigation of scintigraphy as an aid to diagnosis of disorders of the temporomandibular joint. M.D.S. Thesis, University of Manchester, 1985.

85. Bradley, W.G., Jr. and Walluch, V.: Effect of methemoglobin formation on the MR appearance of subarachnoid hemorrhage. Radiology 156:99, 1985.

86. Ettinger, W.H., Jr.: Osteoarthritis. II. Pathology and pathogenesis. Md. State Med. J. 33:10, 1989.

87. Schwartz, R.D.: The role of articular cartilage: Arthroscopic findings of intracapsular pathology. Syllabus from Lecture. State of the Art—1989, A National Multi-Disciplinary Conference on TM Joint Diseases. Sponsored by the Department of Orthopedic Surgery, Hospital for Joint Diseases Orthopedic Institute, N.Y., p 18, 1989.

88. Schwartz, R.D.: The role of articular cartilage: Arthroscopic findings of intracapsular pathology. Syllabus from Lecture. State of the Art—1989, A National Multi-Disciplinary Conference on TM Joint Diseases. Sponsored by the Department of Orthopedic Surgery, Hospital for Joint Diseases Orthopedic Institute, N.Y., 1989.

89. Howell, D.S.: Etiopathogenesis of osteoarthritis. In *Arthritis and Allied Conditions—A Textbook of Rheumatology,* 10th ed. D.J. McCarty (ed.). Lea & Febiger, Philadelphia, 1985.

90. Johnson, R.P. and Brewer, B.J.: Mechanical disorders of the knee. In *Arthritis and Allied Conditions—A Textbook of Rheumatology,* 10th ed. D.J. McCarty (ed.). Lea & Febiger, Philadelphia, 1985.

91. Stedman's Medical Dictionary, 21st ed.: Williams & Wilkins, Baltimore, 1966.

92. Dorwart, B.B., Hansell, J.R., and Schumacher, H.R.: Effects of cold and heat on urate crystal–induced synovitis in the dog. Arthritis Rheum. 17:563–571, 1974.

93. Sokoloff, L. and Hough, A.J.: Pathology of osteoarthritis. In *Arthritis and Allied Conditions—A Textbook of Rheumatology,* 10th ed. D.J. McCarty (ed.). Lea & Febiger, Philadelphia, 1985.

94. Schwartz, R.D.: The role of articular cartilage: Arthroscopic findings of intracapsular pathology. Syllabus from Lecture. State of the Art—1989, A National Multi-Disciplinary Conference on TM Joint Diseases. Sponsored by the Department of Orthopedic Surgery, Hospital for Joint Diseases Orthopedic Institute, N.Y., p 22, 1989.

95. Bell, W.E.: *TM Disorders: Classification, Diagnosis, Management,* 2nd ed. Year Book Medical Publishers, Chicago, 1986.

96. Bell, W.E.: *Orofacial Pains: Classification, Diagnosis, Management,* 4th ed. Year Book Medical Publishers, Chicago, p 302, 1989.

97. Bell, W.E.: *Orofacial Pains: Classification, Diagnosis, Management,* 4th ed. Year Book Medical Publishers, Chicago, p 299, 1989.

98. Bell, W.E.: *TM Disorders: Classification, Diagnosis, Management,* 2nd ed. Year Book Medical Publishers, Chicago, pp 198–201, 1986.

99. Kraus, S.L.: Physical therapy management of temporomandibular joint dysfunction. In S.L. Kraus (ed.). *TMJ Disorders—Management of the Craniomandibular Complex.* Churchill Livingstone, New York, 1988.

100. Bell, W.E.: *TM Disorders: Classification, Diagnosis, Management,* 2nd ed. Year Book Medical Publishers, Chicago, p 205, 1986.

101. Freedman, M.H. and Weisberg, J.: *Application of Orthopedic Principles in Evaluation of the TM Joint.* Physical Ther. 62:597–603, 1982.

102. Chase, D.C., Handler, B.H., and Kraus, S.L.: Spelling relief for TMJ troubles. Patient Care 22:158, 1988.

103. Mahan, P.E.: The TMJ in function and pathofunction. In W.K. Solberg and G.T. Clark (eds.). *TMJ Problems, Biologic Diagnosis and Treatment.* Quintessence Publishing Co., Lombard, IL, 1980.

104. Razook, S.J.: Nonsurgical management of TMJ and masticatory muscle problems. In *TMJ Disorders—Management of the Craniomandibular Complex.* S.L. Kraus (ed.). Churchill Livingstone, New York, 1988.

105. Friedman, M.H. and Weisberg, J.: *Temporomandibular Joint Disorders, Diagnosis and Treatment.* Quintessence Publishing Co., Lombard, IL, 1985.

106. Gershuni, D.H. and Kuei, S.C.: Cartilage deformation following experimental synovitis in the rabbit hip. J. Orthop. Res. 1:3, 1984.

107. Atkinson, T.J., Wolf, S., Anavi, Y., and Wesley, R.: Synovial hemangioma of the temporomandibular joint: Report of a case and review of the literature. J. Oral Maxillofac. Surg. 46:804–808, 1988.

108. Enzinger, F.M. and Weiss, S.W.: *Soft Tissue Tumors.* C.V. Mosby Co., St. Louis, 1983.

109. Thomas, C.F. and Evarts, C.M.: Cavernous hemangioma of the synovial membrane of the knee joint. Report of three cases. Cleve. Clin. Q. 32:223, 1965.

110. Moon, N.F.: Synovial hemangioma of the knee joint. A review of previously reported cases and inclusion of two new cases. Clin. Orthop. Rel. 90:183, 1973.

111. Schwartz, R.D.: The role of articular cartilage: Arthroscopic findings of intracapsular pathology. Syllabus from Lecture. State of the Art—1989, A National Multi-Disciplinary Conference on TM Joint Diseases. Sponsored by the Department of Orthopedic Surgery, Hospital for Joint Diseases Orthopedic Institute, N.Y., p 23, 1989.

112. Kaminishi, R.M.: Intracapsular fibrosis of the TMJ. Syllabus from Lecture. State of the Art—1989, A National Multi-Displinary Conference on TM Joint Diseases. Sponsored by the Department of Orthopedic Surgery, Hospital for Joint Diseases Orthopedic Institute, N.Y., p 85, 1989.

113. Mahan, P.E.: The Temporomandibular joint in function and pathofunction. In W.K. Solberg and G.T. Clark (eds.). *TMJ Problems, Biologic Diagnosis and Treatment.* Quintessence Publishing Co., Lombard, IL, 1980.

114. Bell, W.E.: *Orofacial Pains: Classification, Diagnosis, Management,* 3rd ed. Year Book Medical Publishers, Chicago, pp 186–196, 1985.

115. Benson, F.: TMJ disorders. In *TMJ Disorders—Management of the Craniomandibular Complex.* S.L.

Kraus (ed.). Churchill Livingstone, New York, p 65, 1988.

116. Bell, W.E.: *Orofacial Pains: Classification, Diagnosis, Management,* 3rd ed. Year Book Medical Publishers, Chicago, pp 189, 1985.

117. Friedman, M.H. and Weisberg, J.: *Temporomandibular Joint Disorders, Diagnosis and Treatment.* Quintessence Publishing Co., Lombard, IL, pp 88–92, 1985.

118. Bell, W.E.: *Orofacial Pains: Classification, Diagnosis, Management,* 4th ed. Year Book Medical Publishers, Chicago, 1989.

119. Simkin, P.A.: Synovial physiology. In D.J. McCarty (ed.). *Arthritis and Allied Conditions—A Textbook of Rheumatology,* 10th ed. Lea & Febiger, Philadelphia, 1985.

120. Bell, W.E.: *Orofacial Pains: Classification, Diagnosis, Management,* 3rd ed. Year Book Medical Publishers, Chicago, p 197, 1989.

121. Widmer, C.G.: Evaluation of temporomandibular disorders. In *TMJ Disorders—Management of the Craniomandibular Complex.* S.L. Kraus (ed.). Churchill Livingstone, New York, 1988.

122. Friedman, M.H: Letter to the editor. In Reader's Round Table. J. Prosthet. Dent. 54:5, 1985.

123. Bell, W.E.: *TM Disorders: Classification, Diagnosis, Management,* 2nd ed. Year Book Medical Publishers, Chicago, p 199–200, 1986.

124. White, R.E., Wise, C.M., and Agudelo, C.A.: Post-traumatic chylous joint effusion. Arthritis Rheum. 28:11, 1985.

125. Schumacher, H.R.: Traumatic joint effusion and the synovium. J. Sport Med. 3:3, 1975.

126. Schellhas, K.: Personal communication. Center for Diagnostic Imaging, St. Louis Park, MN, 1988.

127. Weinberger, A. and Schumacher, R.H.: Experimental joint trauma. Synovial response to blunt trauma and inflammatory reaction to intra-articular injection of fat. J. Rheumatol. 8:3, 1981.

128. Pinals, R.S.: Traumatic arthritis and allied conditions. In: *Arthritis and Allied Conditions—A Textbook of Rheumatology,* 10th ed. D.J. McCarty (ed.). Lea & Febiger, Philadelphia, 1985.

129. Gregg, J.R., Nixon, J.E., and De Stefano, V.: Neutral fat in traumatized knees. Clin. Orthop. 132:219–224, 1978.

130. Schmid, K. and MacNair, M.B.: Characterization of the proteins of human synovial fluid in certain disease states, J. Clin. Invest. 35:814, 1956.

131. Kraus, S.L.: Physical therapy management of TMJ dysfunction. In *TMJ Disorders—Management of the Craniomandibular Complex.* S.L. Kraus (ed.). Churchill Livingstone, New York, 1988.

132. Ernest, E.A., III, Kayne, B.S., Montgomery, E.W., et al: Three disorders that frequently cause temporomandibular joint (TMJ) pain: Internal derangement—temporal tendinitis—the Ernest syndrome. J. Neurol. Orthop. Med. Surg. 7:2, 1986.

133. Ernest, E.A.: The Orthopedic influence of the TMJ apparatus in whiplash: Report of a case. Gen. Dent. Mar.-Apr., pp 62–64, 1979.

134. Travell, J.G. and Simons, D.G.: *Myofascial Pain and Dysfunction—The Trigger Point Manual.* Williams & Wilkins, Baltimore, p 64, 310, 1983.

135. Brooke, R., Stenn, P., and Mothersill, K.: The diagnosis and conservative treatment of myofascial pain dysfunction syndrome. Oral Surg. 44:844, 1977.

136. Lim, R.Y.: Carotodynia exposed: Hyoid bone syndrome. South. Med. J. 80:4, 1987.

137. Sicher, H.: Structural and functional basis for disorders of the temporomandibular joint articulation. J. Oral Surg. 13:275, 1955.

138. Brown, I.N.: Hyoid bone syndrome. South. Med. J. 47:1088, 1954.

139. Kopstein, E.: Hyoid syndrome. Arch. Otolaryngol. 101:484–485, 1975.

140. Eagle, W.W.: Elongated styloid process. Arch Otolaryngol. 25:584–587, 1937.

141. Cornell, R.W., Jensen, J.L., Taylor, J.B., and Thyne, R.R.: Mineralization of the stylohyoid-stylomandibular ligament complex. Oral Surg. 48:286–291, 1979.

142. Shankland, W.E., II: Ernest syndrome as a consequence of stylomandibular ligament injury: A report of 68 patients, J. Prosthet. Dent. 57:501–505, 1987.

143. Burch, J.G.: Activity of the accessory ligaments of the temporomandibular joint. J. Prosthet. Dent. 24:621–628, 1970.

144. Spalteholz-Spanner, A.: Handatlas der Anatomie des Menschen, teil I. Scheltema en Holkema NV, Amsterdam-Haarlem, pp 338–339, 1971.

145. Shenoi P.M.: Styloid syndrome. J. Laryngol. Otol. 86:203–211, 1972.

146. Steinmann, E.P.: Styloid syndrome in a case of an elongated process, Acta Otolaryngol. 66:347–356, 1972.

147. Smalloff, R. and Price, D.B.: Distention of the stylomandibular ligament as a cause of styloid pain syndrome. Ear Nose Throat J. 63:23, 1984.

148. Trimble, D.L., Shoenaers, J.A., II, and Stcolinga, P.J.W.: Acute suppurative arthritis of the temporomandibular joint in a patient with rheumatoid arthritis. J. Maxillofac. Surg. 2:92, 1983.

149. Schmid, F.R.: Infectious arthritis. In *Arthritis and Allied Conditions—A Textbook of Rheumatology* 10th ed. D.J. McCarty (ed.). Lea & Febiger, Philadelphia, 1985.

150. Bounds, G.A., Hopkins, R., and Sugar, A.: Septic arthritis of the temporomandibular joint: A problematic diagnosis. Br. J. Oral Maxillofac. Surg. 25:61–67, 1987.

151. Newman, J.H.: Review of septic arthritis throughout the antibiotic era. Ann. Rheum. Dis. 35:198, 1976.

152. Russell, A.S. and Ansell, B.: Septic arthritis. Ann. Rheum. Dis. 31:40, 1972.

153. Mitchell, W.S., Brooks, P.M., Stevenson, R.D., and Buchanan, W.T.: Septic arthritis in patients with rheumatoid disease: A still underdiagnosed complication. J. Rheumatol. 3:124, 1976.

154. Lund, S.: Dizziness and vertigo in the post-traumatic syndrome: A physiological background. Acta Neurochir. Suppl. 36:118–120, 1986.

155. Morgan, D., House, L., Hall, W., and Vamvas, S.: *Diseases of the Temporomandibular Apparatus,* 2nd ed. C.V. Mosby Co., St. Louis, p 214, 1982.

156. Weeks, V.D. and Travell, J.: Postural vertigo due to trigger areas in the sternocleidomastoid muscle. J. Pediatr. 47:315–327, 1955.

157. Libin, B.M.: Otologic and jaw symptoms of TMJ—MPDS. Ear, Nose, Throat J. 61:1, 1982.

158. Myrhaug, H.: The incidence of ear symptoms in cases of malocclusion and temporomandibular joint disturbances. Br. J. Oral Surg. 2:28–32, 1964.

159. Arlen, H.: The otomandibular syndrome, a new concept. Ear, Nose, Throat J. 57:553–556, 1978.

160. Malkin, D.: The Rolf of TMJ dysfunction. Int. J. Orthod. 25:20–21, 1987.

161. Watanabe, I., Kumagami, H., and Tsuda, Y.: Tinnitus due to abnormal contraction of stapedial muscle. An abnormal phenomenon in the course of facial

nerve paralysis and to audiological significance. Oto-rhinolaryngology 36:217–226, 1974.

162. Gibbs, C.H. and Suit, S.R.: Movements of the jaw after unexpected contact with a hard object. J. Dent. Res. 52:810, 1973.

163. Bell, W.E.: *Temporomandibular Disorders: Classification, Diagnosis, Management,* 2nd ed. Year Book Medical Publishers, Chicago, p 70, 1986.

164. Eversole, M.: Temporomandibular joint derangements and disorders. J.A.D.A. 110:69–79, 1985.

165. Benson, F.: Temporomandibular disorders. In *TMJ Disorders—Management of the Craniomandibular Complex.* S.L. Kraus (ed.). Churchill Livingstone, New York, p 71, 1988.

166. Morgan, D., House, L., Hall, W., and Vamvas, S.: *Diseases of the Temporomandibular Apparatus,* 2nd ed. C.V. Mosby Co., St. Louis, p 76, 1982.

167. Meyer, R.A.: Clicking sounds owing to temporomandibular joint injury. J.A.M.A. 248:1, 1982.

168. Speck, J., Ellis, D., and Awde, J.D.: The bite in the temporomandibular joint pain dysfunction syndrome. J. Otolaryngol. 8:3, 1979.

169. Hammersley, N.: Chronic bilateral dislocation of the temporomandibular joint. Br. J. Oral Maxillofac. Surg. 24:367–375, 1986.

170. Schultz, L.: Report of 10-years experience in treating hypermobility of the temporomandibular joints. J. Oral Surg. 5:202–207, 1947.

171. Helman. J., Laufer, D., Minkov, B., and Gutman, D.: Eminectomy as surgical treatment for chronic mandibular dislocation. So. Int. J. Oral. Surg. 13:486–489, 1984.

172. Beckett, H.: Unusual dislocations associated with epileptic fits. Br. Med. J. 288:938, 1984.

173. Weinberg, S. and La Pointe, H.: Cervical extension-flexion injury (whiplash) and internal derangement of the temporomandibular joint. J. Oral Maxilliofac. Surg. 45:653–656, 1987.

174. Wakeley, C.: The Mandibular Joint. Ann. R. Coll. Surg. 2:111, 1948.

175. Gay, J.R. and Abbott, K.H.: Common whiplash injuries of the neck. J.A.M.A. 152:698–704, 1953.

176. Rocabado, M.: *Selected Papers.* Rocabado Institute, Tacoma, Washington, 1981.

177. Dunn, J.: Cervical strain and mandibular whiplash pathomechanics and treatment. Syllabus from Lecture. State of the Art—1989, A National Multi-Disciplinary Conference on TM Joint Diseases. Sponsored by the Department of Orthopedic Surgery, Hospital for Joint Diseases Orthopedic Institute, N.Y., 1989.

178. Bell, W.E.: *Temporomandibular Disorders: Classification, Diagnosis, Management,* 2nd ed. Year Book Medical Publishers, Chicago, p 44, 1986.

179. Eppinger, R.: Personal communication. Department of Crash Worthiness of the National Traffic Safety Administration, May, 1989.

180. Roydhouse, R.H.: Whiplash and temporomandibular joint dysfunction. Lancet 1:394, 1973.

181. Mahan, P.E.: The physiology of occlusion. In *Clinical Dentistry.* J.W. Clark (ed.). Harper & Row, New York, 1976.

182. Robinson, M.J.: The influence of head position on temporomandibular dysfunction. J. Prosthet. Dent. 16:169–172, 1966.

183. Mannheimer, J., Attanasio, R., Cinotti, W.R., and Pertes, R.: Cervical strain and mandibular whiplash: Effects upon the craniomandibular apparatus. Clin. Prev. Dent. 11:1, 1989.

184. Clark, G.T.: Examining temporomandibular disorder patients for craniocervical dysfunction. J. Craniomand. Pract. 2:1, 1984.

185. Friedman, M.H. and Weisberg, J.: The temporomandibular joint. In *Textbook of Physical Therapy: Orthopedic and Sports.* J.A. Gould, et al (eds.). C.V. Mosby Co., St. Louis, 1985.

186. Ommaya, A.K., Backaitis, S., Fan, W., et al: *Automotive Neck Injuries.* National Highway Traffic Safety Administration, 9th International Technical Conference on Experimental Safety Vehicles, 1982.

187. Partyka, S.: *Whiplash and Other Inertial force Neck Injuries in Traffic Accidents.* Mathematical Analysis Division, National Center for Statistics and Analysis, Dec., 1981.

188. National Accident Sampling System: *A Report on Traffic Crashes and Injuries in the United States.* United States Department of Transportation, National Highway Traffic Safety Administration, 1982.

189. Huelke, D.F., O' Day, J., Lawson, T.E., et al: Cervical injuries in automotive crashes. Report no. UM-HSRI-80-40. University of Michigan, Ann Arbor, 1980.

190. Culver, R., Bender, M., and Melvin, J.W.: Mechanisms, tolerances and responses obtained in neck injury by superior-inferior head impact. Report no. UM-HSRI-78-21. University of Michigan, Ann Arbor, 1978.

191. Benham, C.: Unpublished research. Department of Biomathematics and Biophysics, The Mt. Sinai Hospital, New York City, 1989.

192. Hale, R.H.: Treatment of recurrent dislocation of the mandible: Review of literature and report of cases. J. Oral Surg. 30:527–530, 1972.

193. Henry, F.A.: The temporomandibular joint. *Textbook of Oral and Maxillofacial Surgery.* G.O. Kruger (ed.). C.V. Mosby Co., St. Louis, 1979.

194. Patel, A.: Jaw dislocation during anaesthesia. Anaesthesia 34:376, 1979.

195. Bellman, M.H. and Babu, K.V.R.: Jaw dislocation during anaesthesia. Anaesthesia 33:844, 1978.

196. Kim, S. and Kim, K.: Subluxation of the temporomandibular joint: Unusual complications of transoral bronchofiberoscopy. Chest 83:288–289, 1983.

197. Lipp, M., Daubländer, M., Ellmauer, S.T., et al: Changes in temporomandibular joint function following different general anesthesia techniques. Anaesthesist 37:366–373, 1988.

198. Gambling, D.R. and Ross, P.: Temporomandibular Joint Subluxation on Induction of Anesthesia. Anesth. Analg. 67:91–92, 1988.

199. Sosis, M. and Lazar S.: Jaw dislocation during general anesthesia. Canad. J. Anaesth. 34:407–408, 1987.

200. Patane, P., Ragno, J., and Mahla, M.: Temporomandibular joint disease and difficult tracheal intubation. Anesth. Analg. 67:482–490, 1988.

201. Salem, M.R., Mathrubhutham, M., and Bennett, E.J.: Difficult intubation. N. Engl. J. Med. 295:879–881, 1976.

202. Redick, L.F.: The temporomandibular joint and tracheal intubation. Anesth. Analg. 66:675–667, 1987.

203. Clayman, G.L. and Goldberg, J.S.: The incidence of forceps delivery among patients with TMJ problems. J. Craniomand. Pract. 2:1, 1984.

204. Garry, J.F.: Early iatrogenic orofacial muscle, skeletal, and temporomandibular joint dysfunction. In *Diseases of the Temporomandibular Apparatus—A Multidisciplinary Approach,* 2nd ed. D.H. Morgan, L.

House, W. Hall, and S. Vamvas (eds.). C.V. Mosby Co., St. Louis, p 65, 1982.

205. Grosfeld, O., Kretowicz, J., and Brokowski, J.: The temporomandibular joint in children after breech delivery. J. Oral Rehabil. 7:65–72, 1980.

206. Shira, R.B. and Alling, C.C.: Traumatic injuries involving the temporomandibular joint articulation. In L. Schwartz and C.M. Chayes (eds.). *Facial Pain and Mandibular Dysfunction.* W.B. Saunders Co., Philadelphia, 1968.

207. Bell, W.E.: *Temporomandibular Disorders: Classification, Diagnosis, Management,* 2nd ed. Year Book Medical Publishers, Chicago, p 159, 1986.

208. Kaufman, R. (New York State Boxing Commission Consultant): Personal Communication. 1988.

209. Kraus, S.: Cervical spine influences on the craniomandibular region. In *TMJ Disorders: Management of the Craniomandibular Complex.* S. Kraus (ed.). Churchill Livingstone, New York, 1988.

210. Proffit, W.R., Vig, K.W.L., and Turvey, T.A.: Early fracture of the mandibular condyles: Frequently an unsuspected cause of growth disturbances. Am. J. Orthod. 78:1, 1980.

211. Waite, D.E.: Pediatric fracture of jaw and facial bones. Pediatrics 51:551 559, 1973.

212. Rowe, N.L.: Fracture of jaws of children. J. Oral Surg. 27:497, 1969.

213. Gilhuus-Moe, O.: *Fractures of the Mandibular Condyle in the Growth Period.* Scandinavian University Books, Univeristatsforlaget, Stockholm, 1969.

214. Lund, K.: Mandibular growth and remodelling processes after mandibular fractures. Acta Odontol. Scand. 32:64, 1974.

215. Berger, S. and Stewart, R.F.: Mandibular hypoplasia secondary to perinatal trauma: Report of case. J. Oral Surg. 35:578, 1977,

216. Shore, R.M., et al: Sacrococcygeal trauma. Clin. Nucl. Med. 6:124–125, 1981.

217. Bucknill, T.M.: Disorders of the sacrum and coccyx. Practitioner 222:77–81, 1979.

218. Bell, W.E.: *Orofacial Pains: Classification, Diagnosis, Management,* 3rd ed. Year Book Medical Publishers, Chicago, p 148, 1985.

219. Gelb, H.: *Clinical Management of Head, Neck and Temporomandibular Joint Pain and Dysfunction—A Multi-Disciplinary Approach to Diagnosis and Treatment.* W.B. Saunders Co., Philadelphia, p. 244, 1977.

220. Bell, W.E.: *Temporomandibular Disorders: Classification, Diagnosis, Management,* 2nd ed. Year Book Medical Publishers, Chicago, pp 141–144, 1986.

221. Morgan, D.H., House, L., Hall, W., and Vamvas, S.: *Diseases of the Temporomandibular Joint Apparatus—A Multi-Disciplinary Approach,* 2nd ed. C.V. Mosby Co., St. Louis, p 213, 1982.

222. Frankel, V.H., Shore, N.A., and Hoppenfeld, S.: Stress distribution in cervical traction: Prevention of TMJ pain syndrome. Clin. Orthop. 32:114–116, 1964.

223. Mohl, N.D., Zarb, G.A., Carlsson, G.E., and Rugh, J.D. (eds.): *A Textbook of Occlusion,* Quintessence Publishing Co., Lombard, IL, pp 263–267, 1988.

224. Morgan, D.H., House, L., Hall, W., Vamvas, S.: *Diseases of the Temporomandibular Apparatus,* 2nd ed. C.V. Mosby Co., St. Louis, p 65, 1982.

225. Bell, W.E.: *Temporomandibular Disorders: Classification, Diagnosis, Management,* 2nd ed. Year Book Medical Publishers, Chicago, p 160, 1986.

226. Moffett, B.: Histologic aspects of temporomandibular joint derangements. In *Diagnosis of Internal De-*

rangement of the Temporomandibular Joint. B.C. Moffett (ed.). University of Washington, Seattle, pp 17–19, 1984.

227. Radin, E. and Paul, I.: Response of joints to impact loading. Arthritis Rheum. 14:3, 1971.

228. Frankel, V.H. and Nordin, M.: *Basic Biomechanics of the Skeletal System.* Lea & Febiger, Philadelphia, 1980.

229. Bell, W.E.: *Temporomandibular Disorders: Classification, Diagnosis, Management,* 2nd ed. Year Book Medical Publishers, Chicago, p 161, 1986.

230. Bell, W.E.: *Temporomandibular Disorders: Classification, Diagnosis, Management,* 2nd ed. Year Book Medical Publishers, Chicago, p 162, 1986.

231. Zimmerman, N.B., Smith, D.G., Pottenger, L.A., and Cooperman, D.R.: Mechanical disruption of human patella cartilage by repetitive loading in vitro. Clin. Orthop. 229:302–307, 1988.

232. Radin, E.L., Parker, H.G., Pugh, J.W., et al: Response of joints to impact loading. III. Relationship between trabecular microfractures and cartilage degeneration. J. Biomechanics 6:51–57, 1973.

233. Bollet, A.J.: Current comment: An essay on the biology of osteoarthritis. Arthritis Rheum. 12:152–163, 1969.

234. Johnson, G.R., Dowson, D., and Wright, V.: The fracture of articular cartilage under impact loading. Third Leeds-Lyons Symposium on Tribiology, p 113, 1976.

235. Weightman, B.O., Freeman, M.A.R., and Swanson, S.A.V.: Fatigue of articular cartilage. Nature 24:303, 1973.

236. Fengler, H. and Franz, R.: Morphological studies of the articular surface after intermittent impulsive loading in animal experimentation. Acta Univ. Carol. Med. 5:273 279, 1986.

237. Hansson, T.: Temporomandibular joint changes related to dental occlusion. In *Temporomandibular Joint Problems.* W. Solberg and G. Clark (eds.). Quintessence Publishing Co., Lombard, IL, 1980.

238. Kraus, S.L.: Physical therapy management of temporomandibular joint dysfunction. In S.L. Kraus (ed.). *TMJ Disorders—Management of the Craniomandibular Complex.* Churchill Livingstone, New York, p 147, 1988.

239. Lasking, D.M.: Role of the meniscus in the etiology of post-traumatic temporomandibular joint ankylosis. J. Oral Surg. 7:340–345, 1978.

240. Jaffe, F.F., Mankin, J., II, Weiss, C., et al: Water binding in the articular cartilage of rabbits. J. Bone Joint Surg. 56A:1031–1039, 1974.

241. Kuo, Y.S. and Kok, S.H.: Temporomandibular joint changes following mandibular fracture treated by mini plate osteosynthesis in the *Macaca cyclopsis* monkeys, J. Formosan Med. Assoc. 87:358–364, 1988.

242. Palmoski, M.J., Colyer, R.A., and Brandt, K.D.: Joint motion in the absence of normal loading does not maintain normal articular cartilage. Am. J. Rheum. 23:3, 1980.

243. Kraus, S.L.: Physical therapy management of TMJ dysfunction. In *TMJ Disorders—Management of the Craniomandibular Complex.* S.L. Kraus, (ed.). Churchill Livingstone, New York, p 146, 1988.

244. Travell, J.G. and Simons, D.G.: *Myofascial Pain and Dysfunction—The Trigger Point Manual.* Williams & Wilkins, Baltimore, p 644, 1983.

245. Mohl, D.N.: The role of head posture in mandibular function. In *Abnormal Jaw Mechanics: Diagnosis*

and Treatment. W.K. Solberg and G. Clark (eds.). Quintessence Publishing Co., Lombard, IL, 1984.

246. Travell, J.G. and Simons, D.G.: *Myofascial Pain and Dysfunction—The Trigger Point Manual.* Williams & Wilkins, Baltimore, p 264, 1983.

247. Shira, R.B. and Alling, C.C.: Traumatic injuries involving the temporomandibular joint articulation. In *Facial Pain and Mandibular Dysfunction.* L. Schwartz and C.M. Chayes (eds.). W.B. Saunders Co., Philadelphia, p 133, 1968.

248. Mongini, F.: The stomatognathic system: Function, dysfunction and rehabilatation. Quintessence Publishing Co., Lombard, IL, p 150, 1984.

249. Gross, B.D. and Lipke, D.P.: A technique for percutaneous lateral pterygoid electromyography. Electromyogr. Clin. Neurophys. 19:47–55, 1979.

250. Juniper, R.P.: Temporomandibular joint dysfunction: A theory based upon electromyographic studies of the lateral ptyerygoid muscle. Br. J. Oral Maxillofac. Surg. 22:1–8, 1984.

251. Gibbs, C.H., Mahan, P.E., Wilkinsson, T.M., and Mauderli, A.: EMG activity of the superior belly of the lateral pterygoid muscle in relation to other jaw muscles. J. Prosthet. Dent. 51:691–702, 1984.

252. Nilner, M. and Kopp, S.: Distribution by age and sex of functional disturbances and diseases of the stomatognathic system. Swed. Dent. J. 7(5):191–198, 1983.

253. Friedman, M.H. and Weisberg, J.: *Temporomandibular Joint Disorders Diagnosis and Treatment.* Quintessence Publishing Co., Lombard, IL, p 82, 1985.

254. Leonard, M.S. and Anderson, Q.N.: Temporomandibular arthrography as an aid in diagnosis of trauma to the temporomandibular joint in the absence of fracture. In *Maxillofacial Trauma, An International Perspective.* J.R. Jacobs (ed.): Praeger, New York, 1983.

255. Sarno, J.: *Mind Over Back Pain.* Berkley Publishing Group, New York, p 15, 1982.

256. Speculand, B. and Goss, A.N.: Psychological factors in temporomandibular joint dysfunction pain. Int. J. Oral Surg. 14:131–137, 1985.

257. Tanaka, T.T.: Facial pain disorders commonly confused with TMJ dysfunction. CDA Journal, March, 1985.

258. Tanaka, T.T.: A rational approach to the differential diagnosis of arthritic disorders. J. Prosthet. Dent. 56:6, 1986.

259. Solberg, W.K.: Current concepts on the development of TMJ dysfunction. In *Developmental Aspects of Temporomandibular Disorders.* D. Carlson, J.A. McNamara Jr., and K.A. Ribbens (eds.). University of Michigan, Ann Arbor, pp 37–47, 1985.

260. Travell, J.G. and Simons, D.G.: *Myofascial Pain and Dysfunction—The Trigger Point Manual.* Williams & Wilkins, Baltimore, p 169, 1983.

261. Rugh, J.D. and Solberg, W.K.: Psychological implications in temporomandibular pain and dysfunction. In *Temporomandibular Function and Dysfunction.* G. A. Zarb and G. E. Carlsson (eds.). C. V. Mosby Co., St. Louis, p 250, 1979.

262. Rugh, J.D. and Solberg, W.K.: Psychological implications in temporomandibular pain and dysfunction.

In *Temporomandibular Function and Dysfunction.* G.A. Zarb and G.E. Carlsson (eds.). C.V. Mosby Co., St. Louis, p 258, 1979.

263. Rugh, J.D. and Solberg, W.K.: Psychological implications in temporomandibular pain and dysfunction. In *Temporomandibular Function and Dysfunction.* G.A. Zarb and G.E. Carlsson (eds.). C.V. Mosby Co., St. Louis, p 259, 1979.

264. Lapeer, G.L.: Chronic temporomandibular joint pain and litigation. Gen. Dent. July/August, pp 275–276, 1986.

265. Foreman, D.M. and Rolfs, D.A.: *Whiplash and the Jaw Joint.* Book Publishing Co., 1985.

266. Myall, R.W.T., Collins, F.J.V., Ross, A., and Hupp, J.L.: Chronic factitious illness: Recognition and management of deception. J. Oral Maxillofac. Surg. 42:97–100, 1984.

267. Sanders, S.: Personal communication. New York Trial Lawyers Association, New York, 1990.

268. Mendelson, G.: Not "cured by a verdict"—Effect of legal settlement on compensation claimants. Med. J. Austral. 2:132–134, 1982.

269. Bochner, A.K.: Psychiatric aspects of back injuries. In *The Back: A Law-Medicine Problem.* O. Schroeder (ed.). Anderson, Cincinnati, pp 220–234, 1965.

270. Mendelson, G.: Compensation, pain complaints, and psychological disturbance. Pain 20:169–177, 1984.

271. Schutt, C.H. and Dohan, F.C.: Neck injury to women in auto accidents: A metropolitan plague. J.A.J.A. 206:689–692, 1968.

272. Miller, H.: Accident neurosis. Proc. Med. Leg. Soc. Vic. 10:71–82, 1966.

273. *Alexander v. South Australian Gas Co.* (S.A. Supreme Court): Aust. Leg. Month. Dig. July, 2982, 1980.

274. Reed, J.L.: Compensation neurosis and Munchausen syndrome. Br. J. Hosp. Med. 19:314–321, 1978.

275. Lawton, F.: A judicial view of traumatic neurosis. Med. Leg. J. 47:6–11, 1979.

276. *Marinkovich v. Munnoch* (N.S.W. Supreme Court): Aust. Leg. Month. Dig. July, 2419, 1980.

277. Thompson, G.N.: Post-traumatic psychoneurosis: A statistical survey. Am. Psychiatry 121:1043–1048, 1965.

278. Balla, J. and Moraitis, S.: Knights in armour: A follow-up study of injuries after legal settlement. Med. J. Aust. 2:355–361, 1970.

279. Mendelson, G.: Persistent work disability following settlement of compensation claims. Law Inst. J. (Melb.) 55:342–345, 1981.

280. Macnab, I.: The whiplash syndrome. Clin. Neurosurg. 20:232–241, 1973.

281. Goldman, J.R.: Residual symptoms of litigants. Unpublished data, 1988.

282. *Dorland's Illustrated Medical Dictionary,* 27th ed. W.B. Saunders Co., Philadelphia, 1988.

283. Bell, W.E.: *Orofacial Pains: Classification, Diagnosis, Management,* 3rd ed. Year Book Medical Publishers, Chicago, p 315, 1985.

284. Morgan, D., House, L. Hall, W., and Vamvas, S.: *Diseases of the Temporomandibular Apparatus,* 3rd ed. C.V. Mosby Co., St. Louis, p 235, 1982.

Leon A. Assael

CHAPTER 12

Hard Tissue Trauma

When an individual is struck by a sudden external force, the hard tissues sustain and dissipate the load. Although the ability of bone and teeth to resist force is the greatest of any organic structure, their ability to undergo elastic deformation is less than 2%.[1] As a result, externally applied loads that exceed the tolerance of bone result in fracture.

The bones of the face are designed to dissipate force through multiple vectors and thus prevent fracture. A blow to the chin is dissipated via the dental contacts and transmitted to the midface. If the teeth do not come into contact, the load is transmitted to both craniomandibular articulations (Fig. 12–1). The transmission of force may be terminated by a fracture that occurs while the load is being propagated.[2] Such blows to the corpus of the mandible result in fractures at various locations. Of these, about 29% occur in the mandibular condyle.[3]

Because humans are both upright and binocular, the mandible is not well protected from injury when danger is faced. The mandible is vital to the survival of the individual. It protects the integrity of the airway and makes mastication possible. Additionally, the mandible must dissipate externally applied force in a fashion that will prevent fatal brain injury. Hence, the human condyle may have lengthened and weakened when compared with that of our predecessors as a survival mechanism, because the sequelae of a condylar fracture nearly always permit continued function even in the absence of treatment. This characteristic is certainly not typically true of mandibular corpus or temporal bone fractures.

MECHANISM OF CONDYLAR FRACTURE

Fractures of the condyle usually are the result of a blow to the chin. This is an indirect mechanism of fracture. Direct injury to the condyle is unusual because it is well encased in the glenoid fossa. A lateral blow to the body of the mandible most commonly results in a contralateral condylar fracture. A frontally directed blow to the parasymphysis may result in an ipsilateral condylar fracture. A blow to the mentum will likely result in bilateral condylar fractures.[4]

As in other bones, the condyle fractures most easily when tensile forces are applied. Hence, the usual condylar fracture occurs when a tensile force acts along the facial surface of the condylar neck. These fractures are usually propagated inferior to the pterygoid fovea, because the attachment of the lateral pterygoid muscle stabilizes the bone superiorly. A force directed along the long axis of the ramus may result in an intracapsular fracture. This type of injury results from a compressive load being sustained by the condylar head. Fractures through the capsule often result in the shearing away of the medial pole of the condyle, with the lateral pterygoid muscle attachment intact.[5] Intracapsular fracture is more likely in a child in whom the condylar neck is not yet completely formed.

Condylar fractures are often associated with predictable additional fractures of the facial skeleton. Force transmitted through the teeth may result in an associated midface fracture. Fractures of the mandibular symphysis, body, and angle may also occur with a condylar fracture. Subsequent clinical findings may be the result of a combination of injuries.

Considerable anatomic variation in the position of fractured segments may be noted after a condylar fracture. Once separated from the distal segment, the condylar head position is determined by the attachment of the capsular structures and the lateral pterygoid muscle. If the capsular structures are relatively intact, as is often the case with low subcondylar fractures, the condylar head may remain in the glenoid fossa with minimal rotation (Fig. 12–2). If posterior stops exist in the occlusion, there may be little overriding of the segments. If there are additional fractures or no posterior stops in the occlusion the distal segment may tend to override, producing a shortening of the mandibular ramus.

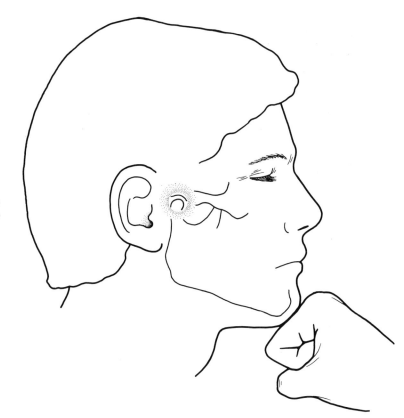

FIGURE 12-1. A blow to the chin. The force is transmitted to the condyles.

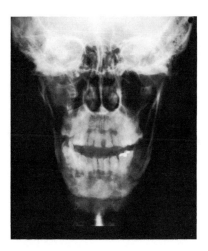

FIGURE 12-2. A subcondyle fracture with minimal displacement of the proximal segment. The condylar head remains in the glenoid fossa with minimal rotation.

Higher energy fractures often result in the disruption of the supporting capsular structures. In this mechanism of injury, tearing of the capsular structures presumably occurs immediately prior to the fracture being propagated. This effect permits the condyle to be displaced from the glenoid fossa, often initially in a lateral and posterior direction, resulting in tympanic plate fracture. Following initial lateral displacment, the attachment of the lateral pterygoid muscle generally pulls the condylar head anterior, medial, and inferior to its preinjury position. Rotation of the position of the condylar head places it into a relatively horizontal position, resulting in a "fracture-dislocation" of the mandibular condyle (Fig. 12–3). If the displacement of the condyle is less severe it may be termed a "fracture-subluxation." Gross disruption of the lateral ligament and disc is a consequence of fracture-dislocation. Although the relationship of the disc to the condyle may be relatively intact, the disc is usually sheared away from the glenoid fossa. The attachment of the disc to the fractured condyle may be due to the firmer capsular attachment to the condylar head when compared with the glenoid fossa capsular attachment.

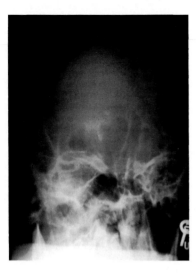

FIGURE 12–3. Fracture dislocation of the condyle. Severe displacement of the proximal segment is observed. The condylar head is out of the glenoid fossa with severe rotation.

DIAGNOSIS OF CONDYLAR FRACTURE

History

The patient with a condylar fracture nearly always offers a history of injury. This history may be masked by several factors, however. If the patient has sustained multiple trauma, attention may not have been drawn to a blow on the face. If the patient lost conciousness or was otherwise impaired at the time of injury, the history may not be accurate. The patient may have personal, social, or legal reasons for intentionally altering the history. In spite of these problems, the history offers the best initial information about where to look for an injury and what its clinical characteristics might be.

In taking the history, it is important to ascertain when the injury occurred. The circumstances of the incident might offer clues as to the type of injury. Did the patient undergo impact once or several times? From what direction did the impact come? What are the patient's symptoms now?

Clinical Findings

Signs and symptoms of a condylar fracture include those in common with all fractures. Tenderness over the site of injury is exacerbated by movement or palpation. Swelling is the result of hemorrhage and edema. Crepitation and interfragmentary mobility may be noted. Spasm in the associated muscle groups will occur. Muscle spasm and interfragmentary mobility result in a functional disability.

The patient with a condylar fracture may exhibit the clinical findings peculiar to this injury. Evidence of trauma will usually be over a site on the mentum or body of the mandible. The patient exhibits preauricular swelling and pain. Ecchymosis is only occasionally present and may be preauricular, retroauricular, or endaural. Evidence of bleeding from the external auditory canal is common.[6] Although trigeminal sensory and facial motor nerve deficits have been reported, these are rare.[7,8] When they occur, consideration should be given to nerve impingement. Dislocation of the condyle into the middle cranial fossae may occur through the roof of the glenoid fossa. The key sign appears to be a severe limitation of jaw movement. Symptoms of central nervous system injury may include a loss of consciousness, a seizure, or a focal neurologic finding.[9]

Derangements of masticatory function are nearly always present in the patient with a condylar fracture. The mandible may be deviated to the side of injury at rest, producing laterognathia and retrognathia (Fig. 12–4). Ipsilateral occlusal prematurity may be observed when maximum intercuspation is attempted. Alternatively there may be no occlusal abnormality

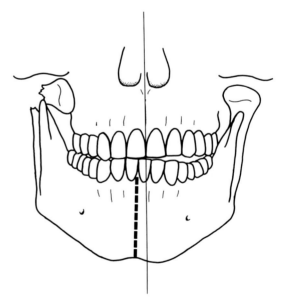

FIGURE 12–4. Deviation after condylar fracture. The mandible is deviated to the side of the injury, producing laterognathism and occlusal prematurity.

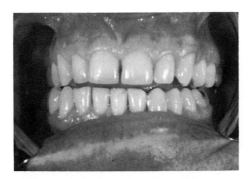

FIGURE 12–5. Attempted right lateral excursion in a patient with a left condylar fracture. A diminished right lateral excursion is seen with a left posterior occlusal prematurity.

at rest. In the usual clinical situation, the mandible deviates to the side of injury on opening. In protrusion, an exaggerated deviation to the side of injury may be noted.

When lateral excursion away from the side of injury is attempted, this movement is normally diminished after condylar fracture. In addition, an occlusal prematurity on the posterior nonworking side may be noted (Fig. 12–5). This finding is due to the inability of the nonworking-side condyle to provide guidance for the clearing of the nonworking-side dental contacts. This premature contact is often on the palatal cusp of the maxillary second molar

on the injured side. Because of the prematurity, the working side contacts may be absent or diminished. This may be noted by the inability of the patient to make a working-side cuspid contact during lateral excursion away from the side of injury.

More rarely, hemarthrosis may produce an ipsilateral posterior open bite and deviation away from the side of fracture (Fig. 12–6). Severe limitation of movement often accompanies this finding. Attempting to place the teeth into occlusion may produce severe pain. Hemarthrosis is most commonly a problem in intracapsular fractures.

Bilateral fractures of the condyle produce many similar clinical findings. In addition, the usual occlusal derangement is an anterior open bite. The open bite is often wedge-shaped, with a single occlusal contact bilaterally. An associated retrognathia is seen, which in its most severe state may be associated with airway impairment. Lateral excursions and mandibular protrusions are usually absent (Fig. 12–7).

Functional occlusal derangements following a condylar fracture are a result of the shortened ramus produced by the fracture and the splinting of the associated muscle groups. Individuals vary in their ability to adapt to these changes in bone position. Hence, clinical findings vary from case to case and they may vary in the same individual during the course of healing (Fig. 12–8).

A patient who has sustained a severe blow to the mandible is at risk for having a cervical spine injury. This may include the spectrum from muscle contusion to fracture dislocation.

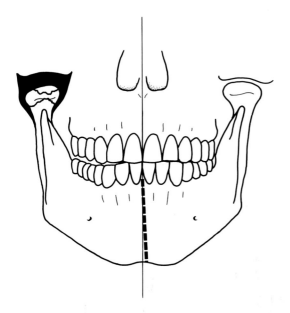

FIGURE 12–6. Deviation away from the side of injury in hemarthrosis. This finding may or may not be associated with a condylar fracture.

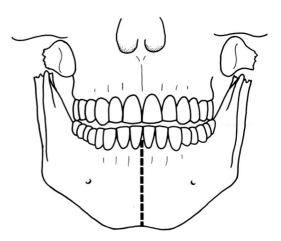

FIGURE 12–7. Bilateral fractures of the condyle. Limited jaw movement, retrognathia, and open bite are observed.

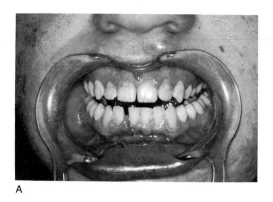
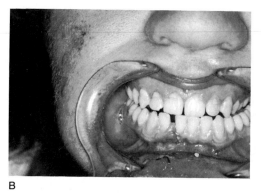

A   B

FIGURE 12–8. Occlusion may vary significantly in patients with condylar fractures during the course of healing. *A,* Patient with bilateral condylar fractures and a symphyseal fracture demonstrates an open bite. *B,* The same patient examined later demonstrates a markedly different occlusion when attempting maximum intercuspation.

Tenderness of the neck, swelling, stiffness, or peripheral neurologic findings are signs that require immediate investigation and the deferment of further clinical examination of the mandible.

Imaging

Diagnostic imaging of condylar fractures can be accomplished sufficiently in most cases with conventional radiography. Although a panoramic film reveals nearly all condylar fractures, it may produce some false-negative findings because of overriding of segments (Fig. 12–9). Towne's projection serves a useful second view, because it demonstrates the medial-lateral position of the condyle and produces a coronal view. Oblique-lateral views of the mandible, transcranial temporomandibular joint (TMJ) views, and submental vertex views produce images in the sagittal and axial planes (Fig. 12–10). As in the conventional radiographic evaluation of any structure, the axiom

of "Use at least two views, preferably at right angles" prevails.

Tomography, either conventional or computerized, offers additional information on the position of condylar fractures (Fig. 12–11). The relationship of the disc and other capsular tissues may be determined on computerized tomography (CT) scanning. The CT scan is also an excellent tool in finding additional occult fractures, particularly of the tympanic plate and glenoid fossa. Direct CT scanning is usually available in multiple planes. The most useful are the axial and coronal views, although occasionally oblique and sagittal views are valuable. Particular concern must be given to the trauma patient to be certain that no cervical spine injury is present before positioning the patient for any examination other than a direct CT axial examination.

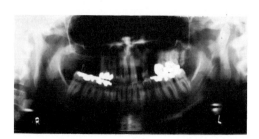

FIGURE 12–9. Panoramic film demonstrating a condylar fracture. This left condylar fracture is well defined by this view.

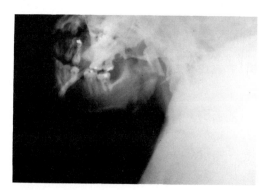

FIGURE 12–10. Oblique lateral of the mandible demonstrating a condylar fracture. As a conventional film this view offers better definition than the panoramic film.

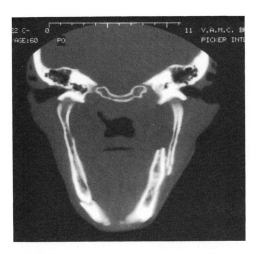

FIGURE 12–11. Computerized tomographic scan of mandible fractures. The position of the condylar segment can be well defined by this method of imaging.

POSTCONDYLAR FRACTURE SYNDROME

Because of the initial clinical findings, late functional occlusal findings, following a condylar fracture, may include a grouping of derangements and adaptations. Although these findings bear some similarity to those seen at the time of injury, they are modified by functional adaptations that have occurred. These vary dependent on the type of injury and the type of therapeutic regimen employed. The entire complex of findings may be termed the "postcondylar fracture syndrome."[10] The patient with postcondylar fracture syndrome has undergone adaptations in order to restore function following the injury.

The late clinical findings that are variably present in these patients include the following:

1. Deviation of the mandible to the side of injury
2. Short ramus on the side of injury
3. Decreased translation of the injured condyle
4. Canting of the occlusal plane and other dental adaptation
5. Loss of condylar guidance with lateral excursion away from the side of injury
6. Functional occlusal abnormalities
7. Muscle adaptation, atrophy, and shortening
8. Internal derangement of the injured joint
9. Growth and development abnormalities.

Deviation of the Mandible to the Side of Injury

This finding will be detectable in frontal view. Soft tissue pogonion will be deviated to the side of injury, often from 5 to 10 mm. An associated canting of the lips and commissure may be noted. On mandibular depression and protrusion, the jaw deviates to the side of injury. If viewed submentally, the entire mandible will be seen to be rotated toward the injured condyle.

Short Ramus on the Side of Injury

The patient demonstrates a shortened ramus when viewed cephalometrically or clinically. This finding may be associated with increased antegonial notching on the side of injury if the injury occurred during growth. The masseter and medial pterygoid muscles are necessarily shortened when this finding is present.

Decreased Translation of the Injured Condyle

The condyle will not translate as effectively. The ratio of hinge motion to translation is altered such that a greater amount of hinge motion per amount of translation occurs on the injured side compared with the normal side. This factor enhances deviation on opening and produces asymmetric lateral excursions. If enhanced, fibroankylosis or ankylosis may result. This finding is due to the derangement in lateral pterygoid function that results from the anterior, medial, and inferior positioning of the muscle attachment after fracture-dislocation.

Canting of the Occlusal Plane and Other Dental Adaptation

As an adaptation to occlusal prematurity on the injured side, orthodontic movement of the teeth results in slow eruption on the side opposite the injury. The loss of cuspid contact in lateral excursion on the side opposite the injury may result in drifting, eruption, or buccoversion of this tooth. The most posterior molar on the side of injury may become periodontally compromised as a result of traumatic occlusion.

Loss of Condylar Guidance with Lateral Excursion Away From the Side of Injury

Pain and limitation of movement may chronically inhibit the role that the injured condyle has in guiding proper mandibular movement. Because the condyle is no longer sliding down the articular eminence in translation, balancing side prematurities may occur. As a result, jaw movements, particularly lateral excursions, may be further deranged.

Functional Occlusal Abnormalities

The patient may be unable to properly tear and grind food on the side opposite the injury. As a result, the patient masticates nearly entirely on the injured side. By chewing only on the side of injury, further cicatrization of the joint and associated muscles may occur.

Muscle Adaptation, Atrophy, and Shortening

The functional abnormalities described in mastication produce changes in muscle function. Muscles that cannot produce physiologic activity atrophy and fibrose. Where the working distance has decreased, muscle length shortens. These adaptations often result in myofascial pain and dysfunction.[11]

Internal Derangement of the Injured Joint

If the capsule is torn at the time of injury, an immediate disc displacement may occur. This finding may not be noted in the initial clinical examination because jaw function is usually splinted by the painful injury. Alternatively, disc displacement may develop as a slow process following condylar fracture and may be fostered by the derangements in masticatory function that result from the injury.

Growth and Development Abnormalities

Subcondylar fracture during active growth at the "condylar site" affects the direction of growth (Fig. 12–12).[12] Disruption of the subcapsular cartilage or its blood supply in a condylar fracture disturbs the amount of growth that occurs. This effect may result in compen-satory changes in the remainder of the facial skeleton.[13] The problems previously delineated may be exacerbated by improperly regulated maxillary and mandibular growth. This may result in a canted maxilla, deviated septum, unequal orbits, and distortion of the mandibular parabolic form. This distortion includes rotation of the entire mandible toward the side of injury. The mandibular plane angle on the side of injury may be higher with increased antegonial notching.

TREATMENT OF CONDYLAR FRACTURE

Surgeons treating condylar fractures agree that treatment is designed to restore masticatory function. Debate is still strong as to the means of providing this result with the most effectiveness and with the least risk for the patient. The avoidance of devastating complications, such as ankylosis and growth disturbance, is an essential part of the treatment planning philosophy. The choices for the treatment of condylar fractures are essentially the same as for any fracture. They are as follows:

1. Closed reduction and immobilization
2. Immobilization without reduction and active physical therapy
3. Active physical therapy as a single modality
4. Open reduction and immobilization
5. Open reduction, stable fixation, and immediate function.

Closed Reduction and Immobilization

The intrinsic value of anatomic reduction of condylar fractures has been historically de-emphasized because of the perceived satisfactory results that have been obtained by closed treatment of these fractures and by the morbidity experienced with open reduction and internal fixation.[14] Manipulation of the fracture has been performed to permit a reduction of the fractured segments, including digital pressure and blind manipulation with probes to reposition the condylar segment.[15] Intermaxillary fixation alone has been seen to reduce the fractured segments.[16] It appears that this method of reduction is useful only in restoring the anatomic position in cases in which the condylar segment is still in the glenoid fossa (Fig. 12–13).[17] In these cases, the goal of treatment is to

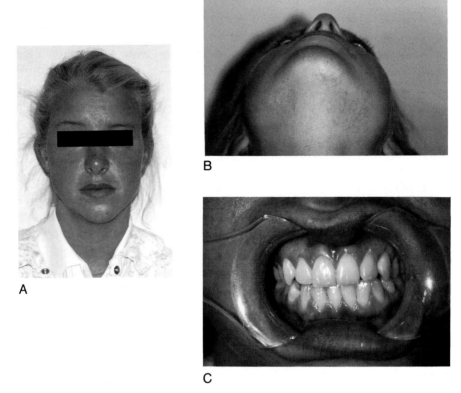

FIGURE 12–12. Postcondylar fracture syndrome. *A,* Full face view showing deviation to the side of injury. *B,* Submental view showing rotation of the entire mandible toward the injured condyle. *C,* Occlusion demonstrates compensatory eruption and deviation.

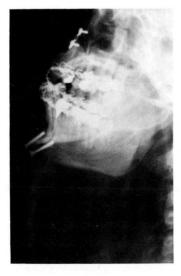

FIGURE 12–13. Closed reduction and intermaxillary fixation of a condylar fracture. Treatment with the condyle upright and in the glenoid fossa has been closed reduction. Other facial fractures were treated with rigid internal fixation in this patient.

restore anatomic form through osteosynthesis of the fracture in an anatomic fashion. Immobilization needs to be for the period of time necessary to permit bony union, often up to 6 weeks. Although the advantage of restoring anatomic form exists, the risk of fibroankylosis rises with the length of the period of immobilization.

Immobilization Without Reduction and Active Physical Therapy

A brief period (1 to 3 weeks) of immobilization followed by active physical therapy is the most common means of treating fracture-dislocation of the condyle. In this method, the goal is to obtain a bony union with the condyle in a new relationship to the glenoid fossa. Pseudoarthrosis at the fracture site rarely if ever occurs.[18] With this method of treatment, postfixation function and physical therapy produce neuromuscular adaptation to restore activity of the joint, teeth, and muscles. As discussed in the findings of postcondylar fracture syndrome, adaptations may have adverse clinical consequences.

Physical therapy is designed to restore the functional movements inhibited by the injury and to assist the compensation that may be produced by changes in tooth position, joint structure, and muscular function. On removal of fixation, there is often an immediate deviation or open bite. Guiding elastics are placed on the arch bars to redirect jaw movement toward maximum intercuspation. Active movement of the jaw is encouraged when the patient is awake. The guiding elastics may be reapplied by the cooperative patient at night. Elastics may be necessary from a few days up to 8 weeks following the removal of fixation.[19] Once the patient is able to maintain normal occlusion, the guiding elastics are discontinued and the arch bars may be removed.

Encouraging the patient to chew on the side opposite the injury promotes translation of the injured condyle, which may assist in restoration of function. The incision of carrots or stick pretzels placed in the canine occlusion opposite the injury also encourages lateral excursions. If the jaw is deviating to the side of injury on opening, it is helpful to direct the patient to open, close, and protrude in front of a mirror with a fist at the side of the jaw to redirect jaw movement.[20] This exercise should be done with 12 repetitions at least three times daily.

If range of motion of the mandible is limited following the initial period after injury, physical therapy specifically designed to restore the mobility of the joint is indicated. Tongue blades, ratchet mouth props, and passive jaw manipulation are all means to restore joint mobility. If jaw mobility appears to be inhibited by a mechanical stop, however, this type of physical therapy may be detrimental.

Active Physical Therapy as a Single Modality

Consideration is often given toward eliminating the immobilization phase and immediately initiating physical therapy. This is a particularly important consideration when the risk of ankylosis is high, as in an intracapsular fracture or a fracture in a child. Intermaxillary fixation is undesirable in epileptic, uncooperative, or edentulous patients.[21] These patients are often treated by the physical therapy regimen previously described.

If prolonged functional therapy is indicated, an orthodontic activator has been employed to give guidance to jaw movement and distract the fracture via an occlusal fulcrum. By opening the bite with an occlusal stop on the posterior side of injury, a rotation with attempted closure distracts the condylar fracture site. Deep lingual guide planes may prevent deviation to the side of injury.[22]

Open Reduction and Immobilization

Open reduction of condylar fractures has been advocated as a means of restoring the preinjury position of the fractured segments in a precise way. Reported indications for open reduction include the following:[23]

1. Displacement into the middle cranial fossa
2. Tympanic plate displacement
3. Inability to obtain adequate occlusion by closed means
4. Lateral extracapsular displacement of the condyle
5. Foreign body (Fig. 12–14)
6. Failure to obtain interfragmentary contact after closed treatment
7. Blocked mandibular excursions
8. Facial nerve paresis secondary to injury
9. Contraindication to intermaxillary fixation
10. Open fracture.

Concern regarding the desirability of the functional adaptations that occur following nonsurgical management of fracture of the condyle has broadened the indications to include a postcondylar fracture syndrome associated

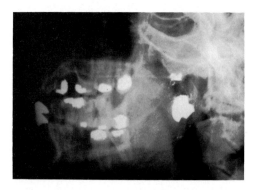

FIGURE 12–14. Gunshot wound to the condyle. Open debridement and reduction are indicated because the foreign body is in the joint.

with anatomic shortening of the ramus[2] and associated post-traumatic internal derangement.[24]

The patient with persistent postcondylar fracture syndrome associated with a short ramus may be condemned to significant dental and skeletal adaptations if open reduction is not performed. Consideration should be given as to whether this adaptation will significantly compromise function in the given clinical situation. The problems of a persistent postcondylar fracture syndrome may be mitigated open reduction. A visibly shortened ramus with associated functional derangements may be a sufficient indication for open reduction.

Doubt may exist as to whether the patient will be able to adequately accommodate to the positional change that results from a condylar fracture. In that case, the decision to perform open reduction may be delayed. Many patients who exhibit functional derangements at the time of injury will have alleviation of these clinical findings during the course of healing. When doubt exists as to whether these adverse clinical findings are the result of a shortened ramus, an initial period of immobilization may be tried. Following this period, active physical therapy may be initiated. If findings of a shortened ramus persist, surgery may be indicated. A decision to perform an open reduction should be made within 3 weeks of injury, because success is less likely after this time.

Data generated by magnetic resonance imaging (MRI) and CT scanning of condylar fractures, arthroscopy, and arthrotomy at the time of injury indicate that disc displacement and dysfunction are important components of the injury in fracture dislocation of the condyle.[24] Attempts at correction of the internal derangement must be combined with anatomic reduction in order to recreate preinjury form.

Initial attempts to perform open reduction of condylar fractures were thwarted by the difficulty of surgical access, potential for severe bleeding, injury to the seventh cranial nerve, and difficulty of producing fixation that would not slip during the course of healing. Rowe and Killey[25] in 1968, stated that "Operative interference is only rarely indicated." Perhaps because of the evolution of thinking that has occurred regarding condylar fracture management, they now state that "Open reduction is logically indicated in certain circumstances."[17] The status of this debate today is that although opinions vary regarding the indications for open reduction, advocates of all

methods, nonoperative and operative, report excellent clinical results. The assiduousness with which post-treatment results are evaluated in the future may determine the optimal mode of treatment for the variety of clinical conditions seen in condylar fractures.

Surgical access to the condyle has been improved by developing a more complete understanding of the anatomy of the region. Protection of the facial nerve through a preauricular approach can now be assured with appropriate dissection.[26,27] Transoral, retromandibular, coronal, submandibular, and retroauricular approaches also offer safe access to the fracture site (Fig. 12–15).[27]

Open reduction of the condyle was first reported without internal fixation.[15] Transosseous suture fixation to improve the stability of reduction was then reported.[5] The difficulties of wire fixation became apparent when the loss of reduction in the postoperative period occurred. Modifications of wire osteosynthesis were developed to improve stability.[28] Additional stability was sought with different methods of fixation including transosseous Kirschner-wire fixation, screw fixation, and external pin fixation.[29,30] None of these methods provided fixation forces sufficient to exceed functional forces. Hence, none of these methods of fixation could reliably permit immediate function.

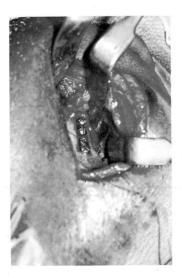

FIGURE 12–15. Surgical access to a condylar fracture. This retroauricular approach will permit safe and aesthetic access that will preserve the facial nerve.

Open Reduction, Stable Fixation, and Immediate Function

Stable internal fixation provides forces that exceed functional forces during the course of healing. This characteristic permits the immediate restoration of function. Immediate function following surgical treatment of condylar fracture offers the advantage of convenience and the lessening of "fracture disease." Fracture disease is the atrophy and fibrosis that occur in muscles and joints once they are immobilized. With immediate restoration of function, the condyle and muscles of mastication more rapidly return to the preinjury mode of function. Whether permanent differences occur in function as the result of this method has not been determined.

Stable internal fixation with immediate function was first performed with a rigid bone plate on the lateral surface of the mandible.[31] Lag screw fixation of condylar fractures has also been reported.[32] Stable fixation of condylar fractures has been accomplished through retromandibular, preauricular, and intraoral approaches.[33]

Plate and screw fixation offers so many advantages that it is the generally preferred method of internal fixation of condylar fractures in current practice (Fig. 12–16). The rigid relationship of the segments may produce

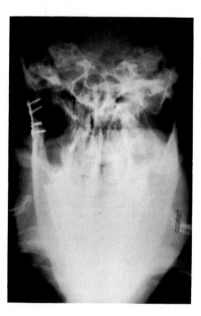

FIGURE 12–16. Plate and screw fixation of a condylar fracture. After this treatment the patient may be placed immediately into function.

problems, however, if there is associated disc displacement. Subsequent clinical findings of internal derangement may be evident. For this reason, advocates of immediate disc repair with open reduction have emerged.[24] Long-term evaluation of results with this option has not yet been accomplished.

CONDYLAR FRACTURE IN THE GROWING CHILD

Most condylar fractures in children result from a fall on the chin. Although chin lacerations are sutured in emergency rooms on a daily basis, many condylar fractures appear to remain undiscovered. Only the late finding of ankylosis or growth disturbance offers evidence of a previous condylar fracture. About 39% of all mandibular fractures in children are in the condyle. Of these, about 25% are intracapsular.[34]

Of all facial fractures in children, condylar fractures have the greatest propensity to produce a growth disturbance.[35] This risk appears to be greatest when the injury is during the first 3 years or during adolescence.[36] Yet, the ability of a child to undergo compensatory growth that decreases the effects of the injury is also the greatest.[37] Fracture dislocation of the condyle in the preadolescent often results in excellent remodeling and function. This period of remodeling and new condylar growth is usually during the first 6 to 12 months following injury. Because of this factor and the higher risks of avascular necrosis and ankylosis, open reduction of a condylar fracture in a child is not widely recommended.[38] On a statistical basis, growth pattern problems can be expected in about 20% of all children with condylar fractures.[39]

Initial management of condylar fractures in children often involves no immobilization. Intense postinjury physical therapy with careful attention to any subsequent growth disturbance is the hallmark of care. Fractures during the period of mixed dentition often demonstrate improved occlusions during the course of healing because of eruption. These may produce a cant of the occlusal plane, however. If the condyle fails to develop translatory ability, greater concern might be expressed about a subsequent growth disturbance. Because the functional activity of the joint is inhibited, the amount and direction of growth in the surrounding structures are changed.[12] Attention to producing translatory movement in the period of postoperative physical therapy is therefore imperative.

Bilateral fractures of the condyle usually require a period of immobilization and guiding elastics, because of the open bite tendency in many of these patients. Bilateral fractures often produce favorable remodeling, according to the same scheme as unilateral fractures.

ANKYLOSIS

Although many patients with ankylosis give a history of trauma, about half of the cases may be due to an inflammatory condition of the joint.[40] Nevertheless, ankylosis is the most severe consequence that can be expected from a condylar fracture. The mechanism of ankylosis is most likely caused by intracapsular injury followed by insufficient jaw movement. The extravasation of blood into the joint along with the disruption of fibrocartilage integrity permits the ingrowth of fibrous connective tissue into the joint, which subsequently results in ossification (Fig. 12–17). The clinical history of a patient who develops ankylosis often reveals a progressive decrease in mobility in the weeks after injury. This is the period when organization of connective tissue is producing decreased mobility. Immobilization during this period enhances the fixation of the joint and promotes ankylosis. The best means of preventing ankylosis is by early and aggressive remobilization of the fracture site.

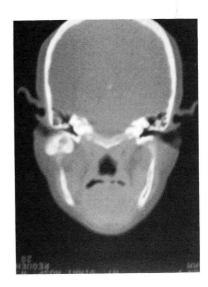

FIGURE 12–18. Computerized tomographic scan demonstrates ossification of the joint following trauma, resulting in ankylosis.

The surgical management of ankylosis is usually the only means of remobilizing the joint. Surgical management can be divided into the procedures that enter the ankylotic section to correct the abnormality and ostectomies in sites remote from the ankylotic section. The ankylosis should be entered and corrected when surgically feasible. In some massive ankyloses, gap ostectomy with interpositional material may be the only practical way of remobilizing the mandible.

If the joint is to be remobilized, attention must be given to the complete surgical removal of the ankylotic segment (Fig. 12–18 and Fig. 12–19). Preoperative CT imaging has provided invaluable assistance in the identification of the

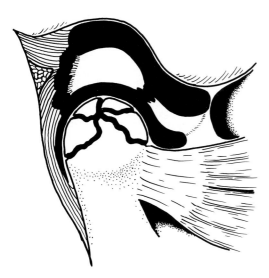

FIGURE 12–17. Intracapsular fracture of the condyle. This finding will increase the risk of ankylosis, especially if treated with immobilization.

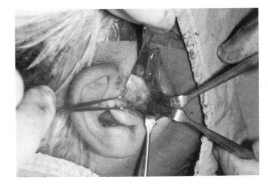

FIGURE 12–19. The appearance of ankylosis at the time of surgery. The ankylotic segment will be removed and replaced with autogenous cartilage.

ankylotic parts. Coronoidectomy may be necessary to complete remobilization in long-standing problems as well as in those associated with zygomatic arch fractures. Bilateral ankylosis may become apparent only after ostectomy on the first side. Hence, the surgeon must be prepared to perform a bilateral procedure. Following remobilization, the jaw should be able to be depressed 35 to 40 mm. Interpositional material to prevent reankylosis is essential.[41] Some alloplastic materials used include Silastic and acrylic. Autogenous materials include costochondral, ear cartilage, and temporal muscle grafts.

Attention to the restoration of the vertical dimension of the mandible is essential in obtaining a favorable result. Interpositional material is best fixed rigidly to permit immediate function. Remobilization of the mandible postoperatively is necessary. Aggressive postoperative physical therapy assures that the gains made at surgery are maintained.

SUMMARY

Condylar fractures are among the most frequent facial injuries. They are important because of the significant functional derangements that may result. Detection of condylar fracture is dependent on a knowledge of the malfunctions that result from this injury. Treatment of condylar fractures is based on the return to the preinjury level of function and the prevention of complications.

REFERENCES

1. Spiessl, B.: *Internal Fixation of the Mandible.* Springer Verlag, Berlin, 1989.
2. Assael, L. and Tucker, M.: Management of facial fractures. In *Contemporary Oral and Maxillofacial Surgery.* L. Peterson (ed.). C. V. Mosby Co., St. Louis, 1988.
3. Olson, R.: Fractures of the mandible. J.O.M.S. 40:23, 1982.
4. Rowe, N. and Williams, J.: *Maxillofacial Injuries.* Churchill Livingstone, Edinburgh, p 8, 1985.
5. Schule, H.: Injuries of the temporomandibular joint. In *Oral and Maxillofacial Traumatology.* W. Schilli and G. Kruger (eds.). Quintessence Publishing Co., Lombard, IL, 1984.
6. Goldberg, M., Aslanian, R., Wright, J., and Marco, W.: Auditory canal hemorrhage. A sign of mandibular trauma. J. Oral Surg. 29:425, 1971.
7. Zielinski, D.: Anaesthesia of the mental nerve secondary to a condylar fracture. J. Oral Surg. 27:227, 1969.
8. Laws, I.: Two unusual complications of fractures of the mandibular condyle. Br. J. Oral Surg. 5:51, 1967.
9. Kallal, R., Gans, B., and Lagrotteria, L.: Cranial dislocation of mandibular condyle. Oral Surg. 43:2, 1977.
10. Assael, L.: Surgical management of condylar fractures. In *Management of Facial Injuries.* P. Manson (ed.). J.B. Lippincott Co., Philadelphia, 1990.
11. Brooke R. and Stenn P.: Postinjury MPD syndrome: its etiology and prognosis. Oral Surg. 45:846, 1978.
12. Enlow, D.: *Facial Growth,* 3rd ed. W. B. Saunders Co., Philadelphia, p 96, 1990.
13. Profitt, W., Vig, K., and Turvey, T.: Early fracture of the mandibular condyle: an unsuspected cause of growth disturbance. Am. J. Orthod. 78:1, 1980.
14. Chalmers, J.: Fractures involving the mandibular condyle: A post-treatment survey of 120 cases. J. Oral Surg. 5:45, 1947.
15. Silverman, S.: New operation for displaced fractures of the mandibular condyle. Int. J. Orthod. 67:876, 1925.
16. Blevins, C. and Gores, R.: Fractures of the mandibular condyloid process: results of conservative treatment in 140 cases. J. Oral Surg. 19:392, 1961.
17. Bradley, P.: Injuries of the condylar and coronoid process. In *Maxillofacial Injuries.* N. Rowe and J. Williams (eds.). Churchill Livingstone, New York, p 355, 1985.
18. MacGregor, A. and Fordyce, G.: Treatment of fractures of the neck of the mandibular condyle. Br. Dent. J. 102:351, 1957.
19. Beekler, D. and Walker, R.V.: Condyle fractures. J. Oral Surg. 27:563, 1969.
20. Gerry, R.: Personal communication, 1981.
21. Spiessl, B.: *New Concepts in Maxillofacial Bone Surgery.* Springer Verlag, Berlin, 1976.
22. Lentrodt, J.: Conservative therapy. In *Oral and Maxillofacial Traumatology.* W. Schilli and E. Kruger (eds.). Quintessence Publishing Co., Lombard, IL, p 71, 1986.
23. Zide, M. and Kent, J.: Indications for open reduction of mandible condyle fractures. J. Oral Maxillofac. Surg. 41.89, 1983.
24. Chuong, R. and Piper, M.A.: Open reduction of condylar fractures of the mandible in conjunction with the repair of discal injury. J. Oral Maxillofac. Surg. 46:262, 1988.
25. Rowe, N. and Killey, H.: *Fractures of the Facial Skeleton,* 2nd ed. Livingstone, Edinburgh, 1968.
26. Al Kayat, A. and Bramley, P.: A modified preauricular approach to the temporomandibular joint. Br. J. Oral Surg. 17:91, 1979.
27. Kent, J., Neary, J., Silvia, C., and Zide, M.: Open reduction of fractured mandibular condyles. Oral Maxillofac. Surg. Clin. North Am. 2:69, 1990.
28. Messer E.: A simplified method for fixation of the fractured mandibular condyle. J. Oral Surg. 30:442, 1972.
29. Brown, A. and Obeid, G.: A simplified method for the internal fixation of the fractured condyle. Br. J. Oral Maxillofac. Surg. 22:145, 1984.
30. Archer, W.: *Oral and Maxillofacial Surgery,* 5th ed. W. B. Saunders Co., Philadelphia, p 1174, 1975.
31. Koberg, W. and Momma, W.: Treatment of fractures of the articular process by functional stable osteosynthesis using miniaturized dynamic compression plates. Int. J. Oral Surg. 7:256, 1978.
32. Petzel, J.: Die chirurgische Behandlung des frakturierten Collum mandibulare durch funktionstabile Zugschraubenosteosynthese. Fortschr. Kiefer. Gesischtschir. 25:84, 1980.
33. Assael, L.: Surgical management of condylar fractures. In *Management of Facial Injuries.* P. Manson (ed.). J.B. Lippincott Co., Philadelphia, 1990.
34. Hall, R., Thomas, G., and Buzowski, G.: Ten-year survey of traumatic injuries to the face and jaws of children, 1970–1979. A computer analysis. Proceedings

from the 8th International Conference on Oral and Maxillofacial Surgery. Quintessence Publishing Co., Lombard, IL, pp 143–150, 1985.

35. James, D.: Maxillofacial injuries in children. In *Maxillofacial Injuries.* N. Rowe and J. Williams (eds.). Churchill Livingstone, New York, 1985.

36. MacLennan, W.: 180 Cases of fracture of the condylar process. Br. J. Plast. Surg. 5:122, 1952.

37. Rowe, N.: Fractures of the jaws in children. J. Oral Surg. 27:497, 1969.

38. Kaban, L.: *Pediatric Oral and Maxillofacial Surgery.* W. B. Saunders Co., Philadelphia, p 251, 1990.

39. Lund, K.: Mandibular growth and remodeling processes after condylar fracture: a longitudinal roentgen cephalometric study. Acta Odont. Scand. (Suppl.) 32:3, 1974.

40. Topazian, R.: Etiology of ankylosis of the temporomandibular joint in 44 cases. J. Oral Surg. 34:227, 1964.

41. MacIntosh, R.: Current spectrum of costochondral grafting. In *Surgical Correction of Dentofacial Deformities.* Bell, W.H., et al (eds.). W. B. Saunders Co., Philadelphia, p 355–410, 1985.

Leon A. Assael

CHAPTER 13

Developmental Disorders

The development of the facial skeleton is dependent on an intricate series of events that must coordinate to produce the correct amount and direction of growth. In this matrix of activity, any structure can be thought of as both an initiator of growth and a responder to growth. The condyle acts as a growth site that will transport adjacent structures into new positions. It stimulates the growth patterns of adjacent structures. The condyle also responds to growth in adjacent structures by growing to accommodate its space in the developing face. The failure of a single component during growth will result in alterations in the amount and direction of growth of the adjacent structures. Nowhere is this more evident than in the case of the condyle that fails to be an appropriate initiator of growth.

EMBRYOLOGY OF THE TEMPOROMANDIBULAR APPARATUS

The first appearance of the human temporomandibular joint (TMJ) is during the eighth week of gestation when two separate areas of mesenchymal organization (blastemas) appear near the eventual location of the condyle and glenoid fossa. During this period, the muscles of mastication and other adjacent soft tissue structures are also undergoing morphogenesis. The condyle develops lateral and superior to Meckel's cartilage. Bone and cartilage are first seen in the condyle at about the tenth gestational week. The developing condyle and glenoid fossa are initially separated but migrate to be in close apposition by the twelfth week.[1-3]

The disc develops as a mesenchymal structure with tissue migrating from the condylar head, temporal bone, and lateral pterygoid tendon.[4] The disc is a highly cellular mesenchymal tissue that becomes progressively fibrous during fetal development.[5] By 14 weeks of gestation, the morphogenesis of the disc has progressed to reveal a thin intermediate zone and a general thickening of the periphery.

A disturbance in the development of the condyle and fossa may occur in utero late in the first trimester. This disturbance may result in agenesis or hypoplasia of the mandibular condyle and its associated soft tissues. The resulting clinical findings, when unilateral, have been termed hemifacial microsomia. Synonyms for this abnormality include otomandibular dysostosis, oculoauriculovertebral dysplasia, and first and second branchial arch syndrome.

HEMIFACIAL MICROSOMIA

Patients who exhibit mandibular deficiencies with associated asymmetries often exhibit signs of hemifacial microsomia. These clinical findings are due to the inadequate development of the TMJ and associated structures. It is the congenital underdevelopment that occurs during growth, as adjacent structures adapt to the altered environment. Patients with hemifacial microsomia present with varying degrees of severity. These are due to the variable expressivity as a congenital finding and the variable adaptations during growth and development.

Hemifacial microsomia is a common congenital lesion occurring in one of every 3500 to 5600 births.[6,7] Because mild forms are often undiagnosed, this number is certainly an underestimation of incidence. Evidence exists that most but not all cases occur in a random fashion. Inherited variants of this lesion have been noted in Goldenhar's syndrome and in instances of successive generations. The mode of inheritance is unknown.[8]

Hemifacial microsomia results from the malformation of the first and second branchial arches. Poswillo[9] hypothesized that damage to the stapedial artery in utero results in this hypoplasia. The extent to which blood supply is lost and the size of the area affected may explain the variability in expression of this phenomenon. Although this explanation is generally accepted, the presence of multiple system problems indicates a more complex etiology. For example, Goldenhar's syndrome is associated with abnormalities of the vertebrae and skin. Cleft lips and palates, renal anomalies, and minor problems in limb development also occur with greater frequency in other noncategorized cases of hemifacial microsomia. Hemifacial microsomia may be evidenced in a heterogeneous group of individuals who have relative degrees of failure in the formation of mesenchyme. This effect may represent a mixed group of inherited and congenital disorders.[10]

Hemifacial microsomia affects the morphology and growth potential of the condyle, ramus, glenoid fossa, ear, and soft tissue of the face. The severity in adjacent structures is generally correlated with the extent of the defect in condylar size and form. All degrees of this congenital deformity result in progressive physical findings during growth and development.

Physical Findings During Growth and Development

The physical findings of hemifacial microsomia become more pronounced as the face grows. Not only are the affected areas malformed, but they fail to grow in proportion to the rest of the face. The seemingly unaffected areas of the face in the infant become progressively deformed, as the affected tissues fail to initiate growth in the associated structures. Hence, the physical findings in hemifacial microsomia are due to a failure to initiate and respond to growth (Fig. 13–1).

The clinician should be familiar with the entire spectrum of physical findings in hemifacial microsomia, although most patients exhibit only some of them. The severity of findings is variable.

The condyle and ramus complex may be only decreased in size, with no substantial morphologic changes in the mildest forms (Fig. 13–2). The small ramus and condyle in the infant result in a generalized retrognathia and deviation of the chin to the affected side. As the child grows, the affected side is impaired in all directions. Decreased anterior growth causes a progressive deviation of the chin; decreased vertical growth causes a short ramus and superior canting of the occlusal plane. Reduced transverse growth results in a constricted dental arch and facial contour deficit. With greater growth potential in the mandibular body than in the ramus, progressive antegonial notching may be noted, with a steep mandibular plane angle (Fig. 13–3).

As the severity increases, the condyle becomes relatively smaller in relation to the ramus. The location of the glenoid fossa and external auditory canal is also substantially affected. These structures are displaced inferiorly. In this circumstance, the coronoid process protrudes superior to the condylar process. A gross increase in the TMJ space may be noted, as the erupted dentition allows for the anterior and inferior displacement of the malformed ramus. Condylar guidance to a functional maximum intercuspation is lost. A large difference between centric relation and centric occlusion is noted. Marked retrusion and devia-

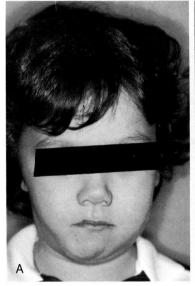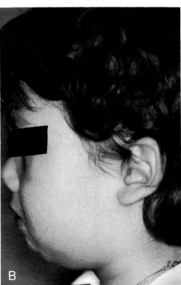

FIGURE 13–1. *A* and *B*, A 3-year-old child with hemifacial microsomia of moderate degree. Associated deficiencies in soft tissue growth are becoming apparent.

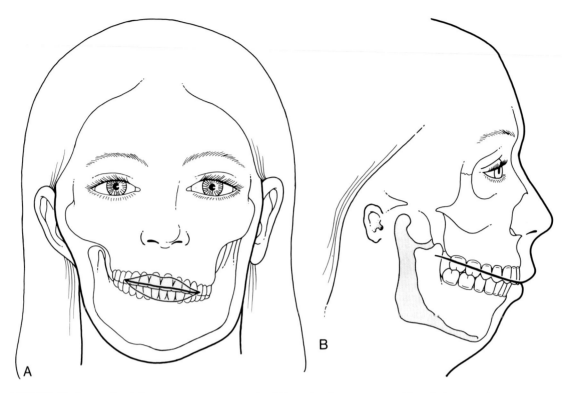

FIGURE 13–2. *A* and *B*, Schematic representation of mild hemifacial microsomia. Although the condyle and fossa are present, they are not well formed. An increased joint space, canting of the lips and occlusal plane, and facial asymmetry are noted.

tion are observed, with hinge axis movement of the mandible.

In the most severe cases, the condyle is entirely absent and the ramus is small and malformed (Fig. 13–4). Canting of the mandible into the defect is more severe. Impaction or agenesis of the permanent dentition on the affected mandibular side is a frequent finding in the severe form. Progressive hypoplasia of the body of the mandible is noted (Fig. 13–5).

The glenoid fossa is also variously malformed in hemifacial microsomia. In the mildest form, there is hypoplasia of the disc, capsule, and articular eminence. Hypoplasia of the tympanic plate may also be noted. In the more severe form, the articular eminence is absent along with the zygomatic arch. The disc is also absent. The glenoid fossa and external auditory canal are inferiorly, medially, and anteriorly placed, resulting in migration of the external ear into the defect. Severe stenosis of the external auditory canal and hypoplasia of the ossicles may result in deafness.

The ear can be inferiorly displaced and prolapsed in the mildest forms of hemifacial microsomia. In more severe forms, preauricular

cartilage tags and absence of the superior portion of the auricle are noted (Fig. 13–6). A cleft in the area in front of the hypoplastic mastoid may also be noted. If the deformity is complete, aplasia of the ear and external auditory canal is found.

The soft tissues are progressively affected. In the mildest forms, only a mild decrease in soft tissue bulk may be noted. The muscles of mastication are smaller and match the deficit in the affected ramus. More severe variants of hemifacial microsomia show hypoplasia or agenesis of the parotid gland. The soft tissues of the orbit may not be well formed, resulting in inferior displacement of the brow and lateral canthus. In the most severe forms, macrostomia or lateral facial clefting occurs. Unilateral microphthalmia may be present.

The dentition is usually morphologically correct in mild to moderate forms. The alveolar processes are less well formed on the affected side. Impaction and crowding of teeth in the deficient alveolus are often noted. In severe forms, partial agenesis of the teeth on the affected side may be observed (Fig. 13–7).

The midface may be normal at birth in the

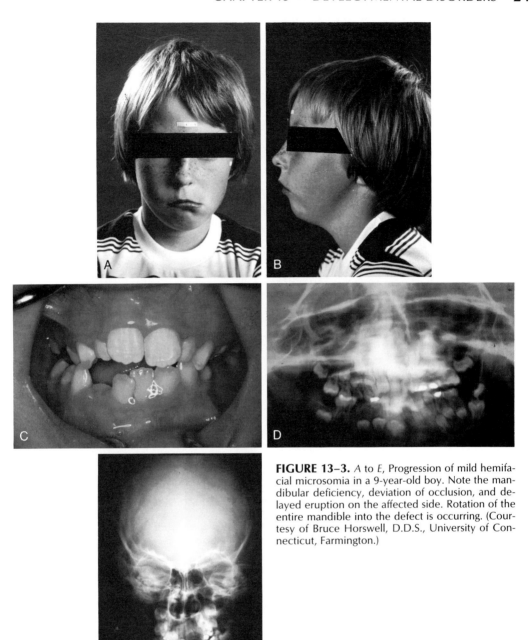

FIGURE 13–3. *A* to *E*, Progression of mild hemifacial microsomia in a 9-year-old boy. Note the mandibular deficiency, deviation of occlusion, and delayed eruption on the affected side. Rotation of the entire mandible into the defect is occurring. (Courtesy of Bruce Horswell, D.D.S., University of Connecticut, Farmington.)

mild and moderate forms. As the child grows, the midface adapts to the deficit in the mandible. This results in a progressive decrease in vertical growth of the maxilla. The nose deviates toward the defect, and the nasal septum may be buckled. The palatal plane is canted, and its transverse dimension is decreased on the hypoplastic side. In severe cases, hypoplasia of the maxilla, orbit, and zygoma may be noted. The zygomatic arch is absent. Failure of midfacial growth is exacerbated by the intrinsic hypoplasia of all these structures.

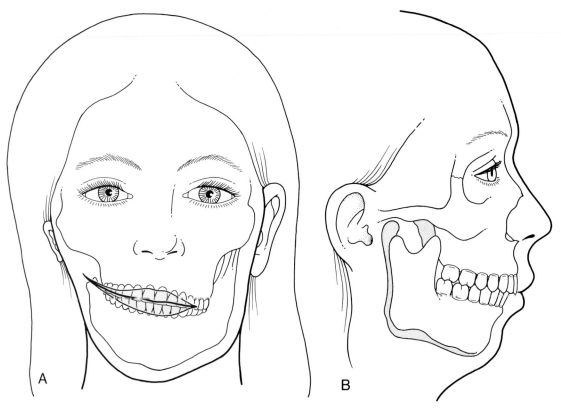

FIGURE 13–4. *A* and *B*, Schematic representation of severe hemifacial microsomia. The condyle is absent, a partial lateral facial cleft is present, and severe retrognathia and canting are present.

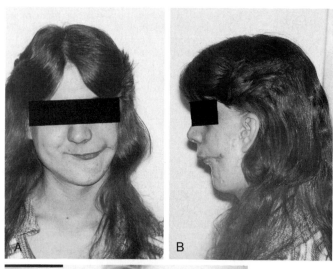

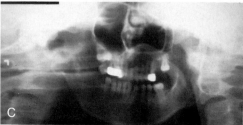

FIGURE 13–5. *A* to *C*, Severe hemifacial microsomia. Absence of the ramus, lateral facial clefting, and associated deformities are noted. Partial anodontia on the affected side and a poorly formed mandibular body are observed.

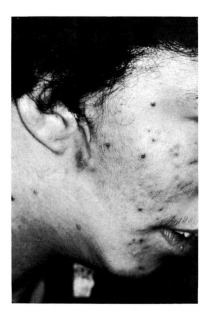

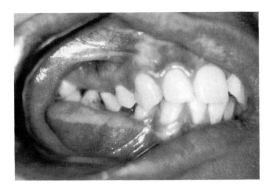

FIGURE 13-7. Dental occlusion in hemifacial micro-somia. Collapse of the alveolar height, width, and projection are noted on the affected side.

FIGURE 13-6. Malformation of the ear in severe hemi-facial microsomia. Preauricular tags, displacement, and hypoplasia are noted.

Treatment

Treatments for hemifacial microsomia may be divided into those that are designed to simply reconstruct the deficits associated with this lesion and those that attempt to mitigate the effects during growth and development. Because the deficits of hemifacial microsomia are progressive, influencing the eventual severity of the clinical findings is an attractive idea. Although interceptive treatment can be helpful, currently it cannot be considered the means to avoid secondary treatment and surgery. Interceptive treatment must not create dental and skeletal compensations that will make subsequent comprehensive reconstructions more difficult. Interceptive treatment should instead promote improved function and maximize

Bilateral expression of hemifacial microsomia can occur and is called mandibulofacial dysostosis or Treacher Collins syndrome (Fig. 13-8). Patients exhibit severe retrognathia, macrostomia, antimongoloid slant of the palpebrae, and colobomas of the lower lids. The findings in the temporomandibular region are usually similar to those of the severest forms of hemifacial microsomia.

FIGURE 13-8. Bilateral severe hemifacial microsomia. Lateral facial clefting and absent rami are noted. Muscles of mastication are rudimentary.

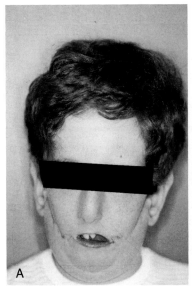

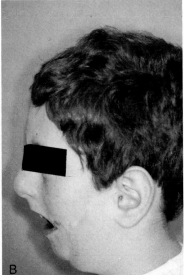

A

B

harmonious growth of the condyle and adjacent structures.

In the growing individual, orthopedic-orthodontic appliances are utilized to distract the condyle inferiorly and anteriorly. These appliances are claimed to promote condylar growth. They appear to be of use only with the mild forms of hemifacial microsomia and only with the deciduous dentition.[11]

Surgical correction can first be considered in the preschool child. In particular, costochondral grafting can be considered in deciduous and mixed dentition stages, when the eruption of teeth and the development of facial bones can be influenced by the correction of abnormalities in the condyle. Costochondral grafting should be strongly considered to replace the missing condyle in severe forms of hemifacial microsomia but should also be considered if the condyle is rudimentary. The costochondral graft regains the deficiency in mandibular height and projection. A posterior open bite is often produced on the defective side. The space created can be supported by an acrylic splint that is recontoured as the permanent teeth erupt. This treatment permits more normal eruption of the permanent teeth and thereby decreases the eventual maxillary deformity.[12] Costochondral bone grafting also allows the affected side to grow, although the extent may not be predictable. Overgrowth of the graft may produce additional problems that may require further corrective surgery.

Simultaneous reconstruction of the glenoid fossa may be a necessary part of the procedure in a severe case. This reconstruction may be accomplished by simply recontouring of the fossa[13] or by bone grafting of the cranial base.[14] Failure of condylar guidance postoperatively will be due to the abnormal glenoid fossa and, more importantly, the absence of a lateral pterygoid attachment to permit translation. If a rudimentary lateral pterygoid is present, its attachment to the costochondral graft may be helpful. To improve translation of the joint postoperatively, active physical therapy is indicated.

The determination of the final functional position of the condyle is often problematic after costochondral grafting. In addition, difficulty in developing normal functional movements of the reconstructed joint is often encountered. The occlusion may undergo continuous changes as the graft remodels. Monitoring of masticatory function and intervention with physical therapy, splint changes, and orthodontics is indicated.

Comprehensive skeletal repair of the deformities associated with hemifacial microsomia requires complex orthognathic surgery when growth is nearly complete. The patient is treated when dentition is completed. Preoperative orthodontics is performed to eliminate associated dental compensations. No orthognathic surgery is planned during growth because the future growth pattern is unpredictable.

Comprehensive skeletal correction generally requires Le Fort I osteotomy to correct the canted occlusal plane and the rotation of the maxilla toward the defect. Interpositional bone grafting is usually necessary to correct the vertical deficiency. Surgical expansion of the palatal width may be performed. Sagittal split osteotomy on the unaffected side is necessary to produce rotation and advancement. The affected side may also be treated by sagittal split osteotomy in mild cases. More severe cases, as previously discussed, require costochondral grafting. Genioplasty for augmentation completes the symmetric restoration of the mandible.[15] Secondary rhinoplasty and facial recontouring may be indicated (Fig. 13–9).

Soft tissue correction in hemifacial microsomia requires the initial repair of any facial cleft and is performed in the infant. Correction of deformities of the auricle may be performed during the patient's childhood. Soft tissue augmentation of the face may be performed with alloplasts or with free tissue transfers.

Correction of the psychosocial stigmata of hemifacial microsomia requires careful attention to resolving the functional and aesthetic problems that occur during growth and development. A multidisciplinary approach and careful attention to the timing of clinical and surgical procedures help in obtaining optimal results.

CONDYLAR HYPERPLASIA

During growth of the facial skeleton, equal and coordinated growth of the condyles is necessary to produce a symmetric face and normal dental occlusion. In adulthood, the maintenance of condylar symmetry depends on a variety of functional and biologic factors. Disturbances in the growth pattern of a condyle during the normal growth period or during adulthood may result in condylar hyperplasia. Condylar hyperplasia is generally a slowly developing enlargement of the condyle and condylar neck that results in malocclusion and facial asymmetry (Fig. 13–10).

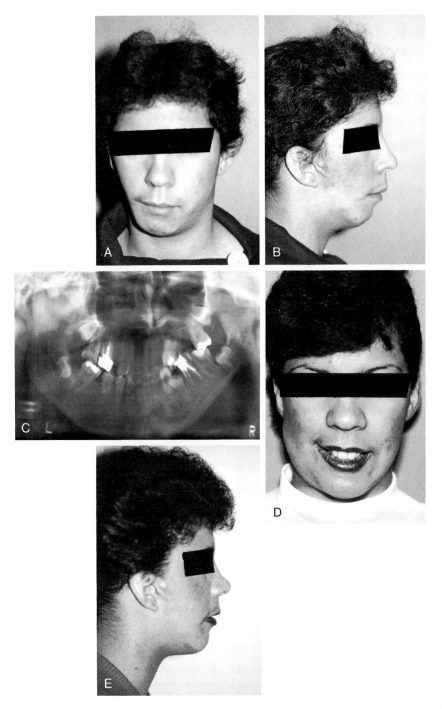

FIGURE 13–9. *A* to *E,* Treatment of hemifacial microsomia. Mandibular and maxillary osteotomies and bone graft augmentation were used to correct the deformity.

Excessive growth of one condyle is only rarely noted in preadolescence. The postpubertal period is a frequent time for asymmetric growth of the condyles, as this is a period when a great deal of vertical growth occurs in the posterior part of the face. Condylar growth in hyperplasia may continue into the third and fourth decades of life.

The differential diagnosis of a developing facial and occlusal asymmetry must include neo-

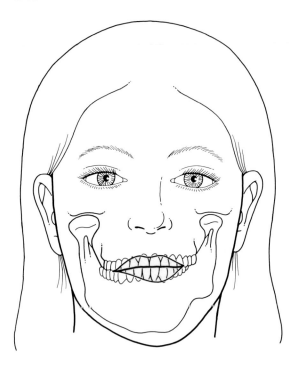

FIGURE 13–10. Schematic of condylar hyperplasia. Note the enlarged condyle and the compensations in mandibular form and asymmetry.

plasm, inflammation, and diseases of the opposite side. These diseases include hemifacial microsomia, hemifacial atrophy, and degenerative joint disease. An overall asymmetric development of the face may also occur without a specific increase in condylar growth activity. As the description of the physical findings in this lesion indicates, the differentiation between primary growth patterns and compensatory changes can be difficult. Imaging of both condyles is necessary to help differentiate these lesions. The use of technetium 99m diphosphonate bone scans may assist in the differential diagnosis by assessing the degree of bone turnover in the affected areas.[16] Active condylar hyperplasia demonstrates increased uptake of radionuclide on the hyperplastic side.

Physical Findings During Growth and Development

The occlusal changes noted in condylar hyperplasia are due to the displacement of the dental arch and the resulting dental compensation. Generally, laterognathia and cross bite on the opposite side occur (Fig. 13–11). A class III malocclusion is usually present on the affected side. An overall class III malocclusion with deviation may represent prognathism with condylar hyperplasia (Fig. 13–12). If hyperplasia is occurring rapidly a posterior open

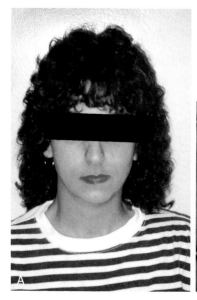
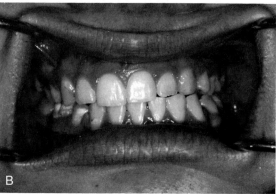

FIGURE 13–11. *A* and *B*, Laterognathia in condylar hyperplasia. Note the deviation of the mandibular dental midline and the cross bite. These correspond to the facial asymmetry.

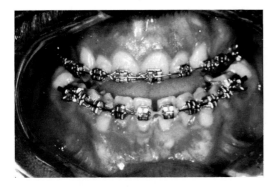

FIGURE 13–12. Deviation prognathism with condylar hyperplasia. Excessive growth of one condyle has occurred within the context of overall mandibular prognathism.

the mandible on the affected side (see Fig. 13–10). Both the maxillary and mandibular occlusal planes are canted.

Skeletally, the chin and mandibular body are deviated away from the hyperplastic side. Canting of the occlusal plane in the maxilla may result in deviation of the nasal septum. Malar hypertrophy may be noted on the affected side. The condyle is generally well formed with only minor morphologic variation. The size of the condylar neck is also relatively increased. If gross abnormality in the condylar form is noted, neoplasm must be suspected.

Treatment

Treatment of condylar hyperplasia depends on when the lesion is detected. If active growth is continuing, the decision toward surgical intervention must include removal of the growth center. If, however, the growth pattern is complete, conventional orthognathic surgical correction can be undertaken. Assessment as to

bite is noted, along with a cant of the mandibular occlusal plane (Fig. 13–13). If growth is slower the teeth erupt into the space being created. This pattern results in a closed bite posteriorly but an increased height of the body of

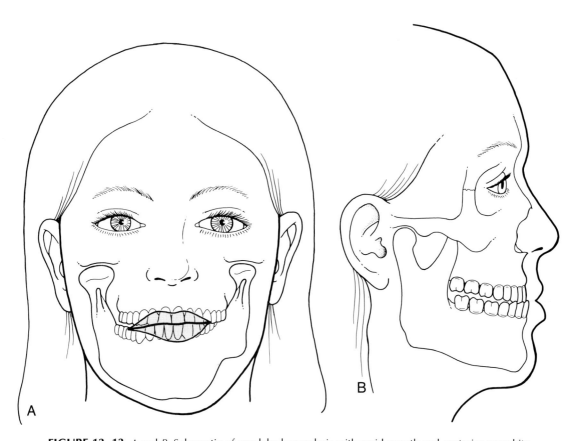

FIGURE 13–13. *A* and *B*, Schematic of condylar hyperplasia with rapid growth and posterior open bite.

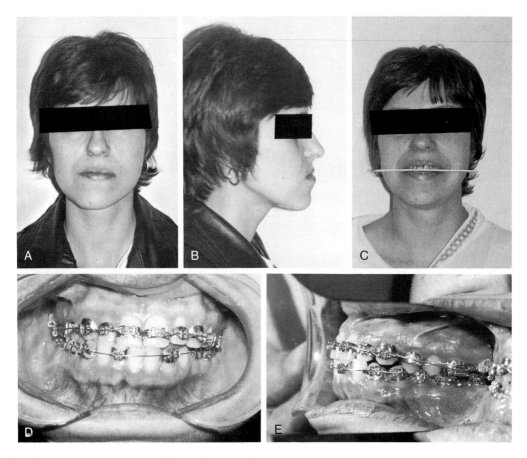

FIGURE 13–14. *A* to *I*, Treatment of condylar hyperplasia. Preoperative orthodontics (*D* to *F*) has eliminated dental compensations in preparation for maxillary and mandibular osteotomies.

whether abnormal growth is continuing is critical in determining the optimal treatment course. The age of the patient does not offer meaningful information as to whether growth is continuing. Long-term orthodontic, cephalometric, and photographic records are helpful in assessing the current status of growth. Bone scanning offers immediate evidence as to the growth activity of the joint.

In the case of continued active growth of the condyle, resection of the condylar head and joint reconstruction may be performed.[17] The degree of resection may be designed to match the extent of hyperplasia, which may offer a partial correction of the associated occlusal deformity.

If the condylar growth is determined to be complete, preoperative orthodontic therapy is initiated to eliminate dental compensations that occurred during the growth period. No

orthodontic treatment is initiated to correct the asymmetry. Correction of jaw position is completed with osteotomies of the jaws (Fig. 13–14). The surgical treatment plan is designed to (1) level the maxilla, (2) correct its midline, (3) place the osteotomized mandible on the leveled and symmetric maxilla in a functional occlusion, and (4) finish the facial symmetry with mandibuloplasty.

SUMMARY

Growth-acquired malformations of the TMJ may be initiated in utero or during the later courses of maturation. Once abnormal growth occurs, the clinical findings that result compromise function and aesthetics. The accurate diagnosis of the abnormality that initiates this cascade of clinical findings will point the way to successful treatment.

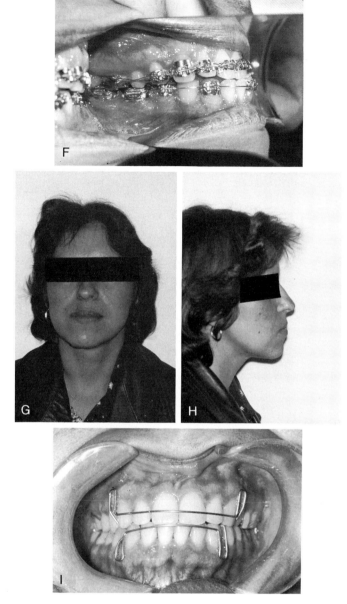

FIGURE 13–14 *Continued* Postoperative examination reveals improvement in occlusion and facial form (*F* to *I*).

REFERENCES

1. Baune, L. and Holy, J.: Ontogenesis of the human temporomandibular joint. 1. Development of the condyles. J. Dent. Res. 41:1327, 1962.
2. Baune, L.: Ontogenesis of the human temporomandibular joint. 2. Development of the temporal components. J. Dent. Res. 49:864, 1970.
3. Yuodelis, R.: The morphogenesis of the human temporomandibular joint and its associated structures. J. Dent. Res. 45:182, 1966.
4. Howerton, D. and Zysset, M.: Anatomy of the temporomandibular joint and related structures with surgical anatomic considerations. Oral Maxillofac. Surg. Clin. North Am. 1:229, 1989.
5. Furstman, L.: Embryology. In *The Temporomandibular Joint.* H. Sarnat and D. Laskin (eds.). Charles C Thomas, Springfield, p 60, 1979.
6. Poswillo, D.: The pathogenesis of the first and second branchial arch syndrome. Oral Surg. 35:302, 1973.
7. Grabb, W.: The first and second branchial arch syndrome. Plast. Reconstr. Surg. 36:485, 1965.

8. Gorlin, R., Pindborg, J., and Cohen, M.: *Syndromes of the Head and Neck,* 2nd ed. McGraw-Hill, New York, p 546, 1976.

9. Poswillo, D.: The pathogenesis of Treacher Collins syndrome (mandibular-facial dysostosis). Br. J. Oral Surg. 13:1, 1975.

10. Johnston, M.: Embryology of the head and neck. In J. McCarthy (ed.). *Plastic Surgery.* W.B. Saunders Co., Philadelphia, p 2491, 1990.

11. Kaban, L.: *Pediatric Oral and Maxillofacial Surgery.* W.B. Saunders Co., Philadelphia, p 278, 1990.

12. Kaban, L., Moses, M., and Mulliken, J.: Surgical correction of hemifacial microsomia in the growing child. Plast. Reconstr. Surg. 82:9, 1988.

13. MacIntosh, B.: Current spectrum of costochondral grafting. In *Surgical Correction of Dentofacial Defor-* *mities, New Concepts.* W. Bell, W. Proffit, and R. White (eds.). W.B. Saunders Co., Philadelphia, 1985.

14. Obwegeser, H.: Correction of the skeletal deformities of otomandibular dysostosis. J. Maxillofac. Surg. 2:73, 1974.

15. Obwegeser, H., Lello, G., and Sailer, H.: Otomandibular dysostosis. In *Surgical Correction of Dentofacial Deformities, New Concepts.* W. Bell, W. Proffit, and R. White (eds.). W.B. Saunders Co., Philadelphia, 1985.

16. Cisneros, G. and Kaban, L.: Computerized skeletal scintigraphy for assessment of mandibular asymmetry. J. Oral Maxillofac. Surg. 42:513–520, 1985.

17. Walker, R.: Condylar hyperplasia. In *Surgical Correction of Dentofacial Deformities, New Concepts.* W. Bell, W. Proffit, and R. White (eds.). W.B. Saunders Co., Philadelphia, 1985.

John E. Fantasia

CHAPTER 14

Neoplasia

Tumors and tumor-like conditions of the temporomandibular joint (TMJ) are extremely rare. Most are presented in the literature as isolated case reports. Further review of the literature, however, leads to a classification schema that reflects the diversity of neoplasia identified at this anatomic site (Table 14–1). Although this classification is not complete, neoplasia arising from any of the various tissues that constitute this synovial articulation is certainly possible, and the schema represents a reasonable formulation that the clinician can use in the workup of the patient.

Symptoms associated with neoplasia of the

TABLE 14–1. Temporomandibular Joint Neoplasia

BENIGN TUMORS AND TUMOR-LIKE CONDITIONS
Osteoma
   (osteoid osteoma)
Chondroblastoma
Chondromyxoid fibroma
Hemangioma
Nonossifying fibroma of bone
Osteochondroma
Synovial chondromatosis
Villonodular synovitis
Central giant cell lesions
Ganglion cyst

PRIMARY MALIGNANT TUMORS
Chondrosarcoma
Synovial sarcoma
Multiple myeloma
   (plasmacytoma)
Malignant germ cell tumor

METASTATIC DISEASE

PRIMARY NEOPLASIA AND METASTATIC DISEASE OF CONTIGUOUS STRUCTURES

NON-NEOPLASTIC CONDITIONS CLINICALLY SUGGESTIVE OF TMJ NEOPLASIA

EXTENSION OF COMMON JAW LESION, WHICH MAY INVOLVE TMJ

joint may include clicking, preauricular swelling, trismus, pain, and jaw deviation. Unfortunately, these symptoms oftentimes are associated with the more common pathologies affecting the joint, such as internal derangements, myofascial pain dysfunction syndromes, arthralgias, arthritides, periarticular angiopathies, traumatic injuries, and infectious processes. Therefore, careful review of the patient's medical history, detailed clinical examination, and use of various diagnostic imaging modalities are often necessary for neoplasia to be included or excluded in the differential diagnosis of temporomandibular disorder.

If neoplasia is a diagnostic consideration biopsy should be carefully planned so as to provide adequate material. Types of biopsy include fine needle aspiration, needle biopsy, incisional biopsy, and excisional biopsy. The type of biopsy done depends on a variety of factors, including location and size of the lesion, medical status of the patient, radiographic interpretation, and index of suspicion for a particular tumor type. A point of caution—because neoplasia of the TMJ is rare and considerable diversity of tumor type exists, fine needle aspiration and needle biopsy are less likely to be representative, thus leading to possible error in diagnosis (e.g., distinction between synovial chondromatosis and chondrosarcoma based on a minimal tissue sample). The surgeon and pathologist should also remember the admonition of Dahlin and Unni,[1] "The pathologist responsible for the diagnosis of osseous lesions is handicapped immeasurably if roentgenographic features are ignored." This certainly applies to TMJ pathology. The surgeon should also consult with the pathologist on the handling of biopsy material because frozen tissue or special fixation may well be indicated for special stains, electron microscopy, and immunohistochemistry of diagnostically challenging cases. Immunohistochemistry is particularly important in assessing metastatic deposits in which the primary lesion is occult or not previously diagnosed.

BENIGN TUMORS

Osteoma

Osteomas are benign tumors of bone that can affect the condyle. Their actual occurrence is debatable, as these lesions are difficult to separate clinically and histologically from enostoses, exostoses, and longstanding osteochondro-

251

mas. Radiologically, these lesions appear as a well-defined radiopacity arising from the condylar head. Papavasiliou and colleagues[2] reviewed the clinical features of 15 cases of osteoma and noted a wide age range and a female predilection. In addition, previous histories of ear infection, surgery, or trauma to the area were reported in seven of the cases. Histologically, the osteoma consists of densely ossified bone that can mimic reactive bony sclerosis. A variant of osteoma, the osteoid osteoma has been reported by Lind and Hillerstrom[3] in the mandibular condyle. The osteoid osteoma consists of a nidus of osteoid trabeculae in a background of fibrovascular tissue. Pain is a frequent clinical finding associated with the osteoid osteoma. The recognized treatment of osteoma of the condyle is condylectomy. Multiple osteoma of the facial bones, including the mandible and maxilla, is a component of intestinal polyposis III (Gardner's syndrome). This syndrome is certainly a diagnostic consideration in any patient who presents with osteoma.

Chondroblastoma

The chondroblastoma is a well-defined benign neoplasm of bone, which is usually located within the medullary cavity. Origin from the cartilage of growth plates has been proposed. Most cases arise in the epiphysis of long bones. However, cases arising in the mandibular condyle[4] and the articular cartilage of the TMJ[5] have been reported. The last example, given by Sparh and colleagues, is of interest because a chondroblastoma associated with a joint without bony involvement had not been previously reported. Too few cases of chondroblastoma of the TMJ have been reported to establish any meaningful clinical data. Histologically, these lesions consist of proliferating chondroblasts with focal zones of chondroid matrix and variable numbers of benign multinucleated giant cells. These lesions can be mistaken for chondrosarcoma, and care must be taken not to misdiagnose this lesion. This tumor is best treated by curettage; however, if the location and anatomy dictate, resection may be indicated.

Chondromyxoid Fibroma

This unusual neoplasm of bone was first described by Jaffe and Lichtenstein in 1948.[6] Review of mandibular involvement has been provided by Grotepass and associates[7] as well as Lustmann and associates.[8] Like many of the cartilage-containing tumors of bone, separation from chondrosarcoma is imperative. The clinical presentation of the mandibular lesions is that of a well-demarcated multilocular radiolucency, with a peak incidence in the second and third decades. Condylar lesions are rare, yet Sellami and coworkers[9] described a chondromyxoid fibroma of the right TMJ in a 32-year-old female, who presented with pain and had evidence of a multilocular condylar radiolucency. The histology of chondromyxoid fibroma is that of loosely arranged, stellate tumor cells within a myxoid background. The overall pattern is characteristically lobulated, with increased cellularity noted at the periphery of the lobules. Treatment should consist of wide excision to include a rim of normal bone. However, too few cases have been reported to be certain of the biologic behavior in the jaws.

Hemangioma

The hemangioma is a vascular neoplasm that commonly involves soft tissues; however, this entity may arise primarily within bone. A specific type of hemangioma, the synovial hemangioma, which most commonly occurs in the knee joint, has been described. This type has been classified as localized and diffuse. Atkinson and colleagues[10] have described such a synovial hemangioma of the TMJ. This lesion was confluent with the synovial membrane in the region of the retrodiscal tissue, extending forward to the posterior pole of the disc. Hemangiomas of bone are usually solitary lesions; however, involvement of overlying soft tissue may sometimes be encountered. Central hemangiomas of bone have been described in the condyle.[11,12] Histopathology of these lesions, be they in bone or soft tissues, demonstrates a proliferation of endothelium-lined channels, which are of varying caliber (e.g., capillary, cavernous, combined capillary/cavernous). Thrombi and phleboliths may be encountered. The presence of the latter is somewhat diagnostic of hemangioma when identified radiographically.

The aforementioned synovial hemangioma was treated with en bloc excision of the mass and discectomy. Because of the degenerative changes of the condyle, a condylectomy was also performed. Surgical excision of the hemangioma is acceptable therapy; however, therapy if any will ultimately be dictated by the size and location of the hemangioma, the medical status of the patient, and the angiographic data. Selective embolization, radiation therapy, sclerosing injections, ligation, and cryosurgery are alternative modalities; yet, the functional aspects of the TMJ limit the use of some of these therapeutic modalities.

Nonossifying Fibroma of Bone

The fibroma of bone typically occurs in the metaphyseal portion of long bone; hence, the synonymous designation of metaphyseal fibrous defect is used. An example in the clavicle has been noted by Dahlin and Unni.[13] The spontaneous resolution of some of these lesions suggests they represent faulty ossification rather than neoplasia. A few of these lesions continue to grow and can cause pathologic fracture. One such fibroma of bone, reported by Nwoka and Koch,[14] caused such a pathologic fracture. This lesion arose in the right condylar head of a 14-year-old male. An additional condylar case has been treated by Toohey;[15] the lesion occurred in a 19-year-old female.

These lesions are composed of a fibroblastic connective tissue arranged in a storiform pattern. Benign multinucleated giant cells may also be seen. Curettage is adequate treatment, yet the extent of a particular lesion may dictate condylectomy. Long bone lesions may be followed radiographically, if clinical and radiographic findings are sufficiently characteristic. However, suspected condylar lesions should be diagnosed and treated. These lesions are exceedingly rare.

Osteochondroma

The osteochondroma or osteocartilaginous exostosis is a common lesion of the axial skeleton. Condylar lesions, as those reported by Loftus and his associates,[16] appear as cartilage-capped exostoses. The most common clinical presentation consists of altered occlusion and development of facial asymmetry. Radiographically, these lesions appear as an irregularly shaped enlargement of the condyle exhibiting varying densities. Grossly, the lesions are lobulated, resulting in deformations of normal condylar morphology. Histologic appearance of the lesion consists of dense spicules of lamellar bone interspersed with fibrous-fatty marrow, with the entire lesion capped by cartilage of varying thickness (Fig. 14–1). Endochondral ossification may be seen. The condylar lesions most typically occur in the third to fifth decades. Males and females are equally affected. Condylectomy is the treatment of choice. Condylar reconstruction may be necessary to normalize mandibular function. Transformation of condylar osteochondroma into chondrosarcoma has not been reported.

Synovial Chondromatosis

Synovial chondromatosis is one of the more commonly reported conditions that affect the TMJ. This condition is characterized by the

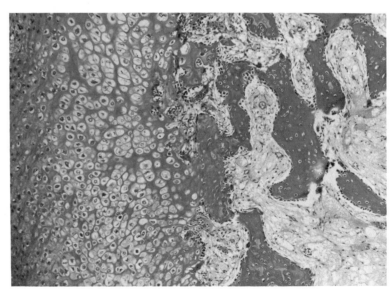

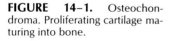

FIGURE 14–1. Osteochondroma. Proliferating cartilage maturing into bone.

formation of multiple foci of hyaline cartilage in synovial and subsynovial connective tissue.[17] The cartilaginous nodules may become detached from the synovium and enter the joint space as loose bodies.[18] The process of synovial chondromatosis is thought to be a metaplastic process rather than true neoplasia. The etiology of this condition is unknown.

Clinical symptoms associated with synovial chondromatosis include preauricular swelling and pain, limited jaw motion, and otalgia.[19] Synovial chondromatosis of the TMJ shows a marked predilection for females in contrast to the male predilection identified in large joint synovial chondromatosis.

Radiographic evaluation includes the panoramic radiograph, which would show cartilaginous nodules if sufficiently calcified. Computerized tomography and magnetic resonance imaging[20] more accurately delineate bone, cartilage, and soft tissues of this pathologic process. The microscopy of synovial chondromatosis exhibits nodules of cartilage, which may be cellular and contain binucleate cells. These nodules are surrounded by a thin layer of synovium. Areas of chondrometaplasia are sometimes identified within the synovial tissues. The cartilaginous loose bodies can undergo calcification or ossification. These loose bodies are nourished by the synovial fluid and can lead to degenerative arthritis. The cartilage of synovial chondromatosis was thought to arise from metaplasia of cells of the synovial membrane, but ultrastructural studies indicate that it arises from metaplasia of the synovial fibroblasts.[21] Microscopically these lesions can be misinterpreted as chondrosarcoma[22] or even as benign mixed tumor of salivary gland origin.[23] It has been reported in the literature that longstanding synovial chondromatosis can undergo malignant transformation.[24] Such malignant transformation, however, is extremely rare and most often reported in the knee, where synovial chondromatosis most commonly occurs.

Several cases of synovial chondromatosis of the TMJ with intracranial extension have been reported.[25,26] In one such case,[26] the patient presented with facial nerve paralysis and anakusis. The facial nerve dysfunction was thought to be secondary to direct neural compression. Treatment of synovial chondromatosis consists of the removal of loose bodies and synovectomy.

Pigmented Villonodular Tenosynovitis

Villonodular synovitis is a rare tumor of the TMJ,[27] most commonly occurring in the knee and hip. Some investigators, however, consider this lesion to be reactive rather than neoplastic and related to similar lesions of bursa and to nodular tenosynovitis (giant cell tumor of the tendon). Repeated intra-articular bleeding and trauma have been suggested as etiologic factors. A localized and diffuse form exists—the localized form being extra-articular, whereas the diffuse form in most instances represents extra-articular extension of a primary intra-articular process.[28] This condition usually affects young adults and has no distinct sex predilection. A palpable mass, accompanying mild pain, and restricted mouth opening are the usual clinical findings.

Radiographically, these lesions may or may not exhibit bone erosion. Computerized tomography with contrast medium demonstrates the extent of this benign disorder of the synovium. Histologically, villous and nodular projections are noted, with a cellular stroma consisting of clusters of oval or rounded cells separated by thickened fibrous connective tissue bands. Multinucleated giant cells and foamy macrophages are common. Abundant hemosiderin is also a consistent finding. Enzinger and Weiss[29] caution that pigmented villonodular synovitis can mimic the inflammatory or xanthomatous forms of malignant fibrous histiocytoma.

A case of TMJ villonodular synovitis has been diagnosed by fine needle aspiration cytology.[30] Two TMJ cases of villonodular synovitis have been reported,[31,32] which occurred simultaneously with synovial chondromatosis.

Central Giant Cell Lesions

The giant cell granuloma is a benign process that occurs almost exclusively in jaw bones.[33] Cases that involve the condylar head have been reported.[14,34] Some of these cases have been called giant cell tumors.[14] However, most investigators believe that giant cell tumor is a distinct entity from giant cell granuloma—the giant cell tumor only rarely affecting the jaws. Care should be taken to distinguish these two different entities, as the giant cell tumor exhibits a more aggressive biologic behavior.

Radiographically, the central giant cell granuloma may be multilocular or less commonly unilocular. The margins of the lesion, however, can sometimes be indistinct. The central giant cell granuloma is composed of spindle-shaped mesenchymal cells in a fibrous stroma. Numerous multinucleated giant cells are a prominent feature, with extravasated red blood cells, hemosiderin, and osteoid scattered throughout the stroma (Fig. 14–2). The treatment of giant cell granuloma is curettage, with removal of the peripheral bony margins. The giant cell granuloma is identical to the giant cell lesions that are associated with hyperparathyroidism. Therefore, evaluation of serum calcium and phosphorus levels, and possibly parathyroid hormone values, is indicated in a patient diagnosed with giant cell lesion of bone.

Interestingly, Sawyer and his associates[35] considered a giant cell granuloma of the condyle in the skeletal remains of a pre-Columbian mummy in Chile that was more than 700 years old.

Ganglion

A ganglion is a cystic structure arising subcutaneously usually in association with tendon sheaths or joints. The wrist is the most common location for this lesion. Barnes[36] emphasizes the distinction between ganglia and synovial cysts. Ganglia are the result of myxoid degeneration of para-articular connective tissue. The resultant cystic lesion is lined by dense fibrous connective tissue and does not communicate with the joint space. Synovial cysts are true cysts lined by synovial cells and may or may not communicate with the joint cavity. Therefore, ganglia and synovial cysts differ in origin and microscopic features.

A ganglion of the TMJ area will most often appear as a relatively painless preauricular swelling.[37,38] Parotid neoplasia, sebaceous cyst, neurofibroma, and lipoma are frequently included in the differential diagnosis. Fluctuation in size can be clinically suggestive of a ganglion. A true synovial cyst of the TMJ has been reported by Shiba and colleagues.[39] This too appeared as a parotid tumor. Surgical excision is the treatment of choice;[40] however, recurrences of ganglia in sites other than the TMJ have been reported. Recurrences are apparently associated with external compression and aspiration not with surgical excision.

PRIMARY MALIGNANT TUMORS
Chondrosarcoma

Chondrosarcoma of the head and neck region is rarely encountered with only a few cases of the TMJ reported.[41–43] This malignant neoplasm may arise from previously normal bone, cartilage, or periosteum, i.e., primary chondrosarcoma, or may develop within a pre-existing benign tumor, i.e., secondary chondrosarcoma. Jaw and TMJ chondrosarcomas are almost always of the primary type.

The clinical symptoms are those of an enlarging mass. A history of rapid growth and pain are also suggestive of a malignant neoplasm. However, mild headache and temporomandibular dysfunction–like symptoms may be the only presenting complaints. Unilateral hearing loss has also been noted as a presenting symptom. Age range is quite variable for the reported condylar chondrosarcomas.

The radiographic appearance of chondrosarcoma is not pathognomonic, as a spectrum of changes can be identified from a widened TMJ

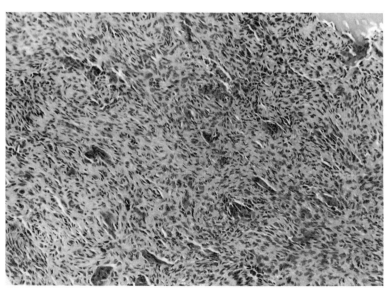

FIGURE 14–2. Central giant cell granuloma. Multinucleated giant cells with proliferating fibroblasts.

space without visible bony erosion to a distinct mass with bone erosion and involvement of surrounding structures. Magnetic resonance imaging and computerized tomography are imperative in the workup of a patient with suspected or biopsy-proven chondrosarcoma. Histologically, the chondrosarcoma can have a well-differentiated appearance with cartilaginous areas, which can be mistaken for an enchondroma or a synovial chondromatosis. In this situation, the clinical behavior, radiographic evidence of destruction, and histologic evidence of invasion are necessary to arrive at a diagnosis of malignancy. Less differentiated chondrosarcomas exhibit varying degrees of cellular hyperchromasia and pleomorphism, with foci of malignant cartilage. Focal calcifications and binucleate cells are also frequent findings (Fig. 14–3). The degree of differentiation appears to influence prognosis. Metastasis to lung is common. Wide resection of the entire lesion is necessary. Adjuvant radiotherapy, chemotherapy, or both have been proposed, particularly if the anatomy of the area precludes as radical a procedure as needed. A thorough review of chondrosarcomas of the jaws has been presented by Garrington and Collett,[44,45] yet specific reference to TMJ chondrosarcoma is not made in their analysis of 37 cases, thus emphasizing the rarity of this tumor in the TMJ area.

Synovial Sarcoma

Synovial sarcoma is a disease that arises in the deep soft tissues, most commonly in the lower extremities. Yet, cases have been reported in the head and neck region, most involving cervical and parapharyngeal sites.[46] DelBalso and colleagues[47] reported a synovial sarcoma that arose in the TMJ of a 22-year-old male. They detailed an approach to diagnostic imaging of the patient who presents with joint dysfunction. An additional case involving the TMJ has also been reported by Dieckmann.[48] Paradoxically, most synovial cell sarcomas occur at sites distant from synovium-lined spaces. Consequently, involvement of the TMJ is most unusual for this rare malignant neoplasm. These lesions most typically occur in young adult males. Orofacial cases most commonly involved the soft tissues of the cheek. Some cases occurring in the parotid region do not appear to arise from the TMJ capsule.[46]

Clinical symptoms include pain, tenderness, and over time a gradually enlarging mass. Radiographically, DelBalso's group[47] stated that their patient with synovial sarcoma exhibited a soft tissue mass in the temporomandibular space extending laterally into masseter muscle and medially around the condyle. At surgery this lesion was found to be adherent to the glenoid fossa. Histologically, synovial sarcoma has a characteristic biphasic pattern consisting of a fibrosarcomatous-like spindle cell population adjacent to epithelioid areas. These epithelioid areas may exhibit gland-like formations. Occasionally, a monophasic histologic pattern might be observed, which leads to confusion with an adenocarcinoma or a fibrosarcoma, depending on which type predominates. Focal zones of microscopic calcifications may also be

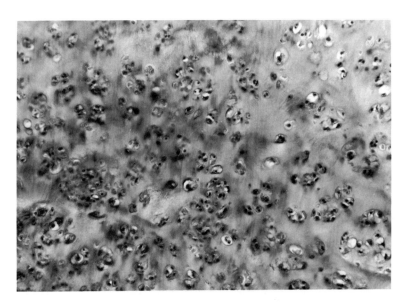

FIGURE 14–3. Chondrosarcoma. Hyaline cartilage containing malignant cells.

identified. Wide surgical excision is the preferred treatment; too few cases make assessment of radiotherapy and chemotherapy difficult. The review of orofacial lesions by Smookler and coworkers[46] emphasizes the extremely aggressive biologic behavior of this malignant neoplasm.

Multiple Myeloma

Myeloma represents a monoclonal proliferation of plasma cells, appearing as a lytic lesion of bone. Soft tissue involvement can also occur. Solitary lesions are referred to as plasmacytoma, but about 70% of patients who have what seems to be a solitary focus eventually develop multiple lesions. Therefore, multiple myeloma is considered a systemic malignant proliferation of plasma cells. These tumors produce abundant immunoglobulin and light chains (kappa or lambda) of the immunoglobulin molecule, which are identifiable in the serum or urine of affected patients. This disease is primarily seen in adults with a peak incidence in the seventh decade.

Pain in the involved bones is the chief clinical symptom. Skull and facial bones are affected in over half the cases, with jaw and TMJ involvement reported on occasion.[49,50] Radiographically, an isolated lytic lesion or multiple lytic lesions of involved sites are appreciated. Sometimes, an osteoporotic radiographic pattern is seen, which can mask the true nature of the causative lesion. Histologically, sheets of well- or poorly differentiated plasma cells are identified. The neoplastic cells have the characteristic features of plasma cells—an eccentric nucleus and an abundant pale basophilic cytoplasm. An amyloid-like substance can be present within the myelomatous infiltrates. The treatment of choice in biopsy-proven cases is primarily chemotherapy. Radiation therapy to an involved area alleviates painful symptoms.

Malignant Germ Cell Tumors

Germ cell tumors represent a diverse group of tumors that primarily occur in infants and children. A review of malignant germ cell tumors of the head and neck region has been presented by Stephenson and colleagues.[51] They reported four such lesions in children, ranging in age from 2 to 44 months. The types of tumors reported were a malignant teratoma with neuroblastoma component, a malignant teratoma with nephroblastoma (Wilms's) component, and two yolk sac carcinomas (endodermal sinus tumors). One of these cases occurred in the TMJ region and extended laterally to the infra-auricular region. The patient was a 23-month-old female.

Metastasis from a gonadal primary teratoma should be ruled out before accepting a head and neck primary teratoma as the diagnosis. Within a teratoma, a variety of mature and identifiable tissues are present, such as skin, bone, smooth muscle, cartilage, and other differentiated tissues. Approximately 5% of head and neck teratomas contain malignant elements; therefore, it is imperative that a teratoma be adequately sampled by the pathologist so as to histologically identify any small foci of malignant germ cell tissue, which may exist and thus adversely affect the prognosis.

Those lesions with malignant features are sensitive to both chemotherapy and irradiation. Complete surgical excision is indicated initially to arrive at the appropriate histopathologic diagnosis. Treatment modality will ultimately be dictated by specific tumor subtype.

METASTATIC DISEASE

Metastatic disease of the TMJ primarily involves the condyle. Symptoms of temporomandibular dysfunction, such as pain, swelling, trismus, or deviation of the mandible, with radiographic evidence of a destructive lesion should suggest the possibility of a malignant process. Metastatic disease should always be considered. A review of the literature by DeBoom and colleagues[52] found 15 such cases, with an additional case of their own. Since this review, additional cases have been reported.[53-58] Most cases of metastatic disease to the condyle are carcinomas, in particular adenocarcinoma. Malignancies of the prostate, breast, lung, colon, and thyroid have the propensity to involve bone. Given the frequency with which these neoplasms occur, they should be considered in the appropriate clinical setting.

Histologic examination of metastatic lesions (Fig. 14–4) does not always result in identification of a primary site.[58] However, with the use of immunohistochemistry, accurate determination of the primary site can sometimes be made. DeBoom's group reported positive identification of a prostatic adenocarcinoma by using immunohistochemical stains for prostate-specific antigen. Such specificity is not always possible, however. As new tumor markers

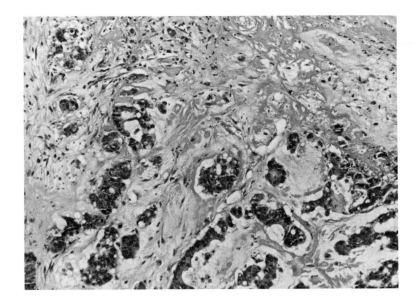

FIGURE 14–4. Metastatic adenocarcinoma. Neoplastic cells exhibiting ductal differentiation.

are identified, greater accuracy of predicting primary sites will be possible in the patient who initially presents with metastatic disease.

Radiographically, an osteolytic lesion is most typical; yet, some metastatic deposits may lead to osteosclerosis. Bone scanning, computerized tomography, or magnetic resonance imaging should be employed to determine the extent of metastatic disease. In most patients with metastatic disease, chemotherapy or irradiation to control pain or localized disease is usually employed. Webster[57] discusses the possible mechanisms of metastasis to bone. A more detailed discussion of the cellular basis for site-specific tumor metastasis has been presented by Zetter.[59]

PRIMARY NEOPLASIA AND METASTATIC DISEASE OF CONTIGUOUS STRUCTURES

Primary neoplasia or metastatic disease of the soft and hard tissues that surround the TMJ must also be considered in the patient with myofascial pain symptoms. A report of neurofibromatosis involving the joint capsule resulting in TMJ dysfunction has been made by Pasturel and colleagues.[60] Sites and cases, which are emphasized, include parotid gland neoplasia[61,62] and temporal bone neoplasia.[63] Tumors that involve these sites may be benign, primary malignancies, or metastases from distant sites.

Correct diagnosis of lesions arising in contig-

uous structures may be difficult in the early stages. Consultations with various specialists and careful followup examinations[61] may be necessary before a diagnosis is made. Tashiro and his associates[64] have reported a case of malignant paraganglioma that manifested itself as pain in the TMJ. Because of the extensiveness of the tumor, the origin could not be confirmed with certainty, yet origin from the glomus jugular was suspected. Har-El and colleagues[65] have reported an angioblastic meningioma. The patient presented with pain in the TMJ. A possible mechanism for such pain based on neuronal pathways was offered. Sinus carcinoma,[66] nasopharyngeal carcinoma,[67,68] tonsillar pillar carcinoma,[68] and perineural invasion by adenoid cystic carcinoma[69] have been reported to cause temporomandibular symptoms.

In addition, jaw claudication and its various causes,[70] geriatric headache,[71] periarticular angiopathies,[72] and traumatic neuroma[73] may appear as temporomandibular symptoms suggestive of neoplasia. Conversely, neoplasia of the TMJ can certainly be misinterpreted as any of the aforementioned conditions.

Multicentric reticulohistiocytosis is a rare disease that is characterized clinically by the combination of polyarthritis and numerous nodules of the skin and mucosa. This condition and its oral manifestations have been reviewed by Katz and Anderson.[74] A case report by Yoshimura and coworkers[75] details the temporomandibular manifestations of this condition.

CONDITIONS CLINICALLY SUGGESTIVE OF TEMPOROMANDIBULAR JOINT NEOPLASIA

This category consists of several related non-neoplastic conditions, which may suggest neoplasia of the TMJ and associated surrounding structures. A case that best exemplifies some of these clinical situations is that of the gouty tophus in the TMJ reported by Faas.[76] This gouty tophus caused destruction of the TMJ and displaced the upper pole of the parotid and impinged on the eustachian tube, causing conduction-type deafness.

Zemplenyi and Calcaterra[77] reported a similar clinical situation caused by chondrocalcinosis. This condition is characterized by deposition of calcium pyrophosphate dehydrate crystals. Arthropathy due to pyrophosphate deposition as a tumor simulating disease of the TMJ has likewise been reported by Sailer and Makek.[78]

EXTENSION OF COMMON JAW LESIONS

Common jaw lesions that typically involve the body or the ramus, or both, of the mandible could extend to and involve the condyle as well. These types of lesions include ameloblastoma, odontogenic keratocyst, central giant cell granuloma, traumatic bone cyst, bone hemangioma, osteoporotic marrow defect, and eosinophilic granuloma (Langerhans's cell granulomatosis). Teeth have also been reported in the condyle.[79]

Additional reviews on the subject of TMJ neoplasia have been presented by Thoma[80,81] and by Gorlin and Goldman.[82] Readers are referred to these reviews for an historical perspective on this topic.

REFERENCES

1. Dahlin, D. and Unni, K.: *Bone Tumors,* 4th ed. Charles C Thomas, Springfield, IL, p 4, 1986.
2. Papavasiliou, A., Sawyer, R., Lund, V., and Michaels, L.: Benign conditions of the temporomandibular joint: a diagnostic dilemma. Br. J. Oral Surg. 21:222–228, 1983.
3. Lind, P. and Hillerstrom, K. Osteoid osteoma in the mandibular condyle. Acta Otolaryngol. 57:467, 1963.
4. Goodsell, J. and Hubinger, H.: Benign chondroblastoma of mandibular condyle: Report of a case. J. Oral Surg. 22:355–363, 1964.
5. Spahr, J., Elzay, R., Kay, S., and Frabble, W.: Chondroblastoma of the temporomandibular joint arising from articular cartilage: A previously unreported presentation of an uncommon neoplasm. Oral Surg. Oral Med. Oral Pathol. 54:430–435, 1982.
6. Jaffe, H. and Lichtenstein, L.: Chondromyxoid fibroma of bone. A distinctive benign tumor likely to be mistaken especially for chondrosarcoma. Arch Pathol. 45:541–551, 1948.
7. Grotepass, F., Farman, A., and Nortje, C.: Chondromyxoid fibroma of the mandible. J. Oral Surg. 34:988–994, 1976.
8. Lustmann, J., Gazit, D., Ulmansky, M., and Lewin-Epstein, J.: Chondromyxoid fibroma of the jaws: A clinicopathologic study. J. Oral Pathol. 15:343–346, 1986.
9. Sellami, M., Doyon, D., Deboise, A., and Laudenbach, P.: Chondromyxoid fibroma of the temporomandibular joint. Apropos of a case report. J. Radiol. 65:97–100, 1984.
10. Atkinson, T., Wolf, S., Anavi, Y., and Wesley, R.: Synovial hemangioma of the temporomandibular joint: Report of a case and review of the literature. J. Oral Maxillofac. Surg. 46:804–808, 1988.
11. Maclennan, W.: Haemangioma of the mandibular condylar process. Br. Dent. J. 105:93, 1958.
12. Uotila, E. and Westerholm, N.: Hemangioma of the temporomandibular joint. Odontol. T. 74:202, 1966.
13. Dahlin, D. and Unni, K.: *Bone Tumors,* 4th ed. Charles C Thomas, Springfield, IL, p 151, 1986.
14. Nwoku, A. and Koch, H.: The temporomandibular joint: A rare localisation for bone tumors. J. Maxillofac. Surg. 2:113–119, 1974.
15. Toohey, M.: Personal communication, 1990.
16. Loftus, M., Bennett, J., and Fantasia, J.: Osteochondroma of the mandibular condyles. Oral Surg. Oral Med. Oral Pathol. 61:221–226, 1986.
17. Forssell, K., Happonen, R., and Forssell, H.: Synovial chondromatosis of the temporomandibular joint. Report of a case and review of the literature. Int. J. Oral Maxillofac. Surg. 17:237–241, 1988.
18. Norman, J., Stevenson, A., Painter, D., et al: Synovial osteochondrosis of the temporomandibular joint. An historical review with presentation of 3 cases. J. Craniomaxillofac. Surg. 16:212–220, 1988.
19. Cannon, C.: Osteochondrosis of the temporomandibular joint presenting as an apparent parotid mass. Ann. Otol. Rhinol. Laryngol. 96:330–332, 1987.
20. Dolan, E., Vogler, J., and Angelillo, J.: Synovial chondromatosis of the temporomandibular joint diagnosed by magnetic resonance imaging: Report of a case. J. Oral Maxillofac. Surg. 47:411–413, 1989.
21. deBont, L., Liem, R., and Boering, G.: Synovial chondromatosis of the temporomandibular joint: A light and electron microscopic study. Oral Surg. Oral Med. Oral Pathol. 66:593–598, 1988.
22. Murphy, F., Dehlin, D., and Sullivan, C.: Articular synovial chondromatosis. J. Bone Joint Surg. 44:77–86, 1962.
23. Thompson, K., Schwartz, H., and Miles, J.: Synovial chondromatosis of the temporomandibular joint presenting as a parotid mass: Possibility of confusion with benign mixed tumor. Oral Surg. Oral Med. Oral Pathol. 62:377–380, 1986.
24. Perry, B., McQueen, D., and Lin, J.: Synovial chondromatosis with malignant degeneration to chondrosarcoma. Report of a case. J. Bone Joint Surg. 70A:1259–1261, 1988.
25. Nokes, S., King, P., Garcia, R., et al: Temporomandibular joint chondromatosis with intracranial exten-

sion: MR and CT contributions. Am. J. Radiol. 148:1173–1174, 1987.

26. Daspit, C. and Spetzler, R.: Synovial chondromatosis of the temporomandibular joint with intracranial extension. Case report. J. Neurosurg. 70:121–123, 1989.

27. O'Sullivan, T., Alport, E., and Whiston, H.: Pigmented villonodular synovitis of the temporomandibular joint. J. Otolaryngol. 13:123–126, 1984.

28. Barnes, L.: *Surgical Pathology of the Head and Neck,* vol 2. Marcel Dekker, New York, pp 891–892, 1985.

29. Enzinger, F. and Weiss, S.: *Soft Tissue Tumors,* 2nd ed. C.V. Mosby Co., St. Louis, pp 638–658, 1988.

30. Dawiskiba, S., Eriksson, L., Elner, A., et al: Diffuse pigmented villonodular synovitis of the temporomandibular joint diagnosed by fine-needle aspiration cytology. Diagn. Cytopathol. 5:301–304, 1989.

31. Raibley, S.: Villonodular synovitis with synovial chondromatosis. Oral Surg. Oral Med. Oral Pathol. 44:279–284, 1977.

32. Takagi, M. and Ishikawa, G.: Simultaneous villonodular synovitis and synovial chondromatosis of the temporomandibular joint. Report of a case. J. Oral Surg. 39:699–701, 1981.

33. Stewart, J.: Benign non-odontogenic tumors. In *Oral Pathology. Clinical-Pathologic Correlations.* J. Regezi and J. Sciubba (eds.). W.B. Saunders Co., Philadelphia, pp 379–382, 1989.

34. Kochan, E.: Reparative giant cell granuloma: J. Oral Surg. 21:390–395, 1963.

35. Sawyer, D., Wood, N., and Allison, M.A.: Condylar tumor from pre-Columbian Chile: A case report. Oral Surg. Oral Med. Oral Pathol. 66:400–403, 1988.

36. Barnes, L.: *Surgical Pathology of the Head and Neck,* vol 2. Marcel Dekker, New York, pp 892–893, 1985.

37. Copeland, M. and Douglas, B.: Ganglions of the temporomandibular joint: Case report and review of the literature. Plast. Reconstr. Surg. 81:775–776, 1988.

38. El-Massry, M. and Bailey, B.: Ganglion of the temporomandibular joint. Case report and literature survey. Br. J. Oral Maxillofac. Surg. 27:67–70, 1989.

39. Shiba, R., Suyama, T., and Sakoda, S.: Ganglion of the temporomandibular joint. J. Oral Maxillofac. Surg. 45:618–621, 1987.

40. Gray, L.: Ganglions of the temporomandibular joint [Letter]. Plast. Reconstr. Surg. 83:574, 1989.

41. Richter, K., Freeman, N., and Quick, C.: Chondrosarcoma of the temporomandibular joint: Report of a case. J. Oral Surg. 32:777–781, 1974.

42. Nortje, C., Farman, A., Grotepass, F., and Vanzyl J.: Chondrosarcoma of the mandibular condyle. Report of a case with special reference to the radiographic features. Br. J. Oral Surg. 14:101–111, 1976.

43. Morris, M., Clark, S., Porter, B., and Delbecq, R.: Chondrosarcoma of the temporomandibular joint: Case report. Head Neck Surg. 10:113–117, 1987.

44. Garrington, G. and Collett, W.: Chondrosarcoma. I. A selected literature review. J. Oral Pathol. 17:1–11, 1988.

45. Garrington, G. and Collett, W.: Chondrosarcoma. II. Chondrosarcoma of the jaws: Analysis of 37 cases. J. Oral Pathol. 17:12–20, 1988.

46. Smookler, B., Enzinger, F., and Brannon, R.: Orofacial synovial sarcoma. A clinicopathologic study of 11 new cases and a review of the literature. Cancer 50:269–276, 1982.

47. DelBalso, A., Pyatt, M., Busch, R., et al: Synovial cell sarcoma of the temporomandibular joint. Computed tomographic findings. Arch. Otolaryngol. 108:520–522, 1982.

48. Dieckmann, J.: Malignant synovioma of the temporomandibular joint. Deutsche Zahnaerztl Zeit. 27:853–857, 1972.

49. Hereb, I., Gyenes, V., and Szabo, G.: Multiple myeloma involving the temporomandibular joint. Fogorv. Sz. 77:105–108, 1984.

50. Ferrari-Parabita, G., Derada-Troletti, G., Soardi, C., and Zane, A.: Il plasmocitoma solitario dei mascellari. Descrizione di un caso a localizzazione mandibolare. Minerva Stomatol. 34:263–269, 1985.

51. Stephenson, J., Mayland, D., Kun, L., et al: Malignant germ cell tumors of the head and neck in childhood. Laryngoscope 99:732–735, 1989.

52. DeBoom, G., Jensen, J., Siegel, W., and Bloom, C.: Metastatic tumors of the mandibular condyle. Review of the literature and report of a case. Oral Surg. Oral Med. Oral Pathol. 60:512–516, 1985.

53. Sailer, H. and Makek, M.: Metastatic arthropathy of the temporomandibular joint. Schweiz. Monatsschr. Zahnmed. 95:377–389, 1985.

54. Hecker, R., Noon, W., and Elliot M.: Adenocarcinoma metastatic to the temporomandibular joint. J. Oral Maxillofac. Surg. 43:629–631, 1985.

55. Owen, D. and Stelling, C.: Condylar metastasis with initial presentation as TMJ syndrome. J. Oral Med. 40:198–201, 1985.

56. Sokolov, A., Klimenko, V., Anisimova, L., and Khorakhorina, S.: Metastasis of adenocarcinoma of the breast to the temporomandibular joint. Two cases. Vopr. Onkol. 32:95–96, 1986.

57. Webster, K.: Adenocarcinoma metastatic to the mandibular condyle. J. Craniomaxillofac. Surg. 16:230–232, 1987.

58. Rubin, M., Jui, V., and Cozzi, G.: Metastatic carcinoma of the mandibular condyle presenting as temporomandibular joint syndrome. J. Oral Maxillofac. Surg. 47:507–510, 1989.

59. Zetter, B.: The cellular basis of site-specific tumor metastasis. N. Engl. J. Med. 322:605–612, 1990.

60. Pasturel, A., Bellavoir, A., Cantaloube, D., et al: Temporomandibular joint dysfunction and neurofibromatosis. Apropos of a case. Rev. Stomatol. Chir. Maxillofac. 90:17–19, 1989.

61. Kaplan, A., Som, P., and Lawson, W.: The coexistence of myofascial pain dysfunction and mucoepidermoid carcinoma of the parotid gland. Report of case. J. Am. Dent. Assoc. 112:495–496, 1986.

62. Grace, E. and North, A.: Temporomandibular joint dysfunction and orofacial pain caused by parotid gland malignancy: Report of case. J. Am. Dent. Assoc. 116:348–350, 1988.

63. Worthington, P.: Secondary malignant tumor of the temporal bone presenting as jaw joint dysfunction. J. Laryngol. Otol. 97:1157–1161, 1983.

64. Tashiro, M., Nagase, M., Nakajima, T., et al: Malignant paraganglioma. Report of a case and review of the Japanese literature. J. Craniomaxillofac. Surg. 16:324–329, 1988.

65. Har-El, G., Calderon, S., and Sandbank, J.: Angioblastic meningioma presenting as a pain in the temporomandibular joint. J. Oral Maxillofac. Surg. 45:338–340, 1987.

66. Christiansen, E., Thompson, J., and Appleton, S.: Temporomandibular joint pain/dysfunction overlying more insidious diseases: Report of two cases. J. Oral Maxillofac. Surg. 45:335–337, 1987.

67. Roistacher, S. and Tanenbaum, D.: Myofascial pain associated with oropharyngeal cancer. Oral Surg. Oral Med. Oral Pathol. 61:459–462, 1986.

68. Cohen, S. and Quinn, P.: Facial trismus and myofascial pain associated with infections and malignant disease. Report of five cases. Oral Surg. Oral Med. Oral Pathol. 65:538–544, 1988.

69. Goss, A., Speculand, B., and Hallet, E.: Diagnosis of temporomandibular joint pain in patients seen at a pain clinic. J. Oral Maxillofac. Surg. 43:110–114, 1985.

70. Goodman, B. and Shepard, F.: Jaw claudication. Its value as a diagnostic clue. Postgrad. Med. 73:177–183, 1983.

71. Rapoport, A., Sheftell, F., and Baskin, S.: Geriatric headaches. Geriatrics 38:81–83, 1983.

72. Hardt, N. and Paulus, G.: Periarticular angiopathies and tumors as the cause of chronic pain in the temporomandibular joint area. Schweiz. Monatsschr. Zahnmed. 94:409–418, 1984.

73. Chau, M., Jonsson, E., and Lee, K.: Traumatic neuroma following sagittal mandibular osteotomy. Int. J. Oral Maxillofac. Surg. 18:95–98, 1989.

74. Katz, R. and Anderson, K.: Multicentric reticulohistiocytosis. Oral Surg. Oral Med. Oral Pathol. 65:721–725, 1988.

75. Yoshimura, Y., Sugihara, T., Kishimoto, H., and Na-gaoka, S.: Multicentric reticulohistiocytosis accompanied by oral and temporomandibular joint manifestation. J. Oral Maxillofac. Surg. 45:84–86, 1987.

76. Faas, I.: A gouty tophus in the temporomandibular joint and on the eustachian tube. Laryngol. Rhinol. Otol. Stuttg. 62:574–577, 1983.

77. Zemplenyi, J. and Calcaterra, T.: Chondrocalcinosis of the temporomandibular joint. A parotid pseudotumor. Arch. Otolaryngol. 111:403–405, 1985.

78. Sailer, H. and Makek, M.: Arthropathy due to pyrophosphate deposition as a tumor-simulating disease of the temporomandibular joint. Schweiz. Monatsschr. Zahnmed. 96:594–603, 1986.

79. Yusuf, Y. and Quayle, A.: Intracondylar tooth. Int. J. Oral Maxillofac. Surg. 18:323–324, 1989.

80. Thoma, K.: Tumors of the condyle and temporomandibular joint. Oral Surg. Oral Med. Oral Pathol. 7:1091–1107, 1954.

81. Thoma, K.: Tumors of the temporomandibular joint. J. Oral Surg. 22:157–163, 1964.

82. Gorlin, R. and Goldman, H.: *Thoma's Oral Pathology,* 6th ed. C.V. Mosby Co., St Louis, pp 594–596, 1970.

Michael J. Bergstein
William Lawson
Peter Som

C H A P T E R   1 5

Diseases That Mimic Temporomandibular Disorders

In the past several years, temporomandibular (TM) disorders have received much attention in the public media and in medical and dental literature. This has increased awareness, resulting in many nonspecialized medical and dental practitioners' treating patients with otalgia for presumed TM disorders without adequate evaluation.[1-3] Radiologic examination of the temporomandibular joint (TMJ), although a necessary part of the evaluation, results in negative findings in 86% of cases.[4] Consequently, it is imperative that the clinician obtain a comprehensive medical history as well as perform a thorough physical examination in a patient in whom the diagnosis of a TM disorder is entertained.

It is very common for the dentist or oral and maxillofacial surgeon to be referred a patient who is already labeled as having a "TMJ syndrome." As the dentist is often the final link before treatment is instituted in such a patient, the clinician must understand the various diagnostic possibilities.

The variety of diseases that may masquerade as TM disorders serves as an obstacle to establishing a correct diagnosis.[5] The syndrome originally described by Costen[6,7] involves tinnitus, TMJ clicking, periauricular pain, headache, trismus, and aural fullness. Others have added hearing loss and vertigo to the constellation of symptoms.[8-10] A great number of diseases manifest themselves with these symptoms and thus mimic TM disorders.

It is our purpose in this chapter to provide a differential diagnosis that must be considered when evaluating a patient who presents with these signs and symptoms. Clinicians must develop a planned and systematic approach to patients with complaints of TMJ pain, otherwise they risk overlooking more serious conditions, which carry increased morbidity and, in some instances, mortality.[2,11,19] Accordingly, if it hasn't already been done, the consulting dentist should be able to perform a comprehensive examination or should refer the patient for further evaluation when warranted. This should include a complete otologic evaluation with a view of the external auditory canal and tympanum, looking for vesicular eruptions or middle ear pathology (e.g., otitis media). In addition to a complete oral cavity and oropharyngeal examination, the nasopharynx, hypopharynx, and larynx should be inspected to rule out lesions that might be responsible for referred pain to the ear.

The dentist should be capable of performing an adequate neck examination, looking for signs (e.g., lymphadenopathy) that may herald the presence of an occult malignancy. A paucity of neurologic and physical findings often is the experience in these patients, making a careful and detailed history of symptoms an invaluable aid in determining the correct diagnosis.

REFERRED PAIN

Pain is considered referred if the origin of the irritative lesion is some distance from the site at which the pain is perceived. The anatomic basis for this phenomenon is that pain is referred from one region to another by sensory nerves that share a common segment within the grey matter of the spinal cord.[20]

Knowledge of the neural innervation of this region is necessary to understand the pathways by which pain is referred in extra-articular disorders. The sensory innervation of the region surrounding the TMJ is supplied by four cranial nerves (V, VII, IX, and X) and two cervical nerves (C1, C2). Trigeminal pain is referred to the region anterior to the tragus by way of the auriculotemporal branch of the third division. Lesions involving the floor of the mouth, teeth, mandible, anterior two thirds of the tongue, palate, paranasal sinuses, and infratemporal fossa can result in pain directed to this same region by the trigeminal nerve.[13,21,24]

Pain involving the sensory branch of the facial nerve is transmitted by way of the nervus intermedius. The pain is felt in the external au-

262

ditory canal and postauricular regions. Patients with lesions involving the geniculate ganglion (e.g., Ramsay Hunt syndrome) as well as tumors of the seventh nerve have reported pain in the TMJ region.[21,25]

Glossopharyngeal referred pain travels from the region of the tonsils, eustachian tube, posterior base of the tongue, and nasopharynx to the petrosal ganglion and down through the nerve of Jacobson to the middle ear.[25] Careful evaluation of these regions is necessary to be certain that they are devoid of a lesion.

Pains arising in the regions of the head and neck innervated by branches of the vagus nerve are also referred to the external auditory canal. The superior laryngeal nerve is responsible for sensation to the hypopharynx, larynx, and trachea. Pain travels via the nodose ganglion, with the auricular branch of the vagus nerve (Arnold's nerve) being responsible for referral to the ear.

Pain involving the cervical region is referred to the posterior aspect of the pinna and mastoid region through the greater auricular nerve and lesser occipital nerve, both of which are branches of C2,C3. Myalgic and arthritic as well as neoplastic diseases involving the cervical region must be considered in the evaluation of the patient with TMJ pain.

DIFFERENTIAL DIAGNOSIS

A knowledge of the differential diagnosis of the disorders that can appear as a TM disorder is essential for the dentist. Temporomandibular joint pain may be due to pathology in a contiguous site or may be referred from a remote site. The patient is capable only of identifying the site where the pain is felt and not the location of its source.[27] Therefore, a comprehensive and careful search of the head and neck is necessary to ascertain the correct diagnosis.

Vascular Syndromes

Carotidynia. Carotidynia is a not uncommon cause of head and neck pain. It is considered a variant of migraine, and a history of migraine often can be elicited from the patient or family.[28] The patient generally presents with recurrent throbbing and facial and neck pain that usually lasts for several weeks, with some episodes even lasting months. Some patients experience only one episode of pain, whereas others experience recurrent episodes of pain with symptom-free intervals, lasting weeks to months.[29]

The most common physical finding is marked tenderness at the bifurcation of the common carotid artery and often along the external carotid artery.[29] The artery may be enlarged, occasionally with edema of the ipsilateral neck. Palpation over the artery often reproduces the patient's pain. The etiology of this condition is unknown, but the pain is believed to be secondary to vasodilation of the artery and nonspecific arteritis.[28] The syndrome is usually a self-limiting one with the patient showing a good response to medical therapy with salicylates and steroids.

Temporal Arteritis. Temporal arteritis, also called giant cell and cranial arteritis, is a vascular inflammatory disease of unknown etiology.[3,21,30] The disease has a predilection for whites over the age of 55 years, with a female-to-male predominance of 2:1.[31]

Patients usually present with constitutional symptoms of fever, fatigue, prostration, and weight loss.[3] Headache is the most common complaint and the initial symptom in two thirds of all patients.[32] In half the cases, the presenting symptom is painful mastication.[33] Pain often also occurs in the ear, mandible, teeth, scalp, and neck.[33] Physical examination reveals a prominent, tortuous, very tender, and enlarged temporal artery.[30,31] In most cases, there is an elevated erythrocyte sedimentation rate (ESR), often greater than 100 mm/hr. Yet, in some cases of documented temporal arteritis, the ESR has persistently remained at normal levels.

Partial or complete loss of vision is the most dreaded consequence of temporal arteritis and occurs in at least one third of all cases.[21,30] The blindness is secondary to occlusion of the retinal artery, with ischemia of the optic nerve. Visual loss, once it occurs, is permanent. Its occurrence is often not preceded by other ocular symptoms. Selsky and colleagues[3] described an elderly white female with complaints of otalgia. She was treated, despite persistent pain for 3 months, presuming a diagnosis of a TM disorder. One morning, the patient awoke with sudden and complete bilateral visual loss. The diagnosis of temporal arteritis was eventually confirmed.

Although biopsy of the temporal artery is confirmatory, therapy should not be delayed in cases in which a high index of suspicion exists. Treatment avoids this potential and catastrophic complication of vision loss. Therapy should be initiated, as soon as the diagnosis is made, with prednisone—40 to 60 mg daily. Prednisone alleviates the patient's symptoms and prevents ocular complications.

Eagle's Syndrome

Eagle originally described this syndrome in patients who develop oral and facial pain after tonsillectomy.[35,36] Typically, patients describe a vague facial pain, referable to the ipsilateral ear. Other symptoms include dysphagia, pain on turning the head or opening the mouth, a foreign body sensation in the throat, and headache.[36–38]

On physical examination, digital palpation of the tonsillar fossa on the affected side elicits the pain. The clinician may also be able to detect a firm, immobile bony point in the tonsillar fossa. Radiographs disclose an elongated styloid process. This elongation is secondary to mineralization of the stylohyoid-stylomandibular complex.[37] Only 4% of the population have an elongated styloid process, and only 4% of these patients develop symptoms referable to this area.[39]

Correll and Wescott[37] described a patient who was treated extensively by multiple medical and surgical specialists for 3 years for a presumed "TMJ-myofascial syndrome." The true diagnosis was finally achieved when palpation of a bony structure in the tonsillar fossa elicited the same pain. In other cases, the similarity of this pain to that produced by impacted teeth has led to needless extractions, in the hope of alleviating the pain.[40]

Treatment of this condition is by excision of the styloid process. However, symptomatic improvement has been reported with steroid and lidocaine injections into the tonsillar fossa.[41]

Neuralgic Pain

Neurogenous pain from a pathologic change in the nerves of the head and neck must be considered if all other sources of referred pain have been eliminated. The major neuralgias in the head and neck region are trigeminal, glossopharyngeal, sphenopalatine, and atypical facial.

Most neuralgias share the following common features:[27,28]

1. A "trigger area" or region where light stimulation produces severe pain in the sensory distribution of that nerve.
2. Pain that is paroxysmal in nature.

3. Pain that does not awaken the patient at night from sleep.
4. Pain that is unilateral.

Trigeminal Neuralgia. Trigeminal neuralgia—tic douloureux—is one of the most painful of all conditions known to humankind.[27,38,42] A misdiagnosis of dental disease is very commonly made and is responsible for many patients' having unnecessary dental extractions early in treatment.[42]

The pain is unilateral but in time may become bilateral; however, initial bilateral involvement is almost never seen. At the onset, the attacks of pain are described as burning, shock-like, and shooting,[43] with frequent radiation of pain to the ear, jaw, and TM region. The pain is paroxysmal and recurrent, usually lasting seconds to minutes. Periods of spontaneous total remission occur, which may span several months or even years. With time, the attacks increase in frequency, leaving the patient with a persistent dull pain even between remissions.[31,42] The pain usually begins in one division of the fifth cranial nerve and proceeds to involve the other branches. The condition is most common in middle and older age, with a slight predominance in females. The etiology is currently unclear.

The clinical diagnosis of trigeminal neuralgia is based on several distinguishing features as follows:[44]

1. The "half-inch test" in which the patient, when asked to demonstrate where the pain begins, will avoid touching the trigger zone by one-half inch for fear of precipitating an attack.
2. Clinically negative neurologic examination findings.
3. Alleviation of the pain and abolishment of the trigger point by administration of a local anesthetic to block the involved trigeminal nerve division.

Glossopharyngeal Neuralgia. By comparison with trigeminal neuralgia, glossopharyngeal neuralgia is an uncommon condition.[38] The disease is characterized by paroxysms of pain that radiate from the pharynx and tonsillar fauces to the TM region, ear, and tympanum. The pain is described as burning, lancing, and stabbing, occurring with swallowing, chewing, talking, or yawning.[31] The tonsillar and pharyngeal regions are trigger zones. This condition is commonly confused with a TM disorder because of the masticatory action that is required to stimulate the pain.[27]

A diagnosis of glossopharyngeal neuralgia may be made by inducing the pain by stimulation of the pharynx and tonsillar fossa. One can also abolish the trigger zone responsible for initiating the pain by topically anesthetizing the pharyngeal mucosa.

Medical treatment involves the use of carbamazepine and phenytoin (Dilantin). This treatment is not nearly as efficacious as it is with trigeminal neuralgia. Surgical section of the ninth nerve may be performed in the patient who is refractory to medical therapy.

Sphenopalatine Neuralgia. Sphenopalatine neuralgia, although an uncommon cause of TMJ pain, must be included in the differential diagnosis. Originally described by Sluder,[45] in 1908, the pain may take the form of a headache or, more often, discomfort located deep in the orbit and at the root of the nose. The pain radiates to the mandible, zygoma, and ear.[38] It is typically unilateral and episodic, with extension to the postauricular and mastoid regions. Attacks are associated with nasal mucosa edema, and other symptoms include rhinorrhea and nasal obstruction. The etiology of this condition, as with most neuralgias, is unclear. The diagnosis rests on immediate cessation of the pain after cocainization of the sphenopalatine ganglion during an attack. Sphenopalatine ganglionectomy is curative.

Atypical Facial Neuralgia. Atypical facial neuralgia is a poorly defined condition that is described as a vague, continuous, nonlocalized pain, which may last hours to days.[31,42] The history does not aid the clinician. No evidence of a trigger zone is found, and the pain is not limited to any one specific anatomic distribution. The regions most often involved are those innervated by the fifth and ninth cranial nerves as well as C1 and C2.

Findings of a complete physical examination, involving medical, dental, neurologic, and otorhinologic consultations, are often normal. When the clinician is managing a patient with atypical facial pain, a search should begin for evidence of associated depression or anxiety.[31,42] Gibilisco[4] retrospectively studied 100 patients classified as having atypical facial pain and found that more than half had associated depressive conditions.

Treatment of this condition includes drug therapy, biofeedback, and psychologic counselling.

Herpes Zoster Oticus (Figures 15–1 and 15–2). Herpes zoster oticus, also referred to as Ramsay Hunt syndrome, is an uncommon

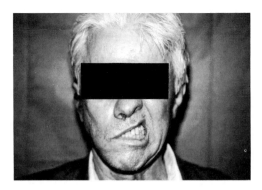

FIGURE 15–1. Facial paralysis secondary to herpes zoster oticus.

acute infectious disease that affects the sensory and motor branches of the facial nerve. Pain is the most common initial symptom and is typically intense, steady, and burning and may be associated with paresthesias over the involved area.[38,46] Within 2 to 3 days, the pain is followed by the onset of an ipsilateral facial nerve paralysis.[21] Within 10 to 14 days, vesicular eruptions appear on the skin of the external auditory canal and concha containing the sensory cutaneous distribution of the seventh nerve. The eruption peaks within 10 days, with the vesicles becoming dry, crusted, and hemorrhagic.[62] The vesicular crusting usually disappears within 4 weeks. Occasionally, examination of the oral cavity reveals a vesicular eruption along the ipsilateral soft palate and anterior tonsillar pillar. Other associated symp-

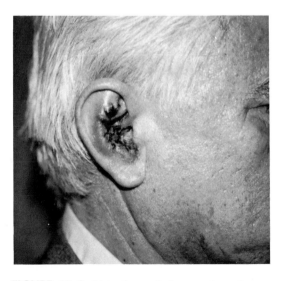

FIGURE 15–2. Note the vesicular eruptions that are classically crusted and hemorrhagic.

toms that may occur with this condition include sensorineural hearing loss, tinnitus, and vertigo.

Facial nerve testing and clinical assessment are extremely important in the management of these patients. If the patients are seen within the first 10 to 14 days of facial nerve paralysis, a short course of high-dose prednisone is advocated by some.[62] Although the management of this condition is generally conservative, Fisch advocates surgical decompression of the facial nerve if testing reveals greater than 90% axonal degeneration.[46]

Sinusitis

A paranasal sinus infection is seldom considered a source of referred pain to the TMJ region.[47] Specifically, it is the maxillary sinus that most often causes the pain that is interpreted as a TM disorder.

Acute and chronic infections of the maxillary sinus can often be diagnosed utilizing the complete history and physical examination. Antral inflammatory disease commonly causes a dull, throbbing pain that is felt in the eyes, cheeks, and teeth.[48] Not uncommonly, the patient experiences pain radiating to the TMJ. Other associated symptoms include profuse nasal and postnasal discharge that may be malodorous and may cause an unpleasant taste. Pain is increased by Valsalva's maneuver or by lowering the head.[48]

Physical examination reveals the nasal mucosa to be both erythematous and edematous. If the nasal mucosa is vasoconstricted with phenylephrine (Neo-Synephrine), a purulent exudate from the middle meatus is often seen. Rihani[5] noted that the pain elicited on palpating the posterior superior portion of the buccal vestibule in a patient with acute sinusitis is very similar to that elicited on palpating the lateral pterygoid muscle in the "TMJ-pain dysfunction syndrome." This finding often leads to a misdiagnosis.

In a prospective study of 111 patients, Lindahl and coworkers[47] found that the diagnosis of "TMJ-pain dysfunction syndrome" was confused with chronic maxillary sinusitis in 20%. Accordingly, the diagnosis of maxillary sinusitis must be given serious consideration in evaluating any patient with the symptom of TMJ pain.

Headaches

The clinician virtually daily is evaluating patients with complaints of pain referable to the head. Headaches can represent the final common pathway for a number of disorders ranging from intracranial lesions to the more common conditions of anxiety, tension, and stress.

Headaches may be broadly classified into traction-inflammatory, vascular, and muscle-contraction types. Although vascular headaches receive the most attention in the literature, the muscle-contraction headache is actually more common and comprises about 90% of the cases.[49]

Headache pain is often paroxysmal and may produce diffuse facial pain as well as pain that is referred to the temporal and auricular regions.[50] A thorough evaluation, including radiologic imaging, is essential in establishing the correct diagnosis before instituting treatment in a patient with the complaint of headache.

The discussion that follows is intended to highlight the most salient features of the more common conditions that appear with headache pain.

Migraine Headaches. Common migraine is a vascular pain syndrome that causes severe, unilateral, dull, or throbbing pain in the supraorbital, frontal, and temporal regions. The pain often remains unilateral but may also involve the opposite side of the head. Typically, the pain lasts for 1 to 2 days. The peak onset of this form of headache is generally in the second and third decades, although episodes beginning before the age of 10 years are not uncommon.[51] The female to male ratio is 3:1, with a strong familial tendency present in the majority of cases.[53] A close association with hormonal changes (e.g., menstruation, oral contraceptives) has been noted as a possible precipitating factor in migraine headaches.

Classic migraine is a less common variant of migraine that is associated with a prodromal phase or an aura. Typically, the prodromes last 15 to 20 minutes and include (1) visual disturbances (e.g., scotoma, hemianopia), (2) paresthesias, and (3) visual or auditory hallucinations.

Treatment involves an effort on the part of the patient to decrease all stimuli, particularly visual ones. The patient often retires to a dark, quiet room to rest. Medical therapy at the time of attack includes ergotamines as well as analgesics. Some patients may require long-term treatment with propranolol (Inderal) because of the frequency and intensity of attacks.

Cluster Headaches. Cluster headaches, also known as histamine headaches, or Horton's syndrome, are characterized as headaches that are intense, unilateral, and recurrent and of short duration.[31] This excruciating pain often occurs at night, awakening the patient from sleep. The pain is classically described as "boring" in character and is located deep in the orbit and temple. Common associated symptoms include tearing and congestion of the ipsilateral eye as well as nasal obstruction with rhinorrhea.[54]

The pain terminates as quickly as it commences. The attacks occur in a series of clusters that may last from 6 to 12 weeks. The patient may go into remission and be symptom-free for several months or even years. About 80% of the patients are males between the ages of 20 and 50.[31] Unlike migraine, no prodrome or associated hereditary history is noted. Unlike neuralgias, there are no trigger zones and the pain is not confined to any particular cranial nerve distribution.

An association with increased blood histamine levels has been noted by some workers but has not been confirmed by others.[55] Vasoactive substances are known to precipitate attacks and are rigorously avoided by patients. These substances include alcohol, nitroglycerine, and histamine. Additionally, behavior modification techniques have been found useful. Patients should avoid changes in the sleep-wake cycle, prolonged anger, and excessive physical activity.[54]

An acute attack once initiated is of high intensity and brief duration, making adequate medical treatment difficult. Therefore, treatment is aimed at the prevention of an episode.

Prophylactic medical therapy includes the use of methysergide, steroids, and ergotamine.

Muscle-Contraction Headaches. These are the most common types of headaches and most likely to be associated with a TM disorder. They usually are initiated by stress, depression, anxiety, fatigue, or emotional conflict.[56] Frequently, disorders of the cervical spine are responsible for pain being referred to the head. The onset of the headaches generally begins between the ages of 20 and 40, with a female predominance noted.[56] The most frequently affected anatomic sites include the supraorbital, occipital, and temporal regions. The pain is most commonly bilateral, short in duration, and varied in intensity. The etiology is believed to be a "neuromuscular skeletal imbalance," causing sustained contraction of the skeletal muscles with resulting pain.[49]

The treatment varies with the suspected etiology of the disorder. Muscle relaxants, e.g., benzodiazepines (Valium), and compounds containing barbiturates, e.g., Fiorinal, are often prescribed with good results. Specific treatment of TM disorders is discussed elsewhere in this text.

Acoustic Neuroma
(Figures 15–3 and 15–4)

Acoustic neuroma is an uncommon, benign, slow-growing tumor of Schwann-cell origin that arises from the vestibular portion of the

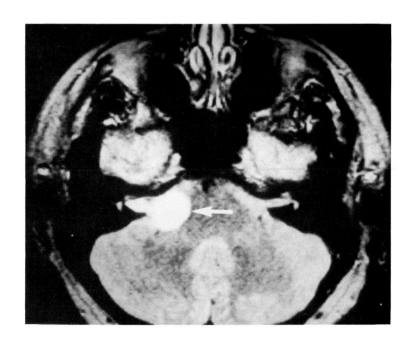

FIGURE 15–3. Acoustic neuroma. Axial magnetic resonance T2-weighted image shows a high signal intensity mass filling and widening the right internal auditory canal and bulging into the posterior fossa (arrow).

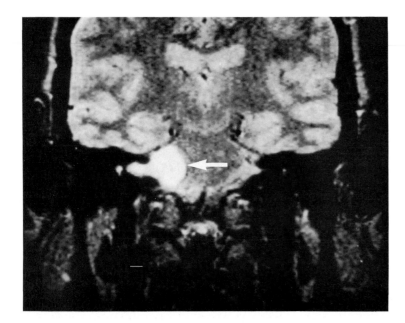

FIGURE 15–4. Acoustic neuroma. Coronal magnetic resonance T2-weighted image as described in Figure 15–3.

eighth cranial nerve.[57] The symptom duration until diagnosis ranges from 3 to 10 years. Unilateral hearing loss is the most common initial symptom. Hearing loss with tinnitus is the initial symptom in over 75% of patients and is present at the time of diagnosis in over 90% of patients. Although true whirling vertigo is uncommon, dizziness and unsteadiness eventually develop in 80% of cases.

The trigeminal nerve is the second most common cranial nerve involved by acoustic neuromas. Facial hypesthesia and occasionally periauricular pain are the most common symptoms secondary to trigeminal involvement.

Physical evaluation should include an otoscopic examination to rule out local disease (e.g., middle ear disease). A complete neurologic examination is essential. The patient should also undergo cochleovestibular testing (e.g., audiometry, electronystagmography, brain stem–evoked response testing) to rule out a central lesion.

Gibilisco[4] described a patient with periauricular and TMJ pain who was followed for 2 years. The patient had undergone dental extractions and several root canal treatments. After further evaluation, a history of unilateral hearing loss was elicited, which suggested the possibility of an acoustic neuroma. A computerized tomography (CT) scan of the temporal bones confirmed the diagnosis.

Confirmation of the presence of an acoustic neuroma is by contrast-enhanced CT scanning or magnetic resonance imaging (MRI). Treatment is by surgical excision of the tumor.

Ear Disease

Pathologic conditions of the ear may masquerade as TM disorders. Patients with TMJ pain often may have symptoms similar to those of true ear pathology. Therefore, disease within the ear must be considered and excluded as a source of TMJ pain.

Weinberg and Lager[58] found on evaluating 138 patients with "TMJ syndrome" that half had experienced tinnitus and vertigo. Curtis[10] stated that otologic symptoms, such as aural fullness, subjective hearing loss, tinnitus, and vertigo, were commonplace in patients having "TMJ syndrome." Consequently, a thorough history including questions regarding hearing loss, previous ear disease, otorrhea, and itching of the ear canal, as well as vertigo and tinnitus, should be obtained to exclude ear pathology as the source of pain.

In addition to eliciting a complete history, examination of the ear is essential in order to arrive at the correct diagnosis. The examination should begin with inspection of the auricle and external auditory canal, looking for the presence of erythema, ear protrusion, tenderness, previous surgical incisions, ecchymosis, or vesicular eruptions. The examination may then proceed to the tympanic membrane where otoscopy with insufflation is essential. Without the ability to insufflate it is difficult to accurately assess the state of the middle ear cavity.

When viewing the tympanic membrane, one must assess whether or not a tympanic membrane perforation exists. If there is a perforation this would be an important clue that the pain may be of otologic origin. If otorrhea exists it is important to note color, odor, and consistency. One should try to determine if the drainage comes from the external auditory canal or from a perforation in the tympanic membrane.

An assessment of ear disease is incomplete without an evaluation of the patient's hearing status. A 512 Hz tuning fork should be used in Weber and Rinne tests to help determine whether any auditory pathology exists. If there is an asymmetric response, this should arouse the clinician's suspicion that primary ear pathology is responsible for the patient's ear pain.

The following conditions represent the most common ear disorders that may mimic a TM disorder.

Diffuse External Otitis. Diffuse external otitis[59,60] is most commonly seen during the summer when there is constant exposure to water and high humidity. The patient initially notes itching of the ear canal. When the patient then scratches, trauma to the skin surface ensues, predisposing to the entry of bacteria with subsequent infection.

Clinically, pulling on the auricle, tragus, or both often elicits tenderness. The skin of the external auditory canal becomes edematous and erythematous. The itching and pain increase and are often associated with a purulent, foul-smelling, grey-green discharge. *Pseudomonas* species are most commonly cultured, but *Staphylococcus aureus, Streptococcus,* and

Proteus species may also be isolated. Otomycosis is a fungal infection of the external auditory canal that can become superimposed on a chronic bacterial infection. *Aspergillus* species are most commonly seen.

Treatment involves mechanical cleansing of the ear canal; application of topical antibiotic drops, acidifying solutions, or both; and maintenance of a dry environment. In more advanced cases, edema may totally occlude the canal, precluding visualization of the tympanic membrane. In such an instance, a wick is inserted into the canal, which is moistened by astringent, steroid, and antibiotic-containing eardrops. Upon removal of the wick after 12 to 24 hours, the canal is patent and allows adequate cleansing, visualization of the tympanic membrane, and routine application of the antibiotic drops.

Malignant External Otitis (Figures 15–5, 15–6, and 15–7). Malignant or necrotizing otitis is a destructive bacterial infection of the external auditory canal that is most often observed in diabetic and immunocompromised patients. The infection may initially appear as a common external otitis, with the symptoms of aural discharge and otalgia. However, physical examination generally reveals the presence of granulation tissue. This finding should alert the clinician to the correct diagnosis. The disease can often quickly progress to involve contiguous portions of the temporal bone, destroying both cartilage and bone. Intracranial extension with caudal cranial nerve palsies and seventh nerve paralysis are not uncommon complica-

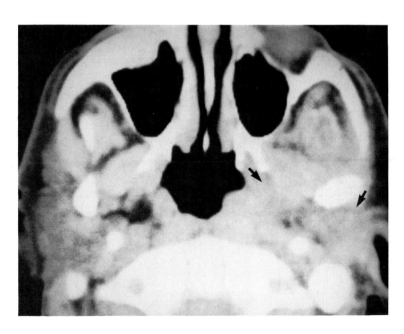

FIGURE 15–5. Malignant external otitis. Axial computerized tomographic scan shows an infiltrating soft tissue mass that extends into the left periauricular region and the parapharyngeal space (arrows). Slight medial deviation of the left nasopharyngeal wall is noted.

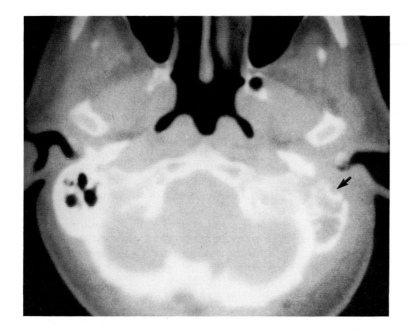

FIGURE 15–6. Malignant external otitis. Axial computerized tomographic scan at bone window setting shows soft tissue thickening of the left external auditory canal and focal erosion of the anterolateral cortex of the mastoid tip (arrow). The mastoid cells are also filled with soft tissue density material.

tions in cases involving delayed diagnosis or inadequate treatment.

Treatment involves extensive debridement of the ear canal with removal of all granulation tissue and prolonged (6 to 10 weeks) intravenous antibiotic therapy directed against *Pseudomonas aeruginosa,* the primary causative pathogen. These agents include synthetic penicillins (e.g., ticarcillin), third generation cephalosporins (e.g., ceftazidime, cefoperazone), and ciprofloxacin.

Bullous Myringitis. Bullous myringitis[59,60] is characterized by the sudden onset of severe ear pain, which is often accompanied by a viral respiratory tract infection. Otoscopy reveals hemorrhagic bullae or vesicles located solely on the tympanic membrane. *Mycoplasma pneumoniae* has often been implicated as the etiologic agent in this condition. Spontaneous or surgical rupture of the vesicles causes a precipitous decrease in the aural pain. Additional therapy includes oral analgesics and anodyne

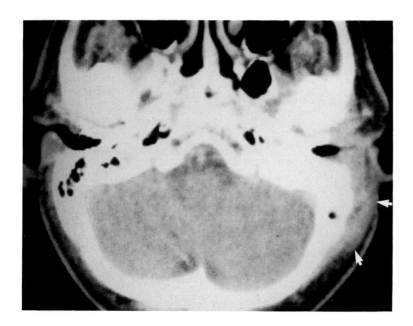

FIGURE 15–7. Malignant external otitis. Axial computerized tomographic scan shown at soft tissue window setting illustrates the soft tissue thickening in the left external auditory canal and postauricular region (arrow).

ear drops (e.g., Auralgan) as well as the oral administration of antibiotics (e.g., erythromycin) in cases with associated otitis media.

Acute Otitis Media. Acute otitis media[59,60] is a bacterial infection of the middle ear that often accompanies an upper respiratory tract infection or follows barotrauma. Patients complain of a deep-seated, throbbing pain, often with an associated hearing loss. This conductive hearing loss is secondary to the accumulation of purulent fluid in the middle ear space. Otoscopy reveals a dull and erythematous tympanic membrane that has lost its normal landmarks and has limited mobility.

The most common etiologic agents implicated are *Streptococcus pneumoniae, Haemophilus influenzae, Branhamella catarrhalis,* and *Staphylococcus aureus.* Treatment includes analgesics and oral antibiotics. Currently, the antibiotics of choice are cefaclor (Ceclor), sulfamethoxazole (Septra), and amoxicillin (Augmentin). Complications of inadequately treated disease include chronic otomastoiditis, cholesteatoma, petrositis, and epidural or brain abscess.

The diagnosis of nasopharyngeal carcinoma must always be considered in any adult who develops otitis media not precipitated by an upper respiratory infection that is refractory to medical treatment. The pathogenesis of this condition is obstruction of the eustachian tube orifice by the nasopharyngeal mass. Such cases of recurrent or refractory serous otitis media require nasopharyngoscopy and CT scanning of the nasopharynx to rule out a mass lesion.

Chronic Otitis Media. In contrast to acute otitis media the pathogenesis of disease in chronic otitis media[64–66] is insidious and slow to progress. The patient's symptomatology is almost uniformly that of a mild nature with symptoms of otorrhea or dull pain in the affected ear. It is not uncommon for a patient with chronic otitis media to have had a history of acute ear disease, which may have either failed to resolve completely or progressed to otitis media with effusion. The ear develops a dampened response to long-term antibiotics, and the middle ear mucosa begins to undergo changes often leading to a state of frank granulation tissue with a concomitant mucopurulent discharge. This condition results in a middle ear space devoid of the capacity to ventilate itself, possibly setting the stage for progression to a chronic tympanic membrane perforation. Hearing loss or atelectasis of the tympanic membrane results with ossicular erosion and the possibility of further progression to cholesteatoma.

Schuknecht[66] described a cholesteatoma as "an accumulation of exfoliated keratin in the middle ear or other pneumatized area of the temporal bone arising from keratinizing squamous epithelium." This ingrowth of squamous epithelium is in the pars tensa or pars flaccida portion of the tympanic membrane. On physical examination, the cholesteatoma appears as a pearly white-grey mass often located at the posterior superior aspect of the tympanic membrane or in the region of the attic.

These pockets of desquamated epithelium result in the capacity of the cholesteatoma to destroy bone. This bone destruction may occur by two mechanisms: (1) proteolytic enzymatic digestion and (2) pyogenic osteitis resulting in bone necrosis. The ability to destroy bone makes cholesteatoma a dangerous condition because of the potential for otologic as well as intracranial complications. Otologic complications include (1) hearing loss, (2) labyrinthine fistula, (3) labyrinthitis—serous or toxic, and (4) facial nerve paralysis. Intracranial complications include (1) epidural abscess, (2) meningitis, (3) brain abscess, and (4) sigmoid sinus thrombophlebitis.

Because of the significance of the possible complications listed, the primary treatment of this condition is surgical. More modest treatment, e.g., suction removal, is reserved for the high-risk patient only (Fig. 15–8).

Malignancies

Malignancies, both regional and metastatic, can manifest themselves as TMJ pain and must always be considered in every differential diagnosis of TMJ pain.[1,2,11,17] Most malignant tumors that involve the TMJ are usually secondary to contiguous spread from neoplasms of the skin, parotid gland, ear, and nasopharynx.[11] However, metastatic disease from the breast, prostate, colon, and lung has also been reported.[11] As alluded to previously, the complex neural innervation of the TMJ region allows for primary pharyngeal and laryngeal malignancies to manifest themselves as ear pain (Fig. 15–9).[19]

Initially, malignancies may appear with trismus, facial pain, and mandibular deviation, all symptoms of TM disorders.[2,18] However, several distinguishing features of malignancies should alert the clinician to perform a more comprehensive diagnostic evaluation.

Hypesthesia. Most disorders of the TMJ do not cause facial or aural numbness; however, malignancies can cause sensory alterations of

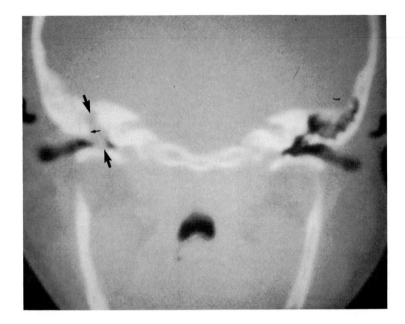

FIGURE 15–8. Cholesteatoma. Coronal computerized tomographic scan shows a soft tissue mass in the right middle ear and mastoid antrum (large arrows). Erosion and beveling of the lateral attic wall and scutum are noted (small arrow).

the mandibular and maxillary divisions of the trigeminal nerve. Most commonly, tumors of the nasopharynx lead to sensory changes in the distribution of the fifth nerve, but many tumors, including those of the infratemporal fossa, maxillary sinus, and the meninges, are known to cause fifth nerve hypesthesia.[10,14,15,19] Often, patients have been treated many months for persistent pain in the TMJ region before fifth nerve symptoms occur. It is during this time, when conventional therapy has been without effect, that an alternate diagnosis should be entertained,[1] and definitive studies performed. The literature is replete with case reports of patients whose tumors enlarged during this critical period and for whom only subsequent palliative therapy could be offered.

Otalgia. In the absence of ear pathology, otalgia unrelated to masticatory function must be viewed with great suspicion, especially when the pain is progressive, very intense, and continuous in nature.[61] Even with other findings

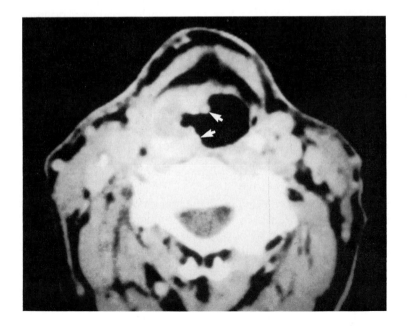

FIGURE 15–9. Pyriform sinus carcinoma. Axial computerized tomographic scan shows a nodular mucosal thickening of the right pyriform sinus with extension into the right supraglottic larynx (arrows).

consistent with a TM disorder, this type of presentation should cause the clinician to search for a tumor.

Tumors of the head and neck in general are often difficult to detect early in their course. Therefore, the patient with this suspicious pain profile must have constant reassessment of the condition performed at regular and frequent intervals, as long as the symptoms remain unabated.[19]

Preauricular Mass. The development of a preauricular mass in a patient with symptoms of TMJ pain should alert the clinician to consider the parotid gland as the primary focus. Parotid masses most often represent tumor within the gland itself.[67]

The parotid gland is located anteriorly to the ear. Its borders are the masseter muscle anteriorly, the zygomatic bone superiorly, the lateral pterygoid muscle medially, the external auditory canal and mastoid process posteriorly, and the sternocleidomastoid muscle and posterior belly of the digastric muscle inferiorly.

The parotid gland is divided by the facial nerve into a superficial lobe, which forms 80% of the gland, and a deep lobe, which forms the remaining 20%. The majority of parotid tumors occur in the superficial lobe, whereas the incidence of deep lobe tumors is approximately 10%.[68]

Although parotid tumors are characterized by a wide variety of histopathology and biologic behavior, the majority (80%) of tumors within the gland are benign.[69] The most common clinical presentation of a benign tumor is that of a firm, mobile, and nontender mass.[70]

A number of clinical features of parotid tumors indicate an increased likelihood of malignancy as follows:

1. *Pain* is often associated with a higher incidence of malignancy. Additionally, pain is often an indicator of a poor prognosis.[70]

2. *Facial nerve paralysis* generally indicates malignant disease. Adenoid cystic carcinoma is well known for tendency toward perineural invasion.[69]

3. *Hardness* and *fixation* of the mass are associated with a 30 to 50% incidence of malignancy.[70]

A complete physical examination of the oral cavity, including bimanual palpation of the parotid gland, must be performed. The skin of the ipsilateral face, scalp, and ear is the primary site of metastatic disease of the parotid gland and therefore must be thoroughly evaluated.

Although radionuclide techniques, ultrasonography, and sialography are applied in the evaluation of parotid masses, CT and MRI scanning are the most useful for evaluating parotid masses (Fig. 15–10).

Surgery at present remains the treatment of choice for parotid tumors, with a superficial parotidectomy and sparing of the seventh cranial nerve being the most common procedures performed.

If the aforementioned conditions exist, further evaluation in consultation with the otolar-

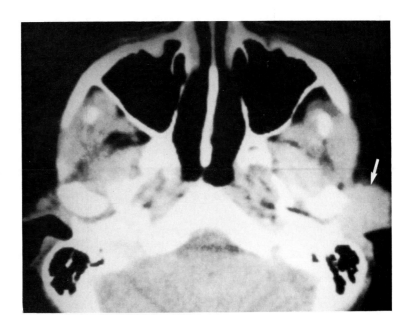

Figure 15–10. Acinic cell carcinoma. Axial computerized scan of a patient presenting with temporomandibular joint (TMJ) complaints shows a mass in the upper pole of the left parotid gland (arrow). The mass abuts the left TMJ.

yngologist, neurologist, and radiologist is required in order that tumor as the etiologic agent is ruled out. Failure to arrive at the correct diagnosis in an expedient manner may result in the rapid demise of the patient.

SUMMARY

The purpose of this chapter is to illustrate the myriad of conditions a patient with symptoms of TMJ pain might suffer from. In order to avoid the pitfalls so common in evaluating patients with TMJ pain, the clinician must perform a complete and critical review of the medical history along with a comprehensive examination. The challenge to the clinician is to know and evaluate the differential diagnosis. Failure to do so can result in a misdiagnosis, which may lead to unnecessary care, long-term therapy without clinical resolution, or a potentially untimely death.

REFERENCES

1. Kaplan, A., Som, P., and Lawson, W.: The co-existence of myofascial pain dysfunction syndrome and mucoepidermoid carcinoma of the parotid gland. J. Am. Dent. Assoc. 112:495–496, 1986.
2. Cohen, S. and Quinn, P.: Facial trismus and myofascial pain associated with infectious and malignant disease. Oral Surg. Oral Med. Oral Pathol. 65:538–544, 1988.
3. Selsky, E. and Nirankari, V.: Temporomandibular joint pain as a manifestation of temporal arteritis. South. Med. J. 78:1249–1251, 1985.
4. Gibilisco, J.: Dental perspective on pain. Postgrad. Med. 76:121–130, 1984.
5. Rihani, A.: Maxillary sinusitis as a differential diagnosis in temporomandibular joint pain dysfunction syndrome. J. Prosthet. Dent. 53:97–100, 1985.
6. Costen, J.: A syndrome of ear and sinus symptoms dependent upon disturbed function of the temporomandibular joint. Ann. Otol. Rhinol. Laryngol. 43:1–15, 1934.
7. Costen, J.: Reflex effects produced by abnormal movement of the lower jaw. Arch. Otolaryngol. 36:548–554, 1942.
8. Bernstein, J., Mohl, N., and Spiller, H.: Temporomandibular-joint dysfunction masquerading as disease of the ear, nose and throat. Trans. Am. Acad. Ophthalmol. Otolaryngol. 73:1208–1217, 1969.
9. Arlen, H.: The otomandibular syndrome. In Clinical Management of Head, Neck and TMJ Pain and Dysfunction: A Multidisciplinary Approach to Diagnosis and Treatment. H. Gelb (ed.). W.B. Saunders Co., Philadelphia, 1977.
10. Curtis, A.: Myofascial pain-dysfunction syndrome: The role of non-masticatory muscles in 91 patients. Otolaryngol. Head Neck Surg. 88:361–367, 1980.
11. Owen, D. and Stelling, C.: Condylar metastasis with initial presentation as TMJ syndrome. J. Oral Med. 40:198–201, 1985.
12. Shapshay, S., Elber, E., and Strong, S.: Occult tumors of the infratemporal fossa appearing as preauricular pain. Arch. Otolaryngol. 102:535–538, 1976.
13. Har-El, G. and Calderon, S.: Angioblastic meningioma presenting as a pain in the temporomandibular joint. J. Oral Maxillofac. Surg. 45:338–340, 1987.
14. Orlean, S., Robinson, N., Ahern, J., et al: Carcinoma of the maxillary sinus manifested as temporomandibular joint dysfunction syndrome. J. Oral Med. 21:127–131, 1966.
15. Christiansen, E., Thompson, J., and Appleton, S.: Temporomandibular joint pain dysfunction overlying more insidious diseases. J. Oral Maxillofac. Surg. 45:335–337, 1987.
16. Hecker, R., Noon, W., and Elliot, M.: Adenocarcinoma metastatic to the temporomandibular joint. J. Oral Maxillofac. Surg. 43:629–631, 1985.
17. Richter, K., Freeman, N., and Quick, C.A.: Chondrosarcoma of the temporomandibular joint. J. Oral Surg., 32:777–781 1974.
18. DeBoom, G., Jensen, J., Siegel, W., and Bloom, C.: Metastatic tumors of the mandibular condyle. Oral Surg. Oral Med. Oral Pathol. 60:512–516, 1985.
19. Roistacher, S. and Tannenbaum, D.: Myofascial pain associated with oropharyngeal cancer. Oral Surg. Oral Med. Oral Pathol. 61:459–462, 1986.
20. Moore K.L. (ed.) Clinically Oriented Anatomy. Williams & Wilkins, Baltimore, 1980.
21. Powers, W. and Britton, B.H.: Nonotogenic otalgia: Diagnosis and treatment. Am. J. Otol. 2:97–104, 1980.
22. Kern, E.B.: Referred pain to the ear. Minn. Med. 55:896–898, 1972.
23. Boles, R: Neuroanatomy for the otolaryngologist. In Otolaryngology, 2nd ed. vol. 1. M.M. Paparella and D.A. Shumrick (eds). W. B. Saunders Co., Philadelphia, 1980.
24. Goethals, P.L.: Referred otalgia, J. Fla. Med. Assoc. 59:26–30, 1972.
25. Hora, J.F. and Brown, H. K. : Obscure otalgia. Laryngoscope 74:122–133, 1964.
26. Paparella, M.M.: Otalgia. In Otolaryngology, 2nd ed., vol. 2. M.M. Paparella and D.A. Shumrick (eds.). W.B. Saunders Co., Philadelphia, 1980.
27. Bell, W.: Category classification of orofacial pains. In Orofacial Pains: Classification, Diagnosis, and Treatment, 4th ed. Year Book Medical Publishers, Chicago, 1989.
28. Murray, T.J.: Carotidynia as a cause of head and neck pain. Can. Med. Assoc. J. 120:441–443, 1979.
29. Raskin, N. and Prusiner, S.: Carotidynia. Neurology 27:43–46, 1977.
30. Acetta, D., Kelly, J., and Tubbs, R.: An elderly black woman with a painful swollen face. Ann. Allergy 55:819–823, 1985.
31. Dalessio, D.: Evaluation of the patient with chronic facial pain. Am. Fam. Physician 16:84–92, 1977.
32. Holenhorst, R.W., Brown, J.R., Wagener, H.P., et al: Neurologic aspects of temporal arteritis. Neurology 10:490–498, 1960.
33. Dalessio, D.J. and Williams, G.W.: Cranial arteritis and polymyalgia rheumatica. In Wolff's Headache and Other Head Pain, 4th ed. D.J. Dalessio (ed.). Oxford University Press, New York, 1980.
34. Ellis, M.E. and Ralston, S.: The ESR in the diagnosis and management of polymyalgia rheumatica/giant cell arteritis syndrome. Ann. Rheum. Dis. 42:168–170, 1983.
35. Eagle, W.W.: Elongated styloid process: Report of two cases. Arch. Otolaryngol. 25:584–587, 1937.

36. Eagle, W.W.: Elongated styloid process. Further observations and a new syndrome. Arch. Otolaryngol. 47:630–640, 1948.

37. Correll, R. and Wescott, W.: Eagle's syndrome diagnosed after history of headache, dysphagia, otalgia and limited neck movement. J. Am. Dent. Assoc. 104:491–492, 1982.

38. Deleon, E.: Facial pain of non-odontogenic origin. J. Oral Med. 23:119–131, 1968.

39. Eagle, W.W.: Elongated styloid process symptoms and treatment. Arch. Otolaryngol. 67:172–176, 1958.

40. Douglas, T.E.: Facial pain from an elongated styloid process. Arch. Otolaryngol. 55:635, 1952.

41. Evans, J.T. and Clairmont, A.A.: The nonsurgical treatment of Eagle's syndrome. Eye, Ear, Nose and Throat Monthly 55:94–95, 1976.

42. Drinnan, A.: Differential diagnosis of orofacial pain. Dent. Clin. North Am. 22:73–87, 1978.

43. Eadie, M.J.: The management of facial pain. Med. J. Austral. 2:224–225, 1975.

44. Moore, D. and Nally, F.: The diagnosis and management of paroxysmal trigeminal neuralgia in association with a temporomandibular joint dysfunction. Oral Surg. 38:874–878, 1974.

45. Sluder, G.: The role of the sphenopalatine ganglion in nasal headaches. N.Y. Med. J. 87:989, 1908.

46. Newton, J. and Fisch, U.: Disorders of the facial nerve. In *Otolaryngology.* G. English (ed.). J.B. Lippincott Co., Philadelphia, 1980.

47. Lindahl, L., Melen, I., Ekedahl, C., and Holm, S.E.: Chronic maxillary sinusitis. Differential diagnosis and genesis. Acta Otolaryngol. 93:1147–1150, 1982.

48. Blitzer, A.: Surgery for infection and benign disease of the maxillary sinus. In *Surgery of the Paranasal Sinuses.* A. Blitzer, W. Lawson, and W. Friedman (eds.). W.B. Saunders Co., Philadelphia, 1985.

49. Markovich, S.E.: Pain in the head: A neurological appraisal. In *Clinical Management of Head, Neck, and TMJ Pain and Dysfunction,* 2nd ed. H. Gelb (ed.). W.B. Saunders Co., Philadelphia, 1985.

50. Bell, W.: Muscle pains. In *Classification of Oral Facial Pains,* 4th ed. W. Bell (ed.). Year Book Medical Publishers, Chicago, 1989.

51. Saper, J.: Migraine: Introduction and clinical features. In *Headache Disorders.* J. Saper (ed.). John Wright Publishing, New York, 1983.

52. Lance, J.: The pathophysiology of migraine. In *Wolff's Headache and Other Head Pain,* 5th ed. D.J. Dalessio (ed.). Oxford University Press, New York 1980.

53. Olesen, J: Some clinical features of the acute migraine attack. An analysis of 750 patients. Headache 18:268–271, 1978.

54. Kudrow, L.: Cluster headache: Diagnosis, management and treatment. In *Wolff's Headache and Other*

Head Pain, 4th ed. D.J. Dalessio (ed.). Oxford University Press, New York, 1980.

55. Anthony, M. and Lance, J.W.: Controlled trials of cimetidine in migraine and cluster headache. Headache 18:261–264, 1978.

56. Diamond, S.: Muscle-contraction headache. In *Wolff's Headache and Other Head Pain,* 4th ed. D. Dalessio (ed.). Oxford University Press, New York, 1980.

57. Gates, G.A. and Chakeres, D.W.: Interpretation of diagnostic tests for acoustic neuroma. In *American Academy of Otolaryngology—Head and Neck Surgery Foundation—Self-Instructional Package,* 2nd ed., The American Academy of Otolaryngology—Head and Neck Surgery Foundation, Washington, D.C., 1984.

58. Weinberg, L.A. and Lager, L.A.: Clinical report on the etiology and diagnosis of TMJ dysfunction pain syndrome. J. Prosthet. Dent. 44:642–653, 1980.

59. Smith, P. and Lucente, F.: Infections of the external ear. In *Otolaryngology Head and Neck Surgery.* L. Harker and C. Cummings (eds.). C.V. Mosby Co., St. Louis, 1987.

60. Sobol, S.M. and Lucente, F.E.: Ear pain. In *Essentials of Otolaryngology.* F.E. Lucente and M.S. Sobol (eds.). Raven Press, New York, 1983.

61. Pearson, B.W.: ENT approach to face pain. Postgrad. Med. 76:133–145, 1984.

62. Senturia, B.H., Marcus, M.D., and Lucente, F.E.: Diseases due to infection. In *Diseases of the External Ear.* F.E. Lucente (ed.). Grune & Stratton, Orlando, 1980.

63. Megoven, F.H.: Medical treatment of facial paralysis. In *Otolaryngology.* G.M. English (ed.). J.B. Lippincott Co., Philadelphia, 1980.

64. Smyth, G.D.L.: Chronic otitis media. In *Otolaryngology.* G.M. English (ed.). J.B. Lippincott Co., Philadelphia, 1980.

65. Neely, J.G.: Treatment of uncomplicated aural cholesteatoma. In *American Academy of Otolaryngology—Head and Neck Surgery Foundation—Self Instructional Package,* 2nd ed. The American Academy of Otolaryngology—Head and Neck Surgery Foundation, Washington, D.C., 1986.

66. Schuknecht, H.F.: *Pathology of the Ear.* Harvard University Press, Cambridge, Massachusetts, 225–228, 1974.

67. Cannon, C.R.: Osteochondrosis of the temporomandibular joint presenting as an apparent parotid mass. Ann. Otol. Rhinol. Laryngol. 96:330–332, 1987.

68. Nigro, M.F. and Spiro, R.M.: Deep lobe tumors. Am. J. Surg. 134:523–527, 1977.

69. Byrne, M. and Spector, J.G.: Parotid masses: evaluation, analysis and current management. Laryngoscope 98:99–105, 1988.

70. Lam, K.H., Wei, W.I., and Law, W.F.: Tumors of the parotid—the value of clinical assessment. N.Z. J. Surg. 56:325–329, 1986.

Kurt P. Schellhas

CHAPTER 16

Influence of TMJ Pathology on Occlusion

The relationship between changing (unstable) disorders of occlusion and temporomandibular joint (TMJ) diseases has been and continues to be the subject of controversy.[1-8] The dental literature is full of theories regarding occlusal disturbances and their accompanying physical signs and symptoms, which are referred to with such terms as "TMJ dysfunction," "craniomandibular syndrome," "myofascial pain dysfunction syndrome," and "TMJ." Although theories differ, a widely accepted one is the concept that occlusal disturbances are responsible for the clinical symptoms and, because TMJ degeneration is generally not considered to be of significance, occlusal adjustment is believed to be therapeutic for "TMJ afflictions."

The suggestion that disease states affecting the TMJ may be irreversible and may lead to "secondary" occlusal disturbances arouses strong emotions in some workers and is considered "heretical" by others. Objective re-examination of currently accepted dogma is needed. Clinical evidence proves the existence of progressive, degenerative states affecting the TMJ, which frequently result in secondary changes in occlusion, acquired facial skeleton deformity, or both.[5-15] Many accepted and widely practiced forms of "TMJ therapy" may aggravate specific types of joint pathology and hasten development of more advanced stages of joint degeneration.[6,8,11,14]

The perfection and clinical use of a reliable technique of two-compartment TMJ arthrography first defined the progressive nature of meniscus derangements and how they lead

to degenerative/adaptive osteocartilaginous changes and resultant occlusal disturbances.[2] Further clinical and laboratory observations with magnetic resonance imaging (MRI) have substantiated and clarified previous observations[6-8,14] and provided additional information regarding the pathophysiology of joint degeneration,[7,14] occlusal disturbances,[6,11-14] and changes in the facial skeleton.[8,11] Internal derangements of the TMJ are often progressive disorders,[7,14] frequently of traumatic origin,[15] and often responsible for the clinical signs and symptoms that continue to be a source of controversy and speculation.

Magnetic resonance imaging has revolutionized the field of diagnostic radiology.[16-22] Details pertaining to the physics of MRI are beyond the scope of this chapter and are described elsewhere.[23] Magnetic resonance imaging provides high contrast multiplanar images of soft tissue structures that could not be comparably defined previously.

NORMAL TEMPOROMANDIBULAR JOINT

The normal TMJ meniscus exhibits a biconcave configuration and a homogeneous low intrinsic signal intensity on T1-weighted, proton density (Fig. 16–1) and T2-weighted, spin echo and multiecho images.[16-19] The bone marrow within the mandibular condyle and temporal bone exhibits high intrinsic signal intensity on short TR/short TE (T1-weighted) and long TR/short TE (proton density) pulse sequences because of the rapid magnetization of normal marrow fat. With long TR/long TE (T2-weighted) images (Fig. 16–2, right), there is decay of normal marrow signal, resulting in lower intensity signal. The normal muscles of mastication are sharply defined on various sagittal, axial, and coronal pulse sequences.[19,24]

TEMPOROMANDIBULAR JOINT DEGENERATION

Traumatic injury appears to be the most frequent cause of TMJ derangement.[7,14,15] Clinical and laboratory investigations have shown that meniscus displacement and degeneration lead to osteocartilaginous remodeling, degeneration, or both, which may result in secondary changes in occlusion and facial contour (Fig. 16–3).[7,8,14,25,26] Joint inflammation, such as might occur with injury or systemic illness, may result in osteocartilaginous degeneration

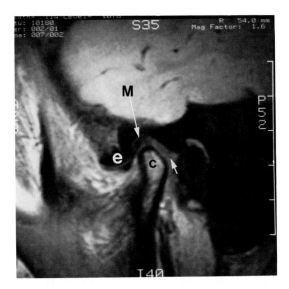

FIGURE 16–1. Normal temporomandibular joint. Closed-mouth, cephalometrically corrected sagittal image produced with a proton density of 2200/20 (TR in msec/TE). The patient in centric occlusion reveals a normal meniscus (M and arrow) atop a mandibular condyle (c). The letter e denotes the articular eminence of temporal bone. The small arrow denotes retrodiscal tissue.

without pre-existing meniscus displacement (Fig. 16–4). Inflammatory arthropathy frequently results in joint pain and acute or unstable occlusal disturbances, or both, such as posterior open bite (Fig. 16–5).[12] With advanced degeneration of the meniscus, perforation of the disc attachments often occurs; this leads to osteocartilaginous erosion and consequent loss of vertical dimension within the joint and the proximal mandibular segment due to remodeling (Fig. 16–6).[7,8,14]

Regressive changes in the TMJ commonly lead to secondary alterations in occlusion, which may be either slow or rapid. With slow progression of joint degeneration, healthy teeth may adapt or "keep pace" with the joint alterations by intruding, erupting, or realigning, or their combination, in order to maintain a comfortable state of occlusion.[8,14] With rapidly progressive joint degeneration, such as may occur with fracture of the condyle or condylar neck (traumatic vs. iatrogenic); osteochondritis dissecans (transchondral fracture); and avascular (aseptic) necrosis (AVN) involving the mandibular condyle; changes in vertical dimension may be too rapid for dental adaptations to accommodate the alterations; major changes in occlusion, facial contour, or both may result (Figs. 16–3, 16–6, and 16–7).

FIGURE 16–2. Early internal derangement of meniscus, hypertrophic mandibular condyle, and normal marrow signal. Closed-mouth sagittal spin echo, multiecho, 2200/20 (left), 80 (right), images reveal slight anterior displacement of the meniscus (solid arrow on left). Note the signal changes in the condylar marrow (open arrows) between proton density (left) and T2-weighted (right) images.

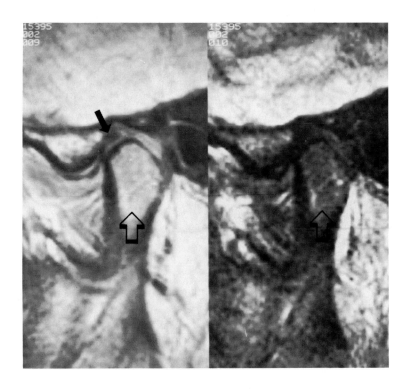

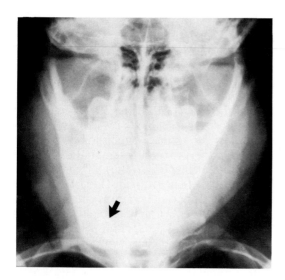

FIGURE 16–3. Skeletofacial deformity and unstable occlusion caused by rapidly progressive degeneration of the right temporomandibular joint. Anteroposterior jaw-protruded radiograph reveals severe displacement of the chin (arrow) toward the degenerated right joint. Lateral tomograms and magnetic resonance images (not shown) revealed severe degeneration of the mandibular condyle, suggesting avascular necrosis.

A variety of conditions may lead to AVN of the mandibular condyle, proximal mandibular segment, or both. However, inflammatory arthropathy due to internal derangement of the meniscus is the most common cause of this serious osteocartilaginous complication.[11,12,27] Both orthodontic occlusal manipulation and orthognathic surgery may aggravate pre-existing TMJ arthropathy and lead to AVN.[6,8,11] Some cases of orthodontics and orthognathic surgery have been and continue to be misdirected at the "symptoms" of joint disease instead of the underlying causal joint pathology, explaining some clinical relapses and therapeutic failures (see Fig. 16–6).[8,11]

Regressive osteocartilaginous remodeling is an adaptive or degenerative process, which occurs in the temporal bone and condyle often in response to meniscus derangement, and is radiologically distinct from osteoarthritis and AVN (Figs. 16–8 and 16–9).[8,11] Regressive remodeling may be either a rapid (see Fig. 16–8) or an insidious process, resulting in the loss of mass and vertical dimension within the mandibular condyle due to meniscus derangement (see Fig. 16–9). Regressive remodeling is often

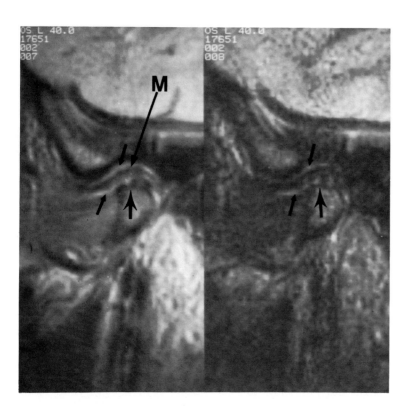

FIGURE 16–4. Pain, joint dysfunction, and occlusal disturbances are due to joint inflammation and osteocartilaginous remodeling. This 28-year-old female sustained a jaw injury 6 weeks prior to the onset of symptoms and 10 weeks prior to imaging studies. Closed-mouth sagittal multiecho, 2200/20 (left), 80 (right), images reveal irregularity of the surfaces of the normally positioned meniscus (M and arrow on left). Note upper and lower joint compartment effusions (small arrows). Note irregularity of the articular surface of the mandibular condyle (large arrows).

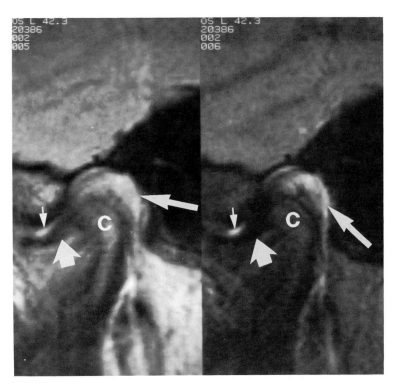

FIGURE 16–5. Acute preauricular pain and ipsilateral posterior open bite are due to inflammatory temporomandibular joint arthropathy. Closed-mouth sagittal, 2200/20 (left), 70 (right), images reveal anterior displacement of the meniscus (large wide arrows) and swelling of the retrodiscal soft tissue (long arrows). Note downward and forward depression of the mandibular condyle (c) compared with that in Figures 16–1 and 16–2. Smallest arrows denote the upper compartment fluid.

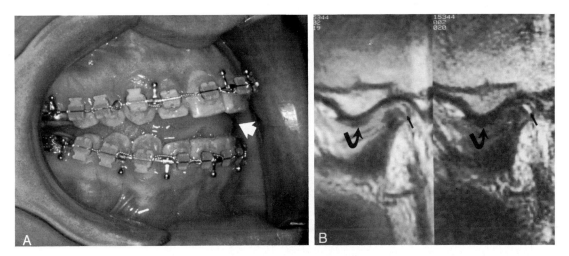

FIGURE 16–6. A and B, Worsening malocclusion and facial deformity despite 6 years of attempted orthodontic "occlusion stabilization" caused by progressive temporomandibular joint degeneration. This 26-year-old female with a 6-year history of progressive anterior open bite and retrognathia was referred for orthognathic surgery (not performed), at which time first imaging studies were performed. A, Oblique photograph of patient in attempted centric occlusion reveals severe anterior open bite (arrow). Note fixed orthodontic appliances. B, Closed-mouth sagittal multiecho, 2200/20 (left), 80 (right), images reveal severe anterior displacement and degeneration of the meniscus (curved arrows) with small joint effusion (small arrows). Note complete absence of condylar marrow signal caused by old avascular necrosis. Compare with Figures 16–1 and 16–2. Note the deformity of the mandibular condyle.

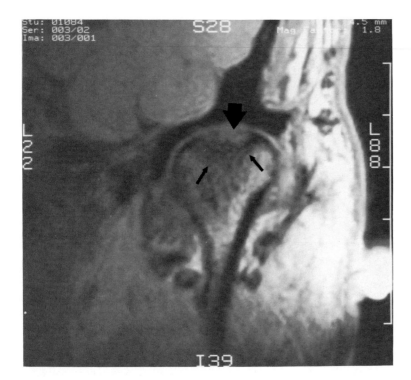

FIGURE 16–7. Osteochondritis dissecans (transchondral fracture) of the mandibular condyle. Coronal T1-weighted, 600/20, image reveals depression of the central articular surface (large arrow) of the condyle, with decreased marrow signal (small arrows) beneath the larger articular defect. At surgery, necrotic articular cartilage and bone were removed from the defect.

accommodated by simultaneous adaptive dental processes, which maintain comfortable occlusion if the joint remodeling is slow.[8]

It is common to see a patient manifesting comfortable occlusion with chin displacement toward the smaller or more degenerated mandibular condyle and TMJ because of regressive remodeling (see Fig. 16–9).[28] In this case, recognition of the underlying "causal" joint pathology may have significant ramifications if therapy is to achieve stable, long-term benefit to the patient.[8]

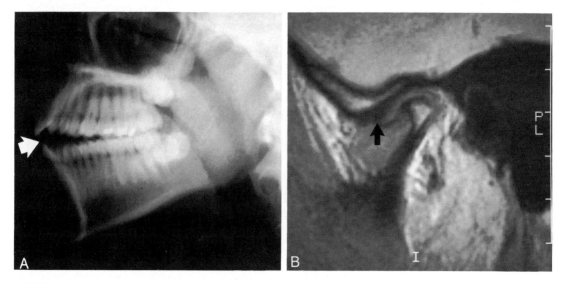

FIGURE 16–8. *A* and *B*, Worsening anterior open bite and unstable occlusion caused by rapidly regressive remodeling of the mandibular condyles and meniscus derangement. This 18-year-old female has a 1-year history of progressive anterior open bite, headaches, and joint dysfunction. *A*, Lateral cephalometric radiograph reveals anterior open bite (arrow). *B*, Closed-mouth sagittal, 2200/25, image reveals severe degeneration of the anteriorly displaced meniscus (arrow). Note the deformity of the small mandibular condyle. Compare with Figure 16–1.

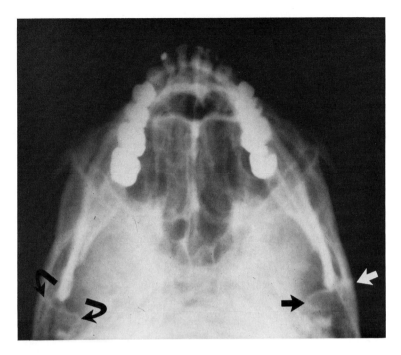

FIGURE 16–9. Regressive remodeling leading to "shrinkage" of the involved mandibular condyle. Submentovertex (base) radiograph reveals a small right mandibular condyle (curved arrows) compared with the normal left condyle (straight arrows). Note slight displacement of the chin toward the degenerated right condyle. Magnetic resonance imaging (not shown) revealed advance-stage meniscus derangement. Patient had a stable occlusion clinically.

In the patient who presents with unstable disturbances of occlusion, acquired changes in facial contour, or both, TMJ imaging should be routine to detect the presence and extent of joint pathology prior to therapeutic endeavors. Unstable occlusion and skeletofacial deformity are generally not recognized as symptoms of joint degeneration; however, these symptoms are common physical signs.[8]

Screening submentovertex and anteroposterior jaw-protruded radiographs of the skull and mandible, along with lateral corrected closed-mouth and open-mouth tomograms, are recommended as basic imaging procedures to detect the presence or absence of joint disease. In cases with accompanying mechanical joint symptoms, pain, or both, MRI should be considered to assess the presence or absence of active joint inflammation and possible marrow pathology.[11,12] If MRI cannot be performed in a patient with abnormal tomograms and highly suspect clinical symptomatology, two-compartment thin-needle TMJ arthrography with videofluoroscopy should be performed without hesitation,[21] as the demonstration and documentation of the type and extent of joint pathology are crucial prior to major therapeutic endeavors.

The advances in our knowledge provided by imaging procedures have produced material impacts in the fields of orthodontics, orthognathic surgery, restorative dentistry, and TMJ therapy. Ultimately, improved patient care has resulted.

REFERENCES

1. Farrar, W.B.: Diagnosis and treatment of anterior dislocation of the articular disc. N.Y. J. Dent. 41:348–351, 1971.
2. Wilkes, C.H.: Arthrography of the temporomandibular joint in patients with TMJ pain-dysfunction syndrome. Minn. Med. 61:645–652, 1978.
3. Wilkes, C.H.: Structural and functional alterations of the temporomandibular joint. Northwest Dent. 57:274–294, 1978.
4. Dawson, P.E.: *Evaluation, Diagnosis and Treatment of Occlusal Problems,* 2nd ed. C.V. Mosby Co., St. Louis, 1989.
5. Schellhas, K.P. and Keck, R.J.: Disorders of skeletal occlusion and temporomandibular joint disease. Northwest Dent. 68:35–42, 1989.
6. Schellhas, K.P.: Unstable occlusion and temporomandibular joint disease. J. Clin. Orthodont. 23:332–337, 1989.
7. Wilkes, C.H.: Internal derangements of the temporomandibular joint: pathologic variations. Arch. Otolaryngol. Head Neck Surg. 115:469–477, 1989.
8. Schellhas, K.P., Piper, M.A., and Omlie, M.R.: Facial skeleton remodelling due to temporomandibular joint degeneration: An imaging study of 100 patients. A.V.R. 155:373–383, 1990.
9. Reiskin, A.B.: Aseptic necrosis of the mandibular condyle: a common problem? Quintessence International 2:85–89, 1979.
10. Schellhas, K.P., El Deeb, M., Wilkes, C.H., et al: Permanent proplast temporomandibular joint implants: MR imaging of destructive complications. Am. J. Radiol. 151:731–735, 1988.

11. Schellhas, K.P., Wilkes, C.H., Fritts, H.M., et al: MR of osteochondritis dissecans and avascular necrosis of the mandibular condyle. A.J.N.R. 10:3–12, 1989.
12. Schellhas, K.P. and Wilkes, C.H.: Temporomandibular joint inflammation: comparison of MR fast scanning to T1- and T2-weighted imaging techniques. A.J.N.R. 10:589–598, 1989.
13. Schellhas, K.P., Wilkes, C.H., and Baker, C.C.: Facial pain, headache and temporomandibular joint inflammation. Headache 29:229–232, 1989.
14. Schellhas, K.P.: Internal derangement of the temporomandibular joint: radiologic staging with clinical, surgical and pathologic correlation. J. Magn. Reson. Imag. 7:495–515, 1989.
15. Schellhas, K.P.: Temporomandibular joint injuries. Radiology 173:211–216, 1989.
16. Katzberg, R.W., Schenck, J.F., Roberts, D., et al: Magnetic resonance imaging of the temporomandibular joint meniscus. Oral Surg. Oral Med. Oral Pathol. 59:332–335, 1985.
17. Harms, S.E., Wilk, R.M., Wolford, L.M., et al: The temporomandibular joint: magnetic resonance imaging using surface coils. Radiology 157:133–136, 1985.
18. Katzberg, R.W., Bessette, R.W., Tallents, R.H., et al: Normal and abnormal temporomandibular joint: MR imaging with surface coil. Radiology 158:183–189, 1986.
19. Schellhas, K.P., Wilkes, C.H., Fritts, H.M., et al: Temporomandibular joint: MR imaging of internal derangements and postoperative changes. A.J.N.R. 8:1093–1101, 1987.
20. Westesson, P.-L., Katzberg, R.W., Tallents, R.H., et al: Temporomandibular joint: comparison of MR images with cryosectional anatomy. Radiology 164:59–64, 1987.
21. Schellhas, K.P., Wilkes, C.H., Omlie, M.R., et al: The diagnosis of temporomandibular joint disease: two compartment arthrography and MR. A.J.N.R. 9:579–588, 1988.
22. Katzberg, R.W., Westesson, P.-L., Tallents, R.H., et al: Temporomandibular joint: MR assessment of rotational and sideways disk displacements. Radiology 169:741–749, 1988.
23. Stark, D.D. and Bradley, W.G.: *Magnetic Resonance Imaging.* C.V. Mosby Co., St. Louis, 1988.
24. Schellhas, K.P.: MR of muscles of mastication. A.J.N.R. 10:829–837, 1989.
25. Debont, L.G.M., Boering, G., Liem, R.S.B., et al: Osteoarthritis and internal derangement of the temporomandibular joint: a light microscopic study. J. Oral Maxillofac. Surg. 44:634–643, 1986.
26. Helmy, E., Bays, R., and Sharawy, M.: Osteoarthrosis of the temporomandibular joint following experimental disc perforation in *Macaca* fascicularis. J. Oral Maxillofac. Surg. 46:979–990, 1988.
27. Sweet, D.E. and Madewell, J.E.: Pathogenesis of osteonecrosis. In *Diagnosis of Bone and Joint Disorders.* D.K. Resnick and G. Niwayama (eds.). W.B. Saunders, Co. Philadelphia, 1988.
28. Boering, G.: Arthrosis deformans van het Kaakgewricht. Een klinisch en rontgenologisch onderzoek. Dissertatie Rijksuniversiteit te Groningen, 1966.

DIAGNOSIS

Andrew S. Kaplan

CHAPTER 17

Examination and Diagnosis

It is not uncommon to see a patient who complains of what seems to be a temporomandibular (TM) disorder, but who in reality suffers from a systemic disease, dental infection, or neoplasia. The practitioner who begins the examination with a presumptive diagnosis of "TM disorder" often looks only for the signs and symptoms that confirm this presumption. This approach can sometimes result in a faulty diagnosis.

Generally the first visit is spent taking a history, followed by a detailed examination. The history is taken for the following purposes:[1]

1. To serve as baseline information, with which treatment outcomes can be compared
2. To alert the practitioner to pertinent medical history or to complications that may be encountered
3. To help establish the etiology of the problem
4. To establish and maintain a legal record
5. To help establish a data base for research.

ORGANIZATION OF THE MEDICAL HISTORY

The history should consist of the following:

1. Personal data
2. Chief complaint
3. History of present illness
4. Past medical history
5. Past dental history.

Personal Data. These include the patient's name, address, and telephone number and any other information needed for bookkeeping purposes. The patient's birth date and sex should also be recorded. It is well known that certain systemic and local disorders have a predilection for certain age groups and genders. Ethnic origin and race should be included for the same reason.

It is useful to have the names, addresses, and telephone numbers of the internist or general practitioner and any other specialist treating the patient, such as chiropractors, osteopaths, physical therapists, and psychologists. The practitioner may wish to confer with these health-care professionals regarding past treatment, clarification of medical history, and collaboration in a multidisciplinary approach. All general dentists and dental specialists should be listed as well.

Chief Complaint. It is often said, "Listen to the patient, for he is telling you the diagnosis." The practitioner should elicit a statement of the main reason the patient has come to the office. This statement should be recorded in the patient's own words, and the patient should be allowed to explain the complaint fully before specific questions are asked. With many patients, the complaint is short and concise. Others relate rather long accounts and may tend to include unrelated information. Nevertheless, it is mainly the effect on the chief complaint that the patient judges the results of treatment.

History of Present Illness. The practitioner should ask for a detailed history, in chronologic order, related to the chief complaint. This approach allows the practitioner to follow and record the course of the disease and the sequence of previously attempted treatment. The practitioner should allow the patient adequate time to tell the story but should also probe for the nature of the pain, the particular health-care professionals seen, and the nature and results of past treatment. With experience, the examiner will gain the expertise needed to direct the conversation to those details important in establishing a diagnosis.

The use of a standard examination and history form is strongly recommended. Several have been published,[2,3] and one I employ is reproduced here (Fig. 17–1). Standard forms insure that pertinent questions are not omitted and that evaluations are uniform for all patients.

The patient should be asked to describe his or her pain in detail, including the date of onset and the specific area that hurts. What kind of pain is it—deep or superficial, sharp or dull, burning or aching? Such details can help the examiner classify the pain as neural, myogenous, or arthralgic. How frequently does the

TEMPOROMANDIBULAR DISORDER EXAMINATION FORM

NAME _____ PATIENT'S PHYSICIAN _____

AGE _____ SEX _____ DATE _____ ADDRESS _____

OCCUPATION _____ _____

ADDRESS _____ PHONE _____

_____ GENERAL DENTIST _____

PHONE (HOME) _____ ADDRESS _____

PHONE (BUS) _____ _____

REFERRED BY _____ ADDRESS _____

CHIEF COMPLAINT _____

_____

_____

Check ( ) all applicable

I. MEDICAL HISTORY

A. Arthritic Disease
    1. Traumatic Arthritis
    2. Osteoarthritis
    3. Rheumatoid Arthritis
    4. Psoriatic Arthritis
    5. Other

B. E.N.T. Disorders
    1. Salivary Gland Disorders
    2. Ear Problems
    3. Nose/Throat Problems
    4. Sinusitis
    5. Cysts
    6. Polyps
    7. Allergies
    8. Other

C. Vascular Disease and Blood Dyscrasias _____

_____

D. Head/Neck Trauma
    Date _____   Description _____

_____

_____

E. Headache/Neuralgia (location, character, frequency, duration) _____

_____

_____

F. Medication (current and past)
    1. Type _____
    2. Allergy to Medication _____

G. Additional Medical Information—Past and Present
    1. Surgery _____
    2. Psychiatric _____
    3. E.N.T. _____
    4. Orthopedic _____
    5. Neurologic _____
    6. Internist _____
    7. Rheumatologic _____
    8. Chiropractic _____
    9. Physical Therapy _____
    10. Endocrine _____
        a. Do your nails break easily?
        b. Is your skin dry?
        c. Do you tire easily?
        d. Does the cold weather bother you?
    11. Osteopathic _____
    12. Other _____
    13. Nutritional State _____

_____

FIGURE 17–1. History and examination form.

II. DENTAL HISTORY

A. Oral Conditions (describe general condition, presence of fixed or removable prosthesis, periodontal problems, and vertical dimension descrepancies)

_____
_____
_____

B. Last Dental Examination and Films _____

C. Recent Dental Treatment _____

D. Previous Orthodontic Therapy Dates _____   Bicuspid Extraction? _____
_____

E. Previous TMJ Treatment and Results (Date/Doctor) _____
_____
_____
_____

F. Pain Symptoms
   1. Date of onset _____
   2. Area of onset _____   Right _____   Left _____
   3. Type: superficial, deep, sharp, dull
   4. Quality: burning, aching
   5. Frequency: _____
   6. Duration: constant, intermittent
   7. Period of greatest intensity _____
   8. Status of pain: increased, decreased, unchanged
   9. Onset: abrupt, gradual
   10. Disappearance: abrupt, gradual
   11. Factors alleviating pain: _____
   12. Triggering devices: eating, yawning, speaking, singing, shouting
   13. Pain in specific teeth: _____
   14. Additional pain information: _____

G. Oral Symptoms (other than pain)
   1. Jaws clenched upon awakening
   2. Clenching and grinding during sleep
   3. Clenching and grinding during waking hours
   4. Muscle fatigue _____

H. Vertigo, Syncope, Meniere's Disease (frequency, duration, circumstances)
_____

I. Ear Symptoms/Joint Noises
   1. Tinnitus—(R) (L)
   2. Popping, clicking, or grating noises on opening and closing—(R) (L)
   3. Stuffiness of ears—(R) (L)

J. Skeletal—Facial Deformity _____
_____

K. Other Complaints _____
_____

III. CLINICAL EXAMINATION

A. Reported Pain
   1. Temporomandibular joint   (R)   (L)
   2. Upper back   (R)   (L)

FIGURE 17–1. *Continued*

3. Middle back	(R)	(L)
4. Lower back	(R)	(L)
5. Scapula area	(R)	(L)
6. Shoulder	(R)	(L)
7. Arm	(R)	(L)
8. Fingers	(R)	(L)
9. Chest	(R)	(L)
10. Occipital area	(R)	(L)

B. Tenderness and Pain on Palpation
   1. Temporalis

a. anterior fibers	(R)	(L)
b. middle fibers	(R)	(L)
c. posterior fibers	(R)	(L)

   2. Masseter

a. zygoma	(R)	(L)
b. body	(R)	(L)
c. lateral surface of angle of mandible	(R)	(L)
3. Digastric	(R)	(L)
4. Posterior cervicals	(R)	(L)
5. Trapezius	(R)	(L)
6. Sternocleidomastoid	(R)	(L)
7. Lateral pterygoid: insertion	(R)	(L)
8. Medial pterygoid: insertion	(R)	(L)
9. Mylohyoid	(R)	(L)
10. Coronoid process	(R)	(L)
11. TMJ lateral aspect	(R)	(L)
Lateral/posterior aspect	(R)	(L)

C. Ear (anterior wall tenderness)   (R)   (L)

D. TMJ Sounds
   (stethoscopic and/or digital palpation)

1. crepitation	(R)	(L)

   2. sagittal opening click:

immediate	(R)	(L)
intermediate	(R)	(L)
full opening	(R)	(L)

   3. sagittal closing click:

immediate	(R)	(L)
intermediate	(R)	(L)
terminal closure	(R)	(L)
4. Nature of click (soft/loud)	(R)	(L)

E. Occlusal Interferences

Left nonworking side   Right nonworking side

Protrusive   Centric occlusion

Occlusion: Angle's class _____
Extruded labial or lingual version teeth _____

FIGURE 17–1. *Continued*

F. Clinical Postural Observation
   1. Head posture (at rest): _____
   2. Range of motion: _____

G. Summary of TMJ Imaging Findings _____
_____

H. Mandibular Movement
   1. Widest interincisal opening _____
   2. Right lateral _____   Left Lateral _____
   3. Pain present with movement? _____

I. Diagnosis _____
_____

J. Plan of Treatment _____
_____

K. Prognosis _____
_____

L. Remarks _____
_____
_____
_____

patient experience the pain? Is it constant or intermittent? Are its onset and disappearance abrupt or gradual? Bell[4] has classified orofacial pain based on clinical characteristics in the flow chart reproduced in Figure 17–2.

It is important to identify pain *patterns.* For example, does the pain occur at certain times of the day? A common pattern would be waking up with a temporal headache or with jaw pain and restriction of movement. Patients sitting for long hours in front of a computer, or leaning over a desk, may complain of headaches occurring late in the afternoon. Such pain can be referred from the trapezius muscle. Pain can also be temporally related to a woman's menstrual cycle or to the performance of certain tasks.

It is useful to find out if the pain has gotten better or worse, or has stayed about the same, since it began. What tends to make the pain worse? If such things as alcohol or certain foods worsen head pain, one might suspect a vasomotor-related pain.

Does mandibular movement exacerbate the pain? Greater pain when chewing hard foods, yawning, or even speaking leads toward a diagnosis of a TM disorder. Does the patient regularly play a musical instrument? Wind instruments and the violin are common culprits for provoking pain. Deep-sea divers biting on rubber oxygen hoses may also provoke or exacerbate temporomandibular joint (TMJ) discomfort. But a TM disorder is unlikely if neither the chief complaint nor the history of present illness relates in some way to mandibular function.

What, if anything, alleviates the pain? If the patient says that alcoholic beverages provide relief, the examiner may suspect that muscle pain may at least be a component, because alcohol relaxes skeletal muscle. It is likewise of benefit to know whether over-the-counter medications, such as aspirin, antihistamines, and anti-inflammatories, alleviate the pain. In addition, many patients discover, on their own, that hot showers, ice packs, and certain forms of exercise make them feel better. The patient with a major stress component to his or her problem may feel better during the weekend or during a vacation.

The patient must be asked if he or she is aware of any *parafunctional* habits. These include bruxism, cheek biting, nail biting, thumb sucking, and pencil chewing. The harmful effects of these habits are the subject of a review by Rugh and Ohrbach.[5] Not all patients are aware of grinding or clenching during the night or even during the day. Many people habitu-

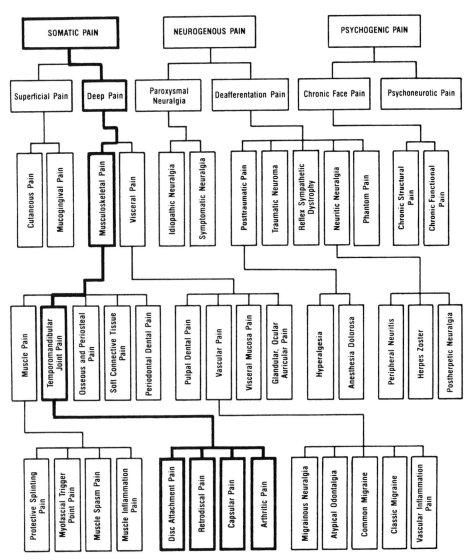

FIGURE 17–2. Orofacial pain syndromes and their relationship to temporomandibular joint disorders. (Reprinted with permission from Bell, W.E.: *Orofacial Pains,* 4th ed. Year Book Medical Publishers, Chicago, 1989.)

ally clench when they are physically exerting themselves, when they are under stress at work, or even when they are sitting in a car in a traffic jam. Queries concerning muscle fatigue in the masticatory muscles can assist in the recognition of bruxism-related symptoms. Patients often deny parafunctional habits during the initial visit. Once their awareness has increased, the report may later become positive.

The patient should be specifically asked if he or she is aware of clicking or popping noises when opening or closing the mouth, or if he or she has noticed any restriction in mandibular movement. Intermittent locking may be a sign that a complete lock is imminent. However,

there are clicks in the head and neck that don't come from the TMJ. In my clinical experience, the most frequently reported of these are a click in the neck when turning the head and a click in the ear when swallowing.

Is there tinnitus or a clogged feeling in the ears? Not all ear symptoms are related to TM disorders.[6] Suspicion should be high if otologic symptoms are not accompanied by other signs and symptoms of TM disorders.

As mentioned, the patient should provide a list of all those from whom treatment has been sought. A description of the treatment provided, along with an assessment of outcome, will assist the clinician in establishing a treatment plan, without repeating failed treatment approaches.

One must be careful to obtain enough information to evaluate the quality of care rendered. For example, it is not sufficient to know that a patient took an anti-inflammatory medication. One must know whether it was taken "as needed" or on a recommended regimen for a specified time, to make a judgment about whether the treatment should be repeated.

Any adverse effects of previous treatment should be noted, especially any TMJ-specific treatment. It is important to learn the type of practitioner who provided the treatment as well as the specific treatment rendered. To find out that splint therapy was attempted and failed is not enough. One must have information regarding the type of splint (repositioning or flat plane), the material (soft rubber or processed acrylic), the time of day the splint was worn, and the number of hours. The same reasoning applies to biofeedback or physical therapy. Without specific details, it is impossible to decide whether a given type of treatment should be tried or retried. If splint therapy has been previously done, the patient should be asked to bring in any appliance he or she may still possess for evaluation.

The patient should also be asked about the *stress* in his or her life. Some patients will readily share this information, whereas others will not. Some patients are unaware of their stressors. Is the patient currently under the care of a psychologist or psychiatrist? A general description of the treatment should be elicited, but the practitioner should *not* attempt to be a psychotherapist.

Does the patient show signs of depression? Chronic pain has a close relationship with depression, although the exact nature of the connection has yet to be established. The eight cardinal signs of depression include loss or increase of appetite, insomnia, loss of energy, anhedonia (decrease or loss of pleasure in usual activities), psychomotor agitation (pacing or slowed speech), feelings of worthlessness, and recurrent thoughts of death or suicide.[7] Presence of any four of these symptoms suggest clinical depression, and psychiatric consultation may be advisable.

The patient should also be given the opportunity to add any information that he or she may believe is important but has not been discussed.

Past Medical History. The American Dental Association medical history form is a good starting point and can be filled out prior to the consultation visit. More information should be elicited, using the TMJ history and examination form (see Fig. 17–1). The examiner must screen for any systemic illnesses that may have affected the structures of the TMJ. These may include arthritides, either local or systemic (see chapter 10); neoplastic disease, either benign or malignant (see chapter 14); and endocrine disorders or vascular diseases.

The medical history should include a detailed description of any head trauma the patient may have sustained, including injuries from accidents, muggings, fights, or sporting accidents. All trauma should be noted, even those in the distant past. It is not unusual for motor vehicle–accident injuries to go unnoticed and undiagnosed for many years.[8]

Details such as the date of occurrence, description of the trauma itself, and post-trauma symptoms should be noted, together with the treatment sought after the incident. Patients who have sustained trauma are often involved in litigation, and the examiner may eventually be asked to provide a detailed report. The practitioner should also be prepared to determine if a true cause-and-effect relationship exists between the trauma and a particular TM disorder.

Has the patient ever suffered from any otolaryngologic disorders? These include chronic sinusitis; ear, nose, or throat pain; and nasal or sinus polyps. A history of known allergies should be taken, especially those to specific food, vegetation, or medication. Common allergens that produce headaches are red wine, cheese, monosodium glutamate (used to heighten food flavor), and chocolate.

If the patient complains of headaches, what are their frequency, anatomic location, and intensity? The relationship between headaches and TM disorders is supported by the literature,[9] and headaches are symptoms often seen in clinical practice. The examiner should be able to differentiate among the three major types of headache: muscle-contraction, migraine, and cluster.[10] The subject of headache is treated in depth elsewhere.[11]

Many causes of headache exist. Not all headaches are caused by or related to TM disorders. Among the causes of headaches are such serious conditions as intracranial bleeding and neoplastic disease. A neurologic consultation may be needed if any doubt exists concerning the cause of chronic headache.

The history of prior hospitalization can yield

valuable information. Has the patient ever undergone surgery? If so, the reason for and type of anesthesia (local or general) should be noted. Patients who have undergone general anesthesia can sustain damage to the TMJ during endotracheal intubation. The examiner must specifically ask about surgical treatment for removal of impacted teeth and periodontal surgery. Patients often don't think of these procedures when asked about "surgery."

Past Dental History. When did the patient last have a thorough dental examination? One must always entertain the possibility that supposed TMD symptoms stem from the teeth or the periodontium. When was the last time a full-mouth radiographic series was taken? If the pain is nonspecific, or the patient feels the pain is coming from the teeth, appropriate radiographs must be taken. In addition, the teeth and periodontium should be examined.

The examiner should also inquire about past orthodontic therapy. Little evidence exists to support an association between orthodontic therapy and TM disorders,[12] but in isolated situations there may be a link (see chapter 23). Furthermore, this possible relationship has led to an increasing amount of malpractice litigation.

An assessment of the patient's dental condition should include noting the presence of full or partial dentures. If the patient wears a removable prosthesis, he or she should be asked if it is worn to bed at night. For some patients, the treatment may be as simple as requesting them to wear the prosthesis while they sleep.

Multiple units of fixed prosthetics should be recorded. The patient should be asked whether he or she has undergone any recent dental treatment. It is common for a patient with a long-term asymptomatic TM disorder to suffer restricted movement, TMJ-related pain, or both, after undergoing an extensive dental procedure that requires the mouth to be open for a long period of time. Such treatment can include endodontic procedures, extensive restoration, or extraction of impacted teeth. Occasionally, patients who have had mandibular nerve blocks can have trismus, with resulting limited opening.

EXAMINATION

Examination for TM disorders differs from the examination of general dentistry. The teeth and periodontium receive less attention than the state of the muscles and joints and the mandibular movement.

The examination is made up of the following components:

1. Observation
2. Masticatory muscle examination (palpitation and resistance testing)
3. Temporomandibular joint examination (palpitation, range of motion, selective joint loading, assessment of joint sounds)
4. Head and neck examination
5. Occlusal analysis
6. Diagnostic anesthetic blocks
7. Cervical spine examination
8. Temporomandibular joint imaging
9. Specialist consultation.

Observation. The examination begins as soon as the patient enters the office. How does the patient walk? Is the gait normal, or does he or she limp or walk excessively slowly or quickly? Does the patient appear to be seriously overweight or underweight? These observations can lead to a suspicion of systemic illness. How does the patient talk? When engaged in conversation is it animated or with flat affect? Does the patient talk excessively fast? Voice changes can suggest anxiety or depression. As more patients are seen, the practitioner develops an appreciation for these kinds of observations, which can lead toward asking appropriate questions.

For the diagnosis of TM disorders, there are several specific observations to be made. Does the patient move the mouth comfortably while speaking or is there evidently "guarding" of mandibular movement? Is there any suggestion of a postural problem? Parafunctional habits sometimes become apparent during the patient interview. Some patients with retrognathia habitually try to protrude the mandible. Others may habitually hold their jaws to one side. Occasionally, patients are chewing gum, which can have more than a small effect on prognosis. Still other patients may have obvious dyskinetic movements of the jaw.

Masticatory Muscle Examination. This is the most important part of the examination. No ideal sequence for muscular palpation exists, but the examiner should adopt a particular order and use it routinely. This strategy insures that parts of the examination are not omitted. This is another reason why the examination and history form should be used.

The recommended technique is simultaneous palpation of the left and right sides, using approximately 3 lb of pressure.[13] I use the following sequence:

1. Temporalis muscles
2. Zygomatic arch
3. Masseter muscles
4. Anterior digastric muscles
5. Cervical spine
6. Trapezius muscle
7. Sternocleidomastoid muscles
8. Medial pterygoid muscles
9. Lateral pterygoid area
10. Coronoid process.

Procedure

Temporalis Muscle. This fan-shaped muscle originates along the superior line of the temporal bone and is inserted at the coronoid process. The muscle can be loosely divided into three sections: anterior, middle, and posterior. These segments are palpated as shown in Figures 17–3 to 17–5. Next, each zygomatic arch is palpated along its lateral aspects (Fig. 17–6). The practitioner should be alert for any abnormality, such as an old fracture that might play a role in problems of mandibular movement.

Masseter Muscle. This muscle is palpated from its origin on the inferior and lateral aspect of the zygomatic arch, to its insertion on the inferior border of the angle of the mandible. The masseter has both a superficial and deep portion. The superficial portion is palpated extraorally against the ascending ramus of the mandible (Fig. 17–7). The deep portion is made accessible by placing the index finger inside the mouth, just anterior to the anterior border of the ascending ramus, and pinching the muscle between the finger and thumb.

Digastric Muscle (Anterior Belly). Before palpating the digastric muscle, it is good practice to palpate the body of the mandible, seeking any abnormalities in bone continuity that might result from old fractures. Mandible body fractures are often accompanied by condylar fractures on the contralateral side. The anterior digastric can be palpated from its origin on the lingual side of the mandible to its tendinous insertion on the hyoid bone (Fig. 17–8). The hyoid bone can also be checked for mobility by manipulating it while asking the patient to swallow.

Sternocleidomastoid Muscle. The sternocleidomastoid muscle is palpated from its dual origin on the sternum and clavicle along its course upward and posteriorly to its insertion on the mastoid process. This muscle is located simply by asking the patient to turn the head to the opposite side (Fig. 17–9).

Cervical Spine (Posterior Cervical Region). The cervical spine is palpated bimanually just to either side of the midline. The practitioner starts at the base of the skull and palpates downward to the seventh cervical vertebra (Fig. 17–10). Soreness of the cervical area is especially common in patients with a forward neck posture (see chapter 5). The practitioner should check especially carefully for signs of pain in this area if there is a history of a motor vehicle accident.

Trapezius Muscle. This muscle is examined from its origin on the acromion process to its insertion along the midline of the spine to the

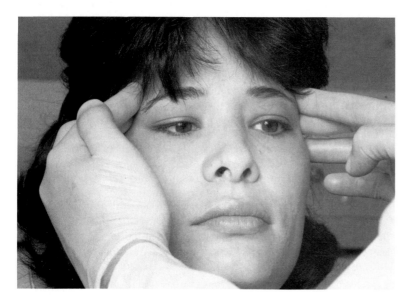

FIGURE 17–3. Palpation of the anterior portion of the temporalis muscle.

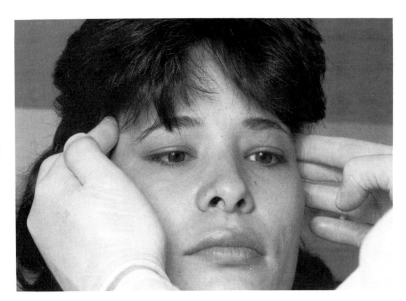

FIGURE 17-4. Palpation of the middle portion of the temporalis muscle.

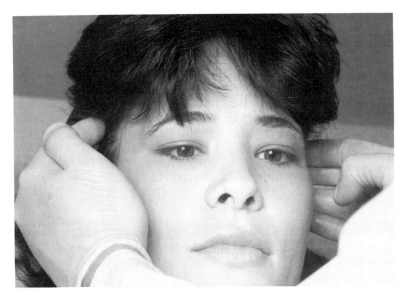

FIGURE 17-5. Palpation of the posterior portion of the temporalis muscle.

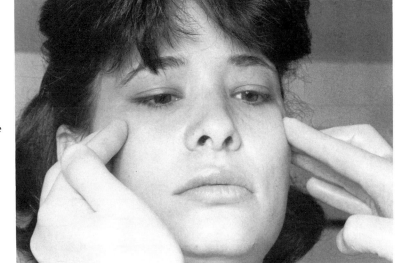

FIGURE 17-6. Palpation of the zygomatic arch.

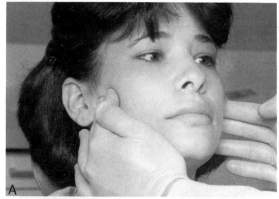

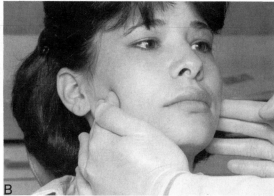

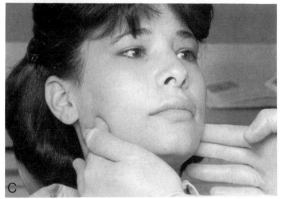

FIGURE 17–7. Palpation of the masseter muscle. *A,* Origin. *B,* Body. *C,* Insertion.

neck posture often have soreness in this muscle.

Lateral Pterygoid Muscle. It has been argued, on the basis of anatomy, that intraoral palpation of the inferior belly of the lateral pterygoid muscle is not possible.[15] Clinicians, nonetheless, make the attempt by sliding a finger along the buccal aspect of the maxillary dentition until the tuberosity region is reached and, then, palpating superiorly and medially (Fig. 17–12). It is likely that the clinician is palpating a portion of the medial pterygoid instead. Because palpation of this region after treatment often shows decreased sensitivity, diagnostic palpation should, in my opinion, continue to be included.

Medial Pterygoid Muscle. The medial pterygoid muscle forms a sling with the masseter muscle around the *ascending ramus* of the mandible. This area is palpated by placing an index finger in the mouth, just medial and posterior to where a mandibular block injection is customarily given (Fig. 17–13). Care must be

base of the skull. The muscle is palpated without difficulty along its superior aspect (Fig. 17–11). The trapezius muscle is perhaps the most common site for muscular trigger points and often refers pain to the base of the cranium and the temporal region.[14] Patients with forward

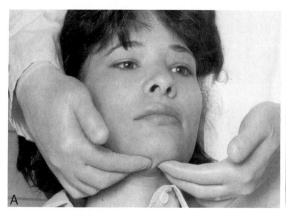

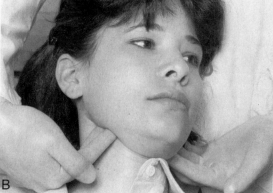

FIGURE 17–8. Palpation. *A,* Anterior digastric muscle. *B,* Posterior digastric muscle.

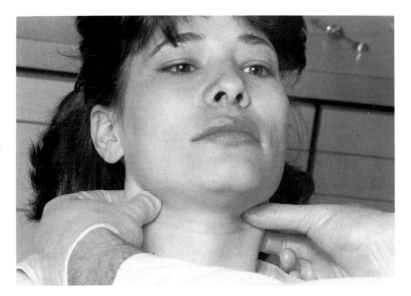

FIGURE 17–9. Palpation of the sternocleidomastoid muscle.

taken as the palpation of this muscle often stimulates a gag reflex.

Mylohyoid Muscle. This muscle forms the floor of the mouth, originating on the lingual aspect of the mandible and inserting at the hyoid bone. It is palpated by placing one finger intraorally and another extraorally as shown in Figure 17–14.

Coronoid Process. The temporalis muscle inserts into the coronoid process of the mandible.

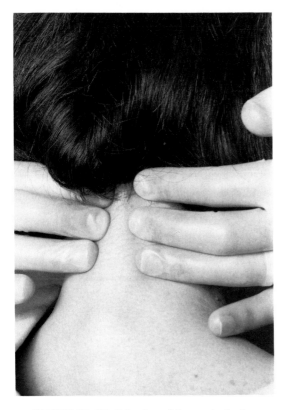

FIGURE 17–10. Palpation of the cervical spine.

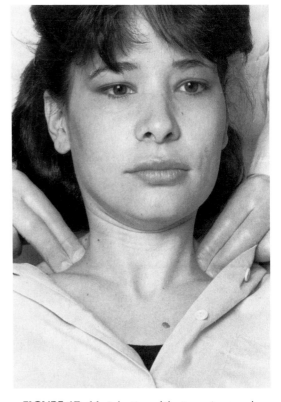

FIGURE 17–11. Palpation of the trapezius muscle.

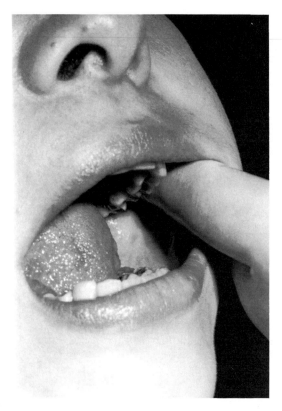

FIGURE 17-12. Palpation of the lateral pterygoid region.

This osseous structure is palpated intraorally. The patient is asked to open his or her mouth, and the clinician then locates the anterior border of the ascending ramus and slides the finger superiorly to the coronoid process (Fig. 17–15).

Muscular Resistance Testing

Friedman and Weisberg[3] have advocated the use of muscular resistance testing. Although these tests cannot replace muscular palpation, they are often helpful in localizing pain and should be done when necessary. It is not mandatory to employ all such tests in the examination of every patient with a possible TM disorder.

Resistive Opening. The clinician places the palm of one hand on the patient's chin. The other hand supports the occiput. The patient then opens against this resistance (Fig. 17–16), and areas of pain or tenderness are noted. This test activates the inferior belly of the lateral pterygoid.

Resistive Closing. The patient is instructed to open the mouth approximately 30 mm. The examiner places two fingers on the incisal edge of the lower anterior teeth, while the other hand steadies the forehead (Fig. 17–17). The patient is instructed to close against this resistance and to point out any areas of pain or sensitivity. This test activates the temporalis, masseter, and medial pterygoid muscles.

Resistive Lateral Movement. The clinician places one hand against the side of the mandible, while the other hand supports the contra-

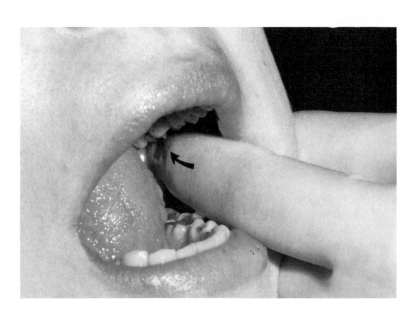

FIGURE 17-13. Palpation of the medial pterygoid muscle.

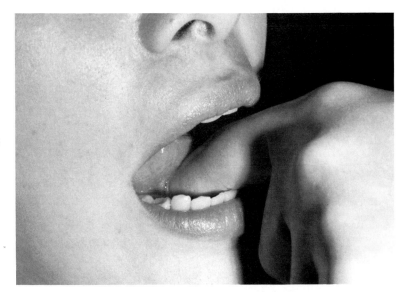

FIGURE 17–14. Palpation of the mylohyoid muscle.

lateral temporal area. The patient is instructed to move the mandible laterally against this resistance. The test activates the lateral and medial pterygoid muscles on the contralateral side (Fig. 17–18).

Resistive Protrusion. One palm is placed against the chin, while the other hand supports the occiput from behind. The patient is told to protrude the mandible against resistance. The test activates the lateral pterygoid (Fig. 17–19).

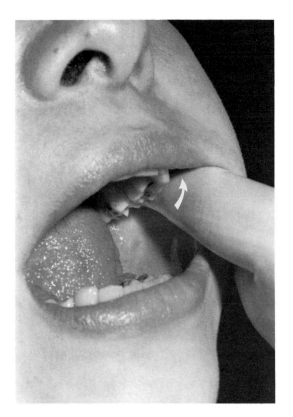

FIGURE 17–15. Palpation of the coronoid process.

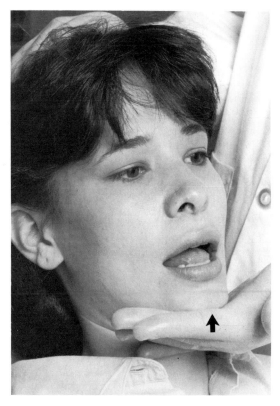

FIGURE 17–16. Resistive opening.

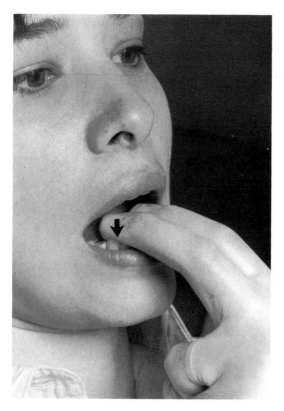

FIGURE 17–17. Resistive closing.

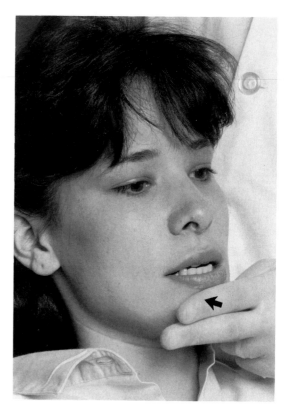

FIGURE 17–19. Resistive protrusion.

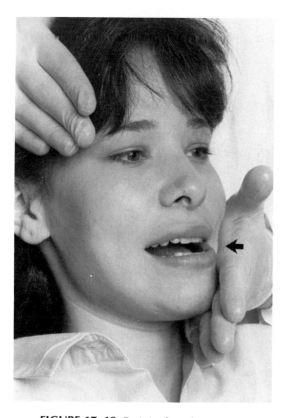

FIGURE 17–18. Resistive lateral movement.

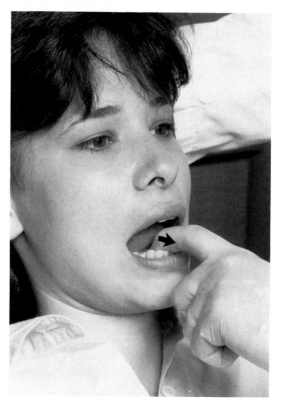

FIGURE 17–20. Resistive retrusion.

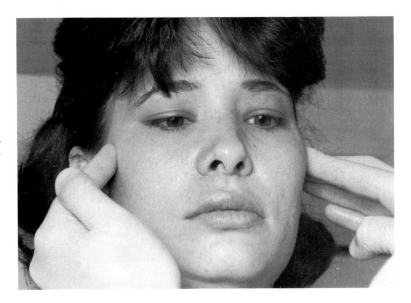

FIGURE 17–21. Palpation of the lateral aspect of the temporomandibular joint and capsule.

Resistive Retrusion. The clinician hooks two fingers behind the lower anterior teeth, while the patient's mandible is protruded. The patient is then instructed to retrude the mandible. This test activates the posterior fibers of the temporalis (Fig. 17–20).

Temporomandibular Joint Examination. The TMJ must be carefully examined in open and closed positions as well as in lateral movement.

The lateral aspect of each joint and capsule is located by *lightly* palpating anterior to the external auditory meatus, while the patient opens and closes (Fig. 17–21). The condyle is felt, as it moves forward and backward. Once

the condyle is located, the patient closes the mouth and any pain is noted. The patient is then told to open the mouth again. The resulting depression posterior to the condylar head is then palpated. This is the posterior-lateral aspect of the condyle and retrodiscal tissue. (Fig. 17–22). The clinician then places a finger in each external auditory meatus and palpates anteriorly, while the patient closes. Any pain is noted.

Range of Motion. The examiner must be thoroughly familiar with the normal movements of the mandible before deviations can be identified. All movements should be smooth and

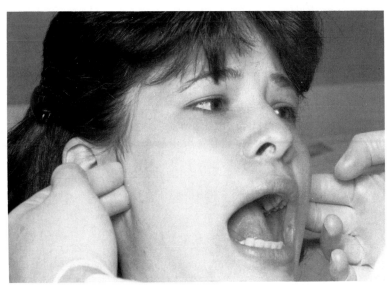

FIGURE 17–22. The patient's mouth is slightly open. Palpation of the posterior aspect of the condyle and lateral aspect of the retrodiscal tissue.

without noise or pain. The mandibular range of motion should be measured at maximal opening, and lateral movement measured bilaterally. Protrusive movement should be checked for freedom of movement, deviation, and pain.

Maximal Interincisal Opening. Maximal interincisal opening should be measured under conditions of both *active* and *passive* range of motion.

Active Range of Motion. This is the extent of voluntary movement in a joint. Normal maximal opening should be between 40 and 50 mm. The patient is asked to open as wide as he or she can, and the opening is measured between the incisal edges of the central incisors (Fig. 17–23).

Passive Range of Motion. This is the maximal movement of a joint when it is manipulated by a clinician and when the patient's muscles are relaxed. Although it is difficult to obtain a reliable reading from a patient with significant muscle splinting, this test will help differentiate between a *muscle-induced* limitation of motion

and a limitation due to other causes. To make the measurement, the patient is placed in a semirecumbent position, with the clinician seated behind and an assistant standing by. The patient is asked to relax the lower jaw as much as possible. The head is cradled in one arm, and both the practitioner's hands are placed in the manner advocated by Dawson[16] and shown in Figure 17–24. When the practitioner opens the patient's mouth, the maximal opening can be measured by the assistant.

Another technique often utilized in physical medicine is the determination of the end feel of a joint. The patient is asked to open the mouth, voluntarily, as wide as possible. If the movement is limited, the practitioner places an index finger on the edge of a mandibular central incisor and the thumb on the edge of the opposing maxillary tooth. In a scissor-like motion, the mandible is opened by sustained pressure (Fig. 17–25), and the practitioner notes the end feel of the movement. A soft, bouncy feeling may indicate muscular or other soft tissue restriction, whereas a hard feeling may in-

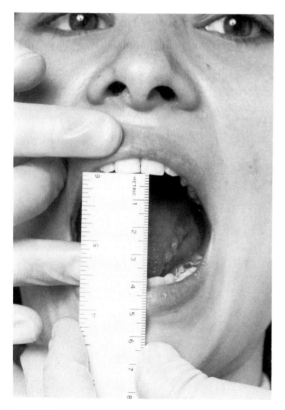

FIGURE 17–23. Measurement of the maximum interincisal distance (active range of motion).

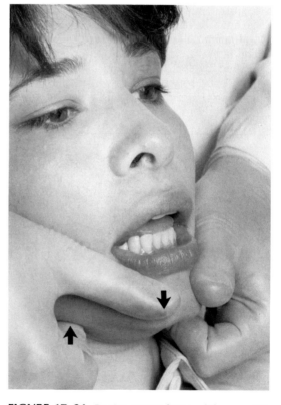

FIGURE 17–24. Passive manipulation of the mandible (passive range of motion).

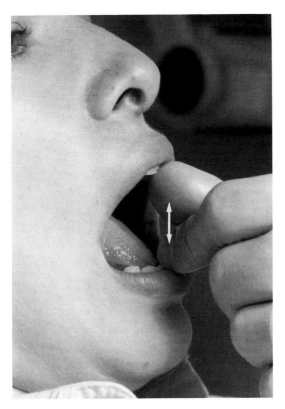

FIGURE 17–25. Sustained pressure on the incisal edges to determine "end feel."

dicate osseous abnormalities, meniscal displacement, or fibrotic contracture.

Lateral Movement. Lateral movement is measured simply by extending a line between the maxillary central incisors, down to the opposing mandibular tooth or teeth. The practitioner demonstrates lateral movement and then asks the patient to imitate the movement as much as possible. The distance is then measured (Fig. 17–26). Normal lateral movement is 8 to 12 mm. Limited lateral movement can indicate a disc displacement without reduction or a muscle problem on the contralateral side. Some patients have difficulty making this movement even with normal TMJs. Patience must be exercised before assuming that there is true limitation.

Protrusive Movement. The patient should be asked to protrude the mandible (Fig. 17–27). Although difficult to measure precisely, this movement should be straight and smooth and should not cause any pain.

Patterns of Mandibular Opening. The particular pattern of mandibular opening should be diagrammed. Limitation and deviation should be noted. Opening and closing deviations are observed simply by taking a small ruler or tongue blade and laying the edge down the midline of the face (Fig. 17–28). While the practitioner "eyes" the straight edge, the patient opens and closes slowly. Deviation can be seen without difficulty and diagrammed. The mandible should open in a straight line without deviation. All movement should be smooth. Limited opening with deviation to one side should arouse the clinician's suspicion for an internal derangement without reduction. Normal opening with deviation to one side in the midrange of opening before returning to midline supports a diagnosis of internal derangement *with* reduction. Some irregular opening or closing movements are difficult to attribute to internal derangement alone and may represent muscular or some other pathology. Figures 17–29 to 17–31 illustrate common patterns of mandibular opening and their interpretation.

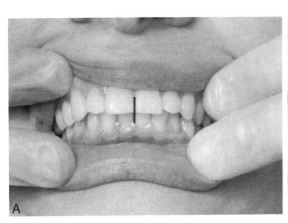

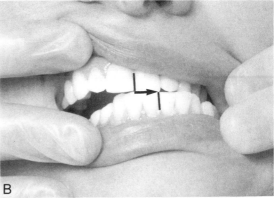

FIGURE 17–26. *A* and *B,* Measurement of maximum lateral mandibular movement.

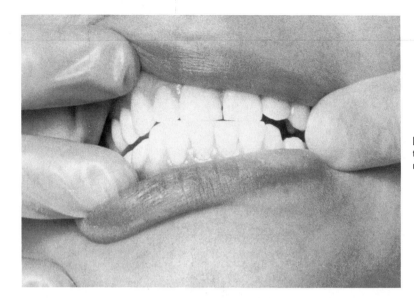

FIGURE 17–27. Observation of the maximal protrusive movement.

Selective Temporomandibular Joint Loading.
The TMJ can be examined by applying specific loads to it. If clenching without anything between the teeth elicits joint tenderness, capsulitis or retrodiscitis can be suspected. The relaxed mandible can also be manipulated posteriorly by the dentist as seen in Figure 17–32. The patient can be asked to bite on an orangewood stick on the ipsilateral side in the posterior region (Fig. 17–33). This should cause the pain to *decrease*. When the patient is asked to bite on the contralateral side, the pain should return.

Not all these loading tests will be useful or necessary for every patient, but practitioners should be familiar with selective loading should difficulties arise in establishing a precise diagnosis.

Head and Neck Examination. A linea alba found on the buccal mucosa, about the level of the occlusal line, is evidence of habitual cheek biting. A scalloped tongue may indicate thrust-

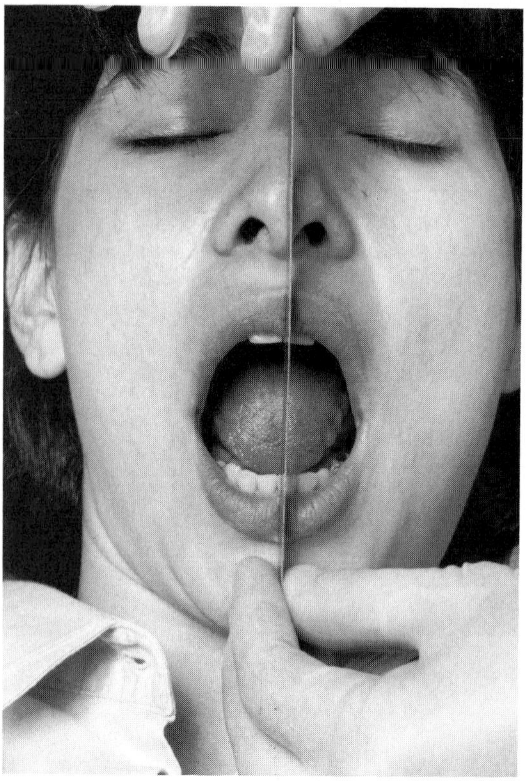

FIGURE 17–28. "Eying" the sagittal opening and closing pattern using a tongue blade.

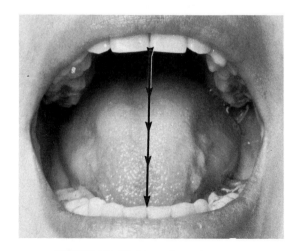

FIGURE 17–29. Normal opening pattern.

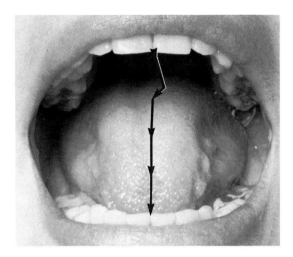

FIGURE 17–30. Opening pattern often seen with internal derangement with reduction.

ing. The patient should be given a thorough head-and-neck examination for palpable nodes, salivary-gland pathology, and neoplastic disease. The procedure is described in detail elsewhere.[1]

Joint Sounds. These are classified as either *clicking* or *crepitus.* Clicking is a brief noise that occurs at some point during opening, closing, or both. Crepitus is a diffuse, sustained sound usually felt throughout a considerable portion of the opening or closing cycle or both. It is often described as a "gravelly" or "grating" feeling in the joint. Clicking has been shown through cadaver studies, arthrography, and open joint surgery to be indicative of disc displacement.[17] The displacement is likely to be in

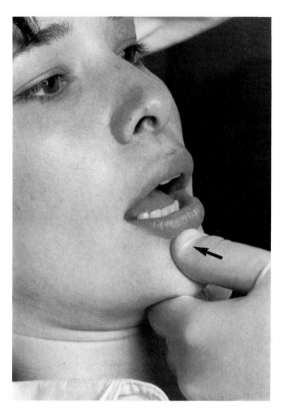

FIGURE 17–32. Selective loading. Posterior temporomandibular joint loading to test for retrodiscal pain and inflammation.

an anterior or a medial direction, or in both. Lateral and posterior displacements have also been reported (see chapter 9).

To evaluate clicking, the practitioner lightly places the hand over each TMJ in turn and asks the patient to open and close. The click may occur early, midway, or late during opening, and early, midway, or late during closing. The later the click occurs during the opening movement the more severe the displacement. Disc displacement is likely to produce a closing click at a smaller interincisal distance than the opening click. Late clicking on opening, and early clicking on closing, may indicate that the condyle is translating over the articular eminence.

Crepitus is evidence of a change in osseous contour. It commonly indicates osteoarthrosis, but other arthritides must be considered as well.

Temporomandibular joint clicking can be rather subtle, and many clinicians listen with a stethoscope (Fig. 17–34). Sonographic analysis of joint sounds has been the subject of research

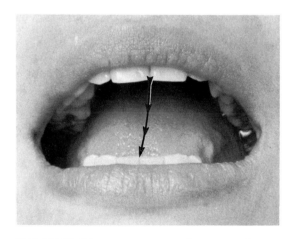

FIGURE 17–31. Opening pattern often seen with internal derangement without reduction.

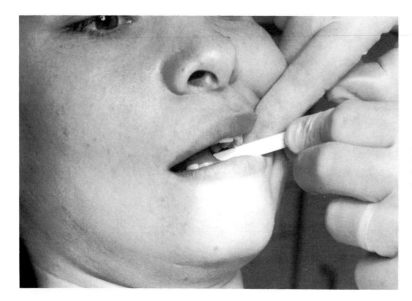

FIGURE 17–33. Selective loading. Biting on an orangewood stick. Biting on the ipsilateral side should relieve pain while biting on the contralateral side should cause pain.

but has not yet found its way into routine clinical practice.[18] Doppler analysis of joint sounds has also been studied.[19]

Occlusal Analysis. The clinician should note the patient's maxillomandibular relationship,

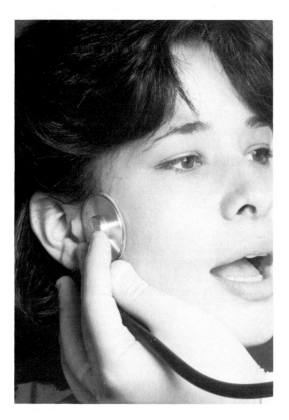

FIGURE 17–34. Listening for joint noises with a stethoscope.

both skeletal and dental. Angle's classification of malocclusion should be used, and extruded teeth and teeth in crossbite should be noted. Nonworking side and protrusive interferences should be recorded. The form of occlusal guidance is noted, and the patient is examined for restorations and prostheses that do not provide adequate support or that cause occlusal prematurities. Occlusion is discussed in detail in chapters 4 and 28.

Diagnostic Anesthetic Blocks. Occasionally, the clinician may have difficulty relating pain to specific anatomic structures or may wish to confirm a clinical suspicion. Bell[4] and Kroening[20] have advocated diagnostic injections of local anesthetic. The suspected source of pain is anesthetized, and the effect on the pain assessed. Only anesthetics that do not contain epinephrine should be given. These include mepivacaine (Carbocaine), lidocaine, and procaine.

The practitioner should use a 25-gauge needle. For extraoral injections, the skin is first swabbed with an alcohol pad. For intraoral injections, the mucosa can be swabbed with a topical anesthetic. Bell[4] has specified the following guidelines for the safe administration of diagnostic injections:

1. Avoid inflamed or infected areas.
2. Use aseptic technique and aspiration with all injections.
3. Be thoroughly familiar with the structures through which the needle will pass.
4. Be thoroughly familiar with the anesthetic and its potential complications.

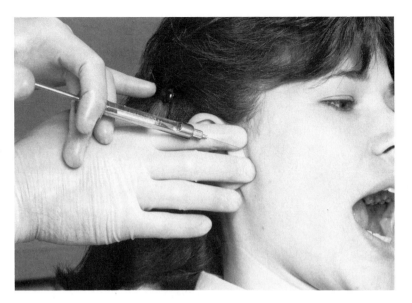

FIGURE 17–35. Diagnostic injection. The temporomandibular joint.

Figures 17–35 to 17–41 illustrate the positioning of the needle for diagnostic injections of the TMJ, as well as the masseter, temporalis, trapezius, sternocleidomastoid, lateral pterygoid, and medial pterygoid muscles. Injections of local anesthetics can be administered in treatment as well as in diagnosis.

Temporomandibular Joint. The joint is innervated by the auriculotemporal nerve as well as by the masseteric branch of the maxillary di-

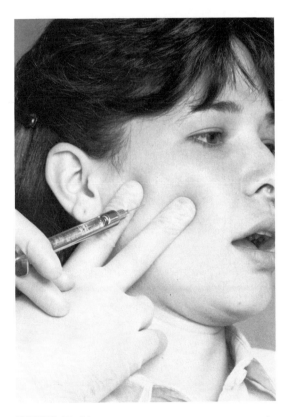

FIGURE 17–36. Diagnostic injection. Masseter muscle.

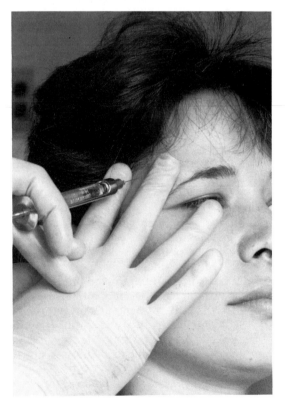

FIGURE 17–37. Diagnostic injection. Temporalis muscle.

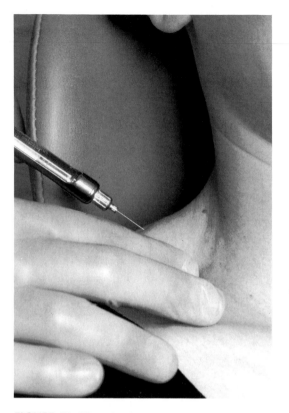

FIGURE 17–38. Diagnostic injection. Trapezius muscle.

into vascular or other structures that pass through the muscle.

Although it is difficult to palpate for specific trigger points in the lateral and medial pterygoids, diagnostic injection still can be attempted. The inferior belly of the lateral pterygoid is anesthetized without difficulty, employing a technique similar to that of the posterior superior alveolar block. The needle should first be bent to an angle of about 45 degrees. The patient is instructed to open the mouth slightly, and the needle is inserted just posteriorly and superiorly over the tuberosity region. The needle should be advanced upward and medially. The solution is deposited, and the needle withdrawn. The medial pterygoid muscle can be anesthetized extraorally in the manner described by Travell and Simons,[14] or intraorally by inserting a needle just posterior to where the needle would be placed for a mandibular block injection. The practitioner should also be familiar with the infiltration of the individual maxillary teeth, the posterior superior alveolar block, the mandibular block, and the mental block for the differentiation of

vision of the trigeminal nerve. The condyle is first located by palpation. The needle is then inserted posterior and superior to it and advanced until the condylar head is felt. The needle is withdrawn slightly while the anesthetic solution is deposited. This injection is generally sufficient to anesthetize the pain emanating from the capsule and the other soft tissues of the joint. If this procedure is not sufficient a slight additional amount of anesthetic should be infiltrated just anterior to the condylar head. *Masseter.* This muscle is palpated extraorally until a trigger point is located. The area is swabbed with an alcohol wipe. The trigger point is localized between the middle and index finger of the nondominant hand. The needle is inserted through the trigger point, slightly withdrawn, and passed through in different directions as described by Travell and Simons,[14] while the anesthetic solution is slowly deposited.

This same technique is used for locating trigger points in the temporalis, trapezius, and sternocleidomastoid muscles. Care must be taken not to inject anesthetic inadvertently

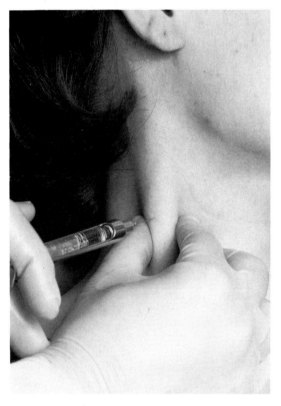

FIGURE 17–39. Diagnostic injection. Sternocleidomastoid muscle.

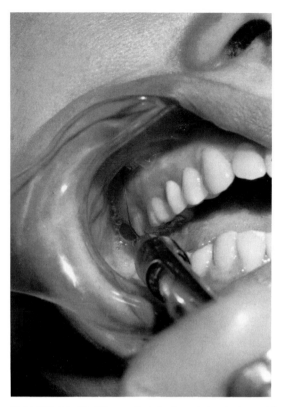

FIGURE 17–40. Diagnostic injection. Lateral pterygoid muscle.

tooth pain, if necessary. These procedures are discussed in detail elsewhere.[21]

Cervical Spine Examination. Dornan and colleagues[22] have suggested that many patients presenting for TMJ evaluations have cervical spine symptoms. It is clinically evident that these problems can act synergistically with TM disorders and, even by themselves, can refer pain as far away as the temporal region. Motor vehicle accident victims in particular often present with both cervical sprain and TMJ injury. Although dental practitioners are not trained to do an in-depth analysis of the upper quarter, they should evaluate these structures generally. If indicated, a referral should be made to a physical therapist, a physiatrist, an orthopedist, or a neurologist.

The evaluation of the cervical spine is straightforward and takes little time. The patient is asked to stand in a relaxed position. The practitioner notes any shoulder asymmetry or deviation of the neck (Fig. 17–42). The patient is then asked to turn sideways and is checked for forward neck posture (Fig. 17–43). Next, the patient is asked to rotate the head to each side (Fig. 17–44). The patient should be able to rotate the head about 80 degrees in each direction. The patient is asked to extend the neck by looking upward (Fig. 17–45) and then to flex the neck by looking downward (Fig. 17–46). Normal movement should be about 60 degrees in each direction. The patient is asked to bend the head to each side (Fig. 17–47). Normal side-bending is approximately 45 degrees. During all these procedures, pain and limitation of movement are noted.

All of these movements are performed utilizing active range of motion. The patient is told to stop if he or she encounters pain. Passive range of motion should be utilized only if the

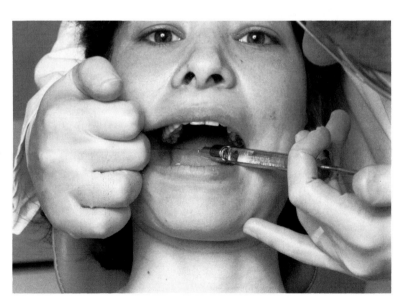

FIGURE 17–41. Diagnostic injection. Medial pterygoid muscle.

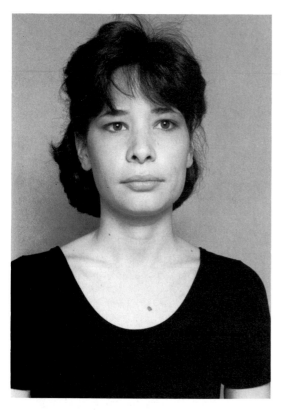

FIGURE 17–42. A patient exhibiting shoulder and neck asymmetry indicating possible cervical problems.

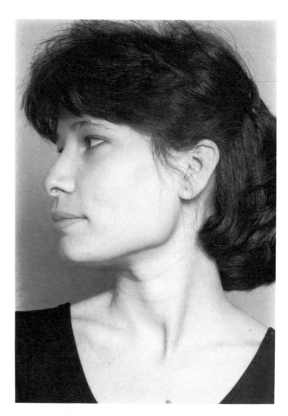

FIGURE 17–44. Cervical range of motion. Rotation.

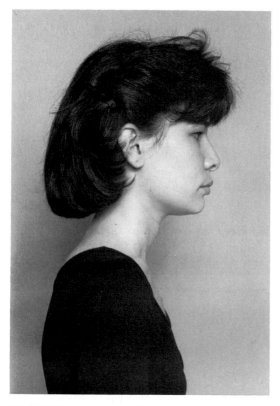

FIGURE 17–43. A patient exhibiting forward neck posture.

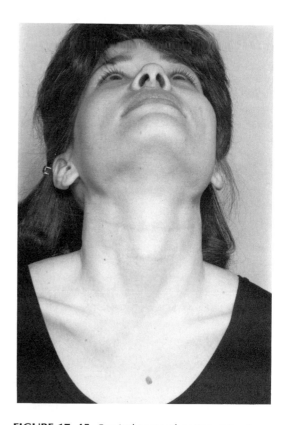

FIGURE 17–45. Cervical range of motion. Extension.

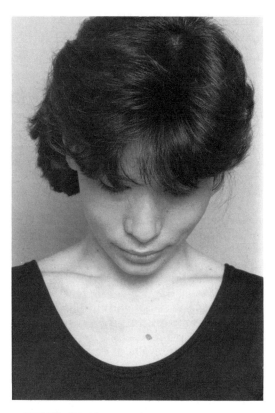

FIGURE 17–46. Cervical range of motion. Flexion.

practitioner is specially trained. Otherwise, it is preferable to refer the patient to an appropriate specialist.

Temporomandibular Joint Imaging. The practitioner has a wide choice of imaging techniques, which are discussed elsewhere in this text. These techniques include not only conventional films of osseous structures but also arthrograms, computerized tomography (CT), and magnetic resonance imaging (MRI), which often give valuable information concerning the soft tissues. These techniques are discussed in detail in chapters 18, 19, and 20.

Panoramic and lateral transcranial projections are helpful only as general screening tools. They may show severe joint pathology but are not sensitive to subtle changes in the osseous contours of the joint. They give little information about meniscal position. Some practitioners had claimed that disc displacement could be deduced from these films,[23] but this practice has largely been abandoned.

Tomograms of the TMJ are somewhat better, because they produce clear radiographic "slices" of the condyle, which clearly show sub-

tle osseous changes. Thus, they make it possible to identify early stages of osteoarthrosis. Joint-space measurements can be made from these films, especially if they are corrected for condylar inclination (see chapter 18). The significance of such joint-space measurements is not clear, however, and no conclusion about meniscal position can be made.

Arthrography requires injection of a radiopaque dye into one or both joint spaces. A fluoroscopic record of joint movement can be recorded on a video cassette. Currently, this is the only technique for visualizing the meniscus during joint movement. It also shows the position of the disc, in relation to the condyle, and the presence of any perforation. The introduction of the needle and dye into the joint may cause increased tenderness for several days. Furthermore, a few patients prove to be allergic to the dye (see chapter 19).

Computerized tomography and MRI are both useful in examining the TMJ. At present, CT is superior for looking at osseous structures, but MRI techniques are constantly improving. Both methods can be applied to locate the po-

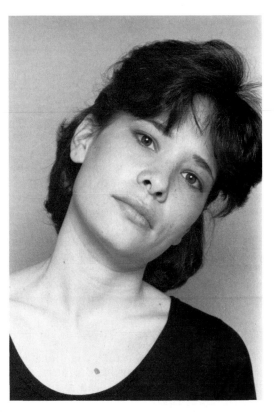

FIGURE 17–47. Cervical range of motion. Side-bending.

sition of the disc, although the ability of CT to do so has been questioned.[24] Magnetic resonance imaging gained favor, as the equipment became more common. Unlike arthrography or CT, MRI has the advantage of not requiring radiation exposure. It is at present the most expensive of the imaging techniques.

Specialist Consultation. If it is possible that the problem is not due to a TM disorder or that it is beyond the training and experience of the practitioner, the patient should be referred to a specialist for further consultation. It is better to have many medical consultations than to treat a patient mistakenly for a TM disorder when a possibly life-threatening disease remains undiagnosed.

In addition, when a TM disorder *is* diagnosed, the practitioner may sometimes wish to recruit the help of one or more other healthcare workers in other fields. These may include other dental specialists, physical therapists, physicians, psychologists, or neurologists.

DIAGNOSIS

Diagnosis is generally established in stages. Based on the history and examination, the clinician establishes a *clinical impression*—the strongest case that can be made based on the information available. Occasionally, a diagnosis is elusive even after repeated visits. It is sometimes necessary to say to a patient "I just don't know what is wrong with you."

Based on the clinical impression, the clinician determines the necessity of further diagnostic tests, usually including some forms of imaging. As mentioned, other specialists may be consulted. Blood workups and other tests may be performed. Possible pathologic findings are discussed in detail in chapters 7 through 16.

After receiving the test results, the practitioner either confirms the clinical impression or re-evaluates the findings to arrive at a *working diagnosis*. From this, a *treatment plan* is decided on and presented to the patient.

TRIAL THERAPY

Throughout therapy, the clinician must continue to monitor the working diagnosis. Inexplicably poor results should lead to re-evaluation. In this respect, all treatment has to be considered trial therapy.

COMPUTER-ASSISTED EXAMINATION AND DIAGNOSTICS

In an attempt to standardize and simplify history-taking procedures at least two groups have developed software packages. Levit and coworkers[26] developed a questionnaire that can be sent to a new patient prior to the first office visit. Known as "The TMJ Scale," Levit's questionnaire relies on patient self-report and is analyzed by computer. The questions are divided into three categories. 1. A global domain predicts if a TM disorder, in fact, exists. 2. A physical domain is comprised of a pain report, perceived malocclusion, palpation pain, and joint dysfunction and motion limitation scales. The patient is asked to palpate extraoral areas and rate the pain. Another scale predicts the possibility that there is a non-TM disorder. 3. The psychosocial domain consists of three factors: psychosocial, stress, and chronicity.

The questionnaires are scored as raw data with reference to previously determined normative data. The results are plotted graphically, and the physical domain scores are rank ordered, according to their severity. These are labeled significant, borderline significant, or not significant. A narrative interpretation of the results can also be generated.

Fricton and Chung[27] developed a computerized questionnaire to "assist in and accurately and efficiently identify and measure the severity of contributing factors for TMJ and craniofacial pain." The patient sits in front of a computer terminal in the clinician's office and over the course of about 1 hour answers questions that generate information regarding medical and illness history, contributing factors, and a preindices and postindices report. Four indices are measured: symptom severity index, illness impact index, life-functioning index, and quality of life index. These indices can be utilized to longitudinally study changes within a patient.

These techniques are helpful research tools and may be convenient in certain practices. They are by no means a necessity for proper diagnosis and examination.

REFERENCES

1. Halstead, C., Blozis, G., Drinan, A., Gier, R.: *Physical Evaluation of the Dental Patient.* C.V Mosby Co., St. Louis, 1982.
2. Gelb, H.: *Clinical Management of Head, Neck and*

TMJ Pain and Dysfunction. W.B. Saunders Co., Philadelphia, 1985.

3. Friedman, M. and Weisberg, J.: *Temporomandibular Joint Disorders, Diagnosis and Treatment.* Quintessence Publishing Co., Lombard, IL. 1985.

4. Bell, W.: *Clinical Management of Temporomandibular Joint Disorders.* Year Book Medical Publishers, Chicago, 1985.

5. Rugh, J. and Ohrbach, R.: Occlusal parafunction. In *A Textbook of Occlusion.* N. Mohl, G. Zarb, G. Carlsson, and J. Rugh (eds.). Quintessence Publishing Co., Lombard, IL, 1988.

6. Uthman, A., Sheth, B., and Gale, E.,: Prevalence of otological symptoms in a clinical setting. J. Dent. Res. 65:385, 1986.

7. Weisman, M. and Myers, J.: Rates and risks of depressive symptoms in a U.S. urban community. Acta Psych. Scand. 57:219–231, 1978.

8. Rogal, O.: *Mandibular Whiplash.* Owen J. Rogal, Philadelphia, 1987.

9. Solberg, W.: Epidemiological findings of importance to management of temporomandibular joint disorders. In *Perspectives in TMJ Disorders.* G. Clark and W. Solberg (eds.) Quintessence Publishing Co., Lombard, IL, 1987.

10. Campbell, A. Cluster headache. J. Craniomand. Disord. 1:21, 1987.

11. Dalessio, D.: *Wolff's Headache and Other Head Pain.* Oxford University Press, New York, 1980.

12. Sadowski, C. and Polson, A.: Temporomandibular disorders and functional occlusion after orthodontic treatment: results of two long-term studies. Am. J. Orthodont. 86:386–390, 1984.

13. Gross, A. and Gale, E.: Evaluation of temporomandibular joint disorders. In *TMJ Disorders: Management of the Craniomandibular Complex.* S. Kraus (ed.). Churchill Livingstone, New York, 1988.

14. Travell, J. and Simons, D.: *Myofacial Pain and Dysfunction. The Trigger Point Manual.* Williams & Wilkins, Baltimore, 1983.

15. Johnstone, D. and Templeton, M.: The feasibility of palpating the lateral pterygoid muscle. J. Prosthet. Dent. 44:318, 1980.

16. Dawson, P.: *Evaluation, Diagnosis, and Treatment of Occlusal Problems.* C.V. Mosby Co., St. Louis, 1988.

17. Helms, C., Katzberg, R. and Dolwick, F.: *Internal Derangements of the Temporomandibular Joint.* Radiology and Research Foundation, San Francisco, 1983.

18. Hutta, J.T., Morris, R., Katzberg, R., et al: Separation of internal derangements of the TMJ using sound analysis. Oral Surg. Oral Med. Oral Path. 63:151, 1987.

19. Davidson, S.: Doppler auscultation: An aid in TMJ diagnosis. J. Craniomand. Disord. 2:128–132, 1988.

20. Kroening, R.: Neural blockade in the differential diagnosis of craniofacial pain. In *Perspectives in TMJ Disorders.* G. Clark and W. Solberg (eds.). Quintessence Publishing Co., Lombard, IL, 1987.

21. Bennett, R.: *Monheim's Local Anesthesia and Pain Control in Dental Practice,* 6th ed. C.V. Mosby Co., St. Louis, 1978.

22. Dornan, R., Clark, G., Greene, E.: Predictors of a serious craniocervical dysfunction in a sample of TMD patients. J. Dent. Res. 66:337, 1987. (Abstract.)

23. Hoppenfield, S.: *Physical Examination of the Spine and Extremities.* Appleton-Century-Crofts, Norwalk, CT, 1976.

24. Weinberg, L.: Correlation of TMJ dysfunction with radiographic findings. J. Prosthet. Dent. 28:519–539, 1972.

25. Fava, C., Gatti, G., Cardesi, E., et al: Possibilities and limits in identifying the TMJ articular meniscus with the CT scanner: A comparative anatomoradiologic study. J. Craniomand. Disord. 2:141–147, 1988.

26. Levit, S., Lundeen, T., and McKinney, M.: The TMJ scale manual. Pain Resource Center, Inc., Durham, North Carolina, 1987.

27. Fricton, J. and Chung, S.: Contributing factors: A key to chronic pain. In *TMJ and Craniofacial Pain: Diagnosis and Management.* J. Fricton, R. Kroening, and K. Hathaway (eds.). Ishiyaku EuroAmerica Inc., St. Louis, 1988.

Andrew S. Kaplan

CHAPTER 18

Plain, Tomographic, and Panoramic Radiography and Radionuclide Imaging

After completing a thorough history and examination, the clinician may choose to image the temporomandibular joint (TMJ). The reason is usually one of the following: (1) to confirm suspected pathology, (2) to screen for unsuspected pathology, (3) to identify the staging of a disease, (4) to evaluate the effects of a given treatment, and (5) to help evaluate the range of motion of the joint.

Radiographic visualization of the TMJ is a challenge to both the dental and medical professional. The major problem is the superimposition of anatomic structures, which obscure the view of the joint.

Radiographic techniques for viewing the osseous portions of the TMJ include plain films, tomography, computerized tomography (CT), and panoramic radiography. To view soft tissues of the TMJ, arthrography and magnetic resonance imaging (MRI) are the techniques of choice. But there is no "ideal" view of the joint.

The choice of a particular technique is determined by the nature of the suspected pathology and by the availability of instrumentation and trained personnel. The patient's physical or mental state may also limit the choices of technique. A patient who is claustrophobic can have serious problems tolerating MRI. A patient with a severe cervical problem may not be able tolerate the head positioning required for a direct sagittal CT scan or a submental vertex (SMV) projection.

Radiographic findings are just one piece of the diagnostic puzzle. Imaging of the TMJ cannot replace a *complete* history and an examination. Diagnosis obtained from an image of the joint alone must be considered incomplete.

This chapter describes plain film techniques, tomography, and panoramic radiography, as they relate to the TMJ. Another technique of imaging the TMJ is also described—radionuclide imaging—not truly a radiographic technique. This occasionally is used to evaluate physiologic activity of the TMJ. These techniques all provide information about the osseous structures of the joint. The following two chapters review arthrography, MRI, and CT scanning.

TRANSCRANIAL RADIOGRAPHY

The transcranial TMJ film, also known as the lateral oblique projection, is commonly employed by dentists. Transcranial radiographs can be taken with relative ease in the dental office during the initial consultation. The time and the equipment cost are the least of all the sagittal imaging techniques. A standard dental x ray unit can be utilized. A head positioning device or craniostat can be purchased from several different manufacturers.

This technique is an aid to the general screening of the osseous structures of the joint. Relatively advanced stages of arthritis and other diseases can be identified. Changes in condylar position as a result of treatment intervention can also be assessed.

The transcranial film has been the subject of much controversy because it can be readily misinterpreted or overinterpreted. The result may be a treatment plan based upon erroneous assumptions and a questionable diagnosis. The difficulty arises from distortion of the osseous structures, superimposition of other anatomic structures, and inability to visualize anything but the lateral third of the condyle and articular fossa.

Distortion

The ideal TMJ radiograph would be taken with the film held perpendicular to the long axis of the condylar head.[1] The x-ray beam would be directed down the long axis of the condyle. Figure 18–1 is a film of a dried con-

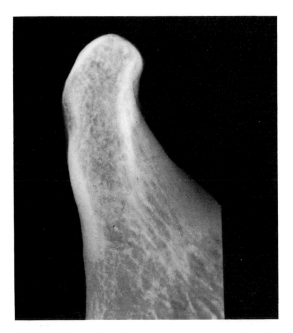

FIGURE 18–1. Film taken through the long axis of the condylar head: dried specimen. Note the distinct cortical margin representing the superior aspect.

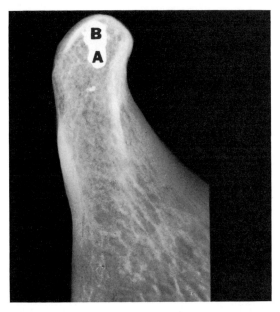

FIGURE 18–2. Film taken through the long axis of the condylar head. Medial (A) and lateral (B) poles identified with radiopaque markers. Note the superimposition of markers.

dylar specimen taken in this manner. Note the clarity of the cortical margin. Anatomically, this margin represents the superior contour of the condylar head. Figure 18–2 shows the same view of the specimen but the medial and lateral poles of the condyle have been identified with radiopaque markers. Note that the markers are almost superimposed. However, in vivo, super-imposition of other structures (see subsequent discussion) makes this "ideal view" clinically impossible.

Most investigators of transcranial techniques recommend angling of the beam anywhere from 15 to 25 degrees above the horizontal plane to prevent superimposition of the ana-tomic structures. Figures 18–3 and 18–4 show both the marked and unmarked specimens viewed at a 20-degree horizontal angle. Note the effect on the positioning of the lateral and medial poles. As the angle is changed, the po-sition of the anatomic landmarks changes. The medial pole is displaced in an inferior direc-tion, and the medial portion of the condylar head is now superimposed on the neck of the condyle.

Most workers also recommend that the beam be displaced in a horizontal plane 10 to 15 degrees. The majority of techniques em-ployed today angle the beam anteriorly.[2] Fig-ures 18–5 and 18–6 show the effect of a 15-de-gree horizontal angulation with a 25-degree vertical angulation on views of the marked and unmarked condyle. The medial pole of the condyle is now displaced in an anterior direc-

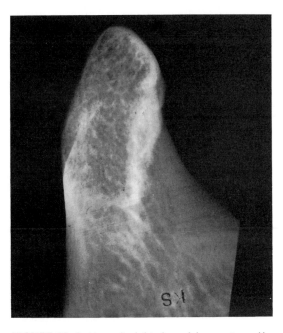

FIGURE 18–3. Unmarked dried condylar specimen film taken at a 20-degree vertical angulation and a 0-degree horizontal angulation.

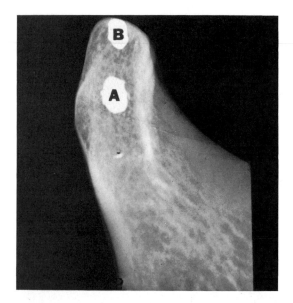

FIGURE 18–4. Marked dried condylar specimen film taken at a 20-degree vertical angulation and 0-degree horizontal angulation. Note the displacement of the medial pole of the condyle (A) from the lateral pole (B).

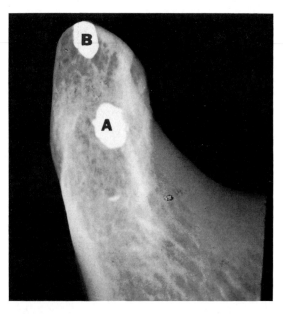

FIGURE 18–6. Marked dried condylar specimen film taken at a 25-degree vertical angulation and a 15-degree horizontal angulation. Note the further displacement of the medial pole (A) and lateral pole (B).

tion but is still superimposed on the neck of the condyle.

Clinically, such angulation is necessary to prevent superimposition of the contralateral TMJ and ipsilateral petrous ridge and zygoma.

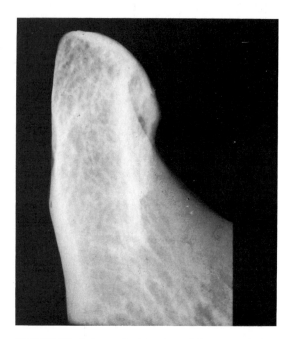

FIGURE 18–5. Unmarked dried condylar specimen film taken at a 25-degree vertical angulation and a 15-degree horizontal angulation.

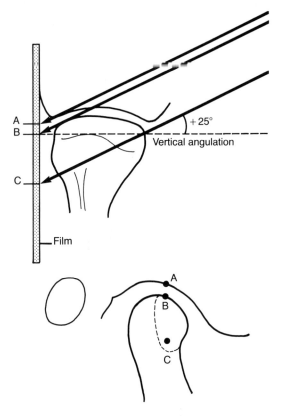

FIGURE 18–7. The necessary angulation of the beam for the transcranial film allows only the lateral third of the joint to be viewed.

The result of the vertical angulation is that only the lateral third of the condyle is clearly visible as diagrammed in Figure 18–7. The clinician must be aware of this limitation, because pathology in the central and medial portions of the condyle may be missed.[3]

Superimposition

According to Rosenberg and Silha,[1] at least four different techniques have been advocated to minimize superimposition. Each requires specific film and x-ray tube positioning. Lindblom,[4] Gillis,[5] and Grewcock[6] suggested positioning the x-ray tube above the contralateral condyle. McQueen[7] advocated the use of an inferior position. Blaschke[2] suggested that a 25-degree horizontal angulation and a 15-degree vertical angulation represent a reasonable compromise. This position is illustrated in Figure 18–8.

Figure 18–9 demonstrates open and closed transcranial views taken in such a position. Although the TMJ is fairly well visualized, superimposition still occurs. The practitioner should be aware that such superimposition is inevitable and should be able to recognize and distinguish the superimposed structures.

In a discussion of this problem, Palla[8] emphasized that the clinician must be able to identify all structures in the radiograph. The external auditory meatus, articular eminence, and condylar head should be clearly visible. Fava and Preti[9] identified structures that are commonly superimposed: the pyramid of the petrous portion of the temporal bone (often only the superior petrosal crest), zygomatic arch, hyperpneumatization of the temporal bone, and double condyle and fossa outlines. Palla[8] also noted that the mastoid air cells and the skull base structures can be superimposed. Examples of transcranial films are shown (Figs. 18–10 and 18–11).

Visualization of Pathology

As previously noted, angling of the x-ray tube results in an oblique image; only the *outer lateral aspect* of the condyle and articular eminence can be visualized.[10,11] Osseous pathology on the superior aspect of the condyle between the lateral and medial poles may be missed. Gonsalves and coworkers[12] placed osseous deformities on dry skull specimens and imaged the TMJs with varying techniques. They reported standardized transcranial views to be the poorest in identifying osseous defects. These researchers also noted that defects, both large and small, are more detectable on the lateral aspects of the condylar head than along the superior aspect.

Eckerdahl and Lundberg[13] compared histologic sections of TMJs with transcranial radiography and tomography of the same specimens. They pointed out that caution must be taken in assuming the absence of pathology in the central and medial aspects when viewing the transcranial oblique radiograph.

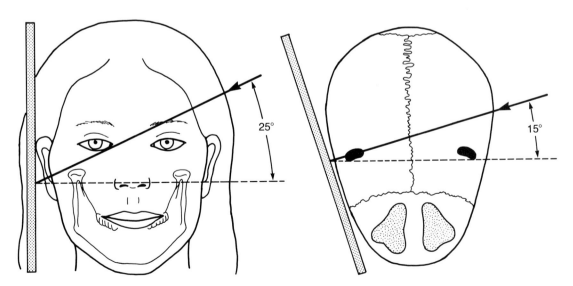

FIGURE 18–8. Recommended tube placement for transcranial radiography. (Redrawn from Rosenberg, H. and Silha, R.: Dent. Radiol. Photog. 55:1, 1982.)

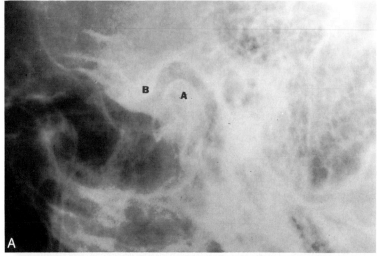

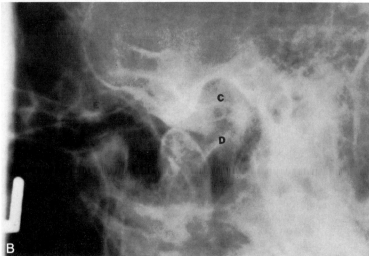

FIGURE 18–9. *A* and *B,* Example of a transcranial film in the open and closed positions. Note the following structures: condyle (A), articular eminence (B), and fossa (C). The superimposed structures include the superior petrosal crest (D) and zygomatic arch (E).

In another study, Jumean and associates[14] compared transcranial radiographs and tomograms with anatomic dissections of the actual specimens. They concluded that transcranial films show only the lateral aspect of the joint. They also found that the tomogram was superior in evaluation of medial and central regions of the condyle. Mongini,[15] in another study comparing transcranial radiographs to tomograms, came to similar conclusions but maintained that the transcranial film is still helpful, if the clinician takes its limitations into account.

Techniques

Several different head positioners or craniostats are commercially available that produce acceptable transcranial TMJ images. Two examples are shown in Figures 18–12 and 18–13.

Most require the patient to be seated. Some employ an angle board placed on a counter top and require that the patient bend the head to the side. According to Tanaka,[16] the upright or seated position is preferable so that mandibular movement is free and unstrained.

Exposures are generally taken while the teeth are in maximal intercuspation and maximal opening. Bell[17] suggests views also be done in maximum lateral excursion and in a closed "unclenched" position. Other practitioners take exposures at the point of clicking. Sufficient information is generally obtained from a fully closed and maximal open position.

Corrected Techniques

Both the horizontal and vertical angulations of the condyles vary from patient to patient and indeed between the right and left sides of

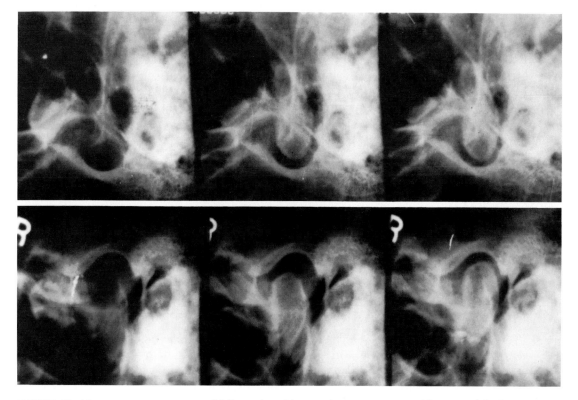

FIGURE 18–10. A six-exposure transcranial film series with normal osseous contours. (Courtesy of the Denar Corporation, Anaheim, California.)

the same patient.[18] For these reasons, several investigators advocate customizing tube angulation for each patient.

Some investigators[19–21] suggest taking an SMV projection first (Fig. 18–14). The resulting view of the condyles allows the vertical angulation of each side to be evaluated (Fig. 18–15 and 18–16). Condylar angulation is determined by the following steps:

1. A reference line is drawn connecting the external auditory meatus. Alternatively, Berrett[18] suggests the midsagittal line as a reference point (Fig. 18–17).
2. Lines are drawn bisecting each condyle from lateral to medial pole, and these lines are extended to the intermeatal line.
3. The resulting angles are measured.
4. The patient's head is rotated by the angle measured.
5. The transcranial exposure is taken.

Interpretation

When analyzing a transcranial radiograph several principles need to be kept in mind as follows:

1. The practitioner should know how the film was taken, including the vertical and horizontal angulations.
2. The practitioner should be familiar with the patient's history and physical examination findings.
3. More meaning than is appropriate should not be given to the film.

The dentist should view the closed-mouth position, locating the external auditory meatus. The TMJ is just anterior. The condyle should be identified and its cortical margin observed. Next, the cortical outline of the glenoid fossa and articular eminence should be viewed. The condyle should have a well-defined, smooth, rounded contour. The cortical margin should be relatively uniform. Slight variations in thickness are not uncommon, particularly on the anterior slope, which is the functional area. The articular fossa and eminence should also have smooth curved surfaces. Their cortical margins should be well defined. The articular eminence may or may not have visible radiolucent air cells.

Pathologic changes that may be visible on the condyle include flattening, lipping, osteo-

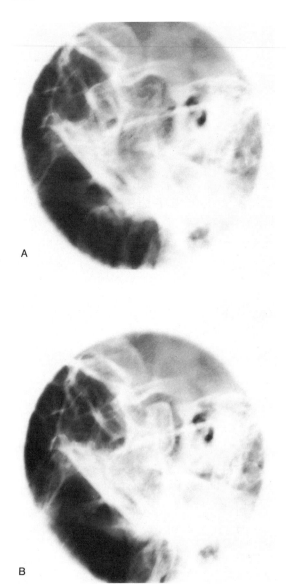

FIGURE 18–11. Open-mouth (*A*) and closed-mouth (*B*) transcranial films with osteoarthrotic changes.

(21%), osteophyte formation (20%), and irregular surface (19%).

The joint space should be well defined. It is not an empty space but contains the meniscus and retrodiscal tissues. If the joint space cannot be seen the reason may be ankylosis, early or advanced osteoarthrosis, or a problem in angulation.

Many practitioners study the transcranial view to analyze the position of the condyle within the fossa. Although the condylar position may be somewhat predictive of disc displacement,[23] it is by no means pathognomonic and should not be considered as a diagnostic entity by itself. This subject is discussed in more detail further on in this chapter.

Additionally, the practitioner should look at views in the open position. The amount of condylar translation should be assessed. Normal movement is evidenced by translation to about the apex of the articular eminence. The clinician can then check for osseous deformities, corroborating what was seen on the view in the closed position. In many transcranial films, the condyle and fossa are more clearly visualized in the open view.

TRANSMAXILLARY AND TRANSORBITAL PROJECTIONS

Because of the limitations of the transcranial TMJ film, supplemental films have been suggested.[24] The most common are transmaxillary and transorbital films. These are taken from an anterior-posterior perspective and provide medial-lateral views of the condyle. These are valuable for identifying osseous pathology on the superior and medial aspects of the joint, which may not be visible with lateral oblique projections.

The transmaxillary film is the more commonly selected of the two. The patient is seated, with the mouth open and the occlusal plane parallel to the floor. The fully translated condyle minimizes superimposition. If the patient is unable to open the mouth the film may be of no value.

As described by Peterson,[25] the beam is directed through the maxillary sinus just below the infraorbital foramen on the contralateral side of the TMJ of interest. Horizontal angulation of the film from the midsagittal plane should be approximately 40 degrees. Vertical angulation is about 10 degrees upward (Fig. 18–18). The film should be placed so that the x-ray beam is perpendicular to it.

phytes, and cortical margin loss. The articular fossa and condyle may show increased radiopacity, which can indicate bony sclerosis characteristic of advanced osteoarthrosis. Severe destruction characteristic of systemic arthritides as well as neoplasia may also be evident. Typical pathologic changes are discussed in detail elsewhere in this text. Bezuur and colleagues[22] studied 89 patients with TM disorders viewing transcranial, SMV, and tomographic films. They found pathology with the following frequency: sclerosis (23%), condylar flattening

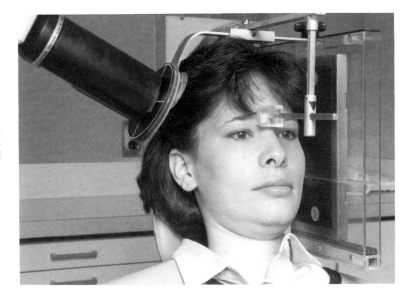

FIGURE 18–12. Farrar positioner and craniostat for temporomandibular joint transcranial films.

The transorbital view is taken in a similar fashion except, as the name indicates, the beam passes through the orbit, with a vertical angulation downward of about 10 degrees. A disadvantage of this projection is that it requires direct radiation of the orbits.

A commercially available positioning device simplifies taking these views in the dental office (Fig. 18–19).

TOMOGRAPHY OR LAMINOGRAPHY

Tomography or laminography overcomes several of the problems inherent in the transcranial oblique projection. In its most simple form, the x-ray source and the film holder move in opposite directions (Fig. 18–20), creating a central point or fulcrum, in the struc-

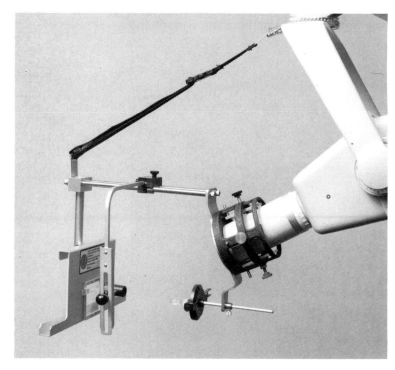

FIGURE 18–13. Denar Accurad head positioner for transcranial films. (Courtesy of the Denar Corporation, Anaheim, California.)

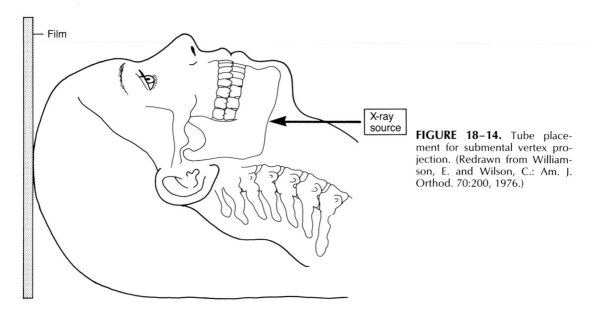

FIGURE 18–14. Tube placement for submental vertex projection. (Redrawn from Williamson, E. and Wilson, C.: Am. J. Orthod. 70:200, 1976.)

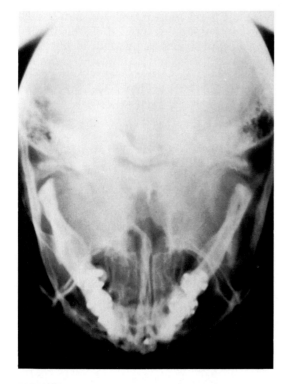

FIGURE 18–15. A submental vertex projection. (Courtesy of Landmark Medical Imaging Incorporated, Decatur, Georgia.)

ture to be imaged. The movement has the effect of blurring out layers of tissue either above or below the layer defined by the fulcrum. This process gives the tomogram "separating capacity",[1] i.e., the ability to picture a single slice of an object (Fig. 18–21). Dramatic decreases are observed in superimposition and distortion.

The movement of the x-ray source and the film describe an angle about the central fulcrum (Fig. 18–22). The size of the angle determines the thickness of the slice. The smaller the angle the thicker the slice—a zero angle being a plain film.

Films taken with exposure angles of 10 degrees or less give a thick section with reduced clarity. Such thick-section tomography is also known as zonography.[1] Exposure angles of 40 to 50 degrees give thin sections. These are the ones most often employed with TMJ tomography. Rosenberg and Silha[1] point out that the source-to-object and object-to-film distances can also affect the thickness of a slice. In practice, however, they are usually kept constant.

The clarity of the structure viewed is called *image quality*. It is of central importance in the diagnostic value of a tomogram. Image quality varies with the path chosen for the x-ray source and film. A particular path is called the *trajectory*. The simplest tomographic trajectory is linear (see Fig. 18–22)—both the source and the film travel in straight lines. Linear tomographic equipment is considerably more expensive than craniostats for transcranial views

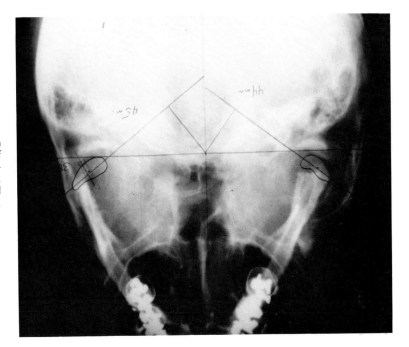

FIGURE 18-16. Lines drawn on a submental vertex for analysis of condylar angulation using the intrameatal line as the reference. (Courtesy of Landmark Medical Imaging Incorporated, Decatur, Georgia.)

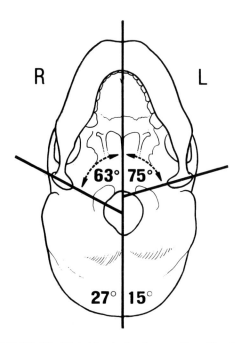

FIGURE 18-17. Midsagittal reference line. (Reprinted with permission from Berrett, A.: Radiology and radiography of the temporomandibular articulation. In *Clinical Management of Head, Neck TMJ Pain and Dysfunction.* H. Gelb (ed.). W.B. Saunders Co., Philadelphia, 1985.)

but is small enough for the dental office. The radiographs produced are of diagnostic quality and offer much greater clarity than transcranial films.

Linear tomograms are slightly obscured by "streaking." These streaks are at their worst when the long axis of the condyle is directly perpendicular to the tube trajectory.[1] In practice, however, streaking detracts little from the diagnostic value of the film.

Linear tomographic units designed for the dental office allow the patient to sit in an upright position. This contrasts with medical equipment that compels the patient to remain prone, with the head turned to one side. As previously noted for transcranial techniques, the sitting position is preferred because it allows for unstrained mandibular movement. Most dental units employ a craniostat device, allowing for duplication of head position for serial imaging (see Fig. 18-22). Depending on the particular equipment, streaking can be horizontal or vertical (Figs. 18-23 and 18-24).

Tomographic slices are usually 1 mm in thickness and taken every 2 mm from one pole to the other. The radiologist will record numbers under each exposure in a given series, indicating the relative depth at which the slice was made. The practitioner must know what views the numbers correspond with, because

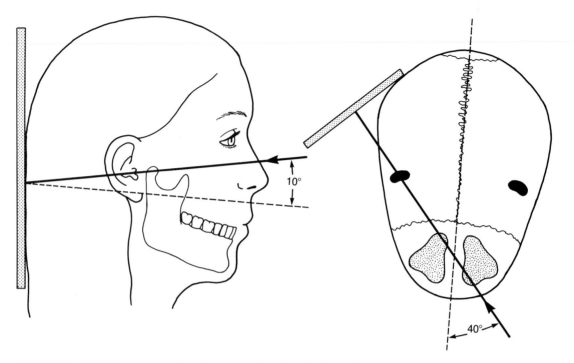

FIGURE 18–18. Tube placement for the transmaxillary film. (Redrawn from Peterson, A. and Nanthaviroj: Odontol. Rev. 27:77–92, 1976.)

slices sometimes start from the medial pole and sometimes from the lateral.[26] Generally, four to six slices are recorded in the open and closed positions.

Separating capacity and, hence, picture definition improve as the complexity of the trajectory increases. At least three other kinds of trajectories have been described: circular, elliptic, and polycycloidal (Figs. 18–25 to 18–27). The complex trajectory of polycycloidal tomography gives the clearest image of all tomographic techniques and eliminates streaking. Figure 18–28 and Figure 18–29 show examples of polycycloidal tomography.

Unfortunately, such elaborate equipment is available only in hospitals and medical imaging centers. Polycycloidal films are always taken with the patient laying down. The use of a craniostat is difficult, although Dunn and associates[27] described such a device. Unfortunately, its use requires the practitioner to be present every time a film is taken or to teach the technique to the medical radiologist and technician. For most dentists, either requirement would be impractical.

In any case, reproduction of the cranial position is important only when it is necessary to make exact joint space measurements and

when it is necessary to take post-treatment films, in order to measure the changes as a result of condylar repositioning techniques.

Corrected Techniques

Some investigators[28] suggest the employment of "corrected tomography," so that the x-ray beam is directed straight down the long axis of the condyle. Otherwise, the tomographic slices are likely to be taken at an oblique angle distorting the image and making it difficult to determine just what portion of the condyle is being viewed. According to Blaschke,[2] three different techniques have been suggested.

1. Nonmeasurement correction: The patient's head is rotated so that the mandible, zygomatic arch, or temple lies flat against the table.

2. Standard measurement correction: The patient's head is rotated a standard amount, usually 15 or 20 degrees, to correct for average condylar angulation.

3. Individualized correction: An SMV film is taken first. Condylar angulation is calculated as previously described, and the patient's head is rotated accordingly.

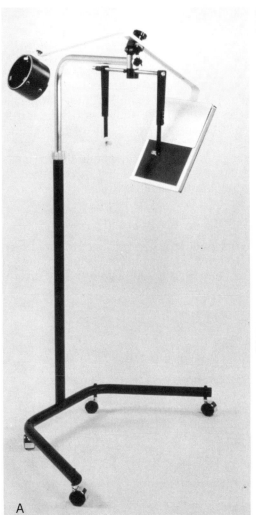

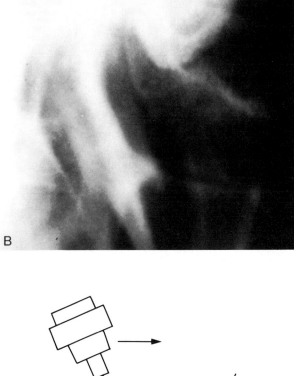

FIGURE 18–19. *A,* Denar head positioning device for transmaxillary films. *B,* Example of a transmaxillary radiograph. (Courtesy of the Denar Corporation, Anaheim, California.)

Rotation of the head is always necessary, but the best technique remains a matter of speculation. For practical purposes, a standardized correction is a reasonable choice.

Interpretation

The tomogram is examined in the same way as a transcranial film. The clinician should first look at the views of the closed position. Usually, four to six images of each side are provided, representing slices from the lateral to the medial poles of the condyle. The cortical outline of the condyle and fossa should be evalu-

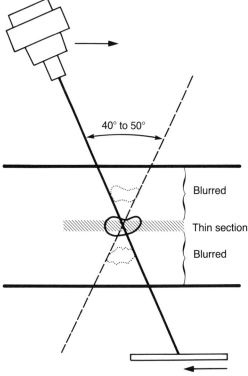

FIGURE 18–20. Linear tomography. Note the plane of focus defined by the fulcrum. The x-ray source and film cassette move in opposite directions.

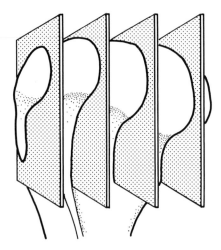

FIGURE 18–21. The concept of tomographic slices through the condyle.

ated for thickening, discontinuity, and changes in shape.

Comparing the slices of each side enables the clinician to pinpoint the location of osseous pathology in the joint. It is also possible to supplement these sagittal slices with images taken in a coronal plane. The kinds of pathologic changes that may be found are the same as those listed in the discussion of transcranial films.

The position of the condyle in the fossa can be accurately determined, but this information has only limited significance.

JOINT SPACE ANALYSIS

The significance of condyle position in relation to the articular fossa has been a subject of much controversy. Although a fruitful area of

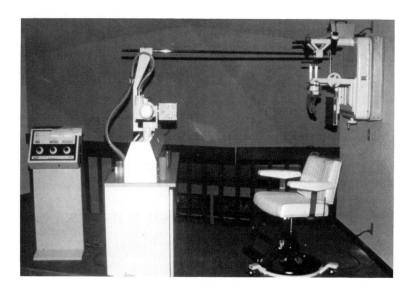

FIGURE 18–22. Linear tomographic equipment. (Courtesy of Landmark Medical Imaging Incorporated, Decatur, Georgia.)

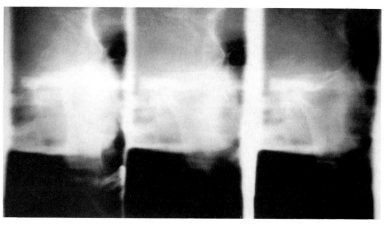

FIGURE 18–23. A normal linear tomogram. Note the linear streaking in the horizontal direction.

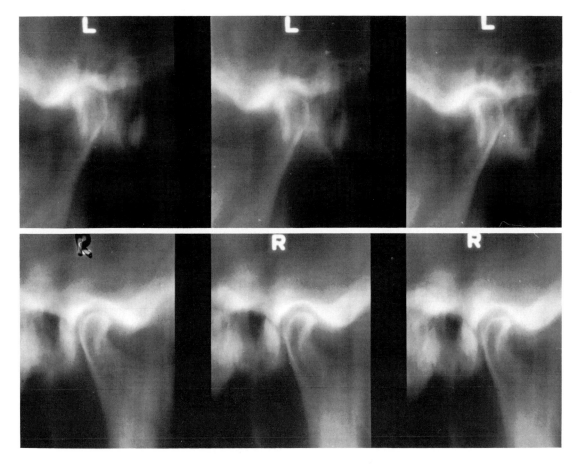

FIGURE 18–24. A linear tomogram. Note the streaking in the vertical direction (six slices).

debate, no agreement exists over optimal condylar position.

Weinberg[36] advocates a concentric position within the fossa. Gelb[37] believes that the condyle belongs in a "4–7 position"—somewhat forward and downward within the fossa (Fig. 18–30). Dawson[38] states the condyle should be located at the most superior anterior position at which the condyles are braced against the medial wall of the fossa. Owen[39] defines a "therapeutic range" between Weinberg's concentric position and Gelb's 4–7. Others have abandoned the concept of an ideal condylar position and give greater importance to the functional relationship of the condyle, disc, and fossa.[40]

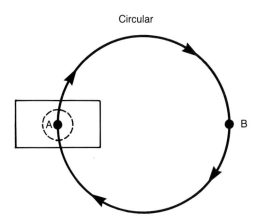

FIGURE 18–25. Circular tomographic trajectory.

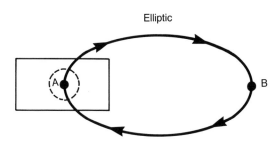

FIGURE 18–26. Elliptic tomographic trajectory.

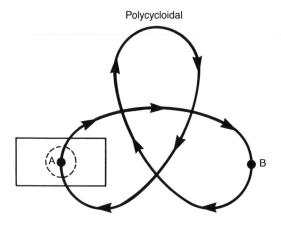

FIGURE 18–27. Polycycloidal tomographic trajectory.

The practitioner must recognize that accepting a particular condylar position as "ideal" can have broad implications in treating TM disorders and, indeed, virtually all other phases of dentistry.

A patient with concentrically located condyles, for instance, would be categorized as normal, according to Weinberg's criteria, but as posteriorly positioned, according to Gelb's and Dawson's. Condyles in the 4–7 position would be too far forward, according to Weinberg's criteria, and would be therapeutically repositioned back to concentricity.

The frequency of various condylar positions in both normal and abnormal populations has been studied. Employing transcranial radiography, Weinberg[41] concludes that the condyle tends to be concentric in asymptomatic individuals, but his data clearly showed a distribution of different positions among the patients studied. Anterior and posterior condylar position occurred with a combined frequency of 60%.

Pullinger and colleagues,[23,42] utilizing tomographic analysis, looked at the frequency of different condylar positions in a group of "supernormal" subjects and a group of patients with TM disorders. They subdivided the patients with TM disorders into two groups: one with myogenous dysfunction and the other with internal derangement.

Supernormal subjects were defined as those without any histories of TM disorders, orthodontic, or occlusal treatment and without any cast molar restoration. This control group was important, because other studies have been criticized for including patients with subclinical diseases.

The results of this study indicate a normal distribution of condylar position among the control group, the most frequent being concentric. The myogenous group also showed a tendency toward concentricity. The internal derangement group showed a higher frequency of

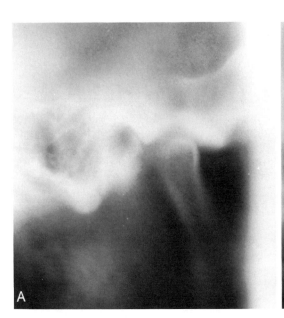
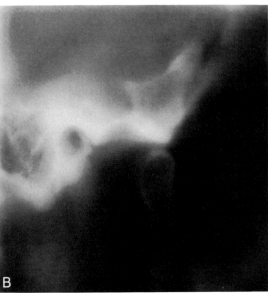

FIGURE 18–28. *A* and *B*, A normal polycycloidal tomogram in the open and closed positions. Note the excellent film clarity and the absence of streaking.

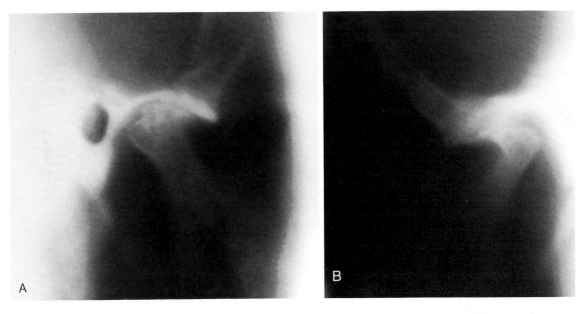

FIGURE 18–29. *A* and *B,* Examples of osteoarthrotic condylar changes as seen on polycycloidal tomography.

posterior position. Within each group, all positions were represented.

Bean and Thomas[43] utilized transcranial radiographs for analysis of condylar position. Their results showed that joint space narrowing bore no correlation to either symptomatic or asymptomatic patients. Ciancaglini and coworkers[44] and Vanden Berghe and coworkers[45] have also published data supporting this position.

Katzberg and coworkers[46] studied the condylar position found in tomograms and its correlation with internal derangement as diagnosed by arthrotomography. They were unable to support the hypothesis that a posteriorly positioned condyle is associated with an internal derangement. Ronquillo and coworkers,[47] in a

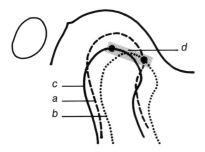

FIGURE 18–30. The "ideal" condylar positions as described by Dawson[38] (*a*), Gelb[37] (*b*), and Weinberg[36] (*c*). Shaded area (*d*) shows the therapeutic range favored by Owen.[39]

study of 143 patients, demonstrated a tendency toward posteriorly displaced condyles in patients with internal derangement with reduction, but a tendency toward concentricity both in patients with internal derangement without reduction and in patients without any meniscal displacement at all.

It appears that enough variability exists to preclude condylar position as a sole diagnostic criterion.

PANORAMIC RADIOGRAPHY

Panoramic radiography equipment is available in the offices of some general dentists and many oral surgeons and orthodontists and in dental schools and hospital dental services. This widespread availability plus the capacity to image the entire maxillomandibular region, including the TMJ, has spurred interest in its use as a screening tool. As with any of the techniques discussed, panoramic radiography is a valuable diagnostic tool, as long as its limitations are understood.

Although considered a separate technique from tomography, it can be likened to tomography that utilizes an elliptic trajectory. Updergrave[29] describes panoramic radiography as "curved surface laminography," because a single anatomic plane is selected and the structures on either side are blurred out. Updergrave,[30] in a later study, described this plane as a "focal trough" (Fig. 18–31). The image pro-

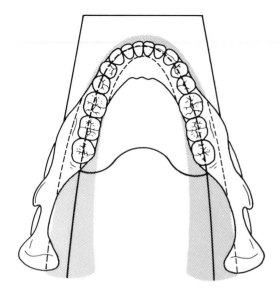

FIGURE 18–31. Focal trough of the panoramic radiographic technique.

duced is a relatively clear depiction of the structures located within the plane. The farther away a structure is from the plane, the poorer the image quality.

To understand the limitations of imaging the TMJ with a panoramic film, one must first understand the inaccuracies in the technique in general. Welander and colleagues[31] identified three inaccuracies as follows:

1. Ghost images: Occasionally, the image of the opposite side of the jaw will appear in the view of the side of primary interest. The ghost image appears reversed and at a higher position on the film.

2. Distortion phenomena: Because the relationship of the x-ray beam and the film is fixed, whereas skeletal structure varies from individual to individual, distortion is inherent in most films. Improper positioning of the patient, moreover, can increase distortion dramatically.

3. Unsharpness: A loss in sharpness will occur as the object to be imaged falls farther outside the focal trough.

In addition, Updergrave[29] pointed out that the radiographic image will be enlarged 7 to 12%. Manson-Hing[32] estimates the enlargement in the Panelipse technique (GE 3000) is a uniform 19%. The Panelipse technique allows the operator to vary the elliptic path of the tube/cassette assembly, permitting adjustment for different size patients and for uniform views of varying planes within the same patient.

Properly taken panoramic projections provide views of the TMJ that are adequate for gross screening. For the identification of certain kinds of joint pathology, the panoramic projection may be the optimal imaging technique. These films can screen for pathology in the ramus and body of the mandible as well as the maxilla and maxillary sinus region. Fractures, luxation, developmental abnormalities, and neoplastic disease, affecting the TMJs, are readily identifiable (Figs. 18–32 to 18–34). In addition, late changes of osteoarthrosis can be seen (Fig. 18–35).

Langland and associates[33] identified several

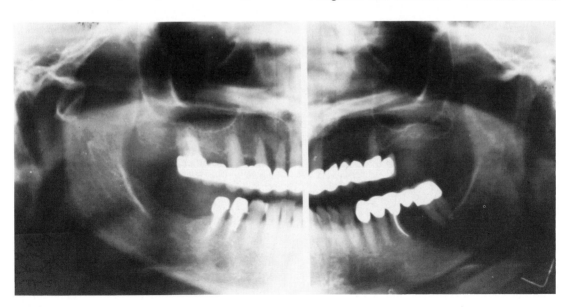

FIGURE 18–32. Condylar fracture as seen on a panoramic projection. (Courtesy of Dr. Arthur Elias, New York, New York.)

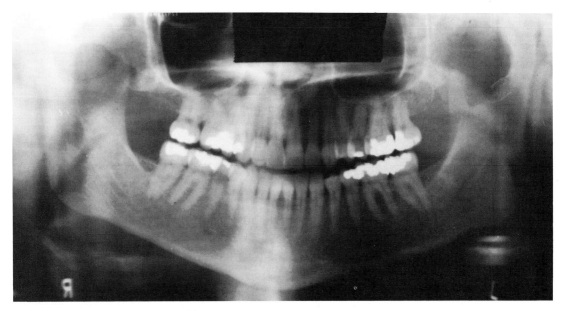

FIGURE 18-33. Hyperplastic condyle as seen on a panoramic projection. (Courtesy of Dr. Arthur Elias, New York, New York.)

normal variations that should be recognized when viewing the TMJ region in a conventional panoramic image. They initially noted that the zygomaticotemporal suture may be mistaken for a fracture line. They also noted that "pseudocystic radiolucencies" may be visualized on the head of the condyle. These are actually cupped-out areas (often of the pterygoid fovea) or anatomic depressions on the condylar head. Last, they observed that a radiolucency is often present at the sigmoid notch.

Panoramic views of the TMJ are subject to distortion for the following major reasons:

1. The condyles of the adult usually are outside the focal trough, causing an unsharp image.
2. The x-ray beam is not shot down the long axis of the condyle, in effect creating an oblique view of the condylar head (Fig. 18–36).
3. The TMJ is subject to the same magnification as the rest of the image.

These limitations have long been recognized, and at least three investigators have suggested techniques of minimizing these shortcomings. All of these techniques involve a change in the usual positioning of the patient.

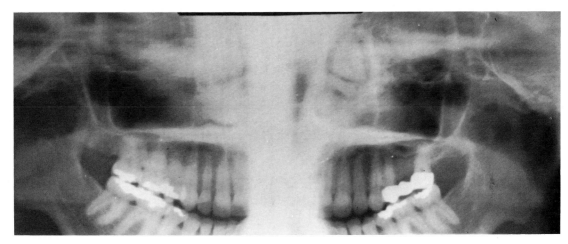

FIGURE 18-34. Severe condylar degeneration as a result of rheumatoid arthritis. (Courtesy of Dr. Arthur Elias, New York, New York.)

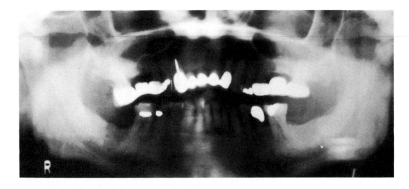

FIGURE 18–35. Arthritis of the temporomandibular joint as seen on a conventional panoramic projection.

Manson-Hing[32] suggested that the chin rest be lowered. This modification results in better visibility of the TMJ region. Unfortunately, it does not address the problem of unsharp images or the fact that the beam passes obliquely through the condyle.

Updergrave[30] noted that the condyle usually lies outside the focal trough. He suggested two different methods for patient positioning to bring the condyle into this crucial plane. He called these techniques "ramus techniques no. 1 and no. 2." These techniques were devised using the GE 3000 panoramic instrumentation. The shape of the focal trough will vary with the model and manufacturer of the equipment.

Technique 1. The film is taken with the patient in an edge-to-edge incisal relationship. The patient positions the mandible slightly anterior to normal positioning on the chin stop. The patient rotates the head away from the TMJ of interest halfway between the center line on the chin rest and the edge nearest the tube head (Fig. 18–37).

Technique 2. This technique is similar to the first, except that the patient's head is rotated so that the midline is aligned with the end of the chin stop. Updergrave believed that this modification brings the condylar head closer to the focal trough and was a good technique for patients with "large heads" (Fig. 18–38).

These two techniques offer at least partial

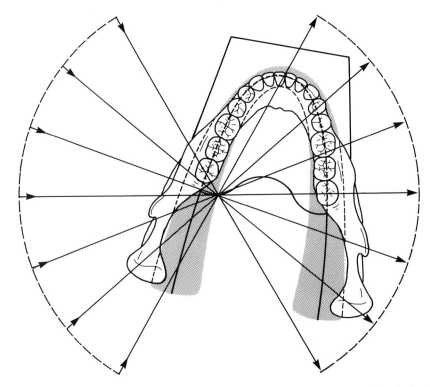

FIGURE 18–36. The oblique angle of the panoramic beam is illustrated, as it passes though the condyle.

poromandibular joint. Dent. Cos. 78:1227–1235, 1936.

5. Gillis, R.: X-rays reveal dysfunction. Dent. Surv. 15:17–26, 1939.

6. Grewcock, R.: A simple technique for temporomandibular joint radiography. Br. Dent. J. 94:152–154, 1953.

7. McQueen, W.: Radiography of the temporomandibular articulation. Minn. Dist. Dent. J. 21:28–30, 1937.

8. Palla, S.: Condyle positions: Determinants and radiographic analysis. In *Abnormal Jaw Mechanics*. K. Solberg and G. Clark (eds.). Quintessence Publishing Co., Lombard, IL, 1984.

9. Fava, C. and Preti, G.: Lateral transcranial radiography of the temporomandibular joints. Part II. Image formation studied with computerized tomography. J. Prosthet. Dent. 59:218, 1988.

10. Eckerdahl, O. and Lunberg, M.: Temporomandibular joint relations as revealed by conventional radiographic techniques: A comparison with the morphology and tomographic images. Dentomax. Radiol. 8:65–70, 1979.

11. Weinberg, L.: What we really see in a temporomandibular joint radiograph. J. Prosthet. Dent. 30:893–913, 1973.

12. Gonsalves, N., et al: Radiographic evaluation of defects created in mandibular condyles. Oral Surg. Oral Med. Oral Pathol. 38:475–489, 1974.

13. Eckerdahl, O. and Lundberg, M.: The structural situation in temporomandibular joints: A comparison between oblique transcranial radiographs, tomography and histological sections. Dentomax. Radiol. 8:42–49, 1979.

14. Jumean, H., Hatjigorgis, C., and Neff, P.: Comparative study of two radiographic techniques to actual dissection of the TMJ. J. Craniomand. Pract. 6:141, 1973.

15. Mongini, F.: The importance of radiography in the diagnosis of temporomandibular joint dysfunction: A comparative evaluation of transcranial radiography and serial tomography. J. Prosthet. Dent. 45:186–189, 1981.

16. Tanaka, T.: Temporomandibular joint radiography. Course syllabus: A diagnostic and therapeutic approach for TMJ disorders—the advanced course. University of San Diego Medical Center, San Diego, 1988.

17. Bell, W.: *Temporomandibular Disorders: Classification, Diagnosis and Management*. Year Book Medical Publishers, Chicago, p 240, 1986.

18. Berrett, A.: Radiology and radiography of the temporomandibular articulation. In *Clinical Management of Head, Neck and TMJ Pain and Dysfunction*. H. Gelb (ed.). W.B. Saunders Co., Philadelphia, p 23, 1985.

19. Oberg, T.: Radiology of the temporomandibular joint. In *Temporomandibular Joint Problems*. K. Solberg and G. Clark (eds.). Quintessence Publishing Co., Lombard, IL, p 49–64, 1980.

20. Omnell, K. and Peterson, A.: Radiography of the temporomandibular joint utilizing the oblique lateral transcranial technique: Comparison of information obtained with a standardized technique and individual techniques. Odont. Rev. 27:77–92, 1976.

21. Williamson, E. and Wilson, C.: Use of submental vertex analysis for producing quality temporomandibular joint laminographs. Am. J. Orthod. 70:200, 1976.

22. Bezuur, L., et al: Recognition of craniomandibular disorders: A comparison between clinical and radiographic findings in 89 patients. J. Oral Rehab. 15:215, 1988.

23. Pullinger, A.: Significance of condylar position in normal and abnormal TMJ function. In *Perspectives in TMJ Disorders*. G. Clark and K. Solberg (eds.). Quintessence Publishing Co., Lombard, IL, pp 89–103, 1987.

24. Peterson, A. and Nanthaviroj, S.: Radiography of the temporomandibular joint utilizing the transmaxillary projection. Odontol. Rev. 27:77–92, 1976.

25. Peterson, A.: What is an optimal temporomandibular joint radiograph? In *Perspectives in TMJ Disorders*. G. Clark and K. Solberg (eds.). Quintessence Publishing Co., Lombard, IL, pp 59–65, 1987.

26. Tanaka T.: *Temporomandibular Joint Radiography*, 1988. (Video Tape.)

27. Dunn, M., Robinov, K., Hayes, C., and Jennings, S.: Polycycloidal corrected tomography of the TMJ. Oral Surg. Oral Med. Oral Pathol. 51:4375–384, 1981.

28. Rozencweig, D. and Martin, G.: Selective tomography of the TMJ and the myofacial pain syndrome. J. Prosthet. Dent. 40:67–74, 1978.

29. Updergrave, W.: The role of panoramic radiography in diagnosis. Oral Surg. Oral Med. Oral Pathol. 22:149–157, 1966.

30. Updergrave, W.: Visualizing the mandibular ramus in panoramic radiography. Oral Surg. Oral Med. Oral Pathol. 31:422–429, 1971.

31. Welander U., McDavid, W., and Tronje, G.: Theory of rotational panoramic radiography. In *Principles and Practice of Panoramic Radiography*. O. Langland, R. Langlais, and C. Morris (eds.). W.B. Saunders Co, Philadelphia, pp 37–54, 1982.

32. Manson-Hing, L.: Advances in dental pantomography: The GE 3000. Oral Surg. Oral Med. Oral Pathol. 31:430, 1971.

33. Langland, O., Langlais, R., and Morris, C.: *Principles and Practice of Panoramic Radiography*. W.B. Saunders Co, Philadelphia, pp 411–443, 1982.

34. Chilvarquer, I., et al: A new technique for imaging the TMJ with a panoramic x-ray machine. Part I. Oral Surg. Oral Med. Oral Pathol. 65:626–631, 1988.

35. Chilvarquer, I., et al: A new technique for imaging the TMJ with a panoramic x-ray machine. Part II. Oral Surg. Oral Med. Oral Pathol. 65:632–636, 1988.

36. Weinberg, L.: Correlation of TMJ dysfunction with radiographic findings. J. Prosthet. Dent. 28:519, 1972.

37. Gelb, H.: *Clinical Management of Head, Neck TMJ Pain and Dysfunction*. W.B. Saunders Co., Philadelphia, p 109, 1985.

38. Dawson, P.: *Occlusal Problems*. C.V. Mosby Co., St. Louis, 1988.

39. Owen, A.: Orthodontic/orthopedic therapy for craniomandibular pain dysfunction. Part A. Anterior disc displacement: review of the literature. J. Craniomand. Pract. 5:358–366, 1987.

40. Farrar, W.B.: Characteristics of the condylar path in internal derangements of the TMJ. J. Prosthet. Dent. 39:319, 1978.

41. Weinberg, L.: Role of condylar position in TMJ dysfunction pain syndrome. J. Prosthet. Dent. 41:636–643, 1979.

42. Pullinger, A., et al: Tomographic analysis of mandibular condylar position in diagnostic subgroups of temporomandibular disorders. J. Prosthet. Dent. 55:723, 1986.

43. Bean, L. and Thomas, C.: Significance of condylar positions in patients with temporomandibular disorders. J. Am. Dent. Assoc. 114:76, 1987.

44. Ciancaglini, M., et al: Valutazione clinico-tomogra-

phica in un campione di soggetti con patologia dell-articolazione temporomandibulare: analisi topographica condilo-temporale. Mondo. Odontostomatologico 229:43, 1987. (Abstract.)

45. Vanden Berghe, L., Deboever, J., and Adriaens, P.: The interpretation of condyle position on radiographs: interexaminer reliability and relationship with clinical parameters. J. Oral Rehabil. 15:211, 1988. (Abstract.)

46. Katzberg, R., Keith, D., Ten Eich, W., and Guralnick, W.: Internal derangements of the temporomandibular joint: An assessment of condylar position in centric occlusion. J. Prosthet. Dent. 49:250–254, 1983.

47. Ronquillo, H., Guay, J., et al: Tomographic analysis of mandibular condyle position as compared to arthrographic findings of the temporomandibular joint. J. Craniomand. Disord. 2:59–64, 1988.

48. Gates, G.: Radionuclide diagnosis. In Oral and Maxillofacial Surgery, vol. 1. D. Laskin (ed.). C.V. Mosby Co., St. Louis, pp 463–545, 1980.

49. Meter, F. and Guiberteau, M. (eds.). Essentials of Nuclear Medicine Imaging. Grune & Stratton, Orlando, 1986.

50. Freeman, L.: Freeman and Johnson's Clinical Radionuclide Imaging. Grune & Stratton, Orlando, 1986.

51. Epstein, J. and Ruprecht, A.: Bone scintigraphy: An aid in diagnosis and management of facial pain associated with osteoarthrosis. Oral Surg. Oral Med. Oral Pathol. 53:1, 1982.

52. Katzberg, R., O'Mara, R., Tallents, R., and Weber, D.: Radionuclide skeletal imaging and single photon emission computed tomography in suspected internal derangements of the temporomandibular joint. J. Oral Maxillofac. Surg. 42:782–787, 1984.

53. Goldstein, H. and Bloom, C.: Detection of degenerative disease of the temporomandibular joint by bone scintigraphy: Concise communication. J. Nucl. Med. 21:928–930, 1987.

54. Pogrel, M.: Quantitative assessment of isotope activity in temporomandibular joint regions as a means for assessing unilateral condylar hypertrophy. Oral Surg. Oral Med. Oral Pathol. 60:15–17, 1985.

55. Keller, D., Jackson, R., Cusumano, J., and Cook, M.: Quantitative radionuclide scanning of the temporomandibular joint. J. Craniomand. Pract. 5:152–156, 1987.

56. Craemer, T. and Ficara, A.: The value of the nuclear medical scan in the diagnosis of temporomandibular joint disease. Oral Surg. Oral Med. Oral Pathol. 58:382–385, 1984.

57. Collier, D., Carrera, C., Messer, E., et al: Internal derangement of the temporomandibular joint: Detection by single photon emission computed tomography. Radiology 149:557–561, 1983.

58. Oesterreich, F., Rossmann, I., Jend, H., and Triebel, H.: Semiquantitative SPECT imaging for assessment of bone reaction in internal derangements of the temporomandibular joint. J. Oral Maxillofac. Surg. 45:1022–1028, 1987.

59. Giancristofaro, M., Del Maschio, A., et al: Direction of temporomandibular joint arthropathy by SPECT compared with conventional computerized tomography. J. Dent. Res. 66:319, 1987. (Abstract.)

Paul A. Danielson

CHAPTER 19

Arthrography

Arthrographic examination of the temporomandibular joint (TMJ) is an important method of imaging to assist in diagnosis and treatment planning. Arthrography of the TMJ was first reported by Norgaard in 1944.[1] Others improved the technical aspects of the procedure and correlated arthrographic findings with clinical, anatomic, and surgical findings.[2-11] Of the various methods of imaging the TMJ, arthrography is indicated for evaluation of the soft tissue components. It is an indirect method of visualizing the intracapsular anatomy of the TMJ. In the patient who presents clinically as having internal derangement or some other meniscal pathology, arthrography provides the clinician with an accurate method of determining the meniscal morphology and the anatomic and dynamic relationship of the meniscus and mandibular condyle.

The basic methodology of arthrographic imaging of the TMJ involves injection of a water-soluble contrast medium (dye) into the lower or upper, or both, joint compartments under fluoroscopic visualization. The dye opacifies the joint space. Intracapsular anatomy affects the shape of the joint space, allowing for indirect visualization of the meniscus or other aspects of intracapsular anatomy. Following injection of the contrast medium, a dynamic evaluation of the patient's joint function can be made using fluoroscopic imaging. A video tape recording of the dynamic phase of the fluoroscopic evaluation allows for multiple viewing of this part of the examination, while minimizing radiation dose. A linear, sagittal, tomographic radiographic series is then taken to image the temporomandibular joint from medial to lateral.

ADVANTAGES

Accuracy. Patients who clinically have symptoms of internal derangement will have positive arthrographic study findings in 85% of the examinations.[12-14]

Visualization. Arthrography allows the clinician to evaluate the two-dimensional anatomic relationship of the meniscus, mandibular condyle, and temporal bone.

Dynamic Functional Assessment. Video tape recording of the arthrofluoroscopic examination of the patient's functioning allows for dynamic evaluation of the joint's components.

Morphologic Evaluation. Arthrography allows for an evaluation of the morphology of the disc, including perforation.

Simplicity. Arthrography is relatively simple to perform and requires equipment available in most radiology departments.

Expense. Arthrography is less expensive than other types of imaging, for example, computerized tomography (CT) and magnetic resonance imaging (MRI).

DISADVANTAGES

1. The procedure is invasive.
2. Substantial radiation dose is needed.
3. Arthrography is less precise than MRI in viewing positional abnormalities.[5]
4. The success of the procedure is partially dependent on the skill level of the arthrographer.
5. Arthrography is an indirect method of evaluating the soft tissue components of the joint.
6. Patients may experience varying degrees of discomfort during and after the procedure.

INDICATIONS

1. Symptoms consistent with internal derangement, such as clicking, popping, and interference.
2. Pain that clinically appears to be intracapsular.
3. Diagnosing loose bodies.
4. Diagnosing adhesions.
5. Diagnosing changes in meniscal morphology.
6. Diagnosing meniscal pathology such as tears and perforations.
7. Evaluating splint therapy (arthrographically guided splint therapy).

8. Evaluation of patients not responding to splint therapy.

9. Documentation of pathology prior to surgical intervention.

CONTRAINDICATIONS

1. Known allergy to local anesthetics, iodine-containing products, or contrast media.

2. Prolonged bleeding time due to congenital dyscrasia or anticoagulant therapy.

3. Infection in the area of needle insertion.

ANATOMIC CONSIDERATIONS

In the normal TMJ, the superior and inferior joint spaces are distinctly separated from each other by the retrodiscal tissues posteriorly, the fibrocartilage articular disc, the medial and lateral ligaments that attach from the disc to the condyle, and the variable attachment of the disc to the superior head of the lateral pterygoid muscle anteriorly.

The disk-condyle-temporal bone relationship varies with condylar position during function. In the fully closed-mouth position, the thicker posterior band of the meniscus lies over the superior aspect of the condyle. The thinner intermediate zone lies anterior to the condylar head, along the posterior aspect of the anterior slope of the glenoid fossa. The anterior band of the meniscus is anterior to the condylar head. The inferior border of the anterior band can vary in its anatomic shape from having a flat inferior margin to a convex shape (Fig. 19–1A).[8]

As the condyle moves forward in the fossa during translation, the posterior band becomes positioned more posteriorly to the condyle, and the intermediate zone lies superiorly to the condylar head. The anterior band remains anterior to the condyle (Fig. 19–1B).

As the patient opens fully, the anterior band becomes superior to the condylar head. It is not uncommon for a patient to be able to open to the extent that the condyle is anterior to the articular eminence and the anterior band of the disc is slightly posterior to the superior crest of the condyle (Fig. 19–1C).

During this process of opening, the shape of the superior and inferior joint spaces changes because of the effect of the movement of the condyle, disc, and ligaments. These movements as well as vascular changes in the retrodiscal tissue result in shifting of the synovial fluid within the joint compartments. In a nor-

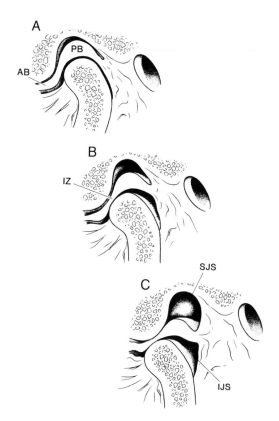

FIGURE 19–1. Closed (A), partially open (B), and open (C) positions of the temporomandibular joint are illustrated. (Anterior band of meniscus = AB; posterior band of meniscus = PB; intermediate zone of meniscus = IZ; superior joint space = SJS; and inferior joint space = IJS.)

mal joint, the inferior joint space contains approximately 0.5 ml of synovial fluid.[16]

The superior joint space has a synovial fluid volume of approximately 1.0 ml.[16] In the fully closed position, the inferior joint space is fairly small and uniform in width. The anterior recess is often teardrop-shaped. As the condyle is translated anteriorly, the anterior recess becomes smaller, and the posterior recess enlarges, accommodating a shifting volume of synovial fluid. This change in relative volume of the posterior and anterior portions of the inferior joint space is significant in arthrographic technique in that having the patient translate the mandible will ease accurate placement of the needle into the inferior joint space (Fig. 19–2A).

A similar shift in synovial fluid is also seen in the superior joint space. As the patient translates the mandible forward slightly, it will also ease placement of the needle into the superior

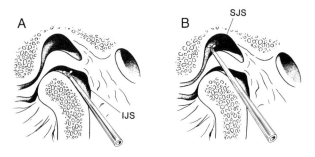

FIGURE 19–2. Needle placement for injection of contrast material into joint spaces. (Inferior joint space = IJS (*A*) and superior joint space = SJS (*B*).)

compartment if both compartments are injected (Fig. 19–2B).

ARTHROGRAPHIC TECHNIQUE

Prior to the initiation of the arthrogram, a medical history is taken that would alert the arthrographer to any allergy, illness, or medical condition that would contraindicate the procedure.

Before the arthrofluoroscopic procedure, lateral closed-mouth and open-mouth linear tomograms are taken to determine any arthritic or osseous changes.

A lead shield is placed on the fluoroscopic table to reduce any radiation to abdominal and chest areas. The patient is then positioned with the side to be examined superior. The head of the patient is rotated toward the table, with the head near or on the table top. Final precise positional changes of the patient can be made after viewing the joint fluoroscopically to allow for the most informative study. Collimation of the x-ray beam should be adjusted to minimize the field of exposure (Figs. 19–3 and 19–4).[17]

If necessary, the patient's hair should be taped to prevent contamination of the field. The preauricular area is then cleansed and the skin surface prepared with an iodine-based solution. The preauricular area is then isolated by either sterile drapes or a plastic ear drape.

A sterile tray is organized for use during the invasive portion of the procedure (Fig. 19–5). Local anesthesia is then given—1% lidocaine with 1:100,000 epinephrine is infiltrated to the TMJ capsule, using a 27-gauge needle. Careful placement of the solution in the region of the joint capsule and the lateral condylar neck minimizes any local discomfort from the actual arthrogram. An auriculotemporal nerve block may also be used to anesthetize the joint.

After injection of the local anesthetic, the patient should be asked if there is any change in the quality of pain. The patient's response is an additional piece of information regarding the source of the pain. If the patient indicates that following the local anesthetic infiltration there is a marked reduction of pain in the area, the clinician not only can proceed with the arthrogram but also has a strong indication that the TMJ is a significant component of the pain.

Prior to injection of the contrast medium,

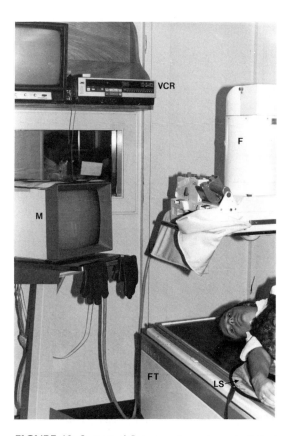

FIGURE 19–3. Typical fluoroscopic equipment. Patient is positioned on the fluoroscopic table (FT). The x-ray beam is emitted from below the patient to the receiving unit (F). Lead shield (LS) minimizes radiation exposure to thorax and abdomen. Video cassette recorder (VCR) and monitor (M) allow for simultaneous and repeated viewing of arthrofluoroscopic study.

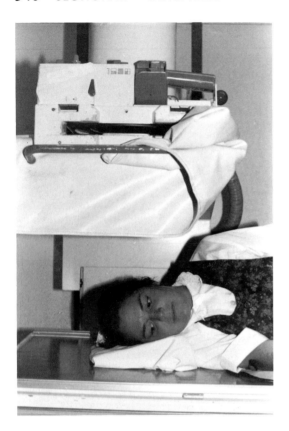

FIGURE 19–4. Positioning of the patient. The patient is placed on the side, with the joint to be examined in the superior position. The top of the patient's head is rotated toward the top of the table and may even need to touch the table. Final position is determined after viewing fluoroscopically.

the regional anatomy is carefully palpated. The patient is instructed initially to occlude the teeth together and then to protrude the mandible. This maneuver allows the arthrographer to establish landmarks for the injection of the contrast medium and to instruct the patient on those jaw positions that will ease the placement of the needle into the desired joint space.

A 3.0-cm long 25-gauge or 27-gauge needle is utilized for injection of the contrast medium into the joint space. This needle is attached to a 10-cc syringe via a standard intravenous extension tube. The extension tube allows for the injection of contrast medium while the joint undergoes fluoroscopy, without exposing the clinician to direct radiation. The contrast medium should be a water-soluble agent, such as methylglucamine diatrizoate (Reno-M 60, Squibb). Some workers recommend adding 0.3 ml of 1:20,000 epinephrine to 3 ml of contrast agent to reduce resorption and elimination of the medium from the joint space, prolonging the time for study of the joint.[12] However, if the arthrotomograms are taken promptly after the video recording of the arthrofluoroscopic examination the epinephrine need not be incorporated into the contrast medium.

With the patient's mouth only slightly open, the needle is directed toward the posterior superior quadrant of the condyle, with the bevel toward the condyle. When the needle engages the condyle, the patient is instructed to protrude the jaw. Movement of the needle confirms the fact that it is in contact with the head

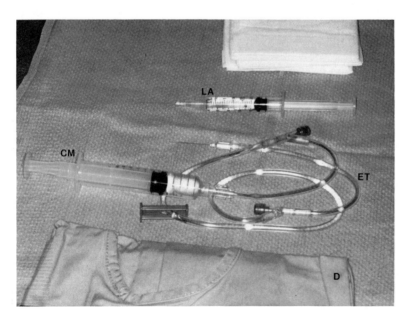

FIGURE 19–5. Sterile tray. Local anesthetic (LA) (1% lidocaine with 1:100,000 epinephrine) is in a 3-cc syringe with a 2.5-cm, 27-gauge needle. Contrast medium (CM) is in a 10-cc syringe with an extension tube (ET) and 27-gauge needle. Ear drape (D) is shown.

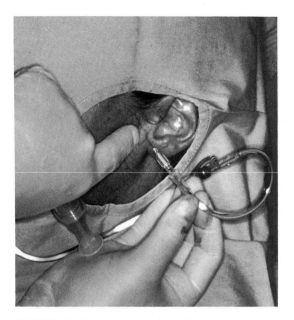

FIGURE 19–6. Placement of needle into the inferior joint space. The condyle is carefully palpated, and the patient is instructed to partially protrude the mandible. The bevel of the needle is directed toward the posterior slope of the condyle. The extension tube allows for injection of the contrast medium under direct fluoroscopic visualization without exposure to the individual conducting the study.

of the condyle. Protrusion of the mandible enlarges the volume of the posterior aspect of the lower joint space, allowing the clinician to advance the needle deeper into the compartment (Figs. 19–2 and 19–6). The position of the needle is confirmed fluoroscopically. A small amount of contrast agent is then injected into the lower joint space. Dye should be clearly visible anterior to the condyle to confirm filling of the compartment (Fig. 19–7). A maximum of 0.8 ml of contrast agent should be used to avoid overdistention of the space. Should dye be observed flowing into both joint spaces on initial injection of the lower space, the study would confirm the presence of a communication, indicative of either a perforation or tear. Rarely is the needle placement itself the cause of the communication.

An x-ray (spot film) may be taken at any time during this study directly on the fluoroscopic table to record a finding (Fig. 19–8).

A video tape recording is made of the entire sequence of the injection of dye into the lower space. Upon completion of the dye injection, the needle is withdrawn, and a video tape recording is made of the arthrofluoroscopic examination of the patient during mandibular

FIGURE 19–7. Monitor image of the injection of the contrast medium. The auditory canal (AC) and articular eminence (AE) are noted. The contrast medium appears black on the screen. Placement of the needle (N) is confirmed as being in the lower joint space. In this case, a simultaneous flow of contrast material into both the superior and inferior joint spaces is seen. The anterior recess of the superior joint space (1) and the anterior recess of the inferior joint space (2) are visualized. The clear area between the two joint spaces indicates the meniscal location (M). In this case, a perforation of the meniscus would be expected, owing to the simultaneous filling of both joint spaces.

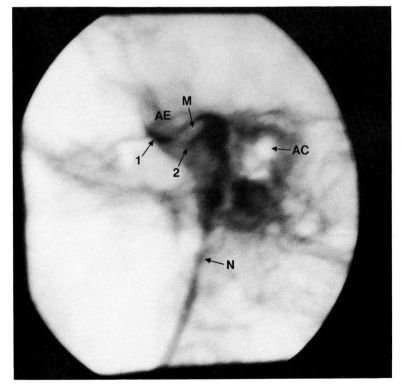

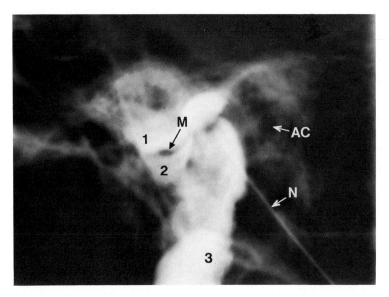

FIGURE 19–8. "Spot" film. A radiographic film can be taken directly on the fluoroscopic table to confirm and record a finding. The contrast material appears white. In this case, the needle (N) can clearly be seen positioned in the posterior aspect of the inferior joint space. The auditory canal (AC) is indicated. The anterior recess of the superior joint space (1) and the anterior recess of the inferior joint space (2) are noted. The meniscus (M) appears anterior to the condyle as a radiolucent area. An area of extravasated contrast agent is observed (3). The simultaneous filling of both joint spaces would be indicative of a communication between the spaces, possibly a perforation or tear. The area of extravasated contrast material (3) far from the needle site would indicate either an area of capsular incompetence or extravasated contrast material from a prior injection.

function (Fig. 19–9). The patient is instructed to bring the teeth into occlusion and then to open to maximum interincisal opening. Protrusion and lateral movement should also be recorded. These should be done in a fairly short amount of time to minimize patient radiation exposure. This portion of the study can provide the clinician with valuable information regarding the functional dynamics of the disc and condyle.

Careful observation of the fluid dynamics of the contrast medium during fluoroscopic examination, while the patient is performing the range of motion activity, and repeated evaluation by reviewing the video tape recording allows for an evaluation of the degree of meniscal displacement. Correlated with clinical evaluation, it can be a great asset in treatment planning and determining the prognosis of various forms of therapy (surgical vs. nonsurgical).

If a satisfactory diagnosis can be made with dye in only the inferior joint space, a superior joint space study need not be completed. In this situation, immediately on completion of the inferior joint space, arthrographic videofluoroscopic recording, closed-mouth and open-mouth linear arthrotomograms are taken at 2- to 3-mm intervals.[18,19]

However, if any additional diagnostic information regarding the morphology of the meniscus is indicated, the superior joint space should be injected with contrast agent at this point.

The patient is instructed to bring the teeth into occlusion, and the needle is directed into the superior joint space along the posterior slope of the anterior wall of the glenoid fossa. The position of the needle is visualized fluoroscopically and contrast medium injected (see Fig. 19–2B). Following infiltration of the superior space, a video tape recording is made of the patient's functioning. The patient should be instructed to open to the maximum interincisal distance, as well as to protrude and move to right and left lateral positions. Upon completion of the video tape recording of the dynamics of joint function, closed-mouth and open-mouth arthrotomograms are taken at 2- to 3- mm intervals from lateral to medial (Fig. 19–10).

The radiation dose for the entire procedure ranges from 1 to 2 R.[6]

COMPLICATIONS

Allergic Reaction. The incidence of allergic reaction to contrast material is rare. Management should be based on the severity of the reaction. For mild reactions characterized by urticaria and rash, subcutaneous epinephrine, 0.2 to 0.5 ml, should be given and repeated at 3-minute intervals. For more severe reactions,

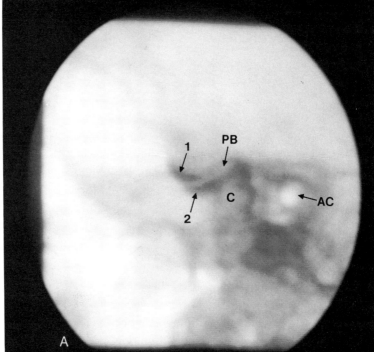

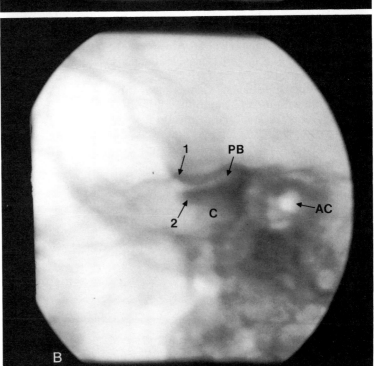

FIGURE 19–9. Videotaped images of arthrofluoroscopic study. *A* and *B* show the videotaped recorded images of a two space arthrofluoroscopic study of the same joint in a closed position (*A*) and a partially open position (*B*).

Auditory canal = AC; mandibular condyle = C; anterior recess of the superior joint space = 1; anterior recess of the inferior joint space = 2; and posterior band of the meniscus = PB.

The PB appears to be slightly anterior to the crest of the condyle in the closed position (*A*). As the condyle translates anteriorly, the posterior band regains a superior position. These findings are consistent with a slightly displaced meniscus anteriorly that reduces on opening. Repeated viewing of the videotape recording will allow for evaluation of the dynamics of the meniscocondylar relationship.

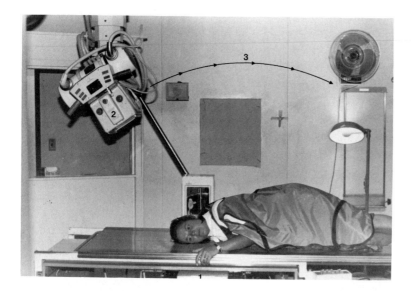

FIGURE 19-10. Arthrotomographic radiographs. Tomographic radiographs taken after completion of the arthrofluoroscopic study allow for accurate visualization of meniscal position and morphology. The film cassette is placed below the table (1). The movement of the x-ray head (2), as represented by the arc (3), produces a limited field of focused exposure that can be varied to study the joint at defined incremental levels as small as 0.5 cm from medial to lateral.

intravenous access should be immediately established to prepare for additional supportive measures.[20,21]

Vagal Reactions. Occasionally, a patient may experience a vagal reaction characterized by bradycardia and hypotension. Atropine, 0.5 mg, intravenously should be given if the hypotension persists.

Extracapsular Injection of Contrast Medium. This complication can be minimized by fluoroscopic visualization of the injection phase. Localized tissue irritation results from this event, causing greater patient discomfort from the procedure. Nonionic contrast agents also reduce pain.[5]

Facial Nerve Weakness. Transient facial nerve weakness can result from the local anesthetic effect on the facial nerve, which is in close approximation to the TMJ. This weakness resolves as the local anesthetic dissipates and is metabolized.

POSTARTHROGRAM INSTRUCTIONS

1. The patient should be informed prior to the procedure that a transient facial nerve weakness due to the local anesthetic may be experienced. The most annoying aspect may be the inability to close the eye for 1 to 2 hours after the procedure.

2. Following the arthrogram, ice should be applied intermittently to the area to reduce swelling for a period of 12 hours. For residual edema after 12 hours, warm moist heat may help reduce the swelling.

3. The patient should also be given ibuprofen, 600 mg qid, for a minimum of 3 to 4 days to reduce any residual inflammation or discomfort. If ibuprofen is contraindicated or is inadequate for pain relief a narcotic should be prescribed.

INTERPRETATION OF ARTHROGRAMS

Initial evaluation of the arthrographic study is made while injecting contrast material under fluoroscopic observation (see Fig. 19-7). When the initial injection of dye is made into the inferior joint space, the dye should remain within the confines of the space forming a crescent around the condylar head. The anterior recess will have a teardrop shape. If contrast material is observed flowing from the inferior to superior space, a perforation should be suspected. Spot films may be taken to record the flow prior to complete filling of both spaces (see Fig. 19-8).

Observations can be made regarding the positions of the posterior band, intermediate zone, and anterior band relative to the condyle. While simultaneous video recording is being made of the fluoroscopic image, the dynamics of the flow of contrast agent will indicate positional shifts of the meniscus during function.

Following injection of the contrast material into the superior space, initial evaluation can

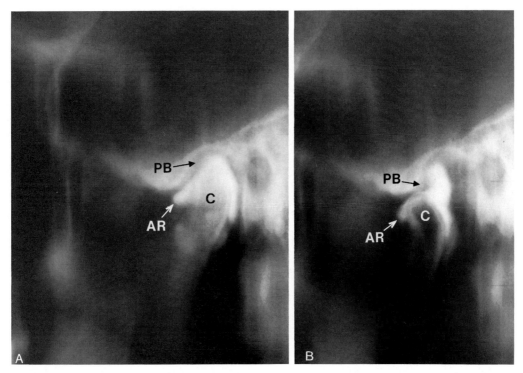

FIGURE 19–11. *A* and *B*, Single space arthrotomogram. Inferior joint space arthrotomogram of the same joint in closed (*A*) and open (*B*) position. The contrast medium is confined to the inferior joint space. In the closed position, the anterior recess (AR) has the "teardrop" shape. The posterior band of the meniscus (PB) is evident by the depression in the contrast material slightly anterior to the crest of the condyle (C). As the condyle translates anteriorly (*B*), there is a reduction in the size of the lower space anterior recess (AR) and the PB depression becomes more clearly visible at the C. Also note the increased volume of the posterior recess of the inferior joint space with the condyle translated. This study's finding is consistent with a slightly anterior displaced meniscus that reduces on opening.

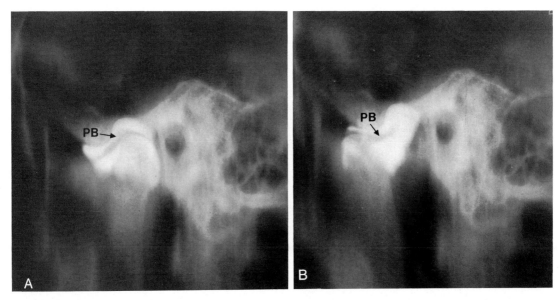

FIGURE 19–12. *A* and *B*, Two space arthrotomogram. This double space study is of a joint with similar pathology to the single space study in Figure 19–11. The contrast medium remains confined to each space. In the closed position (*A*), the anterior recess of the lower space has the "teardrop" appearance. The posterior band (PB) is a clearly defined radiolucent area between the superior and inferior spaces slightly anterior to the crest of the condyle. As the condyle translates anteriorly to the open position (*B*), the PB can be visualized posterior to the condylar head. The meniscus appears normal morphologically. Almost total elimination of contrast material from the anterior recesses of both the superior and inferior joint spaces occurs.

345

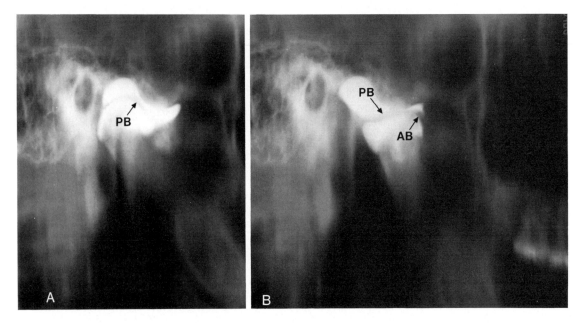

FIGURE 19–13. *A* and *B,* Anterior displaced meniscus with partial (incomplete) reduction: two space study. In the closed position (*A*), the posterior band (PB) lies anterior to the crest of the condyle and the anterior band is not clearly visualized. In the open position (*B*), the PB now is at the crest of the condyle. A small filling defect anterior to the condyle indicates the location of the anterior band (AB).

be made of the morphology of the meniscus. Video recording of the fluoroscopic image allows repeated viewings of the functional dynamics of the condyle-disc-eminence relationship. Specific observations may be made of any changes in disc shape with mandibular movement, such as folding.

ARTHROTOMOGRAPHIC EVALUATION

In a normal TMJ with the patient's mouth closed, the posterior aspect of the inferior joint space is concave anteriorly conforming to the anatomy of the condylar head. On its anterior

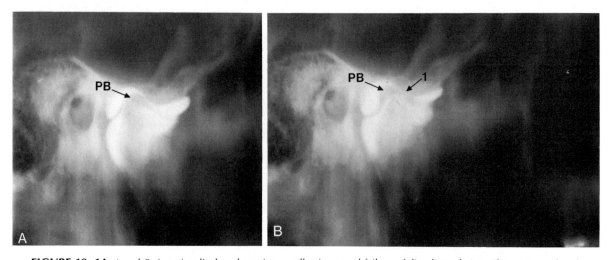

FIGURE 19–14. *A* and *B,* Anterior displaced meniscus, adhesions, and failure of discal translation. The posterior band (PB) appears in the same relative position in both the closed (*A*) and open (*B*) views. In the open view, the lack of contrast material in the superior space in the area of the anterior slope of the glenoid fossa (1) is consistent with adhesions.

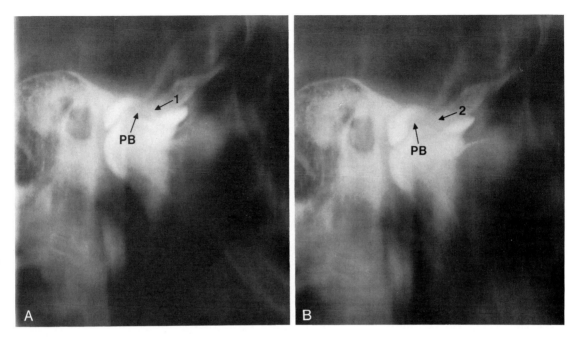

FIGURE 19–15. *A* and *B*, Anterior displaced meniscus with adhesions. In the closed position (*A*), there is incomplete filling of the superior space (1). The posterior band (PB) of the meniscus is anterior to the crest of the condyle. In the open position (*B*), the area void of contrast material (2) appears to be slightly more diffuse and the meniscus remains in the same position, with the translation of the joint taking place in the lower joint space.

border, it is convex conforming to the anatomy of the anterior recess.[11,12,22]

The anterior recess of the inferior joint space extends from the anterior superior peak of the condylar head to the most anterior inferior aspect of the inferior joint space. This region is thin superiorly, widening in a teardrop shape. The superior aspect of the inferior space varies

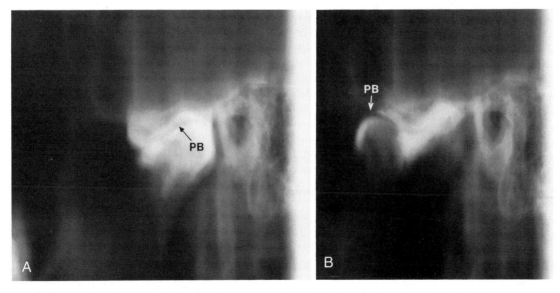

FIGURE 19–16. *A* and *B*, Anterior displaced meniscus with partial reduction. The posterior band of the meniscus (PB) is anterior to the condyle in the closed position (*A*). As the condyle translates anteriorly, the meniscus is also carried anteriorly with the PB only reaching the crest of the condyle in a fully open position (*B*).

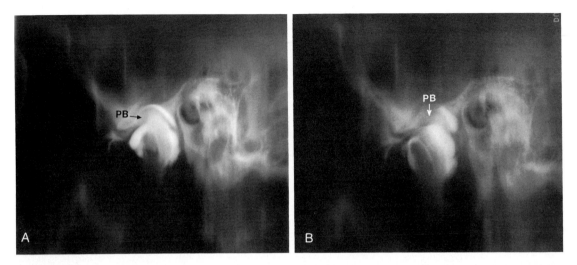

FIGURE 19–17. *A* and *B*, Anterior displaced meniscus, adhesions, capsular incompetence, and restricted range of motion. These arthrotomograms are from a 27-year-old male with a history of trauma to the temporomandibular joint. His clinical symptoms consisted of pain and limited range of motion. The superior joint space shows lack of filling in the anterior recess in the closed position (*A*), which becomes even more defined as the patient attempts to open (*B*). The condyle shows a restricted range of motion, remaining posterior to the articular eminence. Also note the poor definition of the posterior aspect of the inferior joint space, which indicates capsular damage.

being either flat in the majority of patients or concave, owing to the anatomy of the anterior band of the meniscus.

As the condyle translates, a reduction in the size of the anterior recess and an enlargement of the posterior recess occur. The anterior recess tends to become a small crescent-shaped band. In a small percentage of cases, the anterior recess remains large as a result of the anterior band anatomy. Injection of the superior joint space confirms this finding and avoids the misinterpretation of this finding as the posterior band from a displaced meniscus.

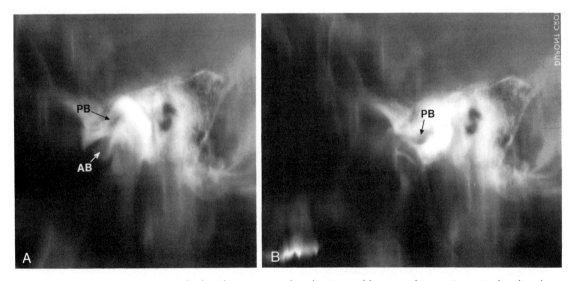

FIGURE 19–18. *A* and *B*, Anterior displaced meniscus with reduction and hypertrophic meniscus. In the closed position (*A*), the posterior band (PB) and the anterior band (AB) of the meniscus are markedly anterior to the condyle. The meniscus appears much thicker than normal indicating a degree of hypertrophy. This finding was confirmed surgically. In the open position (*B*), the meniscus reduces and folding is evident in the area of the PB.

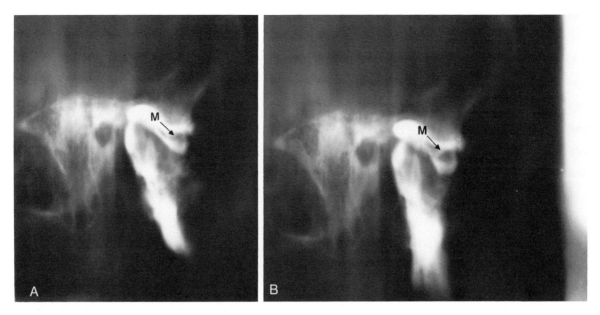

FIGURE 19–19. *A* and *B*, Anterior displaced meniscus without reduction—"closed lock." In the closed view (*A*), a radiolucent void is noted between the two joint spaces anterior to the condyle. As the patient tries to translate the joint (*B*), the defect enlarges and gives the image of the meniscus (M) folding and limiting the normal range of motion of the condyle.

Deviations from these normal findings are indicative of intracapsular pathology. The following examples are representative arthroto-mograms to illustrate different diagnostic findings (Figs. 19–11 to 19–23).

SUMMARY

Arthrography of the TMJ is a method of imaging the joint's intracapsular components. The basic methodology is one of injection of a

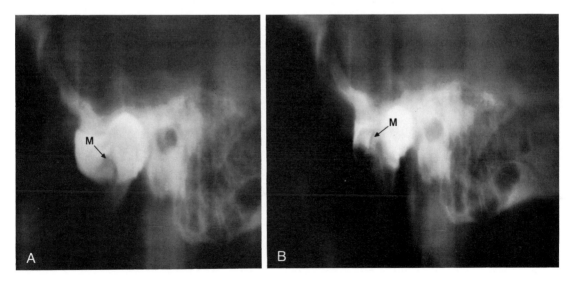

FIGURE 19–20. *A* and *B*, Anterior displaced meniscus without reduction and folding of meniscus. In the closed position (*A*), there is contrast material visible in both joint spaces. The meniscus (M) is anterior to the condyle and appears contorted in morphology. In the open position (*B*), the condylar translation is limited. The contrast agent is eliminated from the anterior recess of the lower joint space. The meniscus appears to remain folded.

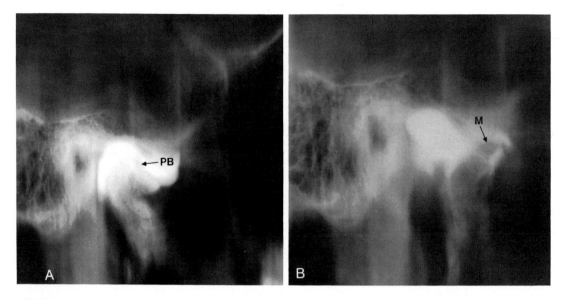

FIGURE 19–21. *A* and *B*, Anterior displaced meniscus without reduction. In the closed position (*A*), the posterior band (PB) is anterior to the mandibular condyle. As the condyle translates anteriorly (*B*), a radiolucent area develops anterior to the condyle that indicates a nonreducing meniscus (M).

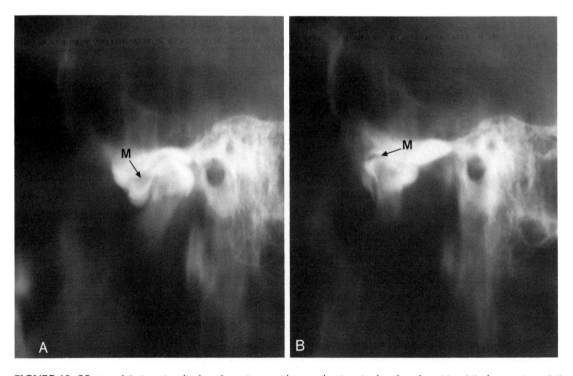

FIGURE 19–22. *A* and *B*, Anterior displaced meniscus without reduction. In the closed position (*A*), the meniscus (M) is anterior to the condylar head. A filling defect appears near the posterior slope of the articular eminence. In the open position (*B*), the filling defect remains at the anterior border of the condyle indicative of continued anterior displacement of the meniscus (M).

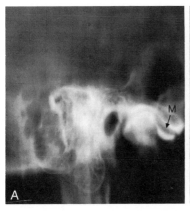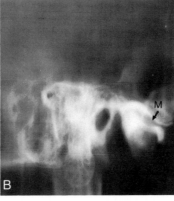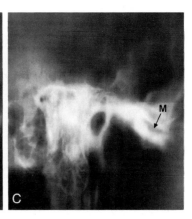

FIGURE 19–23. *A, B,* and *C,* Anterior displaced meniscus causing interference. In the fully closed position (*A*), the meniscus (M) is visualized anterior to the condyle along the posterior slope of the articular eminence. As the patient attempts to translate the joint (*B*), the meniscus interferes with movement and appears to fold anterior to the condyle. With increased effect, the condyle moves past the disc and the meniscus is visualized posterior to the condyle (*C*).

water-soluble contrast medium into either the inferior or the superior joint space using local anesthesia. The contrast agent allows for radiographic evaluation of the anatomy of the joint space compartments; the meniscal morphology, including perforation; and the mandibular condyle-meniscal-temporal bone relationship.

The study is done employing direct fluoroscopic visualization, which allows for a dynamic assessment of the TMJ components. Combined with a video cassette recording of the dynamic phase of the fluroscopic study, repetitive viewings of the dynamics of the soft and hard tissue components of the joint are possible.

Linear sagittal arthrotomographic radiographs provide the clinician and radiologist with highly refined static images for the evaluation of the intracapsular components of the joint and their relationship to the osseous anatomy.

REFERENCES

1. Norgaard, F.: Arthrography of the temporomandibular joint. Acta Radiol. 25:679–685, 1944.
2. Farrar, W.D., and McCarty, W.L., Jr.: Inferior joint arthroscopy and characteristics of condylar paths in internal derangement of the TMJ. J. Prosthet. Dent. 41:548–555, 1979.
3. Blasche, D.D., Solberg, W.K., and Sanders, B.: Arthrography of the temporomandibular joint; review of current status. J. Am. Dent. Assoc. 100:388–395, 1980.
4. Bronstein, S.L., Tomessetti, B.J., and Ryan, D.E.: Internal derangement of the temporomandibular joint:

correlation of arthrographic with surgical findings. J. Oral Surg. 39:572–584, 1981.
5. Katzberg, R.W.: Temporomandibular joint imaging. Radiology 170:297–307, 1989.
6. Bell, K.A. and Walters, P.J.: Videofluoroscopy during arthrography of the temporomandibular joint. Radiology 147:879, 1983.
7. Westersson, P.-L.: Double-contrast arthrography of the temporomandibular joint: introduction of an arthrographic technique for visualization of the disc and articular surfaces. J. Oral Maxillofac. Surg. 41:163–172, 1983.
8. Kaplan, P.A., and Tu, H.K., et al: Inferior joint space arthrography of normal temporomandibular joints: reassessment of diagnostic criteria. Radiology 159:585–589, 1986.
9. Schellhas, K.P., Wilkes, C.H., et al: The diagnosis of temporomandibular disease: two-compartment arthrography and MR. Am. J. Roentgenol. 151:341–350, 1988.
10. Murphy, W.A.: Arthrography of the temporomandibular joint. Radiol. Clin. North Am. 19:365–378, 1981.
11. Kaplan, P.A., and Tu, H.A.: The normal temporomandibular joint: MR and arthrographic correlation. Radiology 165:177–178, 1987.
12. Katzberg, R.W., Dolwick, M.F., Helms, C.A., et al: Arthrography of the temporomandibular joint. Am. J. Roentgenol. 134:995–1003, 1980.
13. Westersson, P.-L., Bronstein, S.L., and Liedberg, J.: Temporomandibular joint: correlation between single-contrast videoarthrography and post-mortem morphology. Radiology 160:767–771, 1986.
14. Bronstein, S.L., Tomasetti, B.T., and Ryan, D.E.: Internal derangement of the temporomandibular joint: correlation of arthrographic with surgical findings. J. Oral Surg. 39:572–584, 1981.
15. DuBrul, E.L.: The craniomandibular articulation. In *Sicher's Oral Anatomy,* 7th ed. C.V. Mosby Co., St. Louis, 1980.
16. Helms, C.A., Katzberg, R.W., and Dolwick, M.F.: Internal derangements of the temporomandibular joint.

Radiology Research and Education Foundation, San Francisco, 1983.

17. Doyle, T.: Arthrography of the temporomandibular joint: a simple technique. Clin. Radiol. 34:147–151, 1983.

18. Dolwick, M.F., Katzberg, R.W., Helms, C.A., and Bales, D.J.: Arthrotomographic evaluation of the temporomandibular joint. J. Oral Surg. 37:793–799, 1979.

19. Katzberg, R.W., Dolwick, M.F., Helms, C.A., et al: Arthrography of the temporomandibular joint. Am. J. Roentgenol. 134:995–1003, 1980.

20. Braunwald, E., et al: *Harrison's Principles of Internal Medicine,* 11th ed. McGraw-Hill, New York, 1987.

21. Wyngaarden, J.B., and Smith, L.H.: *Cecil Textbook of Medicine.* W. B. Saunders Co., Philadelphia, 1982.

22. Dolwick, M.F., Kipton, J.S., Warner, M.R., and Williams, V.F.: Sagittal anatomy of the human temporomandibular joint spaces: normal and abnormal findings. J. Oral Maxillofac. Surg. 41:86–88, 1983.

David L. Milbauer

CHAPTER 20

Magnetic Resonance Imaging and Computerized Tomography

Imaging of the temporomandibular joint (TMJ) for evaluation of possible internal derangement evolved dramatically during the 1980s. During the first half of the decade, arthrographic procedures permitted detailed assessments of the position and configuration of the articular disc and refinements in technique yielded accuracy rates of up to 97%.[1-3] Despite these high diagnostic yields, TMJ arthrography failed to gain widespread popularity. The procedure requires expertise to both perform and interpret. Besides its technical demands, arthrography requires injection of a contrast medium and can be quite painful for the patient. Investigators thus sought alternative imaging methods.

Computerized tomography (CT) scanning was first introduced in the early 1970s and evolved into higher resolution third- and fourth-generation models by the 1980s. As the technology improved, interest in this modality for evaluating temporomandibular disorders (TMDs) grew. Creative methods to permit scanning in the sagittal plane provided the first direct visualization of the articular disc.[4-7] Early reports on both direct sagittal scanning and thin axial scanning with sagittal reformation indicated comparable sensitivity to that of arthrography in detecting anterior disc displacement. Soon the literature reflected a lively competition between the two modalities.[5-10] Computerized tomography was not without drawbacks. Some patients found the positioning required for direct sagittal scanning awk-

ward or difficult to maintain, and the slightest movements were found to seriously degrade reformated sagittal images. Artifacts from dental restorations as well as other limitations resulted in a significant number of technically suboptimal studies. Similar to arthrography, a drawback of CT scanning is that it requires ionizing radiation.

Magnetic resonance imaging (MRI) was introduced in the early 1980s and was relatively crude. Technologic developments rapidly brought this new modality into the radiologic mainstream. As early as 1984, preliminary work appeared illustrating the potential of MRI in evaluating the TMJ.[11] Improvements in surface coil design along with other technologic refinements permitted imaging with high spatial resolution and with improved signal-to-noise ratios. It soon became apparent that MRI could reliably demonstrate the position and configuration of the articular disc. This technique has currently surpassed CT scanning in the evaluation of internal derangements of the TMJs. Arthrography remains an important tool in demonstrating perforations of the disc or its attachments as well as in evaluating joint dynamics with videofluoroscopy (see Chapter 19). Although CT scanning has largely been supplanted by MRI for suspected internal derangements of the TMJ, it remains a useful modality in evaluating the osseous TMJ structures when visualization of fine bone detail is necessary.

COMPUTERIZED TOMOGRAPHIC SCANNING

In the early 1980s, before MRI had evolved to its current level of clinical utility, CT scanning appeared to hold promise as an alternative to arthrography in evaluating TMDs. In 1980, Suarez and coworkers[13] first reported the use of CT in TMJ imaging. In 1981, Katzberg and associates[14] introduced the concept of CT-assisted arthrography. Recognizing the importance of viewing the TMJ in the sagittal plane, Helms, in 1982,[15] reported nine cases of anterior disc displacement diagnosed utilizing sagittal reformation derived from multiple axial sections.

The idea of direct sagittal scanning of the TMJ offered an opportunity to improve both image quality and, potentially, diagnostic capability. However, the CT scanner did not lend itself physically to direct sagittal scanning of the TMJ. Efforts by various radiologists to overcome this barrier resulted in some creative solutions.[16–19] A method for obtaining direct sagittal images was described by Manzione and colleagues, in 1982 (Fig. 20–1).[16] In 1984, Sartoris and coworkers[18] offered an alternative method of direct sagittal imaging utilizing a specially constructed patient-support table situated on the side opposite the normal scanning table (Fig. 20–2). Another method of direct sagittal scanning described by Simon and associates[19] included a head support outfitted with threaded shafts allowing precise incremental adjustments between scans to produce a contiguous "slice" study (Fig. 20–3).

A series by Manzione and colleagues,[17] evaluating 51 TMJs in 47 patients and four cadaver specimens, indicated direct sagittal scanning to be 94% accurate in detecting internal derangements and 96% accurate in detecting bony degenerative changes. Investigators interpreting reformatted sagittal images from axial scanning methods reported generally similar results. Thompson and coworkers[20] reported CT findings in agreement with surgical or arthrographic findings in 13 of 15 joints. In a series of 200 patients evaluated by Helms and associates,[21] using the reformatted technique, a 97% accuracy rate was reported in 75 cases in which surgical and arthrographic followup data were available.

THEORY OF COMPUTERIZED TOMOGRAPHY SCANNING

The CT scanner consists of an x-ray tube and multiple detectors located opposite the tube. A thin collimated x-ray beam is passed through a slice of tissue in the patient's body, and the exiting beam strikes the detectors opposite the tube that measure and record its intensity. As the tube moves around the patient, the sequence is repeated and the resultant data are stored by a computer. By quantitating the amount of radiation received by the detectors for the various exposures, the computer can determine the stopping capability of small portions of tissue in the sampled slice. This value is the "attenuation coefficient" (u), derived through a complex series of simultaneous equations. These values assigned to each small unit of tissue in a given slice matrix may be represented as shades of grey by a cathode ray tube (CRT). The CRT may in turn expose film to produce a hard copy of the finished scan.

Assigning shades of grey values or "windowing" permits the visual differentiation of various tissues having only small attenuation differences. Appropriate selection of window levels and width allows optimal evaluation of soft tissue and bone pathology individually from the same examination slice. Further soft-

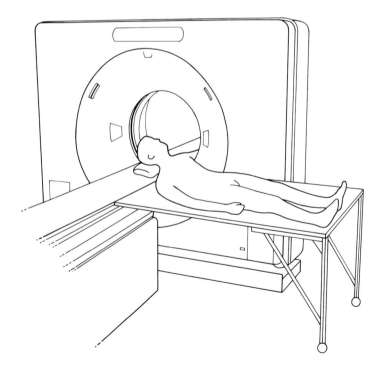

FIGURE 20–1. Direct sagittal computerized tomographic scanning. This early method employed a stretcher that was placed perpendicular to the table alongside the scanning gantry.

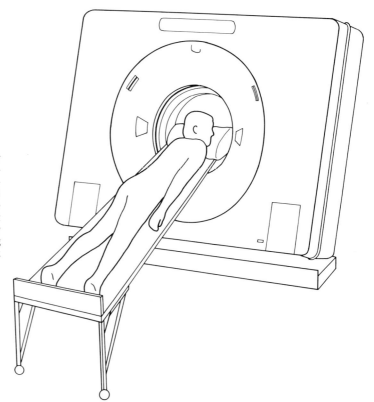

FIGURE 20–2. Alternative method for direct sagittal computerized tomographic scanning. A specially constructed patient-support table is situated opposite the normal scanning table. The combination of an inclined support table and a tilting of the scanning gantry offered greater flexibility in the scanning of a patient with only moderate neck mobility.

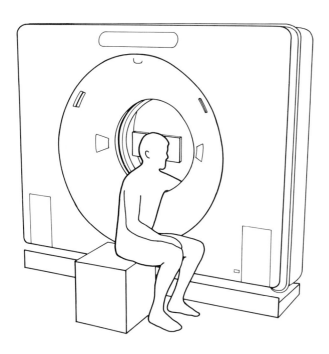

FIGURE 20–3. Method for direct sagittal computerized tomographic scanning devised by Simon and colleagues.[19] The patient's head is supported by a specially designed rest that permits incremental adjustments between scans. These provide contiguous sagittal sections through the entire joint space.

ware display manipulation, such as the "blink mode," aids in the visual detection of the most subtle differences in attenuation values in adjacent structures.

Scanning Techniques

The two techniques for CT scanning of the TMJ are axial scanning with sagittal reformation[15,20,22] and direct sagittal scanning.[15-18] In the first method, conventional axial sections are obtained through the TMJ and the data obtained are processed by a computer to generate images perpendicular to the scan plane. The direct sagittal images are generally superior to those obtained by reformated techniques. However, more patients have difficulty tolerating the direct sagittal methods. Unfortunately, sagittal reformated techniques are particularly prone to image degradation by patient movement.

Axial scanning is performed with 1.5-mm thick sections at 1- to 1.5-mm intervals with the jaw closed.[13,19] Some radiologists advocate scanning with both open-mouth and closed-mouth positions.[20-22] Multiple reformated sagittal images are generated across the condyle (Fig. 20-4). Direct sagittal images, using various accessory devices,[16-19] are obtained, employing 1.5- to 2-mm thick sections (Fig. 20-5). Both the reformated and direct sagittal images may be displayed by a special blink mode designed to highlight small density differences between adjacent tissues (Figs. 20-5 and 20-6).

Image Interpretation

Anterior disc displacement is diagnosed by CT when an abnormal soft tissue density is identified anterior to the condyle (Figs. 20-6 and 20-7). Recognition of the displaced disc is aided by the normal fat tissue present in the precondylar space, which has been termed the "lateral pterygoid fat pad" by Manzione and coworkers.[17] Indirect signs of internal derangement observed by Thompson and associates[20] include (1) remodeling of joint surfaces (Fig. 20-8); (2) osteophytic and other bony degenerative changes (Fig. 20-9); (3) altered joint spaces; (4) asymmetry of the length of the rami, with shortening on the involved side; (5) cephalad migration of the coronoid process on the involved side; and (6) lateral ptygeroid muscle asymmetry.

MAGNETIC RESONANCE IMAGING

Since the first reports on MRI of the TMJ in 1984,[12] improvements in MRI technology have enabled the routine visualization of the articular disc position and configuration with such clarity that MRI has largely supplanted ar-

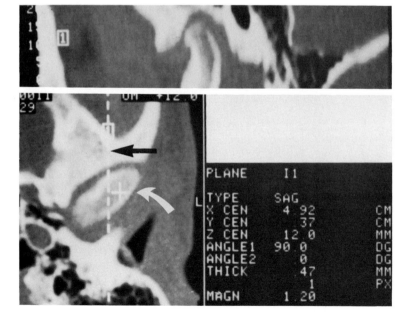

FIGURE 20-4. Sagittal reformated image of the temporomandibular joint (above) obtained from axial scanning (below). The dotted line (straight arrow) indicates the plane of computer reconstruction through the condyle (curved arrow) and glenoid fossa. (Courtesy of Dr. Joel Friedman, Riverdale, N.Y.)

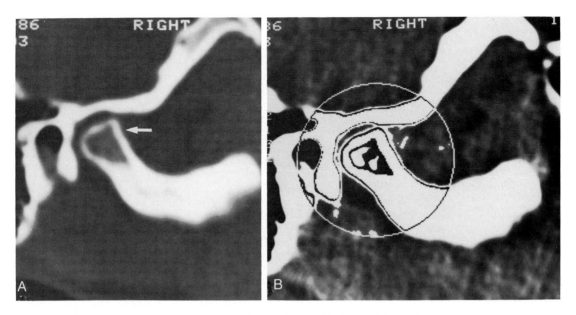

FIGURE 20–5. *A,* Direct sagittal image. Arrow indicates the mandibular condyle. *B,* The same section as in *A* utilizing a "blink mode" that highlights small differences in tissue density. (Courtesy of Dr. Joel Friedman, Riverdale, N.Y.)

thrography and CT in the evaluation of internal derangement.[23–26] With its superb soft tissue contrast resolution and multiplanar imaging capabilities, MRI permits a thorough examination of the joint anatomy not possible with other imaging modalities. Magnetic resonance imaging is noninvasive and does not rely on ionizing radiation, further adding to its overall appeal.

Preliminary works by Roberts and colleagues,[7] in 1985, and Katzberg and colleagues,[29] in 1986, showed good correlation between MRI studies and arthrographic examinations. Among the 67 patients evalu-

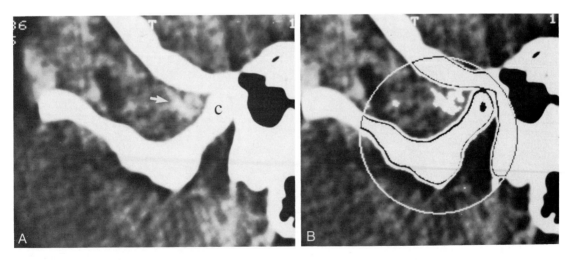

FIGURE 20–6. *A,* Anterior displacement by direct sagittal scan. Note the increased soft tissue density (arrow) anterior to the condyle (C). *B,* Same image as that in *A* using the "blink mode" that highlights the anteriorly displaced disc. (Courtesy of Dr. Joel Friedman, Riverdale, N.Y.)

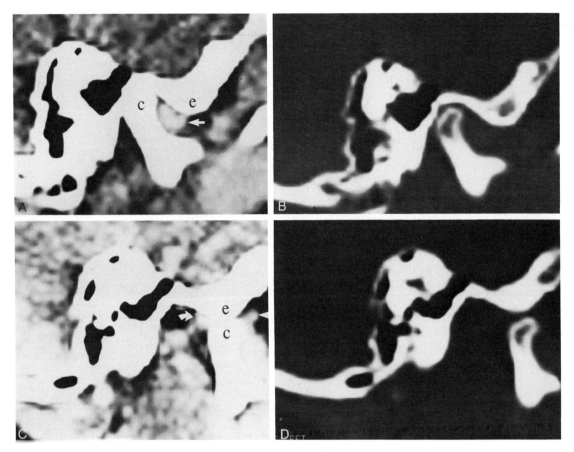

FIGURE 20–7. Anterior disc displacement with reduction. Sagittal closed view with soft tissue (*A*) and bone detail (*B*) technique. Note the anteriorly displaced disc (arrow). *C* and *D,* Sagittal open views. Note the disc reduces to its normal position between the condyle and eminence. The curved arrow indicates the posterior band. (Straight arrow = anterior band; c = condyle; e = eminence.) (Courtesy of Dr. Joel Friedman, Riverdale, N.Y.)

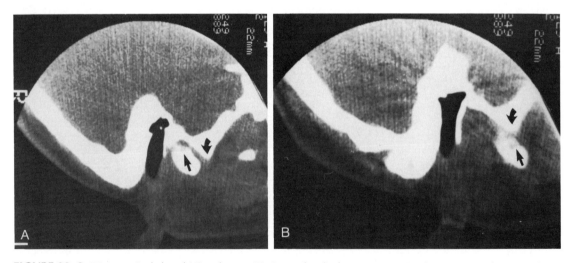

FIGURE 20–8. Direct sagittal closed (*A*) and open (*B*) views of early degenerative joint disease. Note the cortical erosion involving the articular portion of the condyle (straight arrow). Curved arrow indicates the eminence. (Courtesy of Dr. Joel Friedman, Riverdale, N.Y.)

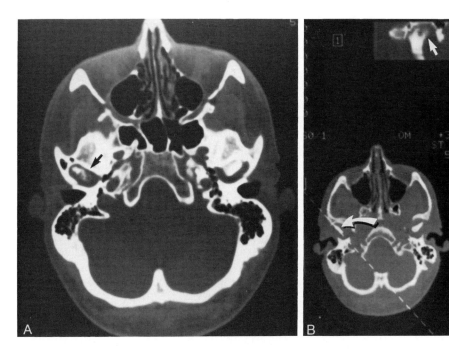

FIGURE 20–9. Degenerative joint disease. Axial image (*A*) demonstrates irregularity of the condyle within the glenoid fossa (arrow). Reformated oblique section (*B*) through the condyle (curved arrow) reveals subchondral cystic degeneration (straight arrow). (Courtesy of Dr. Joel Friedman, Riverdale, N.Y.)

ated by Harms and associates,[4] 15 TMJs with subsequent surgical confirmation all correlated accurately with preoperative MRI findings. By studying autopsy specimens comparing MRI with direct sagittal CT scanning, Westesson and associates[6] found MRI to be superior in depicting soft tissue anatomy of the TMJ and therefore more reliable in demonstrating disc position and configuration compared with CT. In another report correlating autopsy findings[8] with sagittal MR images, there was a 73% accuracy rate in delineating disc position, roughly comparable with the results obtained with single contrast arthrography.[3]

These investigators found the occurrence of mediolateral disc displacement was an important factor in reducing the accuracy of imaging in the sagittal plane alone. They believed that a combination of sagittal and coronal imaging had the potential for matching the 92% accuracy rate reported with double contrast arthrotomography.[2]

Historical Perspective

The phenomenon of nuclear magnetic resonance (NMR) was initially developed independently in the 1940s by Bloch at Stanford and Purcell at Harvard, for which they received the Nobel Prize in physics in 1952. First described as a quantum mechanical phenomenon, NMR soon found application as a new means of spectroscopy and has been used for structural analysis of organic compounds for years. In the early 1970s, Damadian introduced the concept of deliberately modulating the external magnetic field such that a small portion of a sample was in resonance with the incident radiofrequency. Lauterbur, in the same time period, devised a method for modulating the magnetic field to produce a line of sample in resonance. Utilizing back projection techniques similar to those in CT, Lauterbur was able to reconstruct the NMR properties of the specimen. When the magnets were large enough to accommodate a whole body "specimen," MRI became a clinical reality.

Theory

The basis of MRI relies on the property of nuclei with an odd number of protons, neutrons, or both to behave as magnets. Hydrogen, being the most sensitive of the stable nuclei to a magnetic field and the most abundant element in the body, is ideally suited for MRI. The axes of these nuclei, when subjected to a strong magnetic field, align within the field. Radio waves of a specific frequency, termed the "resonant frequency," may be used to excite these nuclei out of alignment with the magnetic field. When the radio wave is turned off, the nuclei tend to realign with the magnetic field, releasing some of the energy absorbed by the incident radio wave. A signal is released in the form of a radio wave of the same frequency as the incident radio wave. The emitted radio wave or signal is received and stored by the MR machine. Through mathematic processes similar to those developed for CT scanning, an image is produced.

The ability to separate incoming information into a three-dimensional picture relies on the concept that the resonant frequency for a given nucleus is determined by the strength of the magnetic field it is subjected to. By slightly changing the strength of the magnetic field across the sample of tissue, the resonant frequency for each nucleus changes accordingly. Thus, a gradient in the magnetic field allows the various signals received by the MR machine to be sorted and traced back to the nuclear source in the tissue sample.

Contrast between different tissues may be manipulated by varying the rate at which radio waves are transmitted. A short repetition time (TR) and echo time (TE) will produce a T1-weighted image, and a long TR and TE will produce a T2-weighted image. T1-weighted images are particularly useful in scanning small anatomic regions, such as the TMJ, where high spatial resolution is desired. T2-weighted images yield a bright signal from fluid and may demonstrate joint effusions and inflammatory changes.

Another method of manipulating tissue contrast is through gradient echo techniques. Sometimes called "Fast Scans," these sequences only partially excite the nuclei in more conventional sequences, resulting in significantly shorter scan times. Some radiologists utilize gradient echo techniques to produce images similar to conventional T2-weighted images when evaluating inflammatory conditions.[27] Others have taken advantage of the short scanning time in gradient echo techniques to obtain multiple images with incremental jaw opening, resulting in a dynamic or motion study.[28]

Instrumentation and Technique

With the advent of improved surface coil designs, most MRI units are capable of satisfactorily imaging the TMJ (Fig. 20–10A). Some MR systems are equipped with dual surface coil capability (Fig. 20–10B), which allows the simultaneous imaging of both TMJs.[30,31] Most investigators agree on scanning protocols, which include sagittal images permitting an assessment of the anterior posterior relationships of the disc, condyle, and glenoid fossa. Some software programs allow oblique sagittal (parasagittal) imaging along the plane of the mandibular rami, which can depict the anterior and posterior disc attachments together. Typically, an axial localizer is initially obtained as a "scout" in order to "prescribe" the sagittal or oblique sagittal sequences (Fig. 20–11A). High resolution sagittal sequences require thin slice thicknesses (3 mm) with small fields of view (12 to 16 cm), which result in a resolving power of approximately 0.5 mm.

Frequently, sagittal images are obtained in both closed- and open-jaw positions. A partial open-jaw position is generally less difficult for the patient to maintain without moving during the scan. The disc is usually better demonstrated in an open view, as it moves forward of the glenoid fossa. Because of the growing awareness of sideways and rotational disc displacements,[32,33] coronal and oblique coronal scanning techniques have become increasingly utilized (see Figs. 20–11B, 20–13, and 20–22B).

Image Interpretation

On T1-weighted images, the fibrocartilaginous disc has a low signal intensity (dark), whereas muscle tissue has a low-intermediate signal intensity or brightness (grey). Marrow elements in medullary bone produce high signal intensity, whereas the more dense cortical bone produces an outline of low-to-no signal intensity (black on all pulse sequences). Fatty connective tissue has a characteristic bright signal on T1-weighted sequences.

In the sagittal plane, the disc has a biconcave shape or bowtie–like configuration, situated between the superior borders of the condyle below and the glenoid fossa above. The ovoid disc has a thicker posterior band averaging 3 mm in thickness and a thinner anterior band and an intermediate zone averaging 2.5 mm

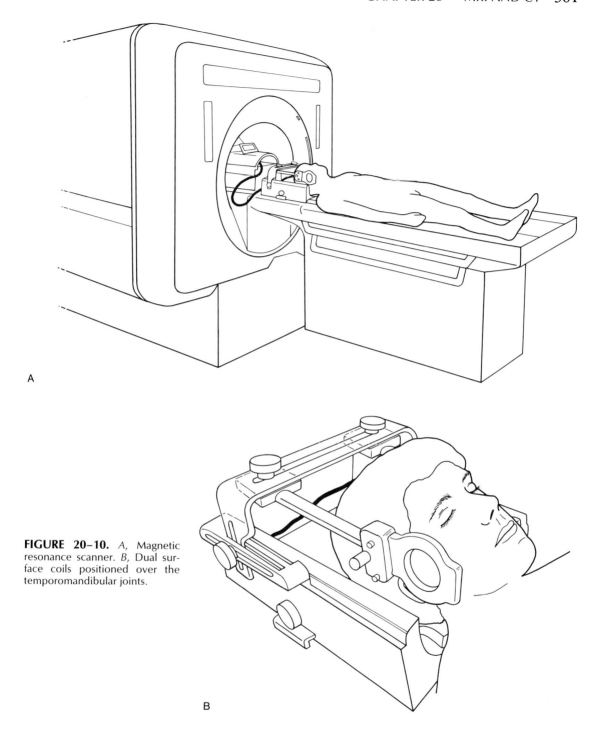

FIGURE 20–10. *A,* Magnetic resonance scanner. *B,* Dual surface coils positioned over the temporomandibular joints.

and 1.5 mm, respectively.[24] The normal disc is sharply delineated from its anterior and posterior attachments. Anteriorly, the disc is continuous with the joint capsule and attaches to at least some of the fibers of the superior belly of the lateral pterygoid muscle, seen as a thread-like structure inserting on the anteromedial lateral aspect of the disc (Fig. 20–12A). The inferior belly of the lateral pterygoid muscle attaches directly to the mandibular condyle at

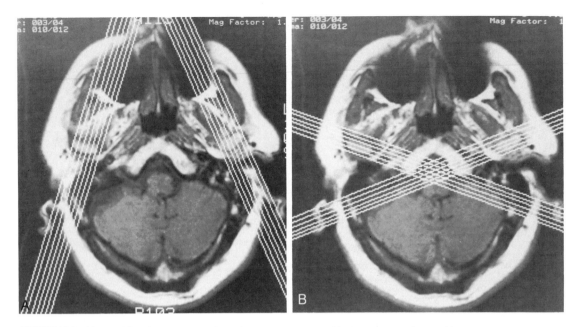

FIGURE 20–11. Axial localizer sections through the temporomandibular joint are obtained to set up a precise series of sagittal (A) or coronal (B) sections through the joint.

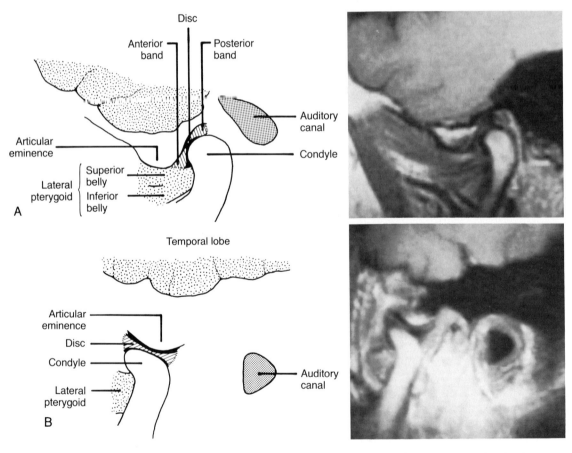

FIGURE 20–12. *A,* Normal sagittal magnetic resonance image (MRI) in closed-mouth position. Note that the disc overlies the condyle with the posterior band in a 12-o'clock position relative to the condyle. *B,* Normal sagittal MRI in open-mouth position. The disc remains interposed between the condyle below and the eminence above.

362

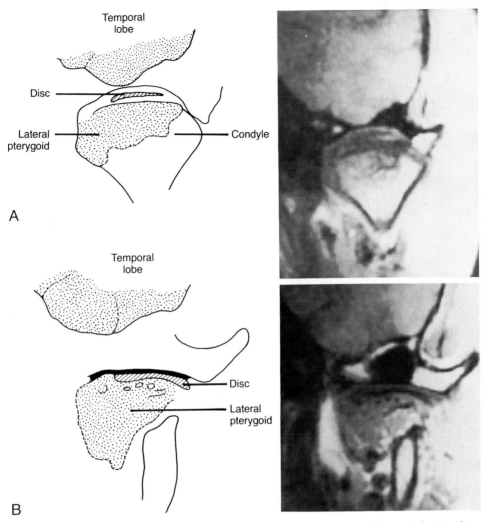

FIGURE 20–13. Normal coronal magnetic resonance image through the midportion of the condyle (A) and just anterior to the condyle (B).

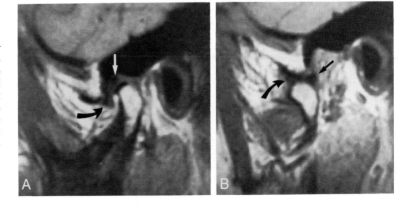

FIGURE 20–14. Mild anterior disc displacement with reduction. In the closed view (A), the posterior band is slightly forward of the top of the condyle (straight arrow). The open view (B) shows the disc in normal relation to the condyle and eminence. The curved arrow indicates the anterior band.

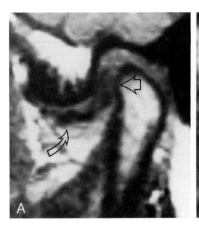
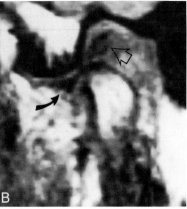

FIGURE 20–15. Moderate anterior disc displacement with reduction. In the closed view (A), the disc is anteriorly displaced with the posterior band (straight arrow) at approximately a 9-o'clock position relative to the condyle. The disc is elongated and slightly deformed. The open view (B) shows reduction of the disc with jaw opening. The curved arrow indicates the anterior band.

the pterygoid fovea. Posteriorly, the disc is contiguous with a loosely organized connective tissue structure, rich in blood vessels and nerve fibers, called the retrodiscal tissue. Fatty elements within this structure produce a higher signal intensity compared with the adjacent disc. Its superior portion is rich in elastin, which is thought to aid disc retraction on jaw closing. The retrodiscal tissue has attachments posteriorly to both the posterior wall of the condylar fossa and the posterior condyle. In the closed position, the posterior band overlies the superior surface of the condyle at the 12 o'clock position. On opening, the disc moves forward remaining interposed between the condyle below and the articular eminence above (Fig. 20–12B).

In the coronal view, the disc has an arc-shaped configuration (Fig. 20–13). The disc tends to be thicker along the medial border and attaches via collateral ligaments to a well-organized capsule laterally and a more loosely organized capsule medially.

Internal Derangements

Of the many disorders that can affect the TMJ, internal derangement is the most commonly diagnosed by MRI studies and may occur in up to 28% of the adult population.[1,3,24,25] Internal derangement may be defined as an abnormal anatomic relationship of the disc, condyle, and articular surface of the temporal bone. The most frequent derangement involves anterior disc displacement, although displacement can occur in all directions.[25,32,33] With anterior displacement, there is elongation of the retrodiscal tissue.

In the early stages of this disorder, opening of the jaw allows the disc to assume a normal relationship between the condyle and articular surface of the temporal bone (Fig. 20–14). This disorder is termed anterior displacement with reduction and is often associated with a well-defined clicking sound. As the disorder progresses, the disc moves farther forward and its configuration may become deformed (Fig. 20–

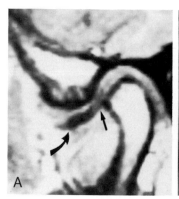
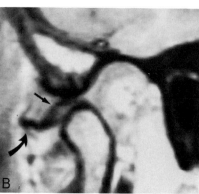

FIGURE 20–16. Anterior disc displacement without reduction. The closed view (A) demonstrates the disc to be forward in position and deformed. The open view (B) shows further anterior displacement of the disc without reduction. The posterior band (straight arrow) remains forward of the condyle. The curved arrow indicates the anterior band.

FIGURE 20–17. Anterior disc displacement without reduction. The closed view (*A*) shows marked anterior disc displacement and deformity of the disc. On opening (*B*), the disc remains anteriorly displaced, folding on itself (arrow).

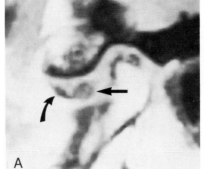

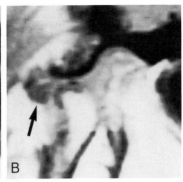

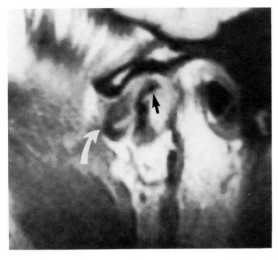

FIGURE 20–18. Anterior disc displacement with limited range of motion. The anteriorly displaced disc (curved arrow) restricts movement of the condyle. Early degenerative changes of the condylar surface are noted (straight arrow).

15A). Reduction occurs at a later phase of jaw opening (Fig. 20–15B), and in general it is thought that the later the clicking sound during mouth opening, the more severe the derangement.[26]

As the displacement progresses, the disc may remain anterior to the condyle in all phases of jaw movement (Fig. 20–16). This condition is referred to as anterior displacement without reduction and is often associated with the disappearance of the clicking sound. The disc configuration becomes elongated, and the normally sharp demarcation between the disc and its posterior attachments may become less distinct (Fig. 20–16A). Not uncommonly, the posterior band becomes progressively thickened and can fold on itself with jaw opening (Fig. 20–17). The disc may become entrapped between the condyle and fossa, limiting jaw movement (Fig. 20–18).

In late stages, the chronically deranged disc may become biconvex (Fig. 20–19). The

FIGURE 20–19. *A* and *B*, Degenerative joint disease associated with anterior disc displacement without reduction. The disc is anteriorly displaced and markedly deformed (straight arrow). Flattening and sclerosis of the condylar surface are evident (curved arrow).

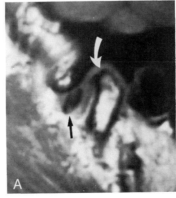

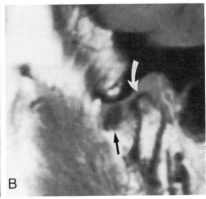

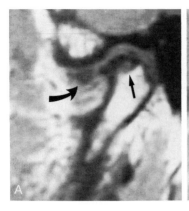
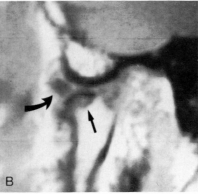

FIGURE 20–20. Osteochondritis dissecans associated with anterior disc displacement without reduction. The closed view (A) shows the disc to be deformed and displaced anteriorly (curved arrow). A sharply defined region of low signal intensity is seen in the superior aspect of the condyle (straight arrow). The open view (B) shows further disc displacement without reduction.

FIGURE 20–21. Advanced degenerative joint disease associated with anterior disc displacement. A prominent osteophyte projects anteriorly from the condyle (straight arrow). Note the disc deformity (curved arrow) without reduction on the open view (B).

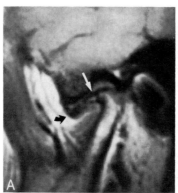
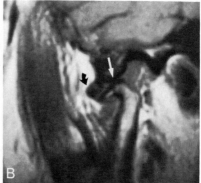

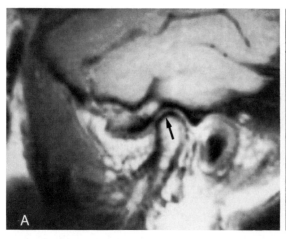
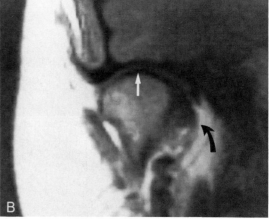

FIGURE 20–22. Medial sideways displacement. The sagittal view (A) shows no visualization of the disc within the glenoid fossa (arrow) in the closed view. The coronal image through the midportion of the joint (B) shows medial sideways displacement of the disc (curved arrow) from its normal position over the condylar head (straight arrow).

chronically displaced and thickened disc cannot function properly, even if it is positioned correctly. Chronic anterior displacement can lead to disc perforation, which usually occurs in the bilaminar zone but may involve the disc itself. Perforation allows direct contact of the

articular cartilage of the condyle and glenoid fossa, leading to degenerative joint disease.

Schellhas and coworkers[34] described the MRI appearance of osteochondritis dissecans and avascular necrosis of the mandibular condyle, often associated with pre-existing internal

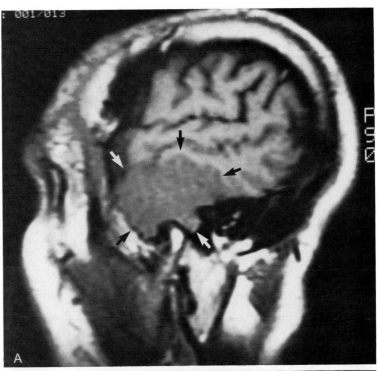
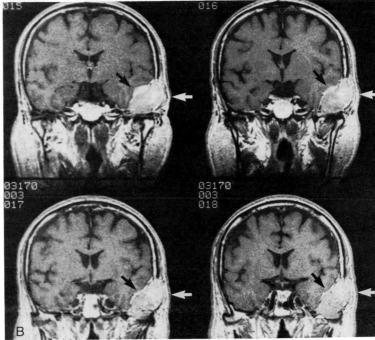

FIGURE 20–23. Plasmacytoma of the temporal bone in sagittal (*A*) and four successive coronal (*B*) planes (arrows).

derangement. Osteochondritis dissecans appears as a focal, sharply defined subchondral region of decreased signal intensity, along the superior aspect of the condyle (Fig. 20–20). Avascular necrosis generally involves a larger area of cortical and medullary infarction, often

resulting in morphologic changes including articular surface collapse, sclerosis, and hypertrophic spurring (Fig. 20–21).

Disc displacements have been noted to occur in all directions, and this fact has been implicated as a major contributor to the false-nega-

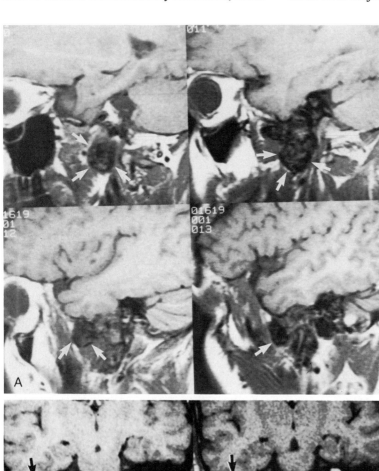

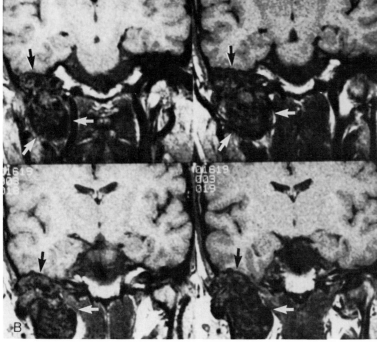

FIGURE 20–24. Giant cell tumor of the mandible in four successive sagittal (*A*) and coronal (*B*) planes.

tive rates in both patient and cadaver studies evaluating internal derangements.[8,25,32] Autopsy specimens have revealed the occurrence of medial and lateral sideways displacements as well as combinations of anterior and mediolateral displacements, which have been termed rotational displacements.[33] Katzberg[25] has devised a classification scheme placing the various displacements into normal, anterior, anteromedial, anterolateral, medial, and lateral subgroups.

The value of coronal imaging has been emphasized to better detect these variations (Fig. 20–22). Katzberg[25] and Westesson and colleagues[8] have reported medial displacements (rotational anteromedial and medial sideways displacements) to be more common than those with lateral components (rotational anterolateral and lateral sideways displacements). Khoury and Dolan,[32] however, found lateral displacements to be more common.

In addition to internal derangements, MRI may be of help in evaluating lesions involving the structures in and around the TMJ. Primary osseous lesions, including tumors, may occur in the temporal bone (Fig. 20–23) or in the mandible (Fig. 20–24). Diseases of the TMJ synovium[35] and masticatory muscles[36] have also been reported.

REFERENCES

1. Bronstein, S.L., Tomasetti, B.J., and Ryan, D.E.: Internal derangements of the temporomandibular joint: Correlation of arthrographic with surgical findings. J. Oral Surg. 39:572–584, 1981.
2. Westesson, P.-L. and Rohlin, M.: Diagnostic accuracy of double-contrast arthrotomography of the temporomandibular joint: correlation with post-mortem morphology. Am. J. Nucl. Radiol. 5:463–468, 1984.
3. Westesson, P.-L., Bronstein, S.L., and Liedeberg, J.: Temporomandibular joint: Correlation between single-contrast video arthrography and post-mortem morphology. Radiology 160:767–771, 1986.
4. Harms, S.E., Wilk, R.M., Wolford, L.M., Chiles, D.G., and Milam, S.B.: The temporomandibular joint: Magnetic resonance imaging using surface coils. Radiology 157:133–136, 1985.
5. Helms, C.A., Gillespy, T., III, Sims, R.E., and Richardson, M.L.: Magnetic resonance imaging of internal derangement of the temporomandibular joint. Radiol. Clin. North Am. 24:189–192, 1986.
6. Westesson, P.-L., Katzberg, R.W., Tallents, R.H., et al: CT and MR of the temporomandibular joint: Comparison with autopsy specimens. Am. J. Radiol. 148:1165–1171, 1987.
7. Roberts, D., Schenck, J., Joseph, P., et al: Temporomandibular joint: Magnetic resonance imaging. Radiology 155:829–830, 1985.
8. Westesson, P.-L., Katzberg, R.W., Tallents, R.H., et al: Temporomandibular joint: Comparison of MR images with cryosectional anatomy. Radiology 164:59–64, 1987.
9. Schellhas, K.P., Wilkes, C.H., Fritts, H.M., et al: Temporomandibular joint: MR imaging of internal derangements and postoperative changes. Am. J. Nucl. Radiol. 8:1093–1101, 1987.
10. Kaplan, P.A., Manzione, J.V., Thompson, J.R., et al: Computed tomography versus arthrography in the evaluation of the temporomandibular joint. Radiology 152:825–827, 1984. [Letter to the editor.]
11. Helms, C.A., Richardson, M.L., Moon, K.L., and Ware, W.H.: Nuclear magnetic resonance imaging of the temporomandibular joint: Preliminary observations. J. Craniomandib. Pract. 2:3, 1984.
12. Helms, C.A., Richardson, M.L., Moon, K.L., et al: Nuclear magnetic resonance imaging of the temporomandibular joint: Preliminary observations. J. Craniomandib. Pract. 2:219, 1984.
13. Suarez, F.R., Bhossry, B.R., Neff, P.A., et al: Preliminary study of computerized tomographs of the temporomandibular joint. Compend. Contin. Ed. Dent. 1:217–222, 1980.
14. Katzberg, R.W., Dolwick, M.F., Keith, D.A., et al: New observations with routine and CT-assisted arthrography in suspected internal derangement of the temporomandibular joint. Oral Surg. 51:569–574, 1981.
15. Helms, C.A., Morrish, R.B., Jr., Kirlos, L.T., et al: Computed tomography of the meniscus of the temporomandibular joint: Preliminary observations. Radiology 145:719–722, 1982.
16. Manzione, J.V., Seltzer, S.E., Katzberg, R.W., et al: Direct sagittal computed tomography of the temporomandibular joint. Am. J. Nucl. Radiol. 3:677–679, 1982.
17. Manzione, J.V., Katzberg, R.W., Brodsky, G.L., et al: Internal derangements of the temporomandibular joint: Diagnosis by direct sagittal computed tomography. Radiology 150:111–115, 1984.
18. Sartoris, D.J., Neuman, C.H., and Riley, R.W.: The temporomandibular joint: True sagittal computed tomography with meniscus visualization. Radiology 150:250–254, 1984.
19. Simon, D.C., Hess, M.L., Smilak, M.S., and Beltran, J.: Direct sagittal CT of the temporomandibular joint. Radiology 157:545, 1985.
20. Thompson, J.R., Christiansen, E.L., Hasso, A.N., and Hinshaw, D.B., Jr., et al: Temporomandibular joints: High resolution computed tomographic evaluation. Radiology 150:105–110, 1984.
21. Helms, C.A., Vogler, J.B., Morrish, R.B., et al: Temporomandibular joint internal derangements: CT diagnosis. Radiology 152:459–462, 1984.
22. Thompson, J.R., Christiansen, E.L., Sauser, D., et al: Dislocation of the temporomandibular joint meniscus: Contrast arthrography versus computed tomography. Am. J. Radiol. 144:171–174, 1985.
23. Schellhas, K.P., Wilkes, C.H., Omlie, M.R., et al: The diagnosis of temporomandibular joint disease: Two compartment arthrography and MR. Am. J. Nucl. Radiol. 9:579–588, 1988.
24. Hasso A.N., Christiansen, E.T., and Alder, M.E.: The temporomandibular joint. Radiol. Clin. North Am. 27:301–314, 1989.
25. Katzberg, R.W.: Temporomandibular joint imaging. Radiology 170:297–307, 1989.
26. Kaplan, P.A. and Helms, C.A.: Current status of temporomandibular joint imaging for the diagnosis of internal derangements. Am. J. Radiol. 152:697–705, 1989.
27. Schellhas, K.P. and Wilkes, C.H.: Temporomandibular joint inflammation: Comparison of MR fast scan-

ning with T1- and T2-weighted imaging techniques. Am. J. Nucl. Radiol. 10:589–594, 1989.

28. Burnett, K.R., Davis, C.L., and Read, J.: Dynamic display of the temporomandibular joint meniscus by using "Fast-Scan" MR imaging. Am. J. Radiol. 149:959–962, 1987.

29. Katzberg, R.W., Bessette, R.W., Tallents, R.H., et al: Normal and abnormal temporomandibular joint MR imaging with surface coil. Radiology 158:183–189, 1986.

30. Hardy, C.J., Katzberg, R.W., Frey, R.L., et al: Switched surface coil system for bilateral MR imaging. Radiology 167:835–838, 1988.

31. Shellock, F.G. and Pressman, B.D.: Dual surface-coil MR imaging of bilateral temporomandibular joints: Improvements in the imaging protocol. Am. J. Nucl. Radiol. 10:595–598, 1989.

32. Khoury, M.D. and Dolan, E.: Sideways dislocation of the temporomandibular joint meniscus: The edge sign. Am. J. Nucl. Radiol. 7:869–872, 1986.

33. Katzberg, R.W., Westesson, P.-L., Tallents, R.H., et al: Temporomandibular joint: MR assessment of rotational and sideways disc displacements. Radiology 169:741–748, 1988.

34. Schellhas, K.P., Wilkes, C.H., Fritts, H.M., et al: MR of osteochondritis dissecans and avascular necrosis of the mandibular condyle. Am. J. Nucl. Radiol. 10:3–12, 1989.

35. Nokes, S.R., King, P.S., Garcia, R., et al: Temporomandibular joint chondromatosis with intracranial extension MR and CT contributions. Am. J. Radiol. 148:1173–1174, 1987.

36. Schellhas, K.P.: MR imaging of muscles of mastication. Am. J. Nucl. Radiol. 10:829–837, 1989.

Michael Gelb

CHAPTER 21

Diagnostic Tests

In the past 40 years or more, there has been an expanding interest within the dental profession toward temporomandibular disorders (TMD). The medical and dental curricula of the 1950s, 1960s, and 1970s devoted few hours to this topic. The surge in popularity regarding TMDs was fueled by many continuing education programs and by the formation of three societies, two journals, and over 80 textbooks on the topic.

The public media coined the term "whiplash of the eighties" and before long, every popular magazine carried articles on the relationship of "TMJ" to headache, earache, dizziness, and "bad bite."

The 1970s also saw the phenomenal growth of the computer industry and the miniaturization of the computer chip. For the first time, complicated electronic equipment could be manufactured at a fraction of the original size. Competition also brought prices down so that many clinicians could now afford to use technology such as electromyography (EMG) and jaw tracking in their offices. The commercialization and promotion of diagnostic methodologies for craniomandibular disorders grew. At one time, over 75 diagnostic devices were on the market for measurement of complicated physiologic responses. Various claims were made, and one of the claims was that TMD could be diagnosed and the correct bite determined after one or two, 3-hour EMG and jaw tracking sessions.

Before long, the American Dental Association (ADA) and neuroscience researchers started investigating these claims. Some popular magazine articles stated that patients were being inappropriately diagnosed and overtreated and that their dentition was being unnecessarily mutilated by dentists who had taken brief courses in how to increase their practice with "TMJ."

An organization was formed dedicated to exposing fraud and quackery in medicine and dentistry, and the journal of the ADA cited TMD as a major area of fraud in dentistry. In fact, it was said that "TMJ" was dentistry's most active area of quackery and unorthodoxy.[45]

The ADA's Council on Dental Materials, Instruments and Equipment drafted a status report on the devices for the diagnosis and treatment of TMD in 1988.[29] The ADA was subsequently sued, and a restraining order was issued to prevent dissemination of this report. The litigation also restrained publication of the 1988 proceedings of a meeting in Chicago—a consensus conference on TMD sponsored by the ADA.

Diagnostic modalities for TMDs are under close scrutiny. Therefore, it is important that the scientific method of clinical decision analysis be applied to diagnostic tests allowing a systemic way of approaching this problem.

This chapter presents the criteria for the acceptance of new diagnostic tests, procedures, and methodologies. In addition, the diagnostic modalities of EMG, jaw tracking, sonography, and thermography are discussed as they relate to temporomandibular disorders and orofacial pain.

CRITERIA FOR ACCEPTANCE

The Food and Drug Administration controls the acceptance of diagnostic instruments for medicine and dentistry. The two primary areas of investigation are safety and efficacy.

Safety

Animal research is required to test the equipment for any electrical, mechanical, or chemical danger. Once animal studies have been approved, human trials usually follow. Government agencies such as the Office of Health Technology Assessment evaluate the safety and effectiveness of new or unestablished medical technologies. No debate exists over the safety of the equipment for diagnosis of craniomandibular disorders. Most of this discussion focuses on the efficacy.

Efficacy

Efficacy is determined by validity and reliability. To measure validity, one asks, "Does the test measure what it says it measures?" The

371

requirements for validity are a testable hypothesis, objective measures, and appropriate control groups. Reliability is concerned with repeatability or how consistently the test shows the same result. Both are over time, on the same patient, and with different clinicians. For a study to be reliable, the methods must be objective and clearly described. The methods should be in adequate detail so that the study can be repeated in at least three separate laboratories to show that the phenomenon is not peculiar to one operation or to one environment. A statistical term, "Kappa," measures how closely data points cluster. It is a measure of reliability. For example, if we call what we are trying to measure a "bull's eye," we can have three outcomes—A, B, and C.

Figure 21–1A represents a test with low reliability and poor validity. The data points are randomly distributed over the target. Figure 21–1B shows high reliability. The data points are very repeatable. Statistically, Kappa is high indicating good clustering. However, this does not measure what it intends to, the bull's eye. This is similar to the "old" centric relation (CR) position in dentistry. The CR position was a terminal hinge position, which was highly repeatable, yet it had low validity in terms of physiologic acceptability.

Figure 21–1C represents the ideal diagnostic test—it has high reliability and high validity. The data points are all clustered near the bull's eye.

Once the validity and reliability of a diagnostic test have been established, an independent "blind" comparison with a "gold standard" must be undertaken. An accepted gold standard of diagnosis, such as biopsy or surgery, is preferably employed to select patients and controls. Once the patients and controls have undergone the diagnostic procedure in question, the results should be interpreted by someone who is "blinded" to whether the subject really had the disease. Afterward, the diagnostic test results should be compared with the gold standard.

The "two-by-two" table is the simplest method of displaying the comparison of a diagnostic test with the gold standard (Fig. 21–2). The gold standard determines which patients have or do not have the disease based on either a positive or negative result.

A gold standard for diagnosis of internal derangement (ID) of the TMJ and myofascial pain and dysfunction (MPD) is still not determined. For ID, surgery, arthroscopy, magnetic resonance imaging (MRI), and arthrography have all been suggested. Palpation, pressure algometry, and thermography have been proposed as gold standards for MPD. Some have suggested chief complaint or subjective report as the best gold standard. Others propose long-term follow-up. The literature is full of TMJ studies with inappropriate gold standards.

Once the gold standard has been established, the diagnostic test in question must be considered. Is it less costly, less risky, less invasive, less uncomfortable? If the test appears to have merit, certain elements must be considered.

For any diagnostic procedure, we want to know how well it identifies individuals with and without the disease. These are the stable properties of a test and are called *sensitivity* and *specificity*. Sensitivity = A / A + C (see Fig. 21–2). Of all the patients who have the disease, how many were identified with positive test results? Another name for this is *true positive*. It gives information about the early detection of a disease.

Specificity = D / B + D (see Fig. 21–2)—of all the patients who do not have the disease, how many had negative test results and were identified correctly? Specificity refers to the ability to select patients with a particular characteristic. They may be normal individuals or a subgroup of patients with TMDs. These patients were referred to as having *true negative* findings.

Hypothetically, if you study 100 people who are healthy and 100 who are sick and subject them to a test, of the 100 who are sick, 80 have positive test findings and 20 have negative find-

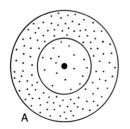 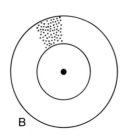 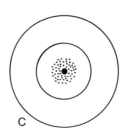

A   B   C

FIGURE 21–1. *A* represents a target with scattered points. This test has low reliability and poor validity. *B* is a target with good clustering and high reliability; however, the points are not near the bull's eye. There is, therefore, low validity. *C* has the best of both attributes: high reliability and high validity. This test is accurate and repeatable.

Fourfold Table Demonstrating "Blind" Comparison with "Gold Standard"

FIGURE 21–2. A 2 × 2 table demonstrating "blind" comparison with a gold standard. The stable properties of sensitivity and specificity are also defined. (Redrawn from Kreig, A.F., Abendroth, T.W., and Bongiovanni, M.B.: Arch. Pathol. Lab. Med. 110:787–791, 1986.)

		Gold standard		
		Patient *has* the disease	Patient *does not have* the disease	
Test result (conclusion drawn from the results of the test)	Positive: Patient appears *to have* the disease	True positive a | b	False positive	a + b
	Negative: Patient appears *not to have* the disease	c | d False negative	True negative	c + d
		a + c	b + d	a + b + c + d

Stable properties:
  a/(a + c) = sensitivity
  d/(b + d) = specificity
Frequency-dependent properties:
  a/(a + b) = positive predictive value*
  d/(c + d) = negative predictive value
  (a + d)/(a + b + c + d) = accuracy
  (a + c)/(a + b + c + d) = prevalence

*Positive predictive value can be calculated other ways too. One of them uses Bayes' theorem:

$$\frac{(prevalence)\ (sensitivity)}{(prevalence)\ (sensitivity) + (1 - prevalence)\ (1 - specificity)}$$

ings. Of the 100 who are healthy, 90 have negative results and 10 have positive results. A two-by-two table is constructed in Figure 21–3. The sensitivity is 0.8, and the specificity is 0.9. This is considered an acceptable test. The cutoff is generally 0.7, but 0.8 or above is preferred.

Electromyographic testing for TMD has shown high sensitivity but, unfortunately, low specificity. Patients with MPD have abnormally high EMG resting levels and are correctly identified as diseased; however, some "normal" individuals also have high EMG resting levels and are incorrectly identified as abnormal as subsequently discussed. This finding is called *false positive*.

Sensitivity and specificity are indices that characterize the test but tell us nothing of its

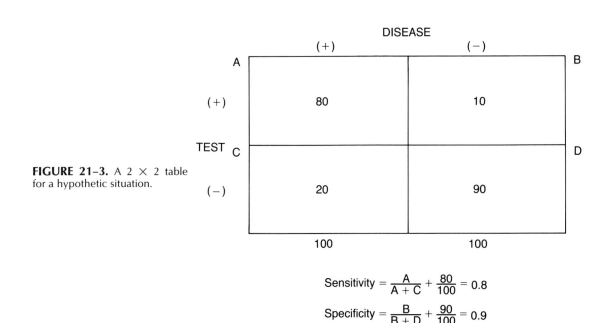

FIGURE 21–3. A 2 × 2 table for a hypothetic situation.

$$Sensitivity = \frac{A}{A + C} + \frac{80}{100} = 0.8$$

$$Specificity = \frac{B}{B + D} + \frac{90}{100} = 0.9$$

usefulness for a particular patient. As clinicians, our task is to determine the presence or absence of disease. If a diagnostic test result is positive, we want to know the probability that the disease is present. The positive value A / A + B tells how well a positive test predicts the presence of disease and is called *positive predictive value*. We also want to know how well a negative test result predicts the absence of disease. This is called *negative predictive value* or D / C + D (see Fig. 21–2).

Using the same aforementioned example for the individual case, if the test finding is positive, the predictive value is A / A + B = 80/90 = 0.88. If the test result is negative, predictive value is D / C + D = 90/110 = 0.81 (Fig. 21–4).

Before utilizing predictive value to decide on ordering a test, the clinician must estimate the prevalence of the disease in the population. The test's sensitivity and specificity are stable properties, already known before any diagnostic workup. For example, given a patient referred for MRI of the TMJ because of TMJ pain, what is the likelihood of ID when the MRI result is positive (posterior band displaced to less than or equal to ten o'clock in closed position, where right is posterior and left is anterior) as well as the likelihood of no ID when the test result is negative? Assume hypothetically a sensitivity or 80% and a specificity of 74% (Fig. 21–5).

Suppose that the dentist assumes the likeli-

hood of ID in patients with TMJ pain to be 50% and orders an MRI to further evaluate the patients. Figure 21–5 shows the calculation of positive and negative predictive value based on an analysis of 1000 patients.

Without any testing, we could guess that 50% of the sample has an ID. However, by applying the known operating characteristics of the MRI to these numbers we have an *incremental ruling-in* gain of 25%, from 50 to 75% when the MRI findings are positive. When the MRI findings are negative, the probability of no ID is 79%—an *incremental ruling-out* gain of 29%.

To demonstrate the importance of the clinician's prior estimate of likelihood of disease on the interpretation of the test result, we can examine Table 21–1.

Consider the following two examples:

An 18-year-old female complains of pain in the left TMJ, difficulty in opening the mouth, and deflection of the jaw to the left on opening. Her jaw began clicking at age 15 when braces were removed. At age 17, the jaw would intermittently lock upon awakening. At present, her jaw has been locked for 2 weeks. With this information, the dentist may consider the likelihood of ID to be about 90%. The positive and negative predictive values for MRI can be found in Figure 21–6.

A 20-year-old male college student complains of jaw and neck pain with a dull, aching quality occurring on and off throughout the day. He is in the mid-

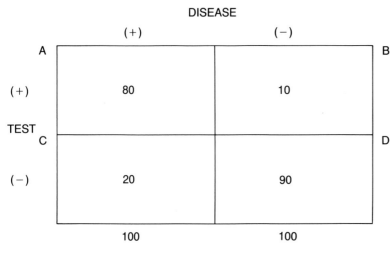

FIGURE 21–4. Positive and negative predictive value for the situation depicted in Figure 21–3.

$$\text{Positive Predictive Value} = \frac{A}{A + B} + \frac{80}{90} = 0.88$$

$$\text{Negative Predictive Value} = \frac{D}{C + D} + \frac{90}{110} = 0.81$$

INTERNAL DERANGEMENT OF THE TMJ

	PRESENT (n = 500)	ABSENT (n = 500)
Positive	**A** 400	**B** 130
Negative	**C** 100	**D** 370

FIGURE 21–5. The probability that the temporomandibular joint (TMJ) pain is due to internal derangement according to the results of magnetic resonance imaging (MRI) when the prior estimate of disease likelihood is 50%.

MRI

Sensitivity = 80%   Specificity = 74%

$$\text{Positive predictive value} = \frac{400}{400 + 130} = \frac{400}{530} = 75\%$$

$$\text{Negative predictive value} = \frac{370}{370 + 100} = \frac{370}{470} = 79\%$$

dle of midterm examinations and believes that he may be grinding his teeth at night. Exercise and alcohol alleviate the pain. There is no history of clicking. In this case, the dentist's prior estimate of the likelihood of ID is 10%. Predictive values are indicated in Figure 21–6.

The usefulness of MRI in both these cases is marginal. In the first patient, a positive MRI finding resulted in an incremental gain of 7% over the already high probability of ID. There would be little need to spend $900 for a result that was already 90% probable. A negative

MRI result would not have markedly reduced the probability of no disease.

In the second case, the likelihood that the student does not have ID increases from 90 to 97% with the test—only a 7% gain.

As stated by Griner and associates,[2] "A test cannot be interpreted properly without considering the prior estimate of the likelihood of disease before the test or procedure result is obtained. When the pretest likelihood of disease is high, a positive result tends to confirm, but an unexpected negative result is not particu-

TABLE 21–1. Incremental Gain Expected from MRI in Confirming or Excluding Internal Derangement of the TMJ According to Prior Estimates of Likelihood of Disease

PRIOR ESTIMATE OF LIKELIHOOD OF DISEASE	TEST POSITIVE		TEST NEGATIVE	
	Predictive Value	Incremental Gain	Predictive Value	Incremental Gain
		%		
90	97	7	29	19
80	92	12	48	28
70	88	18	61	31
60	82	22	71	31
50	75	25	79	29
40	67	27	85	25
30	57	27	90	20
20	43	21	94	14
10	25	15	97	7

Reprinted with permission from Griner, P.F., et al: Ann. Intern. Med. 94:555–570, 1981.

INTERNAL DERANGEMENT

	Present (n = 900)	Absent (n = 100)
MRI Positive	720	26
MRI Negative	180	74

Positive predictive value = 97%
Negative predictive value = 29%

FIGURE 21–6. The positive and negative predictive values of internal derangement based on magnetic resonance imaging when the prior likelihood of internal derangement is about 90%.

larly helpful in ruling the disease out. When the pretest likelihood of disease is low, a normal result tends to exclude but an unexpectedly positive result is not particularly helpful in confirming the disease."

CUTOFF POINTS

Diagnostic test results for a sample of patients can be displayed in either a normal or skewed distribution. An ideal test can separate those with and without disease into separate groups with no overlap (Fig. 21–7A).[2] The gold standard identifies the disease, and the cutoff point defines the parameters of the disease. In Figure 21–7A, line A defines the test cutoff point, above which the result is 100% sensitive and below which the result is 100% specific. There are no false-negative or false-positive test results.

Most tests have a range of results that show some overlap (Fig. 21–7B). "When a test is developed for clinical use and can be measured analytically, it is customary to define the normal range as being limited to 2 standard deviations from the mean. This range encompasses approximately 95% of the test results among subjects without disease. Approximately 2.5% of subjects fall either above or below this arbitrarily defined range."[2] Line A indicates this cutoff point in Figure 21–7B. All values that fall to the right of A are considered to be positive; those to the left are considered negative.

The choice of cutoff point A for this hypothetic test results in high specificity, i.e., 98%, but limited sensitivity, i.e., 60%. Such a cutoff point may be appropriate to confirm a suspected diagnosis but cannot be used to screen

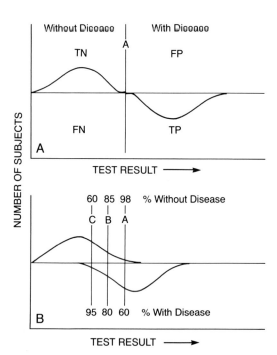

FIGURE 21–7. A, Hypothetic distribution of results of an ideal test (a) and most tests (b) used in clinical medicine. (TN = true negative; FP = false positive; FN = false negative; and TP = true positive.) (Redrawn from Griner, P.F., et al: Ann. Intern. Med. 94:555–570, 1981.)

for or to exclude disease because of its low sensitivity. To employ such a test for these last two purposes, the choice of cutoff point *C* would be appropriate, because almost all patients with disease are identified (sensitivity is 95%; specificity falls to 60%). Point *B* is intermediate between the two (sensitivity 80%; specificity 85%). Each cutoff point thus defines a set of operating characteristics for the test in question. As sensitivity increases, specificity decreases, and vice versa.[2]

By altering the cutoff point of a test, the specificity and sensitivity can be changed. A test with high specificity can *confirm* the presence of a disease. High sensitivity is needed to *screen* for the presence of disease. A given test may be employed to screen as well as to confirm a diagnosis by changing the criteria for a positive test according to the specific purpose for which the test is to be done. There are also other methods for choosing a cutoff point.

In clinical dentistry and medicine, there are three therapeutic alternatives for which a formal model has been constructed[5]: (1) treatment without testing, (2) withholding treatment without testing, and (3) performing a diagnostic test and treating if the results are positive. Decision tree models based on *net utility* and *threshold* can help select appropriate cutoff levels to determine which test results are positive.

Net utility is defined as the "lowest net cost" or highest "net value." In this model,[7] net utility is calculated at each test score. The cutoff level giving the highest net utility is selected.

The threshold is defined as that test score in which the utilities are nearly equal. In this model,[7] relative utilities are calculated at each test score as positive or negative. However, dentists are usually not used to thinking of the utility or value of a particular outcome.

Utilities can be estimated subjectively and objectively. Objective measures are *expected survival, quality-adjusted life years,* and *cost.* Cost-benefit analysis is usually expressed in dollars, whereas cost-effectiveness analysis is expressed in effectiveness and reflects survival, quality-adjusted life years, and personal preference.

Utilities were calculated for temporal artery biopsy in a group of patients with temporal arteritis (TA).[4] The probability of steroid side effects was the major contributor to the expected value of the biopsy. The utility of steroid side effects (U_{sse}) was equal to $1000, the estimated cost of providing medication and treating steroid side effects for 1 year. The utility of temporal arteritis (U_{TA}) was equal to $200,000—the expected court award for the development of bilateral blindness in malpractice litigation, multiplied by 0.25—the likelihood of bilateral blindness in untreated TA.

Kreig and coworkers[7] believe that it is important for investigators to provide raw data on test performance for three reasons:

1. The data can be used in simple decision tree models to identify appropriate cutoff levels.
2. The data can be used to evaluate empirical cutoff levels or decision rules.
3. The data can be used to evaluate optimal cutoff levels for detailed decision trees depicting specific clinical problems.

Fewer that 20% of medical procedures have been shown by scientific evidence to be beneficial.[8] It is difficult to confirm this figure when dealing with diagnostic tests, because the methodology of evaluation has not been standardized. Clinical decision situations are more and more characterized by complexity and uncertainty because of increasing diagnostic and therapeutic possibilities, increasing quality demands by the public, and pressure toward cost-conscious decision making.[6]

Decision analysis is a method for structuring and analyzing the selection diagnostic procedures for individual patients. Three types of decision aids are available as follows:

1. Protocols, or algorithmic flow charts, are the simplest forms. Protocols may be established from the analysis of clinical data bases combined with statistical analysis. Protocols are employed in clinical and hospital practices.
2. Individual clinical decisions can be solved with theoretical techniques involving the decision tree. Computer software programs have been written to help implement this technique into clinical practice.
3. The most promising area of decision support systems may be the field of medical informatics and expert systems. These systems are part of the realm of artificial intelligence. Computer programs can store and compile a vast array of information on a topic such as facial pain. The clinician can then communicate with the computer via interactive software.

Computers are becoming increasingly important to clinical decision analysis. They allow us to store and retrieve hundreds of pieces of information on each patient in a way that is relatively accessible. Relational data bases make it feasible to search a sample of patients for statistical correlations. Computers are helpful with both clinical epidemiology and individual clinical decision analysis. The computer can also provide experts' advice and perform the rapid computations required for decision tree analysis.

An example of a decision tree is seen in Figure 21–8. The relevant probabilities can be ascertained from the literature, experts' opinion, or research and analysis of patient records. Because each practice may have a unique set of patients, the last approach gives the most detailed information.

Clinical decision analysis can be divided into the following four stages:

1. Defining and structuring the clinical problem.
2. Assessing the relevant probabilities and utilities.
3. Calculating the preferred course of action.
4. Formulating the results of the analysis in a clinically relevant way.

A three-stage scenario for the future development of decision analysis can be seen in Table 21–2. "An optimistic scenario of the future role of decision analysis in clinical dentistry would include a decision-consultation department, decision-oriented clinical data bases and medical knowledge bases, research groups for development, testing and updating of clinical strategies, decision analysis courses in all levels of dental and medical education, and decision-oriented clinical textbooks."[6]

University-based TMJ and facial pain clinics as well as private practices need to establish relational data bases and to assess probabilities and utilities. Excellent decision-analytic software continues to be developed.

According to Habbema and coworkers,[6] "The paramount prerequisite for success is that clinicians be prepared to invest time and energy in research programs in collaboration with decision analysts, mathematicians, and computer experts, knowing that it will take a long time before large scale practical results are available."

A balance between empirical and formal decision methods is needed. Development of a decision tree or a knowledge base for a clinical problem is also an effective method of discovering gaps or contraindications in our clinical knowledge.

The state of affairs of EMG, electronic jaw tracking, sonography, and thermography is directly applicable to decision analysis. The development of a national data base with specific methodologic parameters will help clinicians make more effective use of their own clinical experience and that of others.

SPECIFIC ELECTRONIC DIAGNOSTIC TECHNIQUES

Surface Electromyography

More controversy has surrounded the utilization of surface EMG in TMD diagnosis than any other diagnostic modality (Fig. 21–9). Proponents claim that EMG can be used in the following:

1. Determination of rest and "myocentric" occlusal positions
2. Detection of hyperactivity, hypoactivity, spasm, fatigue, and muscle imbalance
3. Treatment of parafunctional habits by biofeedback.

This section briefly reviews the first two categories. The orientation of this analysis is from the view of a clinical scientist. The clinical scientist must be both a neuroscientist and a clinician who manages TMD and craniofacial pain.

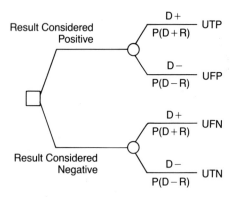

FIGURE 21–8. Decision tree model of relative utilities or thresholds for considering test results as positive or negative. D+ indicates disease present; D−, disease absent; P(D + R), probability of disease present given test score R: P(D − R), probability of disease absent given test score of R; UTP, utility of true positive; UFP, utility of false positive; UFN, utility of false positive; and UTN, utility of true negative. (Redrawn from C.M.A. Journal 24:703–710, 1981.)

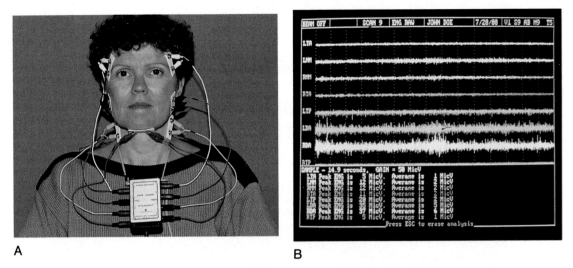

A

B

FIGURE 21-9. *A,* Surface electrodes for electromyography (EMG) of the masseter, anterior and posterior temporalis, and digastric muscles. (Courtesy of Myotronics, Seattle, Washington.) *B,* Color readout from the computer screen of raw EMG data.

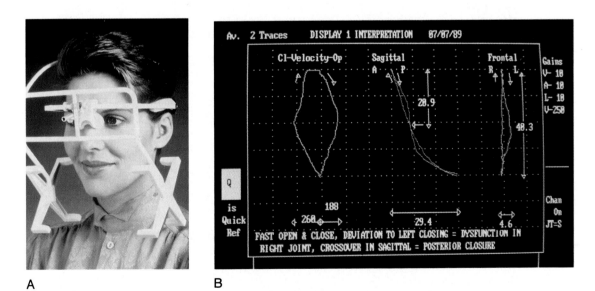

A

B

FIGURE 21-10. *A,* Jaw tracking apparatus, including head set and sensor arrays, with magnet attached to the lower central incisors. *B,* Computer color readout of sagittal and frontal opening and closing patterns as well as the velocity of these movements. (Courtesy of Bioresearch Associates, Milwaukee, Wisconsin.)

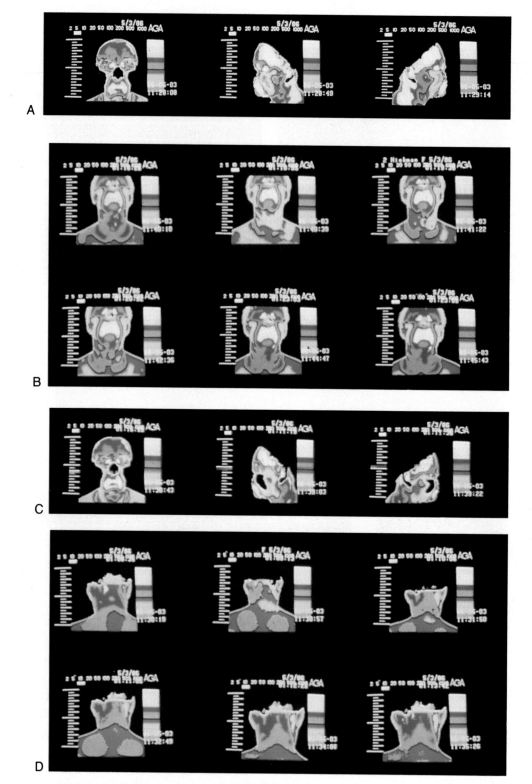

FIGURE 21–12. The Academy of Neuromuscular Thermography has adopted Weinstein's protocol for temporomandibular joint and facial pain electronic infrared thermography. *A,* First of three facial series. *B,* The anterior neck study examines blood flow changes through the carotid territory as well as the sternocleidomastoid musculature. The anterior neck study performed in extension stresses the posterior neck. *C,* The second facial series. Notice the running time. *D,* The posterior cervical trigger point study. The yellow areas have increased heat emission, suggestive of myofascial disease.

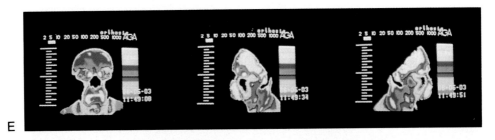

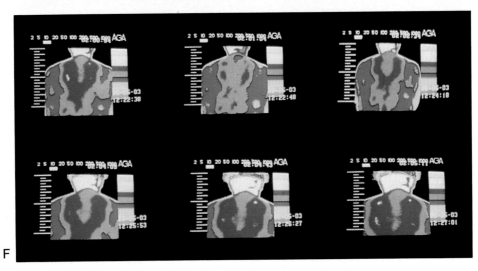

E

F

FIGURE 21–12 *Continued E,* Third facial series. *F,* Interscapular trigger point series.

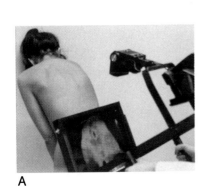

A

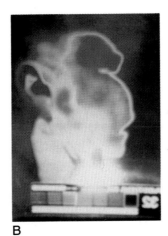

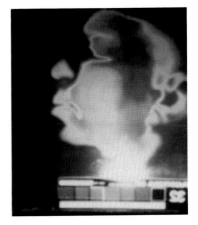

B

FIGURE 21–13. *A,* Liquid crystal thermography equipment with Polaroid camera attachment. (Courtesy of Flexitherm, Westbury, New York.) *B,* Right and left lateral views of liquid crystal plates.

TABLE 21–2. A Three-stage Scenario for the Future Development of Decision-analysis

	STAGE 1 (+/− 1985–1990)	STAGE 2 (+/− 1990–1995)	STAGE 3 (+/− 1995–2000)
Clinical Applications	Applied research groups for analysing clinical problems by decision analysis methods.	Departments for developing testing and updating clinical strategies.	Clinical decision making consultation departments in the main (university) hospitals.
Education	Post-graduate courses in decision analysis.	Complete decision-analysis courses in the medical curriculum. Protocol-based teaching for paramedical professions.	Clinical textbooks written from a decision analytic point of view. Decision techniques become standard in all stages of medical education.
Research and Informatics			
A. Decision Analysis	Research into the assessment and elicitation of probability judgments and utilities.	User-friendly decision analytic software.	Library of basic decision strategies; software for embedding individual patient analysis in a decision strategy.
B. Expert Systems	Research into inference mechanisms. Integration with some aspects of decision analysis.	Development of easy-access knowledge bases for a variety of clinical disciplines.	Large scale testing of expert systems for decision support.
C. Data Bases	Development of research- and decision-oriented clinical data-bases.	Implementation of decision-making oriented data-base systems. Improvement of privacy protection techniques.	Networks for the exchange of patient information for clinical decision making.

Reprinted with permission from Habbema, J.D., et al: Ann. Med. Intern. (Paris) 137:267–273, 1986.

Determination of the Rest Position

It is well accepted that there is some degree of tonicity of the masticatory muscles in the *rest position.*[19–24] This should not be confused with the *clinical rest position of minimal EMG,* which occurs at approximately the 6 to 15-mm interincisal opening.[10]

Rest position was once thought to be immutable. Dental school instructors taught not to violate the freeway space. It is now known that the rest position of the mandible is adaptable,[32] and freeway space can at times be violated. Muscle sarcomere and fiber adaptation can often allow creation of a new freeway space. A low level of postural activity is normal at rest position, and a "neuromuscularly determined rest position" has yet to be shown valid.

"Myocentric" Occlusal Position

The masticatory muscles are multipinnate in nature. Different compartments of the jaw-closing muscles contain different proportions of slow, fast, and intermediate firing fibers. Each compartment has a specific functional role and fires at specific interincisal openings. Age, sex, and facial morphology are variables that have great influence on surface EMG recordings and that can easily confound research results. Because of the complexity and variability of the masticatory muscles, the use of surface EMG to determine the "myocentric" occlusal position is suspect. Belser and Hannam[25] concluded that "No consistent predictable or reproducible associations have been demonstrated between a specific experimental occlusal state and EMG data during normal function."

Most mandibles that are class II, division 2 in both symptomatic and asymptomatic people move down and forward in rest position. A similar position is seen after the electrical pulsing applied in establishing myocentric occlusal position. Some clinicians have stated that the down and forward position is "ideal." This concept has led to a large number of false-positive findings.

Surface EMG and electronic pulsing should, therefore, not be routinely done to determine the ideal occlusal position. In patients who experience refractory facial pain, in whom cervical, neurologic, and psychiatric workups are negative in nature, neuromuscular scans and surface EMGs may prove to be helpful, but more data is still needed.

Detection of Hyperactivity, Hypoactivity, Spasm, Fatigue, and Muscle Imbalance

Surface EMG recordings describing normal mastication have yet to be done. Correlation of occlusal patterns with surface EMG during mastication (see Jaw Tracking) likewise needs to be studied. Therefore, without a definition of *normal,* determination of what constitutes hyperactivity, hypoactivity, spasm, fatigue, and muscle imbalance is speculative at best.

DIAGNOSIS AND TREATMENT OF TEMPOROMANDIBULAR DISORDERS

The criteria discussed in the first part of this chapter must be applied when evaluating surface EMG for the diagnosis of TMJ disorders.

According to the Wozniak report,[29] "The major criticisms of existing surface EMG studies include the lack of adequate control groups, the lack of studies of the reliability and validity of the methods, the inadequate or nonexistent statistical tests, the fact that large variability exists in both normal and patient groups with considerable overlaps between the groups and conclusions that are not based on the results. There is a need for a better description of the normal population; its variability; and the effects of age, sex, weight, and skeletal type on the masticatory muscle EMG parameters."

Belser and Hannam[25] concur in their view of EMG as a diagnostic aid in clinical dentistry. Their conclusions are as follows:

1. A universally recognized terminology should be used to describe and interpret muscle disorders when these are diagnosed electromyographically.

2. Electromyographic techniques and measurements used to evaluate disorders of muscle contraction should conform to those conventionally used in diagnostic neurology. Techniques and measurements employed to evaluate the behavioral use of normal muscles should be based upon established standards of normality for the behavior under test. These should take into account differences due to factors such as craniofacial morphology, age, gender, and attitudinal compliance, as well as methods of recording and data expression.

3. Proponents and users of any clinical diagnostic approach should be able to provide convincing evidence that the method is a valid predictor of a disorder. The conventional manner in which this occurs is the publication of controlled clinical studies in peer-reviewed scientific journals. To proceed otherwise is to invite criticism on ethical grounds.

Most researchers agree that surface EMG can measure a behavioral event, such as bruxing or clenching. With portable EMG devices, relaxation of the masticatory muscles may be attained by the patient via biofeedback at home or at work.

Summary

Routine use of surface EMG for diagnosis of TMDs is not justified by the scientific literature. Our goal over the next few years is to evaluate EMG parameters for normal individuals and for those who belong to specific diagnostic TMD subgroups.

JAW TRACKING

Electronic jaw tracking, axiographic tracing, and pantographic recordings are all attractive diagnostic devices because they record dysfunctional jaw movements commonly present in patients with TMDs (Fig. 21–10).

Border Movement

Range of motion studies with active and passive measurements are part of a standard clinical examination for TMDs (see chapter 17).

Limited jaw opening with deviation and deflection is commonly found in patients so affected. Compromised chewing ability is also seen frequently. Electronic jaw tracking can document these measurements and store them for future reference and comparison. However, the question often asked is, "Does the dentist learn any diagnostically relevant information that could not have been obtained with ruler, paper, and pencil?[72]

Electronic jaw trackers can document (1) amplitude of jaw movements in vertical, horizontal, and anterior posterior directions; (2) reproducibility or consistency of movement; and (3) velocity of movement.

Scientific research is scarce and mostly unreplicated in the linking of jaw motion to TMD diagnosis. Furthermore, the accuracy and repeatability of the measurements have been challenged. Advocates of condylar tracing devices, such as the axiograph and pantograph, criticize incisor tracing devices as being too coarse. These workers prefer measurement of condylar movement.

To the credit of the manufacturers of electronic jaw trackers, sensor array design changes and linearizing software programs have improved accuracy. Variations will always occur from day-to-day and perhaps more so among patients with TMDs. As with other modalities, large clinical data bases are needed to evaluate the claims of the few existing studies.

While clinical data bases are being formed for EMG and jaw tracking, an ethical question is forced upon us. Which patients should have EMG and jaw tracking done and who do we charge? Ethically, routine EMG and jaw tracking should be performed with informed consent and at no charge, for both patients and control subjects, until the diagnostic benefits are clearly established. In patients with mutilated dentitions or multiple treatment failures, EMG and jaw tracking may be indicated at a customary fee.

Axiography is a technique-sensitive method of measuring condylar movement, which holds much promise. Existing research, however, must be translated from German to English, before it can be evaluated. The pantograph may be an overly sensitive, but not specific enough, device. The EMG findings of Cooper and Rabuzzi[27] found 81% of their asymptomatic population as "unhealthy."

In the face of these results, the clinician must realize that health and disease are a continuum. The TMJ triad of predisposition (susceptibility), tissue alteration, and psychologic dependence holds true for many diseases.[28] The degree of predisposition, tissue alteration, and psychologic dependence necessary for precipitation of the "disorder" is unique to the individual. Pain is a subjective phenomenon that varies between individuals and within an individual on a temporal basis.[29]

Data from EMG and jaw tracking may be giving the clinician insight into an individual's predisposition by showing functional alterations. Research that simply looks at EMG or jaw tracking parameters without controlling for other biopsychosocial factors may be equivocal.

Bioresearch Associates (Milwaukee, Wisconsin) have created LEWARTH software to measure electrognathographic parameters of chewing. Further research is required to determine whether patients with a TMD can be distinguished from normal individuals by employing this software (Fig. 21–11).

FIGURE 21–11. Physiologic functions, such as chewing, swallowing, speech, and rest position can be recorded and measured with the jaw tracking apparatus. (Courtesy of Bioresearch Associates, Milwaukee, Wisconsin.)

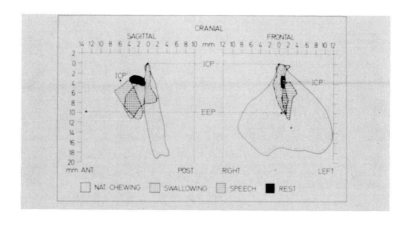

THERMOGRAPHY

Body temperature has been used as a diagnostic tool since medicine was first practiced. In 400 B.C., Hippocrates recognized relative right-left temperature symmetry in healthy individuals and increased heat emission over inflamed areas. He employed his hand as the first temperature-sensing device, and the physician's hand is still often employed today. The thermoscope was invented by Galileo at the end of the 16th century. Over the next two centuries the oral temperature for healthy individuals was established at 98.6°F. In 1840, Sir John Herschel focused the infrared rays of the sun on hard surfaces to record a thermogram. Infrared technology has had wide applications with the military, which has accelerated the development of the modern electronic thermographic devices.

Electronic infrared thermography is a noninvasive method of determining skin temperature by converting thermal energy into electronic signals, which are displayed on a video monitor (Fig. 21–12). Skin temperature is a reflection of the underlying cutaneous blood flow, composing arterial perfusion, venous outflow, and lymphatic drainage, controlled by the autonomic nervous system. Skin temperature changes have been found clinically and experimentally in the presence of neuromuscular disorders (Fig. 21–13). The pathophysiologic basis for the temperature change is likely due to interaction between sympathetic nerve fibers and afferent pathways.[8]

Skin temperature is centrally controlled, and normal changes affect both sides uniformly and simultaneously, resulting in a symmetric thermal pattern. One study of facial and bilateral trunk and extremity segments showed remarkable symmetry in a series of healthy subjects.[9] The overall mean temperature difference is 0.24°C.[10]

Because thermography demonstrates physiology, it may be helpful in documenting the presence of muscle spasm, myositis, and myofascial trigger points (Fig. 21–14). These muscle problems are commonly seen in patients with TMDs.[11,12]

A study in 1970 found that the symptomatic masseter muscle was hotter than the contralateral side in 15 subjects with unilaterally painful masseters.[13] Because these thermographic images were not stable, the results were inconclusive. The study was repeated in 1974 with an improved infrared camera.[14] Of 23 patients with unilateral painful masseters, 14 were hotter on the painful side, five were hotter on the contralateral side, and four showed no difference. In seven symptomatic patients with hot masseters who followed through treatment, six showed temperature symmetry after symptoms had resolved.

These investigators hypothesized that the higher surface temperature was due to inflammation with hyperemia in the tender area of the muscle.[15] In 1983, a group in Sweden measured the surface temperature over 35 normal TMJs and 29 normal masseters.[16] The variability within subjects from right to left was small, 0.3°C to 0.4°C. However, a wide range between subjects was observed—for the TMJ, 32.1°C to 35.5°C, and for the masseter, 30.9°C to 35.7°C.

In 1985, the same team concluded that temperature differences between right and left sides were less than 1°C in 90% of cases (42 subjects) and that the reproducibility after 6 weeks was satisfactory.[17] Absolute temperature compari-

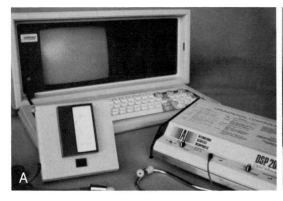 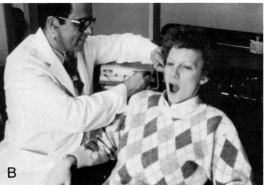

FIGURE 21–14. A, Sonography equipment. (Courtesy of International Acoustics Incorporated (IAI), Chicago, Illinois.) B, Clinician listening to joint noise from microphone in patient's external auditory meatus.

sons appear to be less useful because of great interindividual variation.

In 1986, another group of researchers, utilizing liquid crystal thermography, found the symptomatic masseter to be 0.5°C to 3.0°C cooler than the asymptomatic side.[41] This temperature change was often associated with a hot or cold reading of the TMJ, depending on whether the condition was acute or chronic, respectively. Results indicated symmetry between men and women and between right and left sides in the same individual. No side dominance pattern for chewing was noted. A difference of 0.5°C between sides would account for at least 2 standard deviations of 95% certainty of abnormality.

Gratt[43] also found overall thermal symmetry in the face and neck regions of normal subjects, concluding that electronic thermography has potential as a diagnostic technique in dentistry.

A pilot study on 20 atypical odontalgia patients found an asymmetric increased heat emission in 100% of patients with 88% being site specific.[44] Thermography has been the only test to date positive for this condition.

Because of the relative symmetry of control subjects, future studies on patient subgroups are promising. A study has indicated that chronicity may be measured with thermography.[42] Thermography should be performed according to the standards of the Academy of Neuromuscular Thermography and controlled for examiner and researcher bias.

Liquid crystal thermography may be a useful screening test for cervical and masticatory pathophysiology (see Fig. 21–13); however, more studies are needed.

SONOGRAPHY

Clicking and crepitus are often present in patients with TMDs. Therefore, a device that graphically displays and analyzes joint sounds may have diagnostic value. Sonography and Doppler ultrasound are two techniques that measure the sounds emitted from the TMJ (Fig. 21–15).

Several studies have demonstrated that clicking can occur during reduction of a displaced disc.[31–33] Mahan has described eight joint sounds, which may or may not involve the articular disc. One of these sounds, crepitus, is usually associated with degenerative joint disease in the TMJ. "Although these sounds appear to clearly represent a pathological intracapsular condition, other sources of sounds

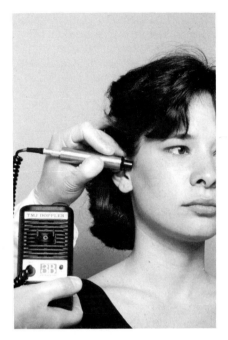

FIGURE 21–15. Doppler ultrasound.

must also be considered, such as clicks attributed to fluid cavitation, clicks associated with sudden movement of ligaments, or mild crepitus associated with the lack of synovial fluid or translatory movement of the condyle over retrodiscal tissues."[34]

Initial claims from one manufacturer of this equipment indicated that anterior disc displacement with reduction could be differentiated from anterior disc displacement without reduction. These two noise patterns could also be distinguished from degenerative joint disease and perforation. Unfortunately, these preliminary studies have been compromised by inadequate control groups and lack of statistical analysis. Therefore, we do not as yet know whether TMJ disorder subgroups have distinctive sound patterns.

Methodologic problems include the following:

1. The high variability of TMJ sounds from day to day[37,38]
2. The inability to detect pertinent sound from artifact, such as room noise, skin and hair noise, respiration, arterial blood flow, and crossover noise from the opposite TMJ[38,39]
3. The variability in the intensity of the sound in different patients.[38]

Sonography research suffers from pitfalls similar to those of EMG and jaw tracking. A large data base, with adequate control groups and examiner bias controls, is needed before routine use is appropriate. It is only with proper scientific method that the diagnostic specificity of sounds for each type of TMJ condition can be clearly established.

REFERENCES

1. Department of Clinical Epidemiology and Biostatistics, McMasters University Health Science Centre: Clinical epidemiology round—How to read clinical journals. II. To learn about a diagnostic test. Cana. Med. Assoc. J., 24:703–710, 1981.
2. Griner, P.F., et al: Principles of test selection and use. Ann. Intern. Med. 94:555–570, 1981.
3. Douglas, C.W. and McNeil, B.J.: Clinical decision analysis methods applied to diagnostic tests in dentistry. J. Dent. Ed. 47:708–714, 1983.
4. Nadeau, S.E.: Temporal arteritis: a decision-analytic approach to temporal artery biopsy. Acta Neurol. Scand. 78:90–100, 1988.
5. Charpak, Y., Blery, C., and Chastang, C.: Designing a study for evaluating a protocol for the selective performance of preoperative tests. Stat. Med. 6:813–822, 1987.
6. Habbema, J.D., Vander Mass, P.J., and Dippel, D.W.: A perspective on the role of decision analysis in clinical practice. Ann. Med. Intern. (Paris) 137:267–273, 1986.
7. Kreig, A.F., Abendroth, T.W., and Bongiovanni, M.B.: When is a diagnostic test result positive? Decision tree models based on net utility and threshold. Arch. Pathol. Lab. Med. 110:787–791, 1986.
8. Pulst, M. and Haller, P.: Thermography assessments of impaired sympathetic function in peripheral nerve injuries. J. Neurol. 226:35–42, 1981.
9. Fulkow, B.: Nervous control of blood vessels. Acta Physiol. Scand. 35:639–663, 1955.
10. Uematsu, S.: Thermographic imaging of cutaneous sensory segment in patients with peripheral nerve injury. Skin-temperature stability between sides of the body. J. Neurosurg. 62:716–720, 1985.
11. Fischer, A.: Diagnosis and management of chronic pain in physical medicine and rehabilitation. In Current Therapy in Physiatry. A.P. Rusk (ed.). W.B. Saunders Co., Philadelphia, 1984.
12. Fischer, A.: The present status of neuromuscular thermography. Academy of Neuromuscular Thermography; First Annual Meeting, May, 1985. Postgrad. Med. 26–33, 1986. (Special edition.)
13. Berry, D.C. and Yemm, R.: Variations in skin temperature of the face in normal subjects and in patients with mandibular dysfunction. Br. J. Oral Surg. 8:242–247, 1970.
14. Berry, D.C. and Yemm, R.: A further study of facial skin temperature in patients with mandibular dysfunction. J. Oral Rehab. 1:255–264, 1974.
15. Berry, D.C. and Yemm, R.: Changes in facial skin temperature associated with unilateral chewing. J. Oral Rehab. 1:127–129, 1974.
16. Kopp, S. and Haraldson, T.: Normal variations in skin surface temperature over the temporomandibular joint and masseter muscle. Scand. J. Dent. Res. 91:308–311, 1983.
17. Kopp, S., Haraldson, T., and Johansson, A.: Reproducibility and variation of the surface temperature over the temporomandibular joint and masseter muscle in normal individuals. Acta Odontol. Scand. 309–313, 1985.
18. American Medical Association on Scientific Affairs: Thermography for selected neurological and musculoskeletal conditions. Scientific Affairs Committee, Am. Med. Assoc., 1990.
19. Moller, E.: Human muscle patterns. In Mastication and Swallowing. B.J. Sessle and A.G. Hannam (eds.). University of Toronto Press, Toronto, 1976.
20. Rugh, J.D. and Drago, C.J.: Vertical dimension: a study of clinical rest position and jaw muscle activity. J. Prosthet. Dent. 45:670–675, 1981.
21. Watkinson, A.C.: The mandibular rest position and electromyograph—a review. J. Oral Rehab. 14:209–214, 1987.
22. Garnick, J. and Ramiford, S.P.: Rest position: an electromyographic and clinical investigation. J. Prosthet. Dent. 12:895–911, 1962.
23. Mongini, F.: The Stomatognathic System. Quintessence Publishing Co., Lombard, IL, 1984.
24. Greenwood, L.F.: The neuromuscular system. In A Textbook of Occlusion. N.D. Mohl, G.A. Zarb, G.E. Carlsson, and J.D. Rugh (eds.). Quintessence Publishing Co., Lombard, IL, 1988.
25. Belser, U.C. and Hannam, A.G.: The influence of altered working-side occlusal guidance on masticatory muscles and related jaw movement. J. Prosthet. Dent. 53:406–413, 1985.
26. American Association of Electromyography and Electrodiagnosis: Glossary of Terms. Muscle and Nerve, vol. 10. [Suppl] 1987.
27. Cooper, B.C. and Rabazzi, D.D.: Myofascial pain dysfunction syndrome: A clinical study of asymptomatic subjects. Laryngoscope 94:68–75, 1984.
28. De Steno, C.: The pathophysiology of TMJ dysfunction and related pain. In Clinical Management of Head, Neck and TMJ Pain and Dysfunction. H. Gelb (ed.). W.B. Saunders Co., Philadelphia, 1985.
29. Wozniak, W.T.: Revised draft status report—Devices for the diagnosis and treatment of temporomandibular disorders. Prepared for the Council on Dental Materials, Instruments and Equipment. American Dental Association, 1988.
30. Oster, C., Katzberg, R., Tallents, R., et al: Characterization of TMJ sounds. Oral Surg. 58:10–16, 1984.
31. Isbeg-Holm, A.M. and Westesson, P.-L.: Movement of disc and condyle in temporomandibular joints with clicking: an arthrographic and radiographic study on autopsy specimens. Acta Odontol. Scand. 40:165–170, 1982b.
32. Isbeg-Holm, A.M. and Westesson, P.-L.: Movement of disc and condyle in temporomandibular joints with clicking: an arthrographic and radiographic study on autopsy specimens. Acta Odontol. Scand. 40:151–164, 1982a.
33. Unsworth, A., Dowson, D., and Wright, V.: "Cracking joints." A bioengineering study of cavitation in the metacarpophalangeal joint. Ann. Rheum. Dis. 30:348–358, 1971.
34. Watt, D.: Temporomandibular joint sounds. J. Dent. 8:119–127, 1980.
35. Gay, T. and Bertolami, C.: The acoustical characteristics of the normal temporomandibular joint. J. Dent. Res. 67:56–60, 1988.

36. Watt, D.: A preliminary report on the auscultation of the masticatory mechanism. Dent. Pract. Dent. Rec. 14:27–30, 1963.

37. Gay, T. and Bertolami, C.: The spectral properties of TMJ sounds. J. Dent. Res. 66:1189–1194, 1987.

38. Delly, J.: The acoustical characteristics of the normal and abnormal TMJ: Diagnostic implications. J. Oral Maxillofac. Surg. 45:397–407, 1987.

39. Heffez, L. and Blaustein, D.: Advances in sonography of the TMJ. Oral Surg. 62:486–495, 1986.

40. Rugh, J. and Johnson, R.: Vertical dimension discrepancies and masticatory pain/dysfunction. In *Abnormal Jaw Mechanics.* W. Solberg and G. Clark (eds.). Quintessence Publishing Co., Lombard, IL, 1984.

41. Finney, J., Holt, C., and Pierce, K.: Thermographic diagnosis of TMJ disease and associated neuromuscular disorders. Postgrad. Med. Proceedings of the Academy of Neuromuscular Thermography, March, 1986.

42. Steed, P.: Academy of Neuromuscular Thermography, Annual Meeting, Orlando, 1989.

43. Gratt, B., Graff-Radford, S., Solberg, W.: Electronic thermography in the diagnosis of atypical odontalgia. (Abstract.) J. Dent. Res. 68: 236, 1989.

44. Gratt, B., Sickles, E., Graff-Radford, S., and Solberg, W.: Electronic thermography in the diagnosis of atypical odontalgia: A pilot study. Oral Surg., Oral Med. Oral Pathol. 68:472–481, 1989.

45. Berry, J.: Questionable care: What can be done about dental quackery? J. Am. Dent. Assoc. 115:679, 1987.

NONSURGICAL THERAPY

Andrew S. Kaplan
Jay R. Goldman

CHAPTER 22

General Concepts of Treatment

The treatment of chronic pain has always been a perplexing problem for both the dentist and physician. Management of orofacial pain and temporomandibular (TMDs) disorders is especially challenging because of complex head and neck anatomy and head and neck interactions and the fact that psychologic stress appears to target these structures.

Often, the lack of formal training to deal with these maladies compounds the problem. Dental school training usually focuses on well-defined pathology with a concrete solution. For the most part, the criteria for both the diagnosis and correction of dental pathology is all or none—100% or 0%. If the pulp of the tooth becomes nonvital, a root canal would be the indicated procedure. If basic steps are followed, a high rate of success may be achieved. The diagnosis and treatment of TMDs are seldom as straightforward. Despite the fact that these disorders have been reported as far back as 300 B.C. by Hippocrates, there are still divergent opinions regarding etiology, pathogenesis, and treatment protocols.

Evaluation of treatment outcome also presents many difficulties. The criteria for evaluating a successful outcome remain varied, presenting further confusion for the clinician and the patient. Inconsistencies are often found between the subjective reporting of symptoms and the objective findings. A given treatment may be effective for some signs and symptoms but not for others. How, then, can one judge when treatment is successful? If pain is eliminated in a patient with an internal derangement, but the clicking persists, is treatment successful? Should a decrease in the frequency of headache be sufficient to label treatment for a patient with myofascial pain dysfunction

(MPD) syndrome successful even in the presence of continued pain on palpation of some of the masticatory muscles? Clinicians answer these questions differently, depending on their education and philosophy. They should exercise caution in applying the criterion for success used for conventional dental procedures to patients with TMDs, for this results in high levels of frustration. The aforementioned difficulties have prompted some clinicians to abandon discussion of the "cure." Instead, they prefer discussing treatment in terms of management. Coping skills and pain management techniques are now often recommended for chronic TMJ disorders.

Temporomandibular disorders, with their predisposing and perpetuating factors, are often multifactorial. They usually include components of occlusion, stress, direct trauma, and systemic disease. The multiplicity of causes is evidenced by the strong clinical opinion that a combination of treatments is more effective than a single treatment.[1] Furthermore, no single treatment has shown a major advantage over others. Complete recovery is reported by only about 60%, whereas another 25% report significant recovery.[2]

Because the causes of TMDs represent a blend, an appropriate treatment plan must be individually designed. The myriad of available treatments add to the confusion. One worker reported that 28 different treatments have been recommended for TMDs.[3] This is probably a conservative estimate. Some of the available treatments are well documented and have overwhelming support for their effectiveness. Other proposed treatments are based on clinical reports or anecdotal evidence and may not be effective.

Academicians, engaged in research, argue that only techniques supported in the literature with long-term follow-up data should be used. Clinicians who utilize scientifically unsupported forms of treatments argue that, historically, the introduction of many valuable treatments in medicine and dentistry have preceded the research and that to withhold treatments until scientific validity is established is wrong.

Both arguments are valid. Although it may be wise to apply the scientific method to new techniques, it does delay clinical application for years. Even without scientifically supported evidence, a large population of patients in pain might significantly benefit, without delay. Two issues are to be addressed here. First, if the technique proposed is noninvasive and can repeatedly and reliably improve treatment or add to diagnostic accuracy, it should be employed. Second, if the fees are not unjustifiably high, the new application should be utilized. In some cases, no fee at all may be appropriate.

A treatment philosophy must be established. However, familiarity with many different approaches is necessary before a reasonable philosophy can be arrived at. Knowledge of anatomy, physiology, pathology, pharmacology, and psychology is a must.

Treatment rendered is often a reflection of the type of specialist consulted. Patients who see an internist, a neurologist, or an otolaryngologist likely receive a prescription, possibly for a muscle relaxant, nonsteroidal anti-inflammatory medication, or tricyclic antidepressant. A patient who sees an oral and maxillofacial surgeon and has evidence of an internal derangement likely has some form of surgery recommended. A patient who sees a general dentist probably has splint therapy recommended. If there is a cervical component, a physical therapist may be consulted. The treatment in this case is a combination of physical medicine modalities, manipulation, and massage. Ideally, the treatment chosen should be the most conservative technique that addresses the given diagnosis and should be independent of the practitioner's training.

SEQUENCE

The first step of any treatment is arriving at an accurate diagnosis. This is preceded by a thorough medical and dental history and a clinical examination (see chapter 17). Based on the clinical impression, diagnostic tests should be ordered. The most common is the radiographic survey. The choice should be based on the nature of the suspected pathology and the technique that would show it to be the best, e.g., computerized tomography (CT) or tomogram for suspected osseous pathology and magnetic resonance imaging (MRI) or arthrogram for soft tissue pathology. If a muscular problem is suspected, the practitioner may want a simple screening film, such as a panoramic or transcranial film, to rule out unsuspected pathology.

Many other diagnostic tests are available (see chapter 21). However, routine use significantly raises the cost of care and may provide little additional information that is clinically valuable.

Before ordering a diagnostic test, the practitioner should ask the following questions:

1. Will the information provided be useful in establishing a diagnosis or ruling out other pathology?
2. Will the information change the proposed treatment plan?
3. Will the information help determine the staging of a disease process and hence be predictive in establishing the clinical course?

If the answer to these questions is no, the diagnostic test should not be done.

After assembling all available information, a working diagnosis should be made. In addition, possible etiology along with predisposing and perpetuating factors should be identified. This process can take several visits, and the true etiology may never be found.

A treatment plan can still be made. It should ideally relate directly to the diagnosis and should also address any limitations imposed by the patient.

Examples of limitations are as follows:

1. Patients who don't believe in taking medication.
2. Patients whose vocations limit them from certain forms of treatment, such as an actress who can't wear an occlusal splint, a singer who can't restrict maximal opening, and a construction worker who can't operate heavy machinery under the influence of certain medications.
3. Patients who refuse to consider surgery under any circumstances.
4. Patients with allergies or other contraindications to certain medications.
5. Patients who have exhibited paradoxical reactions to certain forms of treatment, e.g., splint therapy and physical therapy, which make them feel worse.
6. Patients who have already had properly executed forms of therapy with unknown reasons for failure.
7. Patients who have not been compliant with previous treatment.

If these limitations are so restrictive as not to allow adequate treatment it would be best for the practitioner to discontinue or not start treatment.

After considering the aforementioned limitations, the practitioner should predict the clinical course and formulate a prognosis, based on the diagnosis and knowledge of the clinical behavior of that particular disorder. For example, degenerative joint disease has a clinical course of several months to several years, whereas the clinical course of traumatically induced retrodiscitis is usually a few weeks if treated in a timely fashion.

The length of time the patient has had the problem and the past treatments should be kept in mind. In general, the longer a patient has been in pain and the more treatments he or she has had, which were ineffective, the poorer the prognosis.

CASE PRESENTATION

The diagnosis should be explained to the patient in clear, concise terms. The words should not be too difficult for the patient to understand, yet should be accurate in the description of the diagnosis. Etiologic factors should be pointed out to the patient, especially when not readily evident. *Patients should be told that success in treatment depends on their active participation.*

Visual aids are often helpful in explaining pathology (Figs. 22–1 to 22–3). A skull, schematic diagrams, and simple drawings are very effective. Mounted study casts are valuable when occlusal problems are evident. It is helpful to allow patients to view films of their TMJs with careful explanation of where the pathology exists. A film of normal TMJs can be shown by way of comparison.

The dentist should describe available treatment options to the patient. One option is the treatment preferred by the dentist. But it is also important to describe other treatment options, including surgery. The patient should be given a clear explanation of why a particular treatment is being recommended. The relationship

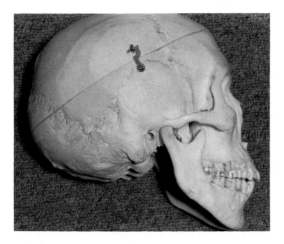

FIGURE 22–1. A skull can be used to point out pertinent anatomic bony structures.

of any given treatment to the diagnosis and the etiology should be readily evident to the patient. The dentist should also remember that no treatment is always a viable option. This especially applies to the asymptomatic click in which often no treatment is indicated.

Possible sequelae of these conditions should be discussed openly. Include those that can occur without treatment and those that can occur despite the best treatment. In particular, the patient with internal derangement with reduction and intermittent locking can later experience the locking phase and will need surgical correction. This can happen with even the best nonsurgical care. Patients also need to understand the chances of success and that, although a majority show improvement, some patients experience treatment failures.

Sometimes, a diagnosis is elusive. It may therefore be appropriate to utilize a stabilization (flat plane) appliance or other treatment modality as a *diagnostic tool.* The rationale for this short-term procedure (2 to 4 weeks) must be clearly explained to the patient.

Patients should also be given an idea of the expected clinical course. Any possible negative effects of the treatment, including side effects of medication, possible shifting of teeth with splint therapy, and reduced range of motion after surgery should be explained.

The patient should also be told of the need for any future treatment, such as surgery, or phase II care, such as orthodontics and prosthetic therapy. Time and costs should be freely discussed.

The patient has to make a commitment when beginning TMD treatment. It must be understood that compliance is necessary so that the clinical course will be as short as possible. This means taking medication, wearing an occlusal appliance, and following up on referral as directed.

The importance of returning for regular followup visits must be emphasized. Failure to follow through on care is negligent, be it on the part of the patient or the dentist. The followup visits allow the dentist to re-evaluate the diagnosis and to alter the course of treatment if needed.

MULTIDISCIPLINARY APPROACH

Most workers recommend a multidisciplinary approach for the treatment of TMDs. Although some patients can be adequately managed utilizing single treatment approaches,

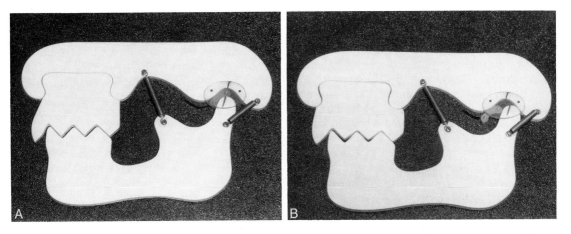

FIGURE 22–2. A commercially available schematic model of the temporomandibular joint is useful for explaining internal derangements. *A,* The disc is in the normal position. *B,* The disc is in an anterior position.

FIGURE 22–3. *A* and *B,* A commercially available flip chart illustrating the various stages of internal derangement. (Reprinted with permission from Higdon, S.J.: *Illustrated Anatomy of the Temporomandibular Joint in Function/Dysfunction.* 1983.)

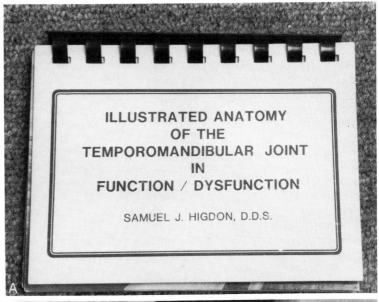

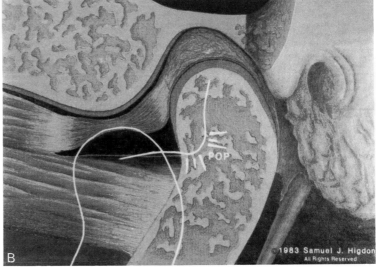

many are best managed by a group of health-care professionals. Because of the multifactorial nature of TMDs, the treatment for any given patient will vary as to the diagnosis and the particular blend of contributing factors. The scope of training is often not diverse enough to enable a dentist alone to provide all phases of care. No one health-care professional is qualified to provide all phases of care. Therefore, the approach has to be multidisciplinary. As stated by Fricton,[4] "A chronic pain problem (then) is conceptualized as having multiple levels of problems that include the pathophysiological with any cognitive, behavioral, social, emotional, environmental, or biological problems. Each level affects each other and impacts on the whole problem. A change in one level will affect a change in at least one other level. Thus, management of all levels of the illness through a team approach has a theoretical basis to facilitate more long-term improvement than a singular approach." The primary group of professionals most often includes a general dentist, an oral and maxillofacial surgeon, an orthodontist, a physical therapist and a psychiatrist or psychologist who play the following roles:

Dentist. The dentist plays the role of diagnostician and usually sees the patient for the initial evaluation. A comprehensive examination and history are completed and appropriate diagnostic tests are ordered. The dentist provides therapy consistent with training, including occlusal splint therapy and appropriate pharmacologic therapy.

Some dentists have adequate training to provide certain physical modalities and trigger point injections. The dentist is also responsible for making appropriate referrals to other members of the health-care team and for periodic monitoring of the patient for progress. The dentist is usually a general dentist but can be an oral and maxillofacial surgeon, periodontist, orthodontist, or prosthodontist. Sometimes, the dentist plays a secondary role; for example, the patient may be referred by a physiatrist or an orthopedist who is managing total patient care.

Oral and Maxillofacial Surgeon. This surgeon acts as a referral source for arthroscopic, open joint, and orthognathic procedures. Surgical correction of dentofacial deformities and neoplastic disease of the TMJ are managed by this health-care professional. The oral and maxillofacial surgeon also performs reconstructive procedures for a patient with severe arthritic destruction.

Orthodontist. He or she acts as a referral source for phase II orthodontic therapy and, in many instances, provides comprehensive phase I treatment.

Physical Therapist. The physical therapist is responsible for evaluation and treatment of the cervical spine and the muscles of the neck as well as the TMJ. He or she must be familiar with problems that affect the cervical spine and must be well versed in TMJ pathology. Treatment provided by the physical therapist includes massage, manipulation, corrective exercises, and various other modalities. These include hot and cold packs, transcutaneous electrical nerve stimulation (TENS) therapy, electrogalvanic stimulation, and ultrasound. In most states, physical therapists, by law, must practice under the prescription of a licensed physician or dentist. In some states, a written diagnosis from the referring physician or dentist is required, but the physical therapist is permitted to employ his or her own treatment plan. The physical therapist plays a pivotal role in presurgical and postsurgical treatment.

Psychiatrist or Psychologist. The psychiatrist should be familiar with TMJ pathology and the applicable psychologic literature. He or she is responsible for evaluating patient anxiety and depression, as they relate directly and indirectly to the TMD. The psychiatrist is in a unique position to probe the social and psychologic aspects of the patient's problem. The psychiatrist must provide psychotherapy, counselling, and behavioral therapy. He or she must also act as emotional support for both the patient and family. The psychiatrist can also assist in managing the patient with pharmacologic therapy. Because antidepressant medications are more commonly used, this role cannot be overstated.

The composition of the primary group may vary, depending on the setting in which care is provided and the availability of trained health-care professionals in a particular area. For example, care provided in the setting of a hospital-based chronic pain center may be directed by a neurologist, psychiatrist, or anesthesiologist, with a dentist having a consultant role.

The primary team has to be supplemented with professionals from other areas of medicine. These professionals include internists, neurologists, otolaryngologists, rheumatologists, physiatrists, and chiropractors.

Internist. The internist rules out the presence of systemic disease and is often the health-care professional who best knows the patient. Working with other practitioners, the internist also approves patients for certain treatment modalities, e.g., the patient with a stomach ulcer needing nonsteroidal antiinflammatory medication. The internist also can provide certain aspects of care, particularly in the patient with systemic illness.

Neurologist. This practitoner first rules out the presence of neurologic disorders and any organic pathology of the cervical spine. He or she diagnoses neurologic disorders. Patients may be referred to the neurologist for non-TMJ–related headache and some forms of facial pain. The neurologist should have an understanding of TMDs because many TMD related headaches need to be considered in the differential diagnosis.

Otolaryngologist. This health-care professional rules out the presence of ear, nose, and throat pathology and assumes primary management of sinus, otologic, and throat-related pathology. Frequent patient complaints of sinus and ear pain underscore the importance of this relationship with TMDs.

Rheumatologist. This practitioner rules out the presence of systemic arthritides. When these diseases are present, he or she assumes the primary management role.

Physiatrist. Physiatry is the branch of medicine concerned with rehabilitation. These physicians work in close conjunction with physical therapists. Some dentists may wish to make a patient referral to a physiatrist because the physiatrist is trained to understand chronic and muscular pain. The physiatrist also can oversee the care given by the physical therapist, can prescribe medication, and can give trigger point and other types of injections.

Chiropractor. Some dentists prefer to make patient referrals to chiropractors for manipulation, massage, and other modalities. Certain chiropractors see many patients with TMDs and likewise make patient referrals to dentists. When working with chiropractors, dentists should be familiar and comfortable with their treatment philosophies. Differing philosophies only confuse the patient with conflicting information and cause a loss of trust.

This group can be either a formal organization located in one center or independent practitioners. One member of the group has to act as the primary caregiver, a "traffic director" making referrals and treatment recommendations in conference with the others. It is important that the patient not receive conflicting information from the different professionals providing care, because as mentioned confusion may cause a patient to lose trust. Appoint-

ments with the various health-care professionals should be scheduled on a convenient basis. Having too many appointments can be stressful in and of itself. Communication between members of the team is essential.

In some dental schools, hospitals and pain centers, it is possible to have some or all members of the primary team present with the patient during initial evaluation and treatment sessions. Members can also meet without the patient and discuss findings and preferred treatment approaches. In this environment, it is simpler to coordinate treatment efforts and track the patient's progress. The hospital environment also lends itself readily for secondary consultations with other specialists and for ordering diagnostic tests, such as blood workups and MRI, CT, or bone scans.

Forms of Treatment

Many different terms are used to categorize varying forms of TMJ treatment. These words are, unfortunately, employed interchangeably by many clinicians but have very different meanings. This practice only adds to the confusion in the treatment of TMDs. The following list clarifies the meaning of several groups of such words:

Surgical vs. Nonsurgical Therapy. Surgery includes those techniques involving correction of abnormalities by physical entry into the joint. These include open joint procedures, arthroscopic procedures, and orthognathic surgery.

Reversible vs. Nonreversible Therapy. Reversible therapy includes those techniques that cause no permanent change in maxillomandibular relationships or tooth position. Flat plane splint therapy has traditionally been considered reversible, but there are occasional examples of unexpected mandibular shifting (see chapter 30).

Nonreversible therapy includes those techniques that cause permanent change in the dentition or maxillomandibular relationships, such as surgery, occlusal adjustment, orthodontics, and prosthetic reconstruction. Repositioning splint therapy in the early stages can be considered reversible but can rapidly cause changes in jaw and tooth relationships. When these occur, orthodontic and prosthetic treatment may be necessary.

Conservative vs. Radical Therapy. Conservative procedures are not necessarily limited to nonsurgical procedures. Conservative therapy is appropriate treatment for a given diagnosis. Radical therapy is inappropriate therapy or overtreatment for a given diagnosis. Flat plane splint therapy can hardly be defined as conservative treatment for a patient with a parotid tumor but some forms of surgery might be. Conversely, full mouth reconstruction for a patient with myofascial pain dysfunction syndrome cannot be considered conservative, when most long-term followup data indicate that flat plane splint therapy and other reversible forms of treatment are as effective.

Phase I and Phase II Therapy. Phase I therapy includes therapy that is considered medical in nature and that attends to symptomatic and functional improvement in joint or muscle function. These approaches include reversible forms, such as physical and psychologic therapy, splint therapy (flat plane and repositioning), and pharmacologic therapy. Phase I care is often all that is needed for many patients.

Phase II therapy includes any necessary dental procedures and is generally irreversible. Both removable and fixed prosthetics and orthodontics are included in this category. Surgery of the TMJ is considered phase II therapy and typically follows unsuccessful or limited phase I therapy. The intent of orthodontic and prosthodontic phase II treatments is to stabilize altered occlusal relationships.

The chapters in Section IV of this book present detailed discussion of nonsurgical treatment, both phase I and phase II. Section V reviews surgical approaches. Despite the organization of each treatment approach into separate chapters, their integration is paramount to successful outcome.

REFERENCES

1. Deardorff, M.W. and Butteworth, J.: Psychometric profiles of craniomandibular pain patients. Part II. A multidisciplinary case report. J. Craniomandib. Pract. 5:367–370, 1987.
2. Okesson, J.: *Management of Temporomandibular Joint Disorders and Occlusion,* 2nd ed. C.V. Mosby Co., St. Louis, 1989.
3. Okesson, J.: Conservative management of masticatory disorders. Proceedings of the American Equilibration Society, 32nd Annual Meeting, Chicago, 1987.
4. Fricton, J., Hathaway, K., and Bromaghim, C.: Interdisciplinary management of patients with TMJ and craniofacial pain: Characteristics and outcome. J. Craniomandib. Pract. 1:115–122, 1987.

Steven G. Messing

CHAPTER 23

Splint Therapy

Occlusal splints are defined as removable interocclusal appliances, which are usually fabricated in hard acrylic. Despite the fact that these appliances are the most commonly prescribed treatment for temporomandibular disorders (TMDs), there is a considerable variety of opinion regarding their specific intended function and design and how and why they are effective. The fact that they are effective has been documented repeatedly in the medical and dental literature.[1-29] This chapter discusses the various theories of splint therapy; the designs of multiple appliances; and the expectations, limitations, and complications of splint therapy. Treatment flow charts found at the end of this chapter illustrate how splint therapy can be used and integrated with other aspects of temporomandibular treatment.

Occlusal splints have been prescribed for the treatment of bruxism and craniomandibular symptoms for almost a century.[30] They have even been reported to effectively treat tinnitus,[31-34] otitis media,[35] hemifacial atrophy with related muscle spasms,[36] sleep apnea,[37,38] fingernail biting,[39] altered taste,[40] and lingual numbness with associated speech impairment.[41] The orthodontic literature contains references that describe occlusal appliances along with their use in eliminating airway obstruction and influencing facial growth and development.[171,172]

In addition to these benefits that have been derived from occlusal splint usage, the TMD treatment objectives of splints have been described as eliminating occlusal interferences, stabilizing tooth and joint relationships, passive stretching of the musculature that reduces abnormal muscle activity, decreasing parafunctional habits, protecting against tooth abrasion, and decreasing joint loading. Splints also function diagnostically as an indirect method of altering the occlusion.[25] This can be applied in the treatment of a patient with temporomandibular joint (TMJ) or muscle symptoms or in a restoration phase after the initial treatment phase has been completed.

Five major theories covering the mechanism of action of splints have been described by Clark[1,18] as follows:

1. Occlusal disengagement therory[3,19]
2. Vertical dimension theory[43-45]
3. Maxillomandibular realignment theory[46-48]
4. TMJ repositioning theory[49-51]
5. Cognitive awareness theory.[11,52]

Each of these theories has multiple proponents, many with variations, and each is discussed.

OCCLUSAL DISENGAGEMENT THEORY

The occlusal disengagement theory proposes that the placement of an appliance with proper occlusal relationships temporarily replaces previously faulty occlusal relationships. This placement eliminates the stimulus causing muscular hyperactivity and, in turn, allows for proper joint and mandibular function.

Carlson and coworkers[53] and subsequently Posselt[54] described the placement of a hard acrylic bite plate overlying the teeth of one or both arches in order to establish balanced articulation. They were primarily interested in "curing bruxism" and in protecting the teeth and periodontium against abrasion and occlusal overloads. Posselt spoke of relieving muscle spasm and TMJ pain. In attempting to explain the effect of the appliance, he stated that occlusal interferences may have initiated the bruxism, and by covering these with an appliance a new pattern of sensory stimuli would be created. He further stated that a flat occlusal surface would allow a conditioned reflex, which is reinforced by improper tooth contact to be prevented or eliminated.

Ramfjord and Ash[3] affirmed these treatment objectives. They differentiated bite plates, which they used to describe the Hawley[55] or Sved[56] appliances, which cover only the anterior segment, from occlusal splints,[54] which cover an entire arch. Ramfjord and Ash believed that bite plates were effective in eliminating occlusal trigger zones (prematurities), but that because they did not cover the entire arch, teeth could move both horizontally and vertically. The occlusal splint, a full arch appliance usually covering all of the maxillary teeth, was the appliance of choice according to these workers.[3] It was constructed to occlude with all opposing teeth in centric relation and was free of occlusal interference in all excursions. Cuspid guidance was advocated in order to assure that balancing prematurities would be avoided. Ramfjord and Ash stated that if this type of splint were properly fabricated, there would be an immediate decrease in muscle tone and associated bruxism.

The maxillary flat hard full coverage appliance, also known as the stabilization splint, Michigan splint, and night guard, remains the most prevalent appliance. Despite its widespread use, there are limited scientific studies to explain its success. (For discussion about this type splint, see Stabilization Splints.)

The theory that improper occlusion is responsible for TMDs, is currently under dispute.[57] At the American Dental Association (ADA) Workship on Craniomandibular Disorders, in 1988,[57] the moderator asked the attendees for a show of hands of those who believed that occlusion played an etiologic role in TMDs. There was an almost unanimous show of hands. Despite this agreement, the panel, in view of the latest literature, expressed doubt that occlusal factors, by themselves, play a large role. Discussions on the subject of occlusion and its adjustment are found in other chapters of this text. In view of its intimate relationship with the occlusal disengagement theory, a brief discussion is appropriate here.

Occlusal prematurity has been defined as "that part of tooth structure that is in the way of harmonious jaw function"[42] and as "occlusal contacts hampering or hindering smooth gliding jaw movements, with the teeth maintaining contact."[43] Description of these types of contacts includes differences between intercuspal and retrusive contact positions, balancing side interferences, and working side interferences.[19,60] Inadequate occlusal contacts are another disturbance, which can be associated with dysfunction and bruxism.[61]

At the turn of the century, in Vienna, Karolyi described tooth adjustment in lateral and protrusive excursions.[62] In the United States, Hutchinson demonstrated occlusal equilibration in 1905 and later wrote about it.[63]

In 1957, Perry[64] stated that alteration of the occlusion was followed by clinical improvement. Shore,[26] in 1959, wrote that traumatogenic occlusions could produce injury to the teeth, supporting structures, neuromuscular

system, and TMJ. He specifically attributed the injury to the occlusion and described at length the principles for occlusal equilibration. Ramjford[65] described prematurities as occlusal trigger areas and stated that they were the cause of bruxism. He further noted that if they were treated by occlusal adjustment, the bruxism would cease. Ahlgren and Posselt[66] and Weisengreen and Elliott[67] found abnormal electromyograms (EMGs) in patients with cuspal interferences and TMJ pain. After occlusal adjustment, the contraction pattern and muscle incoordination improved.

Many other subsequent studies have supported the relationship between occlusion and TMDs. They have included the prevalence of malocclusion in hyperfunction,[68–70] the correlation among occlusal prematurities and pain and dysfunction of the masticatory system,[23,60,71–74] tooth loss and numbers of occluding teeth,[77–78] unilateral tooth loss,[79] and problems of occlusal contacts.[42,59,80] Multiple studies have been carried out concerning the experimental placement of occlusal prematurities.[81–89] Farrer and McCarty,[2] Weinberg,[152–155,158] and Dawson[25] all have discussed the role of occlusal problems and made suggestions on occlusal adjustments. At the ADA Workshop on Craniomandibular Disorders,[57] Mahan discussed distalizing lateral guidance as a possible etiology for TMDs.

Despite all of this scientific evidence supporting the relationship between occlusion and TMDs, an equal volume of contradictory material exists.

In 1961, Kydd and Sander[88] stated that a slide between centric occlusion and intercuspal position was normal and prevalent. Other workers agree.[89–96] Further articles report that this slide is not associated with muscle tenderness.[97–100] Celenza[101] and Farrar[2,127] have observed that when this slide is eliminated by occlusal adjustment it reoccurs.

Multiple studies have been published that conclude that occlusion plays a minor role in TMDs.[59,102–106] Bush and colleagues[99] in their evaluation of 298 dental students found no difference in muscle palpation among class I, class II, or class III malocclusions, nor did they find any correlation in laterotrusive, protrusive, or retrusive prematurities. Kopp[110] found no significant correlation between molar loss, crepitation, and tenderness to palpation. Heloe and Heloe[111] found no occlusal correlations among 406 Swedish patients with TMJ pain and dysfunction. Agerberg and Carlson[77] found no occlusal differences in patients with TMJ dysfunctions when compared with the general population. Several other studies have thoroughly evaluated this relationship. A long-term epidemiologic study on a large population, by Egermark-Erickson and associates,[107] failed to correlate occlusal factors with mandibular dysfunction in children and adolescents.

Roberts and colleagues[108] evaluated 205 patients with known clinical and arthroscopic diagnoses of TMJ internal derangements. These investigators noted horizontal and vertical overlap of the incisors at centric occlusion, Angle's classification,[109] cross bites, tooth wear, lateral and anterior guidance, laterotrusive and mediotrusive occlusal contacts, and deflective contacts between intercuspal and centric relation positions. They correlated these factors with presence and type of internal derangements. Statistical analysis revealed little or no correlation between these occlusal factors and internal derangements.

Seligman and colleagues[97] published a study in 1988 correlating clinical muscle tenderness with occlusion in a large group of dental hygiene students. Relationships between muscle tenderness and occlusion, especially Angle's classification, vertical overlap, cross bite, presence and length of centric relation-centric occlusion slide, and unilateral centric occlusion contacts were evaluated. Significant findings occurred in only highly specific situations, and these workers concluded that the associations were weak ($P<.05$). They further state, "Occlusal interferences exert little influence on muscle pain and tenderness in the absence of other factors," agreeing with the findings of several previous studies.[100,112]

At the ADA Workshop on Craniomandibular Disorders,[57] Mohl, Johnson, Katzberg, and Laskin all stated that occlusion by itself did not play an etiologic role. Mohl discussed the loss of posterior support resulting in increased biomechanical loading, which when accompanied by parafunctional habits increased the amount of degenerative joint disease.

Tanaka[57] discussed that the combination of occlusal prematurities and bruxism may cause damage to the collateral ligaments, allowing for laxity and subsequent internal derangement.

Laskin emphasized the multifactorial nature of TMDs and stated that although occlusion by itself may not cause problems, in combination with other factors it may play a role.

Bell has written, "occlusion may be a predisposing factor that requires activation by other means before it becomes a decisive cause."[24] Zarb and Carlsson[58] have discussed the multifactorial etiology and stated that occlusal prematurities alone may not cause a temporomandibular problem until excessive forces, such as parafunctional habits, are superimposed.

Many questions still remain unanswered. One individual may have an occlusion with marked deviations from normal, yet excellent function, whereas another may have a morphologically ideal occlusion with severe dysfunction.[61] Not all patients with bruxism experience malocclusions, and not all patients with malocclusions experience bruxism.[113]

The issue seems equivocal at this time. Voluminous publications support both points of view. Clearly, more research is necessary concerning the interrelationships between contributing factors. Additional studies addressing the nature of bruxism, and its interrelationship with occlusal factors, are necessary.

VERTICAL DIMENSION THEORY

The vertical dimension theory is based on the premise that it is necessary to restore the proper interarch space in order to achieve proper muscle activity. Christiansen[114] wrote that the treatment appliance should function to restore the vertical dimension that had been lost. The new interarch dimension must be carefully evolved, in order to re-establish the original vertical dimension. By doing so, the muscle function would return to normal.

Shore[26] also discussed the use of occlusal splints to restore lost vertical dimension. Gelb[27,132] and Witzig and Spahl[196] have discussed increasing the vertical dimension to compensate for the vertical height that was never achieved during growth and development. Ito and coworkers[115] measured joint loading under various occlusal conditions. In order to evaluate whether posterior tooth loss caused increased joint loading, five different splint types were evaluated. When posterior support was eliminated, clenching on the anterior segment caused increased joint loading with a superior shift in condylar position.

MacDonald and Hannam[116] have also stated that anterior function without posterior support resulted in increased joint loading. They postulated that a patient with posterior occlusal collapse may be susceptible to increased joint loading and subsequently predisposed to tissue change or damage of the joint area.

Farrar,[49] Bell,[24] and Mongini[119] all have stated that greater joint loading is the most significant clinical finding and may be the cause of other symptoms.

Earlier studies of the vertical dimension theory were concerned mainly with muscle activity. The splint proposed is similar to the stabilization splint utilized in the occlusal disengagement theory (see Stabilization Splints). Further studies focus on joint loading, which may have different splint requirements (see Joint Loading).

Several studies contradict this theory. Goldspink[120] employed rat and cat models to show that striated muscles adapt without difficulty to change in length. Within 3 to 4 weeks, a suitable number of sarcomeres are added to allow adaptation of muscle length. Tallgren[122] utilized dentures of varying thicknesses to show the adaptability of the musculature of subjects.

Several studies have discussed muscular adaptation to the increase of vertical dimension caused by splint insertion.[123–124] Hellsing[125] studied vertical dimension adaptability in ten subjects before, during, and after the removal of occlusal splints. He concluded that the muscle spindles, together with the periodontal receptors, give the neurophysiologic feedback that the system needs to be adaptive. He found that his subjects were extremely adaptive. In all patients, simple closure was sufficient to change interocclusal distance after splint removal.

Drago and associates[126] applied maxillary splints of varying thicknesses to evaluate whether excessive vertical dimension caused hyperactivity. Interestingly, the *thickest* splints had the greatest *decrease* in muscle activity.

Apparently, the craniomandibular system is adaptive and can function in the presence of vertical change. When the change becomes excessive, and the adaptive capacity of the system is overcome, pathology or dysfunction may result.

MAXILLOMANDIBULAR REALIGNMENT THEORY

Several maxillomandibular realignment theories exist. All propose that the mandible is malpositioned relative to the maxilla at the position of maximum intercuspation. Further, all believe that if the mandible is repositioned, a more optimum maxillomandibular relationship can be evolved, and symptoms eliminated. Splints are an intermediary step in the process,

interposing a new interarch relationship that achieves a balanced mandibular position. Three variations of the maxillomandibular realignment theory are proposed.

Centric Relation Jaw Position

Centric relation has been defined as the most superior position of the condyles in the fossae with the discs centrally interposed.[127] Dawson[25,42,128] has written extensively on the subject of centric relation jaw position. He stated that it is critically important to understand that it is a skeletally determined position and that the condyle-disc assemblies are braced medially as well as superiorly.

According to Dawson, "The most common cause of masticatory muscle pain is displacement of the mandible to a position dictated by maximal intercuspation of the teeth. Displacement of the mandible always results in displacement of the condyle-disc assemblies, which in turn can lead to progressive changes in the condyle-disc alignment."[25]

A splint, according to Dawson, is employed as a temporary occluding surface that prevents the existing occlusion from controlling the jaw-to-jaw relationship. Further, it guides the mandible into a braced, ligamentous relationship at which the mandible can function around its condylar hinge axis. This position is determined by bimanual manipulation.[128] In this technique, the mandible is prevented from making any occlusal contact while it is being opened and closed by the patient. When the mandible is hinging freely, firm upward pressure is applied to the lower border of the mandible while thumb pressure keeps the anterior section open. This maneuver forces the condyles superiorly into the desired relationship (Fig. 23–1). This position is subsequently verified by placing firm upward pressure on the mandible, seating the condyles firmly. Dawson believes that physiologically positioned condyles resist pressure with no discomfort. Once this centric relation position is achieved by manipulation, a centric relation occlusal splint can be fabricated.

Similar to the previously mentioned stabilization splint, it does not have occlusal fossa. However, the centric relation occlusal splint is fabricated so that opposing cusp tips all contact the splint surface equally at the centric relation position. Anterior guidance that discloses posterior contact in all excursions is provided. Dawson believes that this is a "permissive

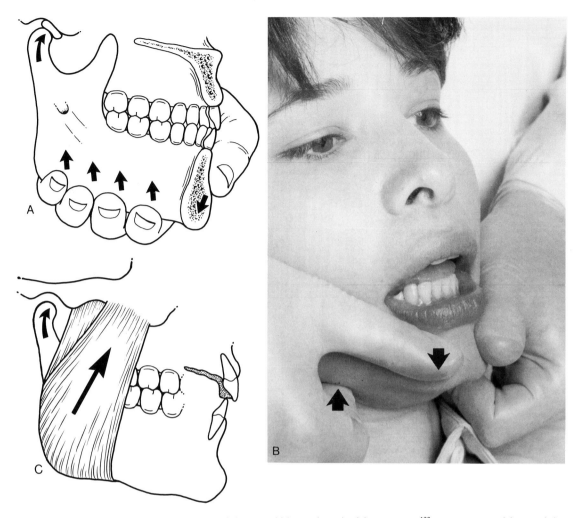

FIGURE 23–1. *A*, Bilateral manipulation of the mandible as described by Dawson.[128] *B*, Direction of force of this manipulation. *C*, Forces acting upon an anterior bite plate as described by Dawson.[128]

splint" rather than a repositioning splint because it allows access to centric relation but does not force the condyle into this position.[25]

Multiple debates have been reported over the validity of this technique. Celenza and associate[101,129,130] and Farrar and associate[2,127] have written that ligamentous border positions, such as centric relation, are not physiologic and that the condyle rarely reaches border positions during function. They have stated that when the condyle is placed at a ligamentous border position, articular remodeling will occur, resulting in the position no longer being a border position (Fig. 23–2).

Gibbs and coworkers[366] measured function utilizing measurements of EMG activity for the masticatory muscles in different mandibular positions. When comparing intercuspal and retruded contact positions, they found a decrease in normal muscle activity of the masseter, temporal, and medial pterygoid muscles associated with clenching in the retruded contact position. They postulated that a slide between intercuspal and retruded contact positions may serve a protective function for the TMJ.

Pullinger, Seligman, and Solberg[367] evaluated occlusal patterns in students and correlated these findings with clinical examinations of TMJ pain and dysfunction. There was a tendency for TMDs to be associated with the lack of a slide between intercuspal and retruded contact positions. Asymmetric slides had greater dysfunction than symmetric slides. These workers agree with Bush,[99] who found

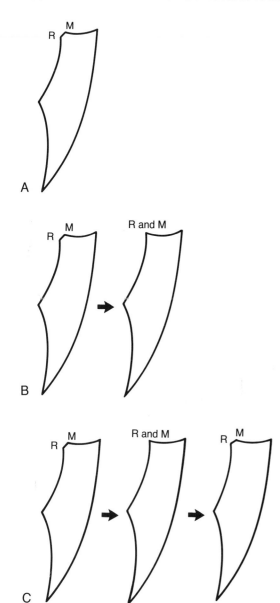

FIGURE 23–2. *A,* The envelope of motion, sagittal view. *B,* Centric relation occlusion eliminates the difference between centric relation and centric occlusion. *C,* Changes in the envelope of motion over time. If a patient is adjusted or restored into centric relation occlusion, a new difference between centric relation and centric occlusion occurs over time. (Redrawn from Celenza, F.V.: Int. J. Periodont. Restor. Dent. 5:2, 1985.)

that all symptomatic subjects with class II and class III occlusions had no slide between intercuspal and retruded contact positions, and class I subjects with tenderness had smaller slides than subjects without tenderness. These studies postulate that a slide between intercuspal position and retruded contact position is protective of the TMJ.

Oral Orthopedics Theory

This theory states that malrelationship of the jaws has an effect on the entire neuromuscular system, involving function of the head, neck, and shoulders.[131] Consequently, occlusion relates to the muscles, the joints, and the surrounding structures as well as to the teeth and jaw.

Leib[131] has described the background of this theory, relating the interrelationships of the jaws to the cervical spine, head posture, and balance. "Improper jaw relationship must mean impaired posture and balance, which is a stress-producing beginning for any function. Where improper jaw relationship exists, many compensatory adjustments must be made by all the parts involved in the activity."[131] Leib then describes anatomic planes of orientation of the correctly developed maxilla and mandible, with the head in proper position. These planes (horizontal, midsagittal, maxillary transverse, molar transverse, cuspid transverse, and auxiliary sagittal) are related to anatomic structures and are traced on dental study casts of the patients to be treated (Fig. 23–3).

The study casts can subsequently be mounted on an articulator, and the lines representing the anatomic planes can be aligned, resulting in the corrected interarch relationship. A splint can then be fabricated, which when placed in the mouth of the patient, guides the mandible to the corrected maxillomandibular relationship (Fig. 23–4).

Gelb has lectured and written extensively on this theory.[27] He has emphasized the multifactorial nature of TMDs and has advocated evaluation of head and neck posture, as well as jaw interrelationships. Gelb suggests ". . . repositioning of the mandible with its condyles to produce an optimum neuromuscular balance as well as bilateral condyle fossae and jaw relationships."[27]

Gelb prepares a wax bite for a patient "try in" and then constructs the study models as described by Leib and fabricates a mandibular orthopedic repositioning acrylic appliance (MORA). Gelb believes that most symptoms should be relieved at the try in stage.[27] The MORA is a hard acrylic appliance that covers the lower posterior teeth only. Gelb cites the

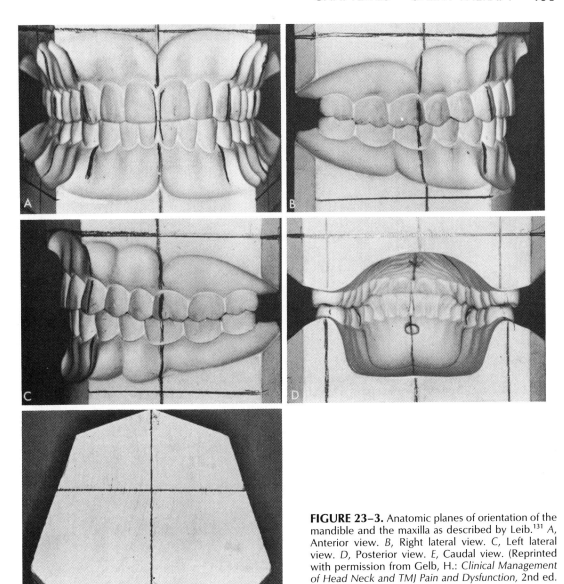

FIGURE 23–3. Anatomic planes of orientation of the mandible and the maxilla as described by Leib.[131] *A,* Anterior view. *B,* Right lateral view. *C,* Left lateral view. *D,* Posterior view. *E,* Caudal view. (Reprinted with permission from Gelb, H.: *Clinical Management of Head Neck and TMJ Pain and Dysfunction,* 2nd ed. W.B. Saunders Co., Philadelphia, 1985.)

advantages of this type of appliance, including ease of construction and adjustment, hygienic, comfortable and inconspicuous, reversible, and phonetically and aesthetically acceptable. Exposure of the anterior teeth in order to provide natural anterior and canine guidance is also advantageous. Unlike the previously discussed stabilization splints, this splint employs occlusal fossa to define a new mandibular position. This type of appliance has been criticized by stating that it results in posterior tooth depression and consequent posterior open bite.[1,125]

Gelb states that when the proper jaw relationship has been achieved, the condylar position within the fossa is halfway down the slope of the eminence, and slightly anterior, in what he calls the 4-7 position (Fig. 23–5). This evaluation of condylar position is based on transcranial radiography. Transcranial radiographs, however, have been shown to be an accurate representation of the lateral pole of the condyle

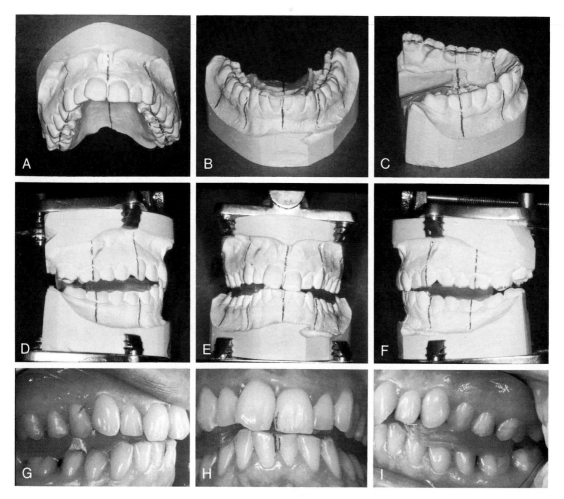

FIGURE 23–4. *A, B,* and *C,* Patient's study casts with guidelines as described by Gelb. *D, E,* and *F,* Study casts mounted on an articulator: guiding planes aligned: wax bite fabricated. *G, H,* and *I.* Wax bite "try-in," anterior and lateral views.

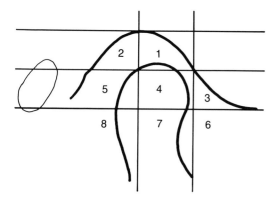

FIGURE 23–5. The 4–7 position as described by Gelb. (Redrawn from Gelb, H.: *Clinical Management of Head Neck and TMJ Pain and Dysfunction,* 2nd ed. W.B. Saunders, Philadelphia, 1985.)

and not an accurate assessment of condylar position within the fossa.[159–163]

Muscle-Determined Position (Myocentric)

This concept of diagnosis and treatment involves a transcutaneous electrical nerve stimulator (TENS) of low frequency to stimulate the fifth and seventh cranial nerves. Stimulation of the motor portion of these nerves causes an automatic involuntary closure, which is independent of muscle tension or inflammation, or proprioceptive occlusal influences. This "... accomplishes a neuromuscularly controlled, balanced muscle contraction that determines a functionally correct occlusal position that is compatible with a continued state of relaxation."[133]

In 1969, Bernard Jankelson with coworkers introduced the electrical device he termed the myomonitor. Subsequent publications have described it further.[133–139]

Jankelson postulated that when malocclusion exists, the teeth guide the mandible to a position that puts greater than normal demand on the posturing muscles. This demand results in chronic tension of these muscles. This chronic tension interferes with proper lymphatic drainage and muscular supply of oxygen to the muscles. The first function of the myomonitor is to cause "normal" muscle contractions in a periodic, rhythmic manner, in order to revascularize the muscles and create their relaxation. A second function of the myomonitor is to control pain via TENS of the A fibers in the central nervous system. A third function of this instrument is to cause a bilateral isotonic neurologically stimulated closure to a position termed "myocentric." It is to this position that splints can be made in an effort to treat chronic muscle spasm and pain.

A computerized system has been introduced to register mandibular movements and position. This procedure, called Computer Mandibular Scanning, provides both a printed and a computer screen image of the mandibular pattern of movement. Robert Jankelson[140]

stated that previously the arc of closure dictated by the myomonitor could be disturbed by the presence of wax or registration material between the teeth at the position of closure. The newer computer-aided models are designed to make the system more accurate and reproducible.

Jankelson[140] describes the provisional deconditioning of patients with TMJ and myofascial pain disorders. The splint is fabricated in the myocentric position, and the affected muscles are given time to relax. "The appliance is used as a flexible medium to respond to necessary changes in vertical, anteroposterior, and lateral position of the progressively equalizing musculature."[140]

The appliance is usually a full arch, mandibular appliance. It is fabricated in hard acrylic, and it too defines a position of the mandible by having definite fossae in the occlusal surface (Fig. 23–6). As with other techniques, there have been studies both supporting and criticizing this technique.

An important point of discussion is whether electrical stimulation causes muscle contraction via nerve stimulation or direct stimulation of the muscle fibers. Choi and Mitani[136] concluded that the contractions were neurally mediated. In another study,[135] intensity duration curve analysis was performed on ten subjects. Stimuli of short duration have been deter-

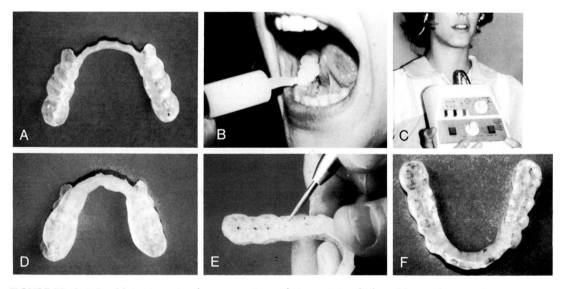

FIGURE 23–6. Splint fabrication using the myomonitor technique. A, Acrylic base fabricated on mandibular model. B, Soft acrylic being added to splint surface intraorally. C, Patient undergoing pulsation using the myomonitor. D, Resulting splint with myocentric occlusion. E, Splint shaped and contoured, leaving cusp tip occlusion. F, Completed splint. (Courtesy of Dr. Robert Jankelson, Seattle, Washington.)

mined to affect only nerve tissue; longer stimuli affect both nerve and muscle tissues. A stimulus that was too brief to directly cause muscle stimulation was applied to these subjects. Muscle contraction suggested that the stimulus responsible was neurally mediated.[135] Williamson and Marshall[141] further confirmed neural mediation by observing the effects of succinylcholine, which blocks neural stimulation at the myoneural end plate. When subjects underwent stimulation using the myomonitor while under the influence of succinylcholine, no muscle contraction resulted.

McMillan and colleagues[142] evaluated activity of muscles at remote sites (ears, nose, and upper lip) as subjects were stimulated with the myomonitor. After examination of branches of the facial nerve on six cadaver specimens, they concluded that anastomoses between buccal branches of the facial nerve were responsible, and that these remote muscle contractions were evidence of the neurally transmitted nature of the myomonitor stimulation.

Several other studies, however, have suggested that the muscle contractions are not neurally mediated but rather are a result of direct muscle stimulation.[143–144] Dao and coworkers[145] evaluated myomonitor stimulation on five subjects. After placement of the myomonitor electrodes as recommended by the manufacturer, hook electrodes were placed in anesthetized areas of the right masseter muscle and connected to a differential preamplifier and a digital storage oscilloscope. The time between onset of stimulation and beginning of EMG response was measured. This time interval was compared with previously determined time intervals for the H reflex (a true muscle contraction reflex that is neurally initiated) or the M response (a result of direct stimulation of individual motor axons before they branch to innervate individual muscle fibers). These investigators conclude that recorded responses were too brief to represent true H reflex contractions but, instead, correspond to the M response characterized by direct muscle stimulation. They therefore believe that the jaw closure created by myomonitor stimulation does not represent neurologically mediated reflex closure and, therefore, cannot establish a physiologic occlusal position.

Feine and coworkers[146] have evaluated the mandibular kinesiograph, which is the forerunner of the previously described computed mandibular scanner. This instrument provided the clinician with a visual display of mandibular movement patterns. These workers compared recordings of opening and closing movements, closure from rest to incusation, and chewing movements on ten normal subjects with seven symptomatic patients. All of the symptomatic group had muscle complaints only, because patients with internal derangements were eliminated from the study. Feine's group concluded that mandibular movements of the symptomatic patients could not be differentiated from the control group and that "application of these invalid criteria to diagnose normal and abnormal function can lead to classification of normal subjects as dysfunctional."[146] Despite the controversy surrounding this equipment, it is used extensively in some craniomandibular practices.

The ADA Council on Dental Materials, Instruments, and Equipment has withdrawn approved status on all EMG equipment. At the ADA Workshop on Craniomandibular Disorders,[57] an ADA representative stated that approval was withdrawn not because of any problem with this equipment, but rather because it was termed experimental because of a lack of controlled scientific studies supporting its use.

It was further stated that because the ADA has no means of evaluating this equipment satisfactorily, the ADA Council on Dental Materials, Instruments, and Equipment chose not to endorse or condemn use of this equipment. Although it is true that at this time there is no conclusive evidence for or against this equipment, it is an area of rapidly expanding attention. In view of the historical lack of objective diagnostic information available on patients with TMDs, efforts to discover scientifically valid and reproducible diagnostic techniques should be encouraged. Clearly, more research is necessary.

TEMPOROMANDIBULAR JOINT REPOSITIONING THEORY

The TMJ repositioning theory proposes that a change in the condylar position within the involved TMJ will improve joint function and relieve symptoms. There are several variations of this theory.

Concentric Positioning Theory

This theory was proposed and extensively written about by Weinberg,[50,147,158] who postulated that proper mandibular function was predicated on being in "functional centric relation."

He stated that the definition of centric relation must include the position of the condyle within the fossa and its correlation with the occlusion.[158] Weinberg defined proper condylar position as concentric in the fossae when the teeth were in maximal occlusion. Evaluation of the condylar position was based on transcranial radiographs, which were believed accurate in their representation of the condylar position in the fossa.[50,147,155] Concentricity was measured by comparing anterior joint space and posterior joint space (Fig. 23–7). Weinberg described variations from the normal, including superior condylar displacement,[151] anterior condylar displacement,[152] and posterior unilateral[154] and bilateral displacements.[153]

Although Weinberg proposed occlusal recontouring to eliminate the deflecting occlusal contacts that caused the deviation from concentricity, he also discussed two types of splints that he used to reposition the condyle to a concentric location. In a situation in which a unilateral superior displacement existed, a unilateral, wedge-shaped repositioning prosthesis was suggested to lower the condylar position into concentricity.[154,158] Bilateral posterior displacement was usually treated by occlusal adjustment, but approximately 20% of posteriorly dysfunctional cases required an "anterior repositioning prosthesis,"[153,158] which was a maxillary appliance covering only the posterior teeth.

This theory has been criticized on the basis of its radiographic diagnosis. Transcranial radiographs have been shown to represent only the lateral third of the condyle. Aquilino and colleagues[159] evaluated three different lateral oblique transcranial techniques and stated that condylar position within the fossa is not constant at different sagittal locations within the joint. This finding agrees with the laminographic evaluation findings by Williamson.[160] It was also believed that joint space dimensions could not accurately be measured based on these lateral transcranial techniques. Other workers have agreed that transcranial views reveal only the relative position of the joint structures and are not direct measurements of joint space.[161–163]

Eckerdal and Lundberg[164] studied sagittally sectioned TMJ autopsy specimens and agreed that joint spaces differ among central, medial, and lateral areas.

Ownell and Peterson[165] took thin tomographic sections over the entire width of 27 TMJs and found variations in joint space and condylar position in 15.

Katzberg and colleagues[166] compared condylar positions between patients with internal derangements and those with arthrographically normal joints. They found no difference in position.

Pullinger and colleagues[167] used bilateral linear tomography on 46 healthy young subjects to assess normal condylar position. Their findings revealed that concentricity was found in only half of the subjects, with a wide range of variability. They concluded that nonconcentricity was not a valid basis for diagnosis. This study confirmed similar findings by Blaschke and Blaschke.[168]

The President's Conference on The Examination, Diagnosis, and Management of Temporomandibular Disorders, sponsored by the ADA in 1982, summarized this discussion by stating that there was insufficient evidence to

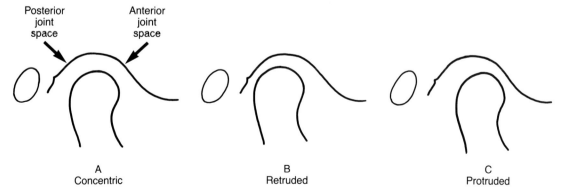

FIGURE 23–7. Normal and abnormal condylar positions as described by Weinberg.[158] *A*, Concentric condylar position. *B*, Retruded condylar position. *C*, Protruded condylar position. (Redrawn from Weinberg, L.A.: Int. J. Periodont. Restor. Dent. 5:11–27, 1985.)

support condylar fossae concentricity as a diagnostic sign of TMDs.[169]

At the ADA Workshop on Craniomandibular Disorders,[57] Mohl stated that there was no correct condylar position, but rather a range of correct positions. Owen has also written on an acceptable range of condylar positions.[173]

Christiansen and colleagues[174] performed computed tomography on 41 TMJs in 25 patients with known internal derangements. Each joint was evaluated at five equidistant sites across the width of the condylar head. Measurements of superior, posterior, anterior superior, and posterior superior joint spaces were performed. They concluded that the location of the condyle and variation of joint space depend on the type, direction, and extent of the meniscus displacement. They observed that decreased joint space can be extremely localized. Normal meniscus position results in constant joint space across the condylar head. Medial displacement results in increased superior joint space. Only anterior medial displacement resulted in an absence of joint space, which occurred most frequently in the lateral two thirds of the condyle.

A study by Jumean and associates[170] has readdressed the accuracy of transcranial radiographs. Seven cadaver heads were radiographed by tomography through the central, medial, and lateral aspects of the condylar head. Transcranial radiographs were subsequently taken. The specimens were then frozen and sectioned corresponding to the tomographic cuts.

The dissection specimens were photographed using black and white film, and these images were the controls. The two types of radiographs were traced by computer cursor, and the data analyzed by computer. When the data were evaluated, there was no significant difference in the lateral aspect of the joints between the tomographic cuts and the transcranial views. Neither radiograph was diagnostic for pathologic changes of the soft tissue of the joints. The tomographs were, however, easier to interpret because of their single plane. This study indicates that transcranial radiographs are an accurate method for evaluating the lateral aspect of the TMJ.

Anterior Repositioning for Treatment of Internal Derangements

Another variation of condylar repositioning theory has been recommended for the treatment of internal derangements. Internal derangements have been defined as "an abnormal relationship of the disc to the condyle when the teeth are in the intercuspal position. Usually the disc is displaced anteriorly and the condyle posteriorly."[175] Internal derangements were first discussed in the British literature in 1887 by Annadale.[176] In the early part of the century, British authors continued to discuss this problem.[177–179] Farrar has written on internal derangements and discussed the use of splints in order to change the mandibular position anteriorly and to normalize the relationship between the condyle and disc.[2,49,127,180]

Farrar and McCarty wrote that up to 80% of painful TMDs are due to internal derangements.[2,181]

Farrar's splint technique for reducing a displaced disc involves the placement of an appliance that has distinct fossa and bracing inclines designed to guide the mandible to a protrusive position in which the normal condyle/disc relationship could be restored (Fig. 23–8). Farrar usually preferred the use of maxillary appliances but used mandibular appliances in cases with severe Spee's curve or multiple missing mandibular teeth.[2] The protrusive position is maintained by the fossa and guiding inclines of the appliance, allowing no other position of closure. This method positions the condyle forward and re-establishes the proper condyle-disc relationship, eliminating the clicking and relieving the condylar pressure on the retrodiscal tissues. This technique is termed "recapturing the disc." The splint has to be worn full time, in order to maintain the disc position on the condyle. Farrar proposed that after a suitable period of healing, the splint could be eliminated and the occlusion corrected either by equilibration, orthodontics, or prosthetic treatment. Dolwick and Riggs[188] stated that anterior repositioning splints function to keep the disc in place so that

1. Soft-tissue healing and tightening of the discal attachments can occur
2. The disc may recontour
3. Osseous remodeling may occur.

Bell and Ware also described internal derangements as abnormal relationships between the condyle and disc and proposed the use of anterior repositioning appliances.[117]

Shortly after Farrar's article on internal derangements,[180] Wilkes published a technique for performing TMJ arthrograms that enabled visualization of the disc displacement.[112] Farrar and McCarty[183] and Katzberg and associates[184] followed with additional arthrographic studies.

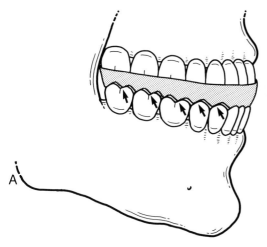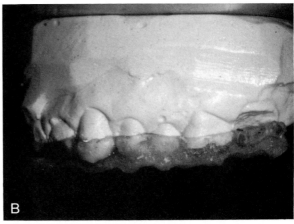

FIGURE 23–8. *A,* Maxillary splint with bracing inclines as described by Farrar and McCarty.[2] *B,* An example of the Farrar-type maxillary splint. (Courtesy of Dr. Bruce Sorrin, Kingston, New York.)

Farrar's technique of treatment of internal derangements by the use of a splint to reposition the displaced disc onto the condyle was made easier and more accurate by arthrography.

Manzione and associates[226] used arthrography to evaluate 56 patients who had previously been diagnosed by other dentists as having internal derangements; they were wearing splints of different types. Twenty-six of these were *not* successfully recaptured by their existing splints. The authors used arthrography to correctly position 23 of these 26 patients in order to successfully reduce their displacements. This important step established arthrography as a treatment tool, as well as a diagnostic instrument. It facilitated accurate mandibular repositioning in order to correctly reposition displaced intra-articular discs. Tallents and coworkers described the technique of arthrography-assisted splint therapy[185] and subsequently reported on its use in treating 82 patients.[186]

Many publications have discussed anterior repositioning appliances and their use in treatment of internal derangements (see Anterior Repositioning Splint Studies).

COGNITIVE AWARENESS THEORY

The cognitive awareness theory states that the presence of any splint in a patient's mouth is a constant reminder to alter previous behavior patterns.

If abnormal muscle activity results in occlusal contact on any type of splint, the intrusion on the patient's conscious awareness may be sufficient to decrease the activity. Wearing a splint may increase the patient's awareness of mandibular position and function, may change the oral tactile stimuli, and may decrease the oral volume, thus influencing the patient's perception about which positions or activities are harmful.[1,11,52]

The placebo effect obtained by wearing a splint may also play a large role. Greene and Laskin reported that some patients showed remission or improvement of their symptoms with the use of a nonoccluding appliance that did not modify the occlusal contacts or alter the mandibular position.[11]

Cassisi and colleagues[266] evaluated the effects of occlusal splints on night bruxism. A patient was fitted with an EMG device that measured bruxing episodes per unit time, as well as duration and amplitude of each episode. A maxillary full arch stabilization splint was compared with a nonocclusal splint and no splint. Interestingly, both splint types produced dramatic and repeated reduction in bruxism when compared with no-splint periods. The authors postulate that the nonocclusal splint reduced bruxism either by placebo means or because of nonocclusal stomatographic alteration, which Young has shown may affect freeway space.[267]

SPLINT USE

It is important to understand that splint therapy is a concept, not merely the introduction of a piece of acrylic. It is not a therapy that functions alone, but within the context of other treatment measures including physical therapy, medication, psychologic counselling, and other branches of dental care including restorative and orthodontic interventions.

Splint therapy should be performed with specific objectives in mind. The ideal splint should be comfortable, noninvasive, reversible, aesthetic, retentive, and functional. It should stabilize jaw relationships, provide desired occlusal patterns, and decrease abnormal muscle activity, parafunctional oral habits, and joint loading.

Unfortunately, no one splint type can satisfy all of these objectives. Many variations have been presented in the literature, each with specific advantages and disadvantages. Proper selection of splint type depends on an individual patient's needs and requests. Aesthetics and phonetics are important to all patients but may play a greater or lesser role depending on a pa-

tient's profession. Occlusal demands vary depending on the class and type of occlusion present. The presence and type of pathology influence the demands on the splint. Parafunctional habits of various types occur at different times of the day and night. The various requirements are often in conflict, and priorities must be discussed with each patient.

Above all else, splint selection depends on an accurate diagnosis. Muscular disorders without joint involvement have different requirements from internal derangements. Internal derangements differ in the extent of meniscus displacement, chronicity, and degree of pathologic tissue change (Figs. 23–9 and 23–10).

Mahan has noted that complex cases have both joint and muscle components and may require clinical trials, with various splints being diagnostic as well as therapeutic.[57]

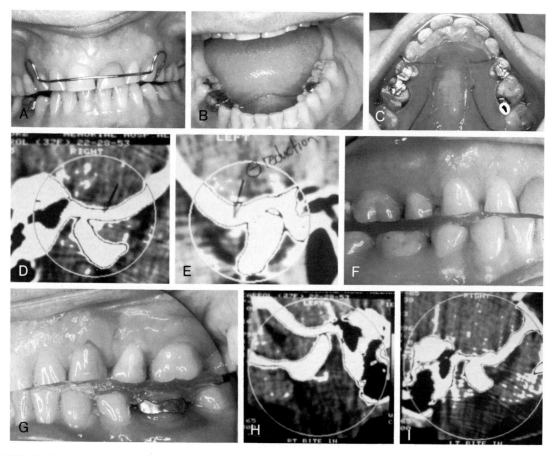

FIGURE 23–9. Patient referred after 10 months of splint therapy using anterior Hawley's and posterior occlusal grinding. *A,* Anterior view. *B,* Open view. *C,* Occlusal view. *D* and *E,* Computerized tomography (CT) of right and left temporomandibular joints (TMJs) reveals that splint therapy has not recaptured displaced discs. *F* and *G,* Right and left views of wax bite, which reduces displacements. *H* and *I,* CT views of TMJs confirm recapture.

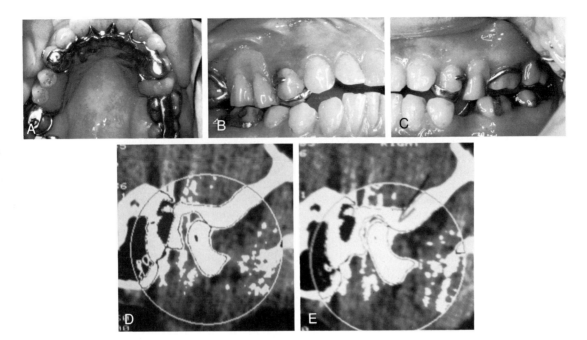

FIGURE 23–10. Patient with maxillary splint of unusual design was referred to evaluate whether discs were recaptured. *A, B,* and *C,* Maxillary splint in place. *D,* Computerized tomographic (CT) view of the left temporomandibular joint (TMJ) without splint reveals disc displacement. *E,* The CT view of the left TMJ with splint confirms recapture.

BRUXISM

Although the etiologic role of occlusion remains a subject of considerable debate, bruxism is generally accepted to be one of the primary contributing factors in TMDs. Pavone[313] has written that bruxism is the most prevalent, complex, and destructive of all dental functional disorders. Shore, and subsequently Ramfjord, postulated that it was occlusal interferences that acted as triggers, stimulating bruxism.[3,26,285,286] They further stated that precise occlusal adjustment would eliminate the habit (Fig. 23–11).

Other studies have indicated that bruxism is not initiated by occlusal factors. Kardachi and colleagues[287] and subsequently Bailey and Rugh[288] performed EMG examinations to evaluate changes in nocturnal bruxism after naturally occurring occlusal prematurities were removed. In both studies, no change in nocturnal bruxism was noted after occlusal adjustment.

Rugh and associates[290] introduced experimental occlusal discrepancies by placing gold

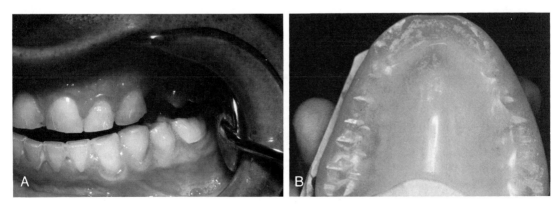

FIGURE 23–11. *A,* Severe bruxism with resulting tooth abrasion. *B,* Severe bruxism with resulting gouging of maxillary night splint.

crowns with deflective contacts on the molars of ten subjects. Nocturnal bruxism was monitored by surface electrode EMG measurements of masseter muscle activity. Nine of the ten subjects experienced a decrease in muscle activity after placement of the crowns.

The investigators agree with Glaros and Rao,[113] who believe that nocturnal bruxism is a sleep disorder related to the patient's waking emotional state. DeBoever[76] also introduced occlusal prematurities in order to create balancing side interferences. These resulted in no significant change in muscle activity. Dubner and colleagues[289] and Carlsson[291] suggested that the important factor is not the presence of occlusal interferences, but rather the patient's response. The very presence of the prematurity does not stimulate the patient to attempt to wear it down. Further, Zarb and Speck[29] suggested that establishing an occlusion that will not cause bruxism is not as important as creating an occlusal scheme that can best withstand the bruxism forces that are placed on it. Other investigators have also suggested that bruxism is not caused by occlusal factors.[293-295]

DeLaat[296] has reported on jaw muscle reflexes and discussed possible physiologic explanations for muscle hyperactivity. Other researchers have supported the view that muscle hyperactivity originates in the central nervous system,[10,297-301] with physical or psychologic stress being the primary cause.[298,302-304] Physical examination of patients with TMDs also demonstrates other known stress-related musculoskeletal, gastrointestinal, and biochemical disorders.[304-305] Experimentally produced stress has also resulted in increased jaw muscle activity.[295,306]

Despite these roles of stress and resulting psychologic distress among patients with TMDs, dentists have been shown to be poor evaluators of patients' psychologic status at clinical examination.[307] Patients are usually not aware of their parafunctional habits.[308-311,313] Unfortunately, practitioners are thus left attempting to control destructive parafunctional habits that are of questionable etiology, that are difficult to predict or measure, and that are often unrecognized by the patients themselves.

Nishioka and Montgomery[320] published a theoretic explanation of the pathophysiologic mechanism by which masticatory muscle hyperactivity may be induced. By evaluating studies of other extrapyramidal movement disorders, such as tardive dyskinesia and orofacial dyskinesias, these workers proposed that masticatory muscle activity (bruxism) is a subclinical imbalance of the neurotransmitter substances in the brain, specifically a dopamine hypersensitivity or hyperactivity or acetylcholine or gamma-aminobutyric acid (GABA) hypofunction. Masticatory muscle hyperactivity is characteristic of orofacial dyskinesias including tardive dyskinesias, as well as TMDs. Pharmacologic evaluation has suggested a neurotransmitter imbalance that is characterized by dopamine preponderance and cholinergic and GABA hypofunction in the basal ganglia. GABA agonists have an inhibitory effect on dopamine-neuron activity,[321] whereas GABA-mimetic drugs have improved the symptoms of tardive dyskinesia.[322-323] GABA agonist therapy (i.e., diazepam) can lower masseter EMG levels in symptomatic patients with TMD who have been diagnosed as having nocturnal bruxism.[324]

Anatomically, different areas of the striatum section of the brain have been identified as being involved with oral licking and gnawing.[328] Medications injected into the ventromedial part of the striatum inhibit gnawing, whereas injections into the anterodorsal portion of the striatum aggravate hyperactivity.[326] Researchers believe that the presence or absence of oral dyskinesia may depend on the biochemical balance between the anterodorsal and ventromedial striatal regions.[320] In addition, other neuroanatomic structures, such as the prefrontal cortex, the nucleus accumbens, and the amygdala, have the potential to regulate the activity of the dopamine system. The amygdala has been implicated in the mediation of stress,[327] and lesions of this structure affect the gnawing syndrome.[328] In addition, electrical stimulation of the amygdala initiates the jaw-closing reflex and stimulation of the sulcal cortex produces the jaw-opening reflex.[329] These workers propose that the amygdala-prefrontal cortex system may be involved in the relationship between stress and the resulting dyskinesias.[320]

Nishioka and Montgomery also believe that the role of occlusion is in concordance with this theory.

Animal research has shown that rats treated with neuroleptic medications exhibit repetitive, high-frequency clonic jaw movements.[330] In these sensitized rats, oral sensory stimuli cause increased muscle activity that has been attributed to increased release of dopamine.[331] One source of these stimuli may be occlusal prematurities. Other factors such as sound, light, and touch have been found to stimulate nocturnal bruxism in patients with symptomatic craniomandibular dysfunction.[332]

This study by Nishioka and Montgomery proposes that bruxism is a central nervous system disorder, which is stimulated in turn by local irritants such as occlusal discrepancies. This hypothesis accounts for both the occlusal theory, which has long been proposed as the etiology of bruxism, and theories that claim that psychologic status and stress are the primary etiologic factors.

Although hyperactivity has long been blamed for muscle symptoms,[316] it was not until 1988 that Wilkinson explained the biomechanics by which bruxism can lead to internal derangements of the TMJ.[312] During incisor clenching, both heads of the lateral pterygoid muscle are activated. When bruxism affects a canine, activation of the contralateral superior head of the lateral pterygoid muscle braces the anterior band of the disc, preventing the disc from rotating back on the condyle as it moves forward, resulting in stretching of the retrodiscal tissue.

In the ipsilateral joint, the disc is braced while the lateral pole of the condyle moves laterally and posteriorly, stretching the lateral discal ligament. This action results in a loosening of the joint and allows for a partial meniscal displacement to the anteromedial, exposing the lateral pole of the condyle, a situation frequently encountered at surgery. This situation explains the correlation between internal derangement and anterior bruxism facets. Wilkinson[312] postulates that anterior clenching may be a major etiologic factor in anterior disc displacement.

Because bruxism is apparently a major etiologic factor in TMDs, practitioners have initiated treatment to relieve symptoms and prevent further injury. Mikami[315] has listed the four treatment objectives for bruxism:

1. Reduce psychic tension
2. Treat signs and symptoms
3. Minimize occlusal irritations
4. Break neuromuscular habit patterns.

Splint placement is designed to fulfill three of these objectives.

Ramfjord and Ash[3] stated that a properly adjusted stabilization splint would reduce nocturnal bruxism. Solberg, Clark, and Rugh used EMG to evaluate patients with bruxism and agreed that splints decreased muscle activity during the period of their use.[280,316–317] Once splint use was discontinued, however, muscle activity returned to prior levels. For this reason, several investigators have recommended indefinite application of a night splint in order to prevent further injury.[187,274] Splint effectiveness at reducing muscle activity has been confirmed by Clark and coworkers,[284] Rugh and Solberg,[316–317] and Nevarro and associates.[318] Kydd and Daly,[319] however, also did an EMG study placing night splints in patients with bruxism and reported no difference in the amount of bruxism. The patients who wore splints did report greater comfort. This relief may be a result of better distribution of forces, as recommended by Zarb and Speck.[292] Another explanation is the decrease in joint loading resulting from the placement of a properly adjusted splint.[115,260–261,268]

STABILIZATION SPLINTS

The stabilization splint is the most commonly recommended type of splint. It has been called the supportive splint, Michigan splint, Ramfjord splint, flat plane splint, autorepositioning splint, and night guard. It is the splint of choice in cases in which the problem is neuromuscular rather than intracapsular. Ash[217] has stated that only stabilization splints are considered highly effective but reversible.

After the use of anterior repositioning for treatment of joint damage, patients are often returned to a stabilization splint for case completion or long-term night maintenance.[257]

Stabilization splints are fabricated to cover the entire arch and occlude with all of the opposing teeth (Fig. 23–12). They usually do not change the maxillomandibular relationship, other than increasing the vertical dimension. Studies have shown that up to 10 to 15 mm of interincisal opening causes rotation between the condyle and the disc, with little or no translation between the disc and eminence.[25,270] For these reasons, they promote stability of the dentition and the joint components and do not create occlusal or intracapsular changes.[57] Their benefits are limited, however, because anterior disc displacement (clicking) is usually not responsive to a stabilization splint.[11,21,271,272]

The ideal stabilization splint is unobtrusive yet strong and able to resist the severe forces imposed on it. It will maintain the stability of the teeth and not break. Thickness should be approximately 2 mm in the molar region.

Retention is achieved by intimate fit of the overlying acrylic with the underlying teeth and may be aided by carefully placed ball clasps.

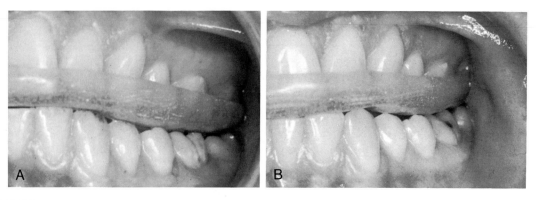

FIGURE 23–12. *A* and *B*, Maxillary stabilization splint as described by Ramfjord and Ash.[3] Maxillary, flat, full arch coverage.

The appliance should be stable, with full seating onto the teeth and no rocking. If the appliance resists seating or is too difficult to remove, the internal surface should be lightly relieved until it seats easily and then relined with a wash of acrylic directly on the teeth. During seating of the acrylic, the appliance should be removed and reseated every 30 seconds to prevent excessive retentive undercuts. Insertion and removal should be easily performed by the patient. During insertion, the splint should snap slightly into place, without excessive pressure on any particular tooth or group of teeth. Removal should be easily performed by the patient, but it should not be too easily dislodged or the appliance will constantly be dropping off the maxilla or raising up off the mandible during speech or function. Stabilization splints may be constructed for either maxillary or mandibular use.

The maxillary stabilization splint is flat, with slight indentations for the buccal cusp tips of the mandibular posterior teeth and lingual edges of the mandibular anterior teeth. Anterior and lateral guidance is created by fabrication of a 3-mm acrylic ramp facial to the lingual edges of the mandibular anterior teeth. The inclines are adjusted to be gradual and smooth, facilitating lateral and protrusive guidance. This arrangement functions to disarticulate the posterior teeth during lateral and protrusive excursion, thereby eliminating balancing or posterior protrusive prematurities. The maxillary stabilization splint has partial palatal coverage to increase strength and rigidity, to distribute clenching forces, and to prevent warping. This design may, however, create difficulty in swallowing or lead to a buildup of saliva under the posterior palatal aspect.

When these problems arise, the palatal aspect may be cut back and thinned until only the anterior third is covered. The maxillary stabilization splint is preferable because all of the mandibular teeth can contact an opposing flat surface. This is especially true when the patient has a considerable incisal overjet. The disadvantages of the maxillary splint are its visibility and effect on phonation (Figs. 23–13 and 23–14).

The maxillary appliance should be adjusted by having the patient close in habitual (centric) occlusion. Contacts should be uniform around the arch, with solid contacts of the opposing mandibular buccal cusp tips and somewhat lighter incisal edges. Protrusive and lateral excursion should smoothly ride up the anterior/canine inclines, resulting in posterior disocclusion. Only point contacts should remain on the posterior aspect of the splint, and all excursive or balancing contacts should be removed.

The patient should next be gently guided to retruded contact position, and the posterior occlusal contact points should also be even. A smooth, flat, anterior posterior slide should be established between the retruded and centric occlusion position. The resulting occlusal table will provide solid, even contact on clenching, access to retruded contact position in the event of bruxism, and anterior and canine-guided posterior disocclusion in the event of protrusive or excursive bruxism.

Maxillary stabilization splints can be fabricated with a palatal ramp, which prevents retrusion during night bruxism. This design is particularly useful following disc recapture or after surgical repair (Fig. 23–15).

The mandibular stabilization appliance is also flat and contacts the opposing palatal

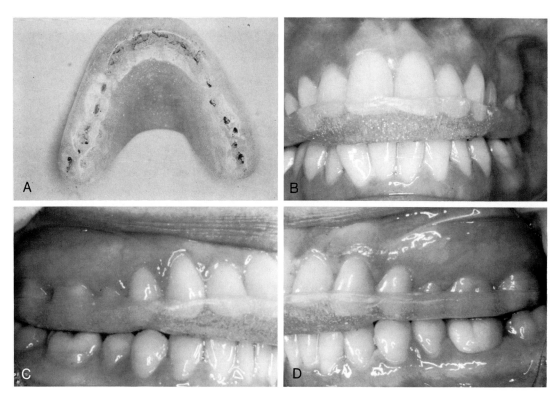

FIGURE 23–13. Maxillary stabilization splint. *A,* Occlusal view. Full arch coverage, flat plane, anterior guidance. *B,* Anterior view. *C,* Right view. *D,* Left view.

cusps of the maxillary teeth. The anterior facial aspect of the splint needs to be built up sufficiently to create lateral and protrusive disocclusion. This design is difficult to construct in cases of anterior overjet. The lingual flanges may be extended to increase strength.

Contours of both the maxillary and mandibular stabilization splints should be adjusted to

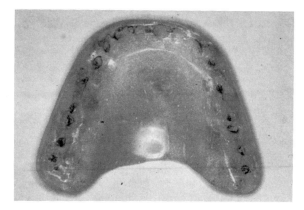

FIGURE 23–14. Maxillary stabilization splint, occlusal view, full arch coverage, flat plane splint, anterior guidance.

minimally affect speech, mastication, and aesthetics. They should extend 1 to 2 mm over the facial surface and be shaped and polished to prevent impingement on the cheeks or the tongue space. The maxillary appliance should be thinned palatally to allow for normal tongue placement, thereby minimizing speech interference and facilitating normal swallowing. The mandibular appliance should be thinned lingually, both anteriorly to facilitate speech and posteriorly to facilitate function. The mandibular lingual flanges can be hollowed out to slight concavity to increase tongue room and retention. Both should be contoured facially to minimize bulk, decrease the patient's awareness, and minimize cheek biting.

The mandibular appliance has a more difficult occlusal pattern because of the overjet of the maxillary anterior teeth. Habitual centric occlusion should result in even posterior contacts of the palatal cusps of the maxillary posterior teeth. Anteriorly, the facial/incisal edge must be brought out sufficiently to achieve slight anterior and lateral contact, enabling protrusive and lateral canine guidance. When there is considerable anterior overjet, this guid-

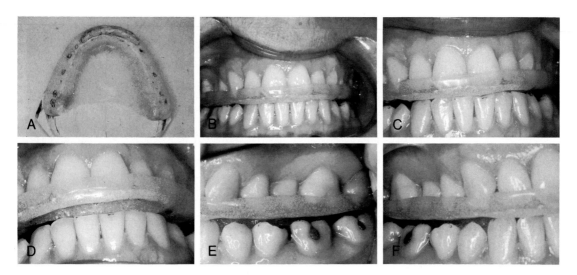

FIGURE 23 15. Maxillary stabilization splint, occlusal view, full arch coverage, anterior guidance, with a palatal ramp. A, Occlusal view. B, Anterior view. C, Protruded view. Note the posterior disocclusion. D, Retruded view. Note the palatal ramp prevents retrusion. E, Right lateral excursion. Note the canine guidance. F, Left lateral view. Note the canine guidance.

ance becomes difficult because a facial shelf must be created to achieve contact. This shelf is often uncomfortable, unsightly, and unacceptable to the patient. For this reason, mandibular splints often are extended only to the mandibular incisal edge and do not achieve anterior guidance with posterior disocclusion. Further, some mandibular appliances do not cover the anterior segment at all.[27] These are the most comfortable splints for patients because all anterior interference with speech, eating, and appearance is eliminated (Figs. 23–16 and 23–17). Because of incomplete arch coverage, however, anterior eruption or posterior depression may result in a change in the patient's occlusion. For this reason, many practitioners recommend the use of multiple appliances, which are less obtrusive during the day and more stabilizing at night (Fig. 23–18).[17,25,90,257,354,355] (See Complications of Splint Therapy.)

The flat occlusal surface of stabilization splints may be utilized to relieve the effects of occlusions that cause posterior mandibular position due to deflective contacts or deep bites with upright incisal inclinations. In these instances, flat splints often result in an anterior shift of mandibular position.

Posselt,[19] Ramfjord and Ash,[3] Laskin,[57] and Tsuga and colleagues[271] have stated that stabilization splints decrease joint loading and pain.

Mahan has described how increased joint loading squeezes the synovial membrane, de-

creasing the lubricating ability of the synovium.[57] The results are inflammation, pain, and stickiness of the joint, which may be etiologic for disc displacement or degenerative joint disease. Stabilization splints have been shown to decrease this joint loading.[115,261,268]

STABILIZATION SPLINT STUDIES

Clark[18] has stated that stabilization splints are the appliances of choice because they maintain and control tooth position. Greene and Laskin[11] treated 40 myofascial pain dysfunction (MPD) patients with stabilization splints and reported a decrease in pain in 65% of the patients. Agerberg and Carlsson[21] treated patients complaining of muscle pain and fatigue with stabilization splints and reported a 71% decrease in symptoms. Carraro and Caffesse[12] used stabilization splints as the only treatment for 27 patients with muscle symptoms; 85% of these patients were cured or improved. Muscle pain was the symptom that responded best to stabilization splint therapy.

Okeson and coworkers[13] treated 33 patients with TMDs employing stabilization splints and reported a decrease in pain in 28 of the 33 patients. They subsequently published another study on 24 patients with muscle and joint pain.[14] The patients were divided into a splint group of 12 patients and a relaxation group of 12 patients. The splint group received maxillary stabilization splints, which were worn at

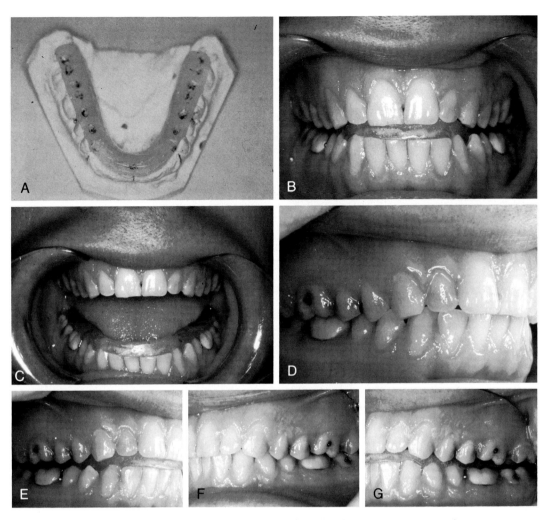

FIGURE 23–16. Mandibular stabilization splint. *A*, Occlusal view, full arch coverage, anterior guidance, posterior cusp tip contact. *B*, Anterior view. *C*, Open view. *D*, Right side, natural occlusion. *E*, Right side, splint in place. *F*, Left side, natural occlusion. *G*, Left side, splint view.

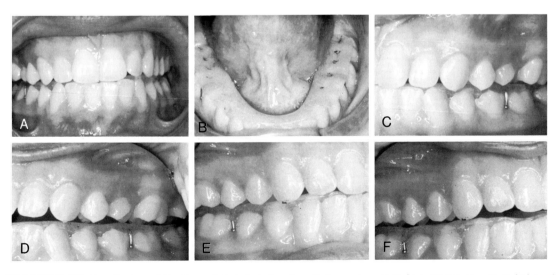

FIGURE 23–17. Mandibular stabilization splint. *A*, Anterior view. *B*, Open view. *C*, Right posterior view. *D*, Right lateral excursion. Note the canine guidance. *E*, Left posterior view. *F*, Left lateral excursion. Note the canine guidance.

415

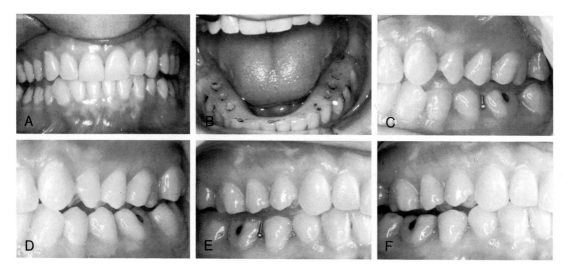

FIGURE 23–18. Mandibular stabilization splint, full arch coverage. *A,* Anterior view. *B,* Open view. *C,* Right posterior view. *D,* Right posterior view without splint. Note the posterior open bite. *E,* Left posterior view. *F,* Left posterior view without splint. Note the posterior open bite. Partial coverage splints have been implicated in causing posterior open bites by tooth intrusion. This case illustrates that a full coverage splint may cause similar changes.

all times except when eating. The second group was given a relaxation audiotape and were asked to listen to it daily. Patients were evaluated weekly for 4 to 6 weeks. The splint group experienced significant decrease in muscle pain and tenderness, as well as significant improvement in maximal opening without pain. The relaxation group showed no significant improvement.

Several long-term studies by Carlsson and associates confirm the effectiveness of stabilization splints. Eighty patients with masticatory disturbances were treated for 1 year.[273] Sixty-three patients received stabilization splints in addition to counselling, exercise, and occlusal adjustment. The remainder did not wear splints. Most splint patients had reduction of muscular signs and symptoms in five visits or less.

A followup evaluation on the same patients after 2½ years showed similar results with a 10% relapse rate.[274] Almost 50% of the patients continued to wear their splints 2½ years later. These investigators concluded that the results indicate ongoing etiology and the need for continued splint use to maintain control of the symptoms.

Another study was performed on 350 patients.[275] After 2½ years, 75% of the patients significantly improved and remained improved, according to a questionnaire that followed after 4 years.[276]

A 7-year study on 154 patients by Mejersjo

and Carlsson[277] showed that the majority of patients had total elimination of signs and symptoms, whereas the remainder had only minimal symptoms. Facial pain was greatly reduced, whereas clicking and crepitus were the symptoms least responsive. Joint noise may be representative of internal derangement and resulting degenerative joint disease. This conclusion agrees with the findings of other studies that state that stabilization splints are not as effective as anterior repositioning splints in treating internal derangements.[7,190,191,227,228]

Another study compared stabilization splints with biofeedback for the treatment of mandibular dysfunction.[278] After 1 year, both subjective and clinical symptoms were reduced in both groups.

Carlsson,[279] who has done extensive research in the field of TMDs, believes that the majority of patients will respond to stabilization splints, although patients with severe internal derangements may require other treatment, such as anterior repositioning or surgery.

Clark and coworkers have performed several studies evaluating the relationship between muscle pain, nocturnal muscle activity, and stabilization splints.[280,281]

In one study by Solberg and colleagues,[280] eight patients with bruxism habits were evaluated by EMG while wearing a stabilization splint at night. In all subjects, a statistically significant reduction in bruxism was noted.

In a subsequent study, Clark[281] treated 25 patients with MPD using maxillary stabilization splints. When evaluated with EMG, 52% had reduced nocturnal muscle activity levels.

Manns and coworkers[282] evaluated the effects of various vertical thicknesses of stabilization splints and the resulting changes in EMG activity. Sixty patients with muscle pain, severe tenderness on palpation, and dysfunction were divided into three groups. Electromyographic activity of the masseter muscles was recorded at baseline levels. All patients had maxillary stabilization splints fabricated. The first group had 1 mm of increased vertical dimension. The second group was raised half the distance between normal occlusion and the height of minimal EMG activity (mean 4.25 mm). The third group was raised to the height of minimal EMG activity (mean 8.25 mm). This approach agrees with a previous study by Rugh and Drago,[283] who found the mean height of minimal EMG activity to be an increase of 8.6 mm. The patients wore the stabilization splints for 3 hours during the day and all night. Electromyographic recordings were performed at five examinations over a 3-week period. The results in groups two and three showed a significant decrease in EMG activity, which declined further over time.

These workers postulated that at the vertical jaw postural position (centric occlusion), a certain amount of muscular tonic activity is necessary and normal. This means that a certain number of muscle fibers are active, and a certain number of sarcomere cross bridges are involved.

"In groups two and three, the increased vertical height of the splints lengthened the masseter muscle near its optimum physiologic elongation, where the highest number of sarcomere cross bridges between thin and thick myofilaments of its muscle fibers are available. Near the optimum muscle length, therefore, a lesser number of muscle fibers are necessary to provide a certain tonic muscle activity. In the muscular length corresponding to the postural mandibular position, there are fewer cross bridges, which means to provide the same tonic muscle activity, more muscle fibers and therefore more motor units must be recruited, thereby determining highest EMG activity."[282]

This explanation accounts for the finding of less EMG activity at increased vertical dimension of the splints. Their observations agree with several other studies that have suggested a decrease in muscle activity at higher vertical dimensions.[124,284]

ANTERIOR REPOSITIONING SPLINTS

The objectives of anterior repositioning splints are to regain the proper relationship between the condyle and the disc and to allow healing of the injured tissues, including the disc attachments.

Like stabilization appliances, anterior repositioning appliances can be fabricated on either arch. The main difference between stabilization and repositioning appliances is found on the occlusal surface. Repositioning appliances employ well-defined fossa, often aided by acrylic flanges or planes, to guide the mandible to a desired occlusion against the maxillary arch. By controlling the maxillomandibular relationship, the joint components can be repositioned with the objective of changing the condylar position relative to the disc, fossa, or both.

In the presence of an internal derangement, the disc is usually located anteriorly or anteromedially to the condylar head at closure. Repositioning appliances attempt to correct this relationship by changing the position to which the mandible closes, thereby also changing the condylar position at closure. The change is usually anterior, with the condyle being guided to a location that repositions it in the central bearing area of the disc.

It is hoped that joint and muscle pain will be diminished by repositioning the mandible to a location that guides the condyle back to a coordinated condyle/disc relationship. Anterior repositioning is maintained for a period of time sufficient for resolution of inflammation and healing. Subsequently, the condyle/disc assembly may be gradually returned to its normal (nonrepositioned) state, with the hope that condyle/disc integrity and coordination during function can be maintained. This approach is not always successful, and dysfunction may recur. Pain, however, does not always return with the dysfunction. Treatment planning decisions may be required regarding living with the nonpainful dysfunction as opposed to dental restoration in the repositioned state. (See the discussion in the treatment planning section at the end of this chapter.)

In order to maintain the recaptured condyle/disc relationship long enough for healing to occur, it is essential that the appliance be used full time, especially during function. For this reason, mandibular repositioning appliances are often chosen for daytime use. The mandibular appliance interferes less with aesthetics,

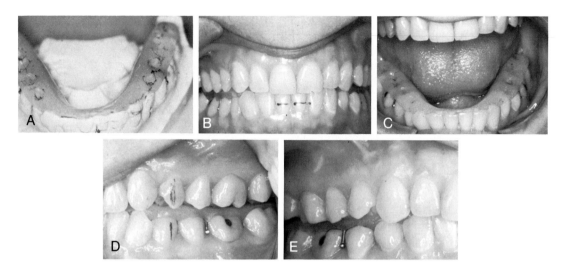

FIGURE 23–19. Mandibular anterior repositioning appliance, full arch coverage. *A,* Occlusal view. Note the deep fossae for repositioning. *B,* Anterior view. *C,* Open view. *D,* Right posterior view. *E,* Left posterior view.

phonetics, and mastication and is generally better tolerated for day use (Figs. 23–19 and 23–20).

Gelb has recommended a MORA, which covers only the posterior teeth.[27] Pertes[354] has suggested modifying this appliance by adding canine coverage, thereby facilitating lateral canine guidance during function. Williamson and Sheffield,[17] Clark,[118] Jankelson,[140] and Okeson[233,240] have recommended full mandibular coverage of all teeth to prevent changes in the occlusal plane and to promote stability of tooth position. The benefits of mandibular re-

positioning appliances are also limiting factors. The unobtrusiveness of the mandibular splint, which is due to its lack of bulk and anterior interference, is also responsible for its limited restrictive ability. During daytime use, the occlusal guidance created is usually adequate to direct the awake patient to the desired mandibular position. During sleep, however, parafunctional habits may result in greater lateral or posterior excursions, with resulting dysfunction and possible reinjury of joint structures.

Maxillary anterior repositioning appliances have the advantages of greater bulk and stabil-

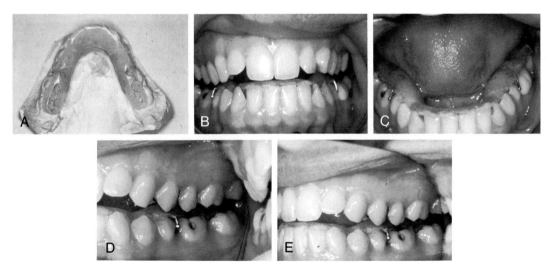

FIGURE 23–20. Mandibular anterior repositioning appliance. *A,* Occlusal view. Note the prominence of the anterior section to achieve guidance. *B,* Anterior view. *C,* Open view. *D,* Right posterior view. *E,* Left posterior view.

ity and therefore greater strength. Because the entire mandibular arch is encompassed, it is possible to fabricate a palatal flange or incline, which prevents retrusion of the mandible during closure. This approach has been recommended by Farrar and McCarty,[2] Mongini,[119] and Tallents and colleagues[185] because it more definitely prevents closure in an undesired position. Its problem, however, is lack of patient compliance due to its interference in daily living (Fig. 23–21).

A practical solution that employs the advantages of each type of appliance is the use of a mandibular splint during the day, in order to promote full-time use and to minimally interfere with the patient's daily activities, and the use of a maxillary splint during the night, to better protect against the potentially harmful effects of bruxism. Dawson,[25] Williamson and Sheffield,[17] Anderson and colleagues,[190] Messing,[257] Pertes,[354] and Nasedkin[355] all have discussed the advantages of this multiple appliance use concept.

The most important step in anterior repositioning therapy is establishing a proper diagnosis. The presence of an internal derangement must be determined, and the type and extent evaluated. Before an anterior repositioning splint can be fabricated, the specific position to which the mandible will be guided must be determined. Because the degree of tissue injury may vary, as well as the extent of tissue metaplasia dependent on the chronicity of the disorder, not all disc displacements are amenable to reduction or recapture. Some displacements may require only slight anterior positioning of the condyle in order to reduce the displacement to a normal condyle/disc relationship, whereas others may not reduce at all, even at maximal opening. When a reciprocal click is demonstrated, it is the closing aspect of the click that is most important in determining the ability to reduce the displacement. Because the closing click represents the displacement of the disc off the condylar head, the later in closure that it occurs, the better the prognosis. Conversely, the earlier in closure that it occurs, the farther the displacement of the disc, the greater the tissue damage, and the poorer the prognosis (Fig. 23–22).

A simply performed clinical evaluation of the suitability of anterior repositioning is to have the patient open widely, past the click indicating reduction of the displaced disc, and then close to an incisal edge-to-edge position. If on opening again clicking is still present, the disc cannot be recaptured at a splint position of edge-to-edge or less, and reduction would require a splint position with an anterior open bite. This situation, although possible, is diffi-

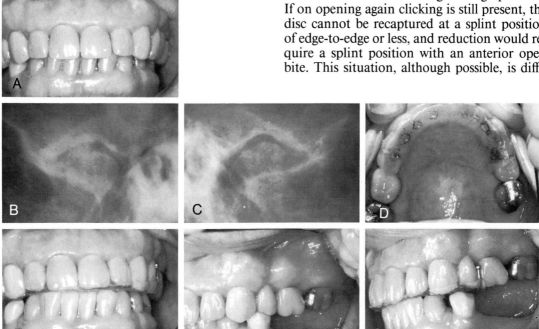

FIGURE 23–21. Maxillary anterior repositioning appliance. Patient would gag severely and couldn't tolerate lower appliance. A, Anterior view without splint. B and C, Transcranial films reveal significant osteoarthritis. D, Occlusal view: splint in place. E, Anterior view. F, Right posterior view without splint. G, Right posterior view with splint.

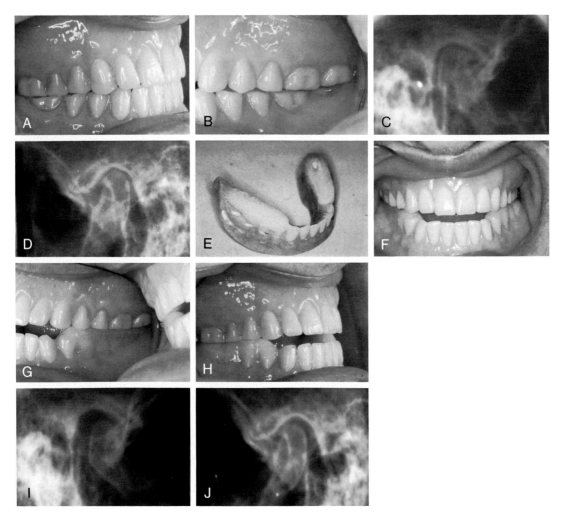

FIGURE 23–22. Mandibular full denture resurfaced as anterior repositioning splint. *A* and *B*, Right and left views of existing dentures. Note the severe posterior wear. *C* and *D*, Transcranial films reveal severe osteoarthritis and posterior/superior condylar position. *E*, Mandibular denture resurfaced to create anterior repositioning. *F*, *G*, and *H*. Denture in place. *I* and *J*, Post-treatment transcranial films. Note the anterior repositioning of the condyles.

cult to manage because of the anterior aesthetics or the possibility of anterior tongue thrusting, with accompanying occlusal changes. This assessment has certain limitations, because patients with deep or retrognathic occlusions have a great deal more condylar translation than prognatic patients or patients with little overjet/overbite. Excessive anterior repositioning may result. This method is, however, a guide that helps determine which patients may be repositioned at an aesthetically and functionally tolerable relationship.

The clinical method used to determine the therapeutic splint position is an extension of this technique. This therapeutic position is the smallest positional change from the centric oc-

clusal position at which the disc will remain in place during function. The patient is asked to open past the click (disc reduction) and subsequently to close on the incisal edges. If no clicking occurs on opening from this edge-to-edge position, then the desired therapeutic position lies somewhere between the original occlusion and the edge-to-edge position. A firm wax bite rim is softened and placed over the occlusal surface of the mandibular arch, and the patient again closes to the edge-to-edge position. The patient is then advised to slowly retrude the mandible, guiding the mandibular incisal edge up the palatal aspect of the maxillary incisors. When the closing click recurs, the patient stops, and the level of the maxillary incisal edge can be marked on the facial aspect of the mandibular incisors. A second line should then be marked 1 mm higher than the line representing the closing click. The wax should now be replaced with a new wax rim, and the patient again is asked to close, stopping at the higher line. If no closing click occurs, the wax bite should be removed, chilled, and replaced so that the position can be evaluated as a possible therapeutic position.

The patient should be able to start from this therapeutic position through all mandibular excursions without dysfunction. If clicking occurs, the bite should be opened additionally and the process repeated until a satisfactory therapeutic position is obtained. The resulting wax bite is used to mount the patient's study models in order to fabricate the desired splint (Figs. 23–23 and 23–24).

There are also difficulties with this technique. A retrognathic mandible with significant overjet will result in excessive condylar translation if the incisors are brought into contact. Patients will state that they feel that their mandible is strained when protruding to that degree. This situation may be solved by closure into the wax rim until a 2-mm thickness exists in the first molar region. The patient can then be "walked" posteriorly, in 1-mm increments, until the click returns. A measurement in millimeters of overjet can be taken and decreased by 1 mm, resulting in the minimal amount of anterior translation necessary to maintain recapture of the displaced disc.

Prognathic patients are the most difficult to treat with an anterior repositioning technique. Because the mandibular incisors are already positioned anteriorly without protrusion, any protrusion results in an aesthetically unsatisfactory situation. If the joint dysfunction cannot be eliminated with a stabilization splint, an attempt can be made to temporarily shift the mandible several millimeters to the contralat-eral side with a repositioning splint, in order to cause translation of the affected condyle and recapture of the displaced disc. This arrangement may be effective for a short time but frequently results in increased muscular symptoms that preclude this asymmetric position. Patients with a class III maxillomandibular relationship may then require surgery—either TMJ surgery to correct the internal derangement or orthognathic surgery to correct the interarch relationship, after which anterior repositioning may again be attempted if necessary.

Although clinically determined anterior repositioning is often effective, studies have revealed that clinical evaluation alone is often not accurate in assuring disc recapture. Techniques using MRI, CT, or arthrography can be employed.

Other situations may occur in which a displaced disc reduces during opening but is not amenable to recapture at a clinically acceptable therapeutic position. This click is then deemed to be nonrecapturable, and a treatment planning decision must be made to proceed with stabilization splint therapy, an attempt to treat "off the disc," or to proceed with TMJ surgery to reposition the displaced disc if possible.

As described in the section on anterior repositioning studies, anterior repositioning splints are effective because they reduce the direct trauma being imposed on the inflamed and edematous retrodiscal tissues, which have resulted from disc displacement. This concept may be extended to other situations in which the meniscus remains in position.

Some patients do not yet demonstrate internal derangements but exhibit posterior and lateral capsulitis, severe joint pain, and accompanying hypermobility indicative of damaged ligaments. These changes may result from chronic microtrauma and represent a stage in breakdown immediately before internal derangement. Apparently, although it is desira-

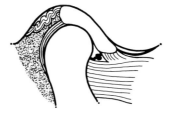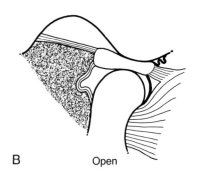

FIGURE 23–23. Normal joint function. *A,* Closed. *B,* Open.

A   Closed   B   Open

ble, it is not always necessary to achieve disc recapture to eliminate the painful symptoms in a patient with internal derangement.

Anterior repositioning for a short period (3 to 4 weeks) may be beneficial concurrent with physical therapy and medication efforts to decrease the inflammation of the joint components. This type of decompression splint is fabricated 1 to 2 mm thick occlusally in the first molar region and 2 mm protruded in order to provide slight condylar translation. When a patient has expressed relief of the severe joint pain, the appliance can be cut flat and resurfaced as a stabilization splint. If eliminating the anterior repositioning results in return of joint pain and inflammation, a maxillary anterior repositioning appliance can be fabricated for night use and for continued stabilization splint use during the day. It will protect the TMJs against harmful trauma resulting from retrusive bruxism at night. The day splint may eventually be eliminated entirely, and the patient maintained on the night appliance.

Although the short-term success of anterior repositioning splint therapy has been well documented, long-term success is more questionable. Clinical estimates made by workers in the field, as well as pilot studies, estimate that only 30 to 40% of displaced menisci are successfully repositioned permanently. Despite this, a much higher percentage of patients have relief of painful symptoms in the presence of ongoing joint dysfunction. This relief is due to the healing or adaptive capacity of the retrodiscal tissues.

IMAGING AS AN ADJUNCT TO ANTERIOR REPOSITIONING THERAPY

Initial therapeutic efforts to recapture displaced menisci with anterior repositioning splints were based on clinical findings. Auscultation and palpation of intracapsular clicking were thought to be diagnostic of condyle/disc dysfunction. Studies have shown, however, that although clinical findings were highly accurate in diagnosing the presence of internal derangements, they were less accurate in determining the type and extent of the displacement and whether or not the proposed splint successfully recaptured the displaced disc (Fig. 23–25).

Messing[356] presented a study in which 60 patients presenting with suspected TMJ internal derangements were evaluated clinically and with transcranial radiographs. After a diagnosis was made, reduction of the internal derangement was attempted utilizing a removable splint. The patients were subsequently referred for single-contrast arthrographic assessment of the repositioning appliance's ability to recapture the displaced disc. Arthrograms revealed that clinical diagnosis regarding the presence of an internal derangement was correct 92% of the time, whereas the type of internal derangement was correct only 76% of the time. Displacements without reduction exhibited joint sounds that were not representative of meniscus reduction, and displacements with reduction often failed to exhibit the anticipated joint sounds. Attempts at reduction of displacements with anterior repositioning splints were successful only 62% of the time. Of those not reduced, an additional 33% were successfully reduced using arthrography as a therapeutic aid. In addition, examples of degenerative joint disease, meniscal perforation and detachment, and ankylosis were diagnosed. This study illustrated that fabrication of an anterior repositioning appliance based solely on clinical findings was successful at recapturing the displaced meniscus only 62% of the time but that it could be greatly improved with arthrography.

Manzione and coworkers[226] published a study that evaluated splints that had been fabricated by various dental clinicians including an oral surgeon, a general dentist, an orthodontist, a periodontist, and a prosthodontist. A total of 56 patients presented for arthrography to evaluate splints that had previously been fabricated to treat craniomandibular symptoms. Of the 56 patients, only 26 (<50%) had successfully had recapture by splint placement. Manzione then described a technique of arthrographically guided splint registration, which was successful at recapturing 22 of the 26 displaced discs that had previously not been recaptured.

Roberts and coworkers[357] evaluated 205 patients clinically and radiographically employing tomography as well as arthrography. Their conclusions agree with those of the previous studies in stating that "clinical findings alone, or clinical findings in conjunction with plain radiographs of the TMJ, are not accurate enough for consistently successful treatment planning." They suggest that an imaging technique that evaluates the soft-tissue structures of the TMJ is necessary for improved success in treatment of internal derangements.

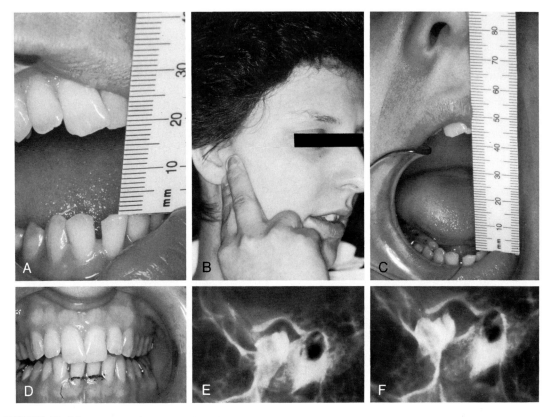

FIGURE 23–25. Patient with anterior disc displacement without reduction. Anterior repositioning splint is used to maintain disc reduction after manipulation. *A,* Severely limited opening. *B,* Manual manipulation results in reduction. *C,* Post manipulation, normal opening. *D,* Splint in place permits normal function. *E,* Arthrogram of locked right temporomandibular joint (TMJ), open view, before splint therapy. *F,* Arthrogram of TMJ after manipulation and placement of anterior repositioning splint. Note the reduction of disc.

Tallents and coworkers described arthrographically assisted splint therapy and reported on success at 6 months and again at 1 to 3 years after splint placement.[186,224,225]

Subsequent to arthrographically guided splint therapy, computed tomography (CT) was proposed as an alternative technique that would be noninvasive, faster, more easily performed, and able to evaluate both hard and soft tissues in one study involving less radiation exposure.

Helms and coworkers[358] initially proposed computer reformatted images of CT in order to create images of the soft tissues within the TMJ. Manzione and coworkers[359] subsequently developed a technique for direct sagittal CT of the TMJ. In a subsequent study, Manzione and colleagues[360] evaluated 51 patients with direct sagittal CT and presented a 94% accuracy rate in evaluating internal derangements. This accuracy was confirmed in a larger study by Manco and others, who evaluated 905 joints in

454 patients and showed a 91.8% sensitivity to joint pathology and an 87.3% accuracy rate in evaluating internal derangements using direct sagittal CT.[361]

Manco and Messing[362] subsequently published a study involving direct sagittal CT to evaluate anterior repositioning appliances. Although CT does not have the ability to observe joint dynamics as does arthrography, serial images allow appliance evaluation. Images are taken of original occlusion, maximal opening to determine if the meniscus reduces, and prospective splint position to evaluate possible splint recapture. If the displaced disc is not reduced at the proposed splint position, an incisal edge-to-edge view is taken to evaluate whether splint reduction is practical at a reasonable maxillomandibular relationship. Manco and Messing[362] evaluated 202 patients who had been referred for radiographic evaluation with anterior repositioning splints that were fabricated to recapture displaced discs. Of the 202 patients, 189 were confirmed to have internal derangements. Of these, 110 (58%) had successfully been reduced, and 79 (42%) were not recaptured. These results confirmed the previous findings, which indicate that clinical findings alone do not give sufficient information for accurate repositioning and illustrated the usefulness of CT in evaluating proper anterior repositioning therapy.

Computed tomography has also been used to evaluate the density of the disc. Manco and co-workers,[361] in their CT study of 905 TMJs, also discussed increased meniscal density in 14 cases that were evaluated histologically after surgery and found to be fibrotic. Two of these cases also showed foci of microcalcification.

Paz and coworkers[363] evaluated 76 discs in symptomatic patients to determine the tissue density of the discs. Density was compared between 52 discs known to be involved with internal derangements and 24 nonderanged discs. A statistically significant increase in tissue density was seen in the discs involved in internal derangements. These investigators postulated that this is representative of histologic change within the disc as described by Scapino,[238] Blaustein and Scapino,[247] and Bessette and coworkers.[365]

Further study may yield clues about which discs have undergone fibrotic changes and may help to predict whether they will respond to anterior repositioning therapy.

A third imaging technique helpful in assessing splint therapy is magnetic resonance imaging (MRI). Katzberg and coworkers[364] initially described the use of MRI to obtain diagnostic images of the TMJs. This technique allows for imaging of hard and soft tissues without exposing patients to radiation. Like the CT technique, it does not permit dynamic joint imaging as in arthrography, but serial visualizations allow images at closed, open, and splinted positions, making it possible to assess pathology in hard and soft tissues as well as possible disc recapture by an anterior repositioning splint.

ANTERIOR REPOSITIONING STUDIES

Farrar and McCarty noted that internal derangements often result in posterior positioning of the condyle, compressing and injuring the retrodiscal tissues.[2,235] This finding has also been described by Weinberg,[153,154] Dolwick,[236] and Eriksson and Westesson.[237] Scapino[238] performed histologic evaluation of three serially sectioned whole TMJs obtained at autopsy and 14 surgically removed menisci from cases of internal derangements. He described pathologic changes in the meniscus itself, including changes in gross form and internal collagen orientation and architecture, as well as pathology of the posterior attachment. Scapino described a compact mass or fibrosis in the anterior part of the posterior attachment, which he postulated was due to remodeling resulting from abnormal condylar loading. The venous channels of the posterior attachment were conspicuously dilated in one of these joint specimens.

Isberg and Isacsson[239] performed a study on monkeys, in which composite and cast gold restorations resulted in retrusive guidance of the mandible. After 5 weeks, histologic evaluation revealed thinning and flattening of the posterior band of the disc similar to that described by Scapino and an increased number of widened endothelium-lined vessels throughout the posterior attachment. These investigators postulated that abnormal condylar pressure on the retrodiscal tissues caused release of biochemical mediators that cause vasodilation.

In a subsequent study, Isacsson and colleagues[240] evaluated the loss of conscious control of mandibular direction found in patients with internal derangements. Fifty patients were evaluated on their ability to move their mandibles laterally to an instructed position. Of the 50 patients, 22 failed to do so. Subsequent arthrographic evaluation revealed that 18 of the 22 had disc displacements without reduction, and the other four had disc displacements that reduced on opening. These workers attributed this loss of control to the fact that mechanoreceptors are not evenly distributed in the TMJ capsule but are concentrated in the anterior and posterior regions.[241] These mechanoreceptors are the principal source of perception of the mandibular position and movement, and they exert coordinated reflex effects on the mandibular muscles.[241-246] Isacsson and coworkers proposed that when internal derangement occurs, the vascularized and innervated posterior disc attachment and posterior capsule are pulled forward between the bony joint components and torn or compressed.[238-240] The resulting tissue damage is likely to include the mechanoreceptors. In several patients, when anterior repositioning was performed, coordination returned.

Blaustein and Scapino[247] further evaluated the remodeling changes that occur subsequent to internal derangement (see Off the Disk Treatment).

McNeil[29] discussed the use of anterior repositioning appliances to properly align the condyle and disc and reduce severe loading of the TMJs. He favored mandibular appliances because of their better aesthetics and greater patient compliance. After a suitable healing period of up to 6 months, McNeil suggested attempting to remove the appliance and performing occlusal adjustment, returning the condyle/disc assembly back into its physiologic position in the fossa.

Graber[189] wrote about the neuromuscular response to anterior repositioning, stating that "the condyle is brought forward in the fossa, and the neuromusculature may adapt to the new position, aided by occlusal interdigitation in habitual maximum contact, a new learned neuromuscular pattern or engram, and the filling in of compressed retrodiscal pad, when it is no longer being traumatized by the condyle."

Clark treated 25 patients with internal derangement using anterior repositioning splints.[7] Of the 14 patients who completed the treatment regimen, 12 patients (86%) reported by questionnaire that they had moderate to highly successful results. Of the 11 patients who discontinued anterior repositioning treatment, six were treated with stabilization-type (nonrepositioning) splints. Only one of these patients reported a moderate to highly successful treatment result. Clark[7] reported that the repositioning appliance therapy was much more successful than the treatment given to patients who did not have successful repositioning.

Anderson and coworkers[190] divided 20 patients with internal derangements into two groups and treated them with maxillary flat plane (stabilization) splints or anterior repositioning splints. After a 90-day period, the patients who had been treated with anterior repositioning splints experienced significant reduction in subjective and objective symptoms of internal derangements. The patients using stabilization splints experienced no significant change in dysfunction level. Two of these patients with nonrepositioning progressed to the closed lock (displacement without reduction) state.

Lundh and associates[191] evaluated 70 patients with internal derangements. Patients were divided into an anterior repositioning group, a flat plane splint group, and a control group without splints. Both splint groups had reduced joint tenderness, but the group with

anterior repositioning had greater reduction in joint dysfunction and greater decrease in muscle tenderness.

Ito and colleagues[192] studied the ability of the anterior repositioning appliance to maintain condyle/disc coordination during chewing. They treated a patient having a unilateral reciprocal click with a maxillary repositioning appliance. Using the Replicator System[193–195] to measure and record condylar motion, they evaluated whether the position of the "recaptured" disc was maintained during chewing fibrous food. When the subject chewed on the side of the healthy joint, the disc remained in place and no dysfunction was observed. When the subject chewed on the side of the internal derangement, dysfunction occurred during 25% of the mandibular closure. This study indicates some of the limitations of anterior repositioning appliances and why they are not always successful. It also emphasizes the need for carefully educating patients about precautions to be taken during splint therapy.

Bewyer[258] has described the intracapsular synovial pathologic changes that accompany internal derangements. Fibrous adhesions limit the normal translatory movement, resulting in decreased sliding movement in the superior joint space and increased rotational movement in the inferior joint space. The meniscus therefore stays more inferior on the slope of the eminence rather than in its normal superior position.

Anterior repositioning may temporarily place the condyle back under the central bearing area of the meniscus. However, if the meniscus is not freely translating with the condylar head, the condyle/disc assembly will not function normally, and dysfunction will be avoided only as long as anterior positioning is maintained. Subsequent attempts to return the condyle/disc assembly superiorly on the slope of the eminence will be unsuccessful because of the lack of meniscal translation.

Williamson and Sheffield[17] evaluated 300 patients who had internal derangements treated with anterior repositioning appliances. After symptoms had been eliminated, the patients were switched to a superior repositioning appliance that guided the condyle/disc assembly back to the superior part of the fossa. Those patients who suffered a relapse were given the choice of continued anterior repositioning or arthroplasty.

Three to 5 years after completion of treatment, patients were asked to grade themselves on pain, dysfunction, and remaining symptoms. The patients were re-examined, and dysfunction was graded by palpation and auscultation. Some 270 patients (90%) stated that they were pain free and in a functionally satisfactory state. Of the remaining 30 patients, 28 were pain free while using the anterior repositioning appliance. Symptoms returned when splint use was discontinued.

Owen has written a series of articles discussing the treatment of internal derangements utilizing anterior repositioning appliances.[173,197,198]

Many other published reports have suggested various anterior repositioning splints in treating patients with internal derangements.[119,199–205]

Lundh and coworkers[210] performed a roentgen stereophotogrammetry study on seven subjects to evaluate changes in the mandibular position relative to the maxilla, after mandibular repositioning to recapture a displaced disc, and over a subsequent 6- to 9-month experimental period. The roentgen stereophotogrammetry technique is an accurate means of studying the motion of bones in three dimensions.[211–213] In this study, cast metal overlays were cemented on the posterior teeth to maintain the position of recapture, rather than an acrylic splint. This was done to assure that any measured movement was actually skeletal, rather than movement of the splint on the teeth. The difference in mandibular position between the untreated and repositioned states was shown to be greatest in the vertical rather than the horizontal direction. A mean change of 2.5 mm was observed in the mandibular vertical direction, whereas only a 0.5-mm protrusive change was seen. These workers postulated that this finding was due to the 3-mm thickness of the posterior band of the disc being successfully interposed between condyle and fossa.

When the subjects were re-evaluated 6 to 9 months later, a large degree of horizontal relapse was observed (70 to 80%), whereas a small change in the vertical plane was observed (12%). This study showed a wide variation in positional changes necessary to reposition a displaced disc. Unlike many previous publications that had emphasized the protrusive component as the most important factor in recapturing the disc, this article identified the significant vertical component and its stability over time. At the end of the study period, five of the seven patients had maintained disc recapture. These investigators attribute the horizontal relapse toward the original mandibular

position to muscle pull, as documented in experiments with adult rhesus monkeys.[206]

Several workers have suggested that excessive anterior repositioning may result in pathologic remodeling of the condyle.[118,152,206–208] Others state that the observed remodeling may be constructive, as seen after orthognathic surgery[214,215] and after healing of a fracture.[216]

McNamara[259] studied rhesus monkeys to evaluate the long-term effects of anterior repositioning on condylar and meniscal tissue. The Herbst appliance was employed to protrude the mandible 3 mm and the osseous and meniscal changes at 3, 6, 12, and 24 months were observed. McNamara observed some adaptive thickening of the condylar cartilage but no pathologic changes of the disc, condyle, or fossa.

Several publications have discussed depression of the posterior teeth as a result of anterior repositioning appliances.[25,217–219] This is most often seen when the appliance does not cover all of the teeth in the arch on which it is worn. Clark[118] has stated that restoration to a functionally acceptable occlusion after mandibular repositioning may be difficult and expensive. Winklestern showed examples of posterior tooth depression and restorative correction of the problem.[220]

Lundh and coworkers[227] employed arthrographic guidance to anteriorly reposition 20 cases of internal derangements. After 6 months of treatment, the repositioning overlays were removed, and all of the patients demonstrated posterior open bites. The patients were followed for several additional months, and in all cases, the open bites gradually decreased and the ongoing intercuspal positions were re-established. These results indicate that the posterior depression is reversible and can be treated by passive eruption. Farrar and McCarty,[2] Gelb,[27] Witzig and Spahl,[196] and Owen[173] have also described passive eruption to close this posterior open bite.

Other researchers study combinations of appliances, alternating day and night use, to prevent posterior tooth depression.

Dawson[25] has written, "It is not acceptable to alter an occlusion to conform to a forwardly positioned condyle. Unless the superior position is achieved and confirmed, the long-term stability will be compromised." This statement is in disagreement with many proponents of the anterior repositioning theory.[2,5,7,27,29,119,131,132,151–158,173,181,196–201,209]

Short-term success of anterior repositioning has been discussed extensively, but long-term results are less clear.

Clark[7] reported 1- to 3-year followup on 14 patients who had been treated with anterior repositioning therapy, and he reported an 86% success rate.

Maloney and Howard[221] reported on 241 patients who had been diagnosed as having internal derangements. After 6 months of treatment, they were weaned off the anterior repositioning splints. Patients who demonstrated bruxism continued to wear stabilization splints at night. Treatment is considered to be successful when patients

1. Are free of pain
2. Have been weaned from the anterior repositioning appliance
3. Are free of clicking, locking, or catching
4. Demonstrate a pain-free range of motion.

Patients were evaluated at 1, 2, and 3 years after treatment. After 1 year, 70% of the patients were symptom free. By the end of the second year, the number of asymptomatic patients had dropped to 53%, and it continued to drop to 36% by 3 years. Correlation of treatment success with length of time of pretreatment clicking revealed that only 8% of patients with a long-term history of clicking (greater than 1 year) had a successful result, whereas 80% of patients whose click was present less than 1 year had a successful result. This effect may be due to the metaplastic changes that occur within the chronically displaced disc.[221–222] Correlation of success with severity of disc displacement also revealed decreased success as the extent of the displacement increased.

Williamson and Sheffield[17] reported on 300 patients 3 to 5 years after the completion of anterior repositioning therapy. Their results were based on a questionnaire in which patients described their present state on a scale of one to ten. Some 79% of the patients described themselves as eight or better, and 90% as six or better (functional and comfortable). Of the 30 patients who had not achieved pain relief, 28 had been asymptomatic while wearing the anterior repositioning appliance.

Tallents and coworkers[186,224] evaluated 51 patients who had previously undergone arthrographically assisted splint therapy. After 6 months, 88% of the patients had successfully maintained the condyle/disc relationship. Two

of the six patients who did not maintain disc recapture had progressed to displacement without reduction (closed lock). Both of these patients had expressed a history of intermittent locking before treatment was initiated. In a subsequent study, Tallents and coworkers[225] followed 68 patients for 1 to 3 years after arthrographically assisted splint therapy of internal derangements. Another 18 patients with displaced discs decided against anterior repositioning therapy and served as untreated controls. Re-evaluation occurred 1 to 3 years after repositioning. Twelve patients (17.7%) progressed to a closed lock state requiring arthroplasty, and four others had recurrent clicking. Two other patients had inadequate resolution of pain. Fifty of the 68 treated patients (73.5%) remained successfully treated. Of the 68 treated patients, 27 (39.7%) stated that they were aware of joint sounds, but there was no sign of disc displacement at followup examination. This finding may be a suggestion of other joint pathology, such as degenerative joint disease. Statistical evaluation revealed that anterior repositioning treatment was significant in reducing TMJ pain, temporal headache, ear pain, and pain in front of the ear, and decreased the possibility of closed lock.

Lundh and coworkers[191] have conducted several studies that give indications of long-term results of anterior repositioning. In one study, 70 patients with internal derangements were divided into an anterior repositioning splint group, a flat stabilization splint group, or an untreated control group. Treatment was limited to 2 months, after which time the splints were eliminated. After the initial treatment period, the anterior repositioning group had superior results in eliminating joint dysfunction and reducing muscle tenderness. Two months after the splints were eliminated, no significant difference was noted between treatment groups or between original and post-treatment symptoms. This may mean that the results lasted only as long as the splint was worn, *or* it may mean that the treatment period did not last long enough for adequate joint healing to occur.

In their previously mentioned stereophotogrammetric study, Lundh and associates[210] allowed anterior repositioning treatment to continue to 6 to 9 months. Despite the relapse in horizontal position, five of the seven patients remained asymptomatic. The longer treatment period or the gradual nature of the return to a more posterior position may be responsible for maintaining the asymptomatic state.

In a third study, Lundh and associates[227] placed 63 patients with known internal derangements into three groups. All were diagnosed using arthrograms. The group with anterior repositioning was positioned arthrographically, in the manner described by Manzione and colleagues[226] and Tallents and coworkers.[185] Cast silver anterior repositioning appliances were placed to capture displaced discs. The second group received flat occlusal splints, as described by Posselt.[19] A third group received only counselling.

After 6 months of treatment, the group with anterior repositioning had significantly less pain and dysfunction than either of the other two groups. Palpable tenderness in both the joints and the musculature was also least in the group with anterior repositioning. No significant difference was observed between the flat splint and control groups. The overlays and splints were removed, and the patients followed for 2 additional months. All symptoms returned in all but one patient during a period of 6 months after the removal of the overlays. Apparently, the increased length of treatment time did not improve the long-term result. The repositioning, however, was abruptly withdrawn, rather than gradually returning to the previous occlusion.

Lundh and Westesson[228] published a report on long-term followup on 15 patients who had been treated to an anterior position 1 to 7 years earlier. All of the patients had been previously diagnosed as having internal derangements. Before anterior repositioning, these patients had been unsuccessfully treated with flat splints, physical therapy, occlusal adjustment, counselling, and medication. Some of the patients had anterior repositioning splints, and others had cast silver onlays placed to define an anterior position. Three of the patients had been diagnosed as having anteriorly displaced discs without reduction; however, during arthrography, the joints were manipulated[2] and the discs successfully repositioned onto the condyle. The anterior repositioning appliance was then fabricated to maintain this position of reduction. The remaining 12 patients had displacements with reduction, and the anterior repositioning devices were fabricated to the therapeutic position of reduction.[185,226]

The patients wore their anterior repositioning devices for a treatment period of 6 to 32 months (mean 10 months). Subsequently, after

symptoms had been eliminated, 11 patients had prosthodontic restoration of their occlusion to the therapeutically derived position, and four patients had occlusions stabilized by orthodontic therapy. The patients were then re-examined at 15 to 86 months (mean 41 months), after completion of treatment. Clinical and radiographic evaluations were performed. Eleven of the 15 patients had corrected sagittal tomography[229,230] and double-contrast arthrography[231,232] performed in order to accurately assess meniscal position and function.

Tomography revealed osseous changes such as flattening, sclerosis, and osteophytes in three patients. Progressive remodeling of the posterior surface of the condyle was seen in two patients. Arthrography revealed that nine of the 11 patients had successfully maintained the therapeutic condyle/disc relationship. One patient had a medial displacement with reduction, and one patient had an anterior displacement without reduction. Neither of these two patients had undergone positioning using arthrography.

Clinically, none of the patients had pain, either subjectively or on joint palpation. Only one patient required occasional use of analgesics. Palpable tenderness of the musculature was greatly reduced from the initial examination. Horizontal and vertical change was measured by incisor overlap. Before repositioning, the median horizontal overlay was 3 mm. This had been reduced to 2 mm (median) by anterior repositioning but had returned to 3 mm at the re-evaluation. Vertical overlap had originally been 5 mm (median), had been reduced to 2 mm (median) by repositioning, and had relapsed slightly to 3 mm (median). These relapse patterns are similar to those of the earlier study.[210] Despite the relapse, condyle/disc integrity was maintained in nine of 11 patients evaluated radiographically, and pain elimination was maintained in all patients. The abrupt return of symptoms previously noted when anterior repositioning was rapidly discontinued was not seen,[191,227] possibly because of the gradual nature of the relapse. In addition, despite the ongoing displacement in two of the patients, their pain symptoms were also relieved by the anterior repositioning. It appears that replacement of the disc onto the condyle may not be absolutely necessary and that a protrusive change in condylar position may be sufficient to give relief of symptoms in some cases.

Okeson conducted a study evaluating longterm followup of patients treated with anterior repositioning.[233] Forty patients with internal derangements were divided into three groups depending on their diagnosis:

1. Those with disc displacement that reduced during opening
2. Those with disc displacement without reduction that could be manually manipulated to reduction
3. Those with disc displacement without reduction that could *not* be manually reduced.

All of the patients were treated with anterior repositioning splints for a period of 8 weeks. Subsequently, the patients were gradually returned to the original occlusal relationship over a 2- to 4-week period. The patients were re-examined after 21 to 48 months (mean 29 months).

Okeson found that after the initial 2-month period of anterior repositioning, 80% of the patients were free of pain, clicking, or catching. When he evaluated the patients 2½ years later, 65% had a return of joint clicking. Despite the clicking, only 25% had pain. Some 48% had reduction of headaches, and tenderness to muscle palpation had been reduced from 65% originally to 30% at followup. Of these patients, 79% showed an increased comfortable range of opening, and only 9% stated that joint pain was worse.

Despite the fact that 65% of the patients had return of joint clicking, only 25% had pain. When the patients were asked whether the treatment had improved or cured their symptoms, 80% responded positively.

Okeson discussed an important question—how do we define success? If success requires elimination of all pain and dysfunction, then the 25% success rate of Okeson agrees with the success rate of Maloney and Howard.[221] This total elimination of all symptoms may represent those patients in whom joint healing had successfully resulted in re-establishment of a healthy condyle/disc assembly at the original occlusal relationship. Farrar stated that he expected this result in only 30% of his cases.[2,127] McNeil[5] estimated 30 to 40% successful recapture of displacements, and Rugh and Solberg[317] predicted 25% long-term success.

If, however, relief of pain and acceptable function are the criteria for success (though clicking may persist), the success rate is much higher. Okeson found that even though only a third of the patients retained the displaced disc, three fourths had pain relief and believed that treatment was successful. Similarly, Lundh and colleagues[210] found that despite the horizontal

rebound in his patients who had undergone repositioning, painful symptoms did not return.

Tanaka[57] reported on 232 patients with internal derangement treated conservatively without success and then undergoing arthroscopy. Subsequent MRI evaluation revealed that 94% of these patients had displaced discs, yet they were pain free.

Apparently, although it is desirable, it is not always necessary to achieve disc recapture to eliminate painful symptoms in patients with an internal derangement.

OFF-THE-DISC TREATMENT

Mohl[248] described the functional anatomy of the TMJ, as well as the histology of the articular structures including the cartilage. With increased loading, the cartilage demonstrates the presence of chondrocytes, lacunae, and proteoglycans characteristic of cartilage matrix. These proteoglycans are responsible for a cushioning effect on articular surfaces. The spatial arrangement of the proteoglycan-collagen network and the ability of the proteoglycans to imbibe and retain extracellular water by osmosis help the load-bearing surfaces resist compressive forces.[249] The proteoglycans responsible for this are sulfated long carbohydrate chains called glycosaminoglycans (GAG). The pressure and amount of GAG relative to its collagen matrix in articular tissues is a measure of the resilience of the tissue and of the location and degree of compressive loading in a joint.[248,250,251]

Kopp, employing special staining techniques, performed critical electrolyte concentration studies on discs and retrodiscal tissues.[252,253] These studies distinguish compression and noncompression areas in soft tissue. In the healthy TMJ, the sulfated GAG were found mainly on the anterior part of the condyle, in the central portion of the disc, and on the articular eminence. They were not characteristic of the posterior attachment area, which is normally not subject to compression.

Blaustein and Scapino[247] evaluated remodeling changes that occur subsequent to internal derangement. They evaluated specimens that consisted of disc and posterior attachment material that had been removed by meniscectomy in patients suffering from internal derangements. Histories, previous treatment records, and arthrotomograms were available on all specimens. The only specimens included were those in which the posterior attachment was confirmed by arthrotomography to be under load as a result of an anteriorly displaced disc. Because remodeling made it difficult to distinguish the normally, clearly defined boundary between the posterior band of the disc and the posterior attachment, specimen areas were identified as the "presumptive posterior attachment" and the "presumptive posterior band." Only those specimens in which the investigators could clearly identify these regions were included in the study.

Evaluation of critical electrolyte concentrations was performed in the manner of Scott and Dorling[254] and Scott.[255] The concentration and location of GAG were determined in each specimen. Similar critical electrolyte concentrations were found in the presumptive posterior band and in the presumptive posterior attachment.

These findings indicate that the retrodiscal tissue, which is not normally under load, when subjected to abnormal compressive loading secondary to anterior disc displacement, may remodel by producing collagen-containing sulfated GAG. The compressive stiffness of the abnormally loaded tissues is thus increased. As the Blaustein and Scapino study states, it is not known whether retrodiscal tissue will always exhibit this remodeling response.

This ability of the retrodiscal tissues to adapt when loaded may be the reason why patients remain pain free after they have been treated with anterior repositioning splints and subsequently returned gradually to a normal mandibular position. It also accounts for the fact that the pain-free state can be maintained in spite of continued joint clicking, indicating ongoing disc displacement. It may also enable patients to be treated off the disc in those cases in which the extent of the disc displacement prevents recapture by anterior repositioning.

Dawson stated, "If an anterior repositioning splint directs the condyles to a joint position that does not align with the disk, it will increase the damage to the connective tissues and do intensified harm to the vascular retrodiskal tissues."[25] Thus Dawson disagrees with others who, in the event that a displaced disc cannot be recaptured, treat off the disc to a slightly protruded position.

Guichet stated that if reduction of a displaced disc cannot be recaptured at the 4-7 position as described by Gelb.[27,132] the patient should be treated to the position of maximum comfort.[256]

Weinberg[158] treated posteriorly displaced condyles by occlusal correction to allow anterior positioning of the mandible without increasing the vertical dimension. He relieved the anterior inclines of the mandibular teeth, the posterior inclines of the maxillary teeth, and the palatal aspect of the maxillary incisors. This method allowed anterior positioning of the mandible but did not recapture the displaced disc. Weinberg nevertheless reported an 80% success rate.

McNeil remarked that it is not necessary to recapture every displaced disc.[5] He described the ability of the retrodiscal tissue to become avascular and noninnervated and to act as articulating tissue both pain free and with relatively normal function. He stated, "There are a large number of patients that can be successfully managed off the disk."[5]

Messing[257] presented a treatment flow sheet describing the steps of splint management for several craniomandibular disorders. In cases of internal derangement in which the disc is not recapturable, the patient is treated off the disc with a decompression splint. Slight anterior repositioning is performed to allow for a healing period so that inflammation may be reduced and healing and adaptation can result.

Okeson's study describing long-term followup of anterior repositioning showed that although 65% of the patients had a return of joint dysfunction after 2½ years, only 25% had pain, and only 9% had pain that was worse.[233] The majority of patients had joints that successfully adapted to the dysfunctional state.

Tanaka discussed the change in shape of the displaced disc, which often makes it impossible to recapture or reposition it. In a study of 232 patients, Tanaka reported that despite resolution of pain, 94% of meniscal displacements remained displaced (see Figs. 23–24 and 23–26 to 23–29).[57]

JOINT LOADING

One factor that plays a role in all splint usage is joint loading. MacDonald and Hannam evaluated occlusal contacts and muscle activity during clenching and determined that anterior contact without posterior support resulted in increased temporal muscle activity and increased TMJ loading.[116,260] As the occlusal contact point moved posteriorly, they observed decreased masseter muscle activity. They postulated that the patient lacking posterior occlusion may be susceptible to increased joint loading and may be predisposed to tissue damage. Further, clenching on a large anterior incisal

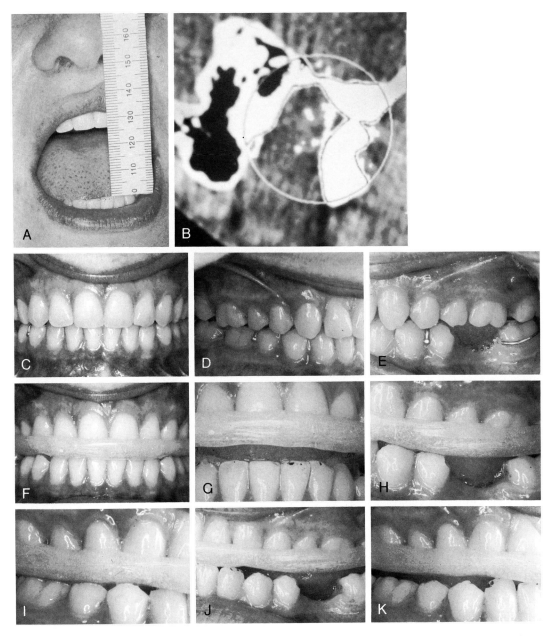

FIGURE 23–26. Patient with anterior displacement of the disc without reduction of the right temporomandibular joint (TMJ). Medical history precluded surgical repair. *A,* Reduced interincisal opening. *B,* Computerized tomographic (CT) view of right TMJ confirms displacement without reduction. *C, D,* and *E,* Mandibular decompression splint (anterior repositioning without recapture). Anterior, right, and left views. *F,* Maxillary anterior repositioning splint for night use, anterior view. *G,* Patient attempting retrusion. Note the palatal ramp of the maxillary anterior repositioning appliance prevents retrusion and resulting trauma to the retrodiscal tissues. *H* and *I,* Right and left posterior views, maxillary appliance. *J* and *K,* Right and left lateral excursions, maxillary appliance. Note the canine guidance.

block resulted in increased muscle activity when compared with a small incisal contact, whereas posteriorly, muscles reached optimum levels with fewer contacts and did not seem to be significantly affected by the number of pos-

terior contacts. This information is important when deciding on which arch to place a splint. Placement on the arch with fewer teeth results in more uniform contact around the arch and decreased joint loading. It also suggests that as

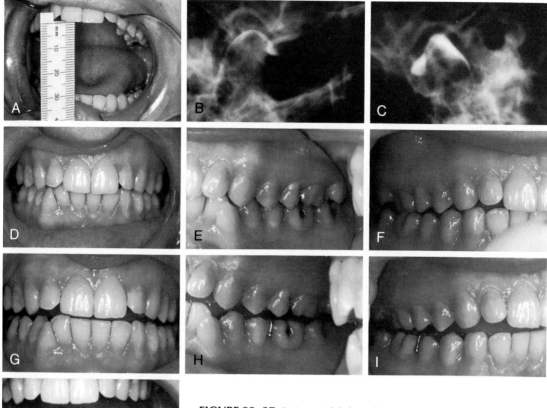

FIGURE 23–27. Patient with bilateral anteriorly displaced discs without reduction. Financial constraints precluded surgical repair. *A,* Reduced interincisal opening with deviation to the left. *B* and *C,* Arthrograms of the right and left temporomandibular joints (TMJs) confirm displacement without reduction. *D, E,* and *F,* Occlusion before treatment. Note the posterior open bite, left side. *G, H,* and *I,* Mandibular decompression splint (anterior repositioning without recapture). *J,* Occlusal view of the final overlay appliance for joint decompression.

long as bilateral posterior occlusal contacts are maintained, contact on *all* teeth is not necessary. This method facilitates the use of appliances that uncover segments of teeth to facilitate eruption. In those cases in which splint use has resulted in posterior open bite due to tooth depression or changes within the joints themselves, selective passive eruption is particularly important.

Hatcher and colleagues[261] developed mechanical and mathematical models to study TMJ loading. Occlusal forces were applied at the areas of the first, second, or third molars, and corresponding TMJ loads were calculated. Muscular-like forces were applied equally to both sides of the mandible and subsequently decreased on one side to represent balancing side function. In all instances, as the occlusal contacts moved posteriorly, the occlusal forces increased and the joint load decreased. When

designing splints, if joint decompression is desirable, bilateral contacts should be achieved as posteriorly positioned as possible.

Ito and coworkers[115] studied loading on the TMJs caused by five different splint designs. The Replicator System[143–145] was used to measure condylar movements when clenching was performed on the following splint types:

1. Stabilization splint (full arch simultaneous contact)
2. Anterior repositioning splint (full arch simultaneous contact in a slightly protruded position)
3. Anterior contact only
4. Bilateral second molar pivot splint
5. Unilateral pivot splint.

No significant condylar movement occurred during clenching on the stabilization splint, the anterior repositioning splint, or the bilateral pivot splint. Anterior contact only resulted in anterior superior movement of both condyles. The unilateral pivot splint resulted in an inferior posterior movement of the condyle on the contact side and an anterior superior movement of the condyle on the balancing side.

The increased TMJ loading indicated by superior condylar movement was greatest with the anterior splint, despite the fact that multiple studies have shown that biting force is less on the anterior teeth than on the posterior teeth.[262-264] The authors agree with other studies that indicate that posterior tooth loss increases TMJ loading and may contribute to osseous and meniscal pathology. Unilateral posterior contact also caused joint loading on the balancing side. Hylander reported similar findings and concluded that "During powerful unilateral biting, forces acting on the balancing side condyle are probably greater than those acting on the working side condyle."[265] This observation reinforces the need for bilateral posterior occlusal contacts in order to prevent potentially damaging joint loading.

DosSantos and colleagues[268] developed two-dimensional mathematical models to evaluate equilibration of forces occurring at the levels of the dentition and the TMJ during incisal contact on a natural dentition, a flat plane splint, and the palatal incline of an anterior repositioning splint. The naturally occurring incisal contact resulted in a higher reaction force in the TMJ than at the level of the dentition, suggesting the presence of uneven distribution of the masticatory load, as discussed previously and in other studies.[241,269]

The flat plane splint model showed increased reaction force at the level of dentition and decreased reaction force at the TMJ. These workers postulated that this finding may explain the relief of TMJ pain obtained from a flat plane splint. Incisal force on the incline of an anterior repositioning splint showed increased force on the TMJ. If the purpose of anterior repositioning is to decompress an injured TMJ and the patient has a retrusive bruxism habit that results in biting on the palatal inclined plane, this joint loading may increase, and the injured joint may thereby be traumatized further rather than decompressed.

A joint with proper condyle meniscus integrity may successfully withstand this joint loading; however, if there is an internal derangement and the disc is not recaptured by the splint, increased joint loading will traumatize the retrodiscal tissue, increasing pain and in-flammation and possibly leading to perforation of the retrodiscal tissues. The type of force distribution and resulting possibility of joint decompression or loading therefore become important in splint selection.

SOFT SPLINTS

In 1942, Matthews[333] proposed the use of soft acrylic or latex rubber in fabricating appliances that could be applied to treat the tooth-grinding habit. Four years later, Kesling[334] described a soft appliance that covered both dental arches in order to maintain a desired interarch relationship.

Shore[26] stated that soft appliances could be abraded or perforated by parafunctional habits and inadvertently become orthodontic appliances. Ramfjord and Ash[3] noted that soft splints were not effective in treating bruxism because the resiliency of the material stimulated the patient to clench or "play" with the appliance. They also believed that soft materials were difficult to adjust and polish and that the resulting irregularities were a trigger for additional bruxism.

Other investigators have favored soft splints, finding them effective at relieving symptoms of craniomandibular disorders.[18,335] Dawson[42] suggested using soft splints to cushion the posterior teeth in treatment of chronic sinusitis.

Singh and Berry[336] studied the effect of mandibular soft splints on the occlusion of ten healthy subjects. Polyethylene appliances were worn for 3-, 5-, and 7-hour intervals, and the subject's occlusion was evaluated before and after each period of use.

Three patients experienced muscle or TMJ pain, all of which resolved after the removal of the splints. Two of these three subjects had worn through the soft splint to create a perforation. Seven of the nine subjects stated that the soft splints were uncomfortable to wear for more than 1 hour, and nearly all of the subjects stated that their teeth did not meet evenly after removal of the soft splints. The investigators concluded that the occlusal changes experienced by the subjects were due to an adjustment of the teeth within the periodontal ligaments in order to adapt to the altered muscular position of the mandible. They also believed that the softness of the appliances was an advantage because the splint would become compressed or worn before the masticatory muscles were overstressed. Although similar changes in occlusion have been confirmed by other studies,[341] the conclusion that the soft material would wear out before the muscles were stressed is not borne out by the fact that these were all healthy subjects, three of whom developed painful symptoms after several hours of soft splint use.

Ahlin and Atkins[337] proposed the temporary use of soft flexible mouthguards in the diagnosis of patients with headache. Forty-two patients with headaches were given soft appliances to wear for a 10-day trial period. Questionnaires were completed before and after the period of splint use. Of these, 83% reported less severity, and 79% reported less frequent headaches. Some 55% reported decreased frequency of medication and 52%, decreased amount of medication. Those patients who expressed symptomatic relief were subsequently fitted with hard acrylic appliances. Those patients who experienced no relief were referred for further neurologic and laboratory testing.

Ahlin[338,339] subsequently reported on the advantages of remoldable thermoplastic appliances to treat craniomandibular disorders. He describes the advantages of low cost, ease of fabrication, and high strength and suggests that exercise of the musculature as experienced with a soft appliance might increase treatment effectiveness.

Okeson[340] utilized EMG to compare the effects of hard with soft appliances on muscle activity. Ten subjects had EMG tracings of masseter muscle activity as they alternated hard, soft, and no splint use. Results showed that mean muscle activity was less in the hard splint group than in the control group, whereas the soft splint group had the highest muscle activity. Eight of the ten subjects had decreased muscle activity while wearing the hard splint, whereas five of the ten subjects had increased muscle activity while wearing the soft splint. Before the study, all subjects were asymptomatic. Six of the ten subjects had pain or aching with the soft splints.

Harkins and coworkers[341] studied the use of soft splints in a symptomatic population. Patients (84) presenting with internal derangements and myalgia were examined and divided into two groups. Half received temporary soft splints, and half acted as untreated controls. After a trial period of 10 to 20 days, the patients were re-evaluated, and hard acrylic splints were inserted in all patients. Symptoms did not change in the control group during the trial period. In the soft splint group, 10% reported elimination of the clicking, 64% re- ported decreased clicking, 7% reported increased clicking, and 19% reported no change. Of these, 74% reported decreased facial myalgia, and 73% reported reduced cervical myalgia while wearing the soft splint. A total of 63% reported less ear pain. All symptoms were not improved, however, because 71% reported greater tinnitus or no change, whereas 79% reported greater vertigo or no change. Transient occlusal changes were reported in 67% of patients who wore soft splints.

These workers believe that the reduction in joint dysfunction and myalgia was due to elimination of occlusal influences. They also state that soft splints could act as neuromuscular deprogrammers, allowing changes in mandibular position. Finally, they stated that relief experienced with soft splint use was a good indication of those patients who would have a good prognosis with hard splint treatment. Of the patients who had relief with a soft splint, 93% had good to excellent results during subsequent use of hard splints.

As with all splints, there are advantages and disadvantages with soft splints. They are inexpensive and easily and quickly fabricated, and therefore especially suited to use as an immediate or emergency splint. If a patient presents in acute distress, a soft splint can be placed for temporary relief until a hard splint can be fabricated. In the case of an acute sprain type of injury, a traumatic blow, or an acute muscle trismus, a soft splint can be worn until joint swelling or severe muscle spasm can be relieved by physical therapy.

Removable soft splints can be applied on a trial basis for diagnostic purposes. Various positions can be tried by heating and remodeling the soft appliance until relief is obtained.

Another useful fabrication is a soft appliance to be worn during athletics. Patients who wear hard acrylic appliances often report clenching with resulting pain and frequent appliance breakage, associated with the intense muscle activity during athletics. The resiliency of a soft appliance acts as a cushion during these periods of intense muscle activity. Larger resilient appliances are recommended for contact sports in order to define the maxillomandibular relationship and prevent both dental and craniomandibular injury.

As with all splints, an improperly adjusted appliance will fail to relieve symptoms and may aggravate the situation. Soft splints are also more difficult to adjust and polish (Fig. 23–30).

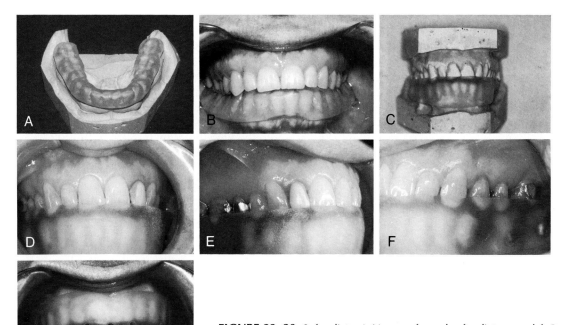

FIGURE 23–30. Soft splints. *A*, Vacuum-formed soft splint on model. *B*, Same vacuum-formed splint in mouth. *C*, Laboratory-processed mandibular soft splint on model. *D*, *E*, and *F*, Same laboratory-processed mandibular soft splint in the mouth. *G*, Interarch soft splint, laboratory processed, maintains interarch relationship.

DIAGNOSTIC SPLINTS IN RESTORATIVE DENTISTRY

In addition to the therapeutic uses of splints in specific neuromuscular or joint disorders, splints are also helpful as a diagnostic step in the restoration of complex dental cases. Although some patients develop painful symptoms or pathology when normal interarch position or proper occlusal relationships are lost, other patients do not. They may gradually evolve unusual relationships characterized by excessive loss of vertical dimension, mandibular shifting in the horizontal plane, or changes in the position of the teeth resulting in the loss of a functional occlusal plane. Extrusion or tilting of teeth may result in a mandibular position that is "locked" into an abnormal maxillomandibular relationship.

Splints provide a method for making indirect and reversible changes in interarch relationships. Dawson[25] stated that "Occlusal splints provide an acceptable surface for reversible occlusal treatment that can be altered as needed."

The initial steps involved in the restoration of badly damaged dentition are diagnostic. Before irreversible steps such as tooth extraction or odontoplasty are performed, teeth can be overlaid with acrylic in the form of removable splints. Proposed changes in vertical dimension or mandibular position can be attempted in a temporary and reversible manner.

Gradual changes in positioning or vertical dimension can be achieved by adjusting the acrylic surfaces, thereby evolving the desired restorative relationships. Once the desired result is obtained and the patient is comfortable for a trial period, temporary restorations can be fabricated to replace the splints. "When extensive restorative dentistry is anticipated, it (splint) can be used diagnostically to test the muscular and articular response to jaw position changes prior to establishing a final maxillomandibular relationship."[118]

POSTSURGICAL SPLINT THERAPY

Splint usage has an important role during the healing period following TMJ surgery. When nonsurgical treatment fails to eliminate the symptoms, TMJ surgery is often prescribed in order to restore proper function. Mahan[57] stated that surgical cases that demonstrate bruxism have a poorer prognosis than those in which there is no indication of parafunction.

Dolwick[175] recommended splint therapy after repair in order to protect the surgical site.

Sanders[342] discussed the use of a stabilization splint to protect against bruxism during the healing period following arthroscopic surgery. Bays[343] discussed surgical repair of perforations and suggested 8 to 12 weeks' use of anterior repositioning appliances in order to prevent direct trauma to the repaired disc and retrodiscal tissues.

Bronstein[344] discussed the morbidity of alloplastic implants placed at meniscectomy. He stated that occlusal stabilization by splint is important in achieving surgical success. Among the factors discussed as predisposing to increased morbidity of alloplastic implants was abnormal joint loading postoperatively, which could increase condylar head resorption or fragmentation of the implant, thereby stimulating a foreign body giant cell reaction.

Alloplastic implants have been shown to be load sensitive, especially to postoperative occlusal stability and splint management.[345] Tissue ingrowth into the implant, which is desirable for viscoelasticity,[346] is decreased by too early or too severe loading.[347] It is concluded that splint use to limit joint loading in a patient displaying parafunctional habits is extremely important. The utilization of alloplastic implants, however, has been discouraged.

McBride[348] described total joint replacement of the TMJ and recommended postoperative splint therapy.

Several reports have discussed postoperative physical therapy after TMJ surgery. Rocabado[349] recommended a joint distraction splint to be worn all night and several hours during the day for 6 months after TMJ surgery. This appliance employs light spring force to cause gentle joint distraction. Uriell and associates[350] also described postoperative management after TMJ arthroscopic surgery. They recommend placement of splints 1 to 2 weeks postoperatively in patients demonstrating clenching or bruxism. In cases of gross occlusal changes postoperatively, splint placement may be necessary immediately.

Ware[357] has also written on the subject of postoperative management. He describes the occlusal changes that occur after surgery and discusses the need for splint therapy with frequent adjustment during the healing period of 6 months.

The objectives of postoperative splint therapy include the following:

1. Control of the etiologic factors that caused the original TMJ injury, such as bruxism or poor occlusal relationships

2. Protecting the operated joint by preventing loading or compression during healing

3. Protecting the nonoperated joint against overloading as a result of changes in the functional patterns during the postoperative period of swelling and altered range of motion

4. Establishing occlusal stability during a period of changing positions, range of motion, and altered proprioception.

In most cases, patients having TMJ surgery have previously undergone splint therapy, and their previous appliance can be resurfaced and used postoperatively. If a patient did not have a previous splint, it is preferable to fabricate one and introduce it before surgery, in order to allow the patient to become familiar with its use.

Immediately after surgery, intracapsular swelling in the operated joint prevents the condyle from seating in its proper position. The condyle, and therefore the entire mandible, is usually displaced toward the opposite side. In addition, if the disc has been successfully repositioned surgically or if it has been removed and an implant placed, a change in mandibular position will result.

The splint is usually inserted 5 to 7 days following surgery, after the initial swelling has subsided. The appliance is resurfaced in the mouth at a passive position, in order to achieve bilateral solid occlusal contact at whatever mandibular position has resulted at that time. The patient is then placed on a 12-week regimen of joint mobilization exercises and physical therapy, in order to restore normal mandibular range of motion. During the healing process, the mandibular position changes frequently as swelling subsides and function gradually returns to normal. Patients are instructed that bilateral solid occlusal support is important and that they should contact the office if they perceive that the bite has changed and no longer feels solid. Typically, the splint is adjusted or resurfaced, 1, 2, 4, 6, 8, and 12 weeks after postoperative insertion. Patients who have undergone arthroscopic surgery usually have less postoperative swelling and require less frequent resurfacing. More extensive surgery results in greater swelling with more frequent occlusal changes as the swelling subsides.

Occlusal changes with subsequent appliance resurfacing usually decrease as healing progresses, and often no further changes occur after 6 to 8 weeks. Physical therapy may continue for 3 to 6 months, however. Definite occlusal therapy whether by occlusal adjustment, orthodontics, or prosthodontic treatment should not begin until all pain and swelling have been eliminated, normal range of motion has been achieved, and no additional occlusal changes are seen on the splint—usually 6 months postoperatively.

After the appropriate healing period, continued use of a stabilization splint at night is recommended in order to prevent reinjury of the operated TMJ by bruxism.

COMPLICATIONS OF SPLINT THERAPY

As with any technique, splint therapy has both positive and negative effects. If the complications are known and understood, they can be included in the treatment planning process and discussed with the patient before treatment begins.

The most common complication of splint therapy is the creation of changes in the patient's occlusion. Occlusal changes resulting from splint therapy have been discussed by many experts.[2,18,25,57,173,198,209,218–220,257,352] Farrar and McCarty discussed the posterior open bite that may follow anterior repositioning and proposed the use of a maxillary Sved appliance[56] in order to allow for posterior eruption and reestablishment of a solid posterior occlusion.[2] Similar techniques have been discussed by Owen,[173,188] Winkelstern,[220] and Lundh and Westesson.[228] Messing described adaptations of the maxillary anterior repositioning appliance that function similarly.[257] Clark[18] and Laskin[57] have expressed concern that re-establishment of a functional occlusion may be difficult and expensive, whereas Tallents and coworkers[209] and Bledsoe[353] have published methods to do so.

The creation of a posterior open bite has been attributed to posterior tooth depression resulting from a lack of full arch coverage[18,42]; however, it is also observed when the entire arch is covered. Other explanations may be equally responsible. Repositioning of the disc between the condyle and fossa changes the vertical dimension on that side and may change occlusion. Of greater importance are the changes that occur within the joint capsule. Many workers have described the pathology that takes place in the retrodiscal tissues following internal derangements.[237–239] When anterior repositioning is performed, the condyle ceases to traumatize these tissues, and healing in the form of fibrosis may occur. When the anterior repositioning splint is removed, the condyle is no longer able to move to its previous posterior position because of the presence of this fibrous tissue, resulting in a posterior open bite.

Regardless of the reasons for their occurrence, posterior occlusal changes remain the most frequent complication of splint therapy. In order to prevent this complication, several authors have proposed the use of multiple splints. Mandibular splints are frequently recommended for day use because of their superior aesthetics and lack of phonetic and functional interference. They do not, however, offer the superior strength and stability of maxillary splints. Anderson and coworkers stated that patients who had internal derangements and slept with a mandibular anterior repositioning splint have reported awakening in a locked position.[190] For this reason, they prescribed a mandibular anterior repositioning splint for day use and a maxillary repositioning night splint. Williamson and Sheffield also recommended mandibular anterior repositioning splints during the day and maxillary repositioning appliances at night.[17] Pertes described alternate-day use of a mandibular repositioning appliance without anterior coverage, with night use of a maxillary anterior resistance splint that contacts only the mandibular anterior teeth.[354] He postulated that this allowed the posterior teeth to "recover and rebound" from any intrusion that occurred from clenching forces on the mandibular splint. Messing,[257] Nasedkin,[355] and Dawson[25] have similarly discussed alternating mandibular splints for day use and maxillary splints at night (Fig. 23–31).

If posterior open bite results despite careful splint monitoring, multiple splint use can establish a new posterior occlusion. Initially, the posterior ends of the mandibular day splint and maxillary night splint are cut back, exposing the most posterior teeth for eruption (usually the second molars). The re-eruption of the mandibular teeth usually proceeds more rapidly than the new eruption of the maxillary teeth, and little change usually occurs in the maxillary occlusal plane. Once the most posterior teeth have erupted into occlusion, the maxillary appliance can be rebuilt to cover these teeth with a thin layer of acrylic, and the remaining posterior teeth are exposed by cut-

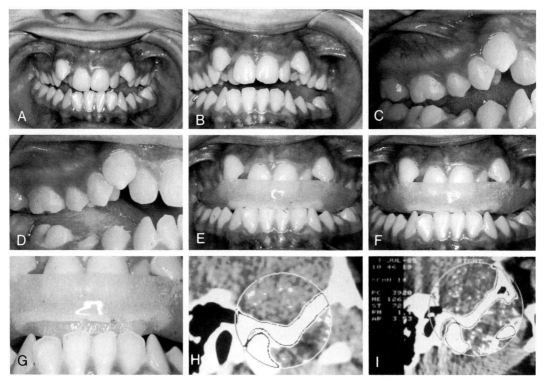

FIGURE 23–31. Double appliance therapy. Teenage patient with tongue thrust, severe malocclusion, and anterior disc displacement with reduction. *A*, Anterior view without splint. *B*, Anterior view with mandibular anterior repositioning splint for day use. *C*, Left posterior view without appliance. *D*, Left posterior view with mandibular anterior repositioning splint. *E*, Maxillary appliance for night use. *F*, *G*, Patient attempting retrusion. Note the palatal ramp prevents mandibular retrusion and resulting disc displacement. *H*, Computerized tomography (CT) of patient's right temporomandibular joint (TMJ) before treatment confirms disc displacement at closure. *I*, CT of right TMJ with splint illustrates disc recapture.

ting out sections of the maxillary appliance. The mandibular appliance can be discontinued, and the resulting maxillary appliance will function similarly to the modified Sved appliance recommended by Farrar, but it can again be resurfaced after the remaining teeth have erupted, to be used as a night splint after active treatment is completed (Figs. 23–32 and 23–33).

Another complication of splint therapy is decay under the splint.[18,352] Emphasis on proper maintenance of oral hygiene under the splint is extremely important in the prevention of caries and gingival inflammation.

A third complication that may occur is degenerative joint remodeling following long-term splint use. McNamara and Carlsson[207] have warned that long-term anterior repositioning may result in osseous remodeling of the joint structures. Goldman[352] has shown severe degenerative joint disease resulting from 2 years of unsupervised use of an anterior positioning device (sagittal appliance).

A more subtle but difficult problem that may result from splint therapy is patients' psychologic "addiction" to the splint. It is sometimes very difficult to convince patients that they no longer need the splint. It is important, before the splint is initially inserted, to review the treatment plan with the patient and emphasize that it is a temporary "crutch" that should be discontinued when it is no longer necessary. Long-term night application of a stabilization splint may, however, be indicated in a patient who has an ongoing bruxism habit.

TREATMENT PLANNING FLOW SHEETS

Any successful course of splint therapy is dependent on an accurate diagnosis. The findings of the history, clinical examination, and diagnostic imaging help to determine whether the diagnosis is neuromuscular, internal derangement, arthritis, or some combination.

Neuromuscular cases may be divided into

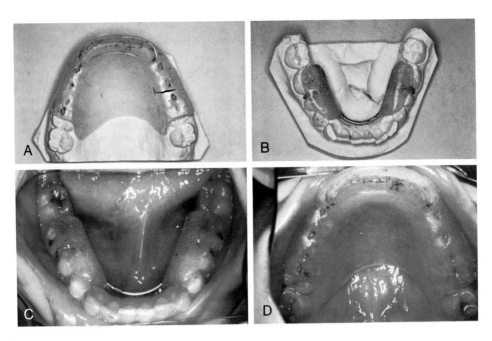

FIGURE 23–32. After posterior occlusal changes have occurred, splints can be cut back to allow for passive eruption. *A* and *B*, Maxillary and mandibular appliances cut back to expose the second molars so that they can passively erupt. *C* and *D*, Splints in the mouth.

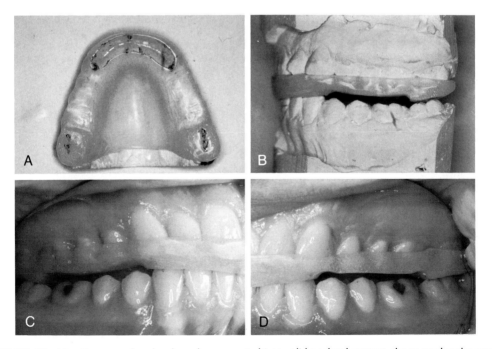

FIGURE 23–33. After the second molars have been erupted into solid occlusal contact, the second molar areas can be rebuilt. The premolar and first molar areas can then be relieved to allow these teeth to erupt. *A*, Occlusal view of maxillary splint. *B*, Lateral view of the maxillary splint with relieved areas for eruption. Note the second molars act as posterior stops. *C*, and *D*, Splint in mouth.

acute—those of brief duration and without joint involvement—and chronic—those of lengthy duration, often associated with joint inflammation, capsulitis, stretched ligaments, and hypermobility.

CHART 1

Acute neuromuscular symptoms are frequently the patient's initial episode of craniomandibular involvement. They are commonly encountered in patients at times of acute emotional stress. Pain is often aching and intermittent but may be more severe, lancinating, and of several days' duration. Treatment involves the placement of a stabilization splint, because the joint is not involved. Patients are instructed in functional restrictions including soft diet and limited opening. Physical medicine in the form of moist heat, massage, high-voltage stimulation, ultrasound, or TENS is performed. Medications such as nonsteroidal anti-inflammatory drugs, muscle relaxants, or analgesics are often prescribed for symptomatic relief. Soft appliances, which are easily made, may be used during the period necessary for fabrication of the stabilization splint. If these measures are not successful at eliminating a patient's symptoms, psychologic counselling should be considered in addition to the other treatment recommendations.

As the patient's symptoms are eliminated, wearing of the stabilization splint may be decreased to night only. If occlusal prematurities have been identified

during the examination, occlusal adjustment may be indicated to help control the contributing factors.

CHART 2

Chronic neuromuscular cases are among the most difficult to treat. In addition to muscular inflammation and pain, patients often have accompanying joint pain and inflammation, stretched ligaments, and hypermobility. The pain pattern differs from the acute type because it is usually intermittent, with periodic episodes that may last hours to several days. Pain may be localized to the muscles of mastication, as well as to the cervical and postural muscles, or may be radiating and include trigger points that refer pain to distant sites. Associated joint pain may be intracapsular, with inflammation of the retrodiscal tissues, or capsular, as in lateral capsulitis. Because of the chronicity, the involved ligaments may be injured repeatedly and become stretched, with resulting hypermobility.

Treatment of the chronic condition is more difficult than the acute manifestations for several reasons. The joint involvement responds quickly to an anterior repositioning appliance because of the decompression effect on the tissues involved. The amount of anterior repositioning may be less than that used to attempt meniscal recapture. Usually 2 mm of protrusion is enough to result in slight condylar translation, which changes the physical pressures on the joint structures. The retrodiscal tissues are subjected to less pressure, and the relationship between the lateral pole of the condyle and the over-

CHART 1   Neuromuscular Case—Acute

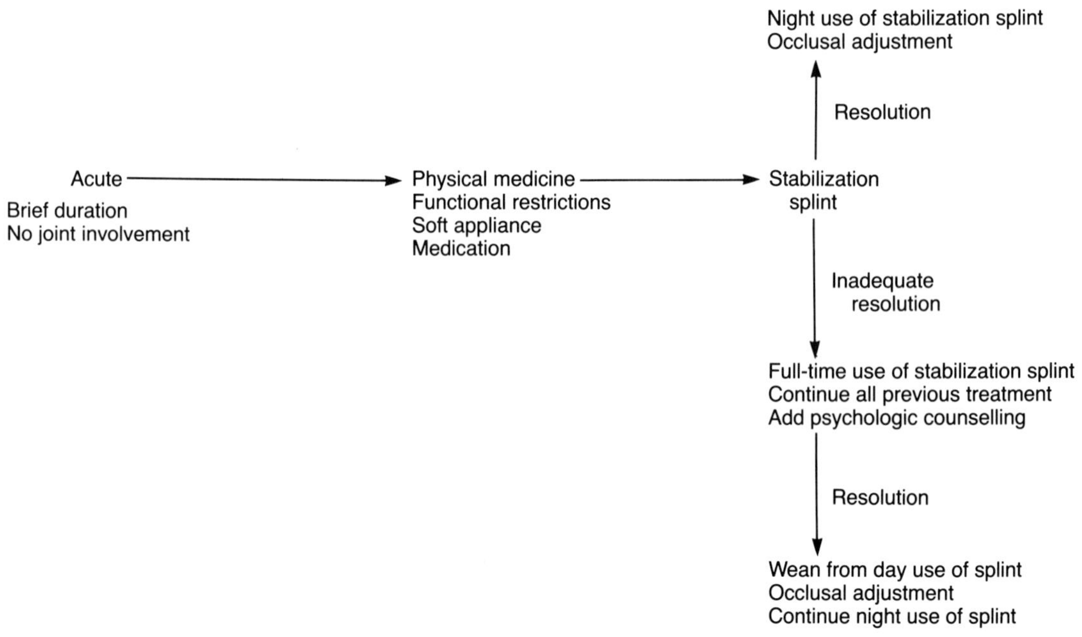

Night use of stabilization splint
Occlusal adjustment

↑ Resolution

Acute ──────────────→ Physical medicine ──────────→ Stabilization
Brief duration   Functional restrictions   splint
No joint involvement   Soft appliance
                        Medication

                                            ↓ Inadequate
                                               resolution

                                            Full-time use of stabilization splint
                                            Continue all previous treatment
                                            Add psychologic counselling

                                            ↓ Resolution

                                            Wean from day use of splint
                                            Occlusal adjustment
                                            Continue night use of splint

CHART 2   Neuromuscular Case—Chronic

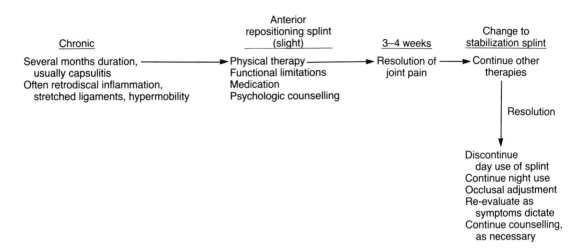

lying capsular tissues is changed sufficiently to interrupt the continual traumatization and allow for resolution of inflammation.

The adjunctive treatments of physical therapy and anti-inflammatory medication act synergistically with the decompression to facilitate resolution of joint inflammation. Severe capsulitis occasionally requires injection of local anesthetic or corticosteroid to relieve severely painful symptoms.

Once the joint pain has been reduced, the anterior repositioning component is eliminated and the splint resurfaced. The splint is converted to a stabilization splint and initially worn full time.

Chronic muscular symptoms are often very difficult to control. Specific diagnostic measures are important, because pain may be referred to distant sites. Distinct trigger points may be identified and require direct treatment with physical medicine modalities such as electrogalvanic stimulation, ultrasound, TENS, vapocoolant spray and stretch, or trigger point injections.

One of the most difficult problems in controlling chronic muscular manifestations is the etiologic role of bruxism. Although splint use and physical medicine are often temporarily successful at relieving the muscular symptoms, the repeated insult to the tissues caused by parafunctional habits such as bruxism causes their return. The resulting seesaw battle between treatment efforts and parafunctional habits can result in intermittent painful symptoms that can continue for years. These patients are often characterized as being in chronic pain. The psychologic aspects of this type of case are extremely important, and treatment success often depends on psychologic counselling as a necessary adjunct to craniomandibular treatment.

As in the acute type of neuromuscular case, once the symptoms have been eliminated, patients can discontinue day use of the stabilization splint. Occlusal adjustment may be performed to eliminate any occlusal prematurities. Night wearing of the stabilization splint should continue, however, because of the likelihood of ongoing bruxism in patients with chronic pain.

CHART 3

Internal derangement requires careful diagnostic evaluation to determine the type and extent of joint pathology. Once a disc displacement is diagnosed, it must be determined whether the displaced disc reduces during opening. If a reducing displacement is noted, is the position of reduction suitable for the fabrication of an anterior repositioning splint, or is the disc displaced to an extent that prevents recapture at an acceptable position for splint therapy? Each of these situations is handled slightly differently.

If a disc displacement is successfully reduced at a position amenable to splint therapy, then an anterior repositioning appliance can be inserted (*1*). Mandibular appliances are more suitable for daytime use because they interfere less with aesthetics and phonetics and can be worn during mastication. Maxillary appliances are used at night because of their strength, stability, and larger flanges, which more successfully define and restrict mandibular position. Successful repositioning splint therapy depends on full-time appliance use.

As with neuromuscular cases, medication, functional restrictions, and physical therapy are prescribed in addition to splint use. In cases of parafunctional activity, patients are referred for psychologic counselling. Physical therapy is helpful both in the elimination of retrodiscal inflammation and swelling, which is facilitated by the use of ultrasound, and in elimination of muscular symptoms, which may be achieved by moist heat, massage, vapocoolant spray and stretch, trigger point injections, electrogalvanic stimulation, or TENS.

CHART 3   Internal Derangements

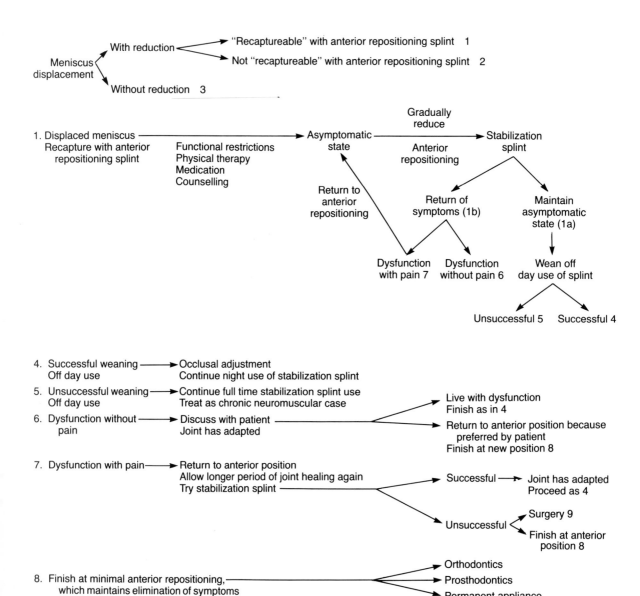

Once the acute symptoms have been controlled and the patient has been comfortable and asymptomatic for 6 weeks, the anterior repositioning aspect of the splint is gradually reduced and eventually changed to a stabilization splint. At this point, the patient will either maintain the asymptomatic state (*1a*) or experience a return of symptoms (*1b*).

(*1a*) Those patients who maintain the asymptomatic state for several weeks are gradually weaned off day use of the splint. Subsequently, they will either remain asymptomatic (*4*) or have a return of symptoms (*5*).

(*4*) Those patients who remain asymptomatic should continue night use to protect against night bruxism. Any occlusal prematurities should be eliminated to prevent traumatic occlusion during daytime function or parafunction.

(*5*) Those patients who have a return of symptoms should return to daytime use of the stabilization splint and should then be treated as a chronic neuromuscular case.

(*1b*) If patients experience a return of symptoms when they are switched from an anterior repositioning splint to a stabilization splint, then these symp-

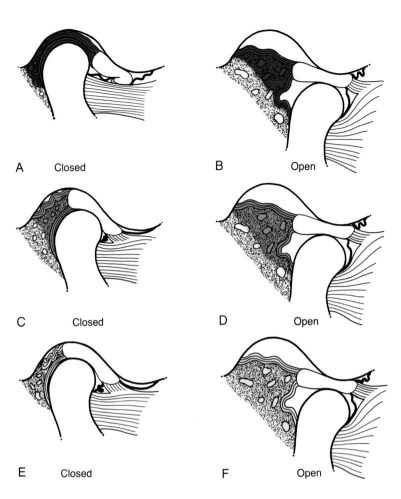

A   Closed   B   Open

C   Closed   D   Open

E   Closed   F   Open

FIGURE 23–24. *A*, Closed view of anteriorly displaced disc with reduction. Note the retrodiscal tissues are being traumatized by condylar impingement (red). *B*, Open view. *C*, The displaced disc has been recaptured by an anterior repositioning splint. Note the resolution of retrodiscal inflammation. *D*, Open view. *E*, Post repositioning therapy. Full-time splint use discontinued. Disc remains in place. Note the healing/fibrosis of the retrodiscal tissue. *F*, Open view.

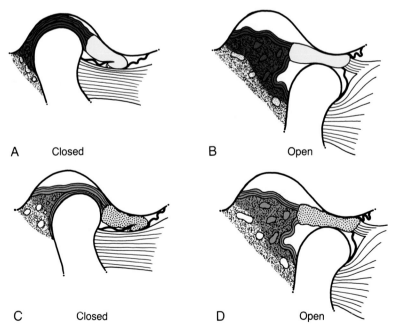

A   Closed   B   Open

C   Closed   D   Open

FIGURE 23–28 *A*, Closed view of severely displaced disc anteriorly with reduction. Note the retrodiscal tissues are being traumatized by condylar impingement (red). *B*, Open view. *C*, The displaced disc *is not* recaptured by an anterior repositioning splint. Note the resolution of the retrodiscal inflammation is achieved by prevention of previous trauma, as the condyle has been anteriorly repositioned. *D*, Open view.

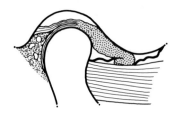

E   Closed

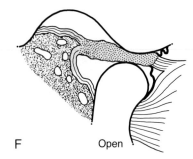

F   Open

FIGURE 23-28 *Continued E,* Post repositioning therapy. Splint use has changed from an anterior repositioning splint to a stabilization splint to a discontinuation of day use. Splint use continues at night. Note the retrodiscal fibrosis/adaptation. *F,* Open view. Note the clicking will continue.

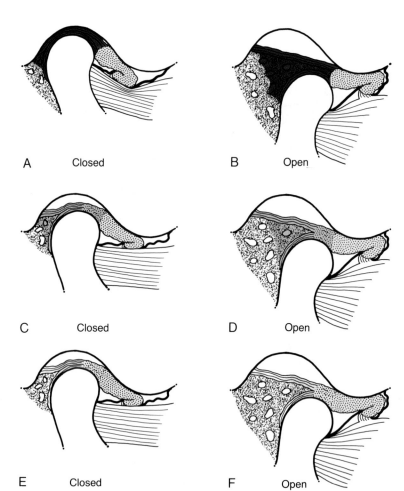

A   Closed

B   Open

C   Closed

D   Open

E   Closed

F   Open

FIGURE 23-29. *A,* Closed view of the anteriorly displaced disc without reduction. Similar to Figure 23-28A, the retrodiscal tissues are traumatized and inflamed. *B,* Open view. *C,* Similar to Figure 23-28C, the disc is not recaptured, but the retrodiscal tissues are decompressed. *D,* Open view. *E,* Gradual elimination of anterior repositioning and, eventually, all daytime splint use has allowed gradual adaptation of the retrodiscal tissues and formation of a pseudodisc. *F,* Open view.

toms will either be nonpainful (dysfunction or clicking only) (*6*) or painful (*7*).

(*6*) Those patients who experience nonpainful dysfunction must make a decision about their preference in treatment. If they are satisfied with elimination of pain and are content to live with a nonpainful click, then treatment can be finished with occlusal adjustment and night appliance use (*4*). If the dysfunction is bothersome to patients and they prefer the anterior position, which was dysfunction free, then they can have restoration to the minimal anterior repositioning at which the dysfunction is eliminated (*8*). Several factors regarding this decision should be discussed with patients, including the extent and expense of the restorative treatment plan, the possibility of the dysfunction progressing to a locked state, and the increased frequency of osteoarthritis experienced by a dysfunctional joint.

(*7*) Those patients who experience the return of painful symptoms should have the previously comfortable therapeutic position restored to allow for a longer period of joint healing or adaptation. After an additional 6 weeks of comfort, the switch to a stabilization splint may again be attempted. If successful, the joint has healed or adapted, and treatment may then proceed with weaning off day use (*4*). If the painful symptoms return again, then patients must make a decision between joint surgery to repair or remove the displaced disk (*9*) or restoration at the therapeutic position of minimal anterior repositioning at which they remain asymptomatic (*8*). Discus-

sion with patients must include the indications and expectations of surgery, contradictions, and possible complications, as well as the extent and expense of the restorative treatment plan.

(*8*) If after discussions with the patient, it is elected to restore to an anterior position, the various phase II possibilities should be discussed, including orthodontic therapy, prosthetic treatment, and overlay appliances.

CHART 4

Although a displaced meniscus may reduce during wide opening, it may not be amenable to recapture using splint therapy. The extent of tissue damage and resulting amount of disc displacement may be too severe to be successfully repositioned at an acceptable craniomandibular relationship. One treatment alternative in this situation is joint surgery to repair, replace, or remove the damaged disc. An alternative, however, is to attempt to treat this joint off the disc (*2*). In addition to functional restrictions, physical therapy, medication, and counselling, treatment includes a splint constructed at slight anterior repositioning sufficient to cause enough condylar translation to decompress the traumatized retrodiscal and lateral capsular tissues. After a suitable period of treatment, patients will either fail to achieve symptomatic relief, in which case they should proceed with joint surgery (*9*), or the painful symptoms

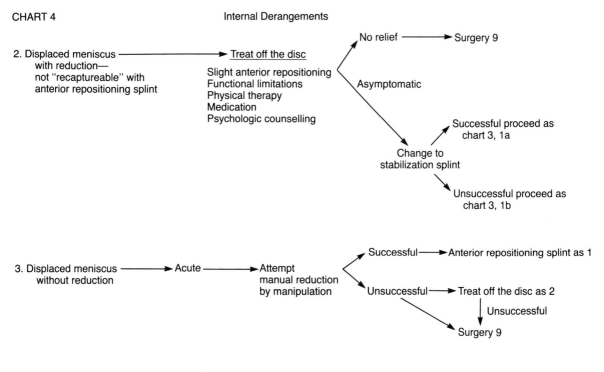

CHART 4   Internal Derangements

will be eliminated. If the pain is eliminated, the splint can be changed to a stabilization splint. If a patient successfully makes the transition to the stabilization splint, proceed as in (*1a*). If a patient has a return of symptoms when switched to the stabilization splint, proceed as in (*1b*).

(*3*) Disc displacements without reduction are either acute or chronic. Acute displacements without reduction are often termed "closed locks" because of their limited opening. These patients are often in severe pain and frequently have intracapsular edema.

Ultrasound and anti-inflammatory medications are used to control intracapsular swelling and inflammation and accompanying muscle spasms. Subsequently, reduction of the displacement by manipulation is attempted in the manner described by Farrar. If manipulation is successful, the patient must immediately be placed on an anterior repositioning splint in order to prevent further displacement and return of locking. Subsequent treatment is the same as for a displacement with reduction (*1*). If manipulation is not successful, the patient is treated off the disc (*2*). If this treatment is not successful, joint surgery may be necessary (*9*).

Chronic disc displacements without reduction are very difficult to diagnose because they often do not have the limitation associated with acute lock. In some cases, the chronic trauma to the displaced disc forces it so far anteriorly that it no longer limits opening, and the patient will not experience limitation, deviation, or clicking. Diagnostic imaging is necessary in this situation in order to arrive at an accurate diagnosis. Chronic displacements without reduction are treated off the disc (*2*).

CHART 5

Occlusal splints play an important supportive role in the treatment of patients who require TMJ surgery. In almost all cases, patients will have undergone a prior period of nonsurgical treatment with the use of a splint. This existing splint can be ground flat and used postoperatively. If a patient has not undergone prior splint therapy, a splint should be introduced before surgery to allow a period of accommodation by the patient.

For the first week following surgery, patients are on a liquid diet, and little or no function is allowed. Postoperative swelling usually develops, and the mandible is displaced slightly to the contralateral side. At 1 week, physical therapy is begun, mobilization exercises are introduced, and a passively positioned splint is inserted. The previously used splint is ground flat and thin and resurfaced in the mouth at a passive position. The splint is adjusted to uniform bilateral contact with a flat occlusal surface. The bilateral posterior contact helps to reduce the pressure on the joints while healing takes place.

Patients are seen regularly for postoperative mobilization and physical therapy. As intracapsular swelling is decreased, mandibular positional changes result, and the splint must be resurfaced to compensate. The postoperative splint is resurfaced at 1, 2, 4,

CHART 5

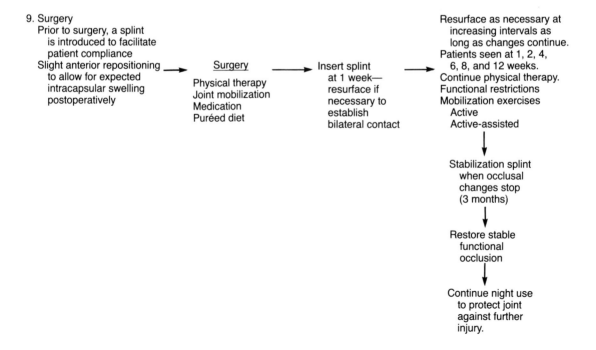

9. Surgery
   Prior to surgery, a splint
      is introduced to facilitate
      patient compliance
   Slight anterior repositioning
      to allow for expected
      intracapsular swelling
      postoperatively

Surgery
   Physical therapy
   Joint mobilization
   Medication
   Puréed diet

Insert splint
   at 1 week—
   resurface if
   necessary to
   establish
   bilateral contact

Resurface as necessary at
   increasing intervals as
   long as changes continue.
   Patients seen at 1, 2, 4,
   6, 8, and 12 weeks.
   Continue physical therapy.
   Functional restrictions
   Mobilization exercises
      Active
      Active-assisted

Stabilization splint
   when occlusal
   changes stop
   (3 months)

Restore stable
   functional
   occlusion

Continue night use
   to protect joint
   against further
   injury.

6, 8, and 12 weeks or until positional and resulting occlusal changes cease. At that time, the splint is again resurfaced and changed to a stabilization splint.

Once joint comfort and adequate range of motion have been achieved, and any muscle symptoms have been eliminated, patients can be weaned from day use of the appliance, and their natural dentition can be evaluated for any postoperative adjustment or restoration. Night use of the splint should be continued to prevent reinjury of the operated joint, which may result from night bruxism.

REFERENCES

1. Clark, G.T.: The President's Conference on the Examination, Diagnosis and Management of Temporomandibular Disorders. American Dental Association, Chicago, 1982.
2. Farrar, W.B. and McCarty, W.L. Jr.: *A Clinical Outline of TMJ Diagnosis and Treatment,* 9th ed. Normandie Publications, Montgomery, AL, 1982.
3. Ramfjord, S.R. and Ash, M.M.: *Occlusion,* 2nd ed. W.B. Saunders Co., Philadelphia, 1971.
4. McNeil, C.: Cranio-facial pain—the TMJ management dilemma. J. Calif. Dent. Assoc. pp. 34–49, March, 1984.
5. McNeil C.: The optimum temporomandibular joint condyle position in clinical practice. Int. J. Periodontics Restorative Dent. 5:71–72, 1985.
6. Laskin, D.M. and Block, S.: Diagnosis and treatment of myofacial pain dysfunction syndrome. J. Prosthet. Dent. 56:75–91, 1986.
7. Clark, G.T.: Treatment of jaw clicking with temporomandibular repositioning: Analysis of 25 cases. J. Craniomand. Pract. 2:263–270, 1984.
8. Kreisberg, M.K.: Headache as a symptom of craniomandibular disorders. II. Management. J. Craniomand. Pract. 4:219–228, 1986.
9. Posselt, U., Odont, D., and Wolff, I.B.: Treatment of bruxism by biteguards and bite plates. J. Can. Dent. Assoc. 23:772–778, 1963.
10. Franks, A.S.: Conservative treatment of temporomandibular joint dysfunction: A comparative study. Dent. Pract. 15:205–210, 1965.
11. Greene, C.S. and Laskin, D.M.: Splint therapy for the myofacial pain-dysfunction (MPD) syndrome: A comparative study. J. Am. Dent. Assoc. 84:624–628, 1972.
12. Carraro, J.J. and Caffesse, R.G.: Effect of occlusal splints on TMJ symptomatology. J. Prosthet. Dent. 40:563–566, 1978.
13. Okeson, J.P., Kemper, J.T., and Moody, P.M.: A study of the use of occlusal splints in the treatment of acute and chronic patients with craniomandibular disorders. J. Prosthet. Dent. 48:708–712, 1982.
14. Okeson, J.P., Kemper, J.T., Moody, P.M., and Haley, J.V.: Evaluation of occlusal splint therapy and relaxation procedures in patients with temporomandibular disorders. J. Am. Dent. Assoc. 107:420–424, 1983.
15. Wenneberg, B., Nystrom, T., and Carlsson, G.E.: Occlusal equilibration and other stomatognathic treatment in patients with mandibular dysfunction and headache. J. Prosthet. Dent. 59:478–483, 1988.
16. Magnuson, T. and Carlsson, G.E.: Treatment of patients with functional disturbances in the masticatory system: A survey of 80 consecutive patients. Swed. Dent. J. 4:145–153, 1980.
17. Williamson, E.H. and Sheffield, J.W.: The treatment of internal derangement of the temporomandibular joint: A survey of 300 cases. J. Craniomand. Pract. 5:120–124, 1987.
18. Clark, G.T.: A critical evaluation of orthopedic interocclusal appliance therapy: Design, theory and overall effectiveness. J. Am. Dent. Assoc. 108:359–364, 1984.
19. Posselt, U.: *Physiology of Occlusion and Rehabilitation,* 2nd ed. F.A. Davis Co., Philadelphia, 1968.
20. Zarb, G.A. and Thompson, G.W.: The treatment of patients with temporomandibular joint pain dysfunction syndrome. J. Can. Dent. Assoc. 41:410–417, 1975.
21. Agerberg, G. and Carlsson, G.E.: Late results of treatment of functional disorders of the masticatory system. J. Oral Rehabil. 1:309–316, 1974.
22. Zarb, G.A. and Thompson, G.W.: Assessment of clinical treatment of patients with temporomandibular joint dysfunction. J. Prosthet. Dent. 24:542–553, 1970.
23. Zarb, G.A. and Speck, J.E.: The treatment of mandibular dysfunction. In *Temporomandibular Joint Function and Dysfunction.* G.A. Zarb and G.E. Carlsson (eds.). Copenhagen, Munksgaard, 1979.
24. Bell, W.E.: *Clinical Management of Temporomandibular Disorders.* Year Book Medical Publishers, Chicago, 1982.
25. Dawson, P.: Occlusal splints. In *Evaluation and Treatment of Occlusal Problems.* C.V. Mosby, St. Louis, 1988.
26. Shore, N.A.: *Temporomandibular Joint Dysfunction and Occlusal Equilibration.* J.B. Lippincott Co., Philadelphia, 1959.
27. Gelb, H.: Effective management and treatment of the craniomandibular syndrome. In *Clinical Management of Head, Neck and TMJ Pain and Dysfunction,* 2nd ed. H. Gelb (ed.). W.B. Saunders Co., Philadelphia, 1985.
28. Anderson, G.C., Schulte, J.R., and Goodkind, R.J.: Comparative study of the treatment methods for internal derangement of the temporomandibular joint. J. Prosthet. Dent. 53:392–397, 1985.
29. McNeil, C.: Non-surgical management. In *Internal Derangements of the TMJ.* C.A. Helms, R.W. Katzberg, and M.F. Dolwick (eds.). Radiology Research and Education Foundation, San Francisco, pages 193–225, 1983.
30. Karolyi, M.: Uber Alveolorpyorrhoe. (Ref. Jahresversammlung des Standesverienes Berliner Zahnarzte, Berlin, 1904.) Oesterr. ungar. Vrtljschr. Zahnh. 21:85, 1905.
31. Bush, F.M.: Tinnitus and otalgia in temporomandibular disorders. J. Prosthet. Dent. 58:495–497, 1987.
32. Gelb, H., Calderone, J.P., Gross, S.M., and Kanton, M.E.: The role of the dentist and the otolaryngologist in evaluating temporomandibular joint syndromes. J. Prosthet. Dent. 18:497–503, 1967.
33. Wedel, A. and Carlsson, G.E.: Factors influencing the outcome of treatment in patients referred to a temporomandibular joint clinic. J. Prosthet. Dent. 54:420–426, 1985.
34. Rubinstein, B. and Carlsson, G.E.: Effects of stomatognathic treatment of tinnitus: A retrospective study. J. Craniomand. Pract. 5:254–259, 1987.

35. Marasa, F.K. and Ham, B.D.: Case reports involving the treatment of children with chronic otitis media with effusion via craniomandibular methods. J. Craniomand. Pract. 6:256–270, 1988.

36. Talacko, A.A. and Reade, P.C.: Hemifacial atrophy and TMJ pain dysfunction syndrome. Int. J. Oral Maxillofac. Surg. 17:224, 1988.

37. Bernstein, A.K. and Reidy, R.M.; The effects of mandibular repositioning on obstructive sleep apnea. J. Craniomand. Pract. 6:179–181, 1988.

38. Clark, G.T. and Nakano, M.: Dental appliances for the treatment of obstructive sleep apnea. J. Am. Dent. Assoc. 118:611–619, 1989.

39. Westling, L.: Fingernail biting: A literature review and case reports. J. Craniomand. Pract. 6:182–187, 1988.

40. Kahn, L.J.: Case report: Altered taste in a 58 year old patient. J. Craniomand. Pract. 4:367–368, 1986.

41. Isberg, A.M., Isacsson, G., Williams, W.N., and Loughner, B.A.: Lingual numbness and speech articulation deviation associated with temporomandibular joint disk displacement. Oral Surg. Oral Med. Oral Pathol. 64:9–14, 1987.

42. Dawson, P.: *Evaluation, Diagnosis and Treatment of Occlusal Problems.* C.V. Mosby, St. Louis, 1974.

43. Costen, J.B.: A syndrome of ear and sinus symptoms dependent upon disturbed function of the temporomandibular joint. Ann. Otol. Rhinol. Larynol. 43:1–15, 1934.

44. Goodfriend, D.J.: Symptomatology and treatment of abnormalities of the temporomandibular articulation. D. Cosmos. 75:844–847, 1106, 1933.

45. Block, L.S.: Diagnosis and treatment of disturbances of the temporomandibular joint, especially in relation to vertical dimensions. J. Am. Dent. Assoc. 34:253–260, 1947.

46. Lerman, M.D.: The hydrostatic appliance: A new approach to treatment of the TMJ pain-dysfunction syndrome. J. Am. Dent. Assoc. 89:1343–1350, 1974.

47. Jankelson, B.: Neuromuscular aspects of occlusion. Dent. Clin. North Am. 23:157–168, 1979.

48. Lieb, M.M.: Oral orthopedics. In *Clinical Management of Head, Neck and TMJ Pain and Dysfunction.* H. Gelb (ed.). W.B. Saunders Co., Philadelphia, 1977.

49. Farrar, W.B.: Differentiation of temporomandibular joint dysfunction to simplify treatment. J. Prosthet. Dent. 28:629–636, 1972.

50. Weinberg, L.A.: The role of condylar position in TMJ dysfunction pain syndrome. J. Prosthet. Dent. 41:636–643, 1979.

51. Gausch, K. and Kilner, S.: The role of retrodisclusion in the treatment of the TMJ patient. J. Oral Rehabil. 4:29–32, 1977.

52. Rugh, J.D. and Robbins, W.: Oral habit disorders. In *Behavioral Aspects in Dentistry.* B. Ingersoll (ed.). Appleton-Century-Crofts, New York, 1981.

53. Carlson, O., Agershov, W., and Krough-Poulsen, W.: Pabidningsskinnen af hardt akrylstof en ny fremstillings metode. Tandlaegebl 69:459–468, 1965.

54. Posselt, U.: *Physiology of Occlusion and Rehabilitation,* Chapter 7, 2nd ed. Blackwell Scientific Publications, Oxford and Edinburgh, 1968.

55. Hawley, C.A.: Removable retainers. Int. J. Orthodont. 5:291, 1919.

56. Sved, A.: Changing the occlusal level and a new method of retention. Am. J. Orthodont. Oral Surg. 30:527, 1944.

57. American Dental Association Workshop on Craniomandibular Disorders, Chicago, November 1–2, 1988.

58. Zarb, G.A. and Carlsson, G.E.: *Temporomandibular Joint Function and Dysfunction.* Copenhagen, Munksgaard, 1979.

59. Carlsson, G.E. and Drokas, B.C.: Dental occlusion and the health of the masticatory system. J. Craniomand. Pract. 2:140–147, 1984.

60. Ingervall, B., Mohlin, B., and Thilander, B.: Prevalence of symptoms of functional disturbances of the masticating system in Swedish men. J. Oral. Rehabil. 7:185–187, 1980.

61. Carlsson, G.E.: Consequences of occlusal interferences. In *Prosthodontic Treatment for Partially Edentulous Patients.* G.A. Zarb (ed.). C.V. Mosby, St. Louis, 1978.

62. Karolyi, M: Beobachtungen uber pyorrhea alveolaris, O. U. V. F. Z. 17:279, 1901.

63. Hutchinson, J.A.F.: Occlusion. J. Am. Dent. Assoc. 14:335, 1927.

64. Perry, H.T.: Muscular changes associated with temporomandibular joint dysfunction. J. Am. Dent. Assoc. 54:664–683, 1957.

65. Ramjford, S.P.: Bruxism, a clinical and electromyographic study. J. Am. Dent. Assoc. 62:21, 1961.

66. Ahlgren, J. and Posselt, U.: Need of functional analysis and selective grinding in orthodontics, a clinical and electromyographic study. Acta Odontol. Scand. 21:187, 1963.

67. Weisengreen, H. and Elliott, H.W.: Electromyography in patients with orofacial pain. J. Am. Dent. Assoc. 67:798–804, 1963.

68. Krough-Polson, W.B. and Olsson, A.: Management of the occlusion of the teeth. In *Facial Pain and Mandibular Dysfunction.* L. Schwartz and C. Chayes (eds.). W.B. Saunders Co., Philadelphia, 1968.

69. Mohlin, B., Ingervall, B., and Thilander, B.: Relation between malocclusion and mandibular dysfunction in Swedish men. Eur. J. Orthod. 2:229–238, 1980.

70. Graham, M.M., Buxbaum, J., and Staling, L.M.: A study of occlusal relationships and the incidence of myofacial pain. J. Prosthet. Dent. 47:549–555, 1982.

71. Wedel, A. and Carlsson, G.E.: Factors influencing the outcome of treatment in patients referred to a temporomandibular joint clinic. J. Prosthet. Dent. 54:420–426, 1985.

72. Williamson, E.H. and Lundquist, P.O.: Anterior guidance: Its effects on electromyographic activity of the temporal and masseter muscles. J. Prosthet. Dent. 49:816–823, 1983.

73. Solberg, W., Woo, M., and Houston, J.: Prevalence of mandibular dysfunction in young adults. J. Am. Dent. Assoc. 98:25–34, 1979.

74. McNamara, D.C.: *Yearbook of Dentistry.* Year Book Medical Publishers, Chicago 1979.

75. Scharer, P., Stallard, R.E., and Zander, H.A.: Occlusal interferences and mastication: An electromyographic study. J. Prosthet. Dent. 17:438, 1967.

76. DeBoever, J.A.: Experimental occlusal balancing contact interference and muscle activity. Paradontologie 23:59, 1969.

77. Agerberg, G. and Carlsson, G.E.: Functional disorders of the masticatory system. II. Symptoms in relation to impaired mobility of the mandible as judged from investigation by questionnaire. Acta Odontol. Scand. 31:335–347, 1973.

78. Helkimo, M.: Studies on function and dysfunction of

the masticatory system. III. Analysis of anamnestic and clinical recordings of dysfunction with the aid of indices. Swed. Dent. J. 67:165–182, 1974.

79. Franks, A.: The dental health of patients presenting with temporomandibular joint dysfunction. Br. J. Oral Surg. 5:157–166, 1967.

80. Woda, A., Vigneren, P., and Kay, D.: Non-functional and functional occlusal contacts: A review of the literature. J. Prosthet. Dent. 42:335, 1979.

81. Griffin, C.J. and Harris, R.: Unmyelinated nerve endings in the periodontal membrane of human teeth. Arch Oral Biol. 13:773–778, 1968.

82. Moller, E.: Action of the muscles of mastication. In *Frontiers of Oral Physiology.* Y. Kawanura (ed.). Karger, New York, 1974.

83. Funakoshi, M., Fujita, N., and Takehana, S.: Relations between occlusal interferences and jaw muscle activators in response to changes in head position. J. Dent. Res. pp. 684–690, July/Aug., 1976.

84. Randow, K., Carlsson, K., Eklund, J., and Oberg, T.: The effect of an occlusal interference on the masticatory system. Odontol. Revy 27:245–255, 1976.

85. Bakke, M. and Moller, E.: Distortion of maximal elevation activity by unilateral premature tooth contact. Scand. J. Dent. Res. 80:67–75, 1980.

86. Riise, C. and Sheikholeslam, A.: Influence of interfering occlusal contacts on the activity of the anterior temporal and masseter muscles during mastication. J. Oral Rehabil. 11:325–333, 1984.

87. Magnusson, T. and Enboni, L.: Signs and symptoms of mandibular dysfunction after introduction of experimental balancing side interferences. Acta Odontol. Scand. 42:129–135, 1984.

88. Kydd, W.L. and Sander, A.: A study of posterior mandibular movements from intercuspal position. J. Dent. Res. 40:419–425, 1961.

89. Ingervall, B.: Retruded contact position of the mandible, a comparison between children and adults. Odontol. Revy 15:130–149, 1964.

90. Hodge, L.C. Jr. and Mahan, P.E.: A study of mandibular movement from centric occlusion to maximal intercuspation. J. Prosthet. Dent. 18:19–30, 1967.

91. Beaton, W.D. and Cleall, J.F.: Cinefluorographic and cephalometric study of class I acceptable occlusal. Am. J. Orthod. 64:469–479, 1973.

92. Calagna, L.J., Silverman, S.I., and Garfinkel, L.: Influence of neuromuscular conditioning on centric registrations. J. Prosthet. Dent. 30:578–604, 1973.

93. Rieder, C.E.: The prevalance and magnitude of mandibular displacement in a survey population. J. Prosthet. Dent. 39:324–329, 1978.

94. Hoffman, P.J., Silverman, S.I., and Garfinkel, L.: Comparison of condylar position in centric relation and in centric occlusion in dentulous subjects. J. Prosthet. Dent. 30:582–588, 1973.

95. Rosner, D. and Goldberg, G.F.: Condylar retruded contact position and intercuspal position correlation in dentulous patients. I. Three dimensional analyses of condylar registrations. J. Prosthet. Dent. 56:230–237, 1986.

96. Zarb, G.A. and Thompson, G.W.: The treatment of patients with temporomandibular joint pain and dysfunction syndrome. Can. Dent. Assoc. J. 41:410–417, 1975.

97. Seligman, D.A., Pullinger, A.G., and Solberg, W.K.: Temporomandibular disorders. III. Occlusal and articular factors associated with muscle tenderness. J. Prosthet. Dent. 59:483–489, 1988.

98. Ingervall, B. and Egermark-Erickson, I.: Function of temporal and masseter muscles in individuals with dual bite. Angle Orthod. 49:131–144, 1979.

99. Bush, F.M., Abbott, D.M., and Butler, J.H.: Occlusal parameters and TMJ facial pain in dental students. J. Dent. Res. 60:529, 1981.

100. Bush, F.M.: Malocclusion, masticatory muscle and temporomandibular joint tenderness. J. Dent. Res. 64:129–133, 1985.

101. Celenza, F.V.: The centric position: Replacement and character. J. Prosthet. Dent. 30:591–598, 1985.

102. Berkowitz, B.K.B., Holland, G.R., and Moxham, B.J.: *A Color Atlas and Textbook of Oral Anatomy.* Wolpe Medical Publishers, London, 1978.

103. Riise, C. and Ericson, S.G.: A clinical study of the distribution of occlusal tooth contacts in the intercuspal position at light and hard tooth contacts in adults. J. Oral Rehabil. 101:473–480, 1983.

104. Kardachi, B.J., Bailey, J.O. Jr., and Ash, M.M. Jr.: A comparison of biofeedback and occlusal adjustment on bruxism. J. Periodontol. 49:367–372, 1978.

105. Droukas, C.B., Lindee, C., and Carlsson, G.E.: Occlusion and mandibular dysfunction in a clinical study of patients referred for functional disturbances of the masticatory system. J. Prosthet. Dent. 53:402–406, 1985.

106. Droukas, C.B., Lindee, C., and Carlsson, G.E.: Relationships between occlusal factors and signs and symptoms of mandibular dysfunction. A clinical study in 48 young adults. Acta Odontol. Scand. 42:277–283, 1984.

107. Egermark-Erikson, I., Carlsson, G.E., and Magnuson, T.: A long term epidemiologic study of the relationship between occlusal factors and mandibular dysfunction in children and adolescents. J. Dent. Res. 66:67–71, 1987.

108. Roberts, C.A., Tallents, R.W., Katzberg, R.W., et al: Comparison of internal derangements of the TMJ with occlusal findings. Oral Surg. Oral Med. Oral Pathol. 63:645–650, 1987.

109. Engle, E.H.: Classification of malocclusion. Dental Cosmos 41:248–264, 1899.

110. Kopp, S.: Clinical findings in temporomandibular joint osteoarthritis. Acta Odontol. Scand. 85:434–443, 1977.

111. Heloe, B. and Heloe, L.A.: Characteristics of a group of patients with temporomandibular joint disorders. Community Dent. Oral. Epidemiol. 3:72–79, 1975.

112. Clarke, N.G.: Occlusion and myofacial pain dysfunction: Is there a relationship? J. Am. Dent. Assoc. 104:443–446, 1982.

113. Glaros, A.G. and Rao, S.M.: Bruxism: A critical review. Psychol. Bull. 84:767–781, 1977.

114. Christiansen, J.: Effect of occlusion raising procedures on the chewing system. Dent. Pract. 20:233–238, 1970.

115. Ito, T., Gibbs, C.H., Marquelles-Bonnet, R., et al: Loading on the temporomandibular joints with five occlusal conditions. J. Prosthet. Dent. 56:478–484, 1986.

116. MacDonald, J.W.C., and Hannam, A.G.: Relationship between occlusal contacts and jaw closing muscle activity during tooth clenching, Part I. J. Prosthet. Dent. 52:718–729, 1984.

117. Bell, W.H., and Ware, W.H.: Management of TMJ pain dysfunction syndrome. Dent. Clin. North Am. 15:487, 1971.

118. Clark, G.T.: The TMJ respositioning appliance: A

technique for construction, insertion and adjustment. J. Craniomand. Pract. 4:37–46, 1986.

119. Mongini, F.: *The Stomatognathic System-Function, Dysfunction and Rehabilitation.* Quintessence Publishing Co., Lombard, IL, 1984.

120. Goldspink, D.F.: The adaptation of muscle to a new functional length. In *Mastication.* D.J. Anderson and B. Mathews (eds.). John Wright & Sons, Bristol, England, 1976.

121. Goldspink, D.F.: Growth of muscle. In *Development and Specialization of Skeletal Muscle.* D.F. Goldspink (ed.). Cambridge Union Press, London, 1980.

122. Tallgren, A.: Changes in adult face height due to aging, wear, and loss of teeth and prosthetic treatment. Acta. Odontol. Scand. (Suppl. 24) 15:1–122, 1957.

123. Kovaleski, W.C. and DeBoever, J.: Influence of occlusal splints on jaw position and musculature in patients with temporomandibular joint dysfunction. J. Prosthet. Dent. 33:321, 1978.

124. Carlsson, G.E., Ingervall, B., and Kocak, G.I.: Effects of increasing vertical dimension on the masticatory system in subjects with natural teeth. J. Prosthet. Dent. 41:284, 1979.

125. Hellsing, G.: Functional adaptation to changes in vertical dimension. J. Prosthet. Dent. 52:867–970, 1984.

126. Drago, C.J., Rugh, J.D., and Barghi, N.: Nightguard vertical thickness effects on nocturnal bruxism. J. Dent. Res. (Special Issue A) 58:316, 1979.

127. Farrar, W.B.: Disk derangement and dental occlusion: Changing concepts. Int. J. Perio. Restor. Dent. 5:36, 1985.

128. Dawson, P.E.: Optimum TMJ condyle position in clinical practice. Int. J. Perio. Restor. Dent. 5:1131, 1985.

129. Celenza, F.V. and Nasedkin, J.W.: *Occlusion: The State of the Art.* Quintessence Publishing Co., Lombard, IL, 1985.

130. Celenza, F.V.: The condylar position: In sickness and health (oh when do we part?). Int. J. Perio. Restor. Dent. 5:38–51, 1985.

131. Leib, M.M.: Oral orthopedics. In *Management of Head, Neck and TMJ Pain and Dysfunction,* 2nd ed. H. Gelb (ed.). W.B. Saunders Co., Philadelphia, 1985.

132. Gelb, H.: The optimum temporomandibular joint condyle position in clinical practice. Int. J. Perio. Restor. Dent. 5:35–61, 1985.

133. Jankelson, B.: The myomonitor: Its use and abuse. Quintessence Int. 2:47–52, 1978.

134. Jankelson, B. and Radke, J.C.: The myomonitor—its use and abuse. Parts I and II. Quintessence Int. 9:1–11, 1978.

135. Jankelson, B., Sparks, S., Crane, P.F., and Radke, J.C.: Neural conduction of the myomonitor stimulus: A quantitative analysis. J. Prosthet. Dent. 34:245–283, 1975.

136. Choi, B.B. and Mitani, H.: On the mandibular position regulated by myomonitor stimulation. J. Jpn. Prosthet. Soc. 17:79, 1973.

137. Jankelson, B.: Neuromuscular aspect of occlusion. Dent. Clin. North Am. 23:157–168, 1979.

138. Dinham, G.A.: Myocentric: A clinical appraisal. Angle Orthod. 3:211–217, 1984.

139. *Myomonitor Instruction Manual.* Myotronics Research, Inc., Seattle, 1984.

140. Jankelson, R.R.: *Neuromuscular Dental Diagnosis and Treatment.* St. Louis, Ishayaku Euro America, 1989.

141. Williamson, E. and Marshall, D.: Myomonitor rest position in the presence and absence of stress. In *Facial Orthopedics and Temporomandibular Arthrography.* E Williamson (ed). Evans, Georgia, 1986.

142. McMillan, A.S., Jablowski, A.B., and McMillan, D.R.: The position and branching pattern of the facial nerve and their effect on transcutaneous electrical stimulation in the orofacial region. Oral Surg. Oral Med. Oral Pathol. 63:539–541, 1987.

143. DeBoever, J. and McCall W.D.: Physiological aspects of masticatory muscle stimulation and the myomonitor. Quintessence Int. 3:57–58, 1972.

144. Bessette, R.W. and Quinlivan, J.T.: Electromyographic evaluation of the myomonitor. J. Prosthet. Dent. 30:19–24, 1973.

145. Dao, T.T., Feine, J.S., and Lund, J.P.: Can electrical stimulation be used to establish a physiologic occlusal position? J. Prosthet. Dent. 60:509–513, 1988.

146. Feine, J.S., Hutchins, M.O., and Lund, J.P.: An evaluation of the criteria used to diagnose mandibular dysfunction with the mandibular kinesiograph. J. Prosthet. Dent. 60:374–380, 1988.

147. Weinberg, L.A.: Correlation of temporomandibular dysfunction with radiographic findings. J. Prosthet. Dent. 28:519, 1972.

148. Weinberg, L.A.: Temporomandibular joint function and its effect on centric relation. J. Prosthet. Dent. 30:176, 1973.

149. Weinberg, L.A.: What we really see in a TMJ radiograph. J. Prosthet. Dent. 30:898, 1973.

150. Weinberg, L.A.: Radiographic investigations into temporomandibular joint functions. J. Prosthet. Dent. 33:672, 1975.

151. Weinberg, L.A.: Superior condyle displacement; Its diagnosis and treatment. J. Prosthet. Dent. 34:59, 1975.

152. Weinberg, L.A.: Anterior condylar displacement: Its diagnosis and treatment. J. Prosthet. Dent. 34:195, 1975.

153. Weinberg, L.A.: Posterior bilateral displacement: Its diagnosis and treatment. J. Prosthet. Dent. 36:426, 1976.

154. Weinberg, L.A.: Posterior unilateral displacement: Its diagnosis and treatment. J. Prosthet. Dent. 37:559, 1977.

155. Weinberg, L.A. and Lager, L.: Clinical report on the etiology and diagnosis of TMJ dysfunction—pain syndrome. J. Prosthet. Dent. 44:642, 1980.

156. Weinberg, L.A.: Definitive prosthodontic therapy for TMJ patients, Part I. J. Prosthet. Dent. 50:544, 1983.

157. Weinberg, L.A.: Definitive prosthodontic therapy for TMJ patients, Part II. J. Prosthet. Dent. 50:690, 1983.

158. Weinberg, L.A.: Optimum temporomandibular joint condyle position in clinical practice. Int. J. Perio. Rest. Dent. 5:11–27, 1985.

159. Aquilino, S.A., Matteson, S.R., Holland, G.A., and Phillips, C.: Evaluation of condylar position from temporomandibular joint radiographs. J. Prosthet. Dent. 53:88–97, 1985.

160. Williamsen, E.H.: Laminographic study of mandibular condylar position when recording centric relation. J. Prosthet. Dent. 39:561, 1978.

161. Brader, A.C.: The application of the principles of cephalometric laminography to the studies of the frontal planes of the human head. Am. J. Orthod. 35:249, 1949.

162. Craddock, R.W.: Radiography of the temporomandibular joint. J. Dent. Res. 32:302, 1953.

163. Bowman, K.: Research studies on the temporomandibular joint: Their interpretation and application to clinical practice. Angle Orthod. 22:154, 1952.
164. Eckerdal, O. and Lundberg, M.: Temporomandibular joint relations as revealed by conventional radiography techniques. A comparison with the morphology and tomographic images. Dentomax. Radiol. 8:65–70, 1979.
165. Omnell, K.A. and Petersson, A.: Radiogrpahy of the temporomandibular joint utilizing oblique lateral transcranial technique. Comparison of information obtained with standardized technique and individualized technique. Odontol. Revy 27:7792, 1976.
166. Katzberg, R.W., Keith, D.A., Ten Eick, W.R., and Guralnick, W.C.: Internal derangements of the temporomandibular joint: An assessment of condyle position in centric occlusion. J. Prosthet. Dent. 49:250, 1983.
167. Pullinger, A.G., Hollender, L., Solberg, W.K., and Petersson, A.: A tomographic study of mandibular condyle position in an asymptomatic population. J. Prosthet. Dent. 53:706, 1985.
168. Blaschke, D.D., and Blaschke, T.J.: Normal TMJ bone relationships in centric occlusion. J. Dent. Res. 60:98, 1983.
169. Blaschke, D.D.: Radiology of the Temporomandibular Joint. Current Status of Transcranial, Tomographic, and Arthrographic Procedures, pp. 64–67. The President's Conference on the Examination, Diagnosis and Management of Temporomandibular Disorders. American Dental Association, Chicago, 1982.
170. Jumean, F., Hatjigiorgis, C.G., and Neff, P.A.: Comparative study of two radiographic techniques to actual dissections of the temporomandibular joint. J. Craniomand. Pract. 6:141–147, 1988.
171. Enlow, D.H., DiGangi, D., McNamara, J.A. Jr., and Mina, M.: An evaluation of the morphogenic and anatomic effects of the functional regulator utilizing the counterpart analysis. Eur. J. Orthod. 10:192–202, 1988.
172. McNamara, J.A. Jr.: Dentofacial adaptations in adult patients following functional regulator therapy. Am. J. Orthod. 85:57–71, 1984.
173. Owen, A.H. III: Orthopedic/orthodontic therapy for craniomandibular pain dysfunction. Part B: Treatment flow sheet, anterior disc displacement and case histories. J. Craniomand. Pract. 6:48–63, 1988.
174. Christiansen, E.L., Thompson, J.R., Zimmerman, G., et al: Computed tomography of condylar and articular disk positions within the temporomandibular joint. Oral Surg. Oral Med. Oral Pathol. 64:757–767, 1987.
175. Dolwick, M.F.: Conference on Temporomandibular Joint Pain and Dysfunction. Plaza Hotel, NY, Sept. 24, 1982.
176. Annadale, T.: Displacement of the interarticular cartilage of the lower jaw and its treatment by operation. Lancet 1:411, 1887.
177. Pringle, J.H.: Displacement of the mandibular meniscus and its treatment. Br. J. Surg. 6:385–389, 1918.
178. Wabely, C.: The causation and treatment of displaced mandibular cartilage. Lancet 2:543–545, 1929.
179. Ireland, V.E.: The problem of clicking jaw. R. Soc. Med. 44:363–372, 1951.
180. Farrar, W.B.: Diagnosis and treatment of anterior dislocation of the articular disc. N.Y. J. Dent. 40:348–351, 1971.
181. McCarty, W.L. Jr.: Diagnosis and treatment of internal derangements of the articular disc and mandibular condyle. In *Temporomandibular Joint Problems.* W.K. Solberg and G.T. Clark (eds.). Quintessence Publishing Co., Lombard, IL, 1980.
182. Wilkes, C.H.: Arthrography of the temporomandibular joint in patients with the TMJ pain-dysfunction syndrome. Minn. Med. 61:645, 1978.
183. Farrar, W.B. and McCarty, W.L. Jr.: Inferior joint space arthrography and characteristics of condylar paths in internal derangements of the TMJ. J. Prosthet. Dent. 41:548, 1979.
184. Katzberg, R.W., Dolwick, M.F., Bales, D.J., and Helius, C.A.: Arthrotomography of the temporomandibular joint: New technique and preliminary observations. A.J.R. 132:949, 1979.
185. Tallents, R.H., Katzberg, R.W., Miller, T.L., et al: Arthrographically assisted splint therapy. J. Prosthet. Dent. 53:235–238, 1985.
186. Tallents, R.H., Katzberg, R.W., Miller, T.L., et al: Evaluation of arthrographically assisted splint therapy in treatment of TMJ disk displacement. J. Prosthet. Dent. 53:836–838, 1985.
187. Dolwick, M.F.: Diagnosis and Etiology of Internal Derangements of the Temporomandibular Joint. The President's Conference on the Examination, Diagnosis, and Management of Temporomandibular Disorders. American Dental Association, Chicago, 1983.
188. Dolwick, M.F. and Riggs, R.R.: Diagnosis and treatment of internal derangements of the temporomandibular joint. Dent. Clin. North. Am. 27:561, 1983.
189. Graber, T.M.: Temporomandibular joint disturbances and the periodontium. Int. J. Perio. Rest. Dent. 6:33, 1984.
190. Anderson, G.C., Schulte, J.K., and Goodkind, R.J.: Comparative study of two treatment methods for internal derangement of the temporomandibular joint. J. Prosthet. Dent. 53:392–397, 1985.
191. Lundh, H., Westesson, P.L., Kopp, S., and Tillstrom, B.: Anterior repositioning splint in the treatment of temporomandibular joints with reciprocal clicking. A comparison with flat occlusal splints and an untreated control group. Oral Surg. Oral Med. Oral Pathol. 60:131–136, 1985.
192. Ito, T., Marquelles-Bonnet, R., Lupkiewicz, M.S., et al: Recommended chewing side with an anterior repositioning splint. J. Prosthet. Dent. 55:610–614, 1988.
193. Gibbs, C.H., Lundeen, H.C.: Jaw movements and forces during chewing and swallowing and their clinical significance. In *Advances in Occlusion.* H.C. Lindeen and C.H. Gibbs (eds.). PSG Publishing Co., Littleton, Mass., 1982.
194. Gibbs, C.H., Lundeen, H.C., Mahan, P.E., and Fujimoto, J.: Chewing movements in relation to border movements at the first molar. J. Prosthet. Dent. 46:308, 1981.
195. Gibbs, C.H., Wickwire, N.A., Jacobson, A.P., et al: Comparison of typical chewing patterns in normal children and adults. J. Am. Dent. Assoc. 105:33, 1982.
196. Witzig, J.W. and Spahl, T.J.: *The Clinical Management of Basic Maxillofacial Orthopedic Appliances.* PSG Publishing Co., Littleton, MA, 1986.
197. Owen, A.H. III: Orthodontic/orthopedic therapy for craniomandibular pain and dysfunction. Part A: Anterior disc displacement; review of literature. J. Craniomand. Pract. 5:357–366, 1987.
198. Owen, A.H. III: Orthodontic/orthopedic therapy for

anterior disk displacement: Unexpected treatment findings. J. Craniomand. Pract. 7:33–45, 1989.

199. Palla, S. and Antonni, C.: Short term treatment outcome of TMJ clicking. J. Oral Rehabil. 12:560–566, 1985.

200. Fox, C.W., Abrams, B.L., Williams, B., and Doukoudakis, A.: Protrusive positioner. J. Prosthet. Dent. 54:258–262, 1988.

201. Stack, B.: Orthopedic/orthodontic case finishing techniques on TMJ patients. J. Funct. Ortho. 2:22–25, 1985.

202. Grummons, D.: Grumzat intermediate appliance. J. Funct. Ortho. 2:36–42, 1988.

203. Keller, D.C.: An anterior maxillary appliance for treating TMJ dysfunction. J. Craniomand. Pract. 3:251–266, 1985.

204. Lynn, J.M.: The biofinisher. J. Funct. Ortho. 2:36–41, 1985.

205. Ricketts, R.M.: Abnormal function of the temporomandibular joint. Am. J. Orthod. 41:435–441, 1955.

206. Ramfjord, S.P. and Enlow, J.J.: Anterior displacement of the mandible in adult Rhesus monkeys: Long term observations. J. Prosthet. Dent. 26:517–531, 1971.

207. McNamara, J.A. and Carlsson, D.S.: Quantitative analysis of temporomandibular joint adaptations to protrusive function. Am. J. Orthod. 76:593–611, 1979.

208. Gianelly, A.A., Ruben, M.P., and Risinger, R.: Effect of experimentally altered occlusal vertical dimensions on temporomandibular articulation. J. Prosthet. Dent. 24:629–635, 1970.

209. Tallents, R.H., Sommers, E., Roberts, C., et al: Occlusal restoration after orthopedic jaw repositioning. J. Craniomand. Pract. 4:369–371, 1986.

210. Lundh, H., Westesson, P.L., Rune, B., and Selvik, G.: Changes in mandibular position during treatment with disk repositioning onlays: A roentgen stereophotogrammetric study. Oral Surg. Oral Med. Oral Pathol. 65:657–662, 1988.

211. Selvik, G.: A roentgen stereophotogrammetric method for the study of kinematics of the skeletal system. Thesis, Lund: University of Lund, Sweden, 1974.

212. Rune, B., Sarnas, K.V., and Selvik, G.: Analysis of motion of skeletal segments following surgical-orthodontic correction of maxillary retrusion: Application of a new stereophotogrammetric method. Dentomaxillofac. Radiol. 4:90–94, 1975.

213. Rosenquist, B., Rune, B., and Selvik, G.: Displacement of the mandible during intermaxillary fixation after oblique sliding osteotomy: A stereometric and cephalometric radiographic study. J. Maxillofac. Surg. 13:254–262, 1985.

214. Hollender, L. and Ridell, A.: Radiography of the temporomandibular joint after oblique sliding osteotomy of the mandibular rami. Scand. J. Dent. Res. 82:466–469, 1974.

215. Edlund, J., Hansson, T., Petersson, A., and Willmar, K.: Sagittal splitting of the mandibular ramus: Electromyography and radiologic follow up study of temporomandibular joint function in 44 patients. Swed. J. Plast. Reconst. Surg. 13:437–443, 1979.

216. Hollender, L. and Lindhal, L.: Radiographic study of articular remodeling in the temporomandibular joint after condylar fractures. Scand. J. Dent. Res. 82:462–465, 1974.

217. Ash, M.M.: Current concepts in the aetiology, diag-

218. Brayer, L. and Erlich, J.: The night guard: Its uses and dangers of abuse. J. Oral Rehabil. 3:181–184, 1976.

219. Berry, D.C.: Occlusion: Fact and fallacy. J. Craniomand. Pract. 4:54–64, 1986.

220. Winkelstern, S.S.: Three cases of iatrogenic intrusion of the posterior teeth during mandibular repositioning therapy. J. Craniomand. Pract. 6:77–81, 1988.

221. Maloney, F. and Howard, J.A.: Internal derangements of the temporomandibular joint. III. Anterior repositioning splint therapy. Aust. Dent. J. 31:36–39, 1986.

222. Scapino, R.D.: Histopathology associated with malposition of the human temporomandibular joint disk. Oral Surg. Oral Med. Oral Pathol. 55:382–397, 1983.

223. Isacsson, G., Isberg, A., Johansson, A.S., and Larsen, I.: Internal derangement of the TMJs; radiographic and histologic changes associated with severe pain. J. Oral Maxillofac. Surg. 44:771–778, 1986.

224. Tallents, R.H., Katzberg, R.W., Macher, D.J., et al: Arthrographically assisted splint therapy: A six month follow up. J. Prosthet. Dent. 56:224–225, 1986.

225. Tallents, R.H., Manzione, J.V., Sommers, E.W., et al: Arthrographically Assisted Splint Therapy: One Year Follow up. Syllabus of the Fifth Annual Meeting on Temporomandibular Joint Pain and Dysfunction, Philadelphia, Nov. 12–14, 1987.

226. Manzione, J.V., Tallents, R., Katzberg, R.W., et al: Arthrographically guided splint therapy for recapturing the temporomandibular joint meniscus. Oral Surg. Oral Med. Oral Pathol. 57:235, 1984.

227. Lundh, H., Westesson, P.L., Jisander, S., and Erikson, L.: Disk-repositioning onlays in the treatment of temporomandibular joint disk displacement: Comparison with a flat occlusal splint and with no treatment. Oral Surg. Oral Med. Oral Pathol. 66:155–162, 1988.

228. Lundh, H. and Westesson, P.L.: Long term follow up after occlusal treatment to correct abnormal temporomandibular joint disk position. Oral Surg. Oral Med. Oral Pathol. 67:2–10, 1989.

229. Omnell, K.A. and Petersson, A.: Radiography of the temporomandibular joint utilizing oblique lateral transcranial projections: Comparison of information observed with standardized technique and individualized technique. Odontol. Revy 26:77–92, 1976.

230. Omnell, K.A.: Radiology of the TMJ. In Current Advances in Oral Surgery, Vol. II. W.B. Irby (ed.). C.V. Mosby, St. Louis, 1980.

231. Westesson, P.L.: Double contrast arthrography and internal derangements of the temporomandibular joint. Swed. Dent. J. (Suppl.) 13:1–57, 1982.

232. Westesson, P.L.: Double contrast arthrography of the temporomandibular joint: Introduction of an arthrographic technique for visualization of the disc and articular surfaces. J. Oral Maxillofac. Surg. 41:163–173, 1983.

233. Okeson, J.P.: Long term treatment of disk interference disorders of the temporomandibular joint with anterior repositioning occlusal splints. J. Prosthet. Dent. 60:611–615, 1988.

234. Rugh, J.D. and Solberg, W.: Psychological implications in temporomandibular pain and dysfunction. In Temporomandibular Joint Function and Dysfunc-

tion. G.A. Zarb and G.E. Carlsson (eds.). Munksgaard, Copenhagen, 1979.

235. Farrar, W.B.: Characteristics of the condylar path in internal derangements of the TMJ. J. Prosthet. Dent. 39:319–323, 1978.

236. Dolwick, M.F.: Normal and abnormal anatomy. In *Internal Derangements of the Temporomandibular Joint*. C.A. Helms, R.W. Katzberg, and M.F. Dolich (eds.). Radiology Research and Education Foundation, San Francisco, 1983.

237. Eriksson, L. and Westesson, P.L.: Clinical and radiological study of patients with anterior disk displacement of the TMJ. Swed. Dent. J. 7:55–64, 1983.

238. Scapino, R.P.: Histopathology associated with malposition of the human temporomandibular joint disk. Oral Surg. Oral Med. Oral Pathol. 55:382–397, 1983.

239. Isberg, A.M. and Isacsson, G.: Tissue reactions of the temporomandibular joint following retrusive guidance of the mandible. J. Craniomand. Pract. 4:143–148, 1986.

240. Isacsson, G., Isberg, A., and Persson, A.: Loss of directional orientation control of lower jaw movements in persons with internal derangements of the temporomandibular joint. Oral Surg. Oral Med. Oral Pathol. 66:8–12, 1988.

241. Klineberg, I.J. and Wyke, B.D.: Articular reflex control of mastication. In *Oral Surgery Transactions*. Kay, L.W. (ed.). IVth International Conference on Oral Surgery, Copenhagen, Munksgaard, 1973.

242. Greenfield, B.E. and Wyke, B.D.: Reflex innervations of the temporomandibular joint. Nature 221:940–941, 1966.

243. Klineberg, I.J., Greenfield, B.E., and Wyke, B.D.: Afferent discharges from the temporomandibular articular mechanoreceptors. Arch Oral Biol. 16:1463–1479, 1971.

244. Thilander, B.: Innervation of the temporomandibular joint capsule in man: An anatomic investigation and a neurophysiologic study of the perception of mandibular position (thesis). Univ. of UMEA, Sweden, 1961.

245. Larsson, L.E. and Thilander, B.: Mandibular positioning; the effect of pressure on the joint capsule. Acta Neurol. Scand. 40:131–143, 1964.

246. Posselt, U. and Thelander, B.: Influence of the innervation of the temporomandibular joint capsule on mandibular border movements. Acta Ondontol. Scand. 23:601–613, 1965.

247. Blaustein, D.I. and Scapino, R.P.: Remodeling of the temporomandibular joint disk and posterior attachment in disk displacement specimens in relation to glycosaminoglycans content. Plast. Reconstr. Surg. 78:756–764, 1986.

248. Mohl, N.D.: Functional Anatomy of the Temporomandibular Joint. The President's Conference on the Etiology, Diagnosis, and Treatment of TMJ Disorder. American Medical Association, Chicago, 1982.

249. Kempson, G.E., Tuke, M.A., Dingle, J.T., et al: The effects of proteolytic enzymes on the membraned properties of adult human articular cartilage. Biochem. Biophys. Acta 428:741–760, 1976.

250. Ingelmark, B.E.: Functionally induced changes in articular cartilage. In *Biomechanical Studies of the Muscle-Skeletal System*. F.G. Evans (ed.). Charles C Thomas, Springfield, IL, 1961.

251. Mathews, B.F.: Collagen/chondroitin sulfate ratio of human articular cartilage related to function. Br. Med. J. 2:1295, 1952.

252. Kopp, S.: Topographical distribution of sulphated glycosaminoglycans in human temporomandibular joint disks. J. Oral Pathol. 5:265–276, 1976.

253. Kopp, S.: Topographical distribution of sulphated glycosaminoglycans in the surface layers of the human temporomandibular joint. J. Oral Pathol. 7:283–294, 1978.

254. Scott, J.E. and Dorling, J.: Differential staining of acid glycosaminoglycans (mucopolysaccharides) by Alcian blue in salt solutions. Histochemistry 5:221, 1965.

255. Scott, J.E.: Affinity, competition, and specific interactions in the biochemistry and histochemistry of polyelectrolytes. Biochem. Soc. Trans. 1:787, 1970.

256. Guichet, H.F.: Clinical management of occlusally related orofacial pain and TMJ dysfunction. J. Craniomand. Pract. 1:60–73, 1983.

257. Messing, S.G.: Splint management and completion. Syllabus of Fourth Annual Meeting—Temporomandibular Joint Pain and Dysfunction. Philadelphia, Nov. 14–16, 1985.

258. Bewyer, D.C.: Biomechanical and physiologic processes leading to internal derangements with adhesion. J. Craniomandib. Disord. Facial Oral Pain 3:44–49, 1989.

259. McNamara, J.A.: Physiologic and Pathologic Adaptation of the TMJ to Altered Function. 14th Annual Meeting of American Academy of Craniomandibular Disorders, Washington, D.C., April 14, 1989.

260. McDonald, J.W.C. and Hannam, A.G.: Relationship between occlusal contacts and jaw closing muscle activity during tooth clenching, Part I. J. Prosthet. Dent. 52:718–728, 1984.

261. Hatcher, D.C., Faulkner, M.G., and Hay, A.: Development of mechanical and mathematical models to study temporomandibular joint loading. J. Prosthet. Dent. 55:377–384, 1986.

262. Mansour, R.M., Reynik, R.J.: In vivo occlusal forces and movements. J. Dent. Res. 54:114, 1975.

263. Helkimo, E., Carlsson, G.E. and Helkimo, M.: Bite force and state of dentition. Octa. Odontol. Scand. 35:297, 1977.

264. Williamson, E.H. and Lunquist, D.O.: Anterior guidance: Its effects on electromyographic activity of the temporal and masseter muscles. J. Prosthet. Dent. 49:816, 1983.

265. Hylander, W.L.: The human mandible: Lever or link? Am. J. Phys. Anthropol. 43:227, 1975.

266. Cassisi, J.E., McGlynn, F.D., and Mahan, P.E.: Occlusal splint effects of nocturnal bruxing: An emergency paradigm and some early results. J. Craniomand. Pract. 5:46–47, 1987.

267. Young, P.A.: Cephalometric study of the effect of acrylic test palatal piece thickness on the physiologic rest position. J. Philipp. Dent. Assoc. 19:5, 1966.

268. Dos Santos, J., Suzuki, H., and Ash, M.M.: Mechanical analysis of the equilibrium of occlusal splints. J. Prosthet. Dent. 59:346–352, 1988.

269. Storey, A.T.: Joint and tooth articulation in disorders of jaw movement. In *Oral-Facial Sensory and Motor Functions*. Kawamura, J. and Dubner, R. (eds.). Quintessence Publishing Co., Lombard, IL, 1981.

270. Gross, M.G.: The effect of increasing occlusal vertical dimension on transcranial radiographic projections of the temporomandibular joints. J. Prosthest. Dent. 60:491–499, 1988.

271. Tsuga, K., Akagawa, Y., Sukaguchi, R., and Tsuru, H.: A short term evaluation of the effectiveness of stabilization type occlusal splint therapy for specific symptoms of temporomandibular joint dysfunction syndrome. J. Prosthet. Dent. 61:610–613, 1989.

272. Clark, G.T.: A critical evaluation of orthopedic interocclusal appliance therapy: Effectiveness for specific symptoms. J. Am. Dent. Assoc. 108:364–368, 1984.

273. Magnussen, T. and Carlsson, G.E.: Treatment of patients with functional disturbances in the masticatory system. A survey of 80 consecutive patients. Swed. Dent. J. 4:145–153, 1980.

274. Magnussen, T. and Carlsson, G.E.: A 2½ year follow up of changes in headache and mandibular function after stomatognathic treatment. J. Prosthet. Dent. 49:398–402, 1983.

275. Wedel, A. and Carlsson, G.E.: Retrospective review of 350 patients, 2½ years after referral to a TMJ clinic. Community Dent. Oral Epidemiol. 11:69–73, 1983.

276. Wedel, A. and Carlsson, G.E.: A four year follow up by means of a questionnaire, of patients with functional disturbances of the masticatory system. J. Oral. Rehabil. 13:105–113, 1986.

277. Mejersjo, C. and Carlsson, G.E.: Long term results of treatment for temporomandibular joint pain-dysfunction. J. Prosthet. Dent. 49:809–815, 1983.

278. Dahlstrom, L. and Carlsson, S.G.: Treatment of mandibular dysfunction: The clinical usefulness of biofeedback in relation to splint therapy. J. Oral Rehabil. 11:277–284, 1984.

279. Carlsson, G.E.: Long term effects of treatment of craniomandibular disorders. J. Craniomand. Pract. 3:337–342, 1985.

280. Solberg, W.K., Clark, G.T., and Rugh, J.D.: Nocturnal electromyographic evaluation of bruxism patients undergoing short term splint treatment. J. Oral Rehabil. 2:215–233, 1975.

281. Clark, G.E.: Nocturnal electromyographic evaluation of myofascial pain dysfunction in patients undergoing splint therapy. J. Am. Dent. Assoc. 99:607–611, 1979.

282. Manns, A., Miralles, R., and Cumsille, M.S.: Influence of vertical dimension on masseter muscle electromyographic activity in patients with mandibular dysfunction. J. Prosthet. Dent. 53:243–247, 1985.

283. Rugh, J. and Dragoo, J.: Vertical dimension and a study of clinical rest position and jaw muscle activity. J. Prosthet. Dent. 45:670, 1981.

284. Clark, G.T., Beemsterboer, P., Solberg, W., and Rugh, J.: Nocturnal electromyographic evaluation of myofascial pain dysfunction in patients undergoing occlusal splint therapy. J. Am. Dent. Assoc. 29:607, 1979.

285. Ramfjord, S.P.: Bruxism. A clinical and electromyographic study. J. Am. Dent. Assoc. 62:21, 1961.

286. Ramfjord, S.P.: Dysfunctional temporomandibular joint and muscle pain. J. Prosthet. Dent. 11:353, 1961.

287. Kardachi, B.J., Bailey, J.O. Jr., and Ash, M.M. Jr.: A comparison of biofeedback and occlusal adjustments on bruxism. J. Periodontol. 19:376, 1978.

288. Bailey, J.O. Jr. and Rugh, J.D.: Effect of occlusal adjustment on bruxism as monitored by nocturnal EMG recordings (abstract). J. Dent. Res. 59:317, 1980.

289. Dubner, R., Sessle, B.J., and Storey, A.T.: The neural basis of oral and facial function. Plenum Press, New York, 1978.

290. Rugh, J.D., Barghi, N., and Drago, C.J.: Experimental occlusal discrepancies and nocturnal bruxism. J. Prosthet. Dent. 51:548–553, 1984.

291. Carlsson, G.E.: Consequences of occlusal interferences. In Prosthodontic Treatment for Partially Edentulous Patients. G.A. Zarb, B. Bergman, J.A. Clayton, and H.F. McKay (eds.). C.V. Mosby, St. Louis, 1978.

292. Zarb, G.A. and Speck, J.E.: The treatment of temporomandibular joint dysfunction: A retrospective study. J. Prosthet. Dent. 38:420, 1977.

293. Holmgren, K. and Sheiksholeslam, A.: Long term study of the effect of an occlusal splint in patients with parafunctional disorders (abstract). J. Dent. Res. 57:341, 1978.

294. Kopp, S.: Pain and functional disturbances of the masticatory system—a review of etiology and principles of treatment. Swed. Dent. J. 6:49–60, 1982.

295. Yemm, R.: Causes and effects of hyperactivity of jaw muscles. In Oral Motor Behaviors—Impact on Oral Conditions and Dental Treatment. P. Bryant, E. Gale, and J. Rugh (eds.). National Institutes of Health, Washington, D.C. Publication No. 79-12845, 1979.

296. DeLaat, A.: Reflexes elicitable in jaw muscles and their role during jaw function and dysfunction: A review of the literature. Part III. Reflexes in human jaw muscles during function and dysfunction of the masticatory system. J. Craniomand. Pract. 5:333–343, 1987.

297. Franks, A.S.: Masticatory muscle hyperactivity and temporomandibular joint dysfunction. J. Prosthet. Dent. 15:1122–1131, 1965.

298. Yemm, R.: Neurophysiological studies of temporomandibular joint dysfunction. Oral Sci. Rev. 2:100–117, 1973.

299. Weinberg, L.A.: Temporomandibular dysfunctional profile: A patient oriented approach. J. Prosthet. Dent. 32:312–325, 1974.

300. Copland, J.: Abnormal muscle tension and the mandibular joint. Dent. Rec. 74:331–338, 1954.

301. Newton, A.V.: Predisposing causes for temporomandibular joint dysfunction. J. Prosthet. Dent. 22:647–651, 1969.

302. Berry, D.C.: Facial pain related to muscle dysfunction. Br. J. Oral Surg. 4:222–226, 1967.

303. Laskin, D.M.: Etiology of the pain-dysfunction syndrome. J. Am. Dent. Assoc. 79:147–153, 1969.

304. Evaskus, D.S. and Laskin, D.M.: A biochemical measure of stress in patients with myofascial pain-dysfunction syndrome. J. Dent. Res. 51:1464–1466, 1972.

305. Gold, S., Lipton, J., Marback, J., and Gurion, B.: Sites of psychophysiological complaints in MPD patients. II. Areas remote from the orofacial region. J. Dent. Res. 480A:165, 1975.

306. Mercuri, L.G., Olsen, R.E., and Laskin, D.M.: The specificity of response to experimental stress in patients with myofascial jaw dysfunction syndrome. J. Dent. Res. 58:1866–1871, 1979.

307. Oakley, M.E., McCreary, C.P., Flack, U.F., et al: Dentist's ability to detect psychological problems in patients with temporomandibular disorders and chronic pain. J. Am. Dent. Assoc. 118:727–730, 1989.

308. Kononen, M., and Siirila, H.S.: Prevalence of nocturnal and diurnal bruxism in patients with psoriasis. J. Prosthet. Dent. 60:238–241, 1988.

309. Reding, G.R., Rubright, W.C., and Zimmerman,

S.O.: Incidence of bruxism. J. Dent. Res. 45:1198–1204, 1966.

310. Magnusson, T. and Carlsson, G.E.: Comparison between two groups of patients in respect of headache and mandibular dysfunction. Swed. Dent. J. 2:85–92, 1978.

311. Egermark-Erickson, I., Carlsson, G.E., and Ingervall, B.: Prevalence of mandibular dysfunction and orofacial parafunction in 7, 11 and 15 year old Swedish children. Eur. J. Orthod. 3:163–172, 1981.

312. Wilkinson, T.M.: The relationship between the disk and the lateral pterygoid muscle in the human temporomandibular joint. J. Prosthet. Dent. 60:715–724, 1988.

313. Pavone, B.W.: Bruxism and its effect on natural teeth. J. Prosthet. Dent. 53:692–696, 1985.

314. Christensen, L.V.: Facial pain and internal pressure of masseter muscle in experimental bruxism in man. Arch. Oral Biol. 16:1021, 1971.

315. Mikami, D.B.: A review of psychogenic aspects and treatment of bruxism. J. Prosthet. Dent. 37:415, 1977.

316. Solberg, W.K. and Rugh, J.D.: Use of biofeedback devices in the treatment of bruxism. J. S. Calif. Dent. Assoc. 40:882, 1972.

317. Rugh, J.D. and Solberg, W.K.: Electromyographic studies of bruxism before and during treatment. J. Calif. Dent. Assoc. 3:56, 1975.

318. Nevarro, E., Barghi, J., and Rey, R.: Clinical evaluation of maxillary hard and resilient occlusal splints (abstract 1246). J. Dent. Res. (Special Edition) 64:313, 1985.

319. Kydd, W.L. and Daly, C.: Duration of nocturnal tooth contacts during bruxism. J. Prosthet. Dent. 53:717–721, 1985.

320. Nishioka, G.L. and Montgomery, M.T.: Masticatory muscle hyperactivity in temporomandibular disorders: Is it an extrapyramidally expressed disorder? J. Am. Dent. Assoc. 116:514–520, 1988.

321. Scatton, B. and Bartholini, G.: Modulation by GABA of cholinergic transmission in the stratum. Brain Res. 183:211–216, 1980.

322. Tamminga, C.A., Crayton, J.W., and Chase, T.N.: Improvement in tardive dyskinesia after muscimol therapy. Arch. Gen. Psychiatry 36:595–598, 1979.

323. Morselli, P.L., et al: On the therapeutic action of SL 76002, a new GABA mimetic agent: Preliminary observations in neuropsychiatric disorders. Brain Res. Bull. (Suppl. 2) 5:411–414, 1980.

324. Montgomery, M.T., et al: Effects of diazepam on nocturnal masticatory muscle activity (abstract 96). J. Dent. Res. 65:180, 1986.

325. Gerlach, J.: Pathophysiological mechanisms underlying tardive dyskinesia. Psychopharmacology (Suppl.) 2:98–103, 1985.

326. Scheel-Kruger, J. and Arnt, J.: New aspects on the role of dopamine, acetylcholine and GABA in the development of tardive dyskinesia. Dyskinesia—research and treatment. Psychopharmocology (Suppl.) 2:46–56, 1985.

327. Scheel-Kruger, J.: The GABA receptor and animal behavior. In *GABA Receptors*. S.J. Enna (ed.). Humana, Clifton, 1983.

328. Carter, C.J. and Pycock, C.J.: 5,7-Dihydroxytrypyamine lesions of the amygdala reduce amphetamine and apomorphine induced behavior in the rat. Naunyn Schmiedebergs Arch. Pharmacol. 312:235–238, 1980.

329. Nakamira, Y. and Kubo, Y.: Masticatory rhythm in intracellular potential of trigeminal motoneurons induced by stimulation of orbital cortex and amygdala in cats. Brain Res. 148:504–509, 1978.

330. Waddington, J.L., Gamble, S.J., and Bourne, R.D.: Sequelae of 6 months continuous administration of cis(2) and trans(e) flupenthixol in the rat. Eur. J. Pharmacol. 69:511–513, 1981.

331. Nieoullon, A., Cheramy, A., and Glowinski, J.: Nigral and striatal dopamine release under sensory stimuli. Nature 269:340–342, 1977.

332. Sato, T. and Harada, Y.: Electrophysiological study on tooth grinding during sleep. Electroencephalogr. Clin. Neurophysiol. 35:267–275, 1973.

333. Matthews, E.: A treatment for the teeth grinding habit. Dent. Rec. 62:154, 1942.

334. Kesling, H.D.: Coordinating the predetermined pattern and tooth positioner with conventional treatment. Am. J. Orthodont. Oral Surg. 32:285, 1946.

335. Wagner, E.P., Crandall, S.K., and Oliver, R.B.: Splints. In *Diseases of the Temporomandibular Apparatus, A Multidisciplinary Approach*. Morgan, D.; House, L.; Hall, W. and Vamvas, S. (eds.). C.V. Mosby, St. Louis, 1982.

336. Singh, B.P. and Berry, D.C.: Occlusal changes following use of soft occlusal splints. J. Prosthet. Dent. 54:711–715, 1985.

337. Ahlin, J.H. and Atkins, G.: A screening procedure for differentiating temporomandibular joint related headache. Headache 24:216–220, 1984.

338. Ahlin, J.H.: The use of a remoldable appliance for diagnosis and treatment of craniomandibular disorders: Two case reports. Functional Orthod. May/June, 1985.

339. Ahlin, J.H.: The theoretical and practical application of a remoldable craniomandibular appliance. Int. J. Orthod. 21:21–23, 1984.

340. Okeson, J.P.: The effects of hard and soft occlusal splints on nocturnal bruxism. J. Am. Dent. Assoc. 114:788–790, 1987.

341. Harkins, S., Marteney, J.L., Cueva, O., and Cueva, L.: Application of soft occlusal splints in patients suffering from clicking temporomandibular joints. J. Craniomand. Pract. 6:71–75, 1988.

342. Sanders, B.: Advances in Arthroscopic Surgery of the TMJ. Presented at the 14th Annual Meeting of the American Academy of Craniomandibular Disorders, Washington, D.C., April 14, 1989.

343. Bays, R.: Repair of bilaminer and discal disorders. Presented at the 14th Annual Meeting of the American Academy of Craniomandibular Disorders, Washington, D.C., April 14, 1989.

344. Bronstein, S.L.: Retained alloplastic temporomandibular joint disk implants, a retrospective study. Oral Surg. Oral Med. Oral Pathol. 64:135–145, 1987.

345. Kent, J.N.: TMJ disorders. Proceedings of the annual meeting of the Colorado Society of Oral and Maxillofacial Surgeons, Vail, Colorado, 1986.

346. Fontenot, M.G., Bloch, M.S., Kent, S.N., and Homsy, C.A.: Comparison of mechanical properties of the human TMJ meniscus and Proplast II laminates. Proceedings, Abstract Session, AAOMS Annual Meeting, Washington, D.C., 1985.

347. Halstead, A., Jones, C.W., and Rawlings, R.D.: A study of the reaction of human tissue to Proplast. J. Biomed. Mater. Res. 13:121–134, 1979.

348. McBride, K.L.: Total reconstruction of the tempo-

romandibular joint with the Vitek-Kent prosthesis. TMJ Update 7 pp. 15–18, 1989.

349. Rocabado, M.: Physical therapy for the postsurgical TMJ patient. J. Craniomand. Disorders Fac. Oral Pain 3:75–82, 1989.

350. Uriell, P., Bertolucci, L., and Swaffer, C.: Physical therapy in the post operative management of temporomandibular joint arthroscopic surgery. J. Craniomand. Pract. 7:27–32, 1989.

351. Ware, O.H.: Post meniscoplasty occlusal management. J. Craniomand. Pract. 7:152–153, 1989.

352. Goldman, S.M.: Uses and Abuses of Appliances. Presented at the 14th Annual Meeting of the American Academy of Craniomandibular Disorders, Washington, D.C., April 13, 1989.

353. Bledsoe, W.S. Jr.: The bonded visible light cured appliance—intermediate splint therapy for the temporomandibular joint patient. J. Craniomand. Pract. 7:126–131, 1989.

354. Pertes, R.A.: Updating the mandibular orthopedic repositioning appliance (MORA). J. Craniomand. Pract. 5:352–355, 1987.

355. Nasedkin, J.N.: TM joint reports: Simplified computer format. J. Craniomand. Pract. 6:271–278, 1988.

356. Messing, S.G.: Clinical Study of 60 Patients Using Transcranial Radiography and Arthrography. Presented at the Third Annual TMJ Radiology and Arthrography Seminar, Montgomery, AL, August 30, 1983.

357. Roberts, C.A., Katzberg, R.W., Tallents, R.H., et al: Correlation of clinical parameters to the arthrographic depiction of TMJ internal derangements. Oral Surg. Oral Med. Oral Pathol. 66:32–36, 1986.

358. Helms, C.A., Morrish, R.B. Jr., Kircos, C.T., et al: Computed tomography of the meniscus of the TMJ;

preliminary observations. Radiology 145:719–722, 1982.

359. Manzione, J.V., Seltzer, S.C., Katzberg, R.W., et al: Direct sagittal computed tomography of the TMJ. AJNR 3:677–679, 1982.

360. Manzione, J.V., Katzberg, R.W., Brodsky, G.L., et al: Internal derangements of the TMJ: Diagnosis by direct sagittal computed tomography. Radiology 150:111–114, 1984.

361. Manco, L.G., Messing, S.G., Busino, L.J., et al: Internal derangements of the TMJ evaluated with direct sagittal computed tomography: A prospective study. Radiology 157:407–412, 1985.

362. Manco, L.G. and Messing, S.G.: Splint therapy evaluated with direct sagittal computed tomography. Oral Surg. Oral Med. Oral Pathol. 61:5–11, 1986.

363. Paz, M.E., Katzberg, R.W., Tallents, R.H., et al: Computed tomography evaluation of the density of the TMJ meniscus. Syllabus of the Fifth Annual Meeting on Temporomandibular Joint Pain and Dysfunction, Philadelphia, PA, Nov., 12–14, 1987.

364. Katzberg, R.W., Schenck, J., Roberts, D., et al: Magnetic resonance imaging of the temporomandibular joint meniscus. Oral Surg. Oral Med. Oral Pathol. 59:332–335, 1985.

365. Bessette, R.W., Katzberg, R.W., Natiella, J.R., et al: Diagnosis and reconstruction of the human temporomandibular joint after trauma or internal derangement. Plast. Reconstr. Surg. 75:192–203, 1985.

366. Gibbs, C., Mahan, P., Wilkinson, T., and Manderli, A.: EMG Activity of the superior belly of the lateral pterygoid muscle in relation to other jaw muscles. J. Prosthet. Dent. 51:681–701, 1984.

367. Pullinger, A., Seligman, D., and Solberg, W.: Temporomandibular disorders II: Occlusal factors associated with TMJ tenderness and dysfunction. J. Prosthet. Dent. 59:363–367, 1988.

John Dunn

CHAPTER 24

Physical Therapy

During the past decade, a multidisciplinary approach to the management of temporomandibular and craniocervical disorders has been advocated by many dental and physical therapy practitioners.[1-7] The growing relationship is based on an understanding of orthopedic concepts relating to the cervical spine and temporomandibular joint (TMJ) and their biomechanical interdependence.

Clinicians have often failed to recognize craniocervical pathology by exclusively examining the muscles of mastication, the occlusion, and the TMJ.[8,9] The presence of craniocervical symptoms and their underlying pathology have neurophysiologic, arthrokinematic, and musculotendinous interactions with the TMJ.[10,11]

The purpose of this chapter is to describe specific pathologies seen by a physical therapist. The pathomechanical basis for cervical spine dysfunction and its influence on the craniomandibular complex are clarified. Soft-tissue involvement in local and referred pain is defined. The detailed methods involved when utilizing modalities to decrease pain and edema and soft-tissue preparation are discussed. Mobilization of soft tissues and joints of the cervical spine and TMJ is a key part of an integrated treatment plan. Techniques for mobilization are described in this chapter. Increases in mobility can be maintained only by a self-mobilization exercise program, also presented. Preoperative and postoperative physical therapy management for arthroscopic and open joint surgery is presented. The goal of this chapter is to provide dentists with insight into physical therapy to better assist their patients.

CERVICAL SPINE INFLUENCE ON THE STOMATOGNATHIC SYSTEM

It is the shared goal of the dentist and physical therapist to posture and align the mastica-tory and craniocervical system within an individual patient's adaptive capability. The relationship between the muscles of mastication, the hyoid bone, and the posterior and anterior cervical musculature during posture is important when considering the effects of head posture and the resting position of the mandible.[29]

Brodie,[12] using a mechanical model, demonstrated that tension in the posterior cervical, anterior cervical, hyoid, and masticatory muscles was affected by head position. He initially documented the resting position of the mandible and showed that it can vary as a function of head posture.

Electromyographic (EMG) studies have supported the relationship between changes in head and neck posture and muscle activity and their influence on resting posture on the musculature attached to the mandible.[13-16] Boyd[15] demonstrated increased anterior temporalis and decreased masseter and anterior digastric activity on backward bending of the head. On forward bending, decreased temporalis activity and increased masseter and anterior digastric activity consistently occurred in all 25 participants in this study.

The mandibular resting position is of particular importance to dentists. The resting position may be defined as the position in which "the stomatognathic structures are in balance."[17] This position exists when the lips are in light contact or slightly apart, the opposing teeth are separated, all masticatory muscles are at rest, and the mandible is passively suspended against gravity.[18,19] Researchers have noted changes in the activity of the masticatory musculature with changes in head position.[13,15,20] These changes in activity have also been shown to influence vertical and horizontal position of the mandible.[21] When abnormal posture creates an imbalance of the head or neck as described by Kendall and colleagues,[22] the forward head posture (FHP) produces slumped and rounded shoulders with concomitant extension of the cervical spine, causing the head to shift anteriorly beyond its normal axis of gravity. This anteriorly adapted position of the cranium may lead to increased gravitational forces on the head[23] and may cause ligament, facet joint, and cervical muscle stress. This posture may alter the neuromuscular influences on the entire masticatory system, thus influencing the resting position of the mandible.[24] Forward head posture has an immediate effect on mandibular closure.[25,26]

Forward head posture influences the resting

vertical dimension of the mandible,[10,16] as Ayub and colleagues[27] and Darling and associates[24] clinically observed. In FHP, the supramandibular muscles may pull the mandible toward the maxilla and cause a decrease in the resting position of the mandible, as well as a more retruded position.[27] This posture causes the suprahyoid and posterior cervical musculature to shorten isometrically while the infrahyoid musculature is stretched[22,23,28,30] (Fig. 24–1), consequently decreasing or eliminating the freeway space. The effects of this abnormal position may lead to an excessive amount of tension in the masticatory musculature, teeth, and supporting structures.[17] Abnormal position may lead to eventual osteoarthrosis and remodeling of the TMJ.[10,31]

The decrease in resting position of the mandible is particularly important to dentists considering orthodontics, prosthetics, or orthognathic surgery.[27] An inaccurate determination of vertical dimension of rest (VDR) in the presence of FHP may result in clenching and grinding of the teeth, remodeling of tissue, TMJ disorders, and aesthetic problems.[14,31–33]

If FHP is present, a dentist may want to consider referring the patient for 4 weeks of physical therapy.[24] Ayub and Darling also found that after approximately 4 weeks of physical therapy there was a decrease in FHP and an increase in the VDR. The improved head position may also decrease the stretch on the anterior cervical musculature, with a resultant decrease in retrusive forces on the mandible. Motion and flexibility on the cervical spine also improved.

The physical therapy consisted of soft-tissue stretching of the suboccipital, supramandibular, and suprahyoid musculature and joint manipulation of the cervical apophyseal joints. Patients could then move to a more ideal head on neck position. They were also instructed in correct posture and given a home exercise program that enabled them to maintain changes of mobility achieved with physical therapy.[24]

PREOPERATIVE MANAGEMENT OF MYOFASCIAL PAIN DYSFUNCTION SYNDROME

Whe considering surgery, it is important to establish whether myofascial pain dysfunction (MPD) syndrome is a contributing factor.[33] Many patients with internal derangement have MPD involving the masticatory and cervical musculature as far down the kinetic chain as the thoracic spine. In a presurgical evaluation, it is important to ascertain whether the MPD preceded an internal derangement or was caused by parafunctional activity or cervical spine dysfunction. Many patients have reciprocal clicking for many years before developing increasing joint pain and decreasing range of motion in the TMJ.[34] This clicking may be typical of an anterior displaced disc with reduction progressing to an anteriorly displaced disc without reduction.[35] While patients are relating their medical histories, it is not uncommon for them to indicate that they have had atypical migraines and neck and shoulder pain for many years.[28] The progression of symptoms may have been a vague facial and neck pain, which may indicate myofascial involvement and may precede internal derangement of the TMJ.

Dental involvement is also extremely important when considering MPD and presurgical physical therapy. The dentist often constructs an occlusal appliance. Most patients who have had splints derived some benefit even if the pathology required surgery. Patients who do not respond may need behavioral relaxation programs such as biofeedback, meditation, and other autogenic training. These programs have been of value in decreasing hypertonicity in the temporomandibular and craniocervical system.[37–39] The relaxation, when coupled with psychologic support, may greatly benefit patients.[40]

COMMON NEUROVASCULAR ENTRAPMENTS INVOLVING FORWARD HEAD POSTURE

One of the common neuroanatomic sequelae involving FHP is suboccipital impingement or entrapment. It may be of insidious onset due to multiple forces of muscle imbalance, which may slowly develop over months or years. In reporting their medical histories, patients often describe transient facial pain, supraorbital pain, pain radiating to the vertex of the skull, and suboccipital pain. Some patients describe tinnitus, dizziness, and a feeling of fullness in their ears.[41–43,45]

The suboccipital region has traditionally been the domain of neurologists, orthopedists, physiatrists, and physical therapists. Dentists have been somewhat unaware of pathologic functioning of the cervical spine musculature and its importance as an etiologic factor in the development of severe headaches in the retro-

FORWARD HEAD POSTURE

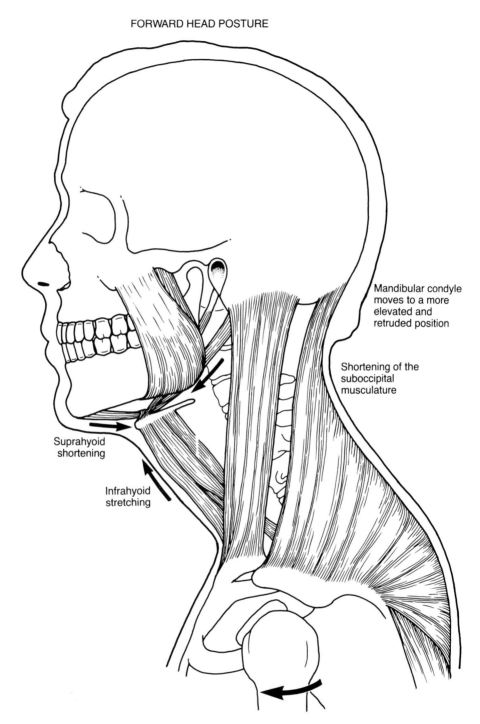

FIGURE 24–1. Forward head posture (FHP). In the presence of FHP, the suprahyoid musculature becomes tightened and shortened, as the head moves forward. Posterior cranial rotation occurs at the occipital atlantal joint. The infrahyoid musculature becomes stretched. Isometric contraction of the suboccipital musculature leads to suboccipital entrapment, with the resultant effect of mandibular elevation and retrusion.

orbital, temporal, and occipital area.[7,46,47] Cervical problems mimic the symptoms associated with TM disorders.

The fine neuroanatomic studies by Bogduk have clarified the numerous possibilities for muscular, osseous, and fascial entrapments of C1, C2, and C3[48] (Fig. 24–2). Of importance is the anatomic description of the communication of the greater occipital nerve with the branches of the supraorbital nerve[48] (Fig. 24–3).

Bogduk[49] demonstrated that neck ache and headache could be completely relieved clinically by serial bupivacaine injections of the cervical nerves, particularly C2 and C3. In patients experiencing short-term relief, radio-frequency denaturation usually destroys the offending nervous structures, producing long-lasting relief.[50]

In patients with temporomandibular disorders, headache is often a primary complaint. These headaches may be influenced by the lower cervical spine when muscle contraction is originating from irritation of the upper cervical nerves. The greater occipital nerve tracks and pierces through the semispinalis capitis and the trapezius, as they attach to the occipital bone.[48] From this point, the nerve courses upward and forward and supplies the dermis of the vertex of the skull. Patients usually experience painful spasm in this area, especially in the trapezius musculature. They generally have pain on palpation of the suboccipital triangle, and trigger points can frequently be found in the trapezius, levator scapulae, and other interscapular musculature.[43] As this musculature goes into spasm and the suboccipital region is brought into further backward bending or posterior cranial rotation, there may be further soft-tissue and bony impingement between the

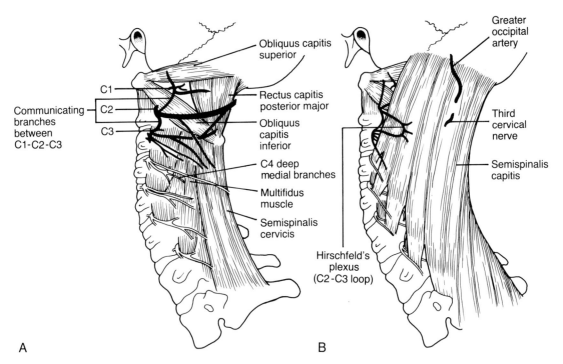

FIGURE 24–2. *A*, Deep plane dorsal rami. A diagramatic view of the dorsolateral anatomy of the cervical spine in its deepest plane. The first cervical nerve is positioned between the posterior arch of the atlas and the vertebral artery (not shown). The nerve then passes through the suboccipital plexus of veins and ascends, curving to enter the suboccipital triangle, which is an area of possible muscle and fascial entrapment. This is found in a patient with forward head posture (FHP). The first three cervical dorsal rami have intercommunicating branches between C1-C2-C3. The stimulation of any one of these posterior rami via compression of the overlying muscle or foraminal encroachment may lead to intersegmental stimulation. This stimulation may fire multisegmentally innervated muscles. (Redrawn from Bogduk, N.: Spine 7:319, 1982.) *B*, Superficial plane dorsal rami. The greater occipital nerve is shown piercing the semispinalis capitis in a more superficial plane. The nerve also pierces the splenius cervicis (not shown). The third occipital nerve pierces the splenius capitis and splenius cervicis. This posterior dorsal ramus may become entrapped during isometric contraction of this musculature in the presence of forward head posture during posterior cranial rotation. Hirschfeld's plexus is further evidence of the communication between C2-C3 and C1 and the possibility of one dorsal ramus stimulating other segments.

COMMON NEUROMUSCULAR ENTRAPMENT

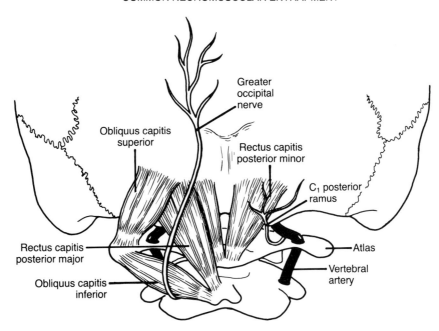

FIGURE 24–3. Common neurovascular entrapments. The C2 dorsal ramus arises from the C2 spinal nerve and moves laterally to the atlantoaxial joint. The ramus curves around the obliquus inferior and tracks laterally to medially beneath the splenius capitis and cervicis as well as the longissimus capitis and semispinalis capitis. As this nerve moves to its most medial position, it receives communicating branches from the third occipital nerve. C2 then tracks dorsally, piercing the semispinalis capitis and running under the trapezius rostrolaterally, as it emerges to the scalp. The nerve then exits through an aperture, with the occipital artery beneath the attachment of the trapezius and the sternocleidomastoid. The intermediate branches terminate as far rostrally as the coronal suture in the dense subcutaneous fascia. There they communicate with the supraorbital nerve.[48] The vertebral artery may also fall prey to compressive forces within the suboccipital triangle.

occiput on C1, C1–2, and C2–3, as well as impingement or entrapment of the vertebral artery (see Fig. 24–3).[41,49,51,52,54,93] Furthermore, ongoing degenerative joint disease may cause traction spurs that encroach on the C1–2 nerve roots.[41,55,56]

The upper cervical neuroanatomy has an intimate interconnection with the spinal nucleus of the trigeminal nerve, which can refer pain sensations to the face and upper three cervical spinal nerves.[43] Many investigators[57–59] have reported a predominance of occipital, suboccipital, and cervical pain associated with referred frontal and retro-orbital pain arising from cervical spine disorders.

A study of patients with limited upper cervical joint mobility noted a high frequency of headaches both unilaterally and centrally. There was a high incidence of positive joint findings of hypomobility in the upper cervical joints, the occiput, C1, C1–2, and C2–3.[60] Below cervical joints C3–4, there was a rapid decrease in positive joint findings.[45] Patients

often described feeling like a tight band surrounded their head or that their head felt heavy.[60]

Steady ocular pain may also result from cervical headache.[62] Feinstein and colleagues[63] were able to produce referred pain to the forehead by stimulating the soft tissue between the occiput and C1. Likewise, stimulation in the upper cervical interspinous space produced occipital headache. Furthermore, stimulation of the dorsal rami of C3 provoked referred pain to the occiput, mastoid region, and forehead.[49] These clinical experiments demonstrate the capability of the upper cervical nerves to produce referred pain in the temporomandibular and craniofacial region.

If the musculoskeletal environment is compromised by FHP, nerve entrapment can initiate noxious mechanoreceptor activity.[51,54,64] The spinal tract of the trigeminal nerve terminates its fibers in the pars caudalis and the first three cervical segments, especially at the C1 and C2 level.[65] At the spinal segment of C1, ascending fibers of C2 and C3 nerves converge with the same nuclear groups of the descending trigeminal fibers. At the C2 segment, ascending fibers of C3 and descending fibers of the trigeminal afferents join[43] (Fig. 24–4). According to Bogduk, this overlapping of the termination of the trigeminal and cervical terminals may be viewed as a combined nucleus.[43] The so-called trigeminocervical nucleus has not been demonstrated anatomically, but its existence has been physiologically observed.[43]

This convergence between the cervical and trigeminal nerves was recorded by Kerr and Olafson.[66] Stimulation of the C1 dorsal root produced pain in the frontal region, the orbit, and the vertex of the cranium. If FHP is clinically present, mechanoreceptor activity may lead to convergence of impulses by stimulating the trigeminal nerves.

A physical therapist's first goal when treating the cervical region is to free up any entrapment of the suboccipital nerves by using myofascial release techniques (discussed later). The second duty is to increase mobility of hypomobile joints, particularly at occiput-C1, C1–2, C2,

and C3. These segments are the most commonly involved in FHP. Mobilization techniques not only free motion but decrease noxious stimuli arising from types I–IV articular receptors of cervical facet joint capsules and adjacent tissues.[64]

Any inflammation, swelling, or change of position may alter the extensibility of the joint capsule, producing mechanical stress. This stress may stimulate mechanoreceptors, producing muscle contraction, which will further malalign the head-on-neck posture. This effect may modulate segmentally, intrasegmentally, and cortically and cause or contribute to pathology of the TMJ, as based on the neurophysiologic relationship between the cervical spine and the trigeminal sensory neurons.[68]

In the TMJ, mechanoreceptors are located in the fibrous capsule, the lateral ligament, and the retrodiscal tissue. They do not exist in the synovial tissue or the central portion of the articular disc.[5] Afferent discharges from these receptor tissues terminate in the deep temporal, masseter, and auriculotemporal nerves, which originate in the mandibular division of the trigeminal nerve.[5] Type IV pain receptors in these articular tissues become activated when they are subjected to mechanical stress and deformation, as well as chemical irritation.[69]

Any noxious mechanical stimuli, such as clicking, arthritis, bruxism, clenching, and internal derangement, may be considered a strain on the joint capsule, as well as on the retrodiscal tissue.[5]

In the presence of decreased capsule extensibility or joint hypomobility, physical therapy mobilization techniques may not only improve the arthrokinematics of the joint but influence decreased mechanoreceptor activity.[5,69] The correct application of various modalities such as ice, ultrasound, and transcutaneous electrical nerve stimulation (TENS) in the appropriate sequence may assist in normalizing mechanoreceptors.[71] This process occurs through the decrease in capsular tension with mobilization, decrease in capsular swelling with ice, collagen bonding with ultrasound, and through mechanically pulsing the elevator muscles with TENS to increase circulation and lymphatic drainage. The resolution of joint tension and joint effusion may then decrease mechanoreceptor activity.[69] Treatment of joint extensibility, effusion, mechanics, and muscle balancing formulates the basis for physical therapy of the craniomandibular and craniocervical system.

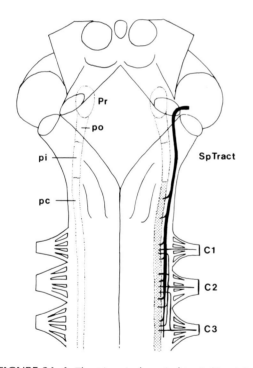

FIGURE 24–4. The trigeminal cervical tract. (Reprinted with permission from Bogduk, N.: Cervical causes of headache and dizziness. In *Modern Manual Therapy of the Vertebral Column.* G. Grieve (ed.). Churchill Livingstone, Edinburgh, 1986.)

PHYSICAL THERAPY

During the past several years, patients referred by dentists have been managed with orthopedic physical therapy modalities and manual treatment techniques.[3] After a complete medical and dental history is taken and a structural and neuromuscular evaluation is made of the upper quarter, an appropriate treatment plan may be formulated. The treatment goal is to restore mobility and function to the TMJ and cervical spine. Pain is usually the reason for referral. It is hoped that in the future, patients will be referred to a physical therapist for correction of dysfunctional posture; mandibular muscle stretching, strengthening, and coordination; and instruction in appropriate mouth breathing and resting position of the tongue.

After the etiologic factors are clarified, the physical therapist selects the most appropriate treatment sequence, which is adjusted in accordance with symptom regression, continued pain reduction, restoration of function, and ongoing preventive education.

Regardless of the approach, selected exercises are usually performed by the patient on a regular basis to maintain muscle strength as well as joint arthrokinematic mobility in both the TMJ and cervical spine. The patient must be willing to carry out these exercises to maintain function and prevent recurrence of symptoms and dysfunction.

The appropriate use of therapeutic modalities such as moist heat, cold packs, vapocoolant sprays, TENS, high-voltage electrical stimulation, noninvasive electroacupuncture, ultrasound, iontophoresis, and phonophoresis has had specific physiologic effects on the temporomandibular and craniocervical system.

PHYSIOLOGIC INDICATIONS FOR MODALITY INTERVENTION

The results of microtrauma and macrotrauma on the cervical spine and TMJs and their associated tissues are well documented.[34,35,47,51] The initial response is often inflammation, as well as mechanical and chemical pain.[72–74] After macrotrauma such as a blow to the TMJ, the response is pain, joint effusion, and reflex muscle guarding. Depending on the degree of insult, this reflex guarding may maintain the capsular and muscular structures in a shortened or tightened state.[29] This response may in turn load the articular surfaces,

adding compressive forces to the joint and further producing increased muscle guarding.[76] Intra-articular adhesions may form between the joint surfaces and the intra-articular disc.[75] If this situation persists, deformation of soft tissue and a dysfunctional adaptive posture can occur.[51,54] If active mandibular or cervical movements are decreased as a result of ligamentous, muscle, capsular, and fascial restriction, excessive nociceptive input will deprive the central nervous system of normal proprioceptive stimulation.[29] Modality intervention using moist heat, ultrasound, and TENS assists in decreasing nociceptive input, edema, and spasm and increases circulation.

If untreated, normal balance between nociceptive and proprioceptive input is lost and constant excitation persists, perpetuating joint and ligamentous structure disorganization. As joint metabolites are retained, nociceptive input increases, further perpetuating the cycle. The trigeminal nerve has a confluence of nerve endings in the substantia gelatinosa that are similar in structure and function and continuous with the dorsal horn of the spinal cord.[43,47,71,79] Increased proprioception from the TMJ may stimulate the proximal fibers of cranial nerves V, VII, IX, and X. These cranial nerves are associated with the trigeminal sensory nuclei and have sympathetic connections with cervical nerves I through III via the nucleus caudalis. The interdependence of the cervical spine and TMJ and its symptoms is based on these neuroanatomic relationships.[43,68,71]

The use of cold, superficial and deep heat, and electrical stimulation can decrease inflammation, improve circulation, and decrease nociceptive input. These modalities are enhanced by soft-tissue and manual joint mobilization techniques at various stages in treatment.[78] Once the neuromuscular compressive forces are reduced, a more appropriate head-on-neck and condyle-to-disc relationship can be achieved.

INDICATIONS FOR CRYOTHERAPY

The most commonly used therapeutic modality following trauma or surgical intervention is cryotherapy. Cold packs, ice massage, or vapocoolant sprays are generally used. Cold is applied to reduce edema, inflammation, and muscle spasm. The mechanism is thought to be "counterirritation" and the production of analgesia.[80,81] The resultant vasoconstriction of cutaneous vessels and diminished heat loss cause stimulation of thermosensors in the skin, leading to reflex excitation of the sympathetic adrenergic fibers and further generalized cutaneous vasoconstriction through the preoptic region of the anterior hypothalamus. Cobbold and Lewis[82] demonstrated that after application of ice packs for approximately 10 minutes to the knee joints of dogs, there was a resultant decrease in blood flow averaging approximately 56%. After 25 minutes, the blood flow returned to the normal precooled rate. Cold also decreases the viscosity of blood, in turn decreasing blood flow.

A hemodynamic increase in flow is caused by vasodilation when heat is applied after ice to help "flush" the area. This "pumping action" aids venous return and removal of excess fluids from the traumatized area.[83] Moore and colleagues[84] suggest that the combination of cold and therapeutic exercise increases circulation, helps elimination of debris, and decreases rehabilitation time.[84]

Application of cold to peripheral nerves alters conduction velocity and synaptic activity.[81] Nerve fibers of different diameters and degrees of myelination appear to have different thresholds of sensitivity to the effects of cold.[85] The small-diameter myelinated fibers or "nociceptive fibers" seem to have greater cold sensitivity, whereas the small-diameter unmyelinated fibers seem to respond the least. Cold can also decrease nerve conduction velocities. Zankel[86] recorded a 6% decrease in motor conduction velocity in eight of ten subjects after cold was applied to the elbow for 5 minutes. In those eight subjects studied, conduction velocity returned to the precooled values within 15 minutes. The longer the application of cold, the greater the decrease in temperature, and in conduction velocity. This effect was demonstrated by Lee and colleagues,[87] who applied ice packs over the ulnar nerve for approximately 20 minutes, resulting in a decrease of motor conduction velocity of 29.4% from precooled values. Thirty minutes after ice pack removal, the conduction velocity was still 8.3% lower than values before ice application.

A primary cause of soft-tissue damage in both the cervical spine and TMJ is muscle guarding leading to spasm. Applications of cold decrease muscle spasm reflexively by breaking up the pain-spasm-pain cycle. Spasm leads to ischemia and compresses intramuscular blood vessels. The ischemia results in tissue damage and liberation of metabolites, stimulating pain fibers, and produces additional pain and muscle spasm. Cold bombards the central pain receptor areas with a barrage of cold impulses, which compete with pain impulses, thus interrupting the cycle of pain and spasm. Once cold has reduced spasm, static stretch and contract-relax techniques can be used to increase range of motion and resting length of the musculature.[80] Spasm caused by exercise can be relieved after 20 minutes of cold pack application and static stretching.[88] The combination of ice application with stretching is probably the most useful technique to decrease muscle spasm and soreness. Many techniques for cold application are available. The commercially sold gel pack, an isopropyl alcohol solution that when put in the freezer does not totally solidify, is extremely useful in therapy because it contours to the facial structures quite well. These packs stay at sufficiently cold temperatures for 15 to 20 minutes. Ice massage is also effective over muscle belly, tendon, and bursa as well as trigger points before deep massage. Belitsky and colleagues[89] found that after 15 minutes of cold application with wet ice, skin temperatures were decreased enough to produce anesthesia and analgesia. Ice massage of the web space between the thumb and index finger of the hand on the same side as the painful region in the face produced a 50% decrease in intensity of dental pain when measured by the Magill pain questionnaire.[90]

The use of vapocoolants such as Fluori-Methane, a nonflammable and nontoxic spray, can be used to rapidly cool the skin and overlying musculature while stretching. Vapocoolant sprays are thought to act as counterirritants, allowing more effective soft-tissue stretching. Travell and Simons[91] believed that trigger points are a result of any dysfunction causing decreased range of motion in either the area of the myofascial trigger point or the referred secondary areas of pain. Trigger points may also result from muscle strains associated with sensitized nerves in areas of increased metabolism and decreased circulation.[91] They can be located by digital pressure over the involved muscles. There may also be associated trigger points in the skin, ligaments, and fascia.[91]

The "spray and stretch technique" is done by placing the affected musculature on passive stretch and spraying a fine spray of vapocoolant at a 30° angle approximately 45 cm from the skin.[91] Spraying is done in unidirectional parallel sweeps along the muscle, over the trigger area first, then over the area of referred pain. If muscle lengthening is needed, then the entire length of the muscle from the proximal to the distal attachment is covered. The skin is generally sprayed two to three times at a rate of 10 cm/second. Figure 24–5 demonstrates spray and stretch of the temporalis muscle. The area can be rewarmed with moist heat, and spray and stretch is repeated as necessary. The postulated mechanism is the stimulation of cutaneous afferents, producing a reflex decrease in gamma motoneuron firing and allowing increased passive stretch of the muscle.

When utilizing vapocoolant sprays near the face, it is important to cover the eyes and avoid inhaling the vapors. Trigger points may also be desensitized by digital acupressure, electronic acupuncture, ice massage, ultrasound, and electrical stimulation[78,92,93] (see Fig. 24–5).

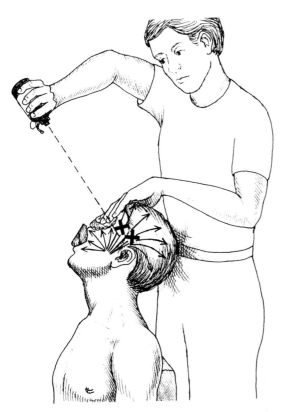

FIGURE 24–5. Spray and stretch technique. (See text for details.) (Reprinted with permission from Travell, J.G. and Simons, D.G.: *Myofascial Pain and Dysfunction: The Trigger Point Manual.* Williams & Wilkins, Baltimore, 1983.)

CONTRAINDICATIONS TO CRYOTHERAPY

Cryotherapy should be avoided in patients with a history of Raynaud's phenomenon, cold urticaria, cryoglobulinemia, and paroxysmal cold hemoglobinurias.[71] Patients with trigeminal neuralgia or postherpetic neuralgia of the trigeminal nerve may have sensory deprivation pain syndromes associated with hypersensitivity. In patients with a history of hypertension, circulatory impairment, and cold intolerance, frosting or blanching of the skin should be avoided.

SUPERFICIAL HEATING AGENTS

The most common superficial heat application techniques use moist heat packs and infrared lamps. Moist heat packs are canvas cases that are usually filled with bentonite, a hydrophilic substance. These packs are generally stored in a heating vat at temperatures of 71° to 79°. The packs are generally wrapped in towels and applied over a patient's symptomatic tissues. The depth of heating is approximately 0.5 to 1 cm through the skin and subcutaneous tissues.[94] Increases in temperature from moist heating produce cutaneous vasodilation, resulting in increased local circulation and speeding removal of inflammatory by-products such as prostaglandins, bradykinins, and histamines by reducing nociceptive activity.[71]

The local effect of moist heat is an elevation of skin temperature that reaches its maximum in approximately 6 to 8 minutes. Hot compresses only slightly increase the temperature of muscle tissue, but this increase can be significant in the facial area, where adipose tissue is very thin. Myospasm is often caused by overuse of the musculature as a result of clenching and bruxism or the protective mechanism of muscle guarding. Superficial heating of the skin may be of value by decreasing the gamma efferent activity.[94] The stretch on the muscle spindle is lessened, thus reducing afferent firing from the spindle. This indirect method may ultimately result in decreased alpha motorneuron firing.[94]

Infrared lamps provide some degree of superficial heating, and depth of penetration is approximately 2 mm below the skin's surface. Infrared is not very effective when used for treatment of TMJ disorders and should only be utilized when a patient's superficial tissues cannot tolerate light touch or the pressure of hot pack application.

DEEP-HEATING AGENTS
Ultrasound

Ultrasound is employed as an adjunct in the management of sort-tissue dysfunctions. These dysfunctions usually include joint capsule tightness, extracapsular tissue contracture, muscle spasm, and pain. The primary effect of ultrasound is thermal. The absorption of ultrasound energy is specific for tissue with high collagen concentration. Muscle, ligamentous, and capsular structures thus are the primary targets of ultrasound energy absorption.[95] Skin and subcutaneous adipose tissue receive little heating. Figure 24–6 demonstrates the application of ultrasound with prolonged stretch.

Ultrasound energy and depth of penetration are frequency dependent. With higher frequency (3 MHz), the concentration of energy is more pronounced in the superficial tissue. In the United States, ultrasound generators function at low frequencies of 800 KHz to 3 MHz.[96] A frequency of 1 MHz is appropriate for deep musculoskeletal dysfunctions such as those of the hip joint. A frequency of 3 MHz, which is more suitable for the TMJ region, has become available.

A physical therapist's goal in the treatment of TMJ and cervical dysfunctions is to increase capsular and periarticular structure extensibility. Ultrasound is the modality of choice for selectively increasing the temperature of these tissues. When collagen is heated to a temperature of 40° to 45°C, collagen bonding is relaxed and becomes less viscous.[71,97] The change in viscosity allows for plastic deformation. Ultrasound is thus an ideal modality both before and during joint and soft-tissue mobilization (see Fig. 24–6). This technique is of great value when working with tightened capsular structures in which extensibility has been lost.

Preheating and simultaneous heating of tissues during passive stretching greatly increase the tissue lengthening produced, with less potential for damage to the tissue.[97] Lehmann and colleagues[98] demonstrated the effectiveness of ultrasound at therapeutic intensities of 1.0 to 2.5 watts/cm^2 for 5 minutes. Applied to the anterior, lateral, and posterior hip, the combination of ultrasound and exercise produced increased range of motion.[99] Bierman[100] reported increased range of motion in patients with scar tissue secondary to lacerations, x-ray burns, and Dupuytren's contracture. Ultrasound was employed at intensities of 1 to 2 watts/cm^2 for 6 to 8 minutes.

Because ultrasound has the ability to increase temperature, it can increase blood flow, help to clear metabolic waste products, and increase cell membrane permeability,[101] leading to quicker healing of soft tissue. Changes in sensory nerve conduction velocity following ultrasound application have been reported by Currier and associates.[102] After 5 minutes of ultrasound application at 1.5 watts/cm^2 over the lateral cutaneous branch of the femoral nerve,

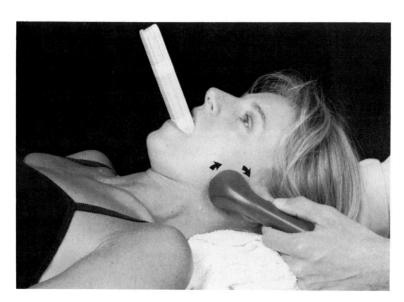

FIGURE 24–6. This patient is receiving ultrasound to the temporomandibular joint while tongue depressors provide continuous stretch. The patient may add more tongue depressors, as the extensibility of the tissues increases over 3 to 5 minutes.

decreased latency was noted with decreased conduction velocity of the peripheral nerve.[102] Pain relief can also be produced by ultrasound heating of peripheral nerves and free nerve endings by increasing their pain threshold.[96]

Ultrasound can be used to drive anti-inflammatory and analgesic agents through the skin, a process known as phonophoresis. Cortisol, dexamethasone, salicylates, and lidocaine are the medications most often used.[103] The ultrasound beam forces medication away from the transducer head[104] and through tissue by increasing skin permeability. Ultrasound has been shown to enhance the effect of hydrocortisone injections[105] and to increase bone healing rates through the piezoelectric effect.[106]

Ultrasound can be delivered via continuous or pulsed modes. Continuous ultrasound is suggested for heat and stretch techniques. Pulsed ultrasound is better suited for enhancing edema reduction, as its mechanical effect is maximized.

CONTRAINDICATIONS TO SUPERFICIAL AND DEEP HEAT

No heat modality used in physical therapy should be directed over the eyes. Superficial or deep heat is generally not applied immediately after trauma or surgical intervention and is not used in the presence of sensory cutaneous loss. Care must be taken not to direct the ultrasound beam toward the eye socket during treatment of the TMJ. Ultrasound is not applied in the presence of malignancy.[71] The epiphyseal growth plates in children should be avoided, particularly intensities greater than 3 watts/cm^2. Evidence of bone demineralization, damage to epiphyseal plates, and retardation of bone growth is noted when a stationary transducer is used for periods of 3 minutes or greater.[96,107] The safety of ultrasound use during pregnancy has not been established.

ELECTROTHERAPY

Interest in electrotherapeutic devices increased after the publication of Dr. Ronald Melzack's gate control theory of pain in 1965.[120] Since that time, electrical stimulation has clinically and experimentally proved valuable as an adjunct for the relief of pain, for reduction of edema, and to decrease muscle spasm and associated inflammatory and metabolic sequelae of temporomandibular and craniocervical disorders. Electrotherapy has become an important part of physiologic manipulation of the soft tissues and nervous structures.

Galvanic Stimulators

The electrical generators most commonly used in physical therapy include high-voltage galvanic stimulators, low-voltage alternating-current generators, interferential stimulators, transcutaneous nerve stimulators, noninvasive acupuncture units, and iontophoretic devices. Each has its own waveform, polarity, and stimulation ranges.

High-voltage galvanic stimulation is used to treat muscle spasm, edema, and joint dysfunction. High-voltage galvanic stimulation in certain modes also works well for pain reduction. High-voltage therapy delivers current in the microampere range; low-voltage units deliver current in the milliampere range. Raising the voltage produces deeper tissue penetration.[108] This deeper penetration is achieved without the significant chemical and thermal effects observed with low-voltage irritation.

Some investigators believe that different electrical polarities produce different physiologic reactions in soft tissue.[108] Positive polarity is thought to produce an acid reaction and cause a coagulation or hardening of tissue protein in addition to increased vasoconstriction.[112,117] Negative polarity produces an alkaline reaction that is thought to soften protein and produce vasodilation.[112,117] These effects can increase or decrease nerve irritability. Clinical application of electrogalvanic stimulation is beneficial for treatment of acute muscle guarding because of its pumping action.[108] Figure 24–7A and B shows electrode placement used to treat cervical spine and TMJ disorders.

Increases in peripheral circulation are thought to be caused by deep penetration of high-voltage current, which stimulates sympathetic neurons, directly causing vasodilation.[110] The healing of decubitus ulcers has also been accelerated by using the negative polarity.[111] The effect of polarity has yet to be scientifically documented.

Interferential stimulation uses two medium-frequency currents around 4000 Hz; these currents, when properly applied, evoke interferential currents between 1 and 100 Hz. The interferential effect occurs when two different unmodulated medium-frequency alternating currents are applied simultaneously to a tissue using two paired electrodes. The problem of loss of penetration due to skin resistance is de-

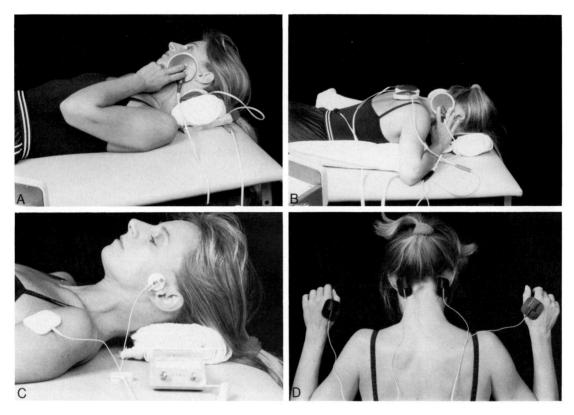

FIGURE 24–7. *A*, Application of electrogalvanic stimulation electrodes to the masticatory and upper cervical musculature. *B*, Electrode placement for spasm located in the posterior cervical musculatures. *C*, The Phoresor II* is utilized to transdermally transport medicinal agents to the temporomandibular joint.

creased with this technique. Better depth and decreased accommodation are produced with this frequency modulation. The technique may be of benefit in decreasing pain and increasing vasodilation in tissues.[109]

Iontophoresis

Iontophoresis is defined as the electrically induced transfer of ions through tissue. Medications can be introduced into the body transdermally using a continuous galvanic direct current of low amperage. The ion solution of a pharmacologic agent is placed under the electrode of the same ion polarity.

Medications such as cortisol, dexamethasone, salicylates, and analgesics have been introduced over inflamed joints and tissues.[103,113] The site of application must be free of anesthesia, cuts, abrasions, and skin eruptions. Some investigators recommend the use of heat or other modalities before iontophoresis.[114] This is probably good advice for treatment of TMJ disorders. Kahn[115] recommended iontophore-

sis with 5% lidocaine (Xylocaine) or 0.5% hydrocortisone ointment under the positive electrode placed over the TMJ. This method produced a decrease in paresthesia, pain, and trismus in patients who underwent TMJ surgery. He also found that following iontophoresis, ultrasound may increase the depth of penetration as compared with electrical stimulation alone. Kahn recommended continuous ultrasound at an intensity of 1 watt/cm^2 for 3 minutes.

Iontophoresis of lidocaine was studied by Russo and associates.[116] They compared the duration and depth of anesthesia produced by lidocaine with physiologic saline using the positive electrode of a Phoresor* (Fig. 24–7*C*). Treatment time was approximately 7 minutes. Various electrical amplitudes were used during that time. This procedure produced local anesthesia for approximately 14.5 minutes as compared with lidocaine infiltration, which

---

*Motion Control, Salt Lake City, UT.

produced anesthesia for 22.2 minutes. The depth of anesthesia penetration was the same with both infiltration and the iontophoresis administration.

This technique may be advantageous for patients who are needle phobics. It also has use in patients who are in severe pain because of inflamed joints and trigger points and may be used before joint mobilization, deep tissue massage, acupressure, or hyperstimulation analgesia with electrotherapeutic devices.

Transcutaneous Nerve Stimulation

The ability of TENS to reduce or eliminate pain has been widely recognized for some time. The literature indicates that the treatment can be beneficial in patients with both acute and chronic pain.[118,119]

Sensory modulation can be altered by various forms of counterirritation. These may include heat, cold, electrical stimulation, various mobilization techniques, and pressure massage.[78] TENS and noninvasive electroacupuncture have attracted much attention since Melzack and Wall[120] developed the gate control theory of pain perception. TENS has been used in athletes,[121] in patients with lower back pain,[122] during childbirth,[123] and in dental procedures.[118,124–127] The use of TENS seems to be limitless in physical therapy. In the management of TMJ disorders, it is used primarily to control pain.

TENS should be used early in TMJ and craniocervical disorders to help hasten recovery. The success of TENS is dependent on the skill of the person assessing the pathology, the local sites of application, and the stimulation mode used. Other modalities such as joint mobilization, transverse friction massage, and contract-relax stretching should be used concurrently with TENS.[28]

The most commonly used mode of TENS features a high rate of frequency, a narrow pulse duration, and moderate intensity—also known as conventional TENS. This mode of TENS reduces pain through selective activation of large-diameter proprioceptive afferents, which inhibit or balance the small-diameter nociceptive input at the dorsal horn,[128] creating a sensation of mild to moderate paresthesia over the painful area. Conventional TENS should not produce muscle contraction and should produce quick pain relief that has a relatively short period of effectiveness.[129] When using conventional TENS, it may sometimes

be necessary to increase the amplitude or pulse width slightly because of rapid accommodation.[128] Wolf[130] used a 100-Hz, 0.25-msec stimulus at an intensity that caused paresthesia. This noxious level of TENS was necessary to modify thermal and mechanical experimental pain. Experimental pain is significantly different from clinical pain, and an uncomfortable level of stimulation is not always required in clinical situations.

Strong, low-frequency (acupuncture-like) TENS requires an induction period of 20 to 30 minutes and must produce a strong, visible contraction in the segmentally related myotome.[128] This mode of stimulation may provide an extended period of pain relief but is often not well tolerated by patients because of strong contraction in a painful area. It may, however, be used as a last-resort method at the dorsal side of the hand bilaterally, where it is easily tolerated. Chapman and colleagues[132] used low-frequency 2-Hz stimulation for 80 minutes, resulting in a strong, throbbing sensation. Tooth pain threshold increased by 187% after 20 minutes of stimulation to the cheek. The threshold remained constant for the remaining period of stimulation. Mannheimer and Carlsson[133] suggest that high-intensity stimulation of an uncomfortable but tolerable quality gives the best pain relief in patients with rheumatoid arthritis. Such stimulation levels are not tolerated as well in the highly innervated and more sensitive craniofacial region.

"Pulse trains," or bursts of stimulation, can be delivered at both high and low intensities. Combined pulse trains provide high-frequency bursts with a low-rate pulse. This mode produces a low repetition rate with high internal frequency. Less current is required than needed for strong low-rate TENS, and this method can also be used as a means of modulating or intensifying conventional TENS.[134] Mannheimer and Carlsson[133] successfully reduced pain in a group of rheumatoid arthritis sufferers using a repetition rate of 3 Hz and an internal frequency of 70 Hz. The current intensity was just below that which would cause pain.

The fourth mode of electrical stimulation using TENS is described as brief and intense. Mannheimer and Lampe[128] suggest a high frequency of approximately 100 to 150 Hz, a high pulse width of 150 to 250 microseconds, and amplitude to the highest tolerable level. The determination of pulse width and amplitude setting with this mode is highly variable. Consideration must be given to the area being treated. In the highly innervated craniofacial region, pulse width level can be set between 100 and 150 msecs. Because the electrodes will be relatively close together, the amplitude setting can be significantly lower than that needed on the extremities, where the interelectrode distance is much greater.

This mode of stimulation combined with correct electrode placement over the superficial aspects of cutaneous nerves will produce a nonrhythmic contraction or tetany of the corresponding musculature and may allow for the performance of gentle manual therapeutic techniques after obtaining an acceptable level of analgesia with 5 to 15 minutes of brief, intense TENS.

The use of brief, intense TENS in the craniofacial region produces strong contraction of the mandibular elevators and simulates trismus. This effect is not helpful, and use of this mode must be considered precautionary. It may be indicated to produce analgesia sufficient for the removal of sutures or other minor dental procedures. However, joint mobilization can only be effectively performed after reducing the strength of the stimulus once analgesic levels have been obtained. Prolonged use of high-intensity TENS also causes ischemia in the area, again limiting its use, especially in postsurgical conditions.

Post-traumatic and postsurgical patients with TMJ disorders often have edema and muscle guarding.[135] Low-rate TENS produces a slow, rhythmic muscle contraction and is the treatment of choice for these patients. The optimal frequency is between 0.7 and 1 Hz (one pulse per second). The principal characteristics of the different stimulation modes are listed in Table 24–1.

Electrode placement for TMJ and upper cervical pain has been described by Mannheimer and Lampe.[128] They recommend placement at the ipsilateral suboccipital fossa and TMJ as the initial choice.

Alternate methods include one electrode on the TMJ and the other on the masseter. Facial electrodes should be of a smaller diameter to minimize overflow of stimulation to the region around the eye. Electrodes of unequal size can also be placed on the dorsal web space and masseter (Fig. 24–8A). The dorsal web space is an area that is anatomically adjacent to that of the head via its location in the somatomotor and somatosensory cortices. Significant activation of this region may allow for inhibition of painful stimuli to the facial area.[128]

Figure 24–8B illustrates the placement of electrodes in the suboccipital fossa and the masseter muscle. This placement is highly effective in stimulating the greater and lesser occipital nerves plus the trigeminal spinal tract, thus reducing cervical spine input and TMJ pain. Figure 24–8B shows electrode placement for the masseter and anterior fibers of the temporalis. A frequent feature of both temporo-

TABLE 24–1. TENS Modes: Optimal Initial Stimulation Parameter Settings

	CONVENTIONAL	STRONG, LOW-RATE (ACUPUNCTURE-LIKE)	HIGH-INTENSITY PULSE-TRAIN (BURST)*	BRIEF, INTENSE
Frequency	50–100 Hz	1–4 Hz	Trains of high-frequency (70–100 Hz) pulses modulated at a rate of 2 Hz	100–150 Hz
Pulse Duration	40–75 μsec	150–250 μsec	100–200 μsec	150–250 μsec
Amplitude	Perceptible, paresthesia up to but not causing significant muscle contraction or fasciculation	To tolerance, giving rise to strong rhythmic muscle contractions	To tolerance; strong, rhythmic contractions plus a background paresthesia	To tolerance, will cause either a tetanic contraction or nonrhythmic fasciculations
	10–30 mA	30–80 mA	30–60 mA	30–80 mA

Note: Pulse duration and amplitude ranges are quite variable and depend a great deal on the quality and distribution of pain, interelectrode distance, number of electrodes utilized, and patient tolerance.

*Pulse-train (burst) parameters can also be delivered at low intensity similar to the conventional mode. When used in this manner, amplitude and pulse width will be in the range of the conventional mode, and the sensation will consist of mild paresthesia plus a rhythmic background pulsing. (Reprinted with permission from Mannheimer, J.S. and Lampe, G.N.: Electrode placement techniques. In *Clinical Transcutaneous Electrical Stimulation.* J.S. Mannheimer, J.S. and Lampe, G.N. (eds.). F.A. Davis Co., Philadelphia, 1984.)

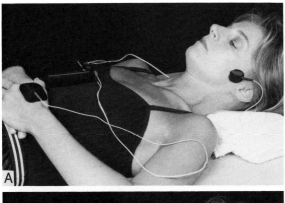
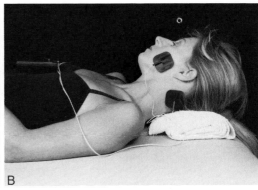
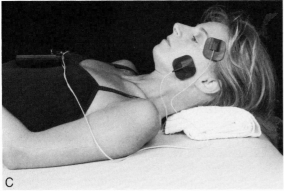

FIGURE 24–8. *A,* The transcutaneous electrical nerve stimulator electrode setup for temporomandibular joint pain. The smaller electrode is placed over the masseter to stimulate the facial and trigeminal nerve branches. The larger electrode is placed over the web space of the ipsilateral hand, which stimulates the superficial radial and musculocutaneous sensory nerves and ulnar motor nerve. *B,* Electrode placement for concomitant temporomandibular and suboccipital pain. This placement stimulates the facial and trigeminal branches and the greater and lesser occipital nerves. *C,* Placement for temporomandibular pain. Electrode placement is over the masseter and anterior fibers of the temporalis. This technique is valuable for temporal headache. *D,* This electrode placement is for bilateral frontal headache, which may result from cervical strain.

mandibular and cervical disorders is headache. TENS with electrode placement in the suboccipital area and web space bilaterally can be used to decrease frontal headache (Fig. 24–8D).

A Pain Suppressor* TENS unit can be used with an electrode pad arrangement stimulating transcranially. Electrodes are placed at each temporal area above and slightly anterior to the ear. Stimulation five to eight times a day is said to produce changes in the metabolite serotonin.[128] This method of stimulation produced mood changes in patients who were treated with it. The pain suppressor unit generates a very low output via an interrupted direct current with a burst frequency of 15 times per second and a carrier frequency of 15,000 cycles per second. This current is delivered at a subthreshold level.

The successful use of TENS depends on proper electrode placement, choice of stimulation mode, and whether the pain is acute or chronic. The first mode of stimulation used is generally conventional TENS. If this mode does not relieve pain, then a strong, low-rate acupuncture-like or pulse train burst mode should be applied. These modes are generally used for patients with chronic pain characterized by deep aching. The goal when using these modes is to produce a strong, rhythmic muscle contraction in segmentally related myotomes, best tolerated away from the region of pain. The stronger the muscle contraction, the greater the pain-relieving effect.[128]

Contraindications to the Use of Electrotherapy

Electrical stimulation, including iontophoresis, high-voltage galvanic stimulation, and TENS, is contraindicated in the presence of open skin lesions, infections, and impaired sensation. Electrical stimulation should not be performed on persons with demand-type cardiac pacemakers or over the carotid sinus, lar-

*Pain Suppression Labs, Inc., Elmwood Park, N.J.

ynx, and pharynx musculature. Patients with a history of transient ischemic attacks, cerebrovascular accidents, and epilepsy should not receive stimulation over the eyes, head, or neck.[71] The safety of electrotherapy during pregnancy has not been established.

BIOFEEDBACK

Many investigators have utilized biofeedback training and other behavior relaxation therapies.[39,136,137] These techniques are useful for treating stress-related temporomandibular disorders and should be part of a comprehensive treatment plan. The physiologic changes of decreased muscle tone, respiratory rate, heart rate, blood pressure, and blood lactic acid levels help to relieve abnormally tight musculature. Biofeedback is discussed in greater detail in chapter 26.

OTHER PHYSICAL THERAPY TECHNIQUES

Techniques such as acupressure have long been utilized by the Japanese and Chinese in the relief of pain in the temporomandibular and craniocervical area.[93,138,139] They work by a mechanism similar to TENS. Noninvasive electroacupuncture has shown effectiveness similar to acupuncture needling.[128] Small hand-held probes are used to generate greater current densities and a pulse rate of 2 to 4 Hz delivered over 30 to 60 seconds of stimulation per site.[71] The mechanism of pain relief in noninvasive electroacupuncture is attributed to endorphin liberation and hyperstimulation analgesia.[128,140]

Contraindications to Pressure Therapy

Acupressure and deep-pressure massage should be avoided over regions of sensory deficit or hypersensitivity or in the presence of circulatory impairment or malignancy. Contraindications to electroacupuncture are the same as for all electrotherapy.

Manual Therapy

Manual therapy is the application of gentle, passive, sustained and oscillating forces to joints or soft tissues to assist in their readapta-

tion. Readaptation is based on the ability of collagen to become plastic through modality preparation and manual therapy technique.[74,75,141] Readaptation may restore joint mobility through lengthening of the muscle, capsule, or fascial structure. Manual techniques are often applied to a hypomobile TMJ, a cervical joint injury, or adapted FHP.[41,42,54,142] Once the tissue is sufficiently flexible and strengthened, the patient can regain a more ideal head-on-neck orthostatic relationship.[27,28,41]

SOFT-TISSUE AND JOINT MOBILIZATION

Comprehensive treatment of temporomandibular and craniocervical disorders can be broken down into three areas: modalities, mobilization, and patient education. The modalities are used early in treatment to control pain and edema and for soft-tissue preparation. The mobilization techniques described here can next be used to assist return of normal, painfree range of motion.

Pain perception often indicates tissue damage and subsequent noxious input. Tissue impingement such as a deranged disc or hyperactive suprahyoid muscle can cause deformation or damage, producing mechanical and chemical pain. Mechanical pain can be constant or intermittent and is influenced by movement and position. Patients with mechanical pain, when in a position of decreased mechanical stress, have periods when they are pain free.[143,144]

Chemical or inflammatory pain, although often accompanying mechanical pain, is usually more constant and less affected by changes in osseous and soft-tissue position.[142] Many patients present with both chemical and mechanical components to their pain. These components may be treated individually or together.[72–74] Treatment of the chemical aspect may ameliorate mechanical deformation as well.[72,142]

The physical therapist, through careful examination, must decide which treatment modality and manual technique are appropriate. An acute inflammatory process should be treated with rest and application of physical agents to enhance the healing process. As the healing process proceeds and inflammation is reduced, dysfunction will appear to be more of a mechanical nature. At this point, treatment shifts to a more mechanical approach—mobilization of the osseous and soft-tissue structures.[72,144,146]

After inflammatory and mechanical pain has been reduced, it is essential to optimize temporomandibular and craniocervical function. Therapy should provide improved muscle strength and flexibility and allow for full body reconditioning, so that the patient can return to normal activity.[147]

Soft-Tissue Mobilization: Temporomandibular Joint

Soft-tissue mobilization techniques include deep pressure point massage, stretching, myofascial release, strain–counterstrain, and craniosacral therapy. The masticatory and cervical musculature is prone to the development of trigger points when shortening, lengthening, or loosening of muscles occurs.[91] Although soft-tissue structures are often tight, a chronically weakened, wasted, and lengthened structure may also be a source of pain and disability.[149] Basmajian indicates that muscle in chronic spasm has decreased myoelectric activity.[148]

Shortening or elongation of structures can change anatomic symmetry in a three-dimensional manner throughout the kinetic chain. Myofascial release is a soft-tissue mobilization technique to improve this three-dimensional deformation.

Myofascial release is a combination of direct, indirect, and reflex neural release procedures. Abnormalities and mechanical asymmetries found by palpation of tissue are signals of altered structure. The pathologic relationship at various levels of tissue can be described as "hard," which indicates restriction of movement of soft-tissue and osseous structures, or "soft," which indicates laxity or hypermobility.[149]

"Tissue barriers" or areas of tightness exhibit decreased motion capability.[150] Assessment of pathology is made as the therapist palpates from superficial to deep tissue. Muscle irritability, evidence of trauma, degenerative change, contraction, contracture, and pain are noted.

The basis of this technique is sensing palpable changes at various levels of tissue and manually directing gentle force to assist in releasing tissues. This alteration of tissue is thought to be mechanical and neuroreflexive.[149]

The technique is accomplished by inducing deformation through gentle compression and traction while simultaneously twisting and shearing hands in opposite directions. Tissue releases are complete when restrictions are no longer apparent. Exercise is critical to maintain the gained extensibility of soft tissue.[41,54]

The technique shown in Figure 24–9 is designed to release a tight masseter. These positions are held for 30 to 120 seconds or longer until a giving way is sensed in the muscle. A modification of this technique, shown in Figure 24–10, simultaneously incorporates the release of the masseter and temporalis complex. When hypertonicity is present in the temporalis, the parietal bone may move in an inferior direction, producing a compression of the tem-

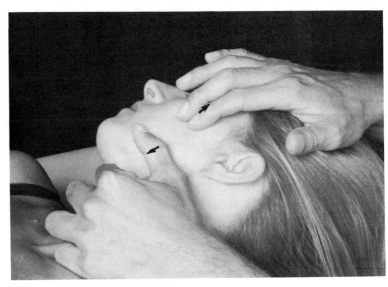

FIGURE 24–9. Masseter release. Tight masseter musculature and surrounding soft tissue may be released using this technique.

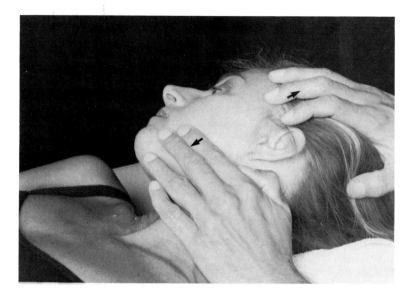

FIGURE 24–10. Temporalis and masseter complex release. This technique incorporates both the masseter and temporalis in a combined release. The technique is valuable for treating patients who chronically clench or who have temporal headache as a significant complaint following surgery.

poroparietal suture.[151] Suture compression may give rise to neurogenic activity and possible intersutural ischemia and headache. Temporalis release may decrease certain kinds of headache, especially when used in conjunction with craniosacral therapy.[151]

The parietal bone may be mobilized in a medial direction by decompressing the temporoparietal suture (Fig. 24–11A). Pressure applied to the parietal bone just above the suture is exerted in a very gentle but sustained motion for 3 to 5 minutes.[151] Once the parietal bones have been decompressed, they may then be moved

in a superior direction to decompress the temporoparietal suture. Another release technique, pictured in Figure 24–11B, has been successful in releasing the temporalis.

Further decompression of the temporal bone and its associated soft tissue may be achieved by the ear-pull technique (Fig. 24–12). Gentle forces are applied in a posterior lateral direction while grasping the pinnae. This is done until the soft tissue and temporal bone appear to "unwind" and move laterally. This technique is helpful for releasing scar tissue around the TMJ after both open and arthroscopic sur-

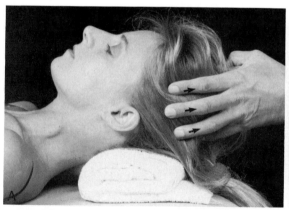
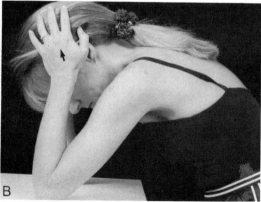

FIGURE 24–11. A, Parietal decompression and lift. The parietal bone must be gently decompressed prior to performing a lift. It must be disengaged from the temporal bone in order to facilitate movement. Finger tip pressure is exerted on the parietal bone for 3 to 5 minutes. Once the temporoparietal suture has disengaged, the parietal bones move superiorly. B, Autorelease of the temporalis. This technique is performed by placing the thenar eminences over the middle fibers of the temporalis bilaterally and applying gentle medial pressure. This technique can be sustained for 3 to 5 minutes for adequate relief of temporal headaches.

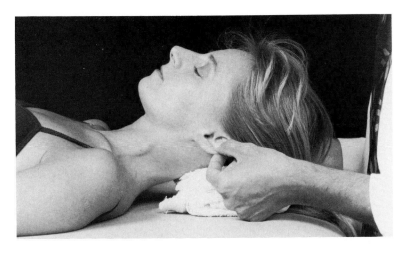

FIGURE 24–12. Ear pull technique. Gentle forces are applied in the posterior lateral direction, while grasping the pinnae. This technique is always done in a bilateral manner until the soft tissue and temporal bones appear to unwind and move laterally. The technique is used for temporal headache and postsurgical scarring of the periauricular tissue of the temporomandibular joint.

gical procedures. Craniosacral techniques have been the subject of much controversy and to date lack scientific documentation. They have, however, been clinically effective.

One of the more common methods used in myofascial release is the bilateral suboccipital release technique (Fig. 24–13), which releases some of the long and particularly the short muscles in the posterior cervical spine. These tissues are often responsible for nerve entrapments, encountered with FHP and posterior cranial rotation. They are frequently injured as a result of whiplash injuries.[51] Entrapment of lesser and greater occipital nerves may cause headache radiating to the occipital-frontal area. Pain can be referred to the TMJ and face through noxious stimuli produced at C1 through C4 synapses in the spinal tract of the trigeminal nerve.[43,48,51,63] Thus, this technique

may be used to treat cervical spine and TMJ disorders concurrently. It is valuable for increasing upper cervical spine mobility and alleviating vague symptoms in many patients, such as blurred vision, dizziness, tinnitus, and craniofacial pain.

Suprahyoid and infrahyoid release techniques (Figs. 24–14 and 24–15) are indicated for patients with lack of craniocervical extensibility. Prolonged periods of FHP following cervical injury can cause dysfunction of the suprahyoid and infrahyoid musculature. These techniques assist relaxation and proper placement of the tongue in patients with abnormal tongue position or swallowing habits and are often used after mandibular and cervical whiplash. FHP can occur after traumatic injuries or over time through maladaptation. FHP straightens the normal cervical spine lordosis,

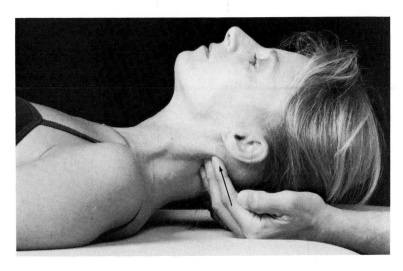

FIGURE 24–13. Bilateral suboccipital release. This technique is particularly valuable when treating a patient with craniofacial and craniovertebral pain. Releasing of the suboccipital soft tissue as well as decompressing of the occipital atlantal joints frequently relieves difficult symptoms to treat, such as dizziness, blurred vision, and tinnitus.

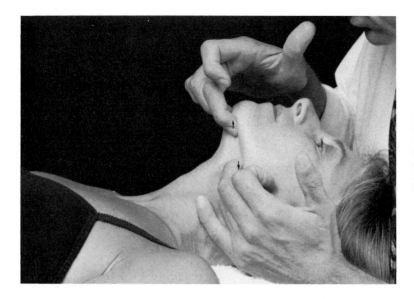

FIGURE 24–14. Suprahyoid release technique. This may be used to free up shortened anterior and posterior bellies of the digastric as well as the stylohyoid muscles. These techniques must be done in a gentle fashion.

which elevates the hyoid bone, shortens the suprahyoids, and stretches the infrahyoid muscle.[51,152]

Soft-Tissue Mobilization: Upper Cervical Spine

Because of the intimate relationship between the upper cervical spine and the TMJ,[147] soft-tissue release techniques can be applied to the cervical spine musculature of the first three cervical segments. Figures 24–16A, B, and C show generalized releases that aid in balancing asymmetries of the maladapted musculature and joints.

The technique pictured in Figure 24–16A brings freedom to the restricted infrahyoid, anterior deep cervical musculature (longus colli, longus capitis), and ligamentous support structures of the anterior spine. Also released are superficial skin, the fascia, the platysma, the sternocleidomastoid, and the anterior division of the scalenes. A vertebral artery test (see Chapter 5) should always be done before this technique. These techniques must be performed gently, because strong force may inhibit release

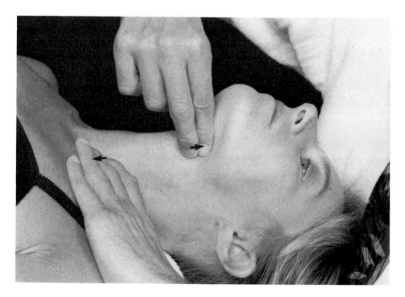

FIGURE 24–15. Infrahyoid release may be used to decrease spasm in the overstretched infrahyoid musculature. This is often seen in the postcervical whiplash patient.

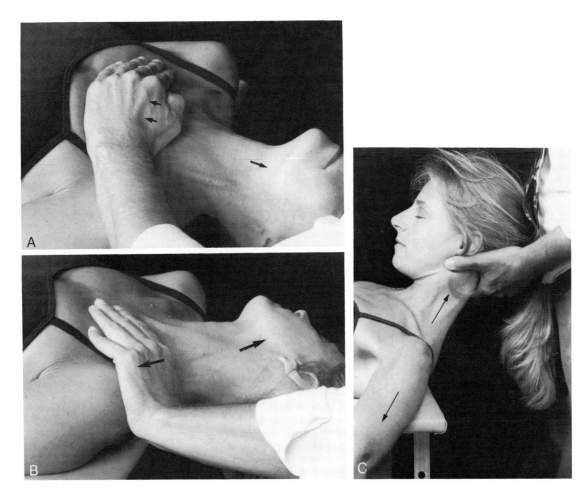

FIGURE 24–16. *A*, Anterior cervical release. This technique is designed to stretch the anterior cervical musculature as well as the ligamentous support structures of the cervical spine. Muscles involved are the longus colli and capitis, platysmas, sternocleidomastoids, and the anterior portions of the scalenes. *B*, Lateral cervical release. The scalenes, sternocleidomastoids, and anterior and lateral ligamentous support structures are released utilizing this technique. *C*, Posterior cervical release. This technique is designed to liberate the trapezius, levator scapulae, splenius capitis, and semispinalis capitis. This musculature is generally shortened because of isometric contraction.

and cause pain during and after treatment. Some patients experience occasional soreness, which may be directly related to the therapist's skill and experience.

The lateral musculature of the cervical spine is attached multisegmentally. The anterior and medial portions of the scalenes are of particular importance in balancing the cranium. Any restriction caused by shortening or spasm may inhibit the movement cephalad in the kinetic chain.[41] These muscles can be released using the technique pictured in Figure 24–16B. Also released in this technique are the sternocleidomastoids, platysmas, and anterolateral ligamentous support structures (see Fig. 24–16B). The posterior cervical musculature (trapezius, levator scapulae, splenius capitis, semispinalis

capitis) is released as shown in Figure 24–16C. These techniques not only stretch muscle but seem to reset important neuroreflexes.[149,153,154]

Joint Mobilization

Joint mobilization techniques are divided into four grades.[143] Each grade successively improves pathologic range of motion of a joint. Grade I, a small-amplitude movement at the beginning of joint range, is used for extremely irritable joints. The technique works through neuromodulation.[155] Grade II is a larger-amplitude oscillation that is partway into the available joint range. Grade III oscillations are large-amplitude movements that move the joint through full available range. Grade IV movements are small-amplitude movements that are performed at the end of joint range. Grades III and IV mobilization are used for joints that are generally stiff and slightly painful.[143] These passive oscillations are performed at a rate of two to three per second. The presenting state of the joint dictates the grade of mobilization to be performed.

Causing pain must always be avoided, and a decision to increase mobilization is based on re-evaluation as therapy progresses. Subjective reports from the patient during the treatment and objective change in range of motion provide the therapist with the information necessary to employ the appropriate technique. These techniques can be used over the spinous processes and transverse processes to produce improved anterior, posterior, and rotational movement.

Manipulation, or grade V mobilization, is distinct from grades I through IV. Manipulation employs a high-velocity, low-amplitude thrust that moves the affected joint beyond its present restricted range.[143] When this technique is used, the patient cannot control the manipulative motion. Grade V manipulation should be used only by physical therapists who have had extensive training and experience in manual therapy. The technique is used when full range of motion has not been achieved

using grades I through IV. Grades I through IV are most often used with the TMJ. Grades I through V are used for treatment of the cervical spine.

Specific Joint Mobilization: TMJ

If mandibular movements are severely limited, a thorough assessment of the masticatory structures involved is necessary.[156] When severe pain, spasm, and marked limitation due to recent trauma are present, extraoral techniques are useful (Fig. 24–17A, B, C). They can help decrease spasm and pain when done in grades I and II oscillations in lateral glide, depression, and protrusion.[157] These mobilization techniques stimulate joint mechanoreceptors that give rise to large myelinated fibers and inhibit small fiber nociceptive input.[155] Conventional TENS used before and during this technique may also activate the large myelinated fibers. Thus, pain relief and rapid restoration of joint function may occur.[128]

As muscle guarding decreases and range of motion increases, restricted soft-tissue structures are more easily assessed and allow the appropriate use of direct intraoral techniques. The primary movement lost to limited capsule extensibility is translation.[29] The "joint play" motions that are also lost are depression and

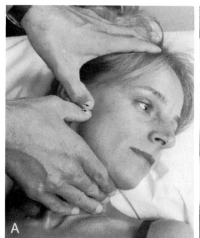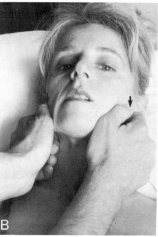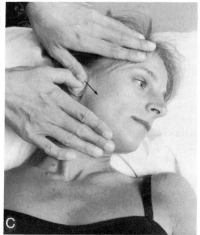

FIGURE 24–17. *A,* Extraoral lateral glide. This technique is performed with the patient's head rotated in the opposite direction of the affected temporomandibular joint. Gentle oscillatory mobilizations are performed over the lateral pole of the condyle, or they may be performed more distally if pain is perceived by the patient. This technique should be done bilaterally in the presence of a unilateral problem. *B,* Extraoral depression of the mandible. The patient lies with the head in a neutral position. The angle of the mandible is grasped with the index finger and thumb bilaterally, and gentle oscillatory pressures are applied in depression. *C,* Extraoral protrusion. The head is rotated to the left maximally. The gliding force of the therapist's thumbs is directed anteriorly. The patient is instructed to actively open during this technique. A decrease in swelling in the retrodiscal tissues may be effected using this procedure.

lateral glide. The technique shown in Figure 24–18 can be used for diagnosis and treatment. Force applied to the molars and the joint must include depression, translation, and side gliding. The examiner senses a "gummy end feel" at the end of the pathologic range of motion in a tight capsular pattern.[29] The patient's pain symptoms should be heeded. A "hard end feel" may indicate an anteriorly displaced disc without reduction. A sharp deflection of the mandible to the ipsilateral side of the displaced disc may be seen.[29]

Once the motion of the TMJ is assessed, treatment is directed at restoring optimal movement. The technique shown in Figure 24–18 is used for reducing an anteriorly displaced disc without reduction; in attempts to reduce dislocated condyles; and for treatment of general loss of joint mobility. This technique should not be used immediately after open joint surgery. The techniques pictured in Figure 17A, B, and C may be used together with the previous technique in the presence of joint effusion, capsulitis, and muscle guarding. Pressure applied should be within the limits of pain.

The desired effect of these mobilization techniques is the deformation of collagen within its elastic range. Clinicians must develop an acute tissue-sensing ability through practice. Active mandibular opening is helpful in increasing the effectiveness of these treatment techniques. If these techniques are used with too much force, increased pain and swelling and decreased mobility may result.

Specific Joint Mobilization: Upper Cervical Spine

Because headache and referred facial pain can originate from C1-3, a discussion of mobilization of the subcranial joints is appropriate. The occiput, C1, C2, and C3 have an intimate osseous relationship.[48] The spinal kinetic chain has a most complex arthrokinematic and neurovascular interaction. Pathology of these segments can influence balance, sight, and occlusion.[41,54] Tongue position may be altered in the presence of FHP.[29,158] Mobilization of the subcranial joints should always be preceded by a vertebral artery test. This test is designed to detect the presence of vascular insufficiency, which may be exacerbated by backward bending, side bending, and rotation of the head.[143,159,160] Symptoms include pupillary changes, nystagmus, dizziness, dysarthria, visual changes, and giddiness.[143,161,162]

The first cervical mobilization technique applied is transverse vertebral pressure, as shown in Figure 24–19A. The gentle force is applied with the thumbs on the lateral tip of the lateral mass of C1. This technique is applied toward and away from the symptomatic side of the upper cervical spine. When it is done appropriately, a decrease in pain, spasm, and joint restriction between the occiput and C1 will occur.

Posteroanterior unilateral vertebral pressure is used when the symptoms are bilateral or unilateral (Fig. 24–19B). This technique should never be done in a way that produces radicular

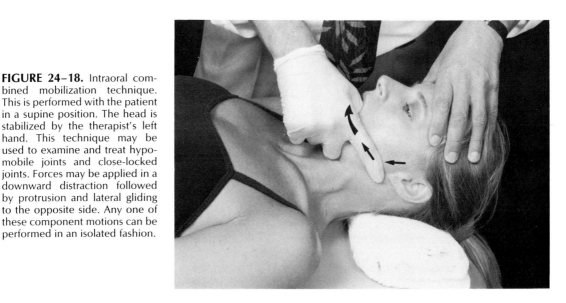

FIGURE 24–18. Intraoral combined mobilization technique. This is performed with the patient in a supine position. The head is stabilized by the therapist's left hand. This technique may be used to examine and treat hypomobile joints and close-locked joints. Forces may be applied in a downward distraction followed by protrusion and lateral gliding to the opposite side. Any one of these component motions can be performed in an isolated fashion.

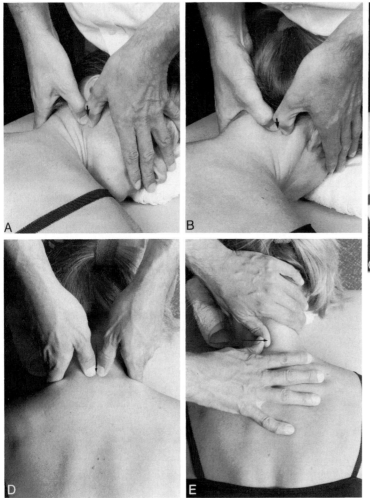

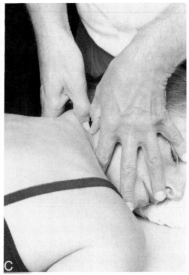

FIGURE 24-19. *A,* Transverse vertebral pressures C1. Patient is in a prone position with the head turned as far to the right as is comfortable. The therapist applies thumb forces over the tip of the right transverse process of the first cervical vertebra. This technique is applied to the first cervical vertebra on the nonpainful side when symptoms are unilateral. In the presence of a bilateral problem, both sides of the cervical spine should be mobilized. *B,* Posteroanterior vertebral pressures in the neutral position. Pressures are applied to the lamina of the vertebra to be mobilized, either at occiput-C1 or C1-C2. At occiput-C1, the primary motions are flexion and extension. At segments C1-C2, the primary motion is rotation. When occiput-C1 is to be mobilized, pressures are applied to C1. When segment C1-C2 is to be mobilized, pressures are applied to the lamina of C2. *C,* Posteroanterior unilateral pressures with rotary enhancement. This technique is applied to the C1-C2 segment with rotation of the head to enhance such mobility. Forces are applied to the lamina of C2. *D,* Posteroanterior central vertebral pressures. This technique can be applied to any spinous process of the cervical spine and is generally used when symptoms are bilateral. *E,* Transverse vertebral pressures (C2-C7). This pressure is applied to the lateral surface of the spinous process of the nonpainful side, directing pressure toward the painful side. This technique can be carried out on vertebrae C2 through C6.

symptoms. At the occipital atlantal joint (O-C1), the primary motions are flexion and extension. When posteroanterior unilateral pressures are used, motion will be increased when the force is directed to the posterior aspect of the lateral mass of the atlas. If it is used at the C1–2 segment, the primary motion will be approximately 40° of rotation. The force is applied to the C2 articular pillar. This movement is further enhanced by rotating the patient's head 30° before applying the technique (Fig. 24–19C), thus taking up the slack at C1–2.[143]

Figures 24–19 *D* and *E* show mobilization techniques used on the middle and lower cervical spine. Motion gained by soft-tissue and joint mobilization will be lost in the absence of a home maintenance program.

PATIENT EDUCATION

Education of patients is a key factor during all phases of physical therapy. Frank discussion of the nature of the pathology and its relationship to posture, pain, and mechanics is necessary. Patients must understand that they are responsible for their problem and its treatment. Professionals must provide support and encouragement. Treatment may require long-term followup to monitor the effectiveness of manual therapy, exercise, and postural re-education. Followup will allow appropriate progression of the program and accurate evaluation of treatment outcome.

Forward head posture with resultant rounding of the shoulders can produce dysfunction of the craniocervical and temporomandibular systems. Postural re-education starts with instruction in relaxed sitting posture. The lumbar lordosis must be supported, and the head-on-neck posture must be balanced and relaxed. This position is adjusted according to an individual's specific needs, such as in work areas, car seats, and home leisure activities. Postural re-education may take much scrutiny and

many adjustments over several months. Architects, keypunch operators, artists, dentists, and computer terminal operators are particularly prone to poor posture.

Patients who sit in FHP over long periods of time are placing the head in a posteriorly rotated position (Figs. 24–20 and 24–21), leading to pathologic changes in the soft tissue of the TMJ, hyoid, and cervical spine. FHP maintained for 15 minutes in normal subjects produced pain in the lower and upper thoracic spine, and pain persisted in some patients for days.[163] Compression forces in the suboccipital region may produce dizziness, nausea, and tinnitus. Cervical headache may be unilateral or bilateral. These headaches may refer pain to the TMJ, retro-orbital, and frontal areas through irritation of the trigeminocervical tract.[45,46]

Adaptive FHP strongly influences the muscle tone and elasticity of the masticatory system. The resting position of the mandible is al-

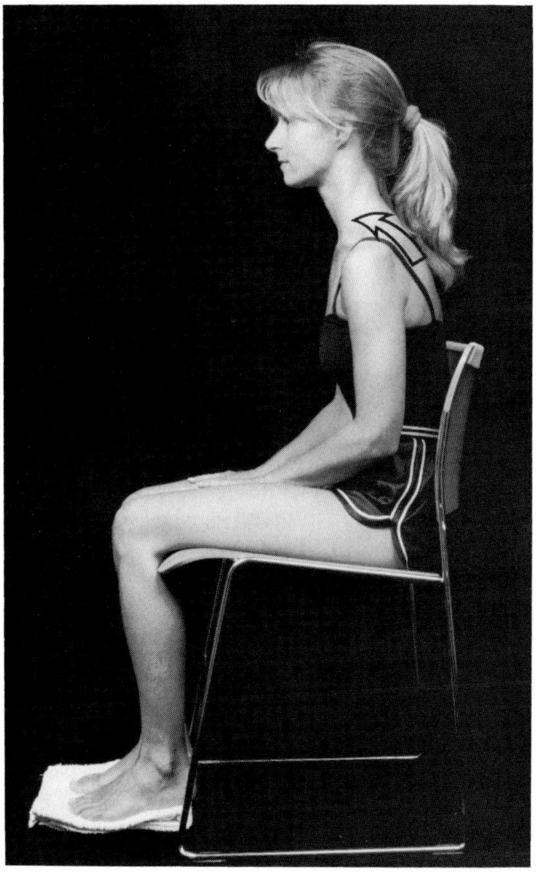

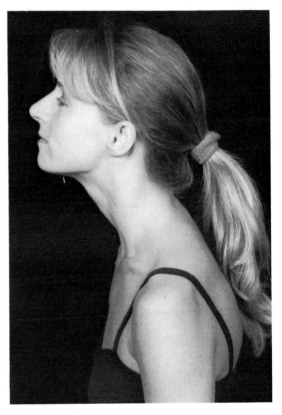

FIGURE 24–20. Inappropriate sitting posture. The patient's lumbar spine has left the back of the chair. This facilitates forward head posture and rounding of the shoulders, as the head goes into a forward position.

FIGURE 24–21. Forward head posture. Please note the increased verticality of the sternocleidomastoid. Tension is produced in the supraclavicular fossa, and posterior cranial rotation occurs. These effects create isometric contraction of the posterior cervical musculature.

tered with prolonged FHP, becoming an elevated and retruded position with increased suprahyoid activity.[164] Suboccipital impingement forces will be further increased. Freeway space may also be influenced.[164] FHP alters breathing and swallowing as a result of decreased airway patency[165] and tongue position. Changes in the hyoid-mandibular tension length relation create widespread pathophysiologic adaptations.[165] FHP has been shown to increase molar contact,[107] causing further stimulation of the trigeminocervical tract and leading to clenching, bruxism, and TMJ loading.

Sitting Posture

FHP is caused by an unsupported lumbar lordosis. When the lumbar spine is flattened by slumped or forward body posture, increased thoracic spine kyphosis, rounding of the shoulders, and posterior cranial rotation result. The pelvis is posteriorly rotated, increasing the lumbar intradiscal pressure. This pressure on the intervertebral discs causes strain and may lead to disc herniation.[166,167]

Chairs with appropriate lumbar support maintain the lumbar lordosis (Fig. 24–22). Proper lumbar support helps balance the forces on the "tripodal system," an intervertebral disc and two osseous facets. It also decreases muscle activity in the upper trapezius and other posterior paraspinal musculature.[168] FHP may lead to increased compressive forces and intervertebral disc degeneration.[163,169]

Chairs with adjustable seat height and lumbar support are preferable. Desks should have adequate leg room. Knees and hips should be in a 90°–90° position with free lateral movement to turn left and right. When the hips are in the 90° position, proper anterior pelvic tilt is maintained, promoting a decrease in lumbar disc pressure and strain and inducing appropriate craniocervical posturing.[170]

Patients using computers must have flexibility in keyboard placement. The monitor should be positioned with a downward gaze angulation of 5° to 20° to the center of the screen. The screen-to-eye distance should be 16 to 24 inches (Fig. 24–23).[171] Sustained postural activities in which acute vision is needed can lead to fatigue and craniocervical pain. Tinted prescription eye glasses for close-up work may decrease eye fatigue at video terminals.

Adjustable desks can decrease severe cervical pain. Architects, for instance, can tilt work tables to a 30° angle, decreasing the stress of for-

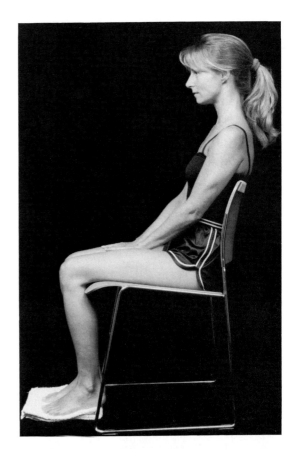

FIGURE 24–22. Appropriate sitting posture. This patient is now maintaining an appropriate lumbar lordosis that is supported. Shoulders are in a neutral position, and the head is in a less forward orientation. This posture may tend to decrease the forces applied to the intervertebral discs of the cervical and lumbar spine and to decrease the muscle hyperactivity in the cervical thoracic area.

ward head bending on the cervical spine. Repeated activities while seated at the desk should be within a 15-inch reach so that the lumbar lordosis is maintained.[172] Patients should be instructed not to have their backs leave the chair. Chairs with arm rests may decrease strain on the trapezius and levator scapulae.

Work at countertops can be particularly fatiguing to the craniocervical musculature from forces placed on the spinal kinetic chain. It causes increased lumbar lordotic flattening, thoracic kyphosis, concomitant rounding of the shoulders, and FHP. Work stations may require redesigning or adaptive devices to assist workers.

Prolonged sitting in an automobile seat with inappropriate lumbar support, complicated by the axial compression of bumps and vibration,

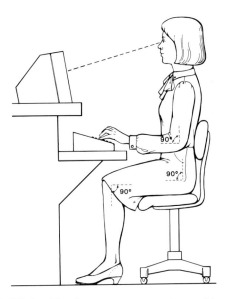

FIGURE 24-23. The appropriate seating position at a video display work station. (Reprinted with permission from Saunders, D.H.: *Evaluation, Treatment and Prevention of Musculoskeletal Disorders.* Viking Press Inc., Minneapolis, 1985.)

can cause increased cervical and lumbar pain. Adaptable cushions to better support the buttocks and lordotic curve are helpful. Airline seats, notorious for their lack of lumbar support and a head rest, force the cranium into FHP. This problem may be remedied by using two airline pillows side to side to maintain the lumbar lordosis.

Patients who continue to sit or stand in abnormal postures will continue to have pain. Patients must maintain proper posture as instructed in order to prevent recurrence of pain. They should always report any change in symptoms, for the better or worse, after postural instruction. An increase in pain may indicate overcorrection or incorrect understanding of postural instruction.

Sleeping Posture

Most people sleep for 6 to 8 hours; therefore, posture while sleeping has the longest duration and is the least easily controlled. Patients should be instructed to avoid lying in a prone position, which stresses the cervical spine by rotating and extending it and places tension on the cervical joints, muscles, and ligamentous structures. The TMJ also receives compressive forces in this position. Patients with waking pain or increased stiffness should have their sleeping posture, pillows, and mattress evaluated.

Appropriate sleep position is lying on the side or back. When lying on the back, the head and neck must be supported by a pillow meeting the patient's biomechanical needs. The pillow should not increase flexion of the head to such a degree as to cause FHP. A pillow that supports the cervical lordosis and the head in a neutral position is recommended. Sleeping with two pillows or a pillow that is too large causes FHP and stretching of the posterior ligamentous structures, increasing stress on the cervical discs and the cervical thoracic junction. Sleeping without a pillow increases posterior cranial rotation, leading to suboccipital tissue impingement. It is critical to maintain the cervical lordosis. Several commercially available pillows have been designed for this purpose. The Wal-Pilo* is designed with head and spine supports that can be positioned for lying on the side or in a supine position. Towels can be rolled and inserted in down pillows to support the cervical lordosis. Figure 24-24 illustrates the supine sleeping position. Note that a pillow under the knees can increase flattening of cervical and lumbar lordosis in some patients.

A side-lying position may produce pressure on the TMJ. The head, spine, and lower extremities should be aligned in a neutral position (Fig. 24-25). This may be accomplished by placing under the head and neck a pillow of sufficient thickness to maintain a neutral position (see Fig. 24-25). A pillow placed between the legs and a firm mattress help prevent abnormal posture. Patients who read in bed should be instructed to use appropriate pillows for support of the lumbar spine in the sitting position. The lumbar lordosis must be maintained. Watching television in bed is best done with the screen elevated above the level of the bed. After balance of cervical and shoulder girdle musculature is established, mandible and tongue position can be optimized.

Postural Position of the Mandible and Tongue

Neuromuscular re-education exercises of the mandible and tongue are used to relax hyperactive muscles. Proper instruction helps patients gain cortical awareness and control. An

---

*Pleasing Patients Unlimited, Beverly Hills, CA.

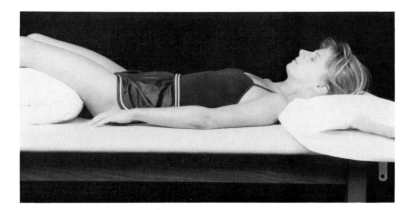

FIGURE 24–24. Supine sleeping position. This patient is appropriately supported at the head and neck by a down pillow. The pillow under the knees is optional and may increase cervical and lumbar flattening that may increase cervical symptomatology and dysfunction.

understanding of the importance of these postural exercises is necessary for the maintenance of masticatory health. Patients must be able to monitor the position of their mandible at rest and during movement. If the position is incorrect, it must be adjusted accordingly.[28] Parafunctional habits such as clenching, lip biting, and abnormal tongue position must be corrected because they all affect the normal resting posture of the mandible and are a source of chronic microtrauma.

The resting position of the tongue provides the foundation for resting muscle tone of the mandibular elevator muscles and establishes resting activity of the tongue musculature itself. The functional coordination between the tongue and mandibular muscles is mediated by the jaw-tongue reflex.[28,173] Patients are instructed to apply the tip of the tongue to the backside of the central incisors and the first half of the tongue to the palate. This is the position that should be maintained by patients while at rest. The teeth should be slightly disoccluded at all times except when swallowing and chewing. This position encourages decreased muscle ac-

tivity of the mandibular elevator muscles. Instructing patients to keep "tongue to the roof, lips together, and teeth apart"[41] helps to overcome parafunctional and functional muscle hyperactivity.

Nasal-Diaphragmatic Breathing

Proper diaphragmatic breathing is also important. In normal breathing, the air is brought in through the nose, helping to slow, warm, moisten, and clean the air of particles before it enters the lungs. Proper resting tongue position helps facilitate nasal-diaphragmatic breathing.[41]

Patients with allergies or nasal obstructions often breathe through their mouths.[165] Mouth breathing increases activity of the scalenes and sternocleidomastoid muscles. Enlargement of the adenoids may lead to forward and downward position of the tongue.[174] Shortening of the scalene and sternocleidomastoid muscles leads to increased posterior cranial rotation. The stylohyoid muscle slackens as the styloid process moves anteriorly toward the mandible, causing the tongue to drop into the lower

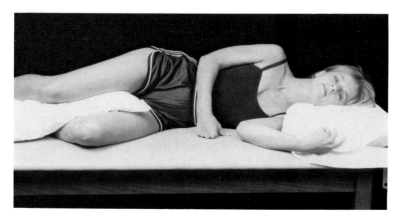

FIGURE 24–25. Side-lying position. The patient's cranium, spine, and lower extremities are positioned neutrally. The head and neck are supported by a down pillow. A pillow is placed between the legs to relieve stress in the lateral musculature of the lumbar spine.

arch.[158] The altered activity of the genioglossi changes the mandibular resting position.[175] The hyoid-to-mandible tension length relationship is thus influenced, increasing the activity and length of the infrahyoid and suprahyoids. As the cranium is pulled further into FHP, activity of the temporalis and masseter muscles increases,[12] causing the mandible to elevate and retrude.[164] These events may eventually influence freeway space, occlusion, and facial morphology and lead to cervical spine pathology.[24,26,27,158,165,175]

Mouth breathers often have difficulty breathing in the supine position during sleep because the tongue may partially obstruct the airway. Patients may need to roll onto their stomach to free their tongue in order to breathe.[158] Mouth breathers should be discouraged from sleeping in a prone position, as this irritates the cervical spine and TMJ.

Diaphragmatic breathing, unlike shallow upper chest breathing, allows for efficient filling of the lungs. Less energy is required for inspiration and expiration, and greater filling allows better oxygenation. People under stress often breathe in a contracted, shallow, and rapid manner that robs them of proper levels of carbon dioxide, which helps to maintain correct body pH.[176] Changes in pH may lead to muscle hypersensitivity, and patients may feel nervous and jittery.[176] Low levels of carbon dioxide may cause vasoconstriction and thus hypoxia, which might be a factor in maintenance of the pain-spasm cycle in the muscles of mastication. Diaphragmatic breathing helps strengthen the diaphragm and intercostal muscles[176,177] and also has a potent relaxation effect. Patients should practice diaphragmatic breathing daily for 5 to 10 minutes until they feel relaxed, then they should remain relaxed for 5 to 10 minutes more. This technique is also valuable for reducing anxiety.

Swallow Sequence

One of the most commonly overlooked problems during treatment of patients with TM and craniocervical disorders is altered swallowing sequence and tongue position. Few other forces can match the tongue's ability to cause occlusal and skeletal deformation.[158] The presence of a residual pediatric tongue thrust or an acquired adult anterior tongue thrust secondary to FHP can affect the response to all other treatment.

The acquired adult tongue thrust is evaluated by palpation of the hyoid bone and suboccipital musculature during swallowing. If the hyoid slowly moves up and down or the suboccipital musculature contracts, the presence of an adult tongue thrust is established. Further confirmation is obtained if head rocking and excessive lip activity are present. Patients indicate that the tip of the tongue presses between or on the lingual surface of the upper and lower anterior teeth.[28] Treatment includes instruction in the normal resting position of the tongue and in proper swallowing. Maintenance of correct head-on-neck posture is also essential. Figure 24–26 shows a water-sipping exercise that is helpful in retraining aberrant swallowing patterns. It can also be used for evaluating facial, hyoid, and cervical musculature.

Patients are shown the normal resting posi-

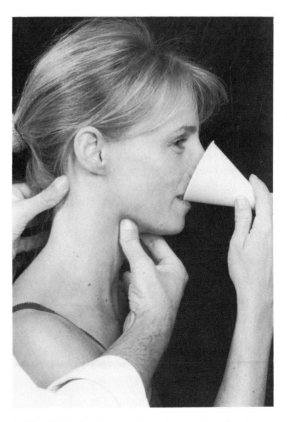

FIGURE 24–26. Examination of altered swallowing sequence. Patients may have long-term residual swallowing sequence problems or adult acquired anterior tongue thrusting. Adult acquired tongue thrusting pathology may be secondary to forward head posture. If so, the hyoid bone may slowly elevate on swallowing. Contraction of the suboccipital musculature may occur during this activity as well. Excessive lip activity may be evident on examination during swallowing.

tion of the tongue. As water is sipped during the initial phase of swallowing, the tip of the tongue should return to its resting position without putting pressure on the posterior teeth. Next, the main force of swallowing should be against the palate and is maintained by the middle third of the tongue. Patients should sense a wavelike motion that starts at the tip and ends with the middle third of the tongue, putting pressure on the most posterior part of the palate.[28,41,158] Completion occurs when the tongue assumes the normal resting position. This exercise requires a lot of reinforcement because a tongue thrust habit is usually well rooted. The exercise should be practiced several times daily.

Self-Mobilization Exercises

Active physical therapy treatment increases range of motion and reduces pain. A self-mobilization program is instituted to maintain joint mobility as well as muscle strength and length, thus preventing recurrence of pain. A stretching program is as important as a musculoskeletal strengthening program. Changes in muscle length are commonly associated with changes in strength.[153,178–180] Overstretched muscle can become weak and painful. Synergists of the lengthened muscle can become shortened and give rise to painful trigger points.[181–183] Treatment is directed at strengthening the overstretched muscles and increasing the length of the shortened muscles to achieve

balance. Maintenance of good posture is accomplished by increasing strength and endurance, allowing for increased functional activity without reinjury from stress and strain.

Passive Stretching: Cervical Spine

Flexibility is a key factor in preventing repeated injury. The following exercises help increase mobility of the cervical joints and musculature. These exercises should be carefully demonstrated, and patients should perform them several times before leaving the physical therapy session. The effects should be evaluated.

The number of repetitions, frequency, and application of home modalities must be determined for each individual patient. Exercises are added slowly, because if several exercises are given at one time, the therapist's ability to assess an increase in pain on subsequent visits is compromised. Patients tend to have better recall if exercises are added slowly. The exercise program is carried out three to six times daily, depending on the specific nature of the pathology. Patients are asked to telephone the therapist if pain or questions should arise.

The major regions requiring stretching are the upper cervical spine, cervical thoracic junction, scalenes, trapezius, levator scapulae, and pectoralis group. Figure 24–27A through G shows exercises used to liberate osseous and soft tissues from the cranium to the midthoracic spine. All exercises should be done without

---

FIGURE 24–27. A, Upper cervical spine retraction. This technique seems to be easier for the patient to sense in the supine position but can be done in the seated position as well. The patient's occiput is supported with a towel. Instructions are given to tuck the chin. This exercise is designed to flex the upper cervical spine, stretching the suboccipital region. B, Rotation with overpressure to the left. This technique enhances upper cervical spine rotation. Hand placement is important and should be above the zygoma so that pressure will not be imparted to the temporomandibular joint. C, Side bending with retraction of the upper cervical spine. Patient applies gentle overpressure to the left side of the cranium. This stretches the scalenes, trapezius, levator scapula, and sternocleidomastoid. D, Nose-to-axilla stretch. The patient rotates her head fully to the right and then brings her nose to the axilla, with the overpressure of the right hand on the cranium. This technique stretches the entirety of the left cervical musculature, including the upper suboccipital musculature (rector capiti group). E, Lower cervical spine extension with overpressure. The patient must be supported appropriately at the thoracolumbar spine in a seated position. Finger pressure over the maxilla provides adequate overpressure. This technique is utilized for restriction in extension at the cervical thoracic junction. F, Anterior shoulder girdle and pectoral muscle stretch. Patient is asked to position herself an adequate distance from the corner, raise her arms, and lean forward into the wall with her chest. This technique may be varied to stretch all portions of the pectoralis and anterior shoulder girdle musculature, as the arms are moved up and down in various positions. G, Lower cervical and thoracic spine stretch in the supine position. This technique should be done only after vertebral artery test findings have proved negative. It is an advanced technique for most patients and should be done in the therapist's office before the patient is given permission to do this exercise at home.

The patient lowers her head to the fully extended position using her arms. This position is maintained for 10 to 30 seconds. The head is then returned to the neutral position on the table, with arms' assisting. The patient is asked to rest there for a short time. This technique may be modified by moving up and down the table to affect segments as far down as the midthoracic spine. As a self-mobilization technique, it is quite valuable when restriction in extension from levels C7 to T6 exists.

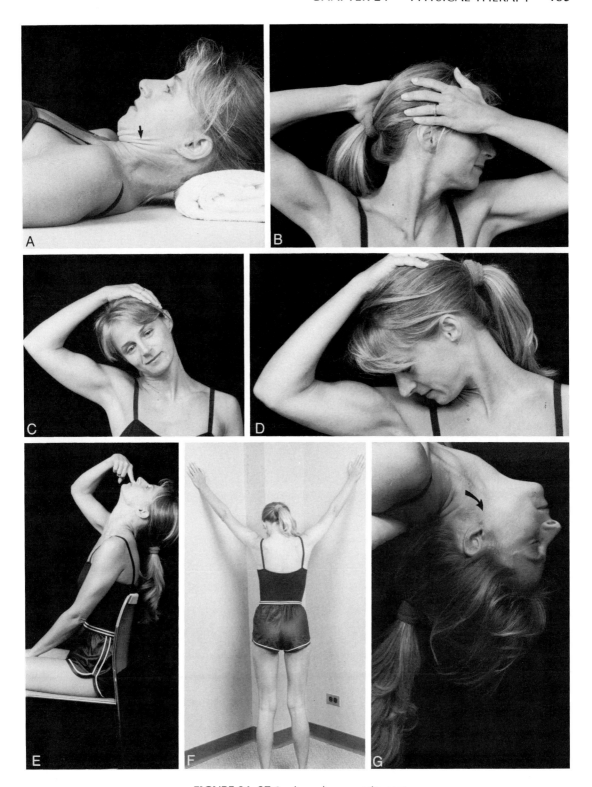

FIGURE 24–27 *See legend on opposite page*

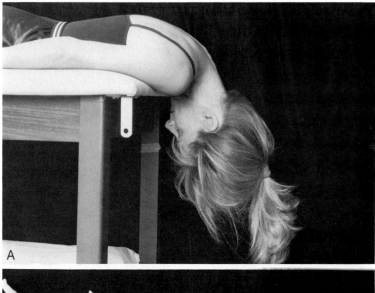

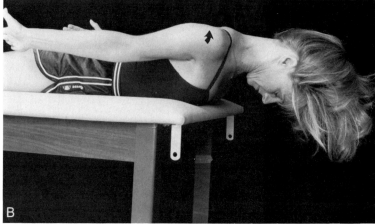

FIGURE 24–28. *A,* Interscapular strengthening technique. This is the starting position for interscapular and upper cervical spine stretching and strengthening. This technique also includes the external rotators of the glenohumeral joint. The patient is positioned with the edge of the table at approximately the nipple line. *B,* The patient is instructed to bring the head and neck to the neutral position with the chin tucked, while externally rotating the shoulder joints and pinching the shoulder blades together. This position may be held 4 or 5 seconds and then released. It is important that upper cervical flexion is maintained during this procedure as well as shoulder retraction and depression.

causing pain. Figure 24–28*A* and *B* shows a useful exercise for strengthening and stretching the weakened upper and middle trapezius and rhomboids. It also stretches the upper cervical extensors and pectoral group of muscles while strengthening the rotator cuff musculature. Other exercises can be used, but a complete discussion is not within the scope of this chapter.

Passive Stretching: Temporomandibular Joint

Passive mobilization of the TMJ is done at home after application of ice or heat. The use of the index finger and thumb between the incisors has proved helpful for stretching the capsule of the TMJ. Figure 24–29 shows a patient actively opening and applying gentle but steady passive force with the fingers to increase mandibular depression.

Active opening is followed by active closure against resistance to the mandible (Fig. 24–30).[4,28,184] These active-passive exercises should be performed three to six times daily. These techniques may be helpful in joint restrictions caused by anterior disc displacement with and without reduction. In the case of a nonreducing disc, it is important to limit interincisal opening to approximately 30 mm to protect the retrodiscal tissue from being overstretched or torn. A ruler or section of tongue blade marked at a length of 30 mm is sent home with the patient as a guide to prevent excessive stretching. These techniques are useful for limited opening due to joint effusion, retrodiscitis, and muscle guarding.[4,28]

Stacked tongue blades can be placed hori-

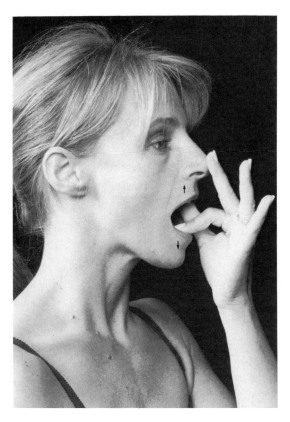

FIGURE 24–29. Active-passive mandibular exercise. The patient is instructed to first actively open as far as possible, then finger pressures are applied to the maxillary and mandibular dentitions. This technique may be performed with both hands.

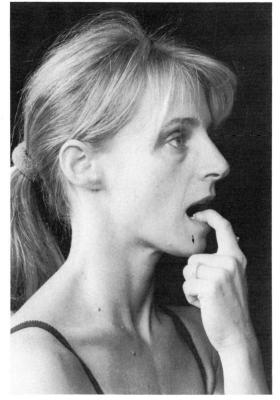

FIGURE 24–30. Active-passive mandibular exercise. The patient is instructed to open as far as possible and then insert a finger on the mandibular dentition and contract against unyielding resistance. The patient then relaxes, and the index finger pulls downward on the mandible.

zontally between the upper and lower incisors to increase mandibular opening. Normal translation begins after 11 mm, or about six tongue blades. With the tongue blades in position, a patient can mobilize the mandible actively into protrusion and lateral excursion (Fig. 24–31).

Neuromuscular Coordination of the Temporomandibular Joint

After joint arthrokinematics have been established through manual therapy and soft-tissue mobilization, balance and coordination of the mandible may be required. Resistive exercises are used to strengthen musculature, correct asymmetric mandibular movement, and decrease spasm.[185]

Weakness of the masticatory musculature is difficult to assess because numerous muscles accomplish the same action. In the past, patients were given isometric exercises for all movements of the TMJ.[4,186] Although the effectiveness of these exercises has never been subjected to formal clinical investigation, they are thought to aid in strengthening, coordinating, and inhibiting muscle spasm. Isometric contractions of the depressors of the mandible cause inhibition of the mandibular elevators, and hence they are useful for patients with masseter and temporalis hypertonicity.

Kraus[28] believes that isometric exercise is beneficial for stretching. Isometric exercises when stretching the mandibular elevators are done by opening the mouth until it is slightly stretched and then contracting the elevator muscles against maximum resistance. The use of isometric exercises may help create better awareness of contraction and relaxation,[28] leading to better muscle relaxation.

Minimal contraction can be used to train

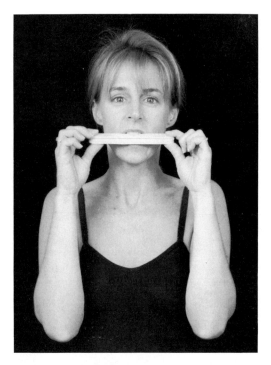

FIGURE 24–31. Active exercise to increase mandibular protrusion and lateral excursion. The patient is given approximately 6 to 7 tongue blades that are placed between the maxillary and mandibular incisors, allowing for approximately 11 mm of opening. The patient is then asked to protrude the mandible at this opening to improve translation. Patients may also improve translation of one side by protruding the mandible and gliding the mandible to the opposite side of the involved joint.

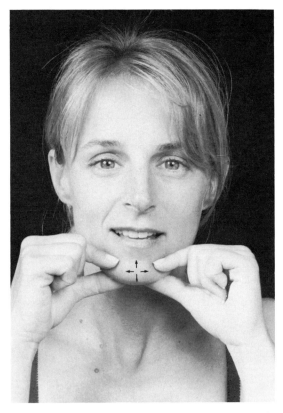

FIGURE 24–32. Isometric coordinating exercises to control excessive translation. The patient is asked to place the tip of the tongue up against the palate. The patient then attempts to move the mandible with light pressure in all directions, using the index fingers.

muscles to relax reflexly, helping coordinate the muscular system. The patient places the tongue on the palate, with the teeth apart, and places the index fingers of both hands on either side of the mandible. Gentle pressures are applied to the mandible for a short time. Pressure is applied in the frontal, sagittal, horizontal, and oblique planes to exercise various muscles and stimulate neuromuscular awareness (Fig. 24–32). A hold-relax technique is used as pressure is applied.[187]

Neuromuscular re-education techniques are important for hypermobility of the TMJ. Some patients have excessive translation, whereas others have translation that occurs too soon on opening. Excessive translation of subluxation occurs when the condyle moves in front of the crest of the articular eminence.[188] This motion may cause overstretching and lead to damage of the retrodiscal tissue and ligamentous and capsular structures, disrupting the condyle-to-disc relationship.[41] Condyle translation occur-

ring before or during the first 11 mm of interincisal opening is premature. Evaluation is performed by palpating the lateral pole of the condyles as they move during opening.

The easiest exercise for regaining control of translation within physiologic range is to have patients place their tongue on the posterior portion of the palate. This exercise maintains pure rotation. Patients then open their mouth while palpating the lateral pole of the condyle with the index finger. Further feedback can be gained by placing the index finger and thumb of the other hand on the chin. (Fig. 24–33). As patients learn to control movement by proprioceptive feedback, they may then attempt rotation on opening without the tongue on the palate (Fig. 24–34). Considerable concentration is needed while performing this exercise.

Isometric and isotonic exercises are helpful in strengthening the masticatory muscles. These include resistive opening and closing, as well as lateral, protrusive, and retrusive move-

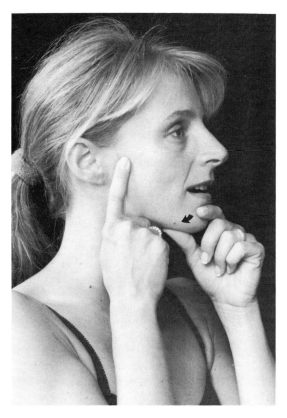

FIGURE 24–33. Neuromuscular re-education for excessive translation. The patient places her right index finger on the lateral pole of the condyle of the temporomandibular joint, while the left thumb and index finger lightly touch the tip of the chin. The patient is asked to open the mouth, keeping the tongue against the palate while palpating the lateral pole. The patient is taught to allow only condylar rotation during this exercise.

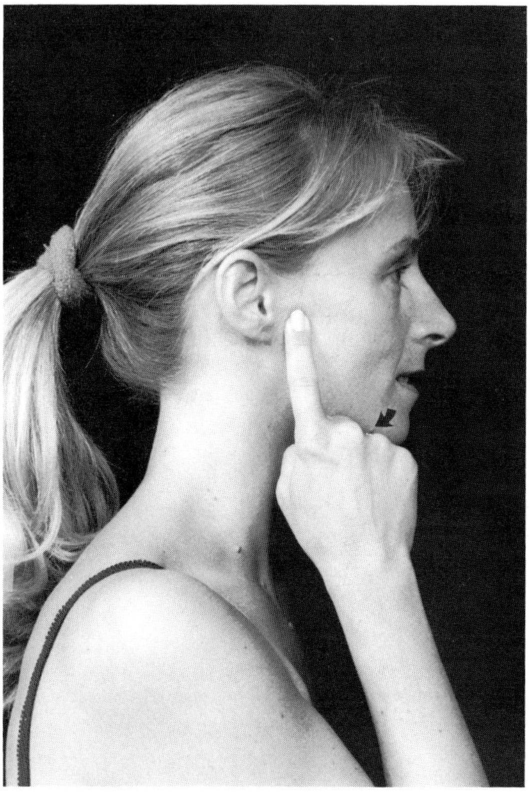

FIGURE 24–34. Neuromuscular re-education exercise #2. As patients are able to control rotation and decrease translation, this technique can be done in a less proprioceptive manner by primarily palpating the lateral condyle with the index finger. This technique may then be progressed to moving the tongue down from the roof of the mouth and attempting opening without translation.

ments. Figure 24–35 shows a resistive exercise in right lateral excursion. Clinical investigation is needed to evaluate the effectiveness of these exercises.

ARTHROSCOPIC SURGERY AND PHYSICAL THERAPY

Arthroscopic surgery of the TMJ has been performed in the United States for approximately 6 years. The procedure is indicated for intracapsular derangement, joint adhesions, and diagnosis.[189] Most surgeons, dentists, and physical therapists believe that pre- and postoperative physical therapy is an integral part of arthroscopic and open joint surgery.[189–200]

Patients should be evaluated within the first 48 hours after an arthroscopic procedure.[189,192,199] Active and passive techniques play a critical

roll in preventing formation of scar tissue (intracapsular adhesions).[33,189] Maintaining joint mobility is the goal.

Preoperative Management of Myofascial Pain Dysfunction

Patients with a MPD component should have physical therapy before the surgical procedure.[33,189,190,200] Physical therapy 3 to 6 weeks before surgery is optimal. Patients who have had decreased joint mobility for several months or even years display hyperactivity of the muscles of mastication, capsular tightness, and generally poor dynamics of the mandible.[190] Patients with internal derangement may have intra-articular adhesions as well as degenerative condyle and fossa changes.[33,201] Many patients with disc derangement also have signifi-

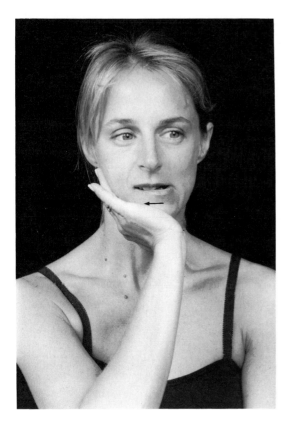

FIGURE 24–35. This is a traditional resistive exercise to strengthen the left lateral pterygoids against a right lateral force provided by the patient's right hand.

cant cervical muscle pain that either preceded the derangement or was a secondary response. If MPD was pre-existing, an arthroscopic procedure may lead to correction of only part of the symptoms. A more favorable result will be achieved if the MPD is treated first.

Ongoing myospasm in the masticatory and cervical musculature produces loss of normal muscle resting length, weakness, and trigger points.[91] Trigger points can be easily located by an aware practitioner. Changes in function and position of the masticatory and cervical musculature lead to muscle fatigue. Fatigue causes ischemia leading to depletion of adenosine triphosphate and metabolic waste retention. This self-perpetuating pain-spasm-pain cycle may be firmly established. Thus, eradication of etiologic components involving the TMJ, occlusion stress, and posture must be identified and addressed before surgery. FHP is a major contributor to MPD.[28,33,41,190,203]

Preoperative Evaluation

A preoperative physical therapy evaluation should include taking a complete medical history describing past medical illnesses, past history of the present illness, and a dental history. A complete craniomandibular evaluation is performed, including measurement of active maximal interincisal opening, lateral movement, and protrusion and retrusion. The quality of the motion is noted as well.

The path of opening, including deflection or deviation, is diagrammed. The cause of mandibular hypermobility or hypomobility must be identified. Masticatory spasm can mimic an anteriorly displaced disc. Passive motion testing in depression, protrusion, and lateral gliding of the TMJ and a notation about the joints' end feel are necessary. Presurgical observation of the condylar rotation and translation is critical for assessing the postsurgical result.

Muscles that are painful to palpation should be recorded. Hypertrophic and atrophic muscles should be identified. Their role in producing abnormal mandibular movement must be established. Palpation of the TMJ is important, as is a brief occlusal analysis. Following a surgical procedure, occlusion will sometimes change.[190,204] Wear facets indicate past or present bruxism. All parafunctional activities and pathologic postural activities are noted. A patient's cervical posture should also be evaluated; painful and restricted segments of the cervical spine may be the source of pain referred to the TMJ region.

Cervical posture and its possible effect on the resting position of the mandible are assessed. Tongue position and swallowing sequence are also evaluated. The presence of painful cervical musculature and myofascial trigger points is noted. Painful areas can be indicated on a pain diagram sheet. All ear pain, face pain, headaches, and vision and balance problems should be evaluated. Neurologic symptoms such as numbness and tingling should be charted according to the dermatomal patterns.

Education of patients and patients' compliance are critical to successful postsurgical physical therapy. At the preoperative visit, patients should be aware of the surgical procedure and what to expect postoperatively. Patients must remain on a liquid or soft diet for 4 to 6 weeks, depending on their ability to tolerate chewing.[196] Handouts listing foods that may aggravate TMJ pain should be provided. The physical therapy program was discussed earlier in this chapter. Patients are shown techniques of pain control to be used immediately after surgery, including cryotherapy, TENS, and active and passive mandibular exercises. They are also instructed in diaphragmatic breathing, which is helpful in decreasing pain and anxiety.

Immediate Postoperative Visit

It is extremely helpful for the physical therapist to have a postsurgical conversation with the oral and maxillofacial surgeon to ascertain the extent of TMJ damage and to note the amount of interincisal opening gained at surgery. The morphology of the disc, the condition of its posterior and anterior attachments, and the condition of the articular surfaces should be specifically discussed. If cauterization of the posterior attachment or anterior band release was done, the physical therapist should be informed. During TMJ surgery, intra-articular bleeding occasionally occurs. It can be significant in predicting the rapidity with which physical therapy techniques can be applied.

After the physical therapist speaks with the oral surgeon, the patient is reevaluated. Swelling in the periauricular area indicates intracapsular edema or extracapsular extravasation of fluid and should be noted. Any changes of occlusion should be observed. Pain and numbness patterns are charted to compare with the pain pattern at the presurgical evaluation. Active movements of the TMJ are recorded, as are the movements of the cervical spine.

An immediate postoperative goal is to maintain the interincisal opening achieved under anesthesia by the surgeon. Postoperative adhesions between the articular surfaces and the disc may reoccur if mobility is not maintained, especially translation. The motion of the upper joint will more likely be maintained if translation is begun within the first 24 hours.[189] Studies have shown that constant mobility following joint trauma or surgery generally causes lysis of blood clots, forestalling organization into connective tissue.[193,205]

Postoperative swelling is decreased with ice during the first 24 to 48 hours. This may be enhanced by TENS application to the masseter and temporalis bilaterally, using a low rate of 0.5 to 1 Hz for 20 to 30 minutes, producing a slow and rhythmic muscle contraction. The pumping action decreases swelling, produces

muscle relaxation, and reduces pain.[71] TENS may be used at home three to four times daily. Patients are instructed to continue diaphragmatic breathing four times a day.

Active exercise helps to stimulate synovial fluid production, remove capsular exudate, and prevent reformation of adhesions. Active exercise is done in an isotonic and isometric manner as previously described, with the mandible in various degrees of opening. The arthrokinematics of both joints are always considered and carefully reassessed. Time and effort should be spent on balancing lateral and protrusive movements. These movements are critical for patients who have had fibrous adhesions for a long time. Patients are given a measured section of a tongue blade that is cut a few millimeters shorter than their gained opening at surgery. It serves as an interincisal guide as well as an immediate feedback device to monitor gained range of motion. Patients gently perform passive mandibular exercises (see Figs. 24–29 through 24–31) without causing pain. They must realize that the home exercise program is a significant part of their rehabilitation process.

Subsequent Physical Therapy Visits

On subsequent visits, the response to previous treatment is evaluated. Patients should be seen three or more times during the first postoperative week and then three times per week for approximately 4 weeks. Ideally, an interincisal opening of 35 mm should be gained and maintained within the first 2 weeks after surgery.

The emphasis of the second and third visits should be on synchronized mandibular movement and the reduction of pain and swelling. Patients should become more aware of neuromuscular control of the mandible during functional movement. They must develop an awareness of opening without deviation. Patients with long-standing mandibular deviation or deflection require both active and passive retraining. Conscious effort is required using both visual and tactile feedback.

As healing progresses, mandibular movement is continually evaluated. If hypomobility develops and the problem is attributed to capsular constriction, ultrasound to heat the connective tissue under the constant force of tongue blades for 3 to 5 minutes may be the treatment of choice.[71] If muscle dysfunction exists, myofascial techniques, proprioceptive neuromuscular techniques, contract-relax exercises, and rhythmic stabilization will help promote relaxation and increase mandibular motion.[28] Resisted isometric contractions of the lateral pterygoids and suprahyoid musculature help to relax the temporalis and masseter by taking advantage of reciprocal inhibition. This technique also can increase maximum interincisal distance.[184,199]

The therapist must further evaluate the cervical spine and abnormal forces placed on the TMJs. FHP has often existed for many years and has resulted in soft-tissue adaptation and deformation of the anterior and posterior structures of the cervical spine. These changes are particularly evident in the suboccipital region, the cervical thoracic junction, and the submandibular musculature.[51,71,203] Continual adaptive forces on the suboccipital region can lead to impingement syndromes of the first and second cervical nerves, causing headache, pain in the suboccipital regions, and referred pain to the vertex of the skull.[45,46] They may also cause trigeminal pain.[43–45] Interscapular pain can be present as a result of isometric contraction of the trapezius, levator scapula, and other interscapular musculature.[91]

The suprahyoid-infrahyoid tension-length relationship influences tongue physiology and the resting position of the mandible.[27,158,164] Many investigators believe that condylar position and the occlusal plane can be affected.[12,24–26] Treatment of the cervical spine is directed at releasing osseous segmental and myofascial restrictions. Proper use of moist heat, electrogalvanic stimulation, ultrasound, and TENS prepares these patients for myofascial release of the soft tissue and mobilization of the osseous structures during healing.[71]

In most patients, by the fourth visit, vigorous passive mobilization of the TMJ in all directions may be achieved. Emphasis is placed on lateral and medial gliding as well as protrusive movement. Combining active and passive techniques is helpful in gaining increased interincisal distance[189] (see Figs. 24–29 and 24–35).

Superficial and deep heating modalities and myofascial release of the cervical and masticatory musculature should be continued. Active exercise and neuromuscular coordination exercises also continue. Strength and synchrony of the masticatory musculature are emphasized during this phase of therapy.

Patients should be followed for 5 to 7 weeks.

Physical therapy can usually be decreased to once a week by the seventh week. The speed at which a patient returns to a normal diet varies and usually is based on chewing tolerance and on the presurgical damage to intra-articular tissues. Most patients continue wearing occlusal splints to decrease the load on the TMJ and to deprogram the masticatory muscles.[204,206] Joint loading must be controlled to allow for unimpaired healing and remodeling of soft tissues and osseous structures.[207]

Physical Therapy Treatment Following Arthrotomy

Arthrotomy (open joint procedures) vary depending on the existing pathology and the technique of the individual oral and maxillofacial surgeon. Most surgeons request that only active motion without resistance be used during the first 3 postoperative weeks. They believe that passive mobilization could disrupt healing, leading to surgical failure.

Some patients with pre-existing hypomobility due to chronic muscle shortening and loss of extensibility of the TMJ capsule and ligaments may progress poorly postoperatively, possibly because of a lack of presurgical physical therapy to stretch the capsular and myofascial structures. The postoperative course for these patients is often poor. Gaining adequate range of motion is difficult, especially if a patient has had prior surgical procedures.

Disc Plication Surgery Protocol

Physical therapy following a disc plication procedure is based on an understanding of revascularization and healing of the involved tissues. Investigators[208] have found that the greatest change in vascularity occurs in the second and third weeks after surgery and that complete healing occurs in 6 weeks. The inhibition of adhesion formation and proper reorientation of collagen fibers after deposition require appropriate motion.[74,208,209] This motion should be active and should apply very gentle pressure. It will decrease scar formation and stimulate glycosaminoglycan synthesis.[75]

Careful early mobilization will prevent the potential loss of mandibular movement associated with immobilization. Early mobilization of the TMJs is helpful in overcoming joint capsule tightness and muscle spasm. The use of grade I mobilization (see Fig. 24–17A through

C) may be helpful in the first 4 weeks postoperatively. These techniques move the joint slightly and are unlikely to put stress on the site of surgical repair.

Conversation between the physical therapist and the surgeon and their clinical judgment and experience form the guidelines for physical therapy. There is no standard postoperative formula. If a patient has had a very tenuous repair or a large perforation of the disc, more caution must be taken in the early stages (1 to 6 weeks) of physical therapy. The physical therapy program should include only gentle active motions. In general, the modalities employed for disc plication are similar to those described for arthroscopic surgery.

The First Postoperative Visit—Days 3 Through 7

The first postoperative visit should be within the first week after surgery. Patients should be managed with modalities to decrease pain and edema. Soft-tissue massage of the cervical and masticatory musculature is important. Gentle rhythmic stabilization exercises should be used for all mandibular movements (see Fig. 24–32). The tongue-to-roof technique facilitates relaxation of the masticatory musculature and rotation of the condyle without translation. In all cases, protrusion is avoided in the early stages. Active lateral gliding should be avoided to the side opposite the surgical site.[194]

Grade I mobilizations over the lateral aspect of the condyle (see Fig. 24–17*A*) have helped improve lateral movement without fear of tissue disruption. This technique is also helpful in decreasing pain and swelling. Depression of the mandible is done in a gentle grade I fashion to neuromodulate pain and increase condylar movement. Utilization of modalities to decrease pain and swelling and gentle mobilization result in a more pain- and edema-free postoperative course during the first few weeks.

Postoperative Days 7 Through 30

Within 30 days, the maximum interincisal opening should be approximately 25 mm.[194] Lateral excursion will be limited to a few millimeters on the side opposite the surgery. Gentle mobilization depressing the condyles is instituted at this time and should be well tolerated. Postoperative swelling should be absent and synovitis somewhat resolved.

Soft-tissue mobilization is critical in normalizing structure and function. Mobilization techniques should be continued to the TMJ and craniocervical spine. Treatment of any existing pathology of the tongue and swallowing sequence should be ongoing. The home therapy and exercise program should be active.

Postoperative Treatment, 4 Through 6 Weeks

By weeks four through six, patients generally obtain 25 to 28 mm of interincisal opening. At this stage, a full active exercise program should be undertaken. Gentle passive mobilization is instituted with great care. Patients may be given active/assistive interincisal opening on their surgeon's recommendation at 6 to 8 weeks (Fig. 24–29). No pain should be felt while stretching is taught. Grade II mobilization techniques are employed at weeks six to eight. Therapy continues toward a goal of an interincisal opening of 32 to 40 mm. Lateral movement of 3 to 7 mm in either direction is acceptable.[194] The goal is to have pain-free functional movement of the mandible; "ideal" movement often cannot be achieved.

Postoperative 6 Weeks to Completion of Rehabilitation

Most patients have completed physical therapy by weeks eight to ten. They should have reached their potential for mandibular movement. It is hoped that the interincisal opening will be 35 to 40 mm and lateral excursion between 4 and 7 mm without deviation.[194] Patients are asked to remain on a soft diet for 4 to 6 months, depending on the extent of the pathology found.

Parafunctional habits such as clenching and bruxism should continue to be monitored, and persistent soft-tissue problems of the upper quarter should continue to be addressed. Activities of daily living that may perpetuate pathology should continue to be evaluated and proper posturing reinforced. Patients need to be encouraged to take part in a full body conditioning program for relaxation and healing.

The oral and maxillofacial surgeon must seek out a physical therapist with expertise in TMD treatment. The working relationship and communication between the physical therapist and the oral surgeon will enhance the benefit to patients.

PHYSICAL THERAPY FOR ARTHROSCOPIC SURGERY OF THE TEMPOROMANDIBULAR JOINT

I. Preoperative evaluation
  A. Subjective
    1. History
    2. Chief complaint of pain in the craniomandibular and craniocervical region
    3. History of trauma to the head and neck
    4. Habits, posturing during work and play, bruxism and clenching, and other parafunctional activities
    5. Ear, nose, and throat symptoms
  B. Objective
    1. Examination of arthrokinematics of the TMJ, interincisal opening, lateral and protrusive movements, gross deviations and deflections, and the pain associated with them
    2. Facial symmetry
    3. Joint sounds on auscultation
    4. Measurement of overbite and overjet and general occlusal examination
    5. Muscle palpation of the temporomandibular and craniocervical musculature
    6. Muscle testing of the entire upper quarter, including the musculature innervated by the fifth and seventh nerves
    7. Complete cervical spine mobility evaluation
      a. General
      b. Segmental
    8. Shoulder girdle evaluation
    9. Postural evaluation
II. Preoperative patient education
  A. Discuss the arthroscopic procedure and different phases of physical therapy treatment
    1. Instruct in a home program for use of ice, massage, and deep breathing to decrease swelling and pain
    2. Describe the use of soft-tissue mobilization to decrease muscle spasm, pain, and swelling
    3. Describe the various uses of modalities such as ultrasound, TENS, electrogalvanic stimulation, and cryotherapy
    4. Discuss diet restrictions for the first 4 weeks of the postoperative course
    5. Discuss the goals of physical therapy during the postoperative course
      a. Neuromuscular control of the TMJ
      b. Decrease in pain and edema
      c. Normalization of mandibular mechanics
    6. Instruct patients in appropriate tongue position with their "lips together, teeth apart, tongue on the roof"
III. Initial postoperative period
  A. Re-evaluation
  B. Initial treatment within 24 to 48 hours
    1. Treat postoperative TMJ mechanics and masticatory muscle splinting
    2. Decrease pain and edema using modalities including electrical stimulation cryotherapy, spray and stretch, TENS, and soft-tissue massage
    3. Begin early TMJ mobilization, including
      a. Distraction
      b. Rotation
      c. Translation
      d. Lateral gliding
    4. Institute mandibular exercises to facilitate increased range of motion and begin passive stretching to achieve an increase in all motions listed earlier; neuromuscular facilitation to centralize mandibular mechanics and create relaxation of splinting muscles of mastication
  D. Immediate postoperative goals
    1. Decrease nociceptive stimulation
    2. Restore normal circulation and lymphatic drainage
    3. Stimulate the removal of intracapsular exudates through fluid mobilization
    4. Prevent reformation of adhesions and capsular scarring
    5. Stimulate synovial fluid production
IV. Postoperative day five
  A. Physical therapy in this postoperative period continues for the next 3 weeks on a three times per week basis. Continue to decrease pain and swelling and to normalize TMJ mechanics
    1. Continue to modulate pain with ultrasound, TENS, electrogalvanic stimulation, and cryotherapy
    2. Continue to mobilize the TMJ in all directions to improve interincisal opening

3. Continue neuromuscular exercises to facilitate centralization of opening and instruct patients in a full program of active exercises to increase endurance, strength, and balancing. Teach passive home mandibular exercise
4. Continue to treat dysfunctions of the craniocervical and shoulder girdle, as well as tongue and mouth breathing pathologies

B. Long-term goals
1. Normalize mandibular mechanics
2. Attain functionally pain-free movement of the mandible
3. Correct and/or reduce potential abnormalities and decrease compressive impingement and entrapment forces on the cervical spine, which can influence TMJ function
4. Increase patient awareness of important postural relationships during work and play activities
5. Implement a home program of exercises and self-management techniques to manage these individual problems

DISC PLICATION SURGERY PROTOCOL

A. Days three through seven
1. Cryotherapy to reduce edema and pain
2. Liquid diet
3. Massage of all appropriate soft tissue as tolerated
4. Electrotherapeutic intervention
5. Controlled active exercise
6. Grade I mobilization in all motions except translation
7. Treat craniocervical components of pain and dysfunction

B. Days seven through thirty
1. Continued pain and edema control, shift to superficial and deep heating modalities
2. Massage and myofascial release technique
3. Electrotherapy as indicated
4. Soft diet
5. Increased active exercise within the limits of controlled rotation
6. Grade I mobilization (avoiding translation)
7. Treat craniocervical, cervical thoracic, and shoulder girdle complex, as well as tongue position and swallowing sequence

C. Weeks four through six
1. Continue pain control
2. Modalities as necessary
3. Soft diet
4. Increase to slight resistance with active exercise in various degrees of available vertical opening; begin active lateral glide to the contralateral side
5. Mobilization in grade I in all motions and grade II in 6 to 8 weeks
6. Continue work on upper quarter mechanics and on adapted, entrapped, and compressed tissues. Continue to address the tongue position, swallow sequence, and mouth breathing pathologies

D. Six to 10 weeks
1. Treatment as before until goals are met

CONCLUSION

This chapter has described the pathologic processes most often encountered by physical therapists. The modalities employed to decrease pain, spasm, and edema and their sequential implementation in a comprehensive treatment program have been discussed. Comprehensive physical therapy of the upper quarter includes all soft tissues and osseous structures, with the goal of regaining normalization of neuromuscular and biomechanical function.

Soft-tissue and joint mobilization techniques constitute the most important part of patient care, helping to restore maladapted tissues and eliminate pain. Once normal function of the TMJs and craniocervical system has been reestablished, a complete self-mobilization program must be maintained. This program, combined with ongoing patient education, should maintain normal function. A physical therapist's commitment to assist in the pre- and postsurgical care will enhance surgical outcomes, ultimately benefiting patients.

REFERENCES

1. Rocabado, M., Johnson, B.E., and Blakney, M.G.: Physical therapy and dentistry: an overview. J. Craniomandib. Pract. 1:96–99, 1982.
2. Gelb, H.: *Clinical Management of Head, Neck and TMJ Pain and Dysfunction.* W.B. Saunders Co., Philadelphia, 1985.

3. Kraus, S.: Temporomandibular joint. In *Evaluation, Treatment and Prevention of Musculoskeletal Disorders.* Saunders, D.H. (ed.). Viking Press, Minneapolis, 1985.

4. Friedman, M.H. and Weisberg, J.: *Temporomandibular Joint Disorders.* Quintessence Publishing Co., Lombard, IL, 1985.

5. Kraus, S.L. (ed): *TMJ Disorders: Management of the Craniomandibular Complex,* New York, Churchill Livingstone, 1988.

6. Friedman, M.H. and Weisberg, J.: Application of orthopedic principles to evaluation of the TMJ. Phys. Ther. 62:597–603, 1982.

7. Danzig, W.N., Van Dyke, A.R.: Physical therapy as an adjunct to TMJ therapy. J. Prosthet. Dent. 49:96, 1983.

8. Clark, G.T.: Examination of temporomandibular disorder patients for cranio-cervical dysfunction. J. Craniomandib. Pract. 2:56, 1983.

9. Kraus, S.L.: Physical therapy in dentistry. Course notes. New York, 1985.

10. Mohl, N.D.: Head posture and its role in occlusion. N.Y. State Dent. J. 42.17–23, 1976.

11. Rocabado, M.: Biomechanical relationship of the cranio, cervical and hyoid regions. J. Craniomandib. Pract. 1:61–66, 1983.

12. Brodie, A.G.: Anatomy and physiology of head and neck musculature. Am. J. Orthod. 36:831, 1950.

13. Funakoshi, M., Fujita, N., and Takehana, S.: Relationship between occlusal interference and jaw muscle activities in response to changes in head position. J. Dent. Res. 55:684–690, 1976.

14. Shpuntoff, H. and Shpuntoff, W.: A study of the physiologic rest position and centric position by electromyography. J. Prosthet. Dent. 6:621–628, 1956.

15. Boyd, C., Sloyle, W., and MaBoyd, C. The effect of head position on EMG evaluation of representative mandibular positioning muscle groups. J. Craniomandib. Pract. 5:55–63, 1987.

16. Prieskel, H.W.: Some observations on the postural position of the mandible. J. Prosthet. Dent. 15:625–633, 1965.

17. Atwood, D.A.: A cephalometric study of the clinical rest position of the mandible. Part II. J. Prosthet. Dent. 7:544–552, 1957.

18. Atwood, D.A.: A review of the fundamentals on rest position and vertical dimension. Int. Dent. J. 9:6–19, 1959.

19. Jarabak, J.R.: An electromyographic analysis of muscular behavior in mandibular movements from rest position. J. Prosthet. Dent. 7:682–710, 1957.

20. Wyke, B.: Neuromuscular mechanisms influence mandibular posture. J. Dent. 2:111, 1972.

21. Lund, P., Nishiyama, T., and Moller, E.: Postural activity in the muscles of mastication with the subject upright, inclined, and supine. Scand. J. Dent. Res. 78:417, 1970.

22. Kendall, H.O., Kendall, F.P. and Boynton, D.A.: *Posture and Pain.* Robert E. Krieger Publishing Co., Huntington, NY, 1952.

23. Calliet, R.: *Neck and Arm Pain,* 2nd ed. F.A. Davis Co., Philadelphia, 1981.

24. Darling, D.W., Kraus, S., and Glasheen-Wray, M.B.: Relationship of head posture and the rest position of the mandible. J. Prosthet. Dent. 52:111, 1984.

25. Goldstein, D.F., Kraus, S.L., Williams, W.B., and Glasheen-Wray, M.B.: Influence of cervical posture

on mandibular movement. J. Prosthet. Dent. 52:421, 1984.

26. McClean, L.F., Brenman, H.S., and Friedman, M.G.F.: Effects of changing body position on dental occlusion. J. Dent. Res. 52:1041, 1973.

27. Ayub, E., Glasheen-Wray, M., and Kraus, S.: Head posture: A case study of the effects of the rest position of the mandible. Orthop. Sports Phys. Ther. 5:179, 1984.

28. Kraus, S.: Physical therapy management of TMJ dysfunction. In *TMJ Disorders: Management of the Craniomandibular Complex.* S. Kraus (ed.). Churchill Livingstone, New York, 1988.

29. Schwarz, A.M.: Positions of the head and malrelations of the jaws. Int. J. Orthod. Oral Surg. Radiol. 14:56–88, 1928.

30. Fish, F.: The functional anatomy of the rest position of the mandible. Dent. Pract. (Bristol) 11:178, 1961.

31. Gattozzi, J.G., Nicol, B.R., Somes, G.W., and Ellinger, G.W.: Variations in mandibular rest position with and without dentures in place. J. Prosthet. Dent. 36:159, 1978.

32. McGee, G.F.: Use of facial measurements in determining vertical dimension. J. Am. Dent. Assoc. 35:342, 1947.

33. Bays, R.A.: TMJ and orthognathic surgery. In *TMJ Disorders: Management of the Craniomandibular Complex.* S. Kraus (ed.). Churchill Livingstone, New York, 1988.

34. Laskin, D.: Etiology of the pain dysfunction syndrome. J. Am. Dent. Assoc. 79:147–153, 1969.

35. Dolwick, F.M., Katzberg, R.W., and Helms, C.A.: Internal derangement of the temporomandibular joint: Fact or fiction? J. Prosthet. Dent. 49:415, 1983.

36. Mongini, F., Ventricelli, F., Conserva, E., et al: Etiology of cranio-facial pain and head in stomatognathic dysfunction. In Proceedings of the 5th World Congress on Pain. R. Dubner, G.F. Gebhart, M.R. Bond (eds.). Elsevier Science Publishers B.V. (Biomedical Div.), Amsterdam, 1988.

37. Rugh, J.D. and Solberg, W.K.: Electromyographic studies of bruxist behavior before and during treatment. J. Calif. Dent. Assoc. 3:56–59, 1975.

38. Clark, G.T., Beemsterboer, P., and Rugh, J.D.: The treatment of nocturnal bruxism using contingent EMG feedback with an arousal task. Behav. Res. Ther. 19:451–455, 1981.

39. Scott, D.S. and Gregg, J.M.: Myofascial pain of the TMJ: A review of the behavioral-relaxation therapies. Pain 9:231–241, 1980.

40. Moss, R.A. and Gramling, M.A.: The role of clinical psychology in the treatment of craniomandibular disorders. J. Craniomandib. Pract. 2:159, 1984.

41. Rocobado, M.: Diagnosis and treatment of abnormal craniocervical and craniomandibular mechanics. Rocobado Institute Course Notes, 1981.

42. Trott, P.H.: Passive movements and allied techniques in the management of dental patients. In *Modern Manual Therapy of the Vertebral Column.* M.G. Grieve (ed.). Churchill Livingstone, New York, 1986.

43. Bogduk, N.: Cervical causes of headache and dizziness. In *Modern Manual Therapy of the Vertebral Column.* G. Grieve (ed.). Churchill Livingstone, New York, 1986.

44. Bogduk, N., Corrigan, B., Kelly, P. et al: Cervical headache. Med. J. Aust. 143:202, 1985.

45. Jull, G.A.: Headaches associated with the cervical

spine—a clinical review. In *Modern Manual Therapy of the Vertebral Column.* G. Grieve (ed.). Churchill Livingstone, New York, 1986.

46. Dugal, G.L. and Anseman, N.E.: The entrapped greater occipital nerves and internal derangement of the TMJ. J. Craniomandib. Pract. 2:52, 1983.

47. Lader, E.: Cervical trauma as a factor in the development of TMJ dysfunction and facial pain. J. Craniomandib. Pract. 1:86, 1983.

48. Bogduk, N.: The clinical anatomy of the cervical dorsal rami. Spine 7:319, 1982.

49. Bogduk, N. and Marsland, A.: The cervical zygapophysial joints as a source for neck pain. Spine 13:610, 1988.

50. Blume, H.G. and Ungar-Sargon, J.: Neurosurgical treatment of persistent occipital myalgia-neuralgia syndrome. J. Craniomandib. Pract. 4:65–73, 1986.

51. Mannheimer, J.S., Attanasio, R., Cinotti, W.R., and Pertes, R.: Cervical strain and mandibular whiplash: Effects upon the craniomandibular apparatus. Clin. Prev. Dent. 11:29–32, 1989.

52. Fast, A., Zinicol, D., and Marin, E.: Vertebral artery damage complicating cervical manipulation. Spine 12:840, 1987.

53. Xiu Qing, C., Bo, S., and Shizen, Z.: Nerves accompanying the vertebral artery and their clinical relevance. Spine 13:1360, 1988.

54. Darnell, M.: A proposed chronology of events for forward head posture. J. Craniomandib. Pract. 1:49, 1983.

55. Jackson, R.: *The Cervical Spine Syndrome,* 3rd ed. Charles C Thomas, Springfield, IL, 1966.

56. Brain, L. and Wilkinson, M.: *Cervical Spondylosis.* W.B. Saunders Co., Philadelphia, 1967.

57. Hunter, C.R. and Maysfield, F.H.: Role of the upper cervical roots in the production of pain in the head. Am. J. Surg. 78:743–749, 1949.

58. Knight, G.: Post-traumatic occipital headache. Lancet 1:6–8, 1963.

59. Edmeads, J.: Headaches and head pains associated with disease of the cervical spine. Med. Clin. North Am. 62:533–544, 1978.

60. Jull, G.: Clinical observations of the upper cervical mobility. In *Modern Manual Therapy of the Vertebral Column.* G. Grieve (ed.). Churchill Livingstone, New York, 1986.

61. Lance, J.W.: *Mechanism and Management of Headache,* 3rd ed. Butterworths, London, 1978.

62. Gayral, L. and Newwirth, E.: Oto-neuro-ophthalmologic manifestations of cervical origin. Posterior cervical sympathetic syndrome of Barre-Lieou. N.Y. State J. Med. 54:1920–1926, 1954.

63. Feinstein, B., Langton, J.N.K., Jameson, R.M., et al: Experiments on pain referred from deep somatic tissues. J. Bone Joint Surg. 36A:981, 1954.

64. Wyke, B.: Neurology of the cervical spinal joints. Physiotherapy 65:72, 1979.

65. Kerr, F.W.L.: Structure of the trigeminal spinal tract to upper cervical roots and the solitary nucleus in the cat. Exp. Neurol. 4:134, 1961.

66. Kerr, F.W.L. and Olafson, R.A.: Trigeminal and cervical volleys. Arch. Neurol. 5:177–178, 1961.

67. Bogduk, N. and Marsland, A.: C3 Headaches. Presented at the International Meeting on Pain and Regional Anesthesia. Australian Pain Society, Perth, February, 1983.

68. Bell, W.E.: *Orofacial Pains: Differential Diagnosis,* 2nd ed. Year Book Medical Publishers, Chicago, 1980.

69. Wyke, B.D.: Articular neurology—a review. Physiotherapy 58:94, 1972.

70. Clark, R.: Neurology of the temporomandibular joints: An experimental study. Ann. R. Coll. Surg. Engl. 58:43, 1976.

71. Mannheimer, J.: Physical therapy concepts in evaluation and treatment of the upper quarter, therapeutic modalities. In *TMJ Disorders: Management of the Craniomandibular Complex.* S. Kraus (ed.). Churchill Livingstone, New York, 1988.

72. Foreman, S. and Croft, A.: *Whiplash Injuries.* Baltimore, Williams & Wilkins, 1988.

73. Hettingia, D.: Normal joint structures and their reaction to injury. J. Orthop. Sport Phys. Ther. Summer, 16–22, 1979.

74. Engles, M.: Tissue response. In *Orthopaedic Physical Therapy.* R. Donatelli and M.J. Wooden (eds). Churchill Livingstone, New York, 1988.

75. Akeson, W.H., Amiel, D., and Woo, S.: Immobilization effects of synovial joints: The pathomechanics of joint contracture. Biorheology 17:95, 1980.

76. Cotta, H. and Phul, W.: The pathophysiology of damage to articular cartilage. Prog. Orthop. Surg. 3:20, 1978.

77. Evans, P.: The healing process at the cellular level: A review. Physiotherapy 66:256, 1980.

78. Mannheimer, J.S. and Lampe, G.N.: *Clinical Transcutaneous Electrical Nerve Stimulation.* F.A. Davis, Philadelphia, 1984.

79. Watson, J.: Pain and nociception—mechanisms and modulation. In *Modern Manual Therapy of the Vertebral Column.* G. Grieve (ed.). Churchill Livingstone, New York, 1986.

80. Michlovitz, S.L.: Cryotherapy: The use of cold as a therapeutic agent. p. 73. In *Thermal Agents in Rehabilitation.* S.L. Michlovitz (ed.). F.A. Davis, Philadelphia, 1986.

81. Knight, K.L.: *Cryotherapy: Theory, Technique and Physiology.* Chattanooga Corp., Chattanooga, 1985.

82. Cobbold, A.F. and Lewis, O.J.: Blood flow to the knee joint of the dog: Effects of heating, cooling and adrenaline. J. Physiol. 132:379, 1956.

83. Cooper, D. and Fair, J.: Contrast baths and pressure treatment for ankle sprains. Phys. Sports Med. 7:143, 1979.

84. Moore, R.J., Nicolette, R.L., and Behnke, R.: The therapeutic use of cold in the care of the athletic injuries. J. Natl. Athletic Trainers Assoc. 6:12, 1967.

85. Douglas, W.W. and Malcolm, J.L.: The effect of localized cooling on conduction in cat nerves. J. Physiol. 130:53, 1955.

86. Zankel, H.T.: Effect of physical agents on motor conduction velocity of the ulnar nerve. Arch. Phys. Med. Rehabil. 47:787, 1966.

87. Lee, J.M., Warren, M.P., and Mason, S.M.: Effects of ice on nerve conduction velocity. Physiotherapy 64:2, 1978.

88. Yackzian, L., Adams, C., and Francis, K.T.: The effects of ice massage on delayed muscle soreness. Am. J. Sports Med. 12:159, 1984.

89. Belitsky, R., Odam, S., and Hubley-Kozey, C.: Evaluation of the effectiveness of wet ice, dry ice, and cryogen packs in reducing skin temperature. Phys. Ther. 57:1080–1084, 1987.

90. Melzack, R., Guite, S., and Gonshor, A.: Relief of dental pain by ice massage of the hand. Can. Med. Assoc. J. 122:189, 1980.
91. Travell, J.G. and Simons, D.G.: *Myofascial Pain and Dysfunction: The Trigger Point Manual.* Williams & Wilkins, Baltimore, 1983.
92. Romer, E.: Acupuncture: A possible therapeutic modality in the treatment of craniomandibular dysfunction. J. Craniomandib. Pract. 7:144–151, 1989.
93. Chin, L.C., Jiang, Y.H., Shen, W.W., et al: Kinesic press-finger compress method for TMJ treatment. J. Craniomandib. Pract. 5:261–267, 1987.
94. Michlovitz, S.L.: Biophysical principles of heating and superficial heating agents. In *Thermal Agents in Rehabilitation.* S.L. Michlovitz (ed.). F.A. Davis, Philadelphia, 1986.
95. Lehmann, J.F., et al: Heating of joint structures by ultrasound. Arch. Phys. Med. Rehabil. 49:28, 1968.
96. Ziskin, M.C. and Michlovitz, S.L.: Therapeutic ultrasound. In *Thermal Agents in Rehabilitation.* S.L. Michlovitz (ed.). F.A. Davis, Philadelphia, 1986.
97. Gersten, J.W.: Effects of ultrasound on tendon extensibility. Am. J. Phys. Med. 34:662, 1955.
98. Lehmann, J.F., Masock, A.J., Warren, C.G., et al: Effect of therapeutic temperatures on tendon extensibility. Arch. Phys. Med. Rehabil. 51:481, 1970.
99. Lehmann, J.F., et al: Comparative study of the efficiency of shortwave, microwave and ultrasonic diathermy in heating the hip joint. Arch. Phys. Med. Rehabil. 40:510, 1959.
100. Bierman, W.: Ultrasound in the treatment of scars. Arch. Phys. Med. Rehabil. 35:209, 1954.
101. Abramson, D.I., et al: Changes in blood flow, oxygen uptake and tissue temperatures produced by therapeutic physical agents. I. Effect of ultrasound. Am. J. Phys. Med. 39:51, 1960.
102. Currier, D.P., Greathouse, D., and Switt, T.: Sensory nerve conduction: Effect of ultrasound. Arch. Phys. Med. Rehabil. 59:181, 1978.
103. Kahn, J.: *Low Volt Technique.* J. Kahn, Syosset, NY, 1983.
104. Antich, T.J.: Phonophoresis: The principles of the ultrasonic driving force and efficacy in treatment of common orthopaedic diagnosis. J. Orthop. Sports Phys. Ther. 4:99, 1982.
105. Newman, M.K., Kill, M., and Frampton, G.: Effects of ultrasound alone and combined with hydrocortisone injections by needle or hydrospray. Am. J. Phys. Med. 37:206, 1958.
106. Dyson, M. and Brookes, M.: Stimulation of bone repair by ultrasound (abstract). Ultrasound Med. Biol. (Suppl. 50)8:50, 1982.
107. Bender, L.F., James, J.M., and Herrick, J.F.: Histologic studies following exposure of bone to ultrasound. Arch. Phys. Med. Rehabil. 35:555, 1954.
108. Binder, S.A.: Applications of low and high voltage electrotherapeutic currents. In *Electrotherapy.* S.L. Wolf (ed). Churchill Livingstone, New York, 1981.
109. Wadsworth, H. and Chanmugan, A.P.P.: *Electrophysical Agents in Physiotherapy.* Science Press, Marrickville, NSW, 1983.
110. Sato, A. and Schmidt, R.F.: Somatosympathetic reflexes: Afferent fibers, central pathways, discharge characteristics. Physiol. Rev. 53:916–947, 1973.
111. Assimacopoulos, D.: Low intensity negative electric current in the treatment of ulcers of the leg due to chronic venous insufficiency. Am. J. Surg. 15:683–687, 1968.

112. Murphy, G.T.: Electrical physical therapy in treating TMJ patients. J. Craniomandib. Pract. 1:68–73, 1983.
113. Kahn, J.: TMJ pain control. Whirlpool 5:14, 1982.
114. Magistro, C.M.: Hyaluronidase by iontophoresis. Phys. Ther. 44:169–175, 1964.
115. Kahn, J.: Iontophoresis and ultrasound for postsurgical temporomandibular trismus and paresthesis. Phys. Ther. 60:307–308, 1980.
116. Russo, J. Jr., Lipman, A.G., Comstock, J.J., et al: Lidocaine anesthesia: Comparison of iontophoresis, injection, and swabbing. Am. J. Hosp. Pharm. 37:843–847, 1980.
117. Kahn, J.: *Principles and Practice of Electrotherapy.* Churchill Livingstone, New York, 1987.
118. Strassburg, H.M., Krainick, J.V., and Thoden, U.: Influence of transcutaneous nerve stimulation on acute pain. J. Neurol. 217:1–10, 1977.
119. O'Neil, R.: Relief of chronic facial pain by transcutaneous electrical nerve stimulation. Br. J. Oral Surg. 19:112–115, 1981.
120. Melzack, R. and Wall, P.D.: Pain mechanisms: A new theory. Science 150.971–979, 1975.
121. Roeser, W.M., Weeks, L.W., Venus, R., et al: The use of transcutaneous nerve stimulation for pain control in athletic medicine. A preliminary report. Am. J. Sports Med. 4:210–213, 1976.
122. Gunn, C.C. and Milbrandt, W.E.: Review of 100 patients with "low back sprain" treated by surface electrode stimulation of acupuncture points. Am. J. Acupuncture 3:224–232, 1975.
123. Augustinsson, L.E., Bohlin, P., Bundsen, P., et al: Pain relief during delivery by transcutaneous electrical nerve stimulation. Pain 4:59–65, 1977.
124. Wessberg, G.A., Carroll, W.L., Dinham, R., et al: Transcutaneous electrical nerve stimulation as an adjunct in the management of myofascial pain dysfunction syndrome. J. Prosthet. Dent. 45:307–314, 1981.
125. Chapman, C.R., Wilson, M.E., and Gehrig, J.D.: Comparative effects of acupuncture and transcutaneous stimulation on the perception of painful dental stimuli. Pain 2:265–283, 1976.
126. Chapman, C.R., Chen, A.C., and Bonica, J.J.: Effects of intrasegmental electrical acupuncture on dental pain: Evaluation of threshold estimation and sensory decision theory. Pain 3:23, 1977.
127. Ihalainen, V., Perkki, K., and Olsarinen, V.J.: The effect of transcutaneous nerve stimulation on tooth pain threshold. Proc. Finn. Dent. Soc. 73:212, 1977.
128. Mannheimer, J.S. and Lampe, G.N.: Electrode placement techniques. In *Clinical Transcutaneous Electrical Stimulation.* J.S. Mannheimer and G.N. Lampe (eds.). F.A. Davis Co., Philadelphia, 1984.
129. Erickson, M.B.E., Sjolund, B.H., and Neilzen, S.: Long term results of peripheral conditioning stimulation as analgesic measure in chronic pain. Pain 6:335, 1979.
130. Wolf, C.J.: Transcutaneous electrical nerve stimulation and the reaction to experimental pain in human subjects. Pain 7:115, 1979.
131. Anderson, S.A. et al: Evaluation of pain suppression effect of different frequencies of peripheral electrical stimulation in chronic pain conditions. Acta Orthop. Scand. 47:149, 1976.
132. Chapman, C.R., Chen, A.C., and Bonica, J.J.: Effects of intrasegmental electrical acupuncture on dental pain: Evaluation of threshold estimation and sensory decision theory. Pain 3:213, 1977.

133. Mannheimer, J.S. and Carlsson, C.A.: The analgesic effect of transcutaneous electrical nerve stimulation TNS in patients with rheumatoid arthritis. A comparative study of different pulse patterns. Pain 6:329, 1979.

134. Eriksson, M.B.E., Sjolund, B.H., and Nielzen, S.: Long term results of peripheral conditioning stimulation as analgesic measure in chronic pain. Pain 6:335, 1979.

135. Markovich, S.E.: Pain in the head: A neurological appraisal. In *Clinical Management of Head, Neck and TMJ Pain and Dysfunction*. H. Gelb (ed.). W.B. Saunders Co., Philadelphia, 1977.

136. Budzynski, T.H. and Stoyva, J.M.: An electro-myographic technique for teaching voluntary relaxation of the masseter muscle. J. Dent. Res. 52:116, 1973.

137. Dohrmann, R.J. and Laskin, D.M.: An evaluation of electromyographic biofeedback in the treatment of myofascial pain-dysfunction syndrome. J. Am. Dent. Assoc. 96:656, 1978.

138. Cherney, J.V.: Acupressure: *Acupuncture Without Needles*. Cornerstone Library, New York, 1974.

139. Duffin, D.: Acupuncture and acupressure. In *Pain: International Perspectives in Physical Therapy*. T.H. Michel (ed.). Churchill Livingstone, New York, 1985.

140. Melzack, R.: Prolonged relief of pain by brief, intense transcutaneous electrical stimulation. Pain 1:357, 1975.

141. Warren, G.C.: The use of heat and cold in the treatment of common musculoskeletal disorders. In *Management of Common Musculoskeletal Disorders*. R.M. Kessler and D. Hertling (eds.). Harper & Row, Philadelphia, 1983.

142. Sprague, R.B.: Mobilization of the cervical and upper thoracic spine. In *Orthopaedic Physical Therapy*. R. Donatelli and M.J. Wooden (eds.). Churchill Livingstone, New York, 1988.

143. Maitland, G.D.: *Vertebral Manipulation*, 4th ed. Butterworths, London, 1977.

144. Grieve, G.P.: *Mobilization of the Spine*. Churchill Livingstone, New York, 1979.

145. Hertling, D.: The temporomandibular joint. In *Management of Common Musculoskeletal Disorders*. R.M. Kessler and D. Hertling (eds). Harper & Row, Philadelphia, 1983.

146. Javinen, M.: Healing of a crush injury in rat striated muscle. Acta Pathol. Microbiol. Scand. (A) 83:269–282, 1975.

147. Passero, P.L., Wyman, B.S., Bell, J.W., et al: Temporomandibular joint dysfunction syndrome. Phys. Ther. Pract. 65:1203–1207, 1985.

148. Basmajian, J.V.: *Muscles Alive, Their Function Revealed by Electromyography*. Williams & Wilkins, Baltimore, 1974.

149. Ward, R.C.: Tutorial CN myofascial release techniques level II. Michigan State University College of Osteopathic Medicine. August 1–3, 1986.

150. Mitchell, F.L., Moran, P.S., and Pruzzo, N.A.: *An Evaluation and Treatment Manual of Osteopathic Muscle Energy Procedures*. Mitchell, Moran and Pruzzo Associates, Valley Park, MO, 1979.

151. Upledger, J.E., Relzlaff, E.W., and Vredevoogd, J.D.: Diagnosis and treatment of the temporoparietal suture head pain. In *Craniosacral Therapy, Appendix G*. J.E. Upledger and J.D. Vredevoogd (eds.). Eastland Press, Chicago, 1983.

152. Rocabado, M.: Biomechanical relationship of the cranial, cervical and hyoid regions. J. Craniomandib. Pract. 1:61–66, 1983.

153. Janda, V.: Muscles, central nervous regulation and back problems. In *Neurobiologic Mechanisms in Manipulative Therapy*. I.M. Korr (ed.). Plenum Press, New York, 1978.

154. Korr, I.M.: *Proprioceptors and Somatic Dysfunction, AAO Yearbook*. American Academy of Osteopathy, Newark, OH, 1976.

155. Wyke, B.: The neurology of joints. Ann. R. Coll. Surg. Engl. 41:25, 1967.

156. Mennell, J.M.: *Joint Pain*. Little, Brown & Co., Boston, 1964.

157. Maitland, G.D.: *Peripheral Manipulation*, 2nd ed. Butterworths, London, 1977.

158. Kraus, S.L.: Influences of the cervical spine on the stomatognathic system. In *Orthopaedic Physical Therapy*. R. Donatelli and M.J. Wooden (eds.). Churchill Livingstone, New York, 1988.

159. Shellhass, K., Latchan, R., Wendling, L., and Gold, L.: Vertebrobasilar injuries following cervical manipulation. J.A.M.A. 244:13, 1980.

160. Dvorak, J. and Dvorak, V.: *Manual Medicine Diagnostics*. Thieme-Stratton, New York, 1984.

161. Tatlow, T.W.F. and Bammer, H.G.: Vertebral artery compression syndrome. Neurology 7:331, 1957.

162. Coman, W.B.: Dizziness related to ENT conditions. In *Modern Manual Therapy of the Vertebral Column*. G.P. Grieve (ed.). Churchill Livingstone, New York, 1986.

163. Harms-Ringdahl, K., Ekblom, J., Schuldt, K., et al: Load moments and myoelectric activity when the cervical spine is held in full flexion and extension. Ergonomics 29:1539, 1986.

164. Daly, P., Preston, C.D., and Evans, W.G.: Postural response of the head to bite opening in adult males. Am. J. Orthod. 82:157, 1982.

165. Tallgren, A. and Solow, B.: Hyoid bone position, facial morphology and head posture in adults. Eur. J. Orthod. 9:1, 1987.

166. Adams, M.A. and Hutton, W.C.: The effect of posture on the fluid content of lumbar intervertebral discs. Spine 8:665, 1983.

167. Kelsey, J.L. Githens, P.B., O'Connor, T., et al: Acute prolapsed lumbar intervertebral discs. Spine 9:608, 1984.

168. Hunting, W., Grandjean, E., and Maeda, K.: Constrained postures in accounting machine operators. Appl. Ergon. 11:145, 1980.

169. Harms-Ringdahl, K. and Ekblom, J.: Intensity and character of pain and muscular activity levels elicited by maintained extreme flexion position of the lower cervical-upper-thoracic spine. Scand. J. Rehabil. Med. 18:117, 1986.

170. Andersson, G.B.J., Murphy, R.W., Ortengren, R., et al: The influence of backrest inclination and lumbar support on the lumbar lordosis in sitting. Spine 4:52–58, 1979.

171. Arndt, R.: Working posture and musculoskeletal problems of video display terminal operators. A review and reappraisal. J. Am. Ind. Hygiene Assoc. 44:437, 1983.

172. Bendix, T., Jessen, F., and Krohn, L.: Biomechanics of forward reaching movements while sitting on fixed forward or backward-inclining or tiltable seats. Spine 13:193, 1988.

173. Moumoto, T. and Kawamura, Y.: Properties of tongue and jaw movements elicited by stimulation of

the orbital gyrus of cat. Arch. Oral Biol. 18:361, 1973.

174. Ricketts, R.M.: Respiratory obstruction syndrome. Am. J. Orthod. 54:495, 1968.

175. Lowe, A. and Johnston, W.: Tongue and jaw muscle activity in response to mandibular rotations in a sample of normal and anterior open bite subjects. Am. J. Orthod. 76:565, 1979.

176. Fried, R.: Healthy breathing. Longevity, May, p. 62, 1989.

177. Krumhansl, B.R. and Nowacek, C.J.: In *Modern Manual Therapy of the Vertebral Column.* G. Grieve (ed.). Churchill Livingstone, New York, 1986.

178. Rocabado, M.: Physical therapy in dentistry. I & II. Course Notes, Orlando, Florida, 1980.

179. Jull, G.: Headaches of cervical origin. In *Physical Therapy of the Cervical Spine and Thoracic Spine.* R. Grant (ed.). Churchill Livingstone, New York, 1988.

180. Janda, V.: Muscles and cervicogenic pain syndrome. In *Physical Therapy of the Cervical Spine and Thoracic Spine.* R. Grant (ed.). Churchill Livingstone, New York, 1988.

181. Travell, J.: Referred pain from skeletal muscle. N.Y. State J. Med. 55:331, 1955.

182. Kraus, H.: Muscular aspects of oral dysfunction. In *Clinical Management of Head, Neck, and TMJ Pain and Dysfunction.* H. Gelb (ed.). W.B. Saunders Co., Philadelphia, 1985.

183. Travell, J. and Rinzler, S.H.: The myofascial genesis of pain. Postgrad. Med. 11:425–434, 1952.

184. Carstensen, B.: Indications and contradictions of manual therapy for TMJ. In *Modern Manual Therapy of the Vertebral Column.* G. Grieve (ed.). Churchill Livingstone, New York, 1986.

185. Zarb, G. and Speck, J.: The treatment of mandibular dysfunction. *Temporomandibular Joint, Function and Dysfunction.* In G. Zarb and G. Carlsson (eds.). C.V. Mosby, St. Louis, 1979.

186. Schwartz, L.: Therapeutic exercises. In *Disorders of the Temporomandibular Joint.* L. Schwartz (ed.). W.B. Saunders Co., Philadelphia, 1959.

187. Shaber, E.P.: Consideration in the treatment of muscle spasm. In *Disease of the Temporomandibular Apparatus* D. Morgan, W. Hall, and J. Vamvas (eds.). *A Multidisciplinary Approach.* C.V. Mosby, St. Louis, 1977.

188. Sheppard, I.M. and Sheppard, S.M.: Range of condylar movement during mandibular opening. J Prosthet. Dent. 15:236, 1965.

189. Vriell, P., Bertolucci, L., and Swaffer, C.: Physical therapy in the postoperative management of temporomandibular joint arthroscopic surgery. J. Craniomandib. Pract. 7:27–32, 1989.

190. Razook, S.: Nonsurgical management of TMJ and masticatory muscle problems. In *TMJ Disorders: Management of the Craniomandibular Complex.* S. Kraus (ed.). Churchill Livingstone, New York, 1988.

191. Bronstein, S.L. and Osborne, J.J.: Mandibular limitation due to bilateral coronoid enlargement: Management by surgery and physical therapy. J. Craniomandib. Pract. 1:58–62, 1984.

192. Hoffman, D., Mannheimer, J.S., Attanasio, R., and Cohen, H.: Clinical update: Management of the temporomandibular joint surgical patient. Clin. Prev. Dent. 2:28–32, 1989.

193. Osborne, J.J.: A physical therapy protocol for orthognathic surgery. J. Craniomandib. Pract. 7:132–136, 1989.

194. Bertolucci, L., Vriell, P., and Swaffer, C.: Postoperative physical therapy in temporomandibular joint arthroplasty. J. Craniomandib. Pract. 7:214–222, 1989.

195. Moriconi, S.E., Popowick, L.D., and Guernsey, H.L.: Alloplastic reconstruction of the temporomandibular joint. Dent. Clin. North Am. 30:307–324, 1986.

196. Dolwick, M.F. and Sanders, B.: Temporomandibular joint internal derangement and arthrosis. St Louis, C.V. Mosby, 1985.

197. Dolwick, M.F.: Surgical management. In *Internal Derangements of the Temporomandibular Joint.* Helms, C., R.W. Katzberg, M.F. Dolwick (eds.). Radiology Research and Education Foundation, San Francisco, 1983.

198. Bell, W., et al: Muscular rehabilitation after orthognathic surgery. Oral Surg. 56.229, 1983.

199. Plante, D.: Postoperative physical therapy. In *Surgery of the Temporomandibular joint.* D.A. Keith (ed.). Blackwell Scientific Publishers, Chicago, 1988.

200. Braun, B.L.: The effect of physical therapy intervention on incisal opening after temporomandibular joint surgery. Oral Surg. Oral Med. Oral Pathol. 64:544–548, 1987.

201. Merrill, R.G.: Historical perspectives and comparisons of TMJ surgery for internal disk derangement and arthropathy. J. Craniomandib. Pract. 4:74–85, 1986.

202. Bonica, J.J.: Management of myofascial pain syndromes in general practice. J.A.M.A. 164:732, 1957.

203. Mannheimer, J.S.: Prevention and restoration of abnormal upper quarter posture. In *Postural Considerations in the Diagnosis and Treatment of Cranio-Cervical-Mandibular and Related Chronic Pain Disorders.* H. Gelb (ed.). Ishiyaku EuroAmerican (in press).

204. Ware, O.H.: Postmeniscoplasty occlusal management. J. Craniomandib. Pract. 7:152–153, 1989.

205. Salter, R.D.: Regeneration of articular cartilage through continuous passive motion. Past, present and future. In *Clinical Trends in Orthopedics.* R. Staub and P.D. Wilson (eds.). Thieme Stratton, New York, 1982.

206. Pertes, R.A.: Updating the mandibular orthopedic repositioning appliance (MORA). J. Craniomandib. Pract. 5:351–355, 1987.

207. Mongini, F.: Remodeling of the mandibular condyle in the adult and its relationship to the condition of the dental arches. Acta Anat. 82:437, 1972.

208. Satko, C. and Blaustein, D.: Revascularization of rabbit temporomandibular joint after surgical intervention: Histological and micro-angiographic study. J. Oral Maxillofac. Surg. 44:871–876, 1986.

209. Akeson, W.H., et al: Collagen cross linking alteration in joint contractures: Changes in reducible crosslink in periarticular connective tissue collagen after nine weeks of immobilization. Connect. Tissue Res. 5:5–19, 1977.

Steven Syrop

CHAPTER 25

Pharmacologic Therapy

Pharmacologic management is an important adjunct to other treatment modalities. As with all therapeutic modalities, establishing a proper diagnosis is crucial to determining the appropriate medication.

Numerous factors must be considered before initiating pharmacologic therapy: proper informed consent, careful analysis of the disorder, selection of suitable medication, proper dispensing of the medication, and appropriate monitoring of the patient.[2]

Whether to take a medication is a decision that patients must make after fully discussing the benefits and risks with their dentist or physician. Patients' attitudes toward medication differ widely. The dentist must educate reluctant patients so that they can make a responsible decision. Patients who are too eager to take medication must be evaluated for potential drug abuse. If an addictive or dependent personality is identifed, drugs with the potential for abuse must be avoided.

Personal demographics of patients must be evaluated to determine the appropriate dosage of a medication with regard to age, environment, heredity, weight, and medical history.

Patients' ages are grouped into three categories: childhood, adult, and elderly. Children may require smaller doses, and certain medications must be avoided completely. Advanced age may bring alterations in metabolism, endocrine function, and drug elimination pathways, necessitating smaller doses or avoidance of certain medications altogether. For example, salicylates (aspirin and related anti-inflammatory agents) should be taken with caution by patients with chronic renal insufficiency, hepatic dysfunction, or peptic ulcer. Older patients are more likely to be taking other medications, making adverse interactions possible.

A patient's lifestyle is an important consideration. What type of work will the patient do while on the medication—driving? working with machinery? studying? Antianxiety medication such as diazepam and muscle relaxants (Flexeril) produce drowsiness, which may adversely affect a patient's daily activities.

Certain hereditary factors allow some persons to metabolize a drug faster or slower than average. Proper therapeutic levels of some medications can only be achieved by titration.

A history of adverse drug response is important to discuss with patients. Especially important is a history of drug allergy. Signs of allergic reaction include skin rash, swelling, urticaria, and difficulty breathing. Many patients confuse a "bad reaction" to a medicine with an allergic reaction. A common adverse reaction is gastritis after taking a nonsteroidal anti-inflammatory drug (NSAID). A medication that provokes an adverse reaction should be avoided, or measures taken to circumvent it. Drug history should include any medications a patient is currently taking. Before a prescription is written, drug interactions should be checked to ensure there will be no conflict with other medicine currently being taken. Patients who are pregnant or nursing should receive the most cautious and conservative drug therapy. Because many drugs pose serious danger to a developing fetus and newborn, it is prudent, if possible, not to prescribe any medication during gestation and lactation. If it is necessary, for instance, to treat an infection, then consultation with an obstetrician is advisable to decide on the most appropriate medication.

Patients should be told how to take the medication, when to take it, and what can be taken with it. Careful instruction is critical not only for safety but for optimal clinical results.

Before prescribing a medication, a clinician should become thoroughly familiar with it. The prescribing physician should know the indications, contraindications, warnings, adverse reactions, and dosage information detailed in the package insert. Patients must be monitored closely while taking a drug to be certain of the effects. The dose may have to be increased or decreased to achieve maximum benefit.

Prescription for generic versus brand name medication is a personal choice. There are two schools of thought on this issue. One claims there is no effective difference between the brand name and generic, whereas the other claims that differences in binding agents, coating agents, and manufacturing standards may reduce the effectiveness of some generic agents. This issue needs further evaluation before it can be resolved.

Pharmacologic management is adjunctive treatment used in combination with other modalities. Some temporomandibular disorders only require acute management. Drug therapy in these cases is short term and may constitute primary treatment. Other temporomandibular disorders are chronic and require long-term administration of medication.

Long-term management may extend throughout a patient's life span and carries a responsibility to monitor the patient for adverse side effects. For example, management of depression may require patients to take antidepressant medication for the rest of their lives. Periodic re-evaluation is necessary with long-term pharmacologic management.

An important rule in prescribing medication to patients with chronic pain is not to prescribe on an as-needed (prn) schedule.[2,3] A prn basis makes patients depend on the pain to receive medication. Pain behavior then becomes rewarded with medication, and patients learn to continue the pain. It is more appropriate to prescribe on a time-dependent schedule, such as four times daily.

One aspect of pharmacologic management is based on science: knowing which medication to prescribe. The other part of pharmacologic management is based on art: knowing each patient in terms of compliance, tolerance, and abuse potential.[4]

Several categories of medications commonly prescribed for patients with temporomandibular disorders are discussed:

1. Anti-inflammatory agents
2. Muscle relaxants
3. Antianxiety agents
4. Antihistamines
5. Narcotics
6. Local anesthetics
7. Dietary supplements
8. Antidepressants.

ANTI-INFLAMMATORY MEDICATION

Inflammation is a complex response induced by a wide variety of stimuli,[3] commonly infection or trauma. Arachidonic acid is stored in membrane-bound phospholipids. The release of arachidonic acid leads to a cascade of derivatives that are prominent in the development of inflammation.[5] These biologically active substances increase vasodilation, increase vascular permeability, and attract neutrophils. This inflammatory cascade is shown in Figure 25–1.

There are two main categories of anti-inflammatory medications: NSAIDs and corticosteroids.

Nonsteroidal Anti-Inflammatory Drugs
Mechanism of Action

The NSAIDs inhibit the formation of cyclo-oxygenase. This action inhibits prostaglandin synthesis from arachidonic acid (see Fig. 25–1).[6–8] Individual agents differ in their mode of inhibition of cyclooxygenase. Decreased prostaglandin biosynthesis diminishes the inflammatory response. Bradykinin, which is the most powerful stimulus of all kinins, is released by the inflammatory process. It becomes a painful stimulus in the presence of prostaglandins. NSAIDs produce analgesia by inhibition of prostaglandins, thereby reducing the painful stimulation by bradykinin.

The NSAIDs consist of six basic groups of compounds, based on chemical structural differences (Table 25–1).

1. Salicylates (aspirin)
2. Propionic acids
3. Acetic acids
4. Fenamates
5. Pyrazolones
6. Oxicams.

Although each category has subtle structural differences, as a group they show equal clinical effectiveness.[9] No one NSAID has been shown to be superior to the others. The primary differences are half-life and degree of gastric disturbance. Some NSAIDs are longer acting, and some cause less gastric irritation. A long-acting NSAID that does not cause gastric disturbance can be tolerated in higher doses and is preferable. Aspirin's long history of safety and use, low cost, and availability make it the standard by which all NSAIDs are measured.[6] Even in the largest tolerated doses, the NSAIDs do not completely arrest the inflammatory response. Common philosophy states that if one NSAID is not producing the desired results, then a change should be made to a different group of NSAIDs. A marked variation occurs in indi-

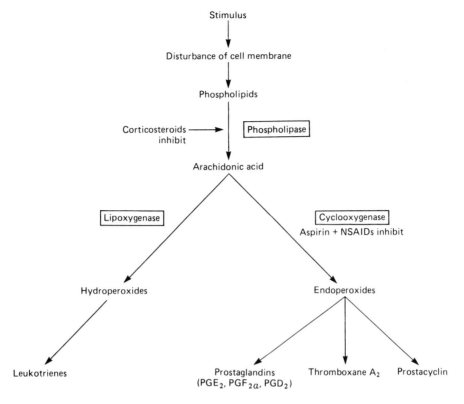

FIGURE 25–1. The inflammatory cascade. (Reprinted with permission from Shearn, M.: Nonsteroidal anti-inflammatory agents. In *Basic and Clinical Pharmacology,* 3rd ed. B.G. Katzung (ed.). Appleton & Lange, East Norwalk, 1987.)

vidual response to different but very closely related compounds. For instance, if aspirin (acetylsalicylic acid) is not effective, a change to naproxen (Naprosyn) may produce a better result.

Indications and Usage

The two primary indications for NSAIDs are reduction of inflammation and control of pain. Because all anti-inflammatory medication is also analgesic, pain control, alone, is an appropriate indication for the use of this category of drugs. Acute synovitis, arthritis, and musculoskeletal pain are the most common uses for NSAIDs.

The antipyretic capacity of aspirin and related compounds is well known. However, because elevated body temperature is not a common symptom of temporomandibular disorders, NSAIDs are generally not prescribed for this reason.

Aspirin is probably the most widely used anti-inflammatory agent. An estimated 10,000

to 20,000 tons are consumed in the United States annually.[10]

Side Effects

One of the most common side effects of the NSAIDs is gastric disturbance. The lining of the stomach becomes irritated as a result of two different mechanisms. Direct contact with the NSAID may cause local irritation of the mucosal lining. Some manufacturers avoid this problem by enteric coating of the product so that it passes through the stomach and dissolves in the small intestine. The second source of gastritis results from a decrease in the action of prostaglandin. Prostaglandin provides a cytoprotective mechanism in the mucosal lining. Because all NSAIDs act on inhibition of prostaglandin synthesis, the protective effect on the gastric mucosal lining is decreased. Even if the NSAID is absorbed in the small intestine, it can have systemic effects on the stomach.

Another side effect of NSAIDs is their influence on clotting. NSAIDs inhibit platelet ag-

TABLE 25–1. Non-Steroidal Anti-inflammatory Agents

CATEGORY	GENERIC	BRAND	HALF-LIFE (HOURS)
Salicylates:			
	Acetylsalicylic acid (aspirin)	Bayer	2.5
	Enteric coated	Ecotrin	2.5
	Aspirin with buffering agent	Bufferin	2.5
	Aspirin with caffeine	Anacin	2.5
	Diflunisal	Dolobid	8–12
	Choline magnesium trisalicylate	Trilisate	9–17
	Salsalate	Disalcid	16
Propionic acid:			
	Ibuprofen	Motrin, Advil, Nuprin, Rufen	1.8–2.5
	Fenoprofen	Nalfon	2–3
	Suprofen	Suprol	2–4
	Naproxen	Naprosyn	12–15
	Naproxen sodium	Anaprox	12–15
Acetic acid:			
	Indomethacin	Indocin	4.5–6
	Sulindac	Clinoril	7.8 (16.4)*
	Tolmetin	Tolectin	1–1.5
Fenamic acid:			
	Meclofenemate	Meclomen	2 (3.3)*
	Mefenamic acid	Ponstel	2
Pyrazolones:			
	Phenylbutazone	Butazolidin	84
Oxicam			
	Piroxicam	Feldene	30–86

*Active metabolite

gregation and can increase bleeding time. Significant variation exists between agents in this regard. With long-term use of NSAIDs, tests for prothrombin and bleeding time should be considered.

Other side effects of NSAIDs include tinnitus and dizziness. These can sometimes be controlled by decreasing the dose. People who take large doses of NSAIDs for many years may develop nephropathy. NSAIDs may affect renal function, because prostaglandins have a role in renal circulation. NSAIDs also have an undesirable effect on male fertility. Men with marginal fertility should not be treated with NSAIDs for any protracted length of time.

Two NSAIDs, indomethacin and phenylbutazone, are more toxic than the rest and should be avoided for long-term use.[3] Indomethacin is associated with untoward symptoms in 35 to 50% of persons who use it.[10] Heachache, dizziness, vertigo, and mental confusion are frequent. Ulceration of the gastrointestinal tract with hemorrhage has been reported. Blood dyscrasias, incluing neutropenia and thrombocytopenia, also result from indomethacin use.

Phenylbutazone is poorly tolerated. Nausea, vomiting, epigastric discomfort, and skin rash are the most commonly reported side effects. Water and electrocyte retention also occurs. Most serious is formation of peptic ulcer with hemorrhage. A number of deaths have occurred, especially from aplastic anemia and agranulocytosis.

The following recommendations can be used for patients prone to gastric irritation:

1. Long-acting NSAIDs should be used to reduce the frequency of oral ingestion. Suggested brands are Dolobid, Disalcid, Naprosyn, Anaprox, Feldene, and Trilisate.

2. NSAIDs that are not absorbed in the stomach can be used. Suggested brands are Ecotrin and Disalcid.

3. NSAIDs should be taken with or after a meal.

4. An antacid medication such as Maalox can be taken before NSAID ingestion.

5. Sucralfate (Carafate) can be prescribed and taken before ingesting a NSAID. Recommended dosage is 1 g taken before ingestion of the NSAID. Sucralfate is a medication prescribed for the treatment of ulcers. It binds with the ulcer site and provides protection from acid, pepsin, and bile salts.

TABLE 25-2. Anti-Inflammatory Potency of Various Corticosteroids

GENERIC	RELATIVE ANTI-INFLAMMATORY POTENCY
Cortisone	0.8
Cortisol	1.0
Prednisone	2.5
Methylprednisolone	4.0

(Reprinted with permission from Metheny, J.L.: Adrenocorticosteroids: Systemic and topical therapy. In *Clinical Pharmacology in Dental Practice*, 4th ed. S.V. Holroyd, R.L. Wynn, and B. Requa-Clark (eds.). C.V. Mosby, St. Louis, 1988.)

6. Patients should be warned of possible side effects and told to discontinue the medication and call the doctor if they occur.

7. NSAIDs should be avoided by patients with ulcerative disease or used in consultation with a gastroenterologist.

Corticosteroids

Mechanism of Action

The corticosteroids have a stronger anti-inflammatory effect than the NSAIDs. Corticosteroids inhibit the formation of arachidonic acid. The entire cascade of chemical reactions is prevented, thereby limiting the formation of prostaglandins, thromboxane, and leukotrienes[6,11] (see Fig. 25-1). This action effectively reduces inflammation. The anti-inflammatory activity of corticosteroids is far superior to that of the NSAIDs.

The corticosteroids vary in anti-inflammatory potency, as shown in Table 25-2.[12]

Indications and Usage

Steroid therapy is indicated to suppress noninfectious inflammation. NSAIDs should be tried first. If they do not succeed in reducing the symptoms, then corticosteroids may be considered. The primary clinical indication is synovitis that is not infectious and has responded poorly to NSAIDs. Steroids have also been used to reduce myositis. Using steroids to decrease muscle inflammation is a less accepted practice than steroid use to reduce joint inflammation.

Corticosteroids used in the treatment of temporomandibular disorders (TMDs) can be administered in various forms:

1. Intra-articular: lavage during arthroscopy; injection
2. Intramuscular: injection
3. Oral: tablets
4. Topical: creams.

Table 25-3 summarizes commonly used corticosteroids and doses.

Injection of steroid into the TMJ is an acceptable treatment when done infrequently. Common dogma does not support long-term repeated intra-articular injections.[13] Repeated injections into the TMJ accelerate joint damage by inducing destructive changes in the fibrocartilage covering of the condyle, followed by repair.[14] Gray and colleagues,[15] in an extensive review of the literature, dispute this notion.

During arthroscopy, steroids are used in two different ways—injection and lavage. Visualization of inflamed retrodiscal tissue allows a surgeon direct access to inject steroid into the area most inflamed. Joint lavage during arthroscopy allows for the continuous flow of steroid through the exposed joint compartment.

Injection of steroid into chronically inflamed muscle is sometimes indicated. Multiple and frequent muscle injections carry the same risks as multiple joint injections. Destructive changes followed by repair and fibrosis may accompany multiple muscle injections.

TABLE 25-3. Common Corticosteroids Used for Temporomandibular Disorders

GENERIC/BRAND NAMES	ORAL FORM	INJECTABLE	TOPICAL
Cortisol (Cortef) (Hydrocortone)	5, 10, 20 mg	25, 50 mg/ml	0.125% to 2.5% cream
Dexamethasone (Decadron) (Hexadrol)	0.25-4 mg 0.5 mg/5 ml elixir	4-24 mg/ml	0.04-0.1% cream
Methylprednisolone (Medrol) (Depo-Medrol)	2-32 mg	20, 40, 80 mg/ml	0.25, 1% ointment

Management of acute noninfectious joint inflammation not responding to NSAIDs may require oral steroid therapy. The author has found the Medrol Dosepak brand of methylprednisolone to be effective and packaged for easy administration. Each tablet is 4 mg; six are taken the first day, five the second day, four the third day, and so on until none is remaining. This 6-day steroid regimen is effective for reducing inflammation. There is little indication for long-term steroid administration in the management of temporomandibular disorders. The risk of side effects outweighs the possible benefits.

Some advocate the use of topical steroids, but cutaneous penetration is usually poor. For example, hydrocortisone has only a 1% absorption rate through the skin.[12] Penetration may be enhanced by trying to "push" the steroid into the joint by a process known as phonophoresis-ultrasound or iontophoresis. Iontophoresis uses electrical current to increase permeability of chemicals through the skin. Ultrasound uses selected wave frequencies to increase absorbtion of chemicals through the skin. It is unknown whether steroid administered in this fashion can penetrate the dense fibrous capsule surrounding the joint.

Side Effects

Corticosteroid administration has many side effects, usually related to dose and duration of treatment. Suppression of the inflammatory response decreases resistance to infection, so dormant infections may be activated. Long-term therapy can cause a redistribution of body fat. There is also a potential for causing electrolyte imbalance and hypertension. Long-term administration of corticosteroids results in suppression of the hypothalamic-pituitary-adrenal axis and may produce a clinical picture similar to Cushing's disease. Osteoporosis is also considered a risk associated with long-term corticosteroid use.[16,17] However, the risk is thought to be minimal at doses less than 7.5 mg/day.[11,16]

MUSCLE RELAXANTS (OTHER THAN BENZODIAZEPINES)

Muscle relaxants consist of two broad categories—centrally acting and peripherally acting agents. Commonly prescribed muscle relaxants used in the treatment of temporomandibular disorders act centrally and are used primarily as sedatives.

Mechanism of Action

Peripheral muscle relaxants work by blocking synaptic transmission at the neuromuscular junction, resulting in blocked muscle contraction. Curare, succinylcholine, and dantrolene (Dantrium) are examples of this group of medications. Baclofen (Lioresal), derived from gamma-aminobutyric acid (GABA), inhibits muscle contraction by its action on the spinal cord. It is used in the treatment of multiple sclerosis to decrease muscle spasm. These peripherally acting agents are not commonly used, but further research is indicated to determine whether this class of drugs has application in the treatment of TMDs.

Centrally acting muscle relaxants, which include methocarbamol (Robaxin), carisoprodol (Soma), and cyclobenzaprine (Flexeril), provide relaxation of muscle tissue by a sedative effect on the central nervous system (CNS).[18] To date, no specific neurotransmitter agent has been identified as responsible for the actions of centrally acting muscle relaxants. They have no direct action on the contractile mechanism of striated muscle, the motor end plate, or the nerve fiber.

One centrally acting muscle relaxant that is different from all of the others is cyclobenzaprine (Flexeril). The structure of cyclobenzaprine is similar to that of the tricyclic antidepressants. This medication provides a strong tranquilizing effect and, if given over a 3- to 4-week period, can have antidepressant activity.

Indications and Usage

Muscle relaxants are indicated for the relief of acute musculoskeletal pain. Muscle pain secondary to anxiety responds well to muscle relaxants because these agents act primarily as sedatives. Hypertonicity of one or two muscles is usually not sufficient justification to prescribe muscle relaxants. However, when multiple muscle groups are involved there is a stronger reason to prescribe a muscle relaxant.

Muscle relaxants are commonly prescribed in conjunction with NSAIDs. Several combination medications contain a muscle relaxant and an NSAID. These fixed-dose preparations may provide suboptimal doses of medication.[18] An example of a fixed-dose combination is Equagesic, combining meprobamate and aspirin. Norgesic and Norgesic Forte combine orphenadrine, aspirin, and caffeine. It is preferable to prescribe medications separately to achieve optimal therapeutic doses of each medicine. In fixed-dose combinations, intolerance to one of the medications may necessitate a decrease in the total dose, providing less effective levels of the other medications. Separate prescriptions allow more flexibility.

Reactions to muscle relaxant medication are highly variable. A dose that may produce strong tranquilizing effects lasting 24 to 48 hours in one person may have no effect on another person. Therefore, individual titration of muscle relaxants is recommended for each patient. Common muscle relaxants are listed in Table 25–4.

Side Effects

By far the most common side effect of muscle relaxants is excessive sedation. As stated earlier, individual titration is important to avoid this. Lightheadedness, dizziness, and nausea are also reported side effects. Most agents in this category are specifically listed as not indicated for children younger than 12 years. Notable exceptions to this are chlorzoxazone (Paraflex) and Parafon Forte, which list specific doses for children.

Cyclobenzaprine (Flexeril), because of its similarity to the tricyclic antidepressants, has greater side effects than other muscle relaxants. The anticholinergic effects manifested as dry mouth, blurred vision, tachycardia, constipation, and urinary retention may accompany its use. Many of these side effects abate after several days with continued use.

ANTIANXIETY MEDICATIONS

Anxiety is recognized by many as an underlying condition that exacerbates symptoms of temporomandibular disorders.[19,20,21] Antianxiety medication is very commonly prescribed in the general population and is consistently one of the ten most prescribed medicines year after year. Valium and Librium have accounted for approximately 75 million prescriptions. The details of the antianxiety agents will be explained later.

There are four categories of antianxiety medications:

1. Propyl alcohol derivatives (meprobamate)
2. Benzodiazepine derivatives (Valium)
3. Diphenylmethanes (antihistamines—Atarax)
4. Buspirone hydrochloride (Buspar).

Meprobamate (Miltown, Equanil) has been available for many years. Its abuse potential is high. Physical dependence is strong, and withdrawal can be complicated. For these reasons, there is little use for meprobamate in patients with chronic temporomandibular disorders. Antihistamines (Atarax and Vistaril; see Table 25–6) can reduce anxiety. They are indicated

TABLE 25–4. Common Muscle Relaxants

GENERIC	BRAND NAME	USUAL DOSAGE MG/DAY DIVIDED DOSES
Carisoprodol	Rela, Soma	1000–1400
Chlorzoxazone	Paraflex	750–3000
	Parafon Forte D.S.C.	
Meprobamate	Miltown, Equanil	1200–1600
Methocarbamol	Robaxin	1500–3000
Cyclobenzaprine	Flexeril	10–30
Orphenadrine	Norflex, Disipal	150–300
Diazepam	Valium	4–40

COMBINATION FIXED DOSAGE		RECOMMENDED DOSAGE
Equagesic	Meprobamate 200 mg	1–2 tabs 3–4 times daily
	Aspirin 325 mg	
Norgesic	Orphenadrine 25 mg	1–2 tabs 3–4 times daily
	Aspirin 385 mg	
	Caffeine 30 mg	
Norgesic Forte	Orphendrine 50 mg	½ to 1 tab 3–4 times daily
	Aspirin 770 mg	
	Caffeine 60 mg	

for elderly patients or for those with a history of drug abuse.[18]

Buspirone hydrochloride (Buspar) is unrelated to the benzodiazepines. It is very selective at reducing anxiety without producing sedation. It lacks muscle relaxant properties. Its action on serotonin transmission—in particular, its high affinity for serotonin receptors—may be related to its effectiveness. However, its exact mechanism of action is unknown.[1]

Benzodiazepines

The benzodiazepines have evolved into numerous derivatives since 1955, when Sternbach first synthesized chlordiazepoxide (Librium). In 1963, diazepam (Valium) was marketed.

Mechanism of Action

The complete mechanism of action of the benzodiazepines has not yet been fully elucidated. There appears to be a specific binding site within the GABA receptor. Benzodiazepines indirectly interfere with GABA-mediated processes.[18] Clinically, benzodiazepines reduce anxiety, have sedative effects, and relax skeletal muscle. Muscle relaxation is due to general sedation rather than direct action on the muscle. Numerous benzodiazepines are more selective than diazepam. Some have increased specificity to target selected disorders, such as Xanax and Klonopin, which are used to treat panic disorders. Newer derivatives also differ in half-life activity. A short-acting benzodiazepine is triazolam (Halcion), prescribed to reduce insomnia. Common benzodiazepines are listed in Table 25–5.

Indications and Usage

Medical opinion is divided regarding the use of benzodiazepines: Some believe that their abuse potential outweighs their benefit. Others believe that their safety margin is so high that the risk of developing problems is very low. Prudent clinicians should re-evaluate the patient and the prescription at 4-month intervals. The benzodiazepines are indicated for reduction of anxiety, insomnia, and hypertonic musculature. Because of their euphoric properties, they have a potential for abuse. They are contraindicated in patients with a history of drug or alcohol dependence. It is not known how large a dose or how long benzodiazepines must be taken before a dependence occurs. Felpel[18] reports that high doses, above therapeutic levels, must be sustained for several months before dependence occurs. When discontinuing benzodiazepines, the dosage should be decreased gradually to avoid withdrawal symptoms. Although there has been concern about the potential for habituation and abuse, some studies suggest that physicians may be too conservative and may even undertreat patients with anxiety disorders.[22]

Side Effects

The most commonly experienced side effect of benzodiazepines is drowsiness. Patients report that they feel lethargic and tired. Some patients react paradoxically, feeling an increase in anxiety, and become irritable. This reaction is not common. In the elderly, confused mental status may result from what would be called a "usual dose" of benzodiazepine.

Clinical toxic reactions are low; there is a

TABLE 25–5. Common Benzodiazepines

DRUG	BRAND	USUAL DOSAGE	HALF-LIFE (HOURS)
Alprazolam	Xanax	0.5 mg 2–3 times/day	12–15
Clonazepam	Klonopin	0.5–1 mg 2–3 times/day	18–50
Chlordiazepoxide	Librium	5–20 mg 3–4 times/day	5–30
Chlorazepate	Tranxene	7.5–15 mg 1–2 times/day	30–100
Diazepam	Valium	2–10 mg 2–4 times/day	20–50
Flurazepam	Dalmane	30 mg at bedtime	2–3
Lorazepam	Ativan	0.5–1 mg 2–3 times/day	10–18
Oxazepam	Serax	10–15 mg 3–4 times/day	5–15
Prazepam	Verstran	10–20 mg 2–3 times/day	30–100
Temazepam	Restoril	15–30 mg at bedtime	10–20
Triazolam	Halcion	0.25–0.5 mg at bedtime	1.5–5

very high safety margin.[22] Complications and even death occur when high doses of benzodiazepines are taken in conjunction with ethanol or other CNS depressants. A few deaths have been reported at doses greater than 700 mg of diazepam or chlordiazepoxide. This is almost 20 times the therapeutic dosage. Treatment of overdose requires support of respiration and cardiovascular function.

Other side effects include skin rash, nausea, headache, impairment of sexual function, and vertigo. Menstrual irregularities have been reported. Women may fail to ovulate while taking benzodiazepines. Benzodiazepines are contraindicated in patients with narrow-angle glaucoma.

ANTIHISTAMINES

Antihistamines block the effects of histamine. They also have other independent actions, which include sedative, antianxiety, and antiemetic effects. In the treatment of temporomandibular disorders, antihistamines are prescribed more for their side effects than for their primary antihistaminic effect.

Histamine has numerous physiologic effects.[23] Its exact mechanism in the body is poorly understood. In most tissues, it is contained in mast cells. In the CNS, it has been implicated as a neurotransmitter. Histamine is released following tissue damage. It is involved in the inflammatory process by producing vasodilation and increased cell permeability.

Antihistamines can be used as sedatives and anxiolytic agents. They are a suitable choice for patients when benzodiazepines are contraindicated, such as for children, the elderly, and potential abusers. Antihistamines can also be used as a diagnostic tool to rule out pain originating from sinusitis. If a sinus problem is present, the patient should be referred to an otolaryngologist. Antihistamines are also used in the management of vertigo, motion sickness, and nausea. Commonly prescribed antihistamines are listed in Table 25–6.

OPIATE-NARCOTIC ANALGESICS

Opiate medications (morphine, codeine) have a strong pain-alleviating effect. They are indicated for short-term relief of acute pain, usually surgically or traumatically induced. There are numerous side effects, most notably respiratory depression. The safety margin of this class of drugs is low, and the abuse potential is high. Because physical and psychologic dependence may develop, opiate analgesics are a generally undesirable choice of medication for most patients with chronic temporomandibular disorders. The risk of dependency and

TABLE 25–6. Common Antihistamines Useful in the Treatment of Temporomandibular Disorders

PURPOSE	GENERIC NAME	BRAND NAME	AVAILABLE FORM	DOSAGE
Sedative to reduce insomnia	Promethazine	Phenergan	Syrup 6.25 mg/5 ml; 25 mg/ml (fortis) Tablets 12.5 mg; 25 mg; 50 mg	Adults: 25–50 mg at bedtime
Sedative for anxiety	Hydroxyzine	Vistaril	Capsules 25 mg; 50 mg; 100 mg Oral suspension 25 mg/5 ml	50–100 mg 4 times/day
		Atarax	Tablets 10 mg; 25 mg; 50 mg; 100 mg Syrup 10 mg/5 ml	50–100 mg 4 times/day
Decongestant	Terfenadine	Seldane	Tablets 60 mg	1 tab 2 times/day
Decrease vertigo	Cyclizine	Marezine	Tablets	1 tab every 4–6 hours
	Meclizine	Antivert	Nonprescription tablets 12.5 mg; 25 mg; 50 mg	25–100 mg in divided dose daily
Antiemetic	Promethazine	Phenergan	Syrup 6.25 mg/5 ml; 25 mg/5 ml (fortis) Tablet 12.5 mg; 25 mg; 50 mg Suppository 12.5 mg; 25 mg; 50 mg	25 mg every 4–6 hours as needed

low safety margin outweigh the benefit in long-term outpatient pain management.

However, in some situations, opiate analgesics are appropriate. It is important to understand this class of drugs, because patients may have had narcotic medications in the past or may currently be addicted to them.

Mechanism of Action

The use of opium as a medicine dates back to the third century B.C.[24] The rather recent discovery of opioid receptors in the CNS and the isolation of morphine-like substances produced in the brain[25] led to enormous advances in understanding how opioid analgesics work. Opiate analgesia is due to action at several different sites within the CNS. Opiate binding sites are located on the axons in the substantia gelatinosa of the spinal cord and in the spinal nucleus of the trigeminal nerve. Drugs acting at these sites are thought to decrease release of neurotransmitters such as substance P, which mediates pain transmission.[24] Other sites within the CNS are affected by opiates. Binding of opiates in the various CNS areas produces the clinical symptoms of analgesia, drowsiness, changes in mood, euphoria, and mental confusion. Pain relief is selective; sensory modalities such as touch, vision, and hearing are not generally affected. Depression of respiration by direct action on the brain stem is a serious complication. There is also direct action on the bowel, resulting in decreased gastrointestinal

motility. Codeine, an important analgesic, is metabolized to form morphine. Approximately 10% of codeine is converted to morphine in this fashion.

Indications and Usage

Acute, postoperative, and trauma-related pain are the most common indications for the opiate narcotic analgesics. Because of serious side effects and dependency potential, long-term administration is contraindicated. Patients in pain may request a specific prescription for narcotic medication, claiming that the pain is so severe they can no longer tolerate it. This demand places a prescribing clinician in a difficult position. Physicians want to help relieve their patients of pain, yet they do not want to risk causing drug dependency. The solution is to reserve narcotic analgesics for specifically indicated conditions such as acute pain from trauma or surgery. Set a limit for the medication by explaining to patients that the prescription will not be renewed when it expires. A specific office policy on narcotic administration should be established and articulated by the practitioner. For example, in my clinical management experience, the rule has been set that patients with chronic pain are never to receive narcotic medications.

Selected narcotic analgesics are listed in Table 25–7. Many of these agents are fixed-dose combinations, combining a narcotic with either acetaminophen or aspirin.

TABLE 25-7. Common Opiate Narcotic Analgesics

BRAND	COMPONENTS	DOSAGE
Tylenol with codeine #3	Codeine 30 mg Acetaminophen 300 mg	1 tab every 4 hours
Fiorinal with codeine #3	Codeine 30 mg Butalbital 50 mg Caffeine 40 mg Aspirin 325 mg	1 or 2 caps every 4 hours, not to exceed 6 caps per day
Darvon	Propoxyphene 65 mg	1 tab every 4 hours
Darvon compound-65	Propoxyphene 65 mg Aspirin 389 mg Caffeine 32.4 mg	1 tab every 4 hours
Darvocet-N 50	Propoxyphene 50 mg Acetaminophen 325 mg	1 tab every 4 hours
Percodan	Oxycodone hydrochloride 4.5 mg Oxycodone terephthazate 0.38 mg Aspirin 325 mg	1 tab every 6 hours
Percocet	Oxycodone hydrochloride 5 mg Acetaminophen 325 mg	1 tab every 6 hours
Dilaudid	Hydromorphone, 1 mg, 2 mg, 3 mg, 4 mg	2–4 mg every 4–6 hours

Side Effects

Opioid analgesics depress respiration by direct action on brain stem respiratory centers. Morphine depresses all aspects of respiration, including rate, minute volume, and tidal exchange. The brain becomes less responsive to carbon dioxide levels. Death due to overdose is secondary to respiratory arrest. Nausea and vomiting, although less serious, are unpleasant side effects caused by direct stimulation of the medulla.

Development of tolerance and physical dependence with repeated use of narcotic analgesics is well recognized. Psychologic dependence also develops. Elimination of the drug is complicated by withdrawal symptoms.

The risk of dependency, increased tolerance, serious side effects, and low safety margin make opiate analgesics a poor choice for chronically ill patients with temporomandibular disorders.

LOCAL ANESTHETICS

Local anesthetics are often used in diagnosis and treatment of temporomandibular disorders. The first local anesthetic discovered was cocaine, first used by the inhabitants of the Andes Mountains in Peru.[26] It was noted that it had a bitter taste and left the tongue numb. Sigmund Freud studied the effects of cocaine in 1884, and in that same year Hall introduced local anesthesia into dentistry.[26] By 1905, the first synthetic substitute was produced, procaine. Today there are many other derivatives. The common local anesthetics used in temporomandibular disorders are listed in Table 25–8.

Mechanism of Action

Local anesthetics prevent generation and conduction of nerve impulses. The main site of action is the cell membrane. Both sensory and motor nerves are equally sensitive to local anesthetics. Small-diameter fibers are blocked more rapidly than larger-diameter fibers.

Local anesthetics are completely reversible without any evidence of structural damage to nerve fibers or cells. How effective the anesthesia is depends in part on the pH of the surrounding tissue. Local anesthetics all are weak bases and are inactive in an acidic medium.

Local anesthestics differ in the length of anesthesia produced, as shown in Table 25–8. Epinephrine-containing anesthetics should not be used for injection into skeletal muscle. Epinephrine causes vasoconstriction and may precipitate a muscle spasm.

Indications and Usage

In diagnosis, an anesthetic block is employed to rule out a particular anatomic location as a source of pain. For example, if a lower molar is suspected as a source of pain, an inferior alveolar injection should block the pain. If the pain continues, it is probably not originating in the tooth, assuming that the block injection provided effective anesthesia. If a second injection is given into the masseter muscle and the pain subsides, it is likely that the muscle was the source of pain.

Local anesthetics are useful to break a muscle spasm. A patient with an inability to open his or her mouth may present as a diagnostic dilemma: Is there an internal derangement or muscle spasm? The suspect muscles can be injected; if the patient can then open wide, the diagnosis of muscle spasm is confirmed. However, negative results do not rule out muscle spasm; they are simply inconclusive.

Muscle injections, especially trigger point injections, have been fully described by Travell.[26] Injecting into a muscle reduces pain by several proposed mechanisms: The needle may disrupt the contractile elements; neural feedback loops sustaining dysfunction may be interrupted;

TABLE 25–8. Common Local Anesthetics Used in Temporomandibular Disorders

ANESTHETICS	CONCENTRATIONS	DURATION OF ACTION (MINUTES)
Procaine	0.5%	20–45
Lidocaine	1%, 2%	60–120
Mepivacaine (Carbocaine)	3%	60–120
Bupivacaine (Marcaine)	0.5%	400–450

and local vasodilation may increase circulation and remove local metabolites.

When thermal agents and stretching exercises have not been successful in alleviating the muscle dysfunction, then injection therapy can be attempted.

Side Effects

Although local anesthetics are reversible with time, they have several serious side effects. As with any injection, allergic reaction, syncope, and intravascular penetration are potential complications. Hypersensitivity is more common with the ester-type anesthetics such as procaine. All anesthetics may cause CNS stimulation, producing restlessness, tremor, and convulsion, although drowsiness is the most common complaint.

Following systemic absorption, cardiac effects may occur. Infiltration of local anesthetic to the carotid bodies near the sternocleidomastoid should be avoided.

DIETARY SUPPLEMENTS

What we eat can affect the way we feel. This intuitive observation has little scientific documentation.

It has been established that certain medications can alter levels of neurotransmitters, which in turn influence behavior.[28] The formation of neurotransmitters depends on brain levels of precursor nutrients.[28] It therefore has been suggested that the composition of the diet and nutrient supplements can influence neurotransmitter levels.[28-30]

Numerous over-the-counter dietary supplements are available to patients. These agents have not received the close scrutiny and testing required of prescription medications. Two neutral amino acids, D-phenylalanine and L-tryptophan, show some promise of clinical effectiveness. However, further research is required, and questions of adverse side effects including death remain unanswered.

D-Phenylalanine acts to inhibit the degradation of endorphins. Enkephalin is an endogenous opioid produced in the spinal cord and diencephalic gray matter in the brain. It is a short-acting opioid, producing strong analgesia. It is rapidly metabolized by enkephalinase. D-Phenylalanine appears to be a very potent inhibitor of enkephalinase,[31] potentiating the opioid analgesia.

An effective clinical dose of D-phenylalanine is 1 to 2 g/day divided into four equal doses.[31]

There is a reported latency period of up to 3 weeks to achieve results. Testing of D-phenylalanine in large clinical trials has yet to be carried out, but the concept of potentiation of the endorphin system to produce endogenous analgesia deserves further study.

Tryptophan is another amino acid that has shown promise in chronic pain management. Serotonin is synthesized from tryptophan and has been implicated as active in the CNS related to depression, sleep, thermal regulation, and pain perception. Tryptophan competes with other amino acids for transport across the blood-brain barrier. To increase tryptophan transport into the brain, subjects consume a special diet that is high in carbohydrate and low in protein. Less protein in the diet decreases amino acid competition with tryptophan to cross the blood-brain barrier.

L-Tryptophan is usually given in a 2-g dose. Seltzer and colleagues,[29,30] in controlled clinical trials, demonstrated increased tolerance to pain following L-tryptophan supplementation and dietary manipulation.

In a well-controlled clinical study, Stockstill and associates[32] refuted the effectiveness of tryptophan and dietary manipulation. They were not able to duplicate the pain reduction reported in other studies.

Because of unexplained morbidity and mortality, L-tryptophan has been taken off the market. The possible causes are under study.

Dietary supplements and diet manipulation may prove to be a helpful adjunct in the treatment of chronic pain. However, at present, insufficient data exist to support routine use.

PLACEBO

Placebo response is a most intriguing medical phenomenon. Placebo response produces symptomatic relief, based primarily on a patient's expectation and belief that the drug or procedure is effective. The placebo response is well documented in the literature.[33] Numerous hypotheses have been set forth to explain the mechanism of action of the placebo response. One claims that placebo treatment reduces anxiety and that reduced anxiety decreases symptoms. It has also been suggested that the effects of a placebo are a result of conditioned response; medications and treatment in the past have been associated with pain relief. Therefore, administration of a placebo medication or treatment can produce a conditioned analgesic response.

A physiologically based hypothesis claims

that placebo stimulates release of endogenous opioids.[34] Placebo responders have increased blood levels of endorphin. Naloxone, a morphine antagonist, has been shown to reverse the placebo effect.[34] Other studies have failed to confirm this.[35]

What is apparent is that placebo treatment is more than simply giving a sugar pill. It elicits a complex psycho-physiologic response. Placebo medication can be inert or active. Inert placebo has no measurable physiologic effect. Active placebo produces a physiologic response that the patient is aware of; this response acts on an organ system unrelated to the pain. An example of an active placebo is one that may cause dry mouth or increased heart rate but has no pharmacologic effect on pain. The overall effectiveness of placebo is between 30 and 60%.[33,36] Successful outcome is often attributed to the medication or treatment when placebo response may have been responsible. Clinicians must be cautious not to jump to the conclusion that successful pain relief was solely the result of the treatment provided. We must realize that a portion of successful pain relief is due to placebo response. The placebo response is critical to testing the efficacy of new drugs. All drugs must be tested against placebo effects. It is interesting to note that not only does a placebo relieve pain, it can also be responsible for untoward side effects such as vertigo and nausea.

In 1859, Quimby stated, "But through a great many mistakes and the prescription of a great many useless drugs, I was led to re-examine the question; and came in the end to the position I now hold: The cure does not depend upon any drug, but simply in the patient's belief in the doctor or the medicine."[37]

Awareness of the placebo response—which is a powerful, widespread, and well-documented effect—should serve to prevent clinicians and health-care professionals from being overly enthusiastic in attributing successful outcome solely to the medication or treatment provided.

REFERENCES

1. Martin, E.W.: *Hazards of Medication.* J.B. Lippincott Co., Philadelphia, 1978.
2. Richlin, D.M. and Brand, L.: The use of oral analgesics for chronic pain. Hosp. Formul. 32–41, 1982.
3. Gregg, T.M.: Pharmacological management of myofascial pain dysfunction. In *The President's Conference On the Examination, Diagnosis, and Management of Temporomandibular Disorders.* D. Laskin, W. Greenfield, E. Gale, et al (eds.). American Dental Association, Chicago, 1983.
4. Syrop, S.B.: Non-surgical management of the patient with facial pain. In *Principles of Oral and Maxillofacial Surgery.* L.J. Peterson (ed.). J.B. Lippincott Co., Philadelphia (in press).
5. Samuelson, B.: An elucidation of arachidonic acid cascade. Drugs (Suppl. 1) 33:2–9, 1987.
6. Shearn, M.: Nonsteroidal anti-inflammatory agents. In *Basic and Clinical Pharmacology,* 3rd ed. B.G. Katzung (ed.). Appleton & Lange, East Norwalk, 1987.
7. Vane, T.: The evolution of non-steroid antiinflammatory drugs and their mechanism of action. Drugs (Suppl. 1) 33:18–27, 1987
8. Simon, L.S. and Mills, J.A.: Non steroidal antiinflammatory drugs. N. Engl. J. Med. 302:21, 1179–1185, 1980.
9. Roth, S.H.: Salicycates revisited. Drugs 36:1–6, 1988.
10. Flower, R.J., Moncada, S, and Vane, J.R.: Analgesics-antipyretics and anti-inflammatory agents. In *Goodman and Gilman's The Pharmacological Basis of Therapeutics,* 8th ed. A.G. Gilman and L.S. Goodman (eds.). Pergamon Press, New York, 1990.
11. Wolfe, C.S. and Hughes, G.R.V.: The optimum management of arthropathies. Drugs 36:370–381, 1988.
12. Methany, J.L.: Adrenocorticosteroids: Systemic and topical therapy. In *Clinical Pharmacology in Dental Practice,* 4th ed. S.V. Holroyd, R.L. Wynn, and B. Requa-Clark (eds.). C.V. Mosby, St. Louis, 1988.
13. Seymour, R.A. and Walton, J.G.: *Adverse Drug Reactions in Dentistry.* Oxford University Press, New York, 1988.
14. Poswillo, D.: Experimental investigations of the effects of intra-articulation hydrocortisone and high condylectomy on the mandibular condyle. Oral Surg. 30:161–173, 1970.
15. Gray, R.G., Tenenbaum, J., and Gottlieb, N.L.: Local corticosteroid injection treatment in rheumatic disorders. Semin. Arthritis Rheum. 10:231–254, 1981.
16. Schreiber, A.M. and Brooks, P.: Immunosuppressive drugs and corticosteroids in the treatment of rheumatoid arthritis. Drugs 36:340–363, 1988.
17. Streeten, D.H.P.: Corticosteroid therapy. II. Complication and theraputic indication. J.A.M.A. 232:1046–1059, 1975.
18. Felpel, L.P.: Antianxiety drugs and centrally acting muscle relaxants. In *Pharmacology and Therapeutics for Dentistry,* 3rd ed. E.A. Neidle, D.C. Kroeger, and Yagiela, J.A. (eds.). C.V. Mosby, St. Louis, 1989.
19. Laskin, D.M.: Etiology of the pain dysfunction syndrome. J. Am. Dent. Assoc. 79:147–153, 1969.
20. Ogus, H.D. and Toler, P.A.: *Common Disorders of the Temporomandibular Joint,* 2nd ed. Wright Publ., Bristol, 1986.
21. Schwartz, L.L.: A temporomandibular joint pain dysfunction syndrome. J. Chronic Dis. 3:284–293, 1956.
22. Baldessarini, R.J.: Drugs and the treatment of psychiatric disorders. In *Goodman and Gilman's The Pharmacological Basis of Therapeutics,* 8th ed. A.G. Gilman and L.S. Goodman (eds.). Pergamon Press, New York, 1990.
23. Holroyd, S.V., Wynn, R.L., Requa-Clark, B., and Roth-Schecter, B.: Histamine and antihistamine. In *Clinical Pharmacology in Dental Practice,* 4th ed. S.V. Holroyd, R.L. Wynn, and B. Requa-Clark (eds.). C.V. Mosby, St. Louis, 1988.
24. Jaffe, J.H. and Martin, W.R.: Opioid analgesics and antagonists. In *Goodman and Gilman's The Pharmacological Basis of Therapeutics,* 7th ed. A.G. Gilman and L.S. Goodman (eds.). Macmillan, New York, 1985.

25. Hughes, J.W., Smith T., Kosterlitz, H., et al: Identification of two related pentapeptides from the brain with potent opiate agonist activity. Nature 255:577–579, 1975.
26. Ritchie, J. and Greene, N.: Local anesthetics. In *Goodman and Gilman's The Pharmacological Basis of Therapeutics,* 8th ed. A.G. Gilman and L.S. Goodman (eds.). Pergamon Press, New York, 1990.
27. Travell, J.O. and Simons, D.G.: *Myofascial Pain and Dysfunction—The Trigger Point Manual.* Williams & Wilkins, New York, 1983.
28. Wurtman, R.J.: Introduction. J. Psychiatr. Res. 17:103–105, 1982–83.
29. Seltzer, S., Stoch, R., Marcus, R., and Jackson, E.: Alteration of human pain thresholds by nutritional manipulation and L-tryptophan supplementation. Pain 13:385–393, 1982.
30. Seltzer, S., Dewart D., Pollack, R.L., and Jackson, E.: Effects of dietary tryptophan on chronic maxillofacial pain and experimental pain tolerance. J. Psychiatr. Res. 17:181–186, 1982–83.
31. Millinger, G.S.: Neutral amino acid therapy for the management of chronic pain. J. Craniomandib. Pract. 4:156–163, 1986.
32. Stockstill, J.W., McCall, W.D.J., Gross, A.J., and Piniewski, B.: The effect of L-tryptophan supplementation and dietary instruction on chronic myofascial pain. J. Am. Dent. Assoc. 118:457–460, 1989.
33. Gaupp, L.A., Flinn, D.E., and Weddige, R.: Adjunctive treatment techniques. In *Handbook of Chronic Pain Management.* C.D. Tollison (ed.). Williams & Wilkins, New York, 1989.
34. Levine, J.D., Gordon, N.C., and Fields, H.L.: The mechanism of placebo analgesia. Lancet 2:654–657, 1978.
35. Posner, J. and Burke, C.A.: The effects of naloxone on opiate and placebo analgesia in healthy volunteers. Psychopharmacology 87:468–472, 1985.
36. Greene, C.S.: Orthodontics and temporomandibular disorders. Dent. Clin. North Am. 32:529–538, 1988.
37. Shapiro, A.K.: A contribution to a history of the placebo effect. Behav. Sci. 5:109–135, 1960.

Steven A. King

CHAPTER 26

Psychologic Aspects

The lack of an identifiable organic etiology and the presence of psychiatric symptoms in many patients with temporomandibular disorders (TMDs) has focused attention on the role of psychologic factors. The relevance of these factors to understanding and treating patients with TMDs is now generally accepted. However, the exact nature of the relationship and the relative significance of these psychologic factors remain controversial. Although some have viewed these factors to be of primary importance, others believe that they have a much smaller role.[1,2] It is unclear which psychologic factors are the most relevant. The etiologic significance of patients' personality characteristics, the presence of associated mental disorders, and response to stress and anxiety have received extensive support and criticism.

Although it is beyond the scope of this chapter to settle these controversies, our goal is to assist readers in understanding the issues involved. To achieve this, the chapter is divided into three sections: (1) theories regarding the relationship between psychologic factors and TMDs; (2) treatment techniques; and (3) recommendations for the clinical evaluation and treatment of TMDs.

THE PROBLEM OF DIAGNOSTIC CLASSIFICATION

A review of the literature on TMDs is complicated by lack of uniform diagnostic criteria and classification.[3,4] Among the diagnoses encountered are TMD, temporomandibular pain disorder (TMPD), temporomandibular joint (TMJ) dysfunction, temporomandibular pain-dysfunction syndrome (TMPDS), myofascial pain dysfunction (MPD), and myofascial pain-

dysfunction syndrome (MPDS). Whether these diagnostic terms refer to the same group of patients, subgroups with essentially similar disorders, or different patient populations is a matter of debate.[5] The diagnostic criteria have also varied: clicking, tenderness of the joint or muscle, pain, and degree of mouth opening. Unfortunately, researchers using the same diagnostic terms have not always used equivalent clinical criteria.

With regard to the role that psychologic factors play in the development of TMDs, several investigators have shown that the differences in diagnostic criteria used play a significant role in the various results reported. Lundeen and colleagues[6] found that patients with masticatory muscle pain reported more stress, depression, and activity impairment than patients who had TMJ pain, leading them to conclude that these two groups of patients may have separate disorders with different etiologies and associated psychologic features. Bush and his colleagues[7] also observed that patients with MPD have more psychologic distress than patients with TMJ syndrome. Kleinkecht and colleagues[8] noted that patients who reported pain only during a TMJ examination were different from those who did not, with the former group demonstrating more interpersonal sensitivity, anxiety, and depression.

The confusion created by the variations in diagnostic terms and criteria is further confounded by the nature of the inquiries into the psychologic states and mental disorders associated with TMDs. With rare exceptions, researchers have failed to use standardized diagnostic criteria for these disorders. In a 1987 review, Dworkin and Burgess[9] were able to identify only one study that applied the diagnostic criteria of the *Diagnostic and Statistical Manual of Mental Disorders, Third Edition* (DSM-III),[10] the standard reference for the diagnosis of mental disorders in the United States. Studies using other standard criteria are also uncommon. Researchers have generally relied on terms such as "depression" and "anxiety," which can refer to either symptoms or mental disorders that vary greatly with regard to etiology, severity, treatment, and prognosis, or have created their own descriptive categories, making cross-study comparisons difficult.

For the sake of clarity, the diagnostic terms employed in the studies reviewed here are retained. When the generic term TMD is used in this chapter, it refers to both masticatory muscle and joint disorders.

THE MIND-BODY INTERACTION

Advances in pain research have blurred the dividing line between mind and body. From the ever growing body of knowledge about the function of the brain and the properties of neurotransmitters and endorphins, it is clear that the mind greatly influences the physiology of the body.

Unfortunately, many patients with pain and the clinicians who treat them still view pain as being "real" (i.e., the result of organic pathology) or "imaginary."[11,12] Anyone who holds such a misconception should remember the following: "Pain occurring in unicorns, griffins and jabberwockies is always imaginary pain, since these are imaginary animals; patients, on the other hand are real, and so they always have real pain."[13]

Rather than placing chronic pain into physiologic and psychologic categories, it is preferable to view it as a separate entity, the chronic pain syndrome (CPS), involving both elements. Black[12] described patients with CPS as suffering from "intractable, often multiple pain complaints, which are usually inappropriate to existing somatogenic problems; multiple physician contacts and many nonproductive diagnostic procedures; excessive preoccupation with the pain problem; an altered behavior pattern with some of the features of depression, anxiety, and neuroticism."

Futhermore, it is important to be aware that patients with similar health problems may adjust to them differently. This has resulted in the concept of "illness behavior," which involves many factors including how a patient perceives pain; decisions regarding whether to seek treatment and, if so, from whom; the meaning of the pain to the patient; the manner in which a patient communicates about pain; and the effect the pain has on a patient's functioning.[14,15]

Among the factors that influence illness behavior are cultural background, socioeconomic status, psychologic functioning, experiences, memory, and learning.[16,17]

Thus it is evident that multiple factors need to be considered when evaluating and treating a patient with chronic pain. Failure to recognize and address these issues result in mismanagement and unsuccessful treatment outcomes.

THEORETIC APPROACHES

During the past 35 years, many theories have been proposed to explain the relationship between psychologic factors and the physical symptoms found in TMDs. These theories have generally fallen into one of three major categories: (1) personality characteristics; (2) psychiatric comorbidity (e.g., mental disorders associated with TMJ problems); and (3) responses to stress and anxiety. Obviously, these categories overlap to a great degree. Therefore, the first two will be discussed together, whereas the third, which has received much attention, will be dealt with separately.

Personality Characteristics and Psychiatric Comorbidity

All of us have basic personality characteristics that define who we are and are reflected in our behavior. Many researchers have sought to determine if there are characteristics that predispose patients to develop TMDs or if these patients are psychologically impaired.

Attempts have been made to explain the psychologic aspects of TMDs through the use of psychoanalytic theory. Lefer[18] believed that many of the symptoms of these disorders are a form of conversion reaction resulting from unconscious conflicts. He also found that many of the patients he studied suffered significant trauma during childhood in the form of the loss of a loved one. Studies on the childhood experience of patients with TMDs that would provide evidence for the psychoanalytic viewpoint are rare, and those that do exist offer contradictory results. Heloe and colleagues[19] discovered that 31% of patients with MPDS reported losing contact with one parent during childhood or early adolescence because of divorce, death, or illness, whereas only 17% of general dental patients described such an experience. However, Salter and associates[2] found different results when they compared 73 patients with TMPDS with a group of patients with facial pain of other identifiable organic origin. Using the Parental Bonding Index, a scale that inquires about childhood experiences and attitudes toward parents, they observed no difference between the two groups.

Lupton[20] was among the first to note that through the use of psychologic tests, certain personality characteristics could be identified among patients with TMDs. He described them as being "distinguished by an extreme emphasis on psychologic and emotional strength and hypernormality." Stenn and colleagues[21] similarly reported that patients with MPDS "appeared to be perfectionistic, organized, concerned about what others thought of them, tended to avoid taking risks, maximized personal safety, and disliked ambiguity in situations."

Other studies have reported the presence of this personality profile in subgroups of their patients rather than all. In a subsequent paper, Lupton[22] found that patients with TMD could be classified into three groups based on their pain tolerance: (1) a "low-tolerance" group, who were willing to "acknowledge the presence of emotional stress in their lives" and were more apprehensive; (2) a "middle-tolerance" group, which the author does not describe except to note that "fewer members [were] willing to accept the 'sick role'"; and (3) a "high-tolerance" or "stoic" group, whose members were "highly defensive."

Shipman and associates[23] observed that the 211 MPD patients they studied could be classified into three categories of psychologic functioning: (1) "hypernormals" who were "physically tense and psychologically rigid people who work to keep their emotional problems hidden and present a normal facade to others"; (2) "psychoneurotics," "emotionally troubled people who are handicapped in life by their personality defects"; and (3) "normals." Pomp[24] was able to classify the 23 MPDS patients he studied into the same categories. Unfortunately, although the authors of both of these studies list the psychologic tests used, it is unclear exactly how patients were categorized.

Using a semistructured psychiatric interview, Heloe and Heiberg[25] similarly categorized MPDS patients into three groups based on what the authors described as the "capacity for interpersonal contact" (CIC). Of the 113 patients studied, 44 were considered to have an "apparently good CIC," 42 a "mildly disturbed CIC," and 27 a "severely disturbed CIC." The three groups of patients differed in a number of areas including the importance of stress factors, their manner of describing their symptoms, the types of symptoms described, and receptivity to a psychiatric evaluation. Heloe and Heiberg believed that the patients who had "apparently good" and "mildly disturbed" CIC correlated with the "hypernormals" described by Shipman and his colleagues. Heloe and Heiberg also reported that when they compared patients with MPDS to other dental patients, the group with MPDS was more likely to demonstrate "restrained aggression" and "tense control of emotions."

Butterworth and Deardorff[26] also identified three subgroups of patients among the 81 patients with TMJ pain that they studied: (1) a "psychologically normal" group of 30% of the patients; (2) another with 44% of the patients with elevations on somatization, depression, and anxiety scales of the Symptom Checklist 90 Revised; and (3) a group of 26% of the patients who showed elevations on a number of the scales on the test, indicating more severe psychopathology. When severity of pain and levels of interference with daily functioning were rated, the first group had the lowest ratings, the second moderate, and the third severe. Other patients who had no pain were closest to the "psychologically normal" pain patients.

Employing a different scale, the West Haven–Yale Multidimensional Pain Inventory, Rudy and colleagues[27] were able to classify 150 patients with TMJ pain into three subgroups that were similar to those defined by Butterworth and Deardorff.[26] Forty-six percent of the patients were identified as being "dysfunctional." These patients had pain that was more severe and interfered with their lives to a greater degree, higher levels of psychologic distress, and decreased perception of their abilities to control their lives. A second group consisting of 22% of the patients deemed "interpersonally distressed" felt that significant people in their lives were nonsupportive. Finally, 32% of the patients were classified as being "adaptive copers." The authors confirmed the difference between the two groups with several other psychologic inventories.

These descriptions of patients with TMD as "hypernormal" or "perfectionistic" are especially interesting in light of work by Blumer and Heilbronn[28] on chronic pain. They believe that chronic pain may frequently be associated with a depression-related disorder that they initially called "pain-prone disorder" and have renamed "dysthymic pain disorder." Among the traits described by them as being present in these patients are denial of conflict and perception of self as highly independent—traits that are similar to those found in patients with TMD described as "hypernormal."

Further connections between the personality characteristics of patients with TMD and other patients with chronic pain have been suggested by other studies. Lupton[22] observed that his "high pain tolerance or stoic patient" group displayed what has been described as the "psychosomatic or conversion-V" or "neurotic triad" profile on the Minnesota Multiphasic Personality Inventory (MMPI),[29] a commonly used psychologic test, with higher scores on the hypochondriasis and hysteria scales and a smaller elevation on the depression scale of this test. Schumann and colleagues[30] found this profile in 61% of patients with TMJ syndrome but in only 26% of healthy controls. However, for most of these patients, the elevated scores were still within the range of normal. The "V" observed by these authors has been described as being a common MMPI configuration among patients with chronic pain, especially those with low-back pain, with the elevations on the hypochondriasis and hysteria scales reflecting the patient's somatic concerns while the lower depression score suggests patients' indifference to these concerns[31] (Fig. 26–1).

Schwartz and associates[32] also found that patients with MPDS scored highest on the hypochondriasis and hysteria scales of the MMPI, whereas Eversole and colleagues[33] noted elevated scores on these two scales and the depression scale. In contrast, when Solbert and coworkers[34] administered the MMPI to 29 patients with TMJ pain and dysfunction and an equal number of control subjects, they found that the TMJ group scored higher on one scale, psychasthenia, which the authors categorized as indicating anxiety. However, in most of the patients who had this elevation, the score was still within normal limits, and the rest of the MMPI score for the majority of patients in both groups also was normal.

Other researchers have focused on the prevalence of the comorbidity of psychiatric disorders in patients with TMJ problems. In one of the first studies to identify a relationship between TMDs and psychiatric disease, Moulton[1] found that only 4 of the 35 patients with TMD could be considered, from a psychiatric standpoint, to be "relatively healthy people." Although 20 of the remaining patients were anxious or tense, 11 others were identified as being "psychotic or prepsychotic," terms that indicate the presence of a severe psychologic impairment. Kydd[35] similarly found that 23 of the 30 patients with TMJ syndrome he studied were "significantly disturbed emotionally." Fine[36] studied the frequency of mental disorders in 50 patients with TMPDS and 50 subjects with facial pain associated with other dental pathology. The patients were assessed by a structured interview administered by a psychiatrist. Of the TMPDs patients, 76% were found to have a psychiatric diagnosis, compared with only 20% of the non-TMJ patients. Most of these TMJ patients were diagnosed as having a "depressive-anxiety reaction," which the author does not define, though he does list the symptoms of depression and anxiety that he found most frequently.

In contrast, when Salter and colleagues[2] compared 73 patients with TMPDS and a control group with facial pain of an identifiable organic etiology, they were unable to find any significant difference between the two groups of patients with regard to the presence of psychologic problems.

Kleinknecht and coworkers[8] observed that although patients with TMD symptoms had higher scores on a psychologic test for depression, the Center of Epidemiologic Studies' Depression Scale, than did people in the general community, their scores were lower than those of acutely depressed psychiatric patients.

In one of the few studies that has attempted to categorize the mental disorders of TMJ patients, Feinmann and Harris[37] used the Clinical Interview Schedule, a semistructured interview

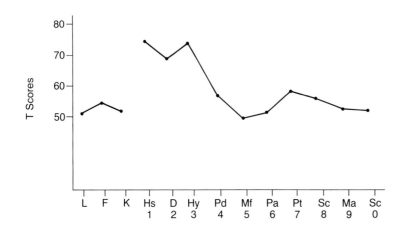

FIGURE 26–1. Minnesota Multiphasic Personality Inventory (MMPI) showing *Conversion V:* scales 1 (hypochondriasis); 2 (depression); and 3 (hysteria).

from which an International Classification of Disease (ICD)-9 diagnosis can be made. Fifty patients with "facial arthromyalgia," which included TMPDS and MPDS, and 43 patients with atypical facial pain were studied. Both groups were found to have relatively similar incidence rates of mental disorders, with 22% of the facial arthromyalgia group and 21% of the patients with atypical facial pain having nondepressive neurosis and 30% of the first group and 42% of the second having a depressive neurosis. Forty-eight percent of the patients with facial arthromyalgia and 37% of the patients with atypical facial pain had no psychiatric illness.

As noted previously, the most frequently used diagnostic classification in this country, DSM-III, has rarely been used in studies of psychologic aspects of dental disorders. Remick and colleagues[38] did apply DSM-III diagnostic criteria to 68 patients with atypical facial pain and found that 68% of the patients fit the diagnostic criteria for a DSM-III psychiatric disorder. Although they found a wide range of psychiatric diagnoses, the most common were the somatoform disorders (18% of the patients). The somatoform disorders are mental disorders such as psychogenic pain and somatization disorders in which there are physical symptoms in the absence of organic pathology.

Patients with these disorders seek frequent medical care for their pain and other symptoms. Because the basis of the symptoms is psychologic rather than physical, these patients are never "cured" by the physical treatments and travel from clinician to clinician seeking the "right" therapy. Unfortunately, in the absence of studies on the prevalence of these disorders in patients with TMDs, one can only speculate on their frequency in this group, but the nature of these disorders and the physical symptoms associated with them suggest their presence in at least some of the TMD patients who have psychologic problems.

Although there is some agreement between these studies, especially with regard to a subgroup of patients with TMDs who appear to be "hypernormal" or otherwise psychologically impaired, there is also a great deal of variability in the amount of psychiatric comorbidity identified. As noted earlier, this may at least partially reflect a nonhomogeneous patient population and the failure by most researchers to use standardized psychiatric diagnostic criteria in their description of mental disorders. Another problem is the questionable reliability

and validity of tests such as the MMPI when used among patients with chronic pain.[39,40] The scoring of many of these tests was developed from populations of physically healthy subjects. It is unclear whether results among patients who report physical suffering can be interpreted in a similar manner. For example, Nailiboff and associates[41] and Watson[42] have suggested that the MMPI conversion-V found by Schumann and coworkers[30] and other pain researchers may actually reflect adjustment to chronic illness and can be found among patients with chronic health problems with or without an identifiable organic etiology.

Stress and Anxiety

Of all the psychologically based theories of the etiology of TMDs, the one that has received the most attention is the relationship between these disorders and stress and anxiety. At the center of this approach is the view that stress can induce muscle hyperactivity or spasm, which in turn causes symptoms of TMD.[43–46]

This approach has raised a number of questions that researchers have sought to answer: Do patients with the TMDs have more environmental stressors? Do they have higher levels of anxiety? Are their responses to stress abnormal?

The first question has been the focus of a great deal of research. Through the use of standardized tests measuring stressful events in patients' lives, a number of researchers have explored this issue.

Several studies have employed the Social Readjustment Rating Scale (SRRS) developed by Holmes and Rahe,[47] a self-administered questionnaire that asks patients about life event changes that have occurred during the previous 1- to 2-year period. These are then weighted according to the relative degree of importance, ranging from loss of a spouse as the most serious to minor violations of the law being of the least importance.

Fearon and Serwatka[48] used this scale to compare 28 patients with temporomandibular symptoms without discernible organic etiology with 28 patients with similar symptoms based on identifiable organicity. They found that when stressful events were measured for the previous 2-year period, the patients whose symptoms lacked an organic cause had significantly higher scores on the SRRS.

When Stein and colleagues[49] employed the same scale to study 16 TMPDS patients and 8 normal controls, he also observed that the former group scored significantly higher. Furthermore, he found a positive correlation between the number of symptoms and their SRRS scores.

Using the Clinical Interview Schedule, a semistructured interview scale, Feinmann and Harris[37] found that 78% of patients with facial arthromyalgia (a category that included TMJDS and MPDS patients) had an adverse life event during the 6 months before the onset of their pain. However, there was no difference between this group and a comparison group of patients with atypical facial neuralgia or its variants.

Speculand and associates[50] measured stressful life events with an alternative questionnaire, the Life Events Assessment. In a study of 85 patients with TMJ dysfunction and an equal number of dental patients used as controls, they found that the patients with TMJ dysfunction reported twice as many stressful events occurring in the 6 months before the onset of their pain as did the controls. The two events that most differentiated the two groups were substantial changes in work conditions and moderate financial difficulties. They also noted that the patients with TMJ dysfunction had other health-related problems and were more likely to report multiple stressful life events.

Heloe and Heiberg[25] found that half of the patients with MPDS they studied reported stressful factors in their lives. They also found that the presence of these factors correlated with their measure of psychologic disturbance, the CIC. Although only one third of the patients with "good CIC" reported stress factors, half of those with a mildly disturbed CIC and three quarters of those with a severely disturbed CIC reported the presence of these factors. They also found that the stress factors reported by the subgroups differed, with the patients with good and mildly disturbed CIC describing stress factors related to their work situation and the severely disturbed reporting factors in several areas including economic and family life.

With the Psychiatric Epidemiology Research Interview Life Events Scale, Marbach and colleagues[51] found somewhat different results. When 151 patients with TMPDS were compared with 139 controls, the two groups showed no difference with regard to the total number of life events that had occurred during the previous year. However, like Speculand and associates,[50] they observed that the patients with TMPDS reported more events relating to physical illness and injury.

Other studies have employed a variety of measurements for stress. Moody and coworkers[52] administered a four-item Subjective Stress Scale to 52 patients with MPDS and an equal number of general dental patients and found that the patients with MPDS had greater levels of stress than the comparison group.

Of the 38 patients with TMJPDS identified by Fine[36] as having a psychiatric diagnosis, 26 reported that the onset of their psychologic symptoms was related to a stressful situation such as bereavement, marital disharmony, a chronically ill relative, a broken engagement, and financial problems. All these subjects reported that their facial problems began within 6 months of the onset of the psychologic symptoms. Of the other 12 patients with a psychiatric diagnosis, 9 believed that their depression and anxiety were related to facial discomfort. In the 12 patients who had no psychiatric diagnosis, 8 reported that their facial problems began shortly after extensive dental treatment.

Marbach and Lipton[53] observed similar results in a study of 170 patients referred to a TMJ clinic. Of the patients, 62% related the onset of their TMJ pain to a specific incident, with dental treatment and stressful life events such as death of a loved one being the most common, occurring in 24% and 23% of the patients, respectively. Furthermore, 31% of the patients reported having had therapy with a mental health professional at some time in their lives.

Although the results of these studies generally indicate that a significant number of patients with TMD are under increased environmental stress, the inferences that can be made from them are limited. Unfortunately, these studies do not delineate the nature of the relationship between the stressful life events and the TMJ symptoms. It is not possible to determine if the life events have what Speculand and colleagues[50] described as a "formative effect" (i.e., they cause the TMJ symptoms) or if the underlying TMD is already present and the stress of the life events causes its symptoms to become manifest. Additionally, the TMD itself may be causing at least some of the life problems reported by the patients. For example, the financial problems faced by these patients may reflect problems at work caused by a reaction to the disorder or even to the medical bills that patients may generate while searching for relief.

Another possible explanation for the increase in stressful events reported by these patients is suggested by results observed by Speculand and associates[54] who found that patients with TMD were less likely to deny the presence of problems in their lives than were other dental patients.

One must also realize that patients' memories for events that occurred 6 months previously or earlier may be faulty or selective. Without the perspective of a prospective study, it is impossible to determine just how accurate each patient's recall is.

However, even when objective measures of stress are sought, the results can be open to various interpretations. For example, Evaskus and Laskin[55] found that patients with MPDS had significantly higher mean urinary levels of 17-hydroxysteroids and catecholamines, suggesting to them that these patients were under greater emotional stress. However, others have noted that the elevation in catecholamines could be caused by increased muscle activity instead of stress.[3]

The increased frequency of health events in patients with TMD observed by Speculand and associates[50] and by Marbach and colleagues[51] has also been found by other researchers. As noted in these two studies, many of the physical disorders described by these researchers as coexisting with the facial problems in their patients are among those that are often considered to have "psychophysiologic" or "psychosomatic" aspects; that is, psychologic factors, especially those related to stress, appear to contribute to the etiology or symptoms of the disorders. Lupton[20] was among the first researchers to theorize that TMD might fit into the category of "psychosomatic illnesses," finding that 80% of the patients with TMD he studied reported a history of these health problems. Others who have noted an association between TMD and psychosomatic illnesses include Berry,[56] who found an increase in incidence of migraine headaches, pruritic skin diseases, hay fever and asthma, and neck, shoulder, and back pain in the more than 100 patients with mandibular dysfunction pain that he studied; Heloe and colleagues,[19] who reported that 68% of the 113 patients with MPDS that they studied complained of recurrent headaches as compared with only 26% of a control group consisting of general dental patients; Feinmann and Harris,[37] who similarly observed that 80% of the patients with facial arthromyalgia and 95% of those with atypical facial pain reported other physical symptoms including headaches, neck and back pain, dermatitis or pruritus, spastic colon, and dysfunctional uterine bleeding; and Gold and coworkers,[57] who noted that patients with MPD were more likely to have back or neck pain, a history of ulcers or colitis, nervous stomach, or asthma than a control group.

Although these studies indicate that TMDs and psychosomatic disorders are in some way associated, the exact nature of the relationship is unclear. It is possible that TMDs could be considered a subgroup of the psychosomatic disorders. However, even if this theory is accepted, it still does not clarify the role that stress has in the development of any of these disorders because their presence could reflect an actual increase in environmental stressors, the way patients with these disorders handle stress, or some other factor that may be unrelated to stress.

Several studies have focused on anxiety in patients with TMD. In the first of two studies, Marbach and colleagues[58] found that the patients with idiopathic facial pain they studied (a group that included patients with MPDS and TMJD) scored no higher on a standardized test to measure anxiety, the State-Trait Anxiety Inventory (STAI), than general hospital medical and surgical inpatients or patients at an outpatient emergency clinic, leading the authors to express doubt about the role of anxiety in the development of facial pain and the benefits of treating the patients with anxiety-reducing methods such as biofeedback or relaxation therapy. In the second study, Marbach and Lund[59] further questioned the role of psychologic factors in TMD, observing that scores of patients with MPDS on various psychologic measurements including the STAI were not significantly different from those of patients with arthritis of the TMJ or trigeminal neuralgia. In contrast, when Gale[60] used another measure for anxiety, the Taylor Manifest Anxiety Scale to study TMD and other facial pain, he found that both groups of patients had higher than normal scores. On followup, the scores of patients with TMD who had been successfully treated in the interim were normal. As a result, the author concluded that the anxiety demonstrated by the patients with TMD was a concomitant of the disorder rather than a cause.

In order to determine if patients with TMD handle stress in a manner different from other people, researchers have observed and measured the responses of patients to experimentally induced stress. Rugh and Montgomery[61] used electromyography (EMG) readings to study the masseter muscle activity at baseline and under stress in 23 patients with TMD and 23 controls. They found that although the patients had significantly higher baseline muscle activity than the controls, when the two groups were given a reaction time task there was no difference between them with regard to elevations in muscle activity or the ability to adapt to the task. They concluded that patients with TMD may have greater levels of stress as reflected by muscle activity but do not differ from others in the way they handle acutely stressful situations.

Although Moss and Adams[62] observed little difference between the masseter EMGs of patients with TMD and of those without this disorder when undergoing laboratory-induced stress, Mercuri and colleagues[63] reported that patients with MPD under similar circumstances had higher masseter and frontalis muscle activity before and after a card-sorting exercise but a control group had greater gastrocnemius activity. Mercuri and colleagues speculated that patients with MPD, unlike other people, have a very specific response to stress resulting in increased activity in the masticatory muscles and that this may be the underlying factor in development of the disorder.

Thomas and coworkers[64] studied the effects of experimentally produced anxiety and frustration. Ten patients with TMD and ten controls were given painful electric shocks that caused anxiety and were asked to complete a puzzle while being subjected to frequent interruptions and harassment to create frustration. Although there was an increase in masseter and temporal muscle tension among the patients with TMD under both conditions, the increase was greater for the frustration-producing task than for the anxiety-provoking one, leading the researchers to suggest that frustration rather than anxiety may play the more significant role in TMJ symptoms. However, Gale and Carlson,[65] using a similar experimental frustration condition, were unable to observe a relationship between frustration and TMJ symptoms.

Scott and Lundeen[66] studied the effects of creating hyperactivity in the lateral pterygoid muscles of healthy subjects by asking them to protrude their mandibles. These exercises created a pain similar to that reported by patients with MPDS, leading the investigators to suggest this as a possible cause of the disorder.

Thus, although patients with TMD appear to have more stress in their lives, the questions of whether they are more anxious or handle stress differently remain unanswered.

TREATMENT TECHNIQUES
Biofeedback and Relaxation Therapy

The importance of stress in the development and maintenance of the symptoms of TMDs has led researchers to focus on methods to alleviate the physical consequences of the stress, especially muscle hyperactivity. Studies in this area have centered on two major forms of treatment: relaxation techniques and biofeedback.

Relaxation techniques include a wide variety of methods used to help a patient relax. In one method using progressive muscle relaxation, subjects learn to relax different muscle groups.[67] For example, a subject is asked to contract and then relax the muscles starting at the feet and progressing to the neck and head.

In biofeedback, electronic equipment is used to measure physiologic functions that a subject is usually unaware of, such as muscle tension through the use of EMG or skin temperature, and to convey this information back to the subject, usually either visually by using a meter or through sound. Biofeedback can enhance the learning of relaxation techniques by offering patients a more concrete gauge for judging how they are proceeding. It can make them aware of an abnormal physiologic activity, such as muscle hyperactivity, and through this awareness allow change to take place. Patients may be given relaxation exercises to perform or may simply be told to try to achieve a certain goal— for example, lowering the pitch of a tone, thus indicating a change in physiologic functioning such as muscle activity.

A number of studies involving patients with TMD have focused on each of these techniques.

Gessel and Alderman[68] observed that 6 of 11 MPDS patients taught progressive relaxation reported benefits with this technique. The five patients who did not improve were found to be suffering from a mental disorder; four had depression, and one the investigators reported as having "the picture of an involutional paranoid reaction." In addition, these patients "demonstrated a submissive attitude toward the therapist" and related to him "as an omnipotent authority figure from whom they openly asked that a 'cure' be administered to them." The researchers concluded that relaxation training was of questionable benefit for patients with TMD with coexisting depression or in patients unwilling to assume an active role in the therapy, although of course this unwillingness could have been a manifestation of depression.

In a study of four patients with MPDS, Reading and Raw[69] observed that all reported a reduction in the frequency and duration of their pain after four weekly relaxation training sessions.

Budyznski and Stoyva[70] were among the first to provide evidence that EMG biofeedback could be used to lower masseter muscle activity and thus could have potential application to TMDs. Their work has led to other studies that have also found this treatment technique to be effective in TMDs. Gessel[71] observed satisfactory control of symptoms in 15 of 23 patients with MPDS treated with EMG biofeedback using the temporalis and masseter muscles. The number of sessions required to achieve this relief ranged from 4 to 14, with a median number of 5. Treatment was terminated after the sixth session unless patients reported improvement in their facial symptoms or exhibited other indicators that the investigator thought correlated with eventual success, including improved awareness of muscle tension, better sleep or mood, or improvement in what he described as "some other tension-related symptom such as dysmenorrhea or gastrointestinal complaints." Gessel also noted that a reduction in these latter complaints was an early indicator that biofeedback would be successful for the facial symptoms. Patients who did not respond to biofeedback were more likely to be depressed, and half of them benefited from subsequent treatment with an antidepressant medication.

Gale and Funch,[72] in a study of patients with chronic TMJ pain treated with biofeedback, relaxation therapy, or a combination of the two, similarly found that patients who benefited from their program were less depressed at the time of the pretreatment evaluation and were more likely to accept control over their own health. Schwartz and colleagues[32] also observed that patients who had MPDS and did not respond to treatment demonstrated a greater degree of emotional stress than those who did improve.

Dohrmann and Laskin[73] reported that masseter muscle EMG biofeedback resulted in pain reduction for all 13 of the patients with MPDS in their study who complained of this symptom and also decreased tenderness and limitations in mouth opening. Furthermore, the symptom reduction was maintained for most of the patients at 1-year follow-up, with only 25% reporting the need for additional treatment during that period after the conclusion of biofeedback.

Carlsson and Gale[74] used masseter muscle EMG biofeedback with relaxation training for 11 patients with TMJ pain of at least 3 years' duration who were refractory to physical treatment. The number of sessions ranged from 6 to 18, with termination after 6 sessions if there was no improvement in ability to relax or reduction in pain. Eight of the patients were observed to be either symptom free or significantly better after treatment and generally continued to maintain this improvement at 1-year follow-up. One patient reported slight improvement, and two denied any effect of the treatment. Curiously, of all the patients studied, these latter two proved to be the best at learning to relax, suggesting to the researchers that their pain may have had a different, nonmuscular etiology than in those who benefited from the treatment.

Clarke and Kardachi[75] researched the effects of temporalis and masseter muscle EMG biofeedback on seven patients during sleep when audio signal indicated bruxism activity and found this technique to be beneficial for the majority of patients studied.

In another two studies, Dahlstrom and colleagues[76,77] studied the effects of biofeedback in 20 patients with mandibular dysfunction; half of the patients had had symptoms for less than 6 months (acute), and the other half had had symptoms for more than this length of time (chronic). Patients were treated with either frontalis or masseter muscle EMG biofeedback for six weekly sessions. Although the patients with mandibular dysfunction were found to have significantly greater muscle activity than controls before treatment, no significant difference was found between the two groups after biofeedback. Patients with both the acute and chronic forms had similar rates of improvement, with six acute and five chronic sufferers reporting a significant reduction in their symptoms. With regard to the difference between the patients who responded to biofeedback and those who did not, the authors found that motivation for improvement was of significance. The patients who did not report improvement were judged to be less motivated, with motivation being based on the patients' attitudes during treatment. No difference was found between the use of masseter and frontalis muscle EMG. Gale and Funch[72] also found that the level of motivation was the most important predictor of treatment success of patients with chronic TMJ pain in their program, which consisted of biofeedback, relaxation therapy, or both.

Dalen and associates[78] also compared frontalis and masseter muscle EMG biofeedback. Patients who had MPDS and were given eight biofeedback sessions over a 4-week period were compared with patients who did not receive this treatment. Patients who demonstrated depression on a standardized test were excluded from the study. The patients using biofeedback were instructed to try to reduce the EMG level, but no specific relaxation techniques were provided. Although there were reductions for both frontalis and masseter EMG during treatment, the masseter levels returned to pretreatment levels after the end of treatment but the frontalis changes remained at 3- and 6-month follow-ups. Patients in both groups reported improvements in pain duration and intensity, although improvement was greater for the patients receiving biofeedback.

Hijzen and coworkers[79] compared the masseter muscle EMG biofeedback with a conservative physical approach (a nightly full-coverage splint) and no treatment. Sixteen patients who had MPD and were symptomatic for at least 1 year but had received no previous treatment for their complaints were assigned to each of these groups, with the biofeedback patients receiving 10 therapy sessions over a 5-week period. At the end of treatment, the biofeedback group reported significantly greater improvements than the other two groups, as reflected by less pain, fewer problems when opening the mouth, increased control of jaw muscles and jaw movements, and increased muscle relaxation. However, when objective measurements were applied, the biofeedback was found to have little lasting effect. The authors suggested that the symptomatic improvement found in these patients may be due more to an increased perception of control provided

by biofeedback rather than to actual physical changes. Splint therapy proved to be no better than no therapy, except for an improvement in joint sounds, which was also the only symptom for which splint therapy was more effective than biofeedback.

Although a number of these studies combined biofeedback and relaxation training without differentiating between their effects, several researchers have compared the efficacy of these two forms of treatment.

Moss and colleagues[80] studied the relative benefits of teaching progressive relaxation exercises by audiotape and masseter EMG biofeedback. Of the five patients with chronic TMJ pain who were studied, three reported better results with the relaxation training, one did best with a combination of the two therapies, and one did not respond to either. They also found that two of the three patients who responded to the relaxation training also reported improvement in physical ailments including back pain, insomnia, and gastrointestinal complaints.

Funch and Gale[81] similarly compared relaxation techniques and biofeedback for a larger number of patients (n = 57) with TMJ pain of at least 2 years' duration. Thirty of the patients received biofeedback of the masseteric area, and 27 received relaxation therapy through the use of an audiotape. Both groups had reductions in their pain following treatment and at 2-year follow-up. The relaxation group tended to have greater pain reduction, although the difference was not statistically significant. Although relaxation techniques and biofeedback have often been considered to be similar approaches to the treatment of pain, Funch and Gale found that there were differences between the patients who maintained improvement due to each of these modes of therapy at 2-year follow-up. The patients in the relaxation group most likely to report continued benefits were those who, at the time of the initial evaluation, reported a history of psychiatric disorders or other physical disorders such as allergies, gastrointestinal complaints, and skin problems, disorders the researchers described as "psychosomatic." Funch and Gale theorized that in patients in whom the TMD is only one of several problems, the generalized benefits of relaxation therapy may be more useful than biofeedback focusing on one part of the body. Among the biofeedback group, the patients who had received treatment with equilibration in the past reported less success at both short- and long-term follow-ups. The authors suggested that equilibration may be associated with bruxism behavior, which does not respond well to biofeedback.

Brooke and Stenn compared the efficacy of biofeedback and relaxation therapy in two separate studies.[21,82] In the first, 11 patients who had MPDS and were symptomatic for more than 1 year and who had not responded to conservative physical treatments were treated with masseter muscle EMG biofeedback, relaxation training, and cognitive behavioral modification focusing on helping the patient deal with specific stressful situations or with just the latter two therapies and no biofeedback. Although both groups reported improvement following treatment, the patients using biofeedback had fewer signs of MPDS than the patients who did not receive this therapy. Although the focus of the biofeedback was on masseter muscle activity, there was no difference between the two groups when this was measured by post-treatment EMG. Like Hijzen and colleagues,[79] these investigators theorized that the greater improvement in the biofeedback group was not due to the direct effect of the biofeedback but rather to a possible expectation by these patients that they had a greater degree of control over muscle tension than did the nonbiofeedback patients.

In the second study, Brooke and Stenn assigned 190 patients with MPDS to one of four treatment modalities: (1) ultrasound, (2) occlusal splint, (3) relaxation training and masseter muscle biofeedback, and (4) relaxation training alone. Groups three and four were treated in seven weekly sessions. At the conclusion of treatment, the biofeedback group and the group receiving only relaxation training had the most patients reporting successful outcomes, with no significant difference between these groups. Each group continued to have approximately the same levels of success at 6-month follow-up. The ultrasound and occlusal splint groups showed additional improvement after this period of time, but the percentage of success was still less than for the two groups receiving relaxation training.

Hypnosis

Another form of treatment frequently used for patients with pain is hypnosis.[83] Although there has been much debate about the exact na-ture of hypnosis and the associated trance state, the following British Medical Association Report[84] definition aptly described it as follows:

"A temporary condition of altered attention in the subject which may be induced by another person and in which a variety of phenomena may appear spontaneously or in response to verbal or other stimuli. These phenomena include alterations in consciousness and memory, increased susceptibility to suggestion, and the production in the subject of responses and ideas unfamiliar to him in his usual state of mind. Further, phenomena such as anaesthesia, paralysis and rigidity of muscles, and vasomotor changes can be produced and removed in the hypnotic state."

Although hypnosis involves a heightened state of relaxation, its usefulness in pain relief goes far beyond this. Patients can be taught various techniques to actually reduce the level of pain. Among the most commonly used hypnotic suggestions for pain relief are anesthetizing the painful area; drawing a visual image of the cause of the pain, for example, a knife sticking in an area of sharp pain, and reversing its effect (e.g., seeing the knife being withdrawn); dissociation of the painful part from the rest of the body; and time distortion.

Unfortunately, despite the widespread use of hypnosis, few controlled studies have investigated its efficacy for pain relief in general or for TMDs. Most reports are anecdotal in nature, such as that by Cohen and Hillis,[85] who examined two cases of TMPDS treated with hypnosis. Although only one patient reported an improvement in symptoms, the authors found that hypnosis was useful in identifying the underlying psychologic factors involved in the second patient's pain, and thus it also benefited the patient. Gerschman and colleages[86] noted the benefits of hypnosis for their clinic patients with orofacial pain, including those with TMPDS.

In one of the few attempts at a controlled study of hypnosis, Stam and associates[87] compared the relative benefits of hypnosis and relaxation therapy. Sixty-one patients with TMPDS were assigned to one of three groups: (1) treatment with hypnosis and cognitive coping skills; (2) treatment with relaxation training and cognitive coping skills; or (3) no treatment. Each of the treatment groups received four weekly sessions. The cognitive coping skills involved ways for the patients to deal with painful episodes. Both treatment groups reported similar levels of improvement in pain and limitations in mouth opening at the conclusion of the treatments. They also observed that patients who responded the most favorably to the therapies were those who were found to be most susceptible to hypnosis before treatment.

Studies on other forms of psychotherapy for the treatment of patients with TMD are also limited. Marbach and Dworkin[89] noted group therapy to be useful both as a treatment modality and as an evaluation method that allowed patients to discuss psychologic issues they may have found difficult to express in the usual clinical setting. Pomp[24] found individual psychotherapy to be of considerable efficacy for patients who had MPD that had failed to respond to other conservative treatments, with complete symptom remission in 15 of 23 patients who completed a 12-session program. Not surprisingly, the patients who responded most favorably to this form of treatment were those who admitted a need for psychotherapy.

Outcome Indicators

In addition to the studies already mentioned, a number of others have sought to identify patients who do benefit from certain forms of therapy.

Speculand and colleagues[54] found that half of the 13% of patients with TMD whom they studied and who did not respond to conservative physical treatments had abnormal illness behavior reflected in their scores on the Illness Behavior Questionnaire.

Lipton and coworkers[90] also searched for indicators of a positive response to nonsurgical treatments among patients with MPDS. They found that the unsuccessfully treated patients were more likely to have experienced their pain for longer than 6 months, had previously consulted three or more clinicians, denied having ever had any relief from their pain, and described "emotional or expressive responses to pain." However, the successfully and unsuccessfully treated patients did not appear to differ with regard to the level of psychologic distress they reported.

In contrast to the results of this study, which suggested that chronicity of pain is a negative outcome factor, Salter and associates[91] were unable to find any relationship between the duration of symptoms and benefits from their program of conservative physical therapy. The authors did observe that the level of psychologic distress as measured by standardized psychologic scales was correlated with outcome in

patients with mild psychologic distress doing best, followed by those who admitted a minimal degree of distress and the patients with severe psychologic distress. These results corresponded to those found earlier by Heloe and Heilberg,[92] who observed that patients with severely disturbed capacities for interpersonal contact and patients who denied any problem in this area were least likely to respond to treatment. Thus, it is not only those patients whose psychologic impairment is obvious who are difficult to treat, but also those who seem to be well adjusted but whose apparent psychologic health reflects an unwillingness or inability to admit to problems. Again, this finding fits with the previously discussed concept of "hypernormality."

Funch and Gale[93] studied the differences between the 54% of patients with chronic TMJ pain who completed their treatment program consisting of biofeedback, relaxation therapy, or a combination of the two, and those who failed to complete it. The only factor that they were able to find that predicted successful outcome was the attitude of family members toward the patient's pain. Patients who viewed family members as being upset with them were more likely to complete therapy than those whose family members were more supportive. The authors observed that these results fit with the important concept of secondary gain, which suggests that certain behavior patterns may be unconsciously maintained if a person receives some benefit from them, even if the behavior itself has an ostensibly negative effect. Thus patients with chronic pain may be less desirous of reducing their level of discomfort if their pain is gaining them sympathy and support from family members. However, if family members are antagonistic, there is less incentive for the patient to continue to have pain. Chronic pain sufferers are often placed in conflict by secondary gain: On one hand, they wish to improve physically; on the other, they desire to maintain the secondary gain. Patients are frequently unaware of the presence of the secondary gain, and it is the task of the treating clinician to bring it to their attention.

CLINICAL EVALUATION AND TREATMENT

As demonstrated by the research discussed in this chapter, the exact nature and importance of psychologic factors in the etiology of TMDs remain the subject of controversy that is unlikely to be resolved in the near future. However, the weight of evidence indicates that these factors play a significant role in TMJ problems presented by many patients. Whether psychologic factors are the cause or result of the TMJ symptoms, especially pain, is open to question; however, there is no question that attention should be paid to these factors for patients to be successfully treated.

Although the dynamic relationship between the TMJ symptoms and psychologic factors is of pre-eminent significance to researchers, it is less relevant to the task of clinicians treating patients with TMDs. What is important to the clinician is detecting the presence of psychologic factors that may be contributing to the TMJ symptoms and determining the most appropriate treatment.

The literature indicates that certain information that can be obtained in the clinical interview should heighten the practitioner's level of awareness regarding the possible influence of these factors. Inquiries should be made about any identifiable stressful events in the recent past that are temporally related to the development of the TMD symptoms. The presence of any psychosomatic disorder such as gastrointestinal disorders, dermatologic conditions, and asthma should be noted. Any patient who presents with a history of unsuccessful treatment with "physical" therapies should be carefully re-evaluated, with special attention focused on the psychologic features. This approach is especially relevant if any irreversible treatment methods are being considered (Table 26–1).

It is essential that clinicians be able to screen for concomitant mental disorders. Studies have shown that a frequent reason for nonresponsiveness to the standard therapies for TMDs is the presence of an underlying psychiatric problem.[68,69] In a study of patients with chronic pain of 25 years or longer duration, Swanson and colleagues[94] found that these patients were more likely to have face and head pain, a diagnosis of depression, and greater elevations on

TABLE 26–1. Clinical Factors Indicating the Presence of Psychologic Elements in Patients with TMDs

1. Stressful life events during the previous year
2. Other "psychosomatic" health problems
3. Coexisting mental disorders
4. A history of multiple unsuccessful therapies for TMJ problems

the MMPI clinical scales than patients who had chronic pain for a shorter period.

Of all the mental disorders, the one most frequently associated with chronic pain is depression. Thus it is important that a clinician who evaluates and treats chronic pain sufferers including those with TMDs, should be able to determine whether the patient is depressed and if the level of depression is sufficient to warrant evaluation of the patient by a mental health professional.

A clinician should observe or inquire about signs and symptoms of depression during the initial examination of the patient. The general appearance of the patient should be noted. Does the patient appear depressed or sad? Does the patient's affect change during the interview—for example, does the patient smile appropriately or does he or she continuously appear sad? Does the patient appear to have lost interest in appearance, as manifested by disheveled dress or lack of care in personal hygiene such as failure to comb the hair or bathe? Are there signs of psychomotor retardation such as slowed speech, decreased amount of speech, and diminished body movements or of psychomotor agitation including inability to sit still and rubbing or pulling at the clothes or other objects.

It is vital to inquire about several areas. A patient's sleep pattern should be determined, because insomnia and hypersomnia are common symptoms of depression. A patient's appetite may also be increased or decreased, with resultant weight loss or gain. Libido is also often reduced in depression. A patient's view of himself or herself is significant. Does the patient feel worthless? Is there a reduction in interest or pleasure in activities?

Because suicide is associated with depression, it is vital to determine the presence of suicidal thoughts in a depressed patient. Unfortunately, many people still cling to the myth that inquiring about suicidal thoughts should be avoided because such questioning might bring to mind the idea of suicide in a person who has not previously considered it. There is no evidence to support this view that may reflect the discomfort that others, including many health-care professionals, have about discussing the topic because of an uncertainty about how to deal with suicidal thoughts. Unless a patient volunteers information about suicidal ideation, a clinician will only learn about it by directly asking.

Although it is impossible to make absolute

predictions about suicide, several factors appear to increase the level of risk: A history of previous suicide attempts, the absence of future-oriented thoughts, and drug or alcohol abuse are three of these factors. Patients who abuse drugs tend to be impulsive, and the chemicals themselves interfere with rational thought. Patients who have actually thought about a way to commit suicide rather than just having vague thoughts about not wanting to live anymore or wishing to be dead are certainly at risk. The method of suicide should be evaluated with regard to lethality and practicality. For example, a patient who has thought of shooting himself or herself and has access to a gun is of more concern than someone who has a similar thought but has never fired a gun and has no idea of how to obtain one. Both would probably be considered to be at more risk than a person who is thinking of a passive method of suicide, such as walking into the street and hoping to be struck by a car.

However, it should be remembered that suicide prediction is not an exact science, and any suicidal thoughts should be taken seriously. A dentist or nonpsychiatric physician who believes that a patient is suicidal should consider the situation a medical emergency that needs to be dealt with immediately by having the patient evaluated by a psychiatrist. If a psychiatrist is not available, arrangements should be made to transfer the patient to a hospital emergency room until a consultation can be performed. As with any potentially lethal medical condition, a clinician should be conservative and err on the side of caution.

It should be remembered that although patients with pain may present with depression, those with depression and other psychiatric disorders may have a chief complaint of pain. For example, Pilling and colleagues[95] found pain to be the most frequent presenting symptom among medical/surgical outpatients referred for a psychiatric consultation. In addition to observing patients for depression and anxiety, clinicians need to be especially attuned to the possible presence of the somatoform disorders, especially somatization disorder and somatoform or psychogenic pain disorder. As noted earlier in this chapter, patients with these disorders present with physical complaints and an unremitting belief that there is something physically wrong with them. These patients do not appear "mentally ill," nor, in most cases, are their symptoms especially bizarre. In fact, the problem a clinician faces is that the symptoms—pain, gastrointestinal or female reproductive problems, shortness of breath, and palpitations—are often those of very common physical disorders. Thus an underlying mental disorder is often considered only after these patients have undergone many workups without an organic cause being identified and after they have had multiple physical treatments without success.

Although the physical complaints may yield secondary gain, these patients are not consciously attempting to mislead the clinician for this purpose, as in malingering. Patients with somatoform disorder are also different from those with factitious disorder with physical symptoms (which has often been called Munchausen's syndrome). These patients intentionally produce or feign physical disorders without the presence of any apparent secondary gain.

Hypochondriasis and conversion disorder are also classified as somatoform disorders and may be associated with pain complaints. In contrast to somatization disorder, patients with hypochondriasis are preoccupied with the fear of having a specific disease or diseases rather than focusing on symptoms. Although there is a great deal of overlap between conversion disorder and somatization and somatoform pain disorders, in conversion disorder the underlying psychologic factors are often more readily apparent. Conversion disorder is rarely encountered in clinical practice today. When a dentist or nonpsychiatric physician suspects that TMD symptoms reflect the presence of any of the somatoform disorders or factitious disorder, referral for a psychiatric evaluation is warranted.

Convincing a patient with TMD or other chronic pain to undergo psychiatric evaluation is often arduous. As Blumer and Heilbronn[28] have noted, "The chronic pain sufferer argues that he or she has no mental problem and needs no psychiatric intervention, that the only real problem is the pain and that the doctors better find out what is wrong where it hurts." Heloe and Heiberg[25] found that patients with MPDS who had the greatest degree of psychologic impairment were also the ones more likely to have a negative reaction to a psychiatric examination. Again, it is vital for clinicians to understand and to convey to their patients that the presence of psychologic factors does not mean that the pain is imaginary.

Determining whether a complaint is due to pain or to depression or some other psychiatric problem is difficult, and, unfortunately, the pain literature provides little assistance. When Blumer and Heilbronn[28] compared patients with major depression with those they diagnosed as having a "dysthymic pain disorder," they observed that those in the pain group had greater impairments in social life, sexual relations, and ability to work and fewer problems with diminished appetite.

Davidson and colleagues[96] found that chronic pain sufferers with major depression were more likely to report early morning awakening, decreased appetite, and reduced libido than those with minor or intermittent depression or no depression. Patients with minor or intermittent depression reported increased appetite more often than those with major depression or no depression.

Studies have noted that patients with chronic pain and depression are more likely to have abnormal results of a dexamethasone suppression test, a neuroendocrine marker for depression, than those with chronic pain alone.[97,98] However, a wide variety of physical conditions and medications can interfere with the results of this test, limiting its clinical usefulness, especially among the medically ill.

Psychologic testing can provide additional information that might be difficult to obtain from a clinical interview or can offer support for a clinician's evaluation of the patient. A multitude of tests are available to assess patients' psychologic status. Among the more commonly used self-administered tests are the MMPI, the Beck Depression Inventory, the STAI, the Symptom Checklist 90 Revised, and the Profile of Mood States. All of these tests have both benefits that make them useful and drawbacks. For example, the MMPI provides a great deal of information but is fairly lengthy, and the results need to be read by a skilled interpreter. In contrast, the Beck Depression Inventory is short (21 questions) and easy to score but provides less information on a patient's psychologic status. There is no one best test that can be recommended above the others, and the decision regarding which one or ones to use depends on the amount and type of information the practitioner wishes to obtain.

Dentists and nonpsychiatric physicians may find the currently available psychologic tests unwieldy because they are long and difficult to interpret. A test that is easy to administer and score and that would provide the clinicians with information on the psychologic status of patients with TMD would be helpful. Gale and Dixon[99] reported the existence of such a test. In a study of 132 patients with TMJD, they found that two questions provided information on anxiety and depression that correlated with the results of seven standard self-administered tests for depression and four such tests for anxiety. The tests—the Single Question Depression Assessment (SQDA) and the Single Question Anxiety Assessment (SQAA)—ask the patients "How depressed are you?" with responses ranging from "never" (0) to "often" (4) and "Do you consider yourself more tense than calm or more 'calm' (0) to 'tense' (4)?" Further studies need to be done to confirm these researchers' findings, but inclusion of these two questions in the interview of patients may be helpful in deciding on treatment. Millstein-Prentky and Olson[100] attempted to develop a 29-item scale on the MMPI to predict treatment outcome for patients with MPDS but were unsuccessful in their efforts. Similar efforts to find measures that predict treatment outcome for chronic pain sufferers in general have also met with mixed results.[101]

A wide range of psychologic tests has also been employed in an attempt to develop an objective method for providing information on the etiology of TMJ and other chronic pain disorders and the relative significance of psychologic factors in the maintenance of symptoms. The variability of results obtained from psychologic testing led the 1982 President's Commission on Temporomandibular Disorders to recommend against the routine use of testing in the clinical evaluation of patients with TMDs.[102,103]

However, several factors suggest that this negative view of psychologic testing should be modified. As noted, testing is quite useful for assessing the psychologic status of patients. Furthermore, though the results appear to be variable, there is a certain degree of consistency in the TMJ literature. For example, several studies using psychologic tests have described a significant number of patients with TMD as being "hypernormal" or "perfectionistic."

At least part of the reason for the wide range of psychologic test results may be variability in the patient populations studied. Furthermore, test scores for chronic pain sufferers have often been interpreted in a simplistic manner. In many studies using these tests, a limited number of scales are isolated and used to make judgments when more complete readings of all results are indicated. It should also be remembered that test results cannot be used to replace a clinical evaluation. Psychologic tests are used as an adjunct to, not in place of, clinical evaluations of patients. Clinicians who rely solely on tests for their information about the psychologic status of patients with TMDs are employing them inappropriately.

Additionally, as with any test used in the medical setting, the information obtained depends to a great degree on the skill of the interpreter. This is especially important when psychologic tests are used among a population different from that for which they were originally developed. As mentioned previously, results of a test such as the MMPI may be a function not only of the psychologic but also the physical status of a patient. Failure to take this into account can cause misinterpretation of the results, generating misunderstandings about the patient.

Studies of TMDs have shown various treatments, both physical and psychologic, to be effective. Again, this may be because of a failure to discriminate between the subgroups of patients who actually have different disorders. However, another explanation is especially relevant to understanding the importance of the psychologic factors involved in these disorders and other chronic pain problems.

Although the treatments in these studies appear to be disparate, there is a common feature to virtually all: the nature of the interaction between the patient and the researchers. By necessity, any attempt to study these patients requires researchers to spend a significant amount of time with them and to offer a nonjudgmental approach while obtaining information. Several authors have noted that, at least with regard to treatments such as biofeedback and relaxation therapies, it is not possible to determine if the benefits found are due to the treatments themselves or to interactions with the researchers.[69,75] It may be that for many patients with TMD, the specific therapy offered is less important than the nature of the interaction between the treating clinician and the patient. In fact, although the 1982 President's Conference on TMDs[102] was unable to determine which form of treatment was most efficacious, it did emphasize "that a warm, positive, and reassuring attitude on the part of the dentist is crucial in the treatment of these disorders." It is also important to keep in mind the experiences that these patients may have had with other practitioners. Moulton[104] noted:

"The most recalcitrant cases were the patients who had found doctors who promised them complete cures, practitioners who seemed to be sure masters of the situation and who assured them that there was a mechanical way to lift the burden of pain. When such a treatment did not give prolonged relief, these patients merely sought another doctor who would hold out hope with a different mechanical method; but as they became increasingly disillusioned and resentful toward dentists, they became less responsive to any treatment."

The importance of the interaction between patient and clinician may also be the reason for the success of placebo treatments reported in a number of studies. Greene and Laskin[105] and Salter and colleagues[91] found placebo treatments to be as effective as the standard physical and psychologic therapies for patients with TMD and MPDS. Goodman and associates[106] observed that 64% of the patients with MPDS whom they studied improved with mock equilibration, and Feinmann and Harris[107] reported that 44% of their patients improved with placebo medication. Laskin and Greene[108] further underscored the significance of the interaction between clinician and patient when they found that 52% of their patients reported improvement with placebo medication that was enthusiastically endorsed by the clinician as compared with the improvement rate of 30% they observed in an earlier study in which the placebo medication was dispensed without such endorsement.[109] They also reported that the symptoms that responded best to placebo therapy were the subjective ones such as pain and tenderness rather than the objective signs of clicking and limitations in mouth opening. Others have demonstrated the importance of the patient's level of motivation in successful treatment.[72,76]

Von Korff and colleagues[110] provided additional evidence that the clinician's belief in the efficacy of a chosen therapy may be more important for a successful outcome than the therapy itself. When they compared two clinics that received TMD patients from a common referral source, they found that although the clinics differed with regard to diagnoses applied to these patients and the forms of treatment they received, each had similar success rates at 1-year follow-up.

Alleviation of pain by a placebo in no way suggests that the pain is more psychologic than organic.[111,112] In fact, in chronic pain in which there is no readily identifiable organic pathology, the placebo treatment may not really be a placebo in the traditional sense of the word. In providing an understanding, compassionate, nonjudgmental approach to the complaints of patients with TMDs, the researchers studying placebo effects may actually be supplying the appropriate and necessary form of treatment for many of these patients.

With regard to psychologically oriented treatment approaches, there is an obvious dearth of information on therapies other than biofeedback and relaxation training. Thus it is difficult to comment on the benefits of the other forms of psychotherapy. Although biofeedback and relaxation training are beneficial for many patients with TMDs, there appears to be a subgroup of patients who do not respond to these or the conventional physical therapies. For some of these patients, this unresponsiveness may be due to the presence of an unrecognized psychiatric problem; therapies such as biofeedback and relaxation training are quite useful for the treatment of TMD symptoms that are stress related but are of much less benefit in the treatment of severe mental disorders such as major depression, which require more intensive psychotherapy and psychotropic medications.

The studies that have attempted to determine whether biofeedback or relaxation training is the better form of treatment have generally found them to be of equal efficacy. Several studies have identified subgroups of TMD patients who are more likely to respond to one form than the other,[81,82] but applicability of these findings to the general population remains unclear.

The lack of clear-cut superiority of either of these two forms of treatment for TMDs is not surprising, considering that their relative benefits for the treatment of chronic pain conditions in general also remain the subject of controversy. Although some experts believe that biofeedback offers benefits beyond those of relaxation training, others believe that biofeedback can actually be detrimental to some patients with chronic pain by focusing on somatic complaints.[113,114] One factor that practitioners must take into account is the cost of biofeedback instrumentation, which can range from a hundred to several thousand dollars depending on the degreee of sophistication. In contrast, relaxation training requires no special equipment.

Each practitioner who treats patients with TMDs must determine how he or she wishes to approach the psychologic aspects. Dentists and nonpsychiatric physicians vary with regard to how comfortable they are in evaluating and treating psychologic problems. It is vital that any clinician who cares for these patients be knowledgeable about these issues or be able to refer patients to a mental health professional who is familiar with TMDs and the psychologic factors associated with them.

CONCLUSION

The literature on TMDs is consistent with other research that has observed an association between chronic pain and the psychologic status of the patient. However, it remains unclear whether personality characteristics, psychiatric comorbidity, and stress and anxiety identified in various studies on TMDs are of etiologic significance, are the result of the facial problems, or are coincidental findings.

It is doubtful that any single psychologic factor can explain all or even most cases of TMDs. The patient population appears to be quite heterogeneous, but future research using stricter diagnostic criteria for both physical and psychologic factors may rectify the current confusion and provide new levels of understanding about this baffling problem.

REFERENCES

1. Moulton, R.E.: Psychiatric considerations in maxillofacial pain. J. Am. Dent. Assoc. 51:408–414, 1955.
2. Salter, M., Brooke, R.I., Merskey, H., et al: Is the temporo-mandibular pain and dysfunction syndrome a disorder of the mind? Pain 17:151–166, 1983.
3. Rugh, J.D. and Solberg, W.K.: Psychological implications in TM pain and dysfunction. In *Temporomandibular Joint Function and Dysfunction.* G.A. Zarb and G.E. Carlsson (eds.). C.V. Mosby, St. Louis, 1979.
4. Moss, R.A. and Garrett, J.C.: Temporomandibular joint dysfunction syndrome and myofascial pain dysfunction syndrome: A critical review. J. Oral Rehabil. 11:3–28, 1984.
5. Greene, C.S., Lerman, M.D., Sutcher, H.D., and Laskin, D.M.: The TMJ pain-dysfunction syndrome: Heterogeneity of the patient population. J. Am. Dent. Assoc. 79:1169–1172, 1969.
6. Lundeen, T.F., Sturdevant, J.R., and George, J.M.: Stress as a factor in muscle and temporomandibular joint pain. J. Oral Rehabil. 14:447–456, 1987.
7. Bush, F.M., Whitehill, J.M., and Butler, J.H.: Temporandibular joint syndrome vs myofascial pain dysfunction: One and the same? (Abstract 1445). J. Dent. Res. (Special Issue) 67:293, 1988.
8. Kleinknecht, R.A., Mahoney, E.R., Alexander, L.D., and Dworkin, S.F.: Correspondence between subject report of temporomandibular disorder symptoms and clinical findings. J. Am. Dent. Assoc. 113:257–261, 1986.
9. Dworkin, S.F. and Burgess, J.A.: Orofacial pain of psychogenic origin: Current concepts and classification. J. Am. Dent. Assoc., 115:565–571, 1987.

10. American Psychiatric Association: *Diagnostic and Statistical Manual of Mental Disorders, Third Edition, Revised.* American Psychiatric Association, Washington, D.C., 1987.

11. Olson, R.E.: Myofascial pain-dysfunction syndrome: Psychological aspects. In *The Temporomandibular Joint.* In B.G. Sarnet and D.M. Laskin (eds.). Charles C Thomas, Springfield, IL, 1979.

12. Black, R.G.: The chronic pain syndrome. Surg. Clin. North Am. 55:999–1011, 1975.

13. Sapira, J.D.: Real pain. In *Hunan Hand and Other Ailments.* S.B. Moskow (ed.). Little, Brown & Co., Boston, 1987.

14. Mechanic, D.: The concept of illness behavior. J. Chronic Dis. 15:189–194, 1962.

15. Pilowsky, I.: Abnormal illness behavior. Br. J. Med. Psychol. 42:347–351, 1968.

16. Marbach, J.J., and Lipton, J.A.: Biopsychosocial factors of the temporomandibular pain dysfunction syndrome. Dent. Clin. North Am. 31:473–486, 1987.

17. Burdette, B.H., and Gale, E.N.: Pain as a learned response: A review of behavioral factors in chronic pain. J. Am. Dent. Assoc. 116:881–885, 1988.

18. Lefer, L.: A psychoanalytic view of a dental phenomenon. Contemp. Psychoanal. 2:135–150, 1966.

19. Heloe, B., Heiberg, A.N., and Krogstad, B.S.: A multiprofessional study of patients with myofascial pain-dysfunction syndrome. I. Acta Odontol. Scand. 38:109–117, 1980.

20. Lupton, D.E.: A preliminary investigation of the personality of female temporomandibular joint dysfunction patients. Psychother. Psychosom. 14:199–216, 1966.

21. Stenn, P.G., Mothersill, K.J., and Brooke, R.I.: Biofeedback and a cognitive behavioral approach to treatment of myofascial pain dysfunction syndrome. Behav. Ther. 10:29–36, 1979.

22. Lupton, D.E.: Psychologic aspects of temporomandibular joint dysfunction. J. Am. Dent. Assoc. 79:131–136, 1969.

23. Shipman, W.G., Greene, C.S., and Laskin, D.M.: Correlation of placebo responses and personality characteristics on myofascial pain-dysfunction (MPD) patients. J. Psychosom. Res. 18:475–483, 1974.

24. Pomp, A.M.: Psychotherapy for the myofascial pain-dysfunction syndrome: A study of factors coinciding with symptom remission. J. Am. Dent. Assoc. 89:629–632, 1974.

25. Heloe, B. and Heiberg, A.N.: A multiprofessional study of patients with myofascial pain-dysfunction syndrome. II. Acta Odontol. Scand. 38:119–128, 1980.

26. Butterworth, J.C. and Deardorff, W.W.: Psychometric profiles of craniomandibular pain patients: Identifying specific subgroups. J. Craniomand. Pract. 5:225–232, 1987.

27. Rudy, T.E., Turk, D.C., Zaki, H.S., and Curtin, H.D.: An empirical taxometric alternative to traditional classification of temporomandibular disorders. Pain 36:311–320, 1989.

28. Blumer, D. and Heilbronn, M.: Depression and chronic pain. In *Presentations of Depression.* O.G. Cameron (ed.). John Wiley & Sons, New York, 1987.

29. Dahlstrom, W.G. and Welsh, G.S.: *An MMPI Handbook,* University of Minnesota Press, Minneapolis, 1960.

30. Schumann, N.P., Zwiener, U., and Nebrich, A.: Personality and quantified neuromuscular activity of the masticatory system in patients with temporomandibular joint dysfunction. J. Oral Rehabil. 15:35–47, 1988.

31. Hanvik, L.J.: MMPI profiles in patients with low-back pain. J. Consult. Clin. Psychol. 15:350–353, 1951.

32. Schwartz, R.A., Greene, C.S., and Laskin, D.M.: Personality characteristics of patients with myofascial pain-dysfunction syndrome unresponsive to conventional therapy. J. Dent. Res. 58:1435–1439, 1979.

33. Eversole, L.R., Stone, C.E., Matheson, D., and Kaplan, H.: Psychometric profiles and facial pain. Oral Surg. 60:269–274, 1985.

34. Solberg, W.K., Flint, R.T., and Brantner, J.P.: Temporomandibular joint pain and dysfunction: A clinical study of emotional and occlusal components. J. Prosthet. Dent. 28:412–422, 1972.

35. Kydd, W.L.: Psychosomatic aspects of temporomandibular joint dysfunction. J. Am. Dent. Assoc. 59:31–44, 1959.

36. Fine, E.W.: Psychological factors associated with non-organic temporomandibular joint pain dysfunction syndrome. Br. Dent. J. 131:402–404, 1971.

37. Feinmann, C., and Harris, M.: Psychogenic facial pain. I. The clinical presentation. Br. Dent. J., 156:165–168, 1984.

38. Remick, R.A., Blasber, B., Campos, P.E., and Miles, J.E.: Psychiatric disorders associated with atypical facial pain. Can. J. Psychiatry 28:178–181, 1983.

39. Naliboff, B.D. and Cohen, M.J.: Frequency of MMPI profile types in three chronic illness populations. J. Clin. Psychol. 39:843–847, 1983.

40. Toomey, T.C., Lundeen, T.F., Mann, J.D., and Abashian, S.: Illness behavior questionnaire: Factor-structure replication & relation to pain (Abstract 1081). J. Dent. Res. (Special Issue) 67:248, 1988.

41. Naliboff, B.D., Cohen, M.J., and Yellen, A.N.: Does the MMPI differentiate chronic illness from chronic pain? Pain 13:333–341, 1982.

42. Watson, D.: Neurotic tendencies among chronic pain patients: An MMPI item analysis. Pain 14:365–385, 1982.

43. Yemm, R.: Neurophysiologic studies of temporomandibular joint dysfunction. Oral Sci. Rev. 7:31–53, 1976.

44. Laskin, D.M.: Etiology of the pain dysfunction syndrome. J. Am. Dent. Assoc. 79:147–153, 1969.

45. Haber, J.D., Moss, R.A., Kuczmierczyk, A.R., and Garrett, J.C.: Assessment and treatment of stress in myofascial pain-dysfunction syndrome: A model for analysis. J. Oral Rehabil. 10:187–196, 1983.

46. Lerman, M.D.: A unifying concept of the TMJ pain-dysfunction syndrome. J. Am. Dent. Assoc. 86:833–841, 1973.

47. Holmes, T.H. and Rahe, R.H.: The social readjustment rating scale. J. Psychosom. Res. 11:213–218, 1967.

48. Fearon, C.G. and Serwatka, W.J.: Stress: A common denominator for nonorganic TMJ pain-dysfunction. J. Prosthet. Dent. 49:805–808, 1983.

49. Stein, S., Loft, G., Davis, H., and Hart, D.L.: Symptoms of TMJ dysfunction as related to stress measured by the social readjustment rating scale. J. Prosthet. Dent. 47:545–548, 1982.

50. Speculand, B., Hughes, A.O., and Goss, A.N.: Role of recent stressful life events experience in the onset

of TMJ dysfunction pain. Community Dent. Oral Epidemiol. 12:197–202, 1984.

51. Marbach, J.J., Lennon, M.C., and Dohrenwend, B.P.: Candidate risk factors for temporomandibular pain and dysfunction syndrome: Psychosocial, health behavior, physical illness and injury. Pain 34:139–151, 1988.

52. Moody, P.M., Calhoun, T.C., Okeson, J.P., and Kemper, J.T.: Stress-pain relationship in MPD syndrome patients and non-MPD syndrome patients. J. Prosthet. Dent. 45:84–88, 1981.

53. Marbach, J.J. and Lipton, J.A.: Aspects of illness behavior in patients with facial pain. J. Am. Dent. Assoc. 96:630–638, 1978.

54. Speculand, B., Goss, A.N., Hughes, A., et al: Temporo-mandibular joint dysfunction: Pain and illness behaviour. Pain 17:139–150, 1983.

55. Evaskus, D.S. and Laskin, D.M.: A biochemical measure of stress in patients with myofascial pain-dysfunction syndrome. J. Dent. Res. 51:1464–1466, 1972.

56. Berry, D.C.: Mandibular dysfunction pain and chronic minor illness. Br. Dent. J. 127:170–175, 1969.

57. Gold, S., Lipton, J., Marbach, J., and Gurion, B.: Sites of psychophysiological complaints in MPD patients. II. Areas remote from the orofacial region (Abstract 480). J. Dent. Res. (Special Issue A) 54:165, 1975.

58. Marbach, J.J., Lipton, J.A., Lund, P.B., et al: Facial pains and anxiety levels: Considerations for treatment. J. Prosthet. Dent. 40:434–437, 1978.

59. Marbach, J.J. and Lund, P.: Depression, anhedonia and anxiety in temporomandibular joint and other facial pain syndromes. Pain 11:73–84, 1981.

60. Gale, E.N.: Psychological characteristics of long-term female temporomandibular joint pain patients. J. Dent. Res. 57:481–483, 1978.

61. Rugh, J.D. and Montgomery, G.T.: Physiological reactions of patients with TM disorders vs symptom-free controls on a physical stress task. J. Craniomandib. Disorders: Facial Oral Pain 1:243–250, 1987.

62. Moss, R.A. and Adams, H.E.: Physiological reactions to stress in subjects with and without myofascial pain dysfunction symptoms. J. Oral Rehabil. 11:219–232, 1984.

63. Mercuri, L.G., Olson, R.E., and Laskin, D.M.: The specificity of response to experimental stress in patients with myofascial pain dysfunction syndrome. J. Dent. Res. 58:1866–1871, 1979.

64. Thomas, L.J., Tiber, N., and Schireson, S.: The effects of anxiety and frustration on muscular tension related to the temporomandibular joint syndrome. Oral Surg. 36:763–768, 1973.

65. Gale, E.N. and Carlsson, S.G.: Frustration and temporomandibular joint pain. Oral Surg. 45:39–43, 1978.

66. Scott, D.S. and Lundeen, T.F.: Myofascial pain involving the masticatory muscles: An experimental model. Pain 8:207–215, 1980.

67. Jacobson, E.: *Modern Treatment of Tense Patients.* Charles C Thomas, Springfield, IL, 1970.

68. Gessel, A.H. and Alderman, M.M.: Management of myofascial pain dysfunction syndrome of the temporomandibular joint by tension control training. Psychosomatics 12:302–309, 1971.

69. Reading, A. and Raw, M.: The treatment of mandib-

ular dysfunction pain. Br. Dent. J. 140:201–205, 1976.

70. Budyznski, T. and Stoyva, J.: An electromyographic feedback technique for teaching voluntary relaxation of the masseter muscle. J. Dent. Res. 52:116–119, 1973.

71. Gessel, A.H.: Electromyographic biofeedback and tricyclic antidepressants in myofascial pain-dysfunction syndrome: Psychological predictors of outcome. J. Am. Dent. Assoc. 91:1048–1052, 1975.

72. Gale, E.N. and Funch, D.P.: Factors associated with successful outcome from behavioral therapy for chronic temporomandibular joint (TMJ) pain. J. Psychosom. Res. 28:441–448, 1984.

73. Dohrmann, R.J. and Laskin, D.M.: An evaluation of electromyographic biofeedback in the treatment of myofascial pain-dysfunction syndrome. J. Am. Dent. Assoc. 96:656–662, 1978.

74. Carlsson, S.G. and Gale, E.N.: Biofeedback in the treatment of long-term temporomandibular joint pain: An outcome study. Biofeedback Self-Regul. 2:161–171, 1977.

75. Clarke, N.G. and Kardachi, B.J.: The treatment of myofascial pain-dysfunction syndrome using the biofeedback principle. J. Periodontol. 48:643–645, 1977.

76. Dahlstrom, L., Carlsson, S.G., Gale, E.N., and Jansson, T.G.: Clinical and electromyographic effects of biofeedback training in mandibular dysfunction. Biofeedback Self-Regul. 9:37–47, 1984.

77. Dahlstrom, L., Carlsson, S.G., Gale, E.N., and Jansson, T.G.: Stress-induced muscular activity in mandibular dysfunction: Effects of biofeedback training. J. Behav. Med. 8:191–199, 1985.

78. Dalen, K., Ellersten, B., Espelid, I., and Gronningsaeter, A.G.: EMG feedback in the treatment of myofascial pain dysfunction syndrome. Acta Odontol. Scand. 44:279–284, 1986.

79. Hijzen, T.H., Slangen, J.L., and Van Houweligen, H.C.: Subjective, clinical and EMG effects of biofeedback and splint treatment. J. Oral Rehabil. 13:529–539, 1986.

80. Moss, R.A., Wedding, D., and Sanders, S.H.: The comparative efficacy of relaxation training and masseter EMG feedback in the treatment of TMJ dysfunction. J. Oral Rehabil. 10:9–17, 1983.

81. Funch, D.P. and Gale, E.N.: Biofeedback and relaxation therapy for chronic temporomandibular joint pain: Predicting successful outcomes. J. Consult. Psychol. 52:928–935, 1984.

82. Brooke, R.I. and Stenn, P.G.: Myofascial pain dysfunction syndrome—how effective is biofeedback-assisted relaxation training? Adv. Pain Res. Ther. 5:809–812, 1983.

83. Hilgard, E.R. and Hilgard, J.R.: *Hypnosis in the Relief of Pain,* revised edition. William Kaufmann, Los Altos, CA, 1983.

84. British Medical Association Report: Medical use of hypnotism. Br. Med. J. (Suppl.) 1:190–193, 1955.

85. Cohen, E.S. and Hillis, R.E.: The use of hypnosis in treating the temporomandibular joint pain dysfunction syndrome. Oral Surg. 48:193–197, 1979.

86. Gerschman, J., Burrows, G., and Reade, P.: Hypnotherapy in the treatment of oro-facial pain. Aust. Dent. J. 23:492–496, 1978.

87. Stam, H.J., McGrath, P.A., and Brooke, R.I.: The effects of a cognitive-behavioral treatment program on temporo-mandibular pain and dysfunction syndrome. Psychosom. Med. 46:534–545, 1984.

89. Marbach, J.J. and Dworkin, S.F.: Chronic MPD, group therapy and psychodynamics. J. Am. Dent. Assoc. 90:827–833, 1975.

90. Lipton, J.A. and Marbach, J.J.: Predictors of treatment outcome in patients with myofascial pain-dysfunction syndrome and organic temporomandibular joint disorders. J. Prosthet. Dent. 51:387–393, 1984.

91. Salter, M.W., Brooke, R.I., and Merskey, H.: Temporomandibular pain and dysfunction syndrome: The relationship of clinical and psychological data to outcome. J. Behav. Med. 9:97–109, 1986.

92. Heloe, B. and Heiberg, A.N.: A follow-up study of a group of female patients with myofascial pain dysfunction syndrome. Acta Odontol. Scand. 38:129–134, 1980.

93. Funch, D.P. and Gale, E.N.: Predicting completion in a behavioral therapy program for chronic temporomandibular pain. J. Psychosom. Res. 30:57–62, 1986.

94. Swanson, D.W., Maruta, T., and Wolff, V.A.: Ancient pain. Pain 25: 383–387, 1986.

95. Pilling, L.F., Brannick, T.L., and Swenson, W.M.: Psychological characteristics of psychiatric patients having pain as a presenting problem. Can. Med. Assoc. J. 97:387–394, 1967.

96. Davidson, J., Krishnan, R., France, R., and Pelton, S.: Neurovegetative symptoms in chronic pain and depression. J. Affect. Disorders 9:213–218, 1985.

97. Atkinson, J., Kremer, E., Risch, S., and Janowsky, D.: Neuroendocrine markers of affective disorders in chronic pain (Abstract 310). Pain (Suppl.) 2:S209, 1984.

98. France, R.D. and Krishan, K.R.R.: The dexamethasone suppression test as a biological marker of depression in chronic pain. Pain 21:49–55, 1985.

99. Gale, E.N. and Dixon, D.C.: A simplified psychologic questionnaire as a treatment planning aid for patients with temporomandibular joint disorders. J. Prosthet. Dent. 61:235–238, 1989.

100. Millstein-Prentky, S. and Olson, R.E.: Predictability of treatment outcome in patients with myofascial pain-dysfunction (MPD) syndrome. J. Dent. Res. 58:1341–1346, 1979.

101. King, S.A. and Snow, B.R.: Factors for predicting premature termination from a multidisciplinary inpatient chronic pain program. Pain 39:201–207, 1989.

102. Griffiths, R.H.: Report of the President's Conference on the Examination, Diagnosis, and Management of Temporomandibular Disorders. J. Am. Dent. Assoc. 106:75–77.

103. Olson, R.E.: Behavioral examinations in MPD. In *The President's Conference on the Examination, Diagnosis and Management of Temporomandibular Disorders*. D. Laskin, W. Greenfield, E. Gale, et al (eds.). American Dental Association, Chicago, 1982.

104. Moulton, R.E.: Emotional factors in non-organic temporomandibular joint pain. Dent. Clin. North Am. 609–620, 1966.

105. Greene, C.S. and Laskin, D.M.: Long-term evaluation of treatment for myofascial pain-dysfunction syndrome: A comparative analysis. J. Am. Dent. Assoc. 107:235–238, 1983.

106. Goodman, P., Greene, C.S., and Laskin, D.M.: Response of patients with myofascial pain-dysfunction syndrome to mock equilibration. J. Am. Dent. Assoc. 92:755–758, 1976.

107. Feinmann, C. and Harris, M.: Psychogenic facial pain. II. Management and prognosis. Br. Dent. J. 156:205–208, 1984.

108. Laskin, D.M. and Greene, C.S.: Influence of the doctor-patient relationship on placebo therapy for patients with myofascial pain-dysfunction (MPD) syndrome. J. Am. Dent. Assoc. 85:892–894, 1972.

109. Greene, C.S. and Laskin, D.M.: Meprobamate therapy for the myofascial pain-dysfunction syndrome: A double blind evaluation. J. Am. Dent. Assoc. 82:587–590, 1971.

110. Von Korff, M.R., Howard, J.A., Truelove, E.L., et al: Temporomandibular disorders: Variation in clinical practice. Med. Care 26:307–314, 1988.

111. Evans, F.J.: The placebo response in pain control. Psychopharmacol. Bull. 17:72–76, 1981.

112. Beck, F.M.: Placebos in dentistry: Their profound potential effects. J. Am. Dent. Assoc. 95:1122–1126, 1977.

113. Schneider, C.J.: Cost effectiveness of biofeedback and behavioral medicine treatments: A review of the literature. Biofeedback Self-Regul. 12:71–92, 1987.

114. Turner, J.A. and Chapman, C.R.: Psychological interventions for chronic pain: A critical review. I. Relaxation training and biofeedback. Pain 12:1–21, 1982.

Robert D. McMullen

CHAPTER 27

Pharmacologic Management of Psychiatric Disorders

Why should a dentist or other nonpsychiatric clinician treating temporomandibular disorders (TMDs) be familiar with the intricacies of psychiatric diagnosis, much less psychopharmacologic treatment? The reasons are not trivial: (1) In our clinic at a tertiary care medical center, perhaps 30% of patients have a psychiatric illness causing or exacerbating pain; (2) the psychiatric illness is often not obvious; (3) considerable skill and patience are needed to induce these patients to have a psychiatric consultation (because of the cost and because it is self-evident to patients that they are seeing you for organic pain, not because they are "crazy" or "imagining" their pain); (4) unfortunately, it often seems that those who are the most psychiatrically ill are the most opposed to a psychiatric evaluation[1]; and (5) perhaps most important, it seems likely that the longer the pain persists, the more likely it is to become refractory to treatment.[2-4]

Even if the pain is in large part caused by a psychiatric illness, allowing the pain to persist for years can cause it to be centralized "phantom pain" and hence resistant to therapy. Also, multiple procedures, including surgery and tooth extraction, can iatrogenically exacerbate the pain, especially if a patient has a diathesis to sprouting neuromas every time a nerve is cut.[5]

Marbach and colleagues[6,7] postulate that "phantom tooth pain" can result from tooth extraction. Thus, it can be critical early in a patient's odyssey that one of the consulted clinicians correctly diagnose the patient's psychiatric illness, if it exists. An early diagnosis may save a patient from a lifetime of misery.

Whether the dentist makes the correct psychiatric diagnosis or is only aware that a patient has significant psychopathology, the advisable next step is referral for a psychiatric consultation. Accomplishing this referral often takes considerable skill and patience.[8] If the patient is new to the dentist and if the condition is not an emergency, the clinician may decide to delay broaching a psychiatric consultation. Also, patients may appropriately wish to see the dentist as their primary caregiver. Trying to send patients to a psychiatrist on the first visit may give the wrong message. One should generally make the referral after establishing a firm alliance with the patient, and then emphasize that it is a *consultation,* not necessarily a referral for long-term treatment—and certainly not a transfer of the patient from the dentist to the psychiatrist.

Because many patients with TMDs will need medication for depression or an anxiety disorder, one might begin, "I would like you to have a consultation with a colleague of mine, Dr. Smith. He is a psychopharmacologist—a psychiatrist by training—who specializes in the treatment of pain and depression. He can help us decide if a medication would be helpful." It is extremely helpful, and often essential, that the dentist indicate that he knows the psychiatrist personally, that he respects him professionally, and that he has sent other patients to him.[9] Telling the patient that you will be calling the psychiatrist to explain the problem may help the patient feel more comfortable going through with the consultation. When feasible, calling the psychiatrist in the patient's presence can be particularly salutary. When, for example, the dentist explains to the psychiatrist on the phone the patient's organic problem, pain problem, and depressive symptoms, the patient is reassured that the dentist is really sending him for this consultation for reasons they have already discussed—and not because the dentist secretly thinks he's crazy.

Patients frequently think that the clinician making the psychiatric referral thinks that (1) their complaints are "imaginary," (2) they are "crazy," and (3) the doctor is trying to get rid of them.[10] All of these fears are particularly common in patients with TMDs because many of them have already seen other dentists and physicians for their condition. A definite organic diagnosis often has not been made during

535

these visits, or patients have been given conflicting diagnoses. A helpful treatment usually has not been found (or patients would not be seeing yet another doctor). Thus, because both the diagnosis and treatment have been vague and because pain is not visible, patients may have received the message from doctors, friends, and family members that their complaints may be imaginary. Patients may already have encountered dentists and physicians who have tried to "get rid of them." A psychiatric referral, therefore, can be loaded with unintended negative meanings for the patient.

It is preferable to deal with patients' fears openly and directly. Ask them why they are reluctant to have the consultation, and then reply to their worries straightforwardly. If they say they are not crazy, ask what they mean by crazy, because it is not a medical term. It may be necessary to explain to some patients that psychiatrists do not deal with only crazy people. They also treat various problems of living, depression, and anxiety disorders. Just as stress and anxiety can exacerbate peptic ulcer disease and coronary artery disease, so can stress, depression, and anxiety exacerbate pain and muscle tension. It may be helpful to ask patients to call the dentist after the psychiatric consultation to relate how it went.

The psychiatric colleague should be expected to render an expeditious report. A written report is not always practicable, but an opinion can be adequately given in a telephone conversation. This opinion should, of course, be conveyed before the patient's next visit to the referring dentist. Do not hesitate to call a psychiatrist who is slow in responding. The psychiatrist does not have to relate all the intimate details of the patient's problems. As with any consultation by a physician, however, the psychiatrist should be expected to render a general report and a recommendation for treatment, if any. For patients with TMDs, select a psychiatric consultant who is particularly adroit with medications (a psychopharmacologist), because their problems more often respond to medication than to intensive psychotherapy. Also, because these patients are usually focused on finding relief from their physical discomfort, a psychiatrist with the style of an avuncular internist is generally more acceptable than one who follows the approach of psychoanalytic psychotherapy.

If the psychiatrist recommends treatment to the patient, the dentist should meet with the patient and reinforce the recommendation. If the patient refuses to be treated by the psychiatrist but is considered a good candidate for drug treatment, the dentist might consider prescribing the medication with the psychiatrist serving in a supervisory capacity. Whether patients have a favorable response to medication or are a treatment failure in initial trials by the dentist, they may eventually, with some encouragement, agree to return to the psychiatrist for followup treatment. A noncritical attitude, gentle insistence, and patience are often all that is necessary to induce patients to seek a psychiatric consultation and to avail themselves of ongoing treatment by the psychiatrist.

The more common drug-treatable psychiatric illnesses that contribute to pain are described individually later. Each description presents the basic diagnostic criteria and the elements of successful treatment. Obvious overt organic disease of the joints, muscles, or nerves frequently coexists with depression and other psychiatric problems.

For more detailed assistance, we suggest perusing of a basic psychiatric text,[11,12] referring the patient to a psychiatrist, or simply establishing a good relationship with a psychiatric colleague who can be called for advice is suggested.

Whether a dentist should proceed with the drug treatment without a consultation is a difficult question. One is often caught in a sort of catch-22 if a patient needs psychiatric treatment but refuses psychiatric consultation. On the one hand, dentists' malpractice liability is minimal if they do not prescribe the psychiatric medication indicated when a patient continues to be ill. Patients may eventually lose a good job, become permanently disabled, or even commit suicide. From a medicolegal standpoint, however, dentists are fairly secure if they urged a patient to go to the proper specialist (a psychiatrist) and the patient chose to refuse. On the other hand, if a dentist proceeds with a psychotropic medication treatment, there are basically three possible outcomes: (1) The patient could get better, (2) the patient could remain the same, and (3) there could be a bad outcome. The third possibility—the bad outcome—is the problem. Patients might have an adverse reaction to a medication. If depressed or psychotic, they might commit suicide. The bad outcome is likely to have no relationship to inappropriate treatment but that might not prevent litigation. A dentist can thus be in a difficult dilemma, in which the ethical choice may be to treat a patient without a consultation but the optimal medicolegal choice may be not to treat but to insist, however unsuccessfully, that the patient see a psychiatrist. Table 27–1 summarizes the medications discussed throughout the chapter.

DEPRESSION

Depression is by far the most common psychiatric disorder in patients with TMDs. It is also exceedingly common in the general population. The purest form of depression associated with facial pain is the *atypical facial pain*

syndrome. In addition to coexisting with the symptoms of depression (see subsequent discussion), the pain is characteristically diffuse rather than focal. A patient does not merely point to the temporomandibular joint (TMJ) in describing it, but describes a widespread, usually unilateral facial pain that may radiate to the frontal, temporomandibular, maxillary, and occipital regions, as well as to the neck and shoulders. It is found more commonly in women and usually between the ages of 30 and 60 years.[13]

However, one should eschew statistical stereotypes. We treated one 75-year-old retired policeman who was psychologically quite sta-

TABLE 27–1. Adult Dosages and Suggested Therapeutic Plasma Level Ranges for Antidepressants

MEDICATION	INITIAL DOSE (MG/DAY)	DOSAGE RANGE (MG/DAY)	SUGGESTED THERAPEUTIC PLASMA RANGE (NG/DAY)
Fluoxetine (Prozac)	5	20–80	—
Trazodone (Desyrel, generic)	50	50–400	—
Bupropion (Wellbutrin)	100	200–450 (divided dose)	
Tricyclics			
Imipramine (Tofranil, generic)	25	50–300	200–300
Amitriptyline (Elavil, generic)	25	50–300	150–250
Desipramine (Norpramin)	25	50–300	150–300
Nortriptyline (Pamelor, Aventyl)	10	30–100	50–150
Protriptyline (Vivactil)	10	50–60	70–240
Maprotiline (Ludiomil, generic)	25	50–250	—
Doxepin (Sinequan, generic)	25	50–300	110–250
Amoxapine (Asendin)	25	50–600	—
Clomipramine (Anafranil)	25	50–300	—
MAO Inhibitors			
Tranylcypromine (Parnate)	10	20–90	—
Phenelzine (Nardil)	15	30–90	—
Selegiline or deprenyl (Eldepryl)	5	10–50	—
Isocarboxazid (Marplan)	10	20–60	—
Pargyline (Eutonyl)	10	200	—

Reprinted with permission from Brotman, Falk, and Gelenberg: Pharmacologic treatment of acute depression subtypes. In *Psychopharmacology The Third Generation.* H. Meltzer (ed.). Raven Press, New York, 1987.

ble but was disabled by diffuse unilateral facial pain and depression. He denied depressed mood yet had all the vegetative symptoms described later. His pain and depression dramatically remitted after 2 weeks on a tricyclic antidepressant.

An initially more confusing collection of patients are those who definitely have an organic muscle or joint problem and depression. Their pain usually seems out of proportion to the mechanical problem. This need not be as confusing as it seems. If patients have *symptoms* of depression, they undoubtedly have depression. The depression reduces patients' pain thresholds and may also increase their clenching. For example, a former professional football quarterback reportedly has bad knees. As far as we know, he has chronic discomfort in his knees. If this ex-athlete ever happened to experience depression, the first thing he would probably do would be to visit his orthopedist to complain that his arthritis had become worse. Actually, his arthritis would not be worse, but his pain threshold would be decreased by the depression, so he would experience more pain. This or a similar example can help clarify the problem to patients.

Patients can almost always benefit from clarification of the nature of depression. It is unfortunate that we use the word depression in lay usage to refer to any feeling of sadness, yet in psychiatric usage to refer only to a state of sadness that is accompanied by certain specific, mostly physical, symptoms. This psychiatric depression is a *physical* illness.

Patients who have for years suffered from depression often refer to it as a "chemical imbalance," which it actually is. The medication is working on something, and the defect appears to be a functional depletion of certain monoamine transmitters, particularly norepinephrine and serotonin.[14] In response to any explanation, however, a patient is likely to say, "Well, who wouldn't be depressed with all this pain?" The clinician can agree that the pain may well have caused the depression, but that it is a physical depression (or "chemical" or "biologic" or "endogenous") with physical symptoms (see subsequent discussion). Although many atypical facial pain syndromes seem to begin after some physical trauma, such as a dental procedure, it is also common with a careful history to find depression preceding the onset of pain.[15]

Whether the depression or the pain came first, if this is even determinable, is for practical purposes inconsequential. In maxillofacial pain with coexisting depression, mechanical intervention in the TMJ is usually not sufficient. An antidepressant is also necessary.[16,17] Except in milder cases, the diagnosis of depression is relatively straightforward, based on criteria from the *Diagnostic and Statistical Manual of Mental Disorders, Third Edition, Revised* (DSM-III-R).[18]

A diagnosis of depression requires that four of eight of the following symptoms be present for at least 2 weeks:

1. *Sleep disturbance,* which is usually middle insomnia (waking up during the night), terminal insomnia (waking up too early in the morning and being unable to return to sleep), or very restless sleep. The symptom may occasionally be excessive sleep (hypersomnia). Patients usually have no difficulty falling asleep. Ask specific questions, such as, "Do you sleep soundly or do you have a restless sleep? Do you wake up at night? How many times do you awaken and for how long are you awake?"

2. *Decreased enjoyment of food,* occasionally with significant weight loss. It is critical to determine whether a patient has any loss of "enjoyment of food." Patients often say that their appetite is fine when, in fact, they are taking no pleasure in food and are eating only because they are hungry. Some depressed patients have increased appetite, especially for sweets, but usually not increased enjoyment of food.

3. *Decreased energy* is often manifested by general tiredness, decreased care of personal appearance, and decreased upkeep of the home.

4. *Decreased concentration* can usually be evaluated by ascertaining whether patients can read articles and books as well as they did in the past and whether their mind wanders when they read. One can also inquire how patients' concentration is at their job.

5. *Pervasive anhedonia* (decreased enjoyment of most things). "Are there any things you used to enjoy that you no longer enjoy?" "Do you still enjoy going out and seeing friends?"

6. *Increased self-blame and self-criticism* are less common with patients with TMD than in other depressed patients, probably because patients with TMD can blame their difficulties on the pain and because TMD-related depression

is often "mild" by psychiatric standards: dysthymia (minor depression) rather than major depression. Other pain-prone patients who have pain elsewhere than the face also tend to have minor depression and therefore tend not to have the excessive feelings of worthlessness, self-reproach, and guilt associated with major depression. However, patients with chronic pain can alternate between major depression and minor depression.[19]

7. *Motor retardation* or *motor agitation.* Motor retardation may only manifest itself in slightly slowed speech, which is difficult to evaluate. The diagnosis of depression is frequently missed in patients with motor agitation, because they do not appear depressed. They are often nervous, talk rapidly, and make continual complaints about their pain as well as their past and present medical/dental care. Such a patient is variously seen as a "crock," as a hypochondriac, as an anxiety-ridden person, or as someone suffering terribly with pain. However, if a clinician asks, patients may describe the other symptoms of depression (e.g., insomnia, decreased appetite, and concentration).

8. *The wish to be dead.* Rather than bluntly asking patients if they are suicidal, it is more diplomatic to ask, "Do you ever feel so depressed and hopeless with your pain that you wish you were dead?" If the answer is yes, then obtain details about what fantasies they have had about killing themselves, the methods they have fantasized using, and how close they feel they have been to suicide. If they have a serious plan of suicide, immediate intervention is indicated (e.g., obtaining a psychiatric consultation immediately, calling the family, having the patient hospitalized).

Treatment of Depression

The treatment of minor depression or major depression is mainly pharmacologic. Cognitive psychotherapy occasionally is helpful for depression[20] but has doubtful usefulness for patients with chronic pain. The first step in treatment is to explain the problem to patients and convince them to accept treatment. Because some highly somatizing patients would scarcely accept an antidepressant, much less see a psychiatrist, there may be little alternative to a dentist's proceeding with the antidepressant treatment without a consultation.

As long ago as 1955, Ruth Moulton,[21] a psychiatrist, advocated that dentists alone treat many of these patients because (1) the patient often adamantly refuses to see a psychiatrist and (2) a rational, conservative intervention is better than allowing the patient to continue seeking someone to perform surgical intervention. Moulton, of course, did not know at that time that antidepressants might be of benefit to these patients, the first such application apparently being reported in 1962.[22]

If in a dentist's professional judgment a patient would balk at any hint of a psychiatric treatment, he or she might proceed by emphasizing to the patient that the medication to be used is to reduce pain. It *is* true that many antidepressants probably have analgesic properties independent of their antidepressant activity,[23,24] although it is frequently argued that the antidepressant effect has the primary action on pain.[25,26] A dentist could add that the medication is also used as an antidepressant and might help improve the patient's mood, concentration, energy, and sleep.

A relatively sophisticated patient can be provided with some detail, explaining that the chronic pain causes a biologic or chemical depression and that the depression reduces the pain threshold, thereby increasing the pain. The depression also causes increased muscle tension and bruxism, thus increasing the pain.[27] The increased pain causes more depression, creating a vicious cycle of pain and depression. If further explanation appears to be helpful to a particular patient, a dentist could draw a diagram and explain how it is thought that norepinephrine and serotonin may be depleted in depression and that antidepressants elevate these transmitters by blocking reuptake, and so on. Such an extended explanation does several things. The time it takes implies concern. Understanding the "what" and the "why" helps compliance. Explaining the medical basis of depression and pain decreases the tendency to see the depression as psychologic, as if it were the patient's fault.

It is advisable to become familiar with the use of at least two to three different antidepressants, preferably from different classes (Table 27–1). The five major classes of antidepressants are (1) fluoxetine (Prozac), (2) various tricyclics, (3) bupropion (Wellbutrin), (4) trazodone (Desyrel), and (5) monoamine oxidase (MAO) inhibitors. In general, nonpsychiatrists should try these medications in the order listed. Trazodone should be avoided in men, because the risk of priapism is between 1:1000 and 1:10,000.[28] Priapism could lead to permanent impotence. The MAO inhibitors are usually tried last because of the dietary restrictions and possible drug interactions.

Fluoxetine (Prozac)

Fluoxetine (Prozac)[29,30] was introduced to the United States market in January, 1988. For many psychiatrists, it has become a common first line of treatment. It should probably be the first antidepressant prescribed by nonpsychiatrists because (1) unlike tricyclics, virtually no orthostatic hypotension is associated with its use, (2) other dangerous side effects are also quite uncommon, and (3) fatal overdose has not occurred even with ingesting 100 to 150 capsules (2000 to 3000 mg). The medication currently is only available in a 20-mg capsule, although smaller doses should be available soon. Advise patients that the most common side effects are (1) jitteriness, as if one had too much coffee; (2) nausea; (3) sedation, drowsiness, and a "spacey" or medicated feeling; and (4) perhaps a pruritic skin rash in 5% of patients.

Patients should be told to discontinue the medication and contact you if they develop a skin rash. The allergic rash is not significantly dangerous, but a patient obviously cannot easily continue a medication that causes a pruritic rash. If the rash is mild and the benefit dramatic, it may be worthwhile continuing the medication (and closely observing the patient) because the rash may remit. The other side effects are worse in the first week or so of treatment. Fluoxetine should be taken with food to reduce the nausea. It should be taken in the morning to avoid significantly disturbing a patient's sleep.

In the uncommon event that it is particularly sedating in an individual patient, it can be taken at bedtime. The therapeutic dose is usually 20 mg/day. The maximum treating dose is 80 mg/day (all in one dose or 40 mg in the morning and 40 mg at noon). However, it is uncommon to need more than 20 to 40 mg/day.

A general principle of treatment with psychotropics is to increase the dose slowly to the therapeutic dose to avoid unpleasant side effects. Thus, it would be reasonable to instruct patients to take 5 mg/day of fluoxetine for the first week, 10 mg/day in the second week, 20 mg every morning in the third week, and to remain on this dose until re-evaluated. Patients should make their weekly increase on their day off (usually Saturday). If they experience excessive side effects, they can either accommodate to them over the weekend or return to the lower dose when they begin work on Monday.

Because fluoxetine is currently available only in 20-mg capsules, tell patients that dispensing 5 mg sounds more difficult than it is. The capsule is easily pulled apart, and the powder inside is water soluble. Demonstrate rolling the opened capsule between your fingers to drop approximately one-fourth capsule into some juice. Fluoxetine will soon be available in a smaller dose, either in tablet form or in liquid suspension.

Many patients have few side effects even when they begin with 20 mg, but comfort and compliance are more certain if patients increase the dose slowly. Obviously, if side effects are minimal, patients could try increasing the dose more rapidly. If the side effects are excessive, the medication can be increased much more slowly. The manner of elevating the dose should be individualized.

Inform patients that there is a 70 to 80% chance that the depression will lift after 4 weeks on 20 mg of fluoxetine. There is a 20 to 30% chance that there will be no benefit. If the latter occurs, the dose of fluoxetine should be gradually increased to 60 mg or even 80 mg if the side effects are tolerable. If a higher dose is not tolerable or if a few weeks on a higher dose yields no improvement, then a different agent should be given. Fluoxetine has such a long half-life that it can be stopped abruptly, but it can be decreased over a few days if that makes patients more comfortable. Note that 5 weeks must elapse after the cessation of fluoxetine before starting an MAO inhibitor.[31] No waiting period is necessary before instituting another antidepressant.

Tricyclics[32–35]

Tricyclics are the old standards and include *nortriptyline* (Aventyl or Pamelor), *desipramine* (Norpramin), *imipramine* (Tofranil), *amitriptyline* (Elavil), and several others. Although very popular with internists, amitriptyline actually has more side effects than most tricyclics, particularly the anticholinergic side effects of dry mouth, constipation, and sedation. It is also more likely to cause orthostatic hypotension, which is the most dangerous side effect. Amitriptyline is probably used frequently because its sedating side effect immediately helps the patient's insomnia, but this benefit may not be worth the other side effects. Maprotiline (Ludiomil) probably should be avoided because it lowers the seizure threshold more than the others.[36]

As with any antidepressant, urge patients to call if they have any questions about dosing or side effects. A few minutes on the telephone can be very helpful. If side effects are truly excessive, the medication can be discontinued. If constipation is encountered, Colace (200 mg—two pills, 100 mg each) can be obtained without a prescription. If dizziness is excessive, the dose can be reduced. If vision becomes blurry, reassurance is in order. If acute eye pain occurs, a rare attack of narrow-angle glaucoma may have ensued, and patients should promptly see an ophthalmologist.

Patients with a history of panic attacks may experience a paradoxical increase in anxiety with a tricyclic or fluoxetine and may have to increase their dose much more gradually—perhaps by 10 mg/week in the case of tricyclics.

For a baseline, take patients' blood pressure while they are sitting and standing and then monitor it, especially standing, as the dose of the tricyclic is increased. Tell patients that the possible orthostatic hypotension is not dangerous in itself—the danger is the fall it could cause. If patients fall and break a hip (a common occurrence in older women, even those not taking medication) or hit their head, they can suffer a worse problem than facial pain and depression. If patients experience dizziness on standing, most commonly in arising from bed in the morning, they should stand up *slowly* while holding on to something until the dizziness remits and call the clinician for guidance.

The only major medical contraindication to a tricyclic is a *left bundle branch block (LBBB),* because tricyclics prolong the QRS interval and can complete the block.[37] This event is more common in elderly patients with a history of cardiac problems. A call to a patient's internist can rule out this possibility. If the patient is older than 50 years and has not recently had a cardiogram (ECG), a visit to the internist for an ECG is probably indicated before taking tricyclics. LBBB is an uncommon problem that in itself is not usually alarming (unless the patient is taking a tricyclic). The ECG should be checked in a casual, matter-of-fact manner, or patients may develop the impression that they are taking a dangerous medication, which they are not. If patients have a cardiac problem,

their physician should be consulted before they start taking a tricyclic. Imipramine and other tricyclics are chemically similar to quinidine and therefore have an effect of reducing premature atrial and ventricular contractions.[38] This can be beneficial in some cardiac cases, but inadvertently taking quinidine and a tricyclic antidepressant together may cause toxicity.

Nortriptyline (Aventyl or Pamelor)

Nortriptyline has become a tricyclic favored by psychiatrists because it usually has the fewest side effects and a lower dose is necessary. Nortriptyline is the first metabolite of amitriptyline (Elavil), so a patient taking amitriptyline is actually taking both amitriptyline and nortriptyline. The usual dose of nortriptyline is 75 to 100 mg/day. As with all psychotropics, a lower dose is usually indicated in elderly patients because of side effects and slower metabolism by the liver. Begin at 10 mg and increase the dose by 10 mg/day to 50 or 75 mg/day. Tell patients that it is available in capsules of 10, 25, 50, and 75 mg, so that they will realize that five or seven 10-mg capsules are not a huge dose. If patients experience too many side effects, they should remain on a lower dose (e.g., 30 mg) until the next visit. The visits should be weekly or biweekly if possible. If administered by a dentist, dental treatment, such as adjustment of a splint, should be made at each visit, particularly for the patient who expects mechanical intervention.

The daily dose should usually be taken all at once for the sake of convenience and compliance. Split doses have no advantage except in uncommon instances when side effects are excessive. Because tricyclics, even nortriptyline, are usually somewhat sedating, the medicine should be taken at bedtime. If the tricyclic actually awakens the patient, then it should be taken in the morning. After patients reach their initial target dose of 75 mg (or 50 mg if the patient is elderly or having excessive side effects), a nortriptyline blood level should be obtained after patients have been on this same dose for at least 1 week. Any laboratory can perform this test. The level should be drawn about 12 hours after the last dose. Tell patients that if they plan to go to a laboratory at 9 A.M., then they should take the medication at 9 P.M. the night before. If they plan to go on their lunch hour, then they should take it at midnight the night before.

Nortriptyline is an interesting medication in that it has a "therapeutic window." It works best when the blood level is between 50 and 150 ng/ml, preferably at least 100 ng/ml. Oddly enough, it often is ineffective if the level is greater than 150 ng/ml. Because of wide variations in individual metabolism, some patients are in the therapeutic range on as little as 30 to 40 mg/day and others require as much as 250 mg.

Desipramine (Norpramin)

Desipramine is the first metabolite of *imipramine (Tofranil)*. The dosing is the same for each. Desipramine has slightly fewer side effects, but imipramine is usually quite tolerable. A major advantage of imipramine is cost; it is available generically in tablets of 10, 25, and 50 mg. The dose to aim for is 200 to 300 mg in younger patients and 100 to 150 mg or even less in elderly patients. How fast the dose is increased depends on a clinician's familiarity with the drug and the patient, as well as the patient's age. For example, in an elderly patient who also is very chary of side effects and who does not know the doctor very well, the dose should be increased particularly slowly. A conservative treatment would be having the patient start at 25 mg at bedtime and increase by 25 mg every 2 days—staying at a lower dose if side effects are excessive, however. If visits are less than weekly, a more gradual increase may be necessary, unless the patient is young and very reliable.

A blood level may be indicated if the patient is taking a maximum dose and shows no improvement after 4 weeks. It is hoped that this maximum dose will be 300 mg in a young patient; however, side effects may limit the dose to much less. The blood level should be obtained in the same way as with nortriptyline— 12 hours after the last dose and only after the patient has been on the same dose for at least a week. The imipramine level is the sum of the imipramine and desipramine levels (the laboratory should determine both levels automatically when an imipramine level is ordered). The desipramine level will be of just desipramine, because it has no significant active metabolite. With either medication, the blood level should be greater than 200 ng/ml and as high as 300 or 400 ng/ml. For example, if the blood level on 200 mg/day of imipramine is less than 200 ng/ml, then the imipramine should be increased somewhat. If this is not possible because of side effects, then consider switching to desipramine, which usually has fewer side effects. This can be done rapidly, dose for dose, because they are so similar and the patient is actually already taking desipramine as well as imipramine. Therefore, imipramine can be decreased by 50 mg/day, while desipramine is increased by 50 mg/day. The dose of desipramine can subsequently be increased with less likelihood of intolerable side effects.

Another alternative would be a switch to nortriptyline, slowly starting it while decreasing imipramine or desipramine. A tricyclic should be discontinued gradually (e.g., 50 mg every 2 or 3 days), because abrupt cessation can cause a slight withdrawal syndrome that can feel like a mild flu. Tricyclics should be used with caution in suicidal patients, because 1500 mg (5 days' supply in some patients) can be fatal. However, leaving serious depression untreated has more risk of fatality than tricyclic therapy.

Bupropion (Wellbutrin)[39]

Bupropion was introduced to the United States market in July, 1989. It is a relatively well-tolerated antidepressant. A common side effect is increased anxiety. It poses a high risk of provoking grand mal seizures in depressed patients with a history of bulimia or anorexia and should be avoided in patients with such a history. Anorexia is here defined as the willful losing of excessive amounts of weight to the point of extreme thinness, not the decreased appetite associated with depression. Anorexic patients obtain this goal by an almost maniacal devotion to counting calories and exercising. Bulimia is an illness characterized by an overwhelming impulse to eat large quantities of food. These binges are usually followed by purging—self-induced emesis or laxative abuse or both.

Seizures are also dose related, so 300 to 450 mg/day should be relatively safe. However, caution is in order with any new medication on the market. Consultation with a psychopharmacologist would be prudent. The 2-year risk of seizures at 450 mg/day is 0.48%.[40] The risk is higher at 600 mg/day. Bupropion is available in 75-mg and 100-mg tablets. Patients can begin with 100 mg the first day, 100 mg twice a day the second day, and 100 mg three times a day on the third day (morning, noon, and afternoon). If patients are excessively anxious or edgy on the medication, lower the dose for a couple of weeks so that they can accommodate to it. Bupropion should be taken in split doses to decrease side effects and risk of seizures. The last dose should not be taken after 4 or 5 P.M., because it may disturb sleep. As with most antidepressants, 3 to 4 weeks of an adequate dose may be necessary for benefit.

Trazodone (Desyrel)[41]

Trazodone, as mentioned, should be avoided in men because of the danger of causing priapism. Proceed with it in a man only if there is no alternative and only with informed consent. Consultation with a psychopharmacologist is advisable if the patient is a man. Unlike other antidepressants, such as the tricyclics, trazodone unfortunately does not seem to have an analgesic action independent of its antidepressant effect.[42] Trazodone is relatively safe in overdose. It has fewer cardiovascular effects than the tricyclics, and hypotension is rarely a problem. The most troublesome side effect is excessive sedation, often making it impossible to reach a therapeutic dose. The maximum dose is 600 mg/day, but only an occasional patient can tolerate a dose approaching that. It is available in tablets of 50, 100, and 150 mg. Begin patients on 50 mg at bedtime and increase by 50 mg every 2 to 3 days until 100 or 150 mg is reached, and then re-evaluate.

A patient occasionally responds to only 50 to 75 mg. As with tricyclics and fluoxetine, patience is necessary. Benefit often takes 4 weeks. If no benefit accrues, further increase may be indicated, which may then be possible because the patient may have accommodated to the sedating side effects. Alternatively, change to another antidepressant.

Monoamine Oxidase Inhibitors

MAO inhibitors often lift a depression in a few days rather than in a few weeks, an enormous advantage in recalcitrant, reluctant, and disbelieving patients. If pain sufferers feel some relief in only a few days, they may become patients rather than "dropouts." A significant history exists of clinicians successfully using MAO inhibitors to treat atypical facial pain. However, being on an MAO inhibitor requires avoiding certain foods, including cheese, and certain medications, especially meperidine (Demerol). Foods with large amounts of tyramine, usually aged foods, can cause massive transient elevations of blood pressure, which could precipitate a stroke or heart attack. Thus, prescription of an MAO inhibitor should usually be initiated by someone who has enough interest to develop expertise with the drugs and who has the time and patience to discuss the diet and other restrictions with the patient. Internists, general practitioners, and dentists rarely prescribe MAO inhibitors. They are primarily prescribed by those psychiatrists who treat many cases of depression.

PANIC DISORDER

Panic disorder is relatively common in society, having a 1-month prevalence of 0.5% and a lifetime prevalence of 1.6% in the general population.[45] That is, in the previous month 0.5% of the United States population suffered from panic disorder. About 1.6% of the population has at some time suffered this disorder. Panic disorder is relevant to our discussion for two reasons: (1) it commonly coexists with depression, and (2) the chronic anxiety often associated with this disorder can exacerbate jaw clenching.[46]

Panic disorder is underreported in the literature of atypical facial pain, probably because it was largely unrecognized in the era before DSM-III, which was published in 1980.[47] (A revised edition appeared in 1987.)[48] In a classic paper on atypical facial pain in 1951, George Engel[49] reported on 20 patients, but only one in detail. In retrospect, in addition to probably suffering from dysthymia, that patient almost definitely had panic attacks.[50] Of the total of 20 patients described, four definitely had panic attacks (suffering hyperventilation) and another five possibly had them (suffering other "syncopal experiences").[51]

Patients (somewhat more commonly women) with panic disorder can present in the office in a number of ways, ranging from calm stability with no sign of a problem to chronic anxiety and somatizing and even overt panic attacks while in the dental chair. The diagnosis is very easy to miss unless one asks specifically if the patient has had any "anxiety attacks" or "panic attacks." For example, severely anxious patients are unlikely to volunteer that they are so anxious (and possibly agoraphobic and somatizing) because of panic attacks. Until they are educated about their condition, they may explain their panic attacks to themselves as occurring because they are anxious and phobic, because they have a heart problem, because they are weak and fragile, because they are on the verge of going crazy, and so on. However, panic attacks are merely discrete, unexpected attacks of massive anxiety, usually lasting only minutes and apparently arising from a hyperexcitable focus in the locus ceruleus of the midbrain.[52] Patients often think that the attacks last much longer than they do because they are so unpleasant and terrifying. Also, patients may remain excessively anxious for hours after an attack.

When the attacks are particularly severe or frequent, patients frequently develop agoraphobia (in Greek, "fear of the marketplace"). Common agoraphobic symptoms are a fear of going outside the home alone; being in elevators or crowded public places; sitting in the middle of a crowded movie theater; and traveling in a car, train, bus, airplane, or subway. Patients often logically conclude that they are having panic attacks because of their phobias. However, a careful history usually reveals that the onset of panic attacks preceded the agoraphobia by a few months. If a patient's history of panic attacks and anxiety is so vague that it precludes a definitive diagnosis, then move on to questions about agoraphobia. If the patient is agoraphobic in several situations, then the patient either has "panic disorder with agoraphobia" or "agoraphobia without history of panic disorder." The last disorder, also an anxiety disorder, may actually be a variant of panic disorder, although with more limited panic attacks.[53]

The basic criteria for a diagnosis of panic disorder according to DSM-III-R[54] requires that "Either four attacks have occurred within a four-week period, or one or more attacks have been followed by a period of at least a month of persistent fear of having another attack." Also, "at least four of the following symptoms developed during at least one of the attacks:

1. Shortness of breath (dyspnea) or smothering sensations
2. Dizziness, unsteady feelings, or faintness
3. Palpitations or accelerated heart rate (tachycardia)
4. Trembling or shaking
5. Sweating
6. Choking
7. Nausea or abdominal distress
8. Depersonalizion or derealization
9. Numbness or tingling sensations (paresthesias)
10. Flushes (hot flashes) or chills

11. Chest pain or discomfort
12. Fear of dying
13. Fear of going crazy or of doing something uncontrolled."

In addition to the common association with depression, panic disorder frequently coexists with mitral valve prolapse, which is usually a relatively benign disorder. (Prophylactic antibiotics occasionally are requested by cardiologists for their patients' dental procedures.) It is not at all clear that prolapse "causes" panic attacks, and it certainly does not preclude the diagnosis of panic disorder.

The association between panic attacks and mitral valve prolapse is unfortunate in some patients, because they become convinced that they have a serious heart problem, particularly because panic attacks commonly cause palpitations, tachycardia, and chest discomfort. Actually, the association between mitral valve prolapse and panic attacks may not be causal but may just be a genetic association, like blue eyes and blond hair.

A common complication of panic disorder is substance abuse, particularly of alcohol and anxiolytics. Alcohol is rather efficient at suppressing panic attacks and anxiety, but it is necessary to keep drinking all day. The result is alcohol dependence and abuse, usually a worse problem than the initial one. Heavy use of benzodiazepines and other anxiolytics is often encountered, although these medications usually alleviate the intercurrent anxiety without completely aborting the panic attacks.

Treatment of Panic Disorder[55,56]

A significant number of patients with chronic pain apparently have anxiety rather than depression as a primary problem.[57] It is important to determine whether a patient's chronic anxiety is secondary to occasional discrete panic attacks, some other anxiety disorder, or depression. Only three benzodiazepines are definitely effective in treating panic attacks: alprazolam (Xanax), clonazepam (Klonopin), and lorazepam (Ativan). Diazepam (Valium), chlordiazepoxide (Librium), and other drugs ameliorate anxiety but may not definitively treat panic attacks.[58]

A number of antidepressants are quite effective in treating panic disorder: the tricyclics, the MAO inhibitors, and fluoxetine.

If patients are not depressed, it is usually simpler to treat them with clonazepam, lorazepam, or alprazolam. The only significant side effect of these medications is sedation, which can usually be managed by lowering the dose or waiting for patients to develop tolerance to the sedating side effects. Patients usually do not become tolerant to the antipanic effect.

Alprazolam has been the standard treatment of panic disorders. However, clonazepam is supplanting alprazolam in the armamentarium of many psychiatrists because (1) it poses less likelihood of withdrawal problems and (2) it has a longer half-life.[59] Twice-daily dosing is usually sufficient with clonazepam, rather than the four or five doses of alprazolam. Abrupt cessation of alprazolam can result in muscle spasms, a dysphoric feeling lasting a few days, and even grand mal seizures, particularly if the dose exceeds 4 to 5 mg/day.[60] Alprazolam is available in scored tablets of 0.25, 0.5, and 1.0 mg. The dose necessary to treat panic disorder varies from 1 to 5 mg or more per day. Patients are usually started on about 0.125 or 0.25 mg four times a day, and the dose is slowly increased until the panic attacks cease or until patients experience excessive sedation and drowsiness. Between 2 and 4 mg/day is usually necessary. When the medication is withdrawn, it should be done slowly (at a decrease of about 0.25 to 0.5 mg/week), especially if a patient has been on a substantial dose for several months.

Clonazepam is effective for panic disorder in approximately the same dose range (2 to 5 mg/day, occasionally more). But it can be given more conveniently in two or three doses a day. It is available in scored tablets of 0.5, 1.0, and 2.0 mg.

OTHER ANXIETY DISORDERS

The highest prevalence (1 month, 7.3%; lifetime, 14.6%) of all mental disorders in the population is found in the anxiety disorders.[61] These include panic disorder (described earlier), social phobia, simple phobia, obsessive-compulsive disorder, post-traumatic stress disorder, and generalized anxiety disorder.[62] It is beyond the scope of this book to detail each of these disorders. A number of these disorders are associated with panic disorder or depression and respond to antidepressants or anxiolytics. With such a high prevalence rate, these disorders are common in any patient population, whether or not their psychiatric disorder contributes significantly to muscle tension or bruxism.

Patients often successfully depend on diazepam or some other benzodiazepine to relieve their anxiety, although it has some albeit overrated abuse potential and can exacerbate depression. It is advisable to establish the precise diagnosis with a psychiatric evaluation, if at all possible, to be able to fit the treatment to the illness.

DELUSIONAL (PARANOID) DISORDER, SOMATIC TYPE

Delusional (paranoid) disorder, somatic type, is not mentioned frequently in relation to atypical facial pain or TMD, although many dentists are aware of it.[63] It is probably more common than recognized, because by the time a dentist realizes that a patient is a more than average somatizer, the patient has often already continued on his or her search for yet another specialist. Of 23 patients with myofascial pain, Pomp[64] describes four as delusional. Of seven cases of "atypical facial neuralgia" reported by Wilson in 1932, two were delusional (cases five and seven) and another (case two) was a paranoid personality at minimum and was possibly delusional.[65] Five of 35 patients seen by Moulton had somatic delusion or schizophrenia or both.[66]

The "essential feature of this disorder is the presence of a persistent, nonbizarre delusion that is not due to any other mental disorder, such as schizophrenia, schizophreniform disorder, or a mood disorder."[67] The onset of the disorder is usually in middle age. It can wax and wane or prove chronic. Although by definition a "psychotic" disorder, it may be difficult to diagnose until the clinician knows the patient quite well. However, the diagnosis is sometimes only made when the patient abruptly becomes flagrantly psychotic.[68] The patient is often appropriate, coherent, and logical on matters other than the delusion. This disorder has also been called "monosymptomatic hypochondriacal psychosis" and has been found to respond relatively well to a particular antipsychotic, pimozide (Orap),[69] which is available only in 2-mg tablets. The dose ranges up to 12 mg, but 2 to 6 mg is usually sufficient. The entire dose can be taken at bedtime.

A variant of delusional disorder, somatic type (or monosymptomatic hypochondriacal psychosis) is dysmorphophobia.[70] This is something of a misnomer because patients are not phobic of dysmorphia. They believe that they have some physical abnormality (usually unattractive), but a clinician can appreciate no significant abnormality.

Patients with Marbach's "phantom bite syndrome" are familiar to TMD clinicians.[71] These patients are obsessed with their bite, are fairly well educated on occlusal problems, and consult specialist after specialist. Phantom bite syndrome, like dysmorphophobia, is probably a subtype of delusional (paranoid) disorder, somatic type. In one of Marbach's cases, the patient's paranoid (psychotic) anger is frighteningly apparent in her plan to use her car to run over the last dentist to discharge her. She did not carry out the plan, "because he never came out of the house. I waited and waited. Some children came out, and I could have run them over but I didn't know if they were his."

When patients obsessively complain that one side of their face is somewhat misshapen or that their abnormal bite has caused all their teeth to shift to one side, a dentist may initially think that they are exaggerating because they are overwrought or eccentric. As time goes on, these patients are found to have a fixed idea that is not true. No amount of logic or explanation can persuade them to look at the situation more flexibly.

One 60-year-old patient with a TMD was convinced in a peculiarly fixed way that her bite was severely abnormal. It was not. She also bitterly complained that noise in her joint was extremely disturbing to her, yet she had only mild crepitus. She had no pain, but she threatened on several occasions to kill herself if the dentists did not correct the problem. One morning at 6 A.M., she made an emergency call to her dentist to tell him that, to her horror, her jaw was about to "drop off," and she pleaded for help. When seen later that day, she was surprisingly calm—as if nothing had happened. When asked about the incident, she revealed that she literally believed her jaw was going to drop down out of the sockets 1 to 2 inches, and no amount of explanation could dissuade her. When an antipsychotic (pimozide 2 mg at bedtime) was added to her regimen (symptoms of depression had already been relieved by an antidepressant), she became much more flexible, her suicidal thoughts ceased, and she could go for hours without thinking of her "dental problem." She said, "Now I can live with it." However, she periodically stopped her antipsychotic medication, suffered a relapse and finally went on to another specialist, still seeking a definitive mechanical or surgical "cure."

One patient who had a delusional disorder of the phantom bite subtype as well as panic attacks and symptoms of a minor depression, was seeing two dentists at the same time, using a different name with each. This was discovered by accident when the two colleagues were consulting each other about an impossibly demanding patient each was treating and then realized it was the same patient using different names. She believed that her bite was malaligned and was convinced that only she knew how to align it. She had a bagful of temporary bridges representing some $20,000 of work by many dentists. She had a paranoid style, felt that all the dentists were ganging up on her, and submitted herself finally to only one psychiatric examination. She also had a fixed idea that her panic attacks were attacks of angina. No amount of explanation of the classic nature of her panic attacks and agoraphobia could sway her. A call to her cardiologist confirmed that she had no cardiac problem and that he too knew they were panic attacks. She continued her hopeless quest for the perfect dentist to align her bite.

As can be seen by these examples, this type of case is often untreatable. However, if a patient is willing to take an antipsychotic, there is some hope for alleviation of symptoms. Unfortunately, antipsychotics or neuroleptics such as pimozide, chlorpromazine (Thorazine), haloperidol (Haldol), and fluphenazine (Prolixin) are difficult to use even in partially willing patients. This type of patient is often very sophisticated and not a little paranoid. Unbeknownst to the clinician, they are very often looking up in the *Physicians' Desk Reference* every medicine they are offered. They can become quite enraged when they read that the main indication is psychosis. Also, at some point patients should be warned of the dangers of developing tardive dyskinesia. Although the risk may be small, especially if the dose is small, patients with paranoid trends who believe nothing is wrong with them psychiatrically are going to balk at taking a medication that may cause a possibly permanent movement disorder. Unfortunately, tardive dyskinesia is more likely to develop in older women,[72] who compose the majority of our patient population.

If patients are destroying their lives (and may even be suicidal), however, the risk is well worth the treatment. As previously mentioned, a psychiatric consultation is highly desirable but not in every case practicable. Consulting a standard text is advisable.[73-76] If the dentist is forced to start treatment using a neuroleptic agent, communication with a psychiatrist in a supervisory capacity is advisable.

Haloperidol can be an apt choice as a neuroleptic, because studies support its use as an analgesic.[77,78] As mentioned, pimozide may be more specific for monosymptomatic delusions.

SCHIZOPHRENIA

Schizophrenia usually entails more bizarre delusions than does delusional disorder, somatic type.[79] Patients may also have hallucinations and loosening of associations. One young schizophrenic patient who complained of severe unilateral facial pain also complained of excruciating pain in the soles of his feet. He firmly believed there was a wire or nerve connecting these two sensations of pain. Other examples of bizarre delusions are believing that one is controlled by outside forces, believing that people can read one's mind, and hearing sounds or voices in one's teeth. This disorder usually requires treatment with a neuroleptic (antipsychotic) medication.

BEYOND PSYCHOTROPICS

Even if patients with atypical facial pain are compliant with medication trials and receive significant benefit, they may still continue to have some pain, especially if the pain was present for many years. At this point, some other psychologic intervention may be indicated, especially if a patient is still dissatisfied or disabled. Referral to a multidisciplinary pain clinic,[80] to biofeedback training, or to some other behavioral or psychotherapeutic modality is then in order.[81-84]

REFERENCES

1. Moulton, R.E.: Psychiatric consideration in maxillo-facial pain. J. Am. Dent. Assoc. 51:408–409, 1955.
2. Lascellos, R.G.: Atypical facial pain and depression. Br. J. Psychiatry 112:651–659, 1966.
3. Lesse, S.: Atypical facial pain of psychogenic origin. In *Masked Depression.* S. Lesse (ed.). Jason Aronson, Northvale, New Jersey, pp. 302–317, 1974.
4. Glaser, M.A.: Atypical facial neuralgia. Arch. Intern. Med. 65:340–367, 1940.
5. Devor, M.: The pathophysiology and anatomy of damaged nerve. In *Textbook of Pain.* P.D. Wall and R.

Melzack (eds.). Churchill Livingstone, New York, 1984.
6. Marbach, J.J.: Phantom tooth pain. J. Endod. 4:362, 1978.
7. Marbach, J.J., Hulbrock, J., et al.: Incidence of phantom tooth pain: An atypical facial neuralgia. Oral Surg. 53:190–193, 1982.
8. Kornfeld, D.S. and Finkel, J.B.: *Psychiatric Management for Medical Practitioners.* Grune & Stratton, New York, pp. 461–466, 1982.
9. Kornfeld, D.S. and Finkel, J.B.: p. 464.
10. Kornfeld, D.S. and Finkel, J.B.: p. 462.
11. Klein, D., Gittelman, R., Quitkin, F., and Rifkin, A.: *Diagnosis and Drug Treatment of Psychiatric Disorders: Adults and Children.* Williams & Wilkins, New York, 1980.
12. Baldessarini, R.J.: *Chemotherapy in Psychiatry.* Harvard University Press, Cambridge, 1977.
13. Lesse, S.: p. 305.
14. Sachar, E.J.: Psychobiology of affective disorders. In *Principles of Neural Science.* E.R. Kandel and J.H. Schwartz (eds.). Elsevier North Holland, New York, 1981.
15. Violar, A.: The onset of facial pain. Psychother. Psychosom. 34:11–16, 1980.
16. Blumer, D. and Heilbronn, M.: Chronic pain as a variant of depressive disease. J. Nerv. Ment. Dis. 170:381–406, 1982.
17. Lesse, S.: pp. 302–314.
18. American Psychiatric Association: *Diagnostic and Statistical Manual of Mental Disorders, Third Edition, Revised.* American Psychiatric Association, Washington, D.C., pp. 235–241, 1987.
19. Blumer, D.: p. 384.
20. Beck, A.T., Rush, J.A., Shaw, B., and Emery, G.,: *Cognitive Therapy of Depression.* Guilford Press, New York, 1979.
21. Moulton, R.E.: Psychiatric considerations in maxillo-facial pain. J. Am. Dent. Assoc. 51:408–414, 1955.
22. Webb, H.E. and Lascelles, R.G.: Treatment of facial and head pain associated with depression. Lancet 1:355, 1962.
23. Watson, C.P., Evans, R.J., Reed, K., and Merskey, H.: Amitriptyline versus placebo in postherapeutic neuralgia. Neurology 32:671–673, 1982.
24. Walsh, T.D.: Antidepressants and chronic pain. Clin. Neuropharmacol. 6:271–295, 1983.
25. Mendel, C.M., Klein, R., Chappell, D., et al: A trial of amitriptyline and fluphenazine in the treatment of painful diabetic neuropathy. J.A.M.A. 255:637–639, 1986.
26. Pilowsky, I.: Pain and illness behavior: Assessment and management. In *Textbook of Pain.* P.D. Wall and R. Melzack (eds.). Churchill Livingstone, New York, 1984.
27. Schwartz, L.: The pain-dysfunction syndrome. In *Disorders of the Temporomandibular Joint.* Schwartz (ed.). W.B. Saunders Co., Philadelphia, 1959.
28. Gelenberg, A.J. (ed.): Biological therapies in psychiatry. Massachusetts General Hospital Newsletter. 10:43–44, 1987.
29. Ayd, F. Jr.: Flouxetine: An Antidepressant with Specific Serotonin Uptake Inhibition. International Drug Therapy Newsletter. 23:2, pp. 5–11, 1988. Ayd, F. Jr. (ed.).
30. Dominguez, R., Goldstein, B., et al: A double-blind, placebo-controlled study on Fluvoxamine and

imipramine in depression. J. Clin. Psychiat. 46:84, 1985.

31. Ayd, F. Jr.: Danger of MAOI therapy after fluoxetine withdrawal. International Drug Therapy Newsletter. 24:8, 1989.
32. Sharav, Y. p
33. Baldessarini, R.J.: pp. 75–125, 1979. (See reference 12.)
34. Klein, D., Gittelman, R., Quitkin, F., and Rifkin, A.: pp. 268–302, 449–462. (See reference 11.)
35. Brotman, A., Falk, W., and Gelenberg, A.: *Psychopharmacology, The Third Generation of Progress.* H. Meltzer (ed.). Raven Press, New York, 1987.
36. Gelenberg, A.J. (ed.): Biological therapies in psychiatry. Massachusetts General Hospital Newsletter. 7:37–38, 1984.
37. Klein, D., Gittelman, R., Quitkin, F., and Rifkin, A.: p. 457. (See reference 11.)
38. Bigger, J., Giardina E., et al: Cardiac antiarrhythmic effect of imipramine hydrochloride. N. Engl. J. Med. 296:206–207, 1977.
39. J. Clin. Psychiatry 44:56–211, 1983.
40. Davidson, J.: Seizures and bupropion: A review. J. Clin. Psychiatry 50:256–261, 1989.
41. J. Clin. Psychopharmacol. Vol. 42, Sec. 2, 1981.
42. Davidoff, G., Guarracini, M., Roth, E., et al: Trazodone hydrochloride in the treatment of dysesthetic pain in traumatic myelopathy. Pain 29:151–161, 1987.
43. Lascelles, R.G.: Atypical facial pain and depression. Br. J. Psychiatry 112:651–659, 1966.
44. Lesse, S.: Psychotherapy in combination with antidepressant drugs in patients with severe masked depressions. Am. J. Psychother. 31:185–206, 1977.
45. Regier, D. and Boyd, J.: One month prevalence of mental disorders in the U.S. Arch. Gen. Psychiatry 45:977–986, 1988.
46. Solberg, W., Flint, R., and Brantner, J.P.: Temporomandibular joint. J. Prosthet. Dent. 28:412–421, 1972.
47. American Psychiatric Association: *Diagnostic and Statistical Manual of Mental Disorders, Third Edition.* American Psychiatric Association, Washington, D.C., pp. 230–32, 1980.
48. American Psychiatric Association: *Diagnostic and Statistical Manual of Mental Disorders, Third Edition, Revised.* American Psychiatric Association, Washington, D.C., pp. 235–241, 1987.
49. Engel, G.: Primary atypical facial neuralgia. Psychosomatics 13:375–396, 1951.
50. Engel, G.: p. 377.
51. Engel, G.: p. 387.
52. Gorman, J., Liebowitz, M., Fyer, A., and Stein, J.: A neuroanatomical hypothesis for panic disorder. Am. J. Psychiatry 146:148–158, 1989.
53. American Psychiatric Association: *Diagnostic and Statistical Manual of Mental Disorders, Third Edition, Revised.* American Psychiatric Association, Washington, D.C., pp. 240–241, 1987.
54. American Psychiatric Association: *Diagnostic and Statistical Manual of Mental Disorders, Third Edition, Revised.* American Psychiatric Association, Washington, D.C., p. 238, 1987.
55. Muskin, P.R. and Fyer, A.J.M.: Treatment of panic disorder. J. Clin. Psychopharmacol. 1:81–90, 1981.
56. Chaturvedi, S.: A comparison of depressed and chronic pain patients. Gen. Hosp. Psychiatry. 9:383–386, 1987.
57. Rickels, K. and Schweizer, E.E.: Current pharmaco-

therapy of anxiety and panic. In *Psychopharmacology: The Third Generation of Progress.* H.Y. Meltzer (ed.). Raven, New York, 1987.
58. Rickels, K. and Schweizer, E.E.: p. 1200.
59. Ayd, F. Jr.: Clonazepam: An alprozolam alternative for panic disorder. International Drug Therapy Newsletter. 22:25–27, 1987.
60. Kantor, S.J.: A difficult alprazolam withdrawal. J. Clin. Psychopharmacol. 6:124–125, 1986.
61. Boyd, G.H.: One month prevalence of mental disorders in the U.S. Arch. Gen. Psychiatry 45:977–986, 1988.
62. American Psychiatric Association: *Diagnostic and Statistical Manual of Mental Disorders, Third Edition, Revised.* American Psychiatric Association, Washington, D.C., pp. 235–253, 1987.
63. Harris, M.: Psychogenic aspects of facial pain. Br. Dent. J. 136:199–202, 1974.
64. Pomp, M.: Psychotherapy for the myofascial pain-dysfunction syndrome: A study of factors coinciding with symptom remission. J. Am. Assoc. 89:629–632, 1974.
65. Wilson, D.: Atypical facial neuralgia. J.A.M.A. 99:813–816, 1932.
66. Moulton, R.: Psychiatric considerations in maxillofacial pain. J. Am. Dent. Assoc. 51:408–414, 1955.
67. American Psychiatric Association: *Diagnostic and Statistical Manual of Mental Disorders, Third Edition, Revised.* American Psychiatric Association, Washington, D.C., p. 199, 1987.
68. Delaney, J.F.: Atypical facial pain as a defense against psychosis. Am. J. Psychiatry 133:1151–1154, 1976.
69. Munro, A.: Monosymptomatic hypochondriacal psychosis. Br. J. Psychiatry (Suppl. 2) 153:37–40, 1988.
70. Birtchnell, S.A.: Dysmorphobia. Br. J. Psychiatry (Suppl. 2) 153:41–43, 1988.
71. Marback, J.J.: Phantom bite syndrome. Am. J. Psychiatry 135:476–479, 1978.
72. Klein, D., Gittelman, R., Quitkin, F., and Rifkin, A.: pp. 181–189. (See reference 11.)
73. Appleton, W.S.: *Practical Clinical Psychopharmacology.* Williams & Wilkins, New York, 1981.
74. Bassuk, E.L., Schoonover, S.C., and Gelenberg, A.J.: *The Practitioner's Guide to Psychoactive Drugs.* Plenum Press, New York, 1988.
75. Baldessarini, R.J.: 1977. (See reference 12.)
76. Klein, D., Gittelman, R., Quitkin, F., and Rifkin, A.: 1980. (See reference 11.)
77. Daw, J. and Cohen-Cole, S.: Haloperidol analgesia. South. Med. J. 74:364–365, 1981.
78. Cavenar, J.O. Jr. and Maltebie, A.: Another indication for haloperidol. Psychosomatics 17:128–130, 1976.
79. American Psychiatric Association: *Diagnostic and Statistical Manual of Mental Disorders, Third Edition, Revised.* American Psychiatric Association, Washington, D.C., pp. 187–198, 1987.
80. Bonica, J.J.: Basic principles in managing chronic pain. Arch. Surg. 112:783–788, 1977.
81. Philips, H.: *The Psychological Management of Chronic Pain.* Springer Publishing Co., New York, 1988.
82. Turner, J.A. and Chapman, R.C.: Psychological interventions for chronic pain: A critical review. I. Relaxation training and biofeedback. Pain 12:1–21, 1982.
83. Turner, J.A. and Chapman, R.C.: Psychological interventions for chronic pain: A critical review. II. Operant conditioning, hypnosis and cognitive behavioral therapy. Pain 12:23–46, 1982.
84. Wall, P. and Melzack, R. (eds.): *Textbook of Pain.* Churchill Livingstone, New York, pp. 776–840, 1984.

Rebecca Castaneda

CHAPTER 28

Occlusal Adjustment

Although the precise role of occlusion in temporomandibular disorders (TMDs) is unclear, dentists are obligated to provide a physiologic occlusion for each patient. An identified "nonphysiologic" occlusion should be carefully evaluated and, if found to be related to or resulting from a TMD, brought back to a physiologic status. The temporomandibular joint (TMJ) should be stabilized, forces should be redistributed over dental and articular structures, and function and comfort should be restored.

When a patient presents with an apparent occlusal problem and complains of joint or muscle pain, a prudent clinician should first attempt reversible therapies. Reversible approaches include splint therapy, medication, and physical therapy. The presence of acute signs and symptoms of dysfunction makes it difficult, if not impossible, to adequately diagnose and therefore properly treat an occlusal problem. As with any other pathology, effective management is dependent on first making an accurate diagnosis, identifying what etiologic factors are involved, and then tailoring treatment based on the diagnosis.

After reversible treatment of acute symptoms with a stabilization appliance, dramatic changes often appear in the occlusion. As the muscles relax and articular structures become less inflamed, the true occlusal malrelationships become evident. Only after successful phase I treatment can a proper occlusal analysis and diagnosis be accomplished. A clinician next must answer two questions:

1. Is definitive occlusal therapy necessary?
2. If it is necessary, will occlusal adjustment, prosthetics, orthodontics, surgery, or a combination be the appropriate solution for the presenting problem?

INDICATIONS AND CONTRAINDICATIONS

Occlusal adjustment has two major indications:

1. As a treatment modality complementary to other major occlusal changes that may or may not be associated with TMDs.[4]
2. To alleviate TMDs clearly associated with a nonphysiologic occlusion, usually after phase I treatment.

The first indication includes occlusal adjustment before extensive restorative procedures to establish a stable intercuspal position; after orthodontic treatment to finalize the occlusion; and before, during, and after periodontal therapy to better distribute occlusal forces.

Occlusal equilibration of a patient with a TMD is indicated when it is certain that occlusal interferences cause discomfort after phase I treatment. It also must be certain that occlusal adjustment will be adequate to create a harmonious relationship between the TMJ and the dentition. Occlusal equilibration may also be indicated for patients who have developed occlusal changes as a result of a TMD. Other indications include correction of minor occlusal problems after orthodontic treatment for TMDs, orthognathic surgery, and TMJ surgery.

Contraindications to occlusal equilibration of the patients with TMD include continued presence of pain or discomfort, unacceptable range of motion, instability in the joints, hyperactive masticatory musculature, and unstable psychologic status after phase I therapy.

SPLINT THERAPY

The most common form of treatment to precede occlusal adjustment in patients with TMD is some form of splint therapy. The two general kinds of splint therapy most commonly in use are the stabilization or flat plane splint and the repositioning splint. Stabilization splints are most often utilized for the treatment of muscular disorders and early internal derangements. They are applied chiefly to promote muscle relaxation. Many clinicians believe that these splints can reversibly test the effects of all the elements of an ideal occlusion, previously discussed. They can be balanced in centric relation (CR), anterior guidance can be created, and interferences can be eliminated without difficulty in the acrylic. Proponents of occlusal theories believe that these appliances can be employed as blueprints for creation of a more ideal occlusion, which later can be reproduced in the dentition via occlusal adjustment. The appliance therefore offers clinicians a means for obtaining maxillomandibular stabilization.

Dentists must realize that splints simultaneously do many different things in the mouth, including increasing vertical dimension, unloading joint structures, and relaxing masticatory musculature. Why a splint has helped a particular patient is not always known. Therefore, it is often difficult to confirm the presence of an occlusal etiology per se. This is why occlusal adjustment is used only in selected patients and only after careful planning.

A repositioning splint is more often selected for the treatment of internal derangement (disc displacement) not successfully treated by a stabilization appliance. These splints are not balanced in CR but position the condyles somewhat forward and downward of CR. The goal is to nonsurgically recapture the disc. Although long-term follow up data on repositioning therapy are scant, patients who must be stabilized in this "therapeutically derived position" and who have relatively minor occlusal changes can undergo occlusal adjustment. Usually, however, the posterior teeth need orthodontic or prosthetic treatment to increase the vertical dimension of occlusion.

Before proceeding to occlusal adjustment or any other irreversible procedure, a clinician should first determine if the patient will remain asymptomatic through nightwear of the splint or can be successfully taken off the splint altogether. Many patients are successfully treated in this way with no occlusal intervention. (Splint therapy is discussed in detail in Chapter 23.)

TREATMENT GOALS

The treatment goals for occlusal adjustment include the following:

1. Correction of interferences in centric relation
2. Elimination of a CR-intercuspal position (ICP) slide
3. Elimination of protrusive, laterotrusive, and mediotrusive interferences
4. Creation of a stable position for the condyle, disc, and fossa that coincides with a stable centric occlusion or therapeutically derived position

5. Redirection of occlusal forces down the long axis of the teeth.

Clark and Adler[3] defined the overall goal of occlusal adjustment "to achieve a stable, atraumatic occlusal contact relationship between maxillary and mandibular teeth in maximum intercuspation and in all functional excursive contact positions" and required that the "TM joints be stable in this maximal intercuspal position."

PREREQUISITES

The prerequisites before starting occlusal adjustment are as follows:

1. Total or dramatic reduction in signs and symptoms and restoration of comfortable function. In general, patients should be symptom free for 3 to 6 months after phase I therapy before the clinician initiates definitive occlusal therapy, if necessary.
2. A relationship should be identified between the presenting signs and symptoms and occlusal instability.
3. It must be clear that occlusal adjustment will be an adequate treatment approach to remedy the occlusal problem.

DETERMINATION OF THE MOST APPROPRIATE FORM OF DEFINITIVE THERAPY

In general, the least invasive form of treatment that can achieve a comfortable, stable, functional occlusion and condylar position will be the most appropriate. Options include occlusal equilibration, fixed and removable prosthodontics, orthodontics, surgery, or any combination. In some situations, occlusal adjustment may be the most appropriate treatment. A final decision of which form of definitive occlusal therapy to use is made after a thorough examination, occlusal analysis, and careful evaluation of the diagnostic casts.

PATIENT WORKUP

As previously noted, definitive occlusal therapy after phase I TMD therapy is generally after a 3- to 6-month symptom-free period. The length of the holding period is a clinical decision based on chronicity, severity, and complexity of the disorder.[5] Taking a careful history helps provide the clinician with the information necessary to meet the most important prerequisite for definitive occlusal therapy, the resolution of symptoms.

The preocclusal correction examination consists of a clinical examination, occlusal analysis with mounted diagnostic casts, imaging of the TMJs, and in some patients mandibular tracking. A thorough clinical examination includes evaluation of the TMJs, mandibular range of motion, masticatory and cervical muscles, oral structures, and occlusion. The clinical findings should agree with the patient's subjective report of symptom status. Any indication of pain or dysfunction reported by the patient or evidenced by the clinical examination should direct the clinician to re-examine the diagnosis and to initiate alternative treatment. Complete remission of joint noise (clicking and crepitus) may not be necessary provided there is no associated pain. In this situation, however, the clinician must recognize that the disc may not be in proper anatomic position, and therefore, a true CR, by definition, will be unobtainable. Occlusal adjustment is then being performed in what may be a compromised situation, and the patient should be so advised.

Occlusal Analysis

An intraoral examination of the occlusion has limitations and should be complemented with mounted diagnostic casts. Careful notes should be made of the intraoral findings and later compared with the mounted casts. Special attention is paid to any slide from centric occlusion to maximum intercuspal position. The direction and magnitude of such a discrepancy are particularly important. Mediotrusive (nonworking), laterotrusive (working), and protrusive contacts and interferences should also be noted.

When evaluating the CR-ICP slide, first place the patient in a reclining position and manipulate the mandible so that the condyles are seated in their CR position. Several techniques to do this have been suggested, including the leaf gauge technique,[6] bimanual manipulation,[7] and the one-handed guidance methods.[5] I prefer the bimanual manipulation technique, although the other techniques are equally effective if done properly. Bimanual manipulation can be selected for evaluating centric occlusion intraorally and for making CR interocclusal records for mounting diagnostic casts. It is impossible to make a careful analysis of the occlusion without the ability to accurately manipulate the patient into CR (Fig. 28–1).

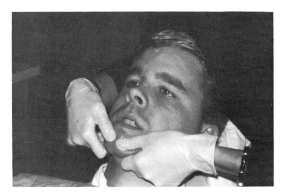

FIGURE 28–1. Demonstration of bimanual manipulation of the mandible into centric relation.

After successful phase I therapy, the relaxed masticatory musculature makes manipulation of the mandible possible with little resistance from the patient. If for some reason the patient has not undergone appliance therapy or is no longer wearing an occlusal appliance, the masticatory muscles can be relaxed or "deprogrammed" by placing cotton rolls between the teeth for approximately 10 minutes (Fig. 28–2). Relaxed masticatory musculature is the sine que non for a proper occlusal analysis and occlusal adjustment.

When the hinging CR position is located, the patient is instructed to stop closure on initial contact. Once the tooth contacts are noted, the patient is asked to close into ICP. The nature of the slide from CR to ICP, if present, is then recorded. Pertinent aspects of the slide include the magnitude and direction. CR-ICP slides can be symmetric (in a straight protrusive direction) or asymmetric (toward the left or right).

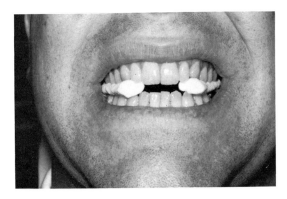

FIGURE 28–2. Deprogramming the masticatory muscles using cotton rolls to disocclude teeth.

The patient is next instructed to slide the mandible forward in a protrusive movement (Fig. 28–3). The presence of posterior tooth interferences should be noted. In addition, the timing of disocclusion of the posterior teeth by anterior guidance should be observed. Lateral excursive movements to the left and right sides are then analyzed for the presence of laterotrusive and mediotrusive contacts. The movements should be of relatively equal angulation and provide for symmetric guidance (Fig. 28–4).

This sequence is repeated to verify the reproducibility of the initial contacts in CR (Fig. 28–5). These contacts are marked with articulating paper, ribbon, and if necessary fine shim stock. The patient is then seated upright and asked to tap the teeth in ICP (Fig. 28–6).

Next, all other evidence of occlusal instability should be recorded, including fremitus and mobility, flared teeth, fractured teeth or restorations, sensitive or painful teeth, and wear facets.

Diagnostic Casts

Choosing the best technique for definitive occlusal therapy is determined by the severity of the malocclusion. Mounted diagnostic casts must be used to better visualize the existing occlusal relationships and to prescribe appropriate treatment. A second set of mounted casts should be made for testing the prescribed occlusal treatment.

The minimal requirements for properly mounting diagnostic casts for occlusal analysis are a semiadjustable arcon articulator, a facebow transfer with an arbitrary hinge axis, and a CR record and a protrusive check bite to set condylar inclination. Whatever the instrumen-

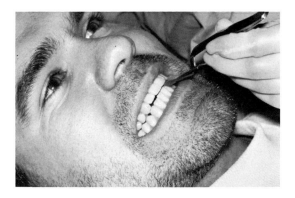

FIGURE 28–4. Recording of laterotrusive and mediotrusive interferences.

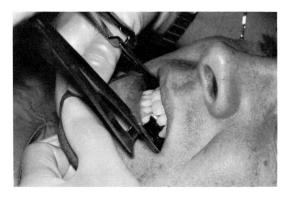

FIGURE 28–5. Recording of centric relation (CR) contacts and verifying the reproducibility of CR.

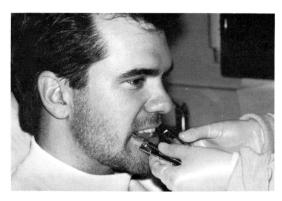

FIGURE 28–6. Recording occlusal contacts in an upright position. The patient is asked to tap the teeth together.

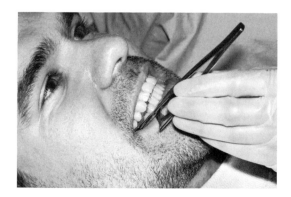

FIGURE 28–3. Recording of posterior interferences in protrusive movement.

tation employed to mount diagnostic casts, it should be remembered that articulators are mechanical devices that approximate but do not reproduce actual mandibular movement. It should also be remembered that anterior guidance has a more immediate and significant effect on mandibular movement in dentate in-

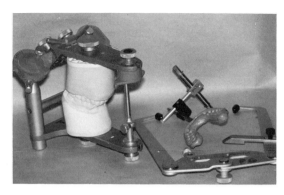

FIGURE 28–7. Semiadjustable arcon articulator and arbitrary hinge axis face-bow.

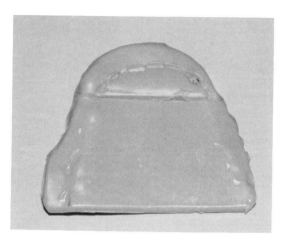

FIGURE 28–9. Delar wax wafer used to register the centric relation. Note the double thickness of the wax in the anterior region.

dividuals than the condylar inclination (Fig. 28–7).

A face-bow transfer should be used to orient the maxillary cast on the articulator (Fig. 28–8). The purpose of the face-bow is to relate the maxillary cast to the articulator and then, together with the CR record, help establish an arc of closure that closely represents that of the patient's. A kinematic face-bow is not necessary and is used primarily in complex restorative cases. The mandibular cast is then related to the maxillary cast with the use of a stable interocclusal record in CR.

Making the Centric Relation Record

As described in the section on occlusal analysis, the mandible is guided into CR, but this time an interocclusal record material is interposed between the teeth and a static registration of the teeth is made.

To do this, the patient is placed in the supine position and the mandible is manipulated into CR several times. I recommend the use of a

single thickness of extra-hard Delar wax posteriorly and a double thickness in the anterior region (Fig. 28–9). With the wax secured on the maxillary teeth, only the mandibular anterior teeth are allowed to register into the double-thickness portion. The wax is then removed from the mouth, chilled, and placed back into the mouth to verify for accuracy. The tooth indentations in the double-thickness portion serve as a guide for the final registration and as a flat anterior stop or jig that helps seat the condyles in CR.

Once the record is verified, it is again removed from the mouth, dried, and lined with a soft wax or registration paste on the mandibular posterior tooth segments and replaced in the mouth (Fig. 28–10). Next, the mandible is guided closed so that the anterior teeth are re-

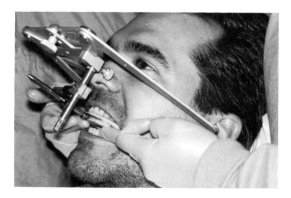

FIGURE 28–8. Face-bow transfer is used to relate the maxillary cast with the articulator.

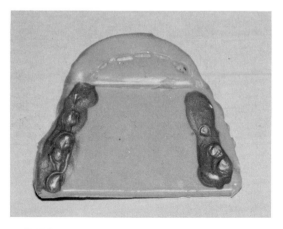

FIGURE 28–10. Completed centric relation record with Aluwax to register the mandibular posterior teeth.

positioned into the wax indentations. The result is a stable CR record that can be utilized to mount both sets of diagnostic casts. Although protrusive records can be employed for setting the condylar inclination, for the purpose of occlusal analysis and diagnostic equilibration, an average setting of 20° is acceptable.

After the diagnostic casts are mounted, the tooth-to-tooth and arch-to-arch relationships are analyzed. A reasonable decision can then be made on the necessity of definitive occlusal treatment and on which technique is most appropriate.

Okeson[4] recommends "the rule of thirds" as a convenient guide in selecting an effective technique. The rule of thirds is based on the severity of the discrepancy of the buccal-lingual tooth and arch relationships (Fig. 28–11).[4]

If the diagnostic casts reveal that centric cusp tips are in close proximity to opposing central fossae or marginal ridges, occlusal adjustment may be an adequate choice to stabilize the occlusion. If the centric cusp tips approach the opposing centric cusp tips, however, orthodontics may be necessary. In extreme situations, combinations of orthodontics, orthognathic surgery, and prosthodontic treatment may be needed. Buccal-lingual tooth relationships between these two extremes can often be adequately treated with fixed prosthodontics alone.

The selected treatment procedure must be tested to predict treatment outcome. With selective grinding, a diagnostic equilibration on a second set of diagnostic casts is mandatory. This exercise helps predetermine the areas and

amount of tooth structure that will need to be removed and the likelihood of dentin exposure, a situation better accepted by patients if planned for in advance.

Other factors, including the condition of the present dentition and periodontium as well as aesthetics, have to be considered in the final treatment plan. If occlusal equilibration is the treatment of choice, the patient must still be prepared for the possibility of treatment complications, in particular, the need for restorations such as crowns and onlays. This possibility should be discussed with the patient before beginning the procedure.

EQUILIBRATION PROCEDURE

According to Dawson,[7] equilibration is divided into four stages:

1. The elimination of tooth surfaces that interfere with CR closure
2. Selective elimination of tooth surfaces that interfere with lateral excursions, depending on the guidance pattern
3. The elimination of posterior tooth surfaces that interfere with protrusive excursions, with some exceptions as in severe class II division II occlusion
4. Harmonization of the anterior guidance.

Dawson's technique assumes that the condylar position is CR, however, following repositioning therapy, the condylar position may be forward of CR in a "therapeutically derived" position. A patient out of necessity is sometimes treated "off the discs." An attempt

A 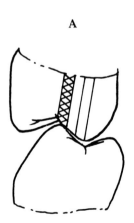   B 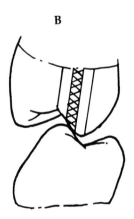   C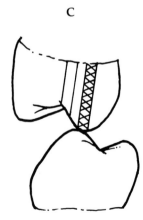

FIGURE 28–11. The rule of thirds. (Reprinted with permission from Okeson, J.: *Fundamentals of Occlusion and TMD,* 2nd ed. C.V. Mosby Co., St. Louis, 1989.

should be made to follow repositioning therapy with a stabilization splint before proceeding with any form of definitive occlusal treatment.

In preparation for occlusal equilibration, patients can be premedicated with an antisialogogue such as scopolamine or an antihistamine. A dry field is critical when using articulating paper or ribbon. If patients are apprehensive about the procedure, a low dose of a sedative such as diazepam can be prescribed before the equilibration appointment. This facilitates manipulation of the mandible by minimizing significant resistance by the patient.

The following is suggested armamentarium for the equilibration procedure:

- Thin marking films of different colors
- Thin articulating paper of various colors
- Articulating paper holders
- Small flame-shaped stones and diamonds of various coarseness
- Small flame-shaped 12-fluted carbide burs
- Polishing stones and rubber points for smoothing contoured enamel and restorations
- Shim stock
- Occlusal indicator wax.

Equilibration by selective grinding is a tedious procedure, and sufficient time must be allocated. Multiple appointments are almost always needed. The length and frequency of appointments should be based on the extent of the equilibration.

Equilibration Sequence

Although some gnathologists advocate first equilibrating eccentric interferences in CR, it is generally agreed that the reverse order minimizes the risk of changing the vertical dimension of occlusion and allows for greater control in redistributing occlusal forces.

Step 1. Interferences to CR Closure. These interferences include those contacts that cause the mandible to shift from CR to a more stable maximum ICP. The goal is to reshape all inclines into either a cusp tip or a convex surface so that the occlusal forces are directed along the long axis of the teeth.[4] Which incline to reshape is determined by which adjustment will direct the occlusal forces more in line with the long axis of the teeth[7] and which adjustment will not eliminate centric holding contacts.

The mandible is guided by the clinician into CR using bimanual manipulation, described earlier, while the dental assistant holds the ar-

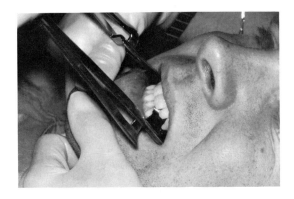

FIGURE 28–12. The dental assistant holds the articulating paper in place while the dentist manipulates the mandible into centric relation.

ticulating paper or ribbon between the dried teeth (Fig. 28–12). Inclines are reshaped into cusp tips or flat surfaces that follow the original natural tooth contour without widening the occlusal table. The goal is to have multiple bilateral simultaneous contacts on posterior teeth and lighter contacts on the anterior teeth (Fig. 28–13).

Step 2. Interferences in Protrusion. Reduction of excursive contacts requires caution so as not to eliminate centric holding contacts. Centric holding contacts should be marked in one color of articulating ribbon; another color ribbon marks excursive contacts (Fig. 28–14). Straight protrusive guidance is established on incisor teeth bilaterally, whereas more lateroprotrusive movements progressively involve opposing cuspids on the same side. For this step in the equilibration process, patients are asked to glide their teeth forward while articulating ribbon is held between the teeth bilaterally.

Step 3. Interferences in Laterotrusion. Cuspid guidance in laterotrusion is established or maintained wherever possible, only if excessive reduction of tooth structure can be avoided. When canine guidance is not achievable, group function is established on buccal cusps of posterior teeth, keeping working group contacts as anterior as possible. Again, use of one color of marking ribbon to mark lateral excursive contacts, followed by another color to identify centric holding contacts, helps to minimize the inadvertent reduction of the CR contacts.

Eliminating working side interferences follows the *b*uccal *u*pper *l*ingual *l*ower (BULL) rule: Interferences are eliminated by adjusting the buccal cusps of upper teeth and the lingual

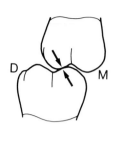
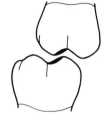
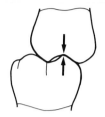

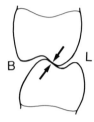
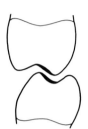
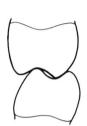

FIGURE 28–13. Occlusal interferences are reshaped into cusp tips or flat surfaces.

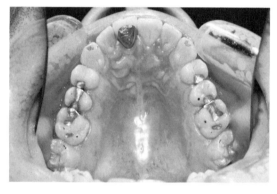

FIGURE 28–14. Centric relation and eccentric tooth contacts are differentiated by using articulating paper of different colors.

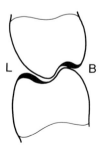

FIGURE 28–15. BULL rule. Interferences are adjusted on the *b*uccal cusps of the *u*pper teeth and *l*ingual cusps of the *l*ower teeth.

cusps of lower teeth (Fig. 28–15). Mediotrusive or nonworking interferences are adjusted on the buccal inclines of maxillary lingual cusps and on the lingual inclines of mandibular buccal cusps. Caution is taken not to adjust cusp tips, but if this becomes necessary, either the maxillary or the mandibular cusp tip alone is adjusted to avoid the loss of CR contacts. Laterotrusive and mediotrusive contacts are alternately evaluated and adjusted, because the elimination of interference of one type may cause an interference in the other.

Parafunctional activity often involves ex-

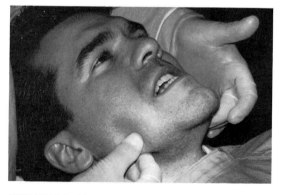

FIGURE 28–16. Parafunctional tooth contacts are best identified by assisting patients through forceful excursive movements.

treme border movements and heavy masticatory forces not evident in the routine dental examination or procedures, so it is critical to identify border movements and extraneous contacts used in parafunctional activities. This is done by assisting patients, through lateral excursive movements with manual, medial force applied on the angle of the mandible and by having them clench in the lateral excursion position (Fig. 28–16). This maneuver mimics parafunctional activity and reveals interferences otherwise not evident.

Finalizing the Equilibration Procedure

The last step in the equilibration process is to evaluate tooth contacts while the patient is in the sitting position. The upright position will change jaw posture and often produces heavier contacts on anterior teeth. Here patients are asked to close on their back teeth while articulating ribbon is held between the teeth (Fig. 28–17). Anterior tooth contacts are carefully adjusted until posterior tooth contacts are felt to be heavier by the patient and then verified with shim stock. This step reduces the likelihood of primary occlusal trauma to the anterior teeth.

Occlusal equilibration should not be done in a single appointment, because patients become fatigued and resistant to manipulation sooner than clinically evident. After each session, the enamel and restored surfaces that have been adjusted should be smoothed and polished with rubber wheels. Leaving rough surfaces on teeth may provoke patients to seek out the rough surfaces and can result in muscle hyperactivity.

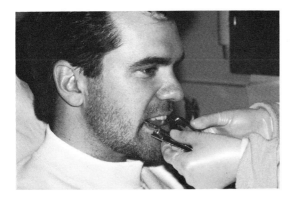

FIGURE 28–17. Final evaluation of tooth contacts in the sitting position.

Equilibration Following Repositioning Appliance Therapy

When repositioning therapy is employed, the resultant mandibular position is commonly anterior and inferior to the CR position. If occlusal equilibration is the treatment chosen to finalize the occlusion, manipulation is not a reliable technique to reproduce the mandibular position determined by the appliance. The procedure for equilibration is to allow patients to close into what has become the therapeutically derived position determined by the appliance. Repeatability of this position is important and should prove stable for a 3- to 6-month period before equilibration. If patients are treated anterior to CR, the anterior position should not be more than 1 mm forward from CR. Equilibration to this position provides for a "long centric."

The same stepwise procedure previously described is used for equilibration in the therapeutically derived position. The appliance is worn by patients between appointments so that the therapeutic position is maintained. Although there is much controversy regarding repositioning therapy, it is indicated in selected patients, usually with internal derangement, when other treatment modalities fail to bring relief. Definitive occlusal therapy after repositioning therapy often involves orthodontics, prosthodontics, or surgery, but equilibration should be employed if possible as the least invasive treatment approach.

Currently, there is insufficient evidence to warrant routine prophylactic equilibration of patients with occlusal interferences.[3,8] Occlusal equilibration is indicated if occlusal trauma has been identified or if occlusal stabilization is supportive of other major prosthodontic or orthodontic therapy. The diagnostic process of occlusal equilibration is the most important part of the treatment, and extreme caution is needed in every step of this procedure.

REFERENCES

1. Mohl, N.D., Zarb, G.A., Carlsson, G., and Rugh, J. (eds.): *A Textbook of Occlusion.* Quintessence Publishing Co., Lombard, IL, 1988.
2. McNeill, C.: The optimal temporomandibular joint condyle position in clinical practice. Int. J. Periodont. Rest. Dent. 6:53–76, 1985.
3. Clark, G.T. and Adler, R.C.: A critical evaluation of occlusal therapy: Occlusal adjustment procedures. J. Am. Dent. Assoc. 110:743–751, 1985.
4. Okeson, J.P.: *Fundamentals of Occlusion and Temporomandibular Disorders.* C.V. Mosby, St. Louis, 1985.

5. McNeill, C.: Presented in a Symposium on Head, Neck and TMJ Pain. Maui, Hawaii, 1989.
6. McHorris, W.H.: Occlusal adjustment via selective cutting of natural teeth. Part I. Int. J. Periodont. Rest. Dent. 5:9–25, 1985.
7. Dawson, P.E.: *Evaluation, Diagnosis and Treatment of Occlusal Problems,* 2nd ed. C.V. Mosby, St. Louis, 1989.
8. Wenneberg, B., Nystrom, T., and Carlsson, G.: Occlusal equilibration and other stomatognathic treatment in patients with mandibular dysfunction and headaches. J. Prosthet. Dent. 59:478–483, 1988.

Donald Tanenbaum

CHAPTER 29

Prosthodontic Therapy

Restoration of the occlusion with fixed or removable prosthodontics has been described as both a cause and a treatment of temporomandibular disorders (TMDs). This chapter discusses both constructive and destructive aspects of prosthodontics. Although there is little scientific documentation on the effects of prosthodontic treatment on the temporomandibular joint (TMJ), there is no shortage of opinion. Throughout the chapter, what can be documented is, and what is clinical observation or opinion is stated as such.

EVALUATION OF PATIENTS BEFORE PROSTHETIC TREATMENT

As common practice, each patient in a dental office should receive at least a screening examination for temporomandibular joint (TMJ) function. This examination should include palpation for muscle tonus, assessment for joint and muscle tenderness, measurement of mandibular range of motion, and palpation for joint sounds. Radiographs of the TMJ are not necessary unless pathology is suspected. Examination procedures are discussed in detail in Chapter 17.

Many patients with subclinical TMJ symptoms may not complain of masticatory pain or altered function at the time of an initial examination. On careful questioning and examination, however, problems with pain and dysfunction may become apparent. Failure, then, to evaluate muscular and TMJ function can potentially compromise the masticatory health of a patient and put the practitioner at risk for accusations of negligence. An example is a patient who presents for treatment with asymptomatic clicking and describes several episodes of intermittent limitation of mandibular movement. An astute practitioner will suspect that these signs might represent a possible intracapsular joint problem that requires further investigation before treatment is begun. Such attention will help establish realistic treatment expectations and define the potential risks of keeping the mouth open for long periods. Understanding this information and sharing it with patients before treatment is critical to proper management. Inadequate planning and explanation may not only lead to a worsening of a patient's physical status, but also strained and potentially litigious clinician-patient relations.

PROSTHODONTIC TREATMENT LEADING TO TEMPOROMANDIBULAR JOINT DISORDERS

Clinical experience has shown that certain aspects of restorative treatment can lead to both self-limited and persistent TMDs. Some are rather obvious, but others are controversial. Long treatment sessions, injection trismus, and "high" restorations all have been known to initiate periods of pain or jaw dysfunctions. Long treatment sessions that require patients to keep their mouths open for extended periods of time can lead to inflammation of the capsule and retrodiscal tissues, as well as muscle pain.[1] These problems can be particularly damaging to the patient with a pre-existing subclinical TMD. Mandibular block injection through the medial pterygoid muscle can result in trismus and a complaint of limited opening that can last for several weeks.

The simplest of occlusal problems and the one that most often creates acute masticatory muscle pain is the failure to properly equilibrate a newly placed restoration. Lack of equilibration is thought to stimulate bruxism in some patients; in others it creates aberrant closing and chewing patterns in an effort to avoid the prematurity.[2]

In addition to these three common and fairly universally agreed on causes, a host of other prosthodontic factors have been implicated in TMDs. These include inadequate molar support, distal bracing and guiding contacts, lateral retrusive canine guidance, insufficient or excessive vertical dimension, gross centric and excursive prematurities, and incorrect maxillary and mandibular anterior tooth relationships.

Among the most controversial is the issue of vertical dimension. On one hand, it has been postulated that insufficient vertical dimension causes distalization of the mandibular condyles, intracapsular tissue loading, ligamentous laxity, and subsequent disc displacement and joint derangement.[3] Clinical testimonials rather than scientific studies support this notion. On the other hand, vertical dimension that is too great has also been implicated in causing TMDs. This concept is based on the premise that excessive vertical dimension can obliterate freeway space, promoting hyperirritability and subsequent pain and dysfunction in the muscles of mastication.[4] Again, scientific documentation for this phenomenon is lacking, but common clinical observation supports this hypothesis.

In fact, most epidemiologic studies have failed to show a definitive correlation between specific occlusal schemes and the presence or severity of mandibular dysfunction. Alternatively, no evidence supports the concept that any specific occlusal pattern offers the greatest therapeutic potential. Any prosthetic dogma that advocates this message is inappropriate.

Clinical observations are consequently very important and should serve as the impetus for clinicians to plan prosthetic therapy based on the pre-existing structural and functional integrity of each individual patient's masticatory system. This approach alone will enable practitioners to successfully handle both normal and compromised clinical situations.

OCCLUSAL THERAPY

Definitive occlusal therapy has been cited as an alternative in the management of temporomandibular disorders. Occlusal equilibration, prosthetic reconstruction, and orthodontics have been advocated.[5-7]

Clinicians and patients are justifiably hesitant to proceed with this kind of treatment, however, for the following reasons:

1. A high probability exists that the body's reparative capacity coupled with assistive and reversible treatment modalities is sufficient to provide pain relief and restoration of function.[8]
2. Uncertainty exists regarding the long-term stability of newly created occlusal/jaw relationships.
3. Considerable time and high cost are necessary to complete treatment.

It is well documented that most patients presenting with TMDs are successfully managed with reversible therapies. Some patients do, however, require prosthetic occlusal stabilization. Most of these patients appear to have one common clinical trait: the presence of irreversible intracapsular tissue injury. These injuries can be due to a recognizable traumatic incident or can be a function of long-standing microtrauma. Structural deficits, functional compensations, and parafunctional activity may play a role in the etiology. Definitive occlusal therapy in patients with TMDs may also be indicated in the following instances:

1. Pre-existing fixed or removable restorations that need to be replaced because of caries, excessive wear, tooth loss, or other reasons
2. Patients who have been treated with repositioning therapy and have a posterior open bite due to maxillomandibular postural changes
3. Patients who have undergone TMJ or orthognathic surgery with resultant occlusal changes
4. An occasional need for prosthetic completion of cases stabilized with orthodontics in which proper supporting occlusion was difficult or impossible to establish.

Three prerequisites for sound clinical care are as follows:

1. Identification of the specific etiologic and perpetuating factors that may have played a causal role
2. Recognition of which tissues have been injured beyond the point of natural healing capacity
3. Appreciation of how the principles of physiologic occlusal stabilization can be used to provide an "adaptive-healing environment" for injured tissues without, at the same time, overloading the periodontium.

It is paramount for clinicians, *before treatment,* to thoroughly evaluate available historical, clinical, and radiographic information and supplement as needed. Aside from helping to formulate a diagnosis, this information helps establish a realistic prognosis. A decision to provide irreversible prosthetic treatment must be based on objective data and careful evaluation rather than on subjective opinion.

ETIOLOGIC AND PERPETUATING FACTORS

Disorders of the temporomandibular joint are usually classified as being myogenous (extracapsular) or arthrogenous (intracapsular).

The pattern of onset, duration of pain, and functional disability experienced are variable.[9] The symptoms commonly are benign, short lived, and resolve with limited supportive therapy. The cause often remains a mystery. In other instances, chronic nonrespondent pain may persist following a single recognizable traumatic incident.

Nevertheless, TMDs can be diagnosed and managed if the parameters of the "etiologic triad" are understood.[10] As with all human pathophysiology, pain and disability result when there is loss of homeostatic balance between the triad components: host resiliency and local structural integrity, intrinsic and extrinsic loading, and emotional reactivity. The greater the loss of homeostatic balance, the greater the potential for irreversible tissue injury, the persistence of associated complaints, and the necessity for more aggressive care.

Because it is not the intent of this chapter to discuss the etiology of TMDs, a full review of this information is not undertaken. Several key concepts, however, should be reviewed as they relate to the issue of tissue injury, repair, and appropriateness of prosthetic therapeutic intervention.

Joint loading can be caused by microtrauma and macrotrauma.[11] Microtrauma is described as insidious and persistent traumatic exposures, whereas macrotrauma is usually related to a single episode. Both can produce irreversible tissue injury, but the continuance of microtrauma can compromise natural healing capacity and the efficacy of treatment modalities. Microtrauma includes parafunctional activity (bruxism, clenching, nail biting) and overuse, which may accompany vocational activities and habitual postural causal factors. If microtrauma cannot be stopped or adequately controlled, compromise must be made and reflected in the approach taken toward prosthetic rehabilitation. The choice of restoration (fixed or removable), material used on the occlusal surfaces, occlusal scheme and morphology, condylar position, and necessity of future appliance wear all are influenced.

A review of the literature also suggests that microtraumatic injury within the masticatory system, in some instances, can be attributed solely to the pre-existing skeletal/occlusal environment.[12–15] Without the presence of parafunction or vocational strain, it has been suggested that structural factors such as inadequate molar support, class II division 2 malocclusions, premaxilla underdevelopment, unilateral cross bite, distal bracing and guiding contacts, lateral retrusive canine guidance, mandibular plane angle, and gross centric and excursive prematurities can produce sufficient soft-tissue and hard-tissue strain and perpetuate irreversible tissue injuries.

These postulates are based on the premise that structural inadequacies or imbalances can produce chronic bodily mandibular displacement. Over time, tissue fatigue and injury result. Whether healing or degeneration occurs often relates to issues of a host's adaptive capacity, which is not well researched at this time.

TISSUE INJURY: HEALING VS. DEGENERATION

Normal functioning of the masticatory system is dependent on the integrity of its investing tissues (muscles, ligaments, tendons, nerves, articular elements) and their compatibility with existing occlusal elements. Abnormal function, mechanical failure, and pain symptoms relate to both muscular dysfunction (see chapter 8) and joint derangement (see chapter 9).[16] The initial appearance and persistence of pain and functional disability are indicative of tissue injury.

In the masticatory system, tissue injury secondary to noxious insult can have the following effects:

1. It can result in healing and a return to physiologic normalcy.
2. It can generate cellular or morphologic adaptive processes capable of sustaining pain-free function (progressive remodeling).
3. It can compromise tissue integrity to the extent that mechanical dysfunction with or without pain persists (regressive remodeling).
4. It can lead to chronic pain and functional disability.

Healing is dependent not only on the nature of the trauma (intensity, duration, frequency) but also on the inherent healing capacity of the specific tissue and secondary involvement of associated structures. Tissues with poor vascularity, low metabolic activity, and high functional demands heal poorly. Ligaments, discs, tendon sheaths, joint capsules, and protective fibrocartilage are such tissues. Because these tissues make up most of the intracapsular environment, the potential for slow or poor healing exists. As the resultant pain or dysfunction persists following an acute injury, secondary tissue changes often occur, compromising adaptive physiologic processes and extending the healing time. These tissue changes are commonly noted after injury to the ligaments of the TMJ. Subsequent disc displacement can provide an environment for change in the retrodiscal tissue, pterygoid musculature, synovial lining, and capsular and osseous networks. These changes increase the likelihood that the primary ligamentous injury will become irreversible.

Tissues with good vascularity and high metabolic activity have excellent capacity for repair as long as injurious loading forces are controlled. Muscular and osseous tissues that have such capacity often heal favorably at the cellular and morphologic level. If these tissues fail to heal, other perpetuating factors must be suspected.

Because the healing potential of a tissue cannot be predicted and the inherent vascular and metabolic potential of tissues cannot be altered, regaining function and eliminating pain are ultimately dependent on controlling loading at the site of injury. Within the masticatory system, mechanical alteration of normal "functional" occlusal or skeletal patterns and control of parafunctional loading may be the key ingredients for success. For this reason, the use of occlusal splints has been advocated.[17,18] Often called *phase I therapy,* the use of these appliances may be all the treatment needed or may be the initial stage or "blueprint" for future prosthetic rehabilitation.

The splint type, the time that it is worn, and the need for subsequent prosthetic stabilization are determined by the nature of the tissue injury (diagnosis), the presence or absence of ongoing loading (parafunction), and the nature of the pre-existing occlusal environment. Splint therapy is discussed in detail in Chapter 24.

Because the focus of this chapter is prosthetic rehabilitation for patients with TMD, further comments address the appliances that serve as blueprints for restorative therapy. These appliances, often called *repositioning splints* (Fig. 29–1), are designed to unload injured intracapsular tissue by distraction or by changing the spatial relationships between the condyle, disc, temporal fossa, and articular eminence. In order to be successful, the unloading must be constant. Full-time wear is required, often creating the need for occlusal rehabilitation because of ligament, disc, osseous, and muscle changes that occur during months of appliance wear. Tooth and maxillomandibular changes

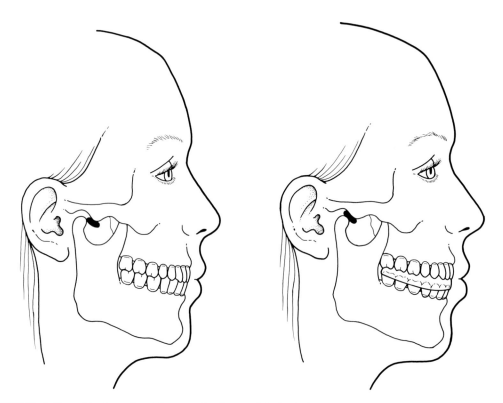

FIGURE 29–1. Repositioning splints. These can be designed for both the maxillary and mandibular arches. The splints change condylar position in the attempt to unload injured joint tissues.

also accompany repositioning therapy. It is hoped that the trade-off is cessation of pain and improved function.

It is my opinion that repositioning therapy is mainly utilized to manage persistent intracapsular tissue pathologies. The associated diagnostic categories include partial or total disc displacement disorders with associated ligamentous and capsular incompetence, retrodiscal tissue distortion, synovial proliferation, and osseous degeneration.

Repositioning therapy must be done in a manner that promotes tissue adaptation and minimizes uncoordinated muscle function and pathologic mandibular displacement. Proper appliance design is essential if painless function is to be achieved.

PRINCIPLES OF PHYSIOLOGIC OCCLUSAL STABILIZATION

A distinguishing feature of a *healthy* TMJ is that it is able to support itself and the teeth, not the converse.

The position, shape, and specific occlusal pattern of the teeth only serve to influence certain postures and *limit* specific movements of the TMJ during functional activity.[19]

In a normal TMJ environment, all excursions of the mandibular condyles are guided by neuromuscular mechanisms during which firm contact is maintained between the articulating components. In addition, border movements are limited by the tautness of the ligaments and, to some extent, by the hard structures. As long as the integrity of these extracapsular and intracapsular tissues exists, there should be no further demands on the dentition.[20]

If irreversible tissue injury occurs, however, the structural mechanisms responsible for condylar guidance, Bennett's side shift, and resting and centric occlusion may be compromised. Confronted with this possibility, a clinician must judge whether or not the dental occlusion can be predictably utililized in specific ways to protect and stabilize these fragile tissues. In considering this possibility, clinicians break down occlusal design into component parts: treatment position, occlusal scheme and morphology, occlusal table, and vertical dimension.[21,22]

Treatment Position

The term *internal derangement* has been used extensively in the literature to describe pathology found in the intracapsular environ-

ment. The specific stages are based on the degree of deviation from normal disc alignment, disc shape, ligament sufficiency, and osseous integrity. Dawson's classification of stages I through V reviews this progression.[23] The three most commonly utilized occlusal positions for prosthetic restoration in patients with TMDs are as follows:

1. Centric relation (CR)
2. Centric occlusion (CO)
3. Therapeutically derived (TD) treatment position.

Centric relation is defined as a border position located at the posterior apex of the envelope of mandibular motion. It exists when the condyles are bilaterally unstrained in their most anterior-superior position. The condyle must be in intimate contact with the intermediate band of the menisci and braced medially against the posterior slope of the eminence at a given vertical dimension. Intact capsular/intracapsular ligaments, nonhyperactive musculature, and a biconcave disc are prerequisites for CR to be a treatment position.[24–26] In the presence of a pathologic intracapsular environment, CR is difficult to obtain and unlikely to remain stable or reproducible.

A CR treatment position may be indicated if the internal derangement is in an early stage (see chapter 9) and thought to be related to an occlusomuscular etiology. For example, the removal of occlusal interferences or the enhancement of posterior occlusal stops may decrease existing mandibular displacement and resulting incoordination, hyperactivity, and joint loading. If the occlusion is optimized in the CR position, progressive remodeling, rather than progressive damage to the articular components, can be expected. The danger is that the disease may be more advanced than the dentist realizes and that intervention creates a therapeutic occlusion that holds the condyles more posteriorly than might be advisable for any but the milder forms of internal derangement.

Management of a pathologic joint that cannot accommodate a CR position requires a choice between CO and a TD treatment position. Both are considered nonborder positions, except where CO is coincident with CR. This is unlikely, however, without previous dental intervention or the presence of distalizing inclines.

In normal and abnormal joints, these nonborder positions provide a range of safety for the structures of the TMJs. They position the condyles away from damaged tissues. A major problem is that among the infinite number of nonborder positions, none except CO in dentulous patients is easily reproducible.

Potential TD positions are neuromuscularly determined and are arrived at arbitrarily or with the use of splint therapy, TMJ radiography, or electronic instrumentation. In addition, TD positions are subject to change in response to alterations in body and head position. For these reasons, it is preferable to use the pre-existing CO position with or without intermittent appliance wear, if at all possible.

Centric occlusion is defined as the position of the mandible when all teeth are fully interdigitated and no tension or imbalance is observable in the masticatory system. This is considered the normal posture that the jaws assume immediately on closing from the rest position. Because resting postures can vary, the path to CO can also vary. Thus, a slide from the first occlusal contact to true CO may be considered to be within the normal range of activity.[27] Centric occlusion is usually inferior to the superior border and lateral to the medial border of the envelope of mandibular movement.[28]

When it is easily reproducible, CO is the position of choice for prosthetic treatment in a patient with damage beyond that which can be improved with repositioning or CR therapy. This is often seen with late stage internal derangement with reduction when surgery is not being considered. In these instances, the intermittent use of a nonrepositioning or stabilization appliance for 8 to 12 hours a day may be necessary and may be the end point in treatment. After some time, remodeling may take place and result in reasonably well functioning and pain-free mandibular movement. Centric occlusion may also be an appropriate position to restore the occlusion in patients who have undergone open joint surgery or arthroscopy.[29]

When neither the CR nor CO treatment position is plausible, the utilization of a TD condylar position may be indicated. The primary indication is the presence of persistent intracapsular tissue injury (i.e., displaced disc that can be consistently recaptured and stabilized). In addition is the presence of a displaced disc, which can be consistently recaptured and stabilized. In addition, the TD position is utilized in situations in which the object is merely to restore the mouth to a position that remains comfortable and stable despite persistence of the internal derangement (Fig. 29–2).

The particular TD position is based on the management philosophy of the clinician. Positioning based on predetermined "ideal" positions has been advocated by various investigators,[30–32] whereas others have arrived at positions using transcranial radiographs,[33] tomograms,[34] arthrograms,[35] mandibular tracking,[36] and electromyography.[37]

A TD position is most often established with a combination of clinical judgment and splint therapy. Currently, the predominant technique is to reposition the mandible so that the meniscus is interposed between the condyle and the eminence during rest and function (see chapter 24). If this is not possible, then one should strive for minimizing the impingement or stretching of injured tissue despite an abnormal disc-condyle alignment. The TD position is generally downward and forward of CO.

Arthrography and roentgen stereophotogrammetric techniques have shown that repositioning therapy and subsequent prosthetic stabilization in TD positions require a change in the relation of the maxilla to the mandible in the sagittal, transverse, and vertical planes. It has been shown that there is considerable relapse toward CO over time, but the TD position continues to be effective in eliminating clicking, intermittent locking, and TMJ masticatory muscle pain.[38] Relapse, in the form of tooth intrusion, occurs because of muscular forces applied to the dentition. This is known to happen when the mandible is maintained in a position other than the habitual one. Despite this gradual movement of the mandible toward CO, recurrence of disc displacement has not been noted.[39] Because the vertical component shows the least relapse, clinicians should attempt to maximize this component when repositioning the mandible to recapture a displaced disc. In addition, long-term use of splint therapy (12 to 18 months) before final occlusal reconstruction is recommended, not only to ensure stability of the disc-condyle relations, but also to minimize the extent of occlusal rebuilding necessary, particularly in the sagittal and transverse planes.

Clinicians have recommended various types and sequences of splint therapy to assist in finding and maintaining the TD position. Mandibular orthopedic repositioning appliances (MORAs), modified Hawley's, with or without inclined planes, full-coverage pivotation maxillary splints, and segmental splints, among others, have been advocated for both general and specific situations. Despite this

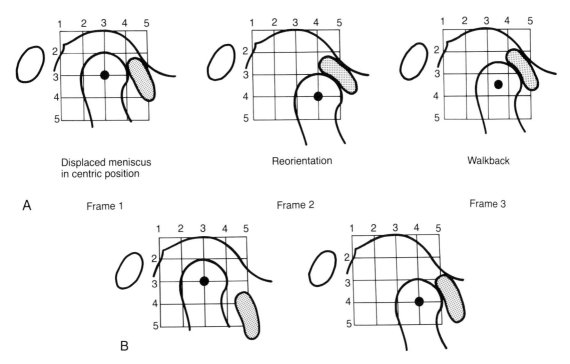

FIGURE 29–2. Therapeutically determined condylar positions. *A*, The intent of condylar repositioning is to re-establish proper orientation of the condylar head, meniscus, and articular fossa *(frame 2)*. A "walkback" technique is often attempted to diminish the degree of condylar movement from the centric occlusion *(frame 3)*. *B*, The intent of condylar repositioning is to minimize the loading of the intracapsular tissues not to reorient the condyle, meniscus, and articular fossa.

variability of design, success of all these appliances relies on achieving certain goals during the course of treatment. In no specific order, these goals include the following:

Decrease Muscle Hyperactivity Especially of the Superior Lateral Pterygoid Muscle. Even though it is difficult to prevent many of the emotional, behavioral, and environmental factors that predispose to muscle overload, elimination of local mechanical strain can be accomplished. Improvement of mandibular overclosure, functional mandibular retrusion, superior luxation of the condyles, and posterior condylar displacement decrease the potential for reactive lateral pterygoid muscle response. Minimizing this muscle hyperactivity reduces the extent of mandibular repositioning necessary to allow the condyles to perform normal rotational function in the lower joint compartment.

Establish Optimal Vertical Dimension. It is necessary to establish vertical dimension without obliterating freeway space and creating unfavorable crown/root ratios. Maximizing the vertical component decreases the need for for-

ward mandibular positioning and may minimize relapse.

Decrease Periodontal Pressoreceptor Activity (Eliminate Posterior Occlusal Triggers). Masticatory electromyographic activity is markedly reduced when posterior teeth are kept apart. Unfortunately, TMJ loading is increased if posterior tooth contacts are removed or minimized. The use of a posterior disocclusion appliance at night, complemented by full posterior occlusal contact potential during the day, is a sensible option.

Decrease Joint Loading and Facilitate Access to the Desired Therapeutic Position. Adequate posterior occlusal contact is needed to decrease joint loading. In order to ensure a consistent occlusal position, guidance of the mandible during closure is achieved through incorporation of distinct occlusal anatomy. This distinct occlusal anatomy must provide maximum occlusal contact and stability in the therapeutic position only.[40] The specific occlusal interdigitation will facilitate neuromuscular adaptation and the creation of a new "N-gram" (occlusal program). Anterior and posterior guide planes are frequently employed to locate a consistent but unlocked occlusal position, at the same time allowing freedom for lateral excursive movement and shallow anterior guidance.

Devise an Occlusal Blueprint That Allows the Teeth and Joints to Share the Load. An attempt should be made to have both components enter into their respective articulations at the same time. In reality, less emphasis is placed on condylar guidance, which is unreliable because of structural deficits, and more emphasis is placed on creating a tooth-guided occlusion.

Once these goals have been achieved and prove to be stable over a period of at least 3 months, the therapeutic position established by the appliance can be transferred to the final restoration.

Occlusal Scheme/Morphology

An occlusal scheme must be designed to be compatible with the compromised environment while at the same time not violate the principles of physiologic occlusal reconstruction. Occlusal design should be guided by the following three considerations:

1. As the chronic nature of internal derangements increases, so does immediate side shift (ISS).

2. Deranged joints are less stable than normal joints. Therefore, deranged joints should be protected and stabilized by some degree of tooth guidance.

3. Deranged joints are subject to remodeling over time and therefore benefit from occlusions that more easily accommodate changes in condylar guidance.

The occlusion that is developed must allow for adequate ISS, which enables the TMJs and the posterior teeth to share the work of guiding the mandible in and out of the treatment position and utilizes deflective occlusal contacts to direct jaw closure to the TD treatment position.

Understanding these prerequisites requires a review of terminology. *Immediate side shift*[42] is defined as a lateral thrust of the mandible. It is regulated by the anatomic configuration of the glenoid fossa and capsular ligament on the nonworking side. During this movement, the nonworking condyle moves medially from its centric position in the fossa, as the teeth leave maximum intercuspation. The maximum amount of movement is determined by

the shape of the fossa, the looseness of the capsular ligaments, and the contraction of the masticatory muscles, primarily the pterygoids.

The greater the side shift, the greater the potential for cusp contact. Therefore, with increasing side shift, cusps are made shorter and fossae grooves should be placed on the occlusal surface in an attempt to minimize deflective tooth contacts during function and parafunction. On maxillary teeth, these grooves are placed more distally, and on mandibular teeth more mesially.[43]

The demands of ISS cannot be accommodated by a "point centric" occlusal scheme, in which cusps function in fossae in a one-to-one tooth arrangement. An occlusal scheme with intercuspation in a small "area" around the treatment position is preferred. Such an occlusal scheme, described as *area centric* (AC), also helps meet the second prerequisite for enabling the TMJs and the posterior teeth to share the work of guiding the jaw in and out of the treatment position (Fig. 29–3).[44]

An AC position allows for multiple tooth contacts over a small area anterior, lateral, and medial to the treatment position. The cusps should glide about on opposing concave surfaces during function and parafunction. Lateral forces are minimized, and occlusal forces are distributed equally over as many teeth as possible. No single posterior tooth should carry any more or less than its share of the occlusal load. Cusps should occlude against marginal ridges in a one-tooth-to-two-teeth relationship. Disocclusion occurs during protrusive movement beyond the AC position.

During lateral movement, disocclusion

Area Centric

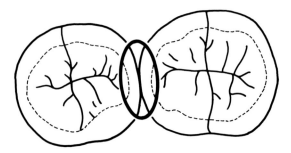

FIGURE 29–3. Area centric. The convex contours of marginal ridges create a "zone" for tooth contacts to be placed, which minimizes lateral forces and distributes occlusal forces while helping guide the jaw in and out of the treatment position.

should be designed to occur against the medial aspect of the canines and the incisor teeth. Disocclusion, however, should not occur immediately. A slight delay before posterior tooth contact is eliminated in lateral and anterior directions reduces reliance on condylar guidance and enables the teeth to guide the jaw in and out of the TD occlusal position. This form of tooth guidance, when coordinated with condylar movement, lends stability to the deranged joint.[45]

Developing an occlusion that accommodates easily to changes in condylar guidance is usually satisfied by ensuring sufficient occlusal contact of the mesial inclines of the maxillary teeth with the distal inclines of the mandibular teeth. This is achieved by placing the mandibular buccal cusps so that they contact the mesial marginal ridges of the maxillary teeth. In addition, a well-developed, nondeflective maxillary incisor cingulum can be utilized to induce reliable anterior vertical stops in the TD position. The cingulum should be complemented by perpendicularly inclined lower incisors.

Vertical Dimension

Once past the incipient stage, intracapsular pathology is best managed by occlusal splints. A common feature of most splints is the increase of vertical dimension. This change is thought to be at least partly responsible for the amelioration of pain and for functional improvement.

Research has shown that increases in the vertical dimension of occlusion (VDO) are well tolerated.[46] Still, care must be taken not to obliterate freeway space. In the absence of freeway space, the muscles remain hyperactive, joint loading is constant, and forces on the periodontium are excessive. If the amount of repositioning necessary to "unload" or "recapture" a disc requires a splint thickness that causes conscious voluntary recruitment of masticatory muscles to maintain tooth clearance, this form of treatment should not be used. Joint healing and stabilization are unlikely to occur under these conditions. In addition, the necessary prosthetic rehabilitation would lead to periodontal breakdown. Care must be taken to avoid creating an occlusal position that will be unobtainable using available restorative/orthodontic techniques.

As previously mentioned, available data suggest that "therapeutic" increases in VDO may be only temporary and often intrude teeth over time.[47] Specific occlusal relationships, however, appear to remain intact. This observation suggests that in a dentate patient, permanent restorations should be delayed as long as practically possible. When free-end partial dentures are indicated, intrusion is unlikely and delay in prosthetic rehabilitation is unnecessary. Dentists must be careful to provide adequate interocclusal space, in order to minimize forces destructive to the residual ridge. Ridge destruction inevitably leads to loss of occlusal stability.

Occlusal Table

In order for the functional requirements to be met, attention must be paid to the dimension and composition of the occlusal table. Clinicians must provide an occlusal table of adequate length and effectiveness. They must also be familiar with the properties of the materials selected for the restoration of the occluding surfaces and their potential for wear during functional and parafunctional activity.

Joint stabilization and unloading rely on adequate posterior support and on the distribution of occlusal contacts. Tooth-supported fixed restorations extending to the molars are the treatment of choice. Premolar occlusion is less desirable unless used in conjunction with a distal extension removable partial denture. Tissue-supported partial dentures are only useful if they are stable and retentive. Inadequate support not only increases joint loading but may increase hyperactivity in the masseter and temporalis muscles. The length of the occlusal table is less important than the positive support gained from each additional tooth. The incorporation of osseointegrated implants to provide posterior support may be a viable option, but no data are available on their use in patients with TMDs.

The materials selected for restoration of occluding surfaces may be gold, acrylic, porcelain, or chrome. These materials may wear unevenly, resulting in loss of vertical dimension, loss of the TD position, and development of occlusal interferences. For this reason, the following factors should be considered: (1) the number of teeth contributing to occlusal support, (2) the material against which the restoration is to occlude, (3) the type of occlusal scheme, and (4) the presence of parafunctional habits.[48]

If possible, at least one natural tooth-to-tooth occlusal contact should be present bilaterally. This is most simply accomplished in a full dentulous patient in the second molar region, by means of passive extrusion or orthodontically guided movement. Minor equilibration is at times necessary to ensure that a broad contact is obtained (Fig. 29–4).

In other instances, anterior contact of the incisors can be obtained in the TD position. If this contact is complemented by sound posterior restorations, the potential for occlusal wear is greatly diminished. Besides lending stability to the final prosthetic reconstruction, the presence of tooth-to-tooth contacts in the TD position reduces the chance of losing the treatment position during the transition from appliance to final restoration.

The favorable occlusal wear properties of gold against gold and gold against acrylic make them the most desirable materials when restoring the occlusion in a fully dentulous patient and when combining fixed and removable prosthetics as part of the treatment. The flexibility to plan, produce, and polish the desired occlusal morphology is an added advantage. Porcelain occluding against gold, enamel, or acrylic shows more wear. For aesthetic reasons, it is practical to consider porcelain restorations in the bicuspid region and incorporate gold into molar restorations. If possible, it is recommended that opposing occlusal contacts be fabricated of the same material. The actual fixed restoration may be in the form of full crown and gold or porcelain onlays, depending on the existing dentition and functional needs (Fig. 29–5).

When utilizing distal extension partial dentures, the selection of porcelain or acrylic teeth and monoplane or semianatomic teeth is dependent on several factors. If the fixed component of the rehabilitation provides stable holding contacts, utilization of monoplane (0°) or semianatomic form (20° to 30°) *acrylic* denture teeth is recommended. Because concern about rapid wear and loss of the therapeutic occlusal relationship is minimized by stable abutment holding contacts, the positive features of acrylic teeth (readily adjusted, contoured, modified, and polished) are an asset. Monoplane or semianatomic teeth are recommended because there is less chance of occlusal prematurities occurring during function and unrestricted horizontal freedom of movement.

If abutment teeth do not provide stable support for a partial denture in the TD position, the distal extension partial must play a greater role. Semianatomic porcelain teeth would likely be most appropriate. The high abrasion resistance and minimal wear characteristics of porcelain help maintain the specific occlusal

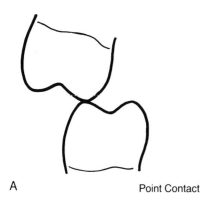

A   Point Contact

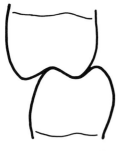

B   Broad Contact

FIGURE 29–4. Extrusion of the most posterior molar to create an occlusal stop in natural tooth structure. Efforts should be made to establish solid and broad occlusal contacts between natural teeth in the posterior molar segments. Point contacts (*A*), which often result from passive extrusion, lead to occlusal instability and lateral interferences. Broad contacts (*B*) should be obtained via equilibration, orthodontically guided movements, or both.

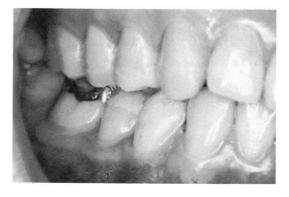

FIGURE 29–5. Combination of porcelain onlays and gold coverage used to restore the therapeutically derived position splint.

position, as long as the underlying basal bone is not overloaded.

In reality, no matter which materials are used or in what combinations (fixed, removable), clinicians must always be aware that alterations in the occlusal scheme can occur as a result of remodeling of the TMJs.

SEQUENCING CLINICAL AND LABORATORY PROCEDURES

After a therapeutic position is established with splint therapy, a period of stabilization is required. This period should last from 3 to 12 months. Several criteria should be met before starting prosthetic treatment:

1. Diminishment or cessation of joint noise
2. Marked reduction in resting and functionally generated pain
3. Normal mandibular range of motion in the sagittal and horizontal planes
4. Stability of the specific occlusal topography created on the appliance.

TRANSFERRING THE REGISTRATION

Control is the key to successfully transferring a TD occlusal relationship from a splint to fixed removable prosthetics. Proper treatment planning is accomplished by studying mounted casts that have been properly oriented by a face-bow registration. Two mountings should be used: one with a cast that was taken with the appliance still in place and the other with casts taken without the appliance and oriented utilizing a transfer jig usually made with quick-cure acrylic (Fig. 29–6). Analysis of these registrations should enable a clinician to determine the following:

1. The additional crown length necessary to support the new TD occlusion
2. How the additional height should be distributed between the upper and lower teeth
3. The most favorable way to create adequate curves of Spee and Wilson
4. Whether the pre-existing anterior tooth relations are adequate to provide sufficient incisal guidance
5. Which arch to rehabilitate first and how to create the initial tooth-to-tooth posterior contacts to stabilize the TD occlusal relationship.

Part of the treatment planning process should include careful examination of the teeth and periodontium. A current set of periapical films should be available for comprehensive evaluation.

In patients with intact dentition, the appliance can first be shortened, uncovering the second molars and allowing for passive eruption. If waiting for passive eruption is impractical or improbable, bonded posterior composite resin or temporary crowns should be considered. Once posterior contacts are established bilaterally, the appliance can be removed to confirm that positional stability has been obtained. At this time, it is wise to encourage the patient to continue wearing the appliance to decrease occlusal forces on the molars and minimize chances of relapse (Fig. 29–7).

After solid posterior contacts are established in the TD position, complementary anterior stops and adequate incisal guidance are created. A bonded composite resin is useful for

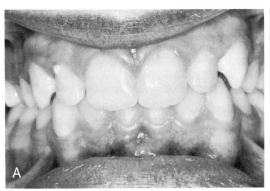
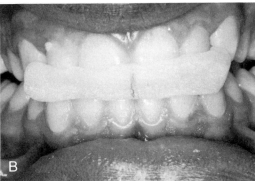

FIGURE 29–6. Self-curing acrylics are often utilized to make sturdy transfer jigs, which can assist in mounting study casts in the therapeutically derived position. *A,* Pre-existing occlusion. *B,* Transfer jig in place.

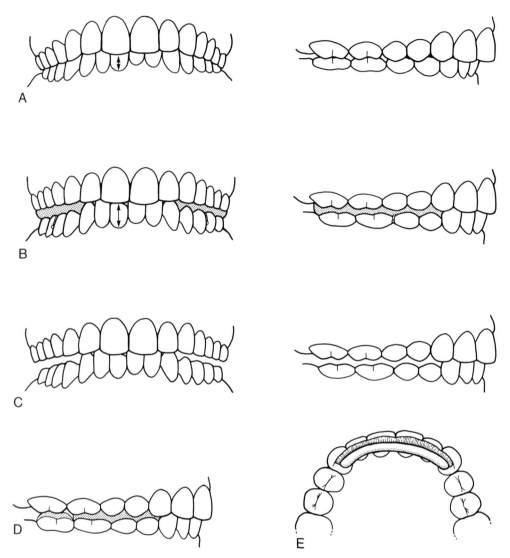

FIGURE 29–7. Case study. *A,* This represents a frontal and lateral view of a class II occlusion, illustrating the amount of overjet and overbite in the centric occlusal position. *B,* This represents the therapeutically derived occlusal position maintained by a mandibular appliance. Note that with the appliance in place, midline relations are maintained but a class I molar relation has been established. In addition, the overbite and overjet relations have been decreased. The appliance is represented by the dotted area. *C,* This represents the therapeutically derived occlusal position, with the appliance having been removed. The representation illustrates the extent of repositioning that has been required. The amount of interocclusal space that must be filled is clearly evident. *D,* This represents the appliance in place after having been shortened in the second molar region. Bonded resin has been placed on the lower second molar to secure the therapeutic position. A temporary acrylic crown could also be used for this purpose. *E,* Intraorally, the placement of bonded resin in the region of the maxillary anterior cingulum is useful to secure the therapeutically derived position with or without the appliance in place. This platform creates a positive stop for the mandibular anterior teeth. This ramp should be placed when deemed necessary, prior to shortening the appliance. Once established, second molar eruption of build-ups can be done with increased predictability. Additionally, the bonded resin can be placed in a fashion to provide adequate incisal and canine guidance.

this purpose because it allows a trial period before making final restorative commitments (see Fig. 29–7). After these initial stabilizing procedures, a new set of study casts is taken. Using a face bow, the case is remounted on a semiadjustable articulator.

This step is of particular help in planning the proper planes of occlusion. Dentists can employ this mounting to diagnostically wax up a functional occlusal pattern on the posterior teeth. Temporary restorations can be fabricated without difficulty.

After posterior and anterior steps are established, the appliance (covering the lower first molar, bicuspids, and canine) can be reduced in thickness. The amount of reduction should correspond to the increased tooth length necessary to restore the maxillary bicuspids and first molars to an adequate plane. Ideally, the appliance's thickness should be reduced in half, leaving an equivalent amount to be restored on the mandibular arch. The thinned appliance can be resurfaced with acrylic after temporization or following placement of the completed restorations (Fig. 29–8).

At this juncture, before restoring the mandibular arch, clinical experience has shown it to be worthwhile to solidify (resurface) the initial tooth contacts, re-examine the patient (range of motion, muscle palpation, joint noises, and so on), and make a new maxillary night guard that eliminates posterior tooth contact during sleep. In addition, several weeks should be allowed to pass before additional changes are made. During this time, the periodontal status of the elongated teeth should be monitored carefully. If structural and functional stability are maintained, moving ahead to the mandibular arch is warranted.

Next, the splint is trimmed to uncover the mandibular first molars. They are prepared and restored to the height of the remaining appliance (Fig. 29–9). Before the mandibular bicuspids and cuspids are prepared, all the maxillary restorations and mandibular first molar restorations should be completed and temporarily cemented. When solid tooth-to-tooth contact has been obtained on the first molars with permanent restorations, second molar restorations, if needed, should be finalized. When long-span maxillary or mandibular posterior bridges are indicated, the maxillary bridge should always be completed before starting the mandibular restorations. Treatment sequencing should always be aimed at maintaining the TD position as the appliance becomes thinner and shorter.

After first and second molar support is established with completed restorations, the remaining appliance usually can be removed and the lower premolars restored (Fig. 29–10). If bonding material was previously placed on intact cuspids to facilitate lateral guidance, bonded porcelain restorations are an appropriate final restoration. If the anterior teeth are in need of complete rehabilitation, single crown restorations or a bridge is now placed. Temporization should be done in a way that minimizes changes in the location and amount of anterior tooth contacts established with the appliance.

After all the restorations have been placed (Fig. 29–11), a maxillary flat plane splint

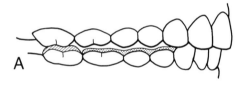

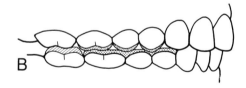

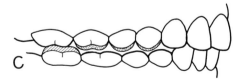

FIGURE 29–8. *A,* Having secured the therapeutic position, the lower appliance is thinned. The degree of reduction is dependent on the length of maxillary restoration needed to create a functional occlusal plane. *B,* Once the maxillary restorations (bonded porcelain, crowns, onlays) are in place, the lower appliance is resurfaced (*C*). This represents the interocclusal space remaining after placement of the maxillary restorations.

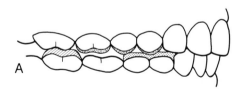

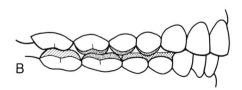

FIGURE 29–9. *A* and *B,* The lower appliance is cut short to expose the lower first molar. Subsequently, a restoration is placed.

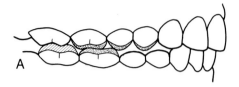

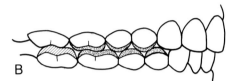

FIGURE 29–10. *A* and *B*, With the remaining appliance removed, the interocclusal distance in the bicuspid region can be appreciated. Appropriate restorations are subsequently placed.

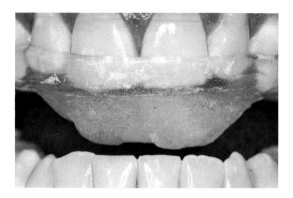

FIGURE 29–12. The final occlusal appliance is designed primarily for night wear. A maxillary stabilization appliance with or without a small palatal ramp is preferred.

should be made and worn indefinitely during sleep. The incorporation of a small palatal acrylic ramp is helpful in preventing mandibular distalization and excessive side shift (Fig. 29–12). If it is used, the clinician must monitor the status of the lower anterior teeth for signs of occlusal trauma.

The treatment sequence employing a maxillary appliance is similar. Anterior contact of the mandibular teeth is maintained on the appliance, not the maxillary teeth, until the posterior restorations are completed. When the posterior restorations are completed, the anterior restorations are placed. There does not appear to be an advantage of maxillary or mandibular splints for facilitating prosthodontic therapy.

REMOVABLE PROSTHETICS

For patients with severe financial constraints but with relatively complete dentition, removable partial overlays are recommended (Fig. 29–13). The need for these restorations on one arch or both is determined after successful

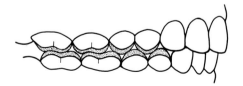

FIGURE 29–11. Completed restorations maintaining the therapeutic position.

splint therapy and analysis of mounted casts as previously described. Long-term use of an acrylic splint is a less desirable option, because it must continually have acrylic added to maintain the TD position. As the splint ages, breakage is also more common.

For patients who have missing posterior teeth and who require removable partial dentures (Fig. 29–14), the TD position is stabilized utilizing the existing anterior teeth with bonding materials or crowns, if possible. Wax bite rims can be employed to transfer the relationship to the articulator. Patients requiring full dentures usually have had quick-cure acrylic added to the existing dentures to establish a TD position. The vertical component is reproduced by measuring the existing VDO with standard techniques.

Depending on what material composes the opposing arch and aesthetic concerns, a restorative material is selected. If possible, noble metals are used because they provide predictable occlusal stability. The transfer from the acrylic appliance to a final removable one is often difficult.

As with fixed restorations, the key to a successful transfer lies in maintaining the therapeutic maxillomandibular relationship with the acrylic appliance out of the mouth. The placement of bonding material or crowns on the anterior teeth before appliance removal helps stabilize the new position. Appropriate bite and face-bow registrations are taken and used to mount the casts on a semiadjustable articulator. Routine laboratory procedures follow. Careful attention when taking the bite assures that only minor final corrections in the mouth will be necessary.

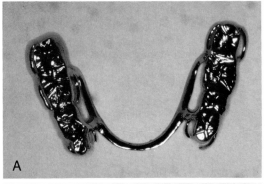
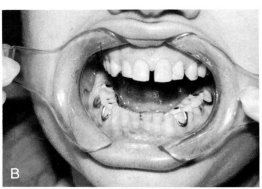
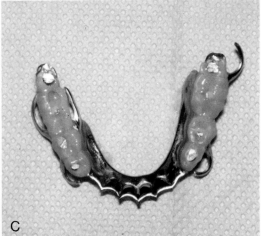

FIGURE 29-13. Removable partial overlays are often used in lieu of fixed restorations to stabilize the therapeutic position. *A,* Chrome cobalt overlay appliance. *B* and *C,* Combination chrome cobalt and composite overlay appliance.

These prostheses should be removed at bedtime and replaced by a maxillary flat plane splint that maintains an acceptable vertical dimension and prevents excessive mandibular distalization or lateral shift.

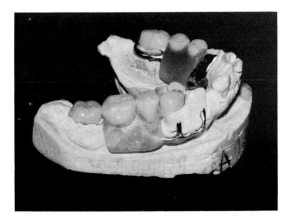

FIGURE 29-14. Removable partial dentures are a viable option when posterior teeth are missing.

CLINICAL HINTS

- Patients with TMDs are subject to trauma from the dental treatment itself and must be cautiously handled.
- Office visits must be kept short (1 to 1½ hours).
- Child-size bite props can be used.
- Ethyl chloride spray and stretch can be used as needed throughout the session (see chapter 22).
- Patients should be encouraged to take a nonsteroidal anti-inflammatory agent 1 day before the visit and for 2 days following.
- Visits should be spaced 7 to 10 days apart.
- Bite registrations should never be taken after a long clinical session. A separate appointment is used to take these registrations in a nonfatigued patient.
- Bite registrations must be taken with the patient in an upright and unstrained position.
- The patient's functional status must be monitored, including range of motion, joint noises, and the presence or absence of mus-

cle or joint tenderness. Subjective complaints should not be ignored.

- Resurfacing the appliance is mandatory after any alteration of the occlusion.
- If a patient becomes symptomatic, it is wise to discontinue active treatment for approximately 3 weeks and encourage a soft diet. Analgesics, anti-inflammatory agents, and muscle relaxants can be judiciously administered.

LIMITATIONS OF PROSTHETIC REHABILITATION AND LONG-TERM FOLLOWUP

As with all restorative treatment, success is dependent on case selection and meticulous attention to detail. Careful attention during splint therapy provides a clinician with valuable insight about whether prosthetic therapy is necessary. Many patients can be maintained using the appliance full or part time as a "crutch" for an indefinite period. Patients having appliance therapy that provides symptomatic relief but simultaneously produces unstable jaw relations, severe malocclusion, periodontal overload, and compromised freeway space will not have a successful prosthetic result.

On the other hand, appliance therapy rarely establishes 100% normalcy. The persistence of joint noise, minor limitations in range of motion, and minor dental asymmetries is acceptable if pain has been eliminated and the patient is able to function at a level acceptable to the patient and dentist.

After completion of prosthetic therapy, patients should be seen regularly to monitor the stability of the newly placed restorations. Careful attention must be paid to the periodontal tissues for signs of overload and deterioration. The importance of follow-up visits must be explained to patients in detail.

REFERENCES

1. Okesson, J.: *Management of Temporomandibular Joint Disorders and Occlusion.* C.V. Mosby, St. Louis, 1989.
2. Bell, W.: *Temporomandibular Joint Disorders.* Year Book Medical Publishers, Chicago, 1986.
3. McNamara, D.: Variance of occlusal support in temporomandibular joint pain dysfunction patients. J. Dent. Res. 61:350, 1982.
4. Okesson, J.: *Management of Temporomandibular Joint Disorders and Occlusion.* C.V. Mosby, St. Louis, 1989.
5. Mongini, F.: *The Stomatognathic System.* Quintessence Publishing Co., Lombard, IL, pp. 255–286, 1984.
6. Clark, G., Mohl N., and Riggs, R.: Occlusal adjustment therapy. In *A Textbook of Occlusion.* N. Mohl, G. Zarb, G. Carlson, and J. Rugh (eds.). Quintessence Publishing Co., Lombard, IL, pp. 285–304, 1988.
7. Zarb, G. and Fenton, A.: Prosthodontic, operative and orthodontic therapy. In *A Textbook of Occlusion.* N. Mohl, G. Zarb, G. Carlson, and J. Rugh (eds.). Quintessence Publishing Co., Lombard, IL, 1988.
8. Solberg, W.: Temporomandibular disorders: Clinical significance of TMJ changes. Br. Dent. J. 160:231, 1986.
9. Bell, W.: *Temporomandibular Disorders: Classification, Diagnosis Management.* Year Book Medical Publishers, Chicago, pp. 172–214, 1986.
10. DeSteno, C.: The pathophysiology of TMJ dysfunction and related pain. In *Clinical Management of Head, Neck and TMJ Pain and Dysfunction.* H. Gelb, (ed.). W.B. Saunders Co., Philadelphia, 1985.
11. Mahan, P.E.: The temporomandibular joint in function and dysfunction. In *Temporomandibular Joint Problems.* W.K. Solberg and G.T. Clark (eds.). Quintessence Publishing Co., Lombard, IL, 1980.
12. Oberg, T., Carlsson, G.E., and Fajers C.M.: The temporomandibular joint: A morphological study on human autopsy material. Acta Odontol. Scand. 29:349–384, 1971.
13. Avant, F.B., Averill, C.J., and Hahn, W.E.: Changes in the temporomandibular joints of rats caused by alterations in the intermaxillary relationship of the teeth. J. Dent. Res. 31:499, 1952.
14. McNamara, J.A.: Neuromuscular and skeletal adaptation to altered function in the oro-facial region. Am. J. Orthod. 64:578, 1973.
15. Mongini, F.: Remodeling of the mandibular condyle in the adult and its relationship to the condition of the dental arches. Acta Anat. 82:437, 1972.
16. Bell, W.: pp. 172–214. (See reference 2.)
17. Clark, G.: pp. 271–284. (See reference 6.)
18. Mongini, F.: pp. 233–252. (See reference 5.)
19. DuBrul, E.L. and Menekratis, A.: *The Physiology of Oral Reconstruction.* Quintessence Publishing Co., Lombard, IL, 21–38, 1981.
20. Solnit, A. and Curnutte, D.: *Occlusal Correction: Principles and Practice.* Quintessence Publishing Co., Lombard, IL, 1988.
21. Young, J.: Successful restorative dentistry for the internal derangement patient. Part I: Treatment position. Mo. Dent. J. Sept.–Oct., 67(5):21–26, 1987.
22. Young, J.: Successful restorative dentistry for the internal derangement patient. Part II: Occlusal scheme, vertical dimension, and occlusal table. Mo. Dent. J. Jan.–Feb., 68(1):25–33, 1988.
23. Dawson, P.: *Evaluation, Diagnosis and Treatment of Occlusal Problems.* C.V. Mosby, St. Louis, 1989.
24. Solnit, A. and Curnutte, D.: p. 49.
25. Dawson, P.: Optimum TMJ condyle position in clinical practice. Int. J. Periodont. Restor. Dent. 3:11–31, 1985.
26. Celenza, F.V.: The condylar position: In sickness and in health. Int. J. Periodont. Restor. Dent. 2:39–51, 1985.
27. DuBrul, E.L. and Menekratis, A.: p. 39.
28. Young, J.: p. 23.
29. Young, J.: p. 26.
30. Dawson, P.: *Evacuation, Diagnosis and Treatment of*

Occlusal Problems, 2nd ed. C.V. Mosby, St. Louis, 1989.

31. Gelb, H.: *Clinical Management of Head, Neck and TMJ Pain and Dysfunction,* 2nd ed. W.B. Saunders Co., Philadelphia, 1985.

32. Owen, A.: Orthodontic/orthopedic therapy for craniomandibular pain dysfunction, Part A: Anterior disc displacement, review of the literature. J. Craniomand. Pract. 5:357–366, 1987.

33. Weinberg, L.: Optimum TMJ condyle position in clinical practice. Int. J. Periodont. Restor. Dent. 2:11–27, 1985.

34. Mongini, F.: The importance of radiology in the diagnosis and TMJ dysfunctions: A comparative evaluation of transcranial radiographs and serial tomography. J. Prosthet. Dent. 45:186, 1981.

35. Tallents, R., Katzberg, R., et al: Arthrographically assisted splint therapy. J. Prosthet. Dent. 53:235, 1985.

36. Mongini, F.: Factors influencing the pantographic tracings of mandibular disorder movements. J. Prosthet. Dent. 48:585, 1982.

37. Cooper, B.: Craniomandibular disorders. In *Management of Facial, Head and Neck Pain.* B. Cooper and F. Lucente (eds.). W.B. Saunders Co., Philadelphia, 1989.

38. Lundh, H., Westesson, P.L., Rune B., et al: Changes in mandibular position during treatment with disk repositioning onlays: A roentgen stereophotogrammetric study. Oral Surg. Oral Med. Oral Pathol. 65:657–662, 1988.

39. Lundh, H., Westesson, P.L., et al.: Long-term followup after occlusal treatment to correct abnormal TMJ disc position. Oral Med. Oral Pathol. 67:2–10, 1989.

40. Lundh, H., Westesson P.L., et al.: Disk repositioning onlays in the treatment of temporomandibular joint disk displacement: Comparison with a flat occlusal splint and with no treatment. Oral Surg. Oral Med. Oral Pathol. 66:155–162, 1988.

41. Young, J.: p. 26.

42. Solnit, A. and Curnutte, D.: p. 67.

43. Solnit, A. and Curnutte, D.: pp. 60–67.

44. Young, pp. 281, Feb., 1988.

45. Solnit, A. and Curnutte, D.: pp. 60–70.

46. Carlsson, G. et al: Effect of increasing vertical dimension on the masticatory system in subjects with natural teeth. J. Prosthet. Dent. 42:284, 1979.

47. Ramjford, S. and Blankenship, J.: Increased occlusal vertical dimension in adult monkeys. J. Prosthet. Dent. 45:74, 1981.

48. Ivanhoe, J. and Vaught, R.: Occlusion in the combination fixed and removable prosthodontic patient. Dent. Clin. North Am. 31:305–322, 1987.

Gordon Gaynor

CHAPTER 30

Orthodontic Therapy

It has always been the goal of orthodontics to establish a proper occlusion within the context of musculoskeletal and facial balance. Aesthetics and function are interchangeable objectives, because the achievement of one most often satisfies the goals of the other. In order to balance the hard and soft tissues that form the matrix for the dentition, orthopedic and orthodontic therapy are combined. Treatment initiated when patients are young allows clinicians to take advantage of a period of accelerated growth, at a time when the bone is more plastic and susceptible to external influences.

This has given rise to the inclusion of functional appliances developed in Europe, such as the activator and the Frankel Functional Regulator, in our storehouse of therapeutic techniques. By harnessing the energies of the muscles and soft elastic tissues surrounding the dental arches and by directing the growth of the bone, we can achieve a more favorable environment for the eruption and placement of the teeth. During the growth stage of the dental arches, the teeth are like passengers on a train, as they are moved from one point to another within the confines of the alveolar bone.

When bone development ceases, however, and the growth of the maxilla and mandible is complete, the situation reverses. Now, the occlusion becomes dominant and directs the mandible into position during the process of interdigitation, and discrepancies in arch shapes and sizes must be accommodated by the dentition. A functional occlusion often develops, producing crossbites and midline shifts. As the teeth seek to find a point of greatest contact, the most bizarre malocclusion can become functional, with the adaptation of the occlusion to an abnormal environment. Orthodontists are often surprised to find individuals so affected masticating well, with healthy pink gingiva. These situations are testimony to the underlying health of our bodies and to their ability to adapt. They also emphasize the importance of proper function without necessarily having proper morphology.

An orthodontist's concern with the relationship of teeth to their skeletal surroundings must be accountable to another entity, the temporomandibular joint (TMJ) and its related structures. This joint differs little from other joints in the body (see Chapter 1) with regard to its composition and function, but it is under a unique control: the dentition. Its parameters of movement are, to some extent, dictated by the position of the teeth, which can limit and direct mandibular movements. The teeth are in control of mandibular function only when an individual occludes or masticates. Once the mandible disengages from the teeth, the condyles are free to move within the confines of the bony fossae, as limited by the ligaments and muscles.

Under normal conditions, the teeth are in occlusal contact only during swallowing and chewing. A bolus of food separates the teeth and acts to cushion the forces transmitted to the skeletal tissues. It would appear unlikely that an individual functioning in such a fashion, no matter how imperfect the occlusion might be, could cause much damage to the supporting systems. Unfortunately, many of us exert a great deal more pressure on our dentition when we indulge in parafunctional activity. The forces transmitted when the teeth are strongly compressed against each other are far in excess of the light pressure exerted during swallowing.

Under stressful conditions, one can produce an almost continuous series of closures, taxing the muscles, ligaments, and joint tissue. Nocturnal bruxism and clenching habits are the most detrimental. Sleep is meant to be a period of rest, when the muscle fibers stretch out and the ligaments elongate. If this recovery period is interrupted by habitual activity, the muscles fatigue and the joint system undergoes undue stress.

No longer are occlusal disharmonies minor interruptions in a closing pattern. With overuse and excessive force, they become jarring forces, which cause a great impact on an already stressed skeletal system. Mandibular shifts caused by arch width discrepancies add to the tension and compression of the ligaments and of the condyle-disc-fossa complex.

The order of treatment for a patient suffering a temporomandibular disorder (TMD) is paramount. Phase I therapy, which is directed at eliminating pain and other symptoms, must be initiated first. Some form of splint therapy, which can change the position of the mandible, may be used. A professional's concern in this regard is to establish a condyle-disc-fossa position that eliminates pain in the muscles and joints. Once a comfortable mandibular position is found and the patients are functioning in that position for approximately 3 months, a phase II treatment plan can be established.

All patients undergoing splint therapy must be informed of the changes in occlusion that may occur and of the possibility of a phase II stage to re-establish the dentition to that new mandibular position. Three modes of therapy are possible, and often they are used together: orthodontics, orthognathic surgery, and prosthodontics.

The key to successful phase II treatment is the maintenance of the therapeutic mandibular position. Therefore, occlusal changes should not be made by an orthodontist on a symptomatic patient with TMD until a skeletal balance between the TMJ and mandible is achieved and maintained for some time. Roth[1] expressed the need for a relaxed neuromuscular response, not only to determine the true maxillomandibular relationship, but also to evaluate the extent of etiologic involvement of the occlusion on the TMD symptoms. Until these conditions are met, any efforts to change the occlusion would be haphazard.

Much of what orthodontists achieve with their young patients can make them less susceptible to later TMD. However, in symptomatic patients with TMD, orthodontic therapy should not be considered as a primary treatment regimen. Only after a patient is stabilized with phase I treatment does the orthodontist have the challenging task of setting the occlusion to a point in space defined by the articulated surface of the plastic splint.

EPIDEMIOLOGY OF TEMPOROMANDIBULAR DISORDERS

A review of epidemiologic studies of TMDs is pertinent in order to give an overview of the magnitude of the disease in a population.

Helkimo[2-4] has established an index to differentiate normal from abnormal mandibular function and has devised a system for measuring the degree of dysfunction. Many researchers have adopted this index in an attempt to standardize results, particularly those in Scandinavian countries.

Despite an investigator's adherence to such an index, some degree of variation can be expected. Anamnestic studies can be skewed by the patients' ability to recollect their history and to verbalize their symptoms and degree of dysfunction and discomfort. Subjective questioning can elicit variable results, based on subjects' understanding of the question, as well as their awareness and interpretation of their symptoms. Clinical examination can evoke different degrees of pain responses, depending on an operator's technique in palpation, as well as a patient's reaction to the examiner and the environment in which the procedure is done. Green and Marbach,[5] in their critical review of epidemiologic studies, discussed some of the areas where discrepancies and misleading data can arise.

Nevertheless, if a reader examines a sufficient amount of data from a large enough number of researchers, the magnitude of TMDs in the population at large becomes apparent.

Table 30–1 lists some of the more important epidemiologic studies conducted during the past 20 years. Although most of the research has been done in Scandinavia, the study by Solberg and others,[6] conducted on a nonpatient population of American college students, is comprehensive and allows comparison with the material from Scandinavia.

Disorders of the TMJ exhibit little regard for age. When the clinical studies[7-9] of the older age-group, exhibiting symptoms in the 73 to 79% range, are compared with the younger population,[10-13] demonstrating symptoms in the 35 to 61% range, there is some diminution in overall clinical symptoms of TMD. The American study[6] of 19- to 25-year-old students revealed one or more symptoms of TMDs in 76% of those examined.

Muscle tenderness was found more frequently, 29%, among the 7- to 14-year-old subjects tested by Nilner and Lassing,[12] compared with the 18% of 15- to 18-year-olds examined by Nilner.[14] These same groups exhibited TMJ tenderness of 39% and 34%, respectively. Solberg and others[6] presented values of 34% and 5% for muscle and TMJ tenderness after ex-

TABLE 30–1. Epidemiologic Studies on the Prevalence of Mandibular Dysfunction in Various Populations

				PREVALENCE OF MANDIBULAR DYSFUNCTION (IN PERCENT)					
				One or More Symptoms		TMJ Sounds		Muscle (M)/TMJ (T) Tenderness	
RESEARCHERS	NUMBER	AGE	POPULATION	Subjective	Clinical	Subjective	Clinical	Subjective	Clinical
Agerberg, Carlsson[16]	1106	65–74	Swedish men/women	68		39		33 M,T	
Agerberg, Osterberg[8]	194	70	Swedish men/women		74		36		36 (M,T)
Hansson, Oberg[9]	63	67	Swedish men/women		73		60		35 (M,T)
Hansson, Nilner[7]	1069	17–73	Swedish men/women		79		65		37 (M) 10 (T)
Ingervall, Hedegard[17]	389	32	Swedish men	12	60				
Helkimo[4]	321	15–65	Finnish Lapps men/women	57	88				
Mohlin[15]	272	20–46	Swedish women	34	25				
Solberg et al[6]	739	19–25	American men/women	26	76	9	28	9 (M) 5 (T)	34 (M) 5 (T)
Mohlin et al[18]	253	18–25	Swedish men	12	28				
Nilner[14]	309	15–18	Swedish teenagers	41		17	14		18 (M) 34 (T)
Grosfeld, Czarneka[10]	250	13–15	Polish teenagers		68				
Grosfeld, Czarneka[10]	250	6–8	Polish children		56				
Williamson[11]	304	13	American children		35				
Nilner, Lassing[12]	440	7–14	Swedish children	36		13	8		29 (M) 39 (T)
Egermark-Eriksson[13]	136 131 135	7 11 15	Swedish children	39 67 74	33 46 61				

amination of their 19- to 25-year-old college student group. In an adult population studied by Hansson and Nilner,[7] 37% of the subjects exhibited muscle tenderness, and 10% TMJ tenderness. Clinical studies of TMJ sounds disclosed a higher incidence in the older adult groups,[7–9] ranging from 36 to 65%, than in the young adult groups,[6] which reported a fre-

quency of 28%. The adolescent subjects[14] evidenced a 14% incidence of TMJ sounds, with the youngest group[12] of 7- to 14-year-olds exhibiting the smallest incidence, only 8%.

Studies utilizing subjective data[12,13,16,17] generally reflected a lower percentage of overall symptoms when compared with studies of similar age-groups in which clinical data[7–10] were obtained. With two exceptions,[13,15] all the subjective data in Table 30-1, when compared with the same investigators' clinical data,[4,6,17,18] disclosed a lower incidence of positive response. Many individuals are not consciously aware of joint sounds or mild muscle soreness. Moreover, a muscle that elicits a painful response on palpation may not be painful during the subject's daily functions.

Pain thresholds are variable and a meaningful percentage of the population is not aware of minor muscle aches. Individuals with lower pain threshold, however, respond dramatically to the slightest muscle tenderness on palpation. These factors stress the importance of subjective data, which are integral not only to an epidemiologic study but to a clinician's overall diagnostic evaluation of a patient. Subjective findings provide an operator with an awareness of a patient's reactive capabilities. Subjective examination is also an individual's self-evaluation and interpretation of his or her personal well-being or relative state of unwellness.

Whether the reader accepts as valid the higher or the lower percentage of these previously mentioned studies or whether a median range appears reasonable is not essential. What is vital is the fact that a large portion of the population is inflicted with some form of TMD, whether it is subclinical or debilitating in intensity. It thus becomes incumbent on practitioners to seek out, if not to treat, patients with TMDs or to see that their patients are directed to appropriate practitioners for care.

RELATIONSHIP OF MALOCCLUSION AND TEMPOROMANDIBULAR DISORDERS

It is difficult to treat a disease having an etiology that is unknown or questionable. Moreover, a patient's ability to understand the problem and accept the prescribed treatment also will suffer. Malocclusion has been historically associated with TMDs and labeled as a causative factor. It would appear reasonable, if problems relating to the TMJ are associated with a form of mandibular dysfunction and the teeth guide the mandible to its final closure, that anything less than an ideal occlusion could predispose the patient to TMD.

A review of the literature tends to negate this premise, with conflicting results and an overall consensus that malocclusion is not a primary etiologic factor in most TMD. Despite the following findings that support this view, the need for a satisfactory functional occlusion is still essential.

An individual may be able to tolerate variations in occlusal form and maxillomandibular relationships, especially as defined by Angle's classification of malocclusion.[19] Nevertheless, a person's ability to function properly should not be compromised. Patients are highly sensitive to the smallest change in their occlusion. Most dentists, for instance, have observed a patient's extreme reaction to a slightly overbuilt restoration; yet so often, an examination will show a patient to have a severe malocclusion but no signs of a TMD. Wide latitude in tissue tolerance is one possible explanation, and a great deal of knowledge is yet to be gained before etiologic factors can be applied to TMDs.

Angle's[19] classification of malocclusion into Class I, Class II, and Class III groups occlusions in the anteroposterior plane. Historically, some of these forms have been included in the etiologic factors that predispose the patient to or cause TMDs.[2,20-22] However, many studies have challenged this direct connection.[15,23-28] Pullinger and others[29] examined 222 freshman dental and hygiene students and found a positive correlation between TMJ tenderness and Class II, division 2 subjects. Riolo and colleagues,[30] in a study of 1342 young people ages 7 to 17 years, found a positive relationship between Class II malocclusions and TMJ sounds, with all other morphologic groups exhibiting no association to other TMJ symptoms.

A correlation between Class III malocclusion and TMJ tenderness was found in Pullinger and associates' study,[29] which agreed with the findings of Mohlin and others[31] in their investigation of 389 Swedish men. Egermark-Eriksson and others[13] could find only a weak connection between TMDs and morphologic malocclusion in their study of 402 children.

Overjet was noted to have a relationship with TMD only in extreme cases of 7 to 9 mm, as reported by Helm and colleagues[28] and Riolo and associates.[30] The latter investigation also reported joint tenderness in subjects with negative overjet (Class III).

Morphologic malocclusion in the vertical plane represents inconclusive evidence when related to mandibular dysfunction. No connection between deep overbite or open bite malocclusions was reported by many researchers.[13,23-27,29] Helm and colleagues[28] and Mohlin and associates[31] reported a higher incidence of TMD symptoms with open bite and no relationship with deep overbites. Riolo and others[30] observed a high degree of muscle tenderness in individuals with an open bite and no correlation with those with a deep overbite. Williamson[11] observed clicking and pain in pretreatment orthodontic patients with deep overbites.

Several studies comparing unilateral and bilateral crossbites with temporomandibular disorders found no relationship.[23–27,29] Mohlin and colleagues[31] observed subjects who had unilateral and bilateral crossbites with mandibular dysfunction, yet no differences in frequency were noted between the two types of crossbites. Egermark-Eriksson[13] agreed with these findings as they pertained to TMJ and muscle tenderness. Riolo and associates'[30] results were at variance with those of Mohlin and Egermark-Eriksson; however, a positive correlation was found between buccal crossbites and TMJ sounds.

Pullinger and others[29] reported no TMJ tenderness associated with crossbites but noted increases in "luxation clicking," particularly in unilateral crossbite subjects. They attributed this finding to laxity of the ligaments supporting the TMJ in crossbite cases, allowing the condyles to advance beyond the articular eminence. Helm and colleagues[28] described a higher frequency of TMJ locking, but without tenderness, in subjects with unilateral crossbite.

Functional shifts from retruded contact position (RCP) to the intercuspal position (ICP) were found to be negatively associated with mandibular dysfunction in Riolo and coworkers'[30] examination of 1342 children and teenagers. Among 298 young adults exhibiting TMJ tenderness, Bush[27] found that no RCP-ICP slide was evident in individuals with Class II and Class III malocclusions. When compared with the asymptomatic group, the Class I subjects had smaller slides. These findings compare favorably with the Pullinger study,[29] in which clicking was more prevalent in subjects who exhibited no slide and decreased as the slide increased. Pullinger and coworkers believe that a symmetric slide may represent a protective mechanism for the TMJ, allowing the condyle to seat more anteriorly as it slides forward from its retruded contact position to its intercuspal position.

An extensive study of the TMJs of 96 cadavers was undertaken by Solberg and others[32] to determine the association of change in joint morphology with various types of malocclusions. Class II and III malocclusions revealed deviations in the temporal and condylar osseus form. Posterior crossbites showed change in all TMJ components, whereas anterior crossbites exhibited deviations in form solely on the articular eminence. Flat condyles and open fossae were observed more frequently with deep overbites. Changes in disc form were more common in patients with abnormal overjet, and extreme overjet was evidenced in disc displacement. Solberg and colleagues concluded that malocclusions were associated with morphologic changes in the TMJ. Increased age was directly related to greater deviation of form, which led these investigators to surmise that the longer the malocclusion exists, the greater impact it has in changes in form of the TMJ.

Morphologic changes in the TMJ do not necessarily correlate with clinical signs and symptoms. Deviation in form is an adaptive change of the TMJ to accommodate inconsistencies in mandibular position, as produced by deviant occlusal patterns. This is an example of the body's protective mechanism working to adapt to an abnormal condition.

RELATIONSHIP OF ORTHODONTIC TREATMENT AND TEMPOROMANDIBULAR DISORDERS

Orthodontic treatment creates changes in both tooth and jaw position. It requires reorientation of periodontal fibers, resorption and apposition of alveolar bone, shortening of some muscle groups, and lengthening of others. The appliances at times cause discomfort and irritation of tissue. Extractions of teeth are at times integral to a successful result. Despite all these drawbacks, orthodontists are able to provide patients with an aesthetic and functional result. All phases of dentistry have unfavorable sequelae, and TMDs have at times been linked to orthodontic treatment.

Franks[33] expressed a positive correlation between orthodontic treatment and TMDs. He reported only a 2% incidence of TMDs in a control group, an incidence that is inconsistent with previously reviewed studies.[4–9,14,31] When comparing TMD symptoms in subjects who had undergone orthodontic treatment, he found that 11% of the 751 patients exhibited positive symptoms. Once again, this figure falls far below the majority consensus of TMD symptoms in a random sample population.

Roth[1] reported a relationship between TMD symptoms and postorthodontic treatment in seven of nine patients who evidenced occlusal and functional discrepancies. When the interferences were removed, the symptoms disappeared. Berry and Watkinson[34] reported a high incidence of mandibular dysfunction an average of 7 years after treatment in patients managed with removable appliances.

These reports notwithstanding, later studies have overwhelmingly discouraged the association between orthodontic treatment (whether of the fixed Begg's[35] or edgewise[36] technique, or of the removable-type[35,36] extraction or nonextraction regimen[37,38]) and TMDs.

Symptoms of TMDs in pretreatment orthodontic patients were reported by Williamson[11] (35%) and Perry[39] (15.5%). Larsson and Ronnermen[36] studied 23 patients 10 years after treatment. Five had undergone nonextraction activator treatment, whereas the other 18 received full banded treatment. In the fixed appliance group, all but one patient with Class II, division 2 malocclusion received extractions. Of these patients, 65% were symptom free, 31% exhibited mild dysfunction, and only 4% (one patient) had severe disturbances. These workers concluded that orthodontic treatment presents little future risk of post-therapeutic TMDs.

Sadowski and Be Gole[40] evaluated 75 former orthodontic patients who had been treated, from 10 to 35 years previously, with full fixed appliances. They were compared with a control group, using subjective findings in the form of questionnaires and clinical evaluations. No differences in the incidence of signs or symptoms of TMD were found between the orthodontically treated and control groups. Both groups exhibited a high degree of mandibular shift from RCP to ICP.

Janson and Hasund[37] investigated 60 patients 5 years out of retention, who were orthodontically treated for Class II, division 1 malocclusions. Thirty were treated with extractions. The other 30 were treated as nonextraction cases. They were compared with an untreated control group of the same age. The incidence of TMDs in the control group compared favorably with the studies by Helkimo.[41] Significantly fewer anamnestic and clinical symptoms were found in the nonextraction group than in the extraction and control groups. Clinically, the group with extraction showed fewer disturbances in the moderate and severe categories but more in the slight disturbance category. Janson and Hasund[37] stated, "The investigation does indicate that systematic orthodontic treatment is not a functional risk to patients with Angle's Class II, division 1 malocclusion."

A 10-year longitudinal study was undertaken by Dibbets and Van der Weele[35] to determine if orthodontic treatment is an etiologic factor in TMDs. Three categories of symptoms were studied: subjective, objective, and radiographic. Further comparisons were made between the Begg's and activator-treated subjects. Three series of data were collected: before treatment, 4 years after retention, and 10 years after initiation of the study. The findings showed that, in all three categories studied, treatment with the Begg's appliance, as compared with activators, does not increase TMD symptoms. The Begg's appliance group did show increases in objective findings soon after retention, but these higher frequencies evened out over the long term (10 years). These investigators attributed these discrepancies to age differences, because the Begg's subjects began treatment later. Thus, it took the activator-treated group a few years to "catch up."

Sadowski and Polson,[38] in two independent clinical studies, evaluated the prevalence of TMDs and the status of occlusal disturbances in former orthodontic patients compared with similar groups of adults exhibiting untreated Class I and Class II malocclusions. No significant differences were found between the treated and untreated groups in eight categories of subjective evaluation, pain and discomfort, or joint sounds.

Sadowski's group, in Illinois, found a statistically significant difference between RCP and ICP shifts in the orthodontic and control groups. In the orthodontic group, 1- and 3-mm shifts were noted in 61% of the subjects and greater than 3-mm shifts in 1%, compared with 70.9% and 6.8%, respectively, of the control group. The Polson study, in Rochester, New York, found no significant differences in shifts. As previously mentioned, the positive or negative impact on the TMJ of an RCP-ICP shift is still undetermined.

In a presentation before the International Association of Dental Research, Jamsa and colleagues[42] discussed their findings, relating occlusal interference and orthodontic treatment to TMD. Two pooled groups comprised of 109 10-year-old and 147 15-year-old children were randomly assigned to an occlusal adjustment treatment or a placebo treatment group. All subjects with orthodontic appliances were placed in a third group, which received no occlusal adjustment. The subjects were examined annually for TMJ symptoms, the younger ones for 6 years and the others for 3 years. At the end of the study, strong statistical relationships were found between occlusal interferences and TMDs in the pooled sample. However, signs of TMDs were somewhat less frequent in the orthodontic treatment group than in the placebo treatment group. The orthodontic patients did not show more interferences than the placebo subjects. The investigators concluded that "Orthodontic treatment with fixed appliances does not usually cause a major risk for TMJ dysfunction."

The many varied concepts regarding the condylar position in the fossa were discussed previously (see Chapter 18). However, there is some question about the effect of various malocclusions and orthodontic treatment on the placement of the condyle in the fossa. Pullinger and others[43] investigated 44 asymptomatic and untreated young adults to determine the effect that occlusion has on condylar position. No relationship was found between the degree of overbite and overjet and the condylar position. Similar findings were registered in correlating RCP-ICP slides. Class II malocclusions revealed a nonconcentric condylar position, with the condyle situated slightly anterior in division 1 cases and slightly posterior in division 2 cases. Some association was found between asymmetric RCP-ICP slides and right-left difference in the position of the condyle in the fossa.

Gianelly and others[44] examined the condylar position of untreated orthodontic patients compared with patients who had undergone four premolar full fixed appliance therapy (20 edgewise and 7 Begg's). It has been hypothesized[45] that patients having had bicuspid extraction tend to force the mandible posteriorly in the fossa, through retraction of the maxillary incisors, predisposing them to disc displacement. No differences in condylar position were found to exist between the treated and untreated patients. The investigators concluded that "Neither four-premolar extraction treatment nor deep bites were associated with posteriorly positioned condyles when visualized by corrected tomograms."

The data on the relationship of malocclusion, occlusal factors, and orthodontic treatment to TMDs are generally negative. A great deal of inconsistency is found within each group and subgroup, clouding any attempt at an overall statement of consensus. This lack of correlation between TMDs and the previously mentioned factors does not mean that the occlusion should be ignored or that the importance and quality of orthodontic care should be compromised. Nothing is black or white, and it is the shade of grey to which we must pay heed. Although one patient may have ability to adjust to an abnormal occlusal condition, another may succumb to symptoms. Establishing a good occlusion, reducing stress, and taking protective measures against parafunctional habits can, in my opinion, make a difference in the health of the TMJ and its related structures.

Moreover, we must consider in an entirely new light the effect of occlusal factors in the healing and adaptive processes of an individual who is recovering from a TMD episode. The results of this relationship are yet to be established. To quote Pullinger,[46] "The objective of any treatment is to promote any residual healing potential and to tilt the balance toward positive adaptation, rather than tissue breakdown. This involves control of adverse loading, stabilizing the joint components, plus stabilizing the end point of mandibular closure."

TREATMENT PLANNING

Prerequisites to Treatment

Orthodontic treatment should not be the primary treatment regimen for TMDs. Patients with acute symptoms should be stabilized in accordance with the therapeutic measures discussed in Chapters 23 through 27. Orthodontists should be satisfied, before starting treatment, that the following prerequisites have been met:

1. The patient is generally free of pain.
2. The patient can function sufficiently to maintain a proper diet, speech, and swallowing.
3. A therapeutic occluding position from which the patient can function has been established.
4. The patient has been maintained in this stable condition for at least 3 months.
5. The patient is willing to continue to be observed by the phase I practitioner during the orthodontic treatment phase.

It is the responsibility of the practitioner who institutes phase I therapy to inform patients of the changes that can occur in the occlusion prior to splint therapy. Even when the mandible is not intentionally repositioned, unexpected changes in occlusion can occur. The occlusal relationship, as well as the profile, can change, and in many instances correction of these changes will require not only orthodontic intervention to restructure the occlusion, but orthognathic surgery as well.

Figure 30–1A,B represents an asymptomatic patient who had a long facial pattern and who had been treated for bruxism and occlusal wear. No prior orthodontic treatment was noted. A maxillary stabilization splint with full

mandibular contact against a flat plane had been employed by his dentist for a period of approximately 6 months. After insertion of the appliance and several adjustment visits, the patient was not seen by the dentist for about 5 months. During that period, the mandible repositioned, resulting in an open bite (Fig. 30–1C,D,E). When the study casts are occluded in maximal intercuspation, the opposing wear facets contact, depicting the presplint occlusion (Fig. 30–1F,G). Orthodontic treatment, with the possibility of orthognathic surgery, was discussed with the patient, who chose not to un-

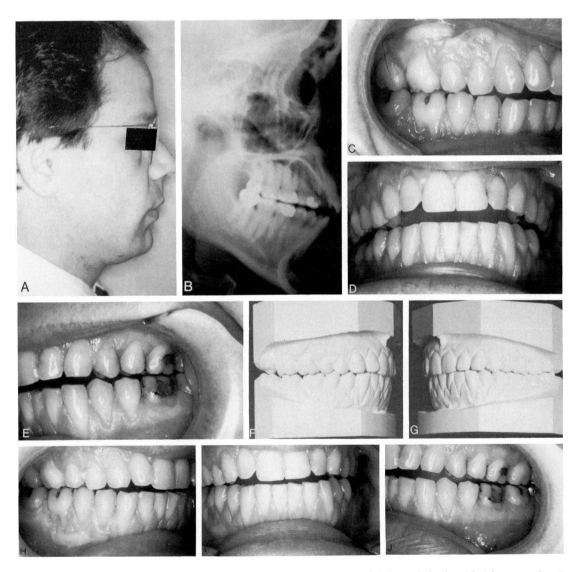

FIGURE 30–1. *A* and *B*, Facial and lateral cephalometric views showing a dolichocephalic (long) facial pattern. *C* to *E*, Intraoral views following splint therapy depicting an open bite. *F* and *G*, Models occluded to maximal cuspal interdigitation reveal opposing wear facets, which are expressive of the presplint occlusion. *H* to *J*, Approximately 1 year following the use of the splint, some closure of the bite is noted.

dergo any further therapy. The splint was discontinued, and the patient was recalled in 1 year. Some reduction in the open bite is noted (Fig. 30–1H,I,J). The patient was functioning well, desired no further treatment, and was dismissed.

The second patient (Fig. 30–2A,B), also a long facial type, was given a similar type of stabilization splint for pain in the maxillary left quadrant, thought to have been caused by bruxism. This individual had, as a child, undergone orthodontic treatment in which four bicuspids were removed. In the course of the 3-month period of splint therapy, the bite opened

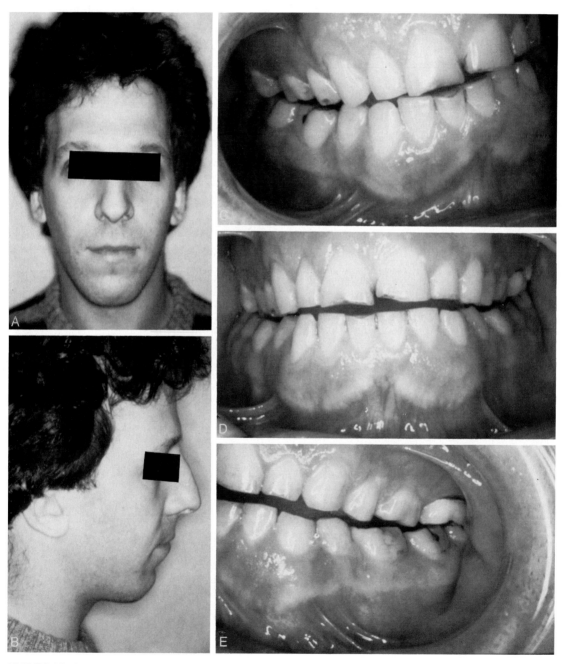

FIGURE 30–2. *A* and *B,* Frontal and side views depicting a long narrow facial pattern. *C* to *E,* Open bite resulting from splint therapy.

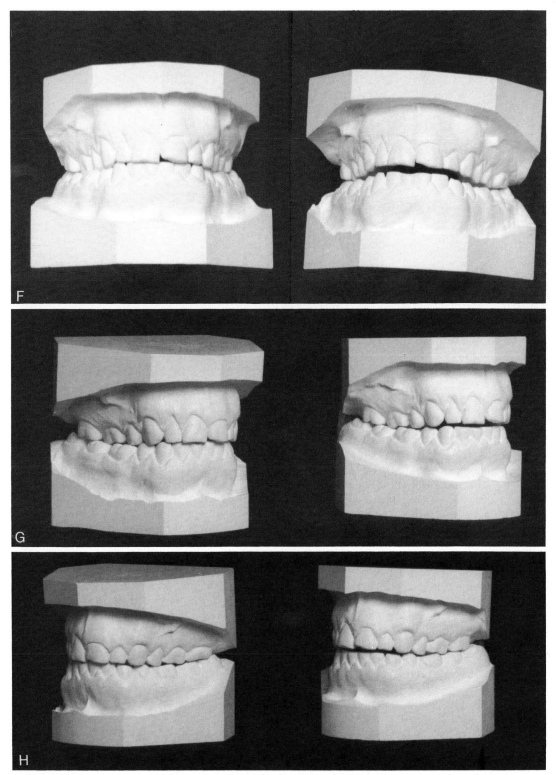

FIGURE 30–2 *Continued F to H,* Study casts taken after orthodontic treatment (left) reveal occlusal contact as compared with study casts taken after splint therapy (right).

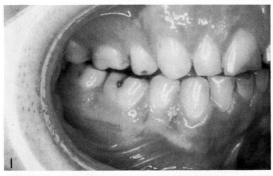

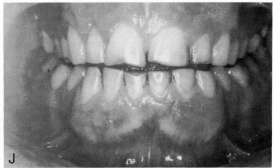

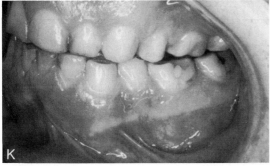

FIGURE 30–2 *Continued I* to *K,* Some of the open bite has been reduced 3 months following the discontinuance of the splint.

(Fig. 30–2C,D,E), causing concern to the patient. Postorthodontic treatment casts revealed adequate cuspal interdigitation when compared with post splint therapy casts. (Fig. 30–2F,G,H). The cause of the pain was found to be of a dental nature; endodontic therapy alleviated the problem. The splint was discontinued, and the patient was examined 3 months later. Some closure of the open bite was observed (Fig. 30–2I,J,K). After declining any further treatment, the patient was dismissed.

Figure 30–3 depicts unwanted changes in mandibular position as a result of splint therapy in a young woman who presented with joint pain, clicking, and muscle soreness. She also had a long, narrow face; the dentition revealed no overjet and little cuspal overlap as the result of severe occlusal wear (Fig. 30–3A,B,C). She had undergone orthodontic treatment as a preteen; four bicuspids were removed as part of the therapy.

A stabilization splint was constructed (Fig. 30–3D,E,F). On her return to the office just 3 weeks later, the bite could be seen to be opening (Fig. 30–3G,H,I). This patient had been made aware of this possibility, and now the probability of further mandibular repositioning and bite opening became real. The patient was strongly opposed to any orthodontic treatment and decided to forego the splint, rather than risk further changes. An occlusal adjustment was made on the posterior teeth to reduce the opening, and the patient was dismissed (Fig. 30–3J,K,L).

These three cases are testimony to the fact that splint therapy is not always reversible. Especially in patients with long facial qualities, there is the possibility that the mandible has been autorepositioned upward and forward in the formative growth period, in an attempt by the individual to maintain occlusal contact while the skeletal components are growing apart. In the cases in which orthodontic therapy was performed, part of the bite closure may have involved vertical elastics on the anterior teeth. In addition to moving the teeth together, this could have caused a mandibular rotation. These repositioned mandibles functioned well for these patients for many years. However, when a splint was inserted, the learned postural mechanisms were eliminated, and the muscles repositioned the mandible at its previous location.

If a patient is not aware of the possible consequences and the ensuing phase II treatment requirements, there may be serious dentolegal implications. Thoughtful and thorough explanations during phase I and phase II consultation visits help to make the treatment proceed smoothly through all stages.

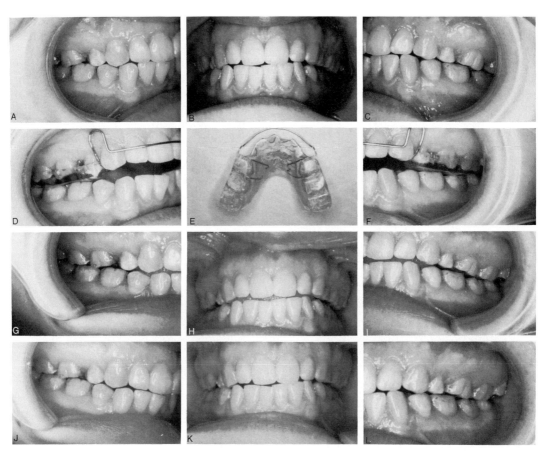

FIGURE 30–3. *A* to *C,* Presplint occlusion with little cuspal interdigitation and edge-to-edge incisal relationship. *D* to *F,* Maxillary posterior occluding splint in place. *G* to *I,* Bite opening after 3 weeks of splint therapy. *J* to *L,* Occlusion after occlusal adjustment.

One of the most important facets of orthodontic treatment planning for the patients with TMDs is communication—with patients at each visit concerning the status of their symptoms and with the phase I dentist who is overseeing them. Better service can be rendered to patients under this two-tier clinician arrangement. The orthodontist has a knowledgeable peer with whom to consult, and there is a feeling of teamwork and shared responsibility. All efforts can be directed to appliance therapy, and, should the patient develop any of the original symptoms, the orthodontist does not have to interrupt the therapy. The patient can be referred to the phase I dentist for evaluation.

The recurrence of symptoms is quite common during orthodontic treatment, and even mild TMJ discomfort can be alarming to patients. The most stable post phase I cases of TMD treatment will have flare-ups from time to time. This, too, should be explained to prospective patients during the orthodontic consultation appointment.

Diagnostic Workup and Evaluation
History and Examination

Before gathering the information that will determine the diagnosis and type of orthodontic treatment indicated, a full report should be requested from the phase I practitioner. This should include pretreatment symptoms, phase I therapy, and the current status of the patient. Familiarity with this information helps orthodontists become acquainted with their patients and aids them in anticipating patients' reactions to treatment. Orthodontists should ask patients to fill out medical and dental questionnaires and should review the TMD history and examination sheet with patients in order to evaluate personally the current status of TMD. Just as orthodontists routinely examine the teeth for discoloration and defects before placing appliances, so they must palpate the musculature to establish a base level of activity. Records need to be maintained for both the orthodontic therapy and the TMD.

Cephalometric Evaluation

Although the literature doesn't support a relationship between malocclusion and TMD (discussed previously), the skeletal characteristics and the relationship of the teeth to each other and their respective bony base are vital to the planning and execution of an orthodontic treatment program. Roentgenographic cepha-

lometry provides orthodontists with a window into the underlying hard tissue that supplies the framework for the overlying soft tissue.

Facial types can be determined cephalometrically using the following formula, which relates posterior face height (PFH) to anterior face height (AFH): posterior face height (S − Go) × 100/anterior face height (N − Me).*

Jarabak determined a mean value of 62 to 65% as a normal range. A lower figure is representative of a shorter posterior face height and more vertical facial growth, whereas a higher figure implies greater posterior face

---

*S = sella; Go = gonion; N = nasion; and Me = menton.

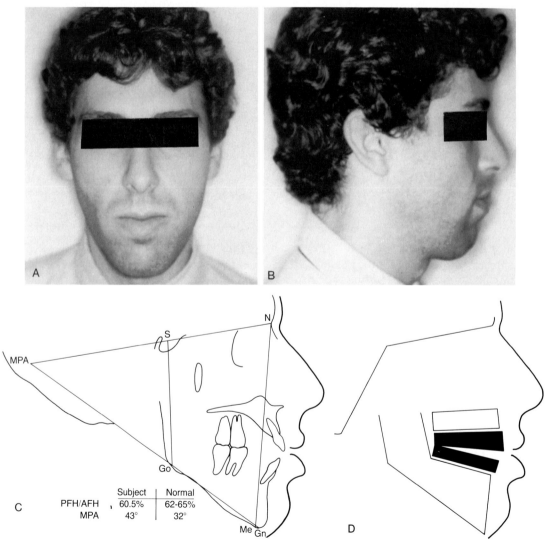

	Subject	Normal
PFH/AFH	60.5%	62–65%
MPA	43°	32°

FIGURE 30–4. *A* to *D*, Representative of a dolichofacial or long facial pattern.

height and a smaller vertical growth component for the face.

Vertical growth direction is also indicated by the size of the mandibular plane angle (MPA). A normal angle is 32°. This angle is composed of the intersecting lines N-S and Go-Gn. The larger the angle, the more vertical a pattern of growth and the greater the tendency for an open bite to develop. A smaller angle denotes a more horizontal growth pattern and an inclination toward a closed bite.

Cephalometric analysis also assists in establishing differences between abnormalities of the skeletal complex and those problems that involve the dentoalveolar structures. Skeletofacial patterns often dictate the parameters for tooth movement. A dolichofacial, or long facial, type represents a more vertical pattern of growth (Fig. 30–4A to D). An orthodontist would have reservations regarding the extent of bite closure that could be achieved in a skeletal open bite malocclusion. Without the aid of cephalometrics, the distinction between a dental and a skeletal pattern is often difficult to detect.

At the other extreme is a brachiofacial pattern, or broad facial type, with a reduction in vertical height (Fig. 30–4E–H). A closed or

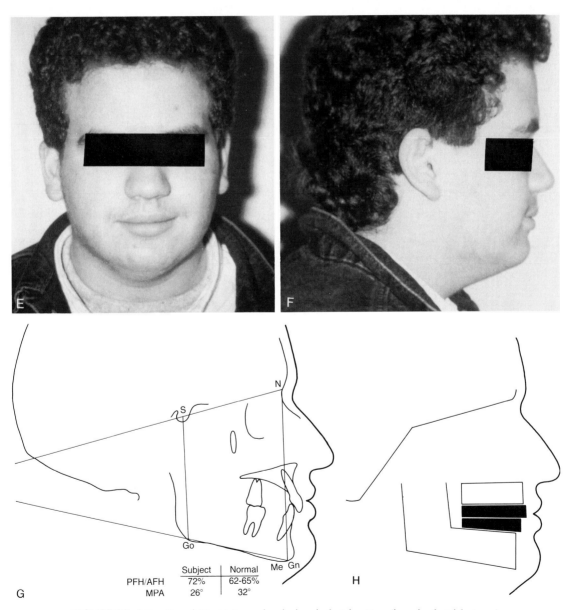

	Subject	Normal
PFH/AFH	72%	62-65%
MPA	26°	32°

FIGURE 30–4 *Continued E to H,* Example of a brachyfacial pattern (broader facial features).

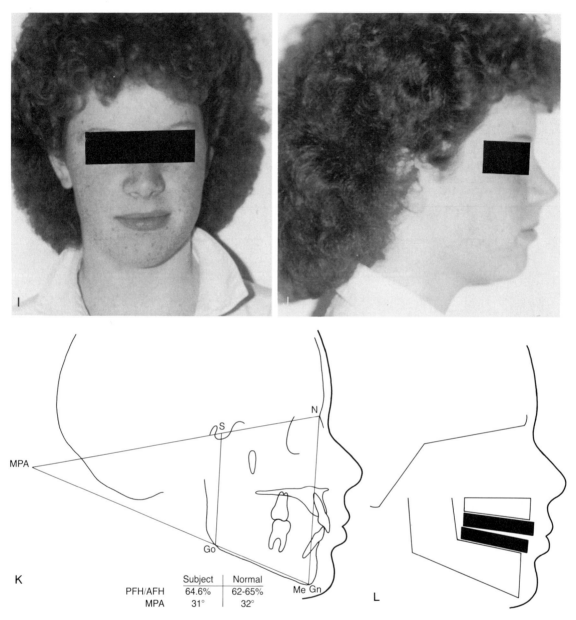

	Subject	Normal
PFH/AFH	64.6%	62-65%
MPA	31°	32°

FIGURE 30-4 *Continued I* to *L*, Well-proportioned facial type. (N = nasion; Me = menton; Gn = gnathion; Go = gonion; S = sella; MPA = mandibular plane angle; PFH/AFH = posterior face height/anterior face height.)

deep overbite condition would be reflective of this skeletal configuration. A downward and backward mandibular growth direction with an obtuse MPA would be indicative of the former facial type (see Fig. 30–4A–D), whereas a more forward mandibular growth direction with a more acute MPA is generally associated with the latter type (see Fig. 30–4E–H). An individual with more balanced facial components is shown in Fig. 30–4I to L. Relative sizes of the

maxilla and mandible, in both length and width, must be determined before tooth movement can be planned.

In Figure 30–5A–D, two types of Class I bimaxillary protrusion are shown. They produce the same effect on the profile, protruding the lips, although the etiologic mechanisms differ. One protrusion (see Fig. 30–5A,B) results from a skeletal abnormality, whereas the other (see Fig. 30–5C,D) is caused by an anterior dis-

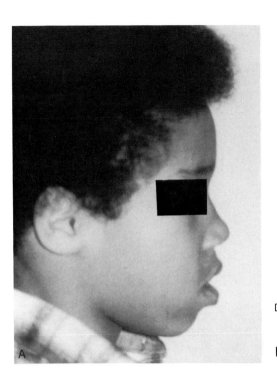

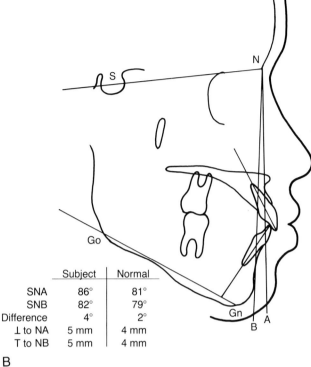

	Subject	Normal
SNA	86°	81°
SNB	82°	79°
Difference	4°	2°
⊥ to NA	5 mm	4 mm
T̄ to NB	5 mm	4 mm

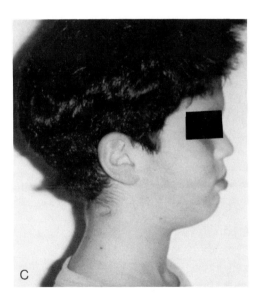

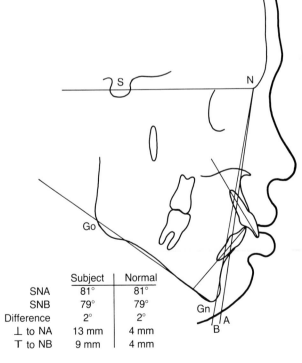

	Subject	Normal
SNA	81°	81°
SNB	79°	79°
Difference	2°	2°
⊥ to NA	13 mm	4 mm
T̄ to NB	9 mm	4 mm

FIGURE 30–5. Class I bimaxillary protrusion type malocclusions with the same basic profile patterns but different etiologic characteristics. *A* and *B* depict a malocclusion due to skeletal dysplasia. Figures *C* and *D* demonstrate malocclusion of a dentoalveolar nature. (S = sella; N = nasion; Go = gonion; Gn = gnathion; B = the deepest point on the concavity of the mandible between the chin and the incisor; A = the deepest point on the concavity of the premaxilla between the anterior nasal spine and the incisor; SNA = angle formed by sella-nasion and nasion, point A; SNB = angle formed by sella-nasion and nasion, point B; NA = nasion, point A; NB = nasion, point B.)

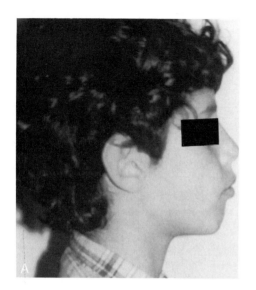

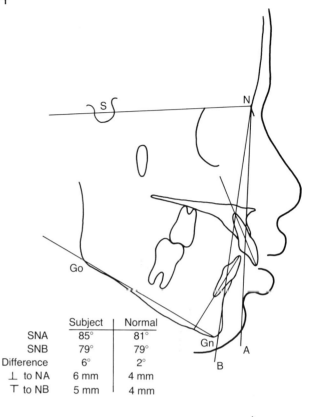

	Subject	Normal
SNA	85°	81°
SNB	79°	79°
Difference	6°	2°
⊥ to NA	6 mm	4 mm
⊤ to NB	5 mm	4 mm

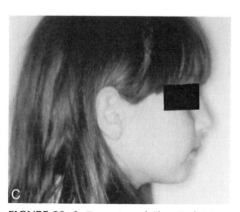

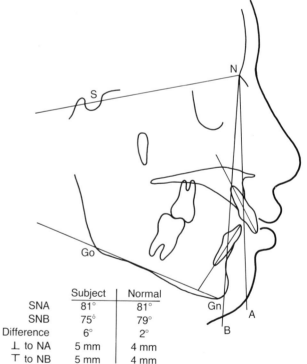

	Subject	Normal
SNA	81°	81°
SNB	75°	79°
Difference	6°	2°
⊥ to NA	5 mm	4 mm
⊤ to NB	5 mm	4 mm

FIGURE 30–6. Two types of Class II, division 1 malocclusions. *A* and *B* are typical of a more normal mandible and protruding maxilla. *C* and *D* typify an underdeveloped and retrusive mandible with a more normal maxilla. (S = sella; N = nasion; Go = gonion; Gn = gnathion; B = the deepest point on the concavity of the mandible between the chin and the incisor; A = the deepest point on the concavity of the premaxilla between the anterior nasal spine and the incisor; SNA = angle formed by sella-nasion and nasion, point A; SNB = angle formed by sella-nasion and nasion, point B; NA = nasion, point A; NB = nasion, point B.)

placement of the teeth. Correction of the dental malocclusion would have a dramatic effect in the latter instance, whereas in the former only a moderate change would occur because of the lack of impact that treatment would have on the basal bone. In the more extreme cases of the Figure 30–5A,B variety, an orthognathic surgical approach may be necessary to fully reduce the dysplasia.

Class II, division 1 type malocclusions also require a differential diagnosis. More often than one suspects, an underdeveloped mandible, not an excessive maxilla, is responsible for the typical overjet seen in these types of cases. Cephalometric evaluation aids in relating one arch to another. Then, by relating each jaw to the overall skeletal complex, one can determine where the growth differential exists.

Figure 30–6A,B shows a Class II, division 1 type malocclusion with a maxillary excess. A mandibular deficiency is noted in Figure 30–6C,D. Successful orthodontic treatment, whether for a child, adult, or phase II patient with TMD, is dependent on a proper cephalo-

metric determination of where the discrepancy lies, so that the mandible can be placed in the correct relationship with the maxilla.

Class II, division 2 malocclusions have been most suspect in contributing to TMDs because these malocclusions tend to force the mandible posteriorly. The lingually inclined maxillary incisors contact the labial surfaces of the lower incisors, and as the individual closes into a deep overbite, the mandible is retruded. Figure 30–7 represents such a situation. The cephalometric analysis reveals a lingual inclination to the mandibular incisors, resulting from the extreme vertical position of the upper incisors. A ramping effect is seen, and a surface, rather than a point, contact is seen to exist between the incisors.

Figure 30–8 depicts two variations of Class III skeletal-type malocclusions. The mandible is so excessive in Figure 30–8A,B that the lower incisors project beyond the labial surfaces of their maxillary counterparts. Closing does not cause any displacement of the mandible because of a complete lack of incisal guidance. In

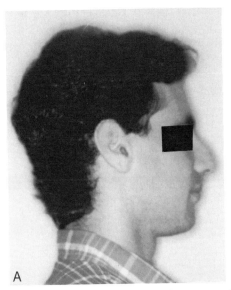
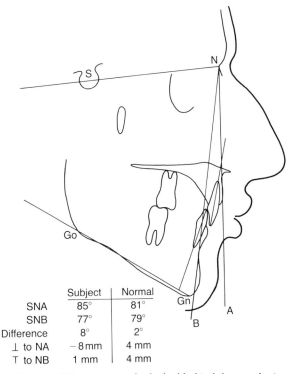

	Subject	Normal
SNA	85°	81°
SNB	77°	79°
Difference	8°	2°
$\perp$ to NA	−8 mm	4 mm
T to NB	1 mm	4 mm

FIGURE 30–7. *A* and *B*, Class II, division 2 malocclusion. The mandible appears to be locked behind the enveloping maxillary incisors. (S = sella; N = nasion; Go = gonion; Gn = gnathion; B = the deepest point on the concavity of the mandible between the chin and the incisor; A = the deepest point on the concavity of the premaxilla between the anterior nasal spine and the incisor; SNA = angle formed by sella-nasion and nasion, point A; SNB = angle formed by sella-nasion and nasion, point B; NA = nasion, point A; NB = nasion, point B.)

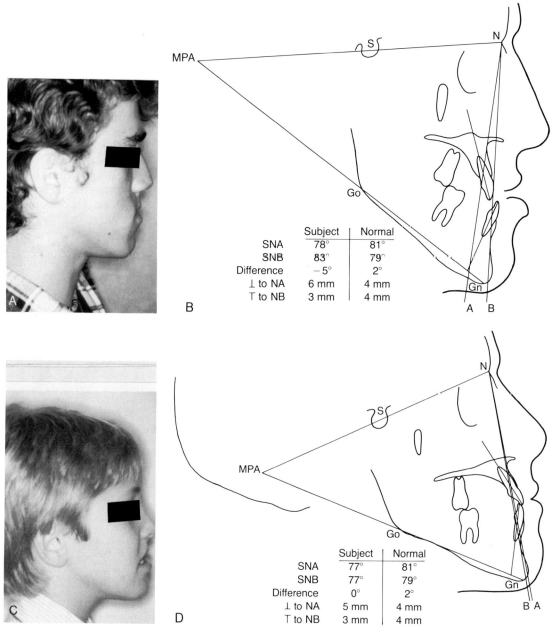

	Subject	Normal
SNA	78°	81°
SNB	83°	79°
Difference	−5°	2°
⊥ to NA	6 mm	4 mm
T to NB	3 mm	4 mm

	Subject	Normal
SNA	77°	81°
SNB	77°	79°
Difference	0°	2°
⊥ to NA	5 mm	4 mm
T to NB	3 mm	4 mm

FIGURE 30–8. Two class III malocclusions of skeletal origin are presented. *A* and *B* characterize a reverse overjet condition with no contact noted between the opposing incisors. *C* and *D* are descriptive of a class III case. A slight overjet due to the lingual inclination of the mandibular incisors exists. (MPA = mandibular plane angle; S = sella; N = nasion; Go = gonion; Gn = gnathion; B = the deepest point on the concavity of the mandible between the chin and the incisor; A = the deepest point on the concavity of the premaxilla between the anterior nasal spine and the incisor; SNA = angle formed by sella-nasion and nasion, point A; SNB = angle formed by sella-nasion and nasion, point B; NA = nasion, point A; NB = nasion, point B.)

comparison, the lingual inclination to the mandibular incisors exhibited in Figure 30–8C,D allows incisal contact. Because of the extreme interincisal angulation, the maxillary incisors can produce a torquing effect on the

lower jaw when closure occurs. In my opinion, the forces on the mandible that are produced in a Class III malocclusion, such as seen in Figure 30–8C,D, differ little from those produced in a Class II, division 2 malocclusion. Both conditions cause posterior displacement of the mandible.

Although there is some evidence in the literature that Class III malocclusions tend to promote TMDs,[29,31] it is my opinion that they are of the variety presented in Figure 30–8C,D. The situation shown in Figure 30–8A,B does not contribute to TMDs.

Anteroposterior cephalometric analysis is helpful in determining skeletal asymmetries (Fig. 30–9). The mandible can be measured for right- and left-side discrepancies, which could explain a jaw shift to one side on opening. The horizontal cant of the occlusal plane can be evaluated for asymmetries, which could result from the ramus on one side being longer than the other. This occlusal tilt could also be the result of one side of the face being longer than the other. The diagnosis of facial asymmetries through frontal cephalometrics can alter the treatment plan to include surgical correction of the skeletal defect before the initiation of orthodontic therapy.

Roentgenographic cephalometrics is also important as a "barometer." It aids in planning therapy, as well as in evaluating the changes that treatment has wrought. In children, growth becomes a dominant factor in treatment, and a cephalostat can give orthodontists some insight into growth potential. Through the use of computers with large patient data banks, growth prediction for an individual is becoming more sophisticated, allowing clinicians to plan therapy more accurately. Advantage can then be taken of a child's ability to grow and an orthodontist's ability to harness and direct that growth to a better end.

Cephalometric evaluation as part of the phase I diagnostic workup can add to the completeness of assessment and helps the dentist achieve more predictable results. Orthodontists frequently do not see patients until after phase I treatment is completed. If no pretreatment cephalostat is made, the changes effected by splint therapy cannot be evaluated, and the patient's pretreatment configuration is lost.

It is not the intent of this chapter to explain cephalometric landmarks or techniques. Interested practitioners can refer to many fine texts on orthodontics, some specifically devoted to cephalometry.[47-53]

Study Casts

More diagnoses have probably been made with the aid of study casts than with any other tools. A study cast replicates the dentition, provides practitioners with a static occlusion, and is simply manipulated. Measurements can be taken to determine tooth size as it relates to available arch length. Interarch and intra-arch relationships can be observed. The ease of fabrication and usefulness of study casts should be appreciated but not abused. Study casts alone

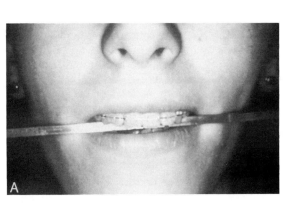
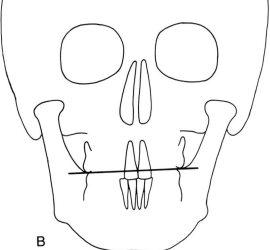

FIGURE 30–9. A and B, Comparison of a full-face photograph with an anteroposterior cephalometric tracing of a patient with a cant to the occlusal plane. Skeletal asymmetry in the length of the midface is evident through cephalometric evaluation.

should not be relied on as a total diagnostic modality. With all their advantages, dental casts are seen outside the facial complex and represent a static position of the dentition. Throughout the years, orthodontists have been taken to task for being overly concerned with providing patients with straight teeth and producing well-occluding final study casts while overlooking the occlusion in function.

In treating the patient with a TMD, function becomes paramount. The goal is first and foremost to provide patients with a well-balanced functional occlusion in a predetermined maxillomandibular position. The orthodontist has to position the teeth not in an ideal cephalometrically designed tracing or a Class I dental relationship, but rather in an arrangement determined by a patient's comfort and function, as defined by a functional condyle-disc-fossa relationship.

When impressions are taken as part of a phase II orthodontic workup, they are best poured twice. One set should be utilized as study casts for starting records and evaluating progress, and the second set should be articulated, employing the splint to establish the therapeutic occlusion.

Even a basic hinge-type articulator helps to provide the orthodontist with dynamic occlusion and allows for functional consideration. Treatment planning for a TMD phase II case is challenging, because practitioners are greatly limited by the specific spatial relationship into which the teeth must be placed. The mandibular position is fixed by the splint. In some instances, a diagnostic setup must be made to determine the feasibility and outcome of one's conditional treatment plan. Resetting segments of plaster teeth in the order of the planned treatment may be tedious, but it is also reassuring to know that one's theoretic concepts can be made functional.

Dental Radiographs

A full series of periapical x-ray films or a panoramic film is a required diagnostic aid for most dental procedures and is no less important for orthodontics. In addition to revealing abnormalities, such as missing and supernumerary teeth, impactions, and displaced teeth, they reveal the condition of the periodontium.

With an increasing number of adults seeking orthodontic treatment, a closer union has developed between orthodontists and periodontists. In young patients, it is rare to see changes in the supporting periodontal structures, despite poor hygiene and acute gingivitis. Children's resistance to periodontitis is high, and any soft-tissue change is usually reversible. However, when an adult patient is treated, the care and concern with the periodontium is increased. Any sign of disease must be attended to, because orthodontic appliances make it more difficult to maintain proper hygienic conditions. When a patient has anything less than healthy supporting tissues, a consultation should be sought, with the periodontist becoming part of the treatment team.

Photographs

Photographs or slides of the patient are also included in the diagnostic workup and are composed of full-face and profile shots, as well as several intraoral exposures. These aids help practitioners evaluate the facial structures, lip lines, profiles, gingival heights, and other aesthetic considerations. They also capture the condition of the enamel, revealing defects and discolorations, as well as positional irregularities of the teeth. Photographs are simple to take and provide an effective chronology of the various stages of treatment, as well as a treatment record.

Additional Diagnostic Material

For patients with internal derangements, diagnostic TMJ films should be available (see Chapters 18, 19, and 20). Most likely, they would have been ordered by the dentist providing phase I therapy. Patients should also be examined for unhealthy habits such as tongue thrusting, nail biting, and placing foreign objects in the mouth. These behaviors can contribute to TMD and can also affect the occlusion.[54] If not corrected, they can have a destabilizing effect on the corrected dentition.

Some orthodontists perform their own myofunctional therapy as part of the overall treatment, whereas others refer their patients to speech pathologists or myofunctional therapists for the necessary repatterning.

Establishing the Diagnosis

A systematic procedure is advised in the evaluation of an occlusion for morphologic and functional discrepancies that compose the elements of a malocclusion. Ackerman and Proffit[55] have devised a classification of five characteristics by which a malocclusion can be diagnosed. This method can be used as a framework within which the diagnosis of the unique elements of phase II TMD can be identified.

FACIAL PROPORTIONS AND AESTHETICS

Facial proportions and aesthetics are evaluated both at the initial examination and during the cephalometric diagnosis. Specific observations should be noted at the time of the initial examination and again during the the preorthodontic examination.

Phase I aesthetic observations include a profile examination, in which the degree of facial convexity is noted. A straight line drawn from the tip of the nose to the chin point reveals the general outline of the lower face. If the lips are behind this line, a concave figuration is noted (Fig. 30–10C), whereas more protrusive lips extend anterior to this plane, revealing a convex profile (Fig. 30–10F). If the line slopes backward, a more retrusive chin position is present. A forward inclination of the facial plane is indicative of a strong chin and a possible prognathic mandibular relationship.

The thickness of the lips and facial tissue should also be observed, both cephalometrically and photographically (Fig. 30–10A,B, C,D,E), because changes in incisal relationships will be more visible on an individual with thinner tissue. The proportions of the head are

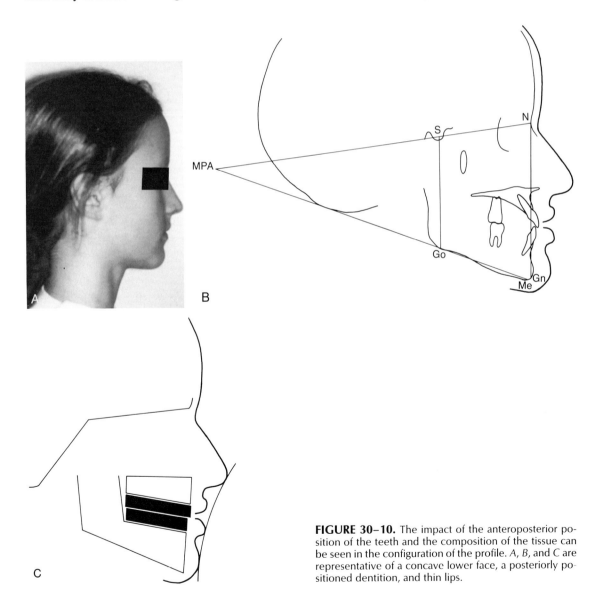

FIGURE 30–10. The impact of the anteroposterior position of the teeth and the composition of the tissue can be seen in the configuration of the profile. *A, B,* and *C* are representative of a concave lower face, a posteriorly positioned dentition, and thin lips.

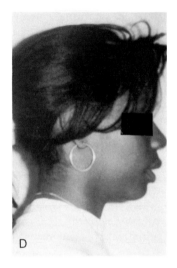

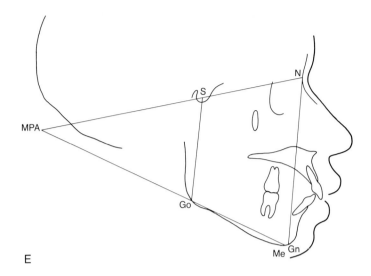

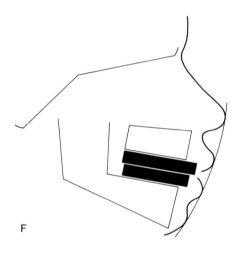

FIGURE 30–10 *Continued D, E,* and *F* depict a convex lower face, forward positioning of the dentoalveolar complex, and full lips. (MPA = mandibular plane angle; S = sella; N = nasion; Go = gonion; Me = menton; Gn = gnathion.)

categorized with regard to upper face, midface, and lower face height. Each should compose approximately one third of the total facial height. Facial typing is evaluated for a long, a broad, or a normal well-proportioned facial type.

A patient's self-image should be discussed as part of the history intake information: What is the individual's attitude toward his or her appearance? Would the changes that may result from mandibular repositioning be acceptable to the patient? The answers to these questions could alter the type of treatment prescribed and, in extreme instances, identify a patient for whom a repositioning splint should not be recommended.

Full-face and profile photographs are very helpful for confirming findings, as well as for presenting to patients an objective image of their appearance.

The second diagnostic aid to aesthetic evaluation is the cephalometric radiograph. It provides orthodontists with the ability to focus in on skeletal configuration and tooth position. When one or more of the standard cephalometric analyses are applied, the various skeletal and dental components can be measured to determine which elements are distorting the facial configuration. Size discrepancies within the skeletal matrix are analyzed, especially with regard to the maxilla and mandible. Spatial relationships between the facial bones are determined; they are then related to the cranial base. The tooth positions and their angulations are added to obtain a true picture of the makeup of facial aesthetics.

Orthodontists must then evaluate the facial changes that will occur as a result of appliance therapy. These changes should be discussed with patients at the time of the consultation. Patients should not harbor any expectations that phase II orthodontic treatment will return the facial features to their original pretreatment position. A careful explanation and description of the various profile changes that can be expected during phase I and phase II therapy allow patients to proceed through treatment with a minimum of anxiety and a maximum of confidence.

ALIGNMENT AND SYMMETRY WITHIN THE DENTAL ARCHES

The alignment of the teeth within each dental arch should be noted. If crowding or spacing exists, an evaluation is made of tooth size and arch length. The discrepancy is recorded, and the space requirements in one arch are compared with those in the opposing arch. In an adult, one cannot incorporate the patient's genetic growth potential; increased arch size must be gained by some sort of expansion, and additional space is obtained through tooth reduction or extraction. Because these procedures have their disadvantages, they must be used in moderation. The ill effects of each individual one are minimized when elements of both options are combined.

The symmetry of the dental arches is examined for aberrations. A line is drawn down the palatal and lingual midlines of both casts. Measurements are recorded from the right and left cusp tip of each cuspid to the midline and posteriorly from the right and left cusp tip of the mesiolingual cusp of the first molar to the midline.

Differences in arch width from one side to the other would indicate asymmetry. Asymmetry in one arch could be reflected in the opposing arch. This asymmetry might be the result of a prior habitual behavior, such as found in students who read while leaning their faces against their open hand. Studious youngsters with this habit in effect use their hand as an orthodontic appliance, affecting the constriction of both the upper and lower dental arches on one side.

EVALUATION OF SKELETAL AND DENTAL RELATIONSHIPS IN THE TRANVSVERSE PLANE OF SPACE

Articulated models are used to examine for any transverse discrepancies. In patients in whom the mandible has been advanced during phase I treatment into a therapeutically derived occlusion, it is not uncommon for a crossbite to exist, even if there was none present prior to splint therapy. When the lower jaw is moved forward, a wider portion of the mandible is brought into contact with a narrower portion of the maxilla. Therefore, some expansion of the upper arch may be necessary.

When a posterior crossbite exists, the buccolingual inclination of the molars should be evaluated. If the upper teeth are inclined lingually and the palatal width is adequate, the crossbite is of a dental nature. In these cases, uprighting the molars is sufficient to correct the crossbite. When a true maxillary arch width insufficiency is noted in an adult, a surgical procedure may be required for palatal expansion.

Patients who exhibit crossbites caused by a palatal insufficiency often close into a normal occlusion on one side and a marked crossbite on the opposite side. This arrangement is common and represents an acquired or habitual occlusion. The mandibular midline shifts to the side of the crossbite, as the mandible is redirected into the functional position.

If the mouth is opened wide, the muscles and ligaments supporting the mandible stretch out to their normal length, causing the mandible to reposition to its normal, unstrained relationship with the maxilla. Therefore, the midlines once again become harmonious in the open position. If the teeth were brought into first contact from a wide-open position in a straight line path of closure, the crossbite would be distributed evenly between both sides. The cusps of the opposing arches would occlude end to end, preventing the patient from attaining a cusp-fossa interdigitation. Because this represents an unworkable relationship, the mandible shifts to one side or the other in an effort to achieve maximum occlusal contact.

Care must be taken to ensure a proper diagnostic evaluation of the crossbite. Lateral shifting of the mandible is translated to the TMJ. On the side of the crossbite, the condyle will be positioned posteriorly and laterally. The condyle is thus positioned more posteriorly, which may increase the likelihood that the disc will displace anteriorly and contact the retrodiscal tissue should microtrauma occur.[56] On the contralateral side, the condyle repositions forward and medially (Fig. 30–11B). The consequences of a lateral shift of the mandible into a crossbite position can be exacerbated during

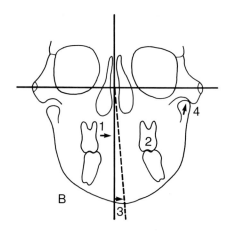

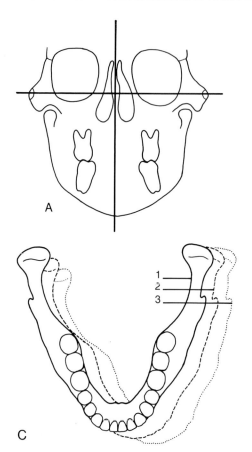

FIGURE 30–11. *A,* Normal transverse occlusal and condylar position. A satisfactory bilateral symmetry is evident. (Courtesy of Dr. Albert H. Owen, III.) *B,* Constricted maxilla (*1*) produces a crossbite (*2*) when the mandible shifts to the side of the crossbite (*3*) and initiates a condylar displacement on the ipsilateral side (*4*). (Courtesy of Dr. Albert H. Owen, III.) *C,* The normal transverse position of the mandible (*1*) is shifted to the left in an acquired centric occlusion (*2*) as a result of a crossbite. Further lateral movement occurs (*3*) when the mandible is in a functioning state.

masticatory or parafunctional activity. On the side of the crossbite, the mandible has assumed a more lateral position, from which it further deviates during functional movements (Fig. 30–11C).

Crossbites most often involve an insufficiency of the upper arch. However, there are instances of mandibular dysplasias, as found in a Class III malocclusion, in which the crossbite is the result of an abnormally large mandible.

EVALUATIONS OF SKELETAL AND DENTAL RELATIONSHIPS IN THE ANTEROPOSTERIOR PLANE OF SPACE

Anteroposterior positions of the maxillomandibular complex often define the parameters of mandibular repositioning. Less flexibility is found in the Class I relationship than in the Class II relationship. In the latter case, a more favorable occlusal interdigitation can be achieved when the mandible is advanced (Fig. 30–12C,D). This is particularly favorable when the Class II malocclusion results from an underdeveloped or posteriorly positioned mandible.

Class I malocclusions, especially of the bimaxillary protrusion variety, offer little leeway in forward movement of the mandible. If the mandible is advanced in a Class I relationship (Fig. 30–12A,B), some tooth reduction is necessary in the mandibular anterior segment. This allows for maintenance of a normal overjet as opposed to an end-on bite. Posteriorly, a tendency toward a Class III molar relationship results.

As previously discussed, there are two basic types of skeletal Class III malocclusions. In one, the mandibular incisors are anterior to the maxillary incisors (Fig. 30–12F); there are no restrictions on the forward movement of the mandible, and no retrusive forces are transmitted to the TMJ by the contacting incisors. In the second type, the mandibular incisors are inclined lingually and maintain a degree of overbite and overjet (Fig. 30–12E). In this instance, the lower incisors can act as a ramp, forcing the condyle backward and upward during the act of closure. When the mandible was growing disproportionately to the maxilla, the lower incisors were caught behind the maxillary inci-

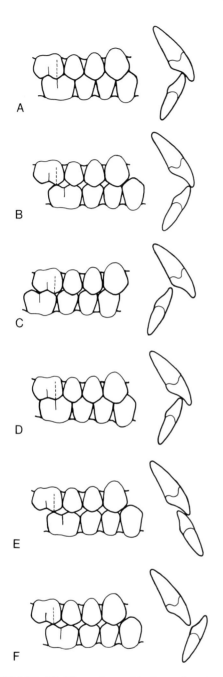

FIGURE 30–12. Effect of repositioning various types of occlusions. *A*, Class I occlusion. *B*, Class I occlusion repositioned anteriorly takes on some of the characteristics of a class III occlusion. *C*, Class II occlusion. *D*, Advancement of the mandible transforms a class II into a class I occlusion. *E*, Class III occlusion with lingually tipped incisors. *F*, No change noted in posterior occlusion, but incisors have been uprighted and unlocked.

sors. As the mandible grew, the incisors were tipped lingually.

This situation occasionally results from orthodontic therapy in which an attempt is made to avoid orthognathic surgery, while providing the patient with a degree of overbite and overjet. To correct this situation, a bilateral osteotomy is necessary to retract the mandible and provide an aesthetic and functional result. Otherwise, the patient must accept a less attractive outcome when the mandibular incisors are uprighted to an even more procumbent position (Fig. 30–12E,F), in an effort by the orthodontist to free the mandible.

EVALUATION OF SKELETAL AND DENTAL RELATIONSHIPS IN THE VERTICAL PLANE OF SPACE

Vertical abnormalities are of two types: open bites and deep overbites. Open bites are either anterior or posterior separations between the teeth in the vertical plane. They can be either developmental, characterized by a skeletal dysplasia, or dental, associated with a particular oral habit. Deep overbites can also emanate from a deviant skeletal pattern or result from various occlusal factors. The latter causes include an increased Spee's curve, a loss of vertical height caused by missing dental components, or severe wear of the occlusal surfaces. Before restoring these cases, the dentist must take careful measurements to evaluate the patient's proper vertical dimension. A reduced vertical dimension causes tension in the elevator muscles and may position the condyle deeper into the fossa.

Both skeletal and dental open bites present challenges to orthodontists during phase II treatment. It is important, however, to differentiate between the two. Cephalometric analysis holds the answer to this diagnostic question. A mild vertical dysplasia with a slight open bite can be corrected orthodontically. In more severe cases, orthodontics, together with an orthognathic surgical approach, should be considered.

Dental open bites exhibit a normal skeletal pattern, but the teeth in the area of the open bite appear depressed and at a lower level than the plane of occlusion. An opening between the posterior teeth, usually in the bicuspid area, typifies a lateral open bite. This type of problem is most often accompanied by a lateral tongue thrust. Myofunctional therapists find this habit the most difficult to correct, and orthodontists should approach it guardedly. Long-term retention, utilizing a lingual tongue guard to prevent the tongue from wedging the posterior teeth apart, should be considered.

Cephalometric evaluation clearly identifies patients with skeletal deep overbite. These patients can present a normal plane of occlusion, but because of the shorter dimensions of the lower face and more vertical pattern of closure, a deep overbite develops. These cases are more difficult to correct and maintain. It is necessary to increase the length of all the posterior teeth in order to establish a greater vertical dimension. In extreme cases, prosthetic therapy is necessary to establish a higher plane of occlusion.

Deep overbites of dental etiology exhibit a more normal skeletal pattern; however, the curve of Spee is abnormally increased. The lower incisors are elevated above the posterior occlusal plane, and the maxillary incisors might appear elongated. Correcting this type of malocclusion is accomplished by leveling or aligning all the teeth to a flatter horizontal plane. The more one levels the occlusal plane, the more one gains in vertical dimension.

Evaluation of Prior Phase I Treatment

Consulting with the Dentist Treating the Temporomandibular Disorder and Planning a Course of Treatment to Stabilize the Phase I Result

Orthodontic treatment for TMDs emanates from the phase I therapy. It is a means of stabilizing the occlusion so that patients can function in a more comfortable mandibular position. Not every patient who undergoes TMJ therapy requires orthodontic treatment. Many patients can function quite well with their pre-existing occlusion, especially when supported by a splint. Occlusal adjustment or prosthodontics is also an option when more minor changes in the occlusion are necessary following phase I treatment.

However, with a great many patients, the discrepancy between the corrected musculo-skeletal position of the mandible and the occlusion is too great for either of the previously mentioned options. In these situations, orthodontic therapy is necessary. A close working relationship among the various members of the TMD team is essential. During the orthodontic appliance phase of treatment, many changes are made in the occlusion, and multiple force mechanisms are employed to move the teeth

into position. There may at times be a recurrence of symptoms; close monitoring by the phase I dentist, as well as the physical therapist, if one is employed, is helpful in returning patients to an asymptomatic state.

All members of the team should be kept informed of a patient's progress. Not only is this helpful to the practitioner, but it reassures patients that their progress is being monitored by all of the therapists involved.

Analysis of Splint Therapy

The product of repositioning splint therapy is often a splint bearing the occlusal blueprint for the most optimal maxillomandibular relationship. It will dictate the proper vertical lower facial height and the anteroposterior and mediolateral positions of the mandible. The splint should be consistent with the appropriate condyle-disc-fossa relationship and should be worn comfortably by patients for several months before the phase II treatment.

In some cases, only an increase in vertical height is necessary to relieve the symptoms of either myofascial pain dysfunction or internal derangement. However, patients may find that without the splint, any attempt to close into the original habitual occlusion at a decreased vertical height may incite a return of the original symptoms. In these cases, the orthodontic treatment is directed toward increasing the lower facial height through eruptive tooth movements. Commonly, mandibular repositioning results in a more forward placement of the mandible, either to recapture the disc or to reduce the condylar loading on the retrodiscal tissue. This requires a more complex series of tooth movements that would vary, depending on the original occlusion or malocclusion. Tooth structure, particularly in the lower arch, is occasionally reduced when the mandible is proclined.

The Treatment Plan
Splint Selection

Splint selection is an important element in both phase I and phase II treatment of patients with TMD. It must serve the therapeutic requirements of the case while preserving the integrity of the dentition. A phase I splint, whether of the stabilization or repositioning variety, should not be an orthodontic appliance and thus should not move teeth. If a patient has parafunctional habits, force can be expected to be transmitted from the splint surface to the opposing teeth.

If only a segment of the dentition contacts the splint, some intrusion of the occluding teeth and extrusion of the teeth not in contact can occur. These cases are best treated with a full-coverage flat plane splint (see Chapter 23). In patients who cannot tolerate a full-coverage splint because it would cause a compromise in their speech or aesthetics, a daytime Gelb-type splint[57] can be employed as an adjunct to the stabilization (full arch) splint, which can be worn at night. This arrangement reduces any unwarranted tooth movement.

The thickness of the acrylic may vary anteroposteriorly, according to the direction of the opening movements of the mandible, which can also be a clue to the direction to which the mandible may reposition. Figure 30–13 shows the three basic opening patterns of the mandible. The corresponding facial types with which they are associated are illustrated in Figure 30–4.

Figure 30–4A to D shows a long, narrow facial type, depicting a more vertical growth pattern. The mandibular plane is tipped downward and backward in a clockwise direction. A small opening in the first molar area would be greatly magnified in the incisor region, and this would be reflected in the thickness of the splint (Fig. 30–13B).

In Figure 30–4I to L, a broader and shorter face is shown. The mandibular plane is more parallel to the palatal plane. When the occlusal plane is opened, the maxillary and mandibular arches remain more parallel, with less of a counterclockwise rotation. The resulting splint would have a more even thickness of acrylic than the splint previously described (Fig. 30–13B).

Figure 30–4E to H depicts a normally proportioned face with well-balanced skeletal components. In this instance, although the anterior thickness of the splint is greater, there is a gradual increase from the posterior to the anterior (Fig. 30–13C).

The splint is usually used throughout orthodontic therapy. When parafunctional habits are absent, the splint can be discontinued when the teeth have been realigned to the therapeutically derived occlusion. Most often, however, supportive splint therapy is continued even after a stable occlusion is achieved.

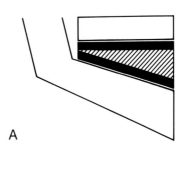

A

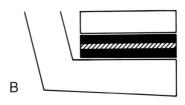

B

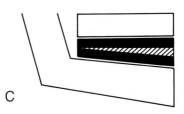

C

FIGURE 30–13. Splint thickness as defined by the facial and opening patterns. *A,* Vertical facial type producing a narrow interocclusal height posteriorly and a wide interincisal height anteriorly when the mandible is opened. *B,* Horizontal facial type with a more even interocclusal and interincisal space when the mandible is opened. *C,* A normal facial type with a gradual increase in interdental height from the molars to the incisors.

TREATMENT

Early Orthodontic Treatment

Orthodontic therapy performed on young people is tantamount to preventive TMD treatment. Mixed dentition intervention is designed to correct skeletal discrepancies or abnormal dental relationships that could affect the normal growth of the jaw. Children are usually treated between the ages of 7 and 10-years, although there is a wide variation of individual growth and development.

A thorough diagnostic evaluation is most important in pinpointing the skeletal areas that are developing abnormally. An appliance is selected to enhance or retard the growth of a particular aspect of the skeleton. Balancing the maxillomandibular components in the mixed dentition stage will provide a healthier environment for the eruption of the remaining permanent teeth and for the proper function of the TMJ and the related musculature.[37]

One of the most common developmental abnormalities of the maxilla is a deficiency in lateral development. This inadequacy can be the result of an overall narrow genetic midfacial development. Habits such as mouth breathing and tongue thrusting have a greater effect on a long, narrow face than on one that is broader. The tongue, instead of transmitting lateral pressure to the palatal bones, drops down to the floor of the mouth. Pressure from the perioral and buccinator muscles is not counterbalanced and the net result is an underdeveloped palate. When the teeth erupt, the maxillary arch is not wide enough to envelop the mandibular arch. The cusp tips make first contact in an edge-to-edge manner (Fig. 30–14B), and the patient adapts to this situation by indiscriminately shifting the lower jaw to the right or left to allow the teeth to deflect into a cusp-fossa contact (Fig. 30–14C).

The side to which the shift occurs exhibits a crossbite, whereas the opposing side appears normal. A learned closing response soon follows, permitting the mandible to close directly into a habitual occlusion and avoiding any cuspal deflection. It must never be assumed that a crossbite is unilateral, no matter how natural the occlusion appears or how normal the closing pattern seems. Maximal opening usually aligns the mandible and corrects the midline, allowing the operator to establish a proper diagnosis.

Treatment for correction of a palatal insufficiency is best initiated during the mixed dentition stage. The sutures of the skull are active, open, and sensitive to any lateral stress exerted on the palate. Palatal expansion appliances are varied in design and can be either fixed or removable.[58,59] Fixed expansion appliances can be of the lingual arch type (Fig. 30–15A) or the type that incorporates a jackscrew device (Fig. 30–15B). Removable expansion appliances utilize the same mechanical devices (Fig. 30–15C), but, because of their ability to be removed, they are less predictable and require greater cooperation by patients.

Fixed expansion appliances are more stable and accomplish the expansion in a shorter time. Figure 30–16A,B,C depicts a young pa-

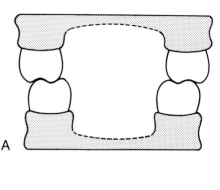
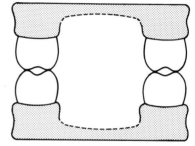
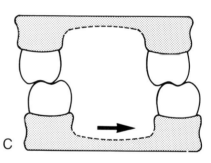

FIGURE 30–14. Lateral shifting of the mandible in response to an arch width discrepancy with the maxilla. *A,* This represents a normal transverse occlusal relationship. *B,* A maxillary lateral insufficiency exists, and the maxillary molars are in a cusp-to-cusp relationship when first occlusal contact is made. *C,* The mandible shifts to one side allowing the molars to achieve a cusp fossa relationship.

tient with a maxillary lateral insufficiency, which results in the mandible shifting into a crossbite position. The off-center (Fig. 30–16B) midline realigns after rapid palatal expansion with a fixed appliance (Fig. 30–16D,E,F) similar to the one shown in Figure 30–15B.

A stepwise radiographic depiction of a rapid palatal expansion procedure is shown in Figure 30–17. In patients with parafunctional habits, therapy to correct the habit should be part of the overall treatment plan[54]; otherwise, the muscle imbalance will continue to act on the

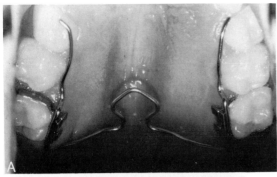
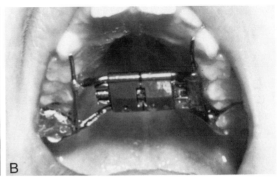
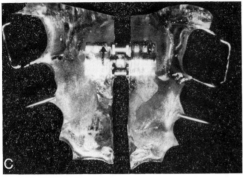

FIGURE 30–15. Example of palatal expansion appliances. *A,* The fixed Wilson lingual expansion arch. *B,* Fixed rapid palatal expansion appliance. *C,* Removable palatal expansion appliance.

developing bones and teeth, destabilizing the results of palatal expansion. Habits do not always affect the dentition, but they should be identified and treated. A habit-free, well-balanced musculature is one way of fortifying a patient against a potential TMD.

Deep overbites and severe overjets should not be treated as individual facets of a malocclusion. Their relationship to each other, as determined by the position of the mandible, is all important. Biteplate therapy to treat a child's overbite may be the correct treatment for the overbite, but it may neglect a more important problem of a retrusive mandible. If this is the case, a functional appliance may be indicated to accomplish both these corrections.

In Class II malocclusions, when the maxilla is too procumbent (see Fig. 30–6A), early treatment is directed toward retarding its forward component of growth. Distal pressure against the maxillary molars is transmitted to the sutural growth centers of the maxilla—pterygopalatine, zygomaxillary, and frontomaxillary—as well as to the spheno-occipital synchondrosis in the skull. Because bone will not grow in an area of compression,[60–62] the forward vector of maxillary growth is slowed, yet all other directional components develop unimpeded. The expectation is for the normally developing mandible to progress forward

and to achieve a Class I relationship with the maxilla.

Class II malocclusions that exhibit normal maxillas and retrusive underdeveloped mandibles require stimulation of condylar growth (see Fig. 30–6B). When the mandible is moved forward by a postural hyperpropulsar type of appliance, tension is transmitted to the condylar head by the pull of the muscles and ligaments. Increased cartilaginous proliferation occurs in response to this tension, resulting in a more rapid period of growth.[63–66] Remodeling of the glenoid fossae allows for accommodation of the repositioned condyles.[67,68]

Controversy exists over the effectiveness of early treatment as preventive therapy for Class III malocclusions. Graber[69] reported a substantial reduction in the growth of the mandible by utilizing retraction therapy, whereas Mitani and Fukazawa[70] found little change between the treated group and the control group.

The most common appliance employed in early Class III treatment is a chin cup attached to headgear. The elastic traction band imparts backward and upward pressure against the chin, forcing the condyles posteriorly and superiorly in the fossa. It would seem that this mode of treatment could predispose patients to many types of joint pathology, but most obviously to anterior disc displacement. Orthodon-

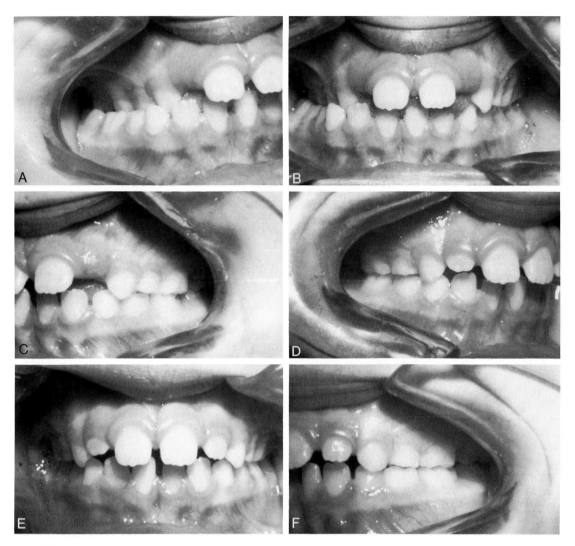

FIGURE 30–16. Correction of crossbite, resulting from a maxillary lateral insufficiency, utilizing a fixed rapid palatal expansion appliance. *A* to *C*, Mandibular shift to the right side into crossbite to accommodate narrow maxilla. Midline is off center. *D* to *F*, Crossbite corrected, and mandible realigns to proper midline position.

tists should try to avoid imposing forces on the mandible that would cause a negative impact on the TMJ.

Class I malocclusion implies a maxillomandibular relationship that is within normal limits. When an arch length deficiency exists, early treatment may concentrate on developing both arches to their greatest morphogenetic potentials. There are instances in which correction of tooth positions is indicated; for example, situations in which a tooth interferes with proper function or normal development, such as in a crossbite. Generally, mixed dentition is not suitable for aligning because the final positions of the the teeth are highly unpredictable. Moreover, additional tooth movement may be indicated when the remaining permanent teeth erupt. By delaying treatment, orthodontists can avoid the need to repeat fixed appliance therapy.

Patient cooperation is paramount. Treating patients in several stages when one could suffice is inefficient and taxing. Thus, when possible, treatment of mixed dentition should be limited to orthopedic correction and the balancing of skeletal components. Comprehensive

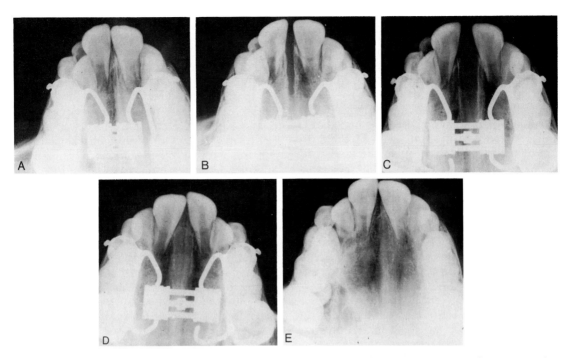

FIGURE 30–17. Radiographic chronology of the changes during rapid palatal expansion. *A,* Appliance inserted. *B,* Initial sutural separation 4 days later. *C,* Final midpalatal expansion 15 days later. *D,* Immature bone formation 6 weeks hence. *E,* Mature bone fill and enlarged maxilla 12 weeks from the time of last appliance activation.

fixed appliance therapy should coincide with a patient's achieving full permanent dentition during the period of treatment.

Functional Appliance Therapy

The 20th century witnessed the coming of age of orthodontics. Parallel but distinct concepts and systems of treatment were evolving in Europe and the United States. Removable appliances (termed *functional appliances*) were being developed in Europe by such pioneers as Andresen,[72] Haupl,[73] Schwarz and Gratzinger,[74] Balters,[75] and Frankel.[76] On this side of the Atlantic, fixed orthodontic appliance systems were being formulated by Angle,[77,78] Case,[79] and Tweed.[80] In Australia, Begg and Kesling[81] were important contributors.

Our main concern in the United States was the establishment of a technique that would produce a consistently satisfactory occlusion—one that would meet certain rigid standards of tooth position and interdigitation. Cephalometric analysis helped orthodontists develop models into which the occlusion was to be conformed.

During the past decades, research into the growth and development of the skull, by such dedicated scientists as Björk,[82,83] Moss,[84] and Graber and colleagues,[85] not only began to change American orthodontists' attitudes toward the European functional appliances, but also provided them with a new approach to their own fixed appliance therapy. Concepts such as the functional matrix therapy,[84,86,87] the genetic capacity of bone growth[66] and the definitive identification of facial and mandibular growth centers,[82,83] defining the roles of sutural[82,88] and cartilaginous[64,89] growth as well as those influential factors that affect them[90] have expanded orthodontists' vistas. Investigators found that by combining the available European appliance techniques with their own, not only could the movement of teeth within their alveolar housing be affected, but the underlying basal bone could also be influenced in growing children.

The 1960s marked the advent of a large segment of American orthodontists incorporating functional jaw orthopedics into their treatment plans.

As orthopedic concepts were developed, appliances were needed to implement these new ideas. Practitioners using fixed appliances were encouraged to examine functional appliances and to evaluate the claims reported by their European counterparts. The result of this evaluation is now apparent in the fusion of functional and fixed concepts by many orthodontists. A combined effort by Graber and colleagues[85] produced a comprehensive text that states that "Functional jaw orthopedics is concerned with permanently altering the position of the mandible by influencing and redirecting the growth process."[85] This process is most effective in young children; its efficacy lessens as children pass through puberty. Skeletal maturity eliminates further influence on the basal bone by functional appliances.

Natural forces from the cheeks, lips, tongue, and supporting muscles affect the direction of the growing bone. In a normal situation, lingual pressure from the tongue is balanced labially by the cheeks and lips. If an imbalance occurs, undue pressure is brought to bear on one or both sides of the arch, upper or lower, causing some distortion in the otherwise symmetric arch development.

In the same manner, orthodontists, through careful diagnosis and appliance design, can eliminate adverse forces and stimulate other positive force systems to discourage or promote bone growth. Orthodontists attempt to provide an environment consistent with the patients' ability to reach the maximal size potential in the most optimal direction.

Two of the early functional orthopedic appliances are Andresen's activator and Frankel's Functional Regulator. Andresen's appliance[72] consists of a rigid block of acrylic for maxillary and mandibular interdigitation at an increased vertical height. A single labial arch wire for the upper anteriors emanates from the acrylic. Expansion was introduced by splitting the two sections. The Harvoltd Woodside's activator is a modification of the original Andresen's appliance (Fig. 30–18A). Because of its bulkiness, this appliance is worn primarily at home and during the night. Balters[75] later streamlined the appliance, now termed a *bionator* (Fig. 30–18B), for longer wear and reduced the acrylic mass with a transpalatal wire. However, some of the original elements were removed as well. Further modifications added a jackscrew and buccal wire extensions to eliminate unwanted muscle pressure. Schwartz and Gratzinger's

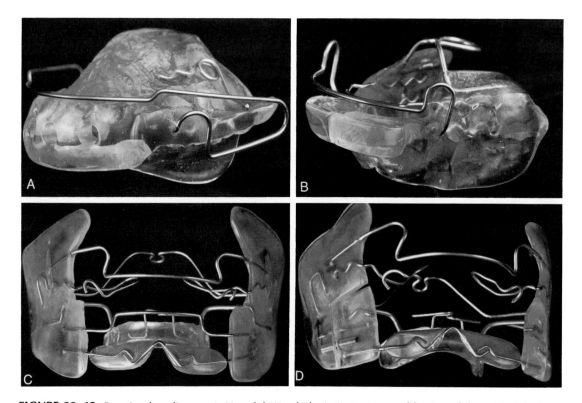

FIGURE 30–18. Functional appliances. *A*, Harvoltd Woodside Activator is a modification of the original Andresen appliance. *B*, Bionator. *C*, Frankel Functional Regulator. *D*, The FRII type.

double plate[74] actually separated the activator into upper and lower sections, joined by intermaxillary wiring. This appliance has great acceptance by patients because it is highly flexible and allows for movement in all directions.

Frankel's Functional Regulator (Fig. 30–18C) has also undergone changes and the overwheming choice is now the FRII type (Fig. 30–18D). It is composed of labial and lingual buccal acrylic shields; transpalatal wire; a labial bow embedded in the buccal shields, extending across the maxillary incisors; crossover wires situated in the embrasure between the permanent maxillary first molars and deciduous second molars and between the maxillary canines and deciduous first molars; a maxillary molar rest on the occlusal surface of the second deciduous molar; and maxillary canine clasps fixed distally in the buccal shields.

This appliance is designed for early treatment in the mixed dentition stage. It is worn nearly full time and is meant for full orthopedic and dental correction. It is unique in that it works from the labiobuccal surface outward, eliminating the forces of the buccinator, mentalis, and perioral muscles. This design allows for maximal lateral arch development. In contrast, other functional appliances depend mainly on lingual pressure from expansion devices to achieve increased lateral arch development.

Figure 30–19 depicts a young boy with a retrognathic, Class II, division 1 type of malocclusion (Fig. 30–19A,B). He was treated during the mixed dentition stage with an Alpern's multipurpose functional appliance, which is hinged anteriorly to allow for independent lateral expansion of both arches (Fig. 30–19C). The mandible was proclined to an edge-to-edge incisal position, and the patient wore the appliance for an average of 18 to 20 hours a day. After 4 months, the patient naturally closed into a forward relationship (Fig. 30–19D), and lateral expansion of the maxilla ensued, activated by a midpalatal jackscrew. One year later (Fig. 30–19E,F), the patient was placed on retention and observed until a more permanent dentition developed and the final stage of fixed edgewise appliance therapy could be initiated. Overlays of the cephalometric tracings reveal a substantial amount of mandibular growth during this phase of functional appliance therapy (Fig. 30–19G).

Both activator and functional regulator appliance systems advance the mandible to stimulate condylar growth. The activators rely on passive extrusion of the posterior teeth for increased vertical size, whereas Frankel's appliance, through the buccal shields, attempts to produce more downward growth of the alveolar ridges.

Two points must be emphasized:

1. These appliances are highly sophisticated and require not only a well-trained orthodontist, but one who is knowledgeable in the construction and use of functional appliances. The fact that they are removable and can be fabricated by a laboratory does not detract from their complexity.

2. Functional orthopedic appliances are designed for growing children. The philosophy of their use and treatment objectives are aimed at achieving a well-balanced occlusion within the framework of a good skeletal relationship.

The bionator has some application for treatment of TMDs. The bionator can act as a repositioning splint; however, because of its rigid establishment of an occlusal position, it should not be selected for patients suffering from myofascial pain dysfunction.

In summarizing the differences between functional jaw orthopedics and TMJ repositioning therapy, one should bear in mind the following concepts: Functional jaw orthopedics attempts to advance the mandible of a growing child in order to achieve the greatest possible growth changes of the mandible within that individual's morphogenetic capacity. In the case of adult patients with TMD, forward repositioning of the mandible is *not* designed to produce any growth changes, although Williamson[91] reported that increases in mandibular length were achieved in patients with anterior disc dislocations after they had been repositioned forward. [91] In addition, McNamara and others[92] and Schneiderman and Carlson[93] noted condylar changes in rhesus monkeys after mandibular repositioning.

Nevertheless, in adults, this new mandibular position is a learned one, based on muscle accommodation. In time, a new proprioceptive mechanism develops and maintains the position. Relapse is always a possible consequence of repositioning therapy. Its success is dependent on a stable, therapeutically derived occlusion with well-functioning movements.

Adult Orthodontic Treatment

Orthodontists' approach to appliance therapy is almost as varied as the number of prac-

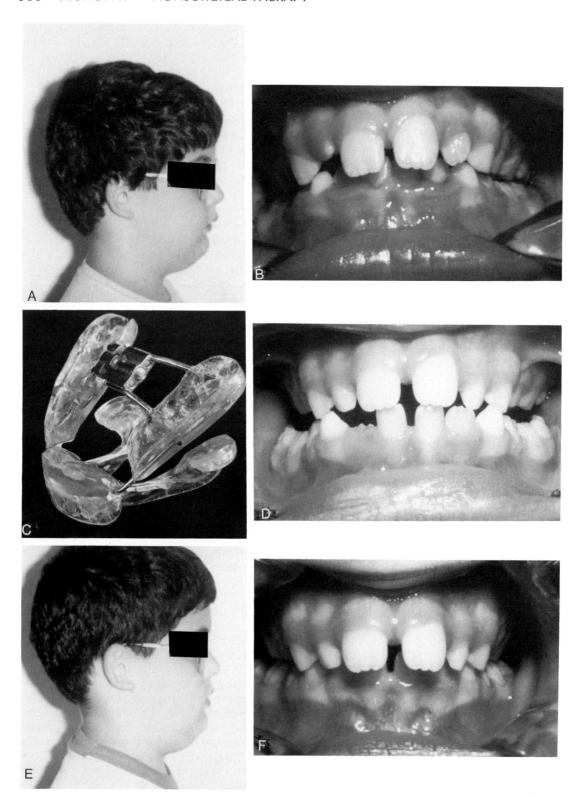

FIGURE 30–19. Early functional appliance treatment with the Alpern multifunctional appliance. *A,* Pretreatment profile showing retrognathia. *B,* Pretreatment intraoral view. *C,* Alpern Multipurpose Functional Appliance. *D,* Mandible advanced to edge-to-edge relationship. *E,* Postfunctional appliance therapy profile reveals more prominence of the mandible and lower lip and greater vertical height. *F,* Maxilla expanded, and posterior occlusion established.

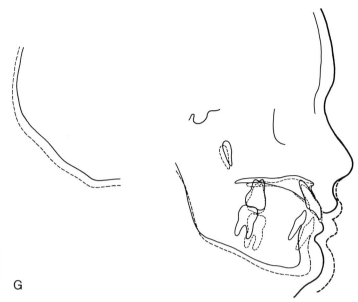

FIGURE 30–19 *Continued* G, Cephalometric comparison of prefunctional (solid line) and postfunctional (broken line) appliance therapy.   G

titioners who treat malocclusions. Several common techniques are used, and the combination of auxiliary appliances that can be associated with them is overwhelming. It is not the purpose of this chapter to describe these techniques; only a few are cited here. For the rest, readers should refer to one of the many textbooks on orthodontics.[47,49,53,74,81,85,94]

Orthodontic treatment for patients with TMD presents some unique problems that require specific approaches and techniques. Nevertheless, standard therapeutic procedures should be employed and basic treatment objectives sought. Patients are referred to an orthodontist after successfully completing phase I therapy. Orthodontists are charged with the establishment of a functional occlusion consistent with the new comfortable mandibular position.

Both the diagnostic workup and the treatment plan are completed, and the appliances necessary to achieve the required tooth movements are selected. Table 30–2 outlines a general step-by-step approach to orthodontic treatment.

Leveling and Alignment

Leveling and alignment of the teeth are the first corrections sought. These are gross movements that produce dramatic results in a short time. Patients are encouraged after this initial stage of treatment, having seen the teeth straightened, but the operator is all too aware

TABLE 30–2. Step-by-Step Approach to Phase II Orthodontic Treatment

I. Leveling and alignment
  A. Remove any exaggerated occlusal curvatures and flatten the occlusal plane
  B. Correct the rotations
  C. Upright the mesiodistally tipped teeth
II. Establishing proper arch width relationships
  A. Upright the teeth in the labiolingual and buccolingual planes
  B. Expand or contract the dental arches
III. Developing the occlusal relationships
  A. Perform vertical tooth movements to achieve interdigitation
  B. Make final alignment for proper functional movements
IV. Occlusal adjustment to refine static and functional occlusion
V. Retention designed for protection of dentition and TMJ mechanism

that the slower and more tedious aspect of treatment is just beginning. This first process occasionally requires interproximal tooth reduction or even extraction to provide the necessary arch length with which to align the teeth.

The cases presented here utilize the edgewise straight wire technique with bracket angulation, as described by Roth.[95–97]

Light, flexible round or multistranded arch wires are employed initially, to be replaced by a stepwise series of thicker round wires. The more accurately the wire fills the rectangular slot, the straighter the teeth become. Tooth position is defined by the angulation of the bracket. Each bracket contains the code for the positioning of each tooth. Tip (mesiodistal angulation), torque (labiolingual crown-root angulation), and in-and-out position (labiolingual position) are incorporated into the bracket slot.

When severe intra-arch malalignment is found, a multistranded or nickel-titanium type of wire is employed. These wires have maximum flexibility and can be engaged into the bracket slots of even the most malpositioned teeth. Loops incorporated into the arch wire can lend similar versatility to a standard stainless steel arch wire and are preferred by some practitioners.

Difficult rotations can require the employment of accessory attachments, such as lingual buttons or rotating wedges. The object of these devices is to concentrate a force in a specific area of the tooth and along a defined vector.

It is important to correct tooth rotations early in treatment, because the longer they are retained, the more stable they become. Unlike lateral tooth movements, in which the tooth is moved through the bone, rotational movement primarily turns a tooth within its socket. A reorientation of the periodontal fibers is necessary to maintain the correction. Fiberotomies, as pioneered by Reitan,[98] are sometimes employed to ensure the reattachment of the transseptal fibers and some of the more superior periodontal fibers for better posttreatment stability.

Establishing Proper Arch Width Relationships

Once rotational malalignments are removed and the dentition is leveled, lateral arch relationships can be addressed.

Limitations exist in the extent to which lateral arch expansion is possible in adults. Lingually inclined molars, bicuspids, and cuspids can be uprighted buccally. Incisors with too vertical a position can be torqued labially. The result of these changes enlarges the circumference of the dental arches.

Further expansion must be approached with caution. Care should be taken not to tip the crowns too far buccally, because that would move the roots beyond the confines of adequate alveolar support. Moreover, excessive expansion can impinge on and displace the labial and buccal muscle bundles, producing inward pressure from the displaced muscles against the teeth. Over time, a lingual collapse

of the arches can occur, undoing the previously achieved results.

Long-term and possibly permanent retention is necessary to retain expansive movements. When significant arch width increases are necessary in the maxilla, a surgical scoring of the alveolus on the buccal and labial surfaces above the root apices of the teeth may be necessary. Freeing these bony plates allows for rapid palatal expansion of the maxilla. This expansion differs from the midpalatal sutural widening one observes in such techniques on children.

The most effective manner of widening the dentition is to employ a lingual expansion appliance, such as a quad helix or Wilson's transpalatal lingual appliance.[99] Although these appliances cause some initial discomfort to the tongue, their effectiveness and aesthetic qualities warrant patients' indulgence.

Because most interarch lateral discrepancies are bilateral, equal expansion of both sides is indicated. However, when asymmetry in arch form occurs, unilateral expansion is required. It is necessary to establish adequate anchorage on the normal side so that it remains stationary while the contralateral side expands. A buttressing effect can be achieved with an expansion lingual arch by torquing the molar roots on the ipsilateral side against the heavy buccal plate of bone. The resultant lateral force causes the contralateral buccal segment to expand. This form of anchorage should not be employed over long periods of treatment.

These multipurpose lingual arches, in addition to their expansion capabilities, can produce other tooth movements, including molar distalizing. An operator skilled in the use of multipurpose lingual arches can achieve all but the final tooth positioning and vertical movements.

As with any tooth movement, expansion will proceed most efficiently if cuspal interferences are eliminated. If a splint is not already in use, it can be effectively employed to disocclude the teeth and to remove unwanted resistance. A splint is particularly advisable when a crossbite exists and the opposing teeth are locked in a malposition of opposing cusps.

Single-tooth crossbites can be corrected with labial, as well as lingual, appliances. The laws of physics dictate that for every action, there is an equal and opposite reaction. For example, when one corrects a lingually displaced maxillary cuspid, the effect of the opposing forces anchoring the corrective mechanics can be unsettling to the whole dentition. Alternating force systems, established in both arches, can provide an effective means of moving the malpositioned teeth while distributing the forces between both arches.

During these first two phases of treatment, leveling and establishing harmonious lateral arch relationships, the splint must be adjusted to keep pace with the changing dentition (Fig. 30–20A,B). Nevertheless, foremost in priorities is the maintenance of mandibular position at the therapeutically derived treatment position.

Developing Occlusal Relationships

The third stage is next instituted to establish the occlusion, primarily through vertical closure of the opposing teeth. The amount of vertical movement is dependent on the thickness of the splint. This procedure establishes a higher occlusal plane and increases the vertical dimension (see Fig. 30–20A). Change is wrought through the application of extrusive forces.

Sections of the splint, beginning with the most posterior segments, are removed. The underlying teeth are exposed, and the opposing teeth are freed from contact with the acrylic surface of the splint. Light, round arch wires are inserted to allow for minimal bracket-arch resistance and ease of tooth movement.

Vertical elastics are then attached to move the most distal molars on one side of the arch into contact (Fig. 30–20C). The splint is then reduced in the bicuspid area (Fig. 30–20D,E) until full occlusion is achieved on the buccal segments of one side (Fig. 30–20F). The same process is applied to the opposite side of the arch until sufficient interdigitation is produced to support the occlusion. The splint, which at this point has been reduced to a small section, can be discarded. Some patients, especially those who exhibit strong parafunctional habits, may require a new splint at this juncture.

In cases of deep overbite (Fig. 30–21A), the thickness of the splint and consequent increase in vertical height are sufficient to accomplish a normal anterior relationship (Fig. 30–21B). The patient requires no vertical repositioning of the incisors. However, when a normal pretreatment relationship exists or an open bite tendency is evident (Fig. 30–21C), any increase in the vertical dimension separates the incisors

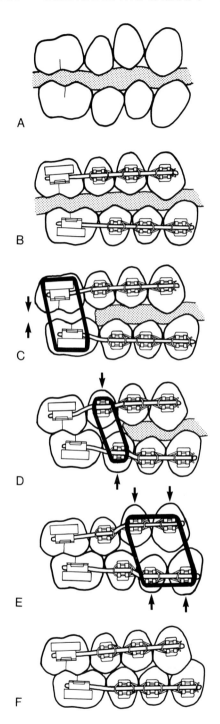

FIGURE 30–20. Vertical bite closure using splint reduction. *A,* Preorthodontic splint in place. *B,* Splint adjusted to accommodate leveling procedure. *C,* Section of splint in molar area is removed, and vertical elastic traction is attached. *D,* Procedure shown in *C* is repeated for second bicuspids. *E,* Procedure shown in *C* is repeated for first bicuspids and cuspids. *F,* Vertical bite closure is completed on one side.

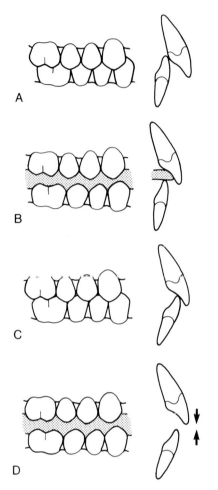

FIGURE 30–21. Effect of splint insertion on overbite. *A,* Deep overbite malocclusion. *B,* Splint increases vertical dimension to a normal overbite. *C,* Normal overbite occlusion. *D,* Splint increases vertical dimension, which produces an anterior open bite.

enough to necessitate closure through elastic traction application (Fig. 30–21D).

With vertical closure complete and cuspal interdigitation effected, final alignment of the teeth is undertaken. Selection of size and composition of the initial finishing wires depends on the amount of displacement that occurred after the leveling process. A nickel-titanium wire, with qualities of high flexibility and memory, may be chosen as a starting point. A more rigid stainless steel rectangular arch wire, approximating the bracket slot size, is eventually inserted for more detailed finishing. Before appliance removal, an orthodontist should discuss with the phase I dentist the requirements for retention and supportive splint therapy.

Occlusal Adjustment

When the appliances are removed, a period of "settling" occurs, during which time the teeth find their most stable positions. Any occlusal adjustment, except for gross discrepancies, should be delayed until after the period of settling. Readers should refer to Chapter 28 for a description of occlusal adjustment procedures.

Retention

In addition to addressing the concern orthodontists have with maintaining the tooth positions they have so diligently achieved, retention following phase II orthodontic treatment must consider factors imposed by the TMJ and its related structures.

Depending on a patient's original diagnosis and accompanying parafunctional habits, an orthodontist, in consultation with the phase I dentist, must construct appropriate retaining appliances. Some kind of splint mechanism is most often incorporated into the retainer. Orthodontists are well equipped to modify retainers to fit the individual requirements of patients with TMD, because these adaptations are similar to ones commonly utilized in practice.

The case presented as Figure 30–22 is a young woman referred for phase II orthodontic treatment after having undergone four months of phase I splint therapy for the alleviation of symptoms arising from an anterior disc displacement. After advancing the mandible to recapture the disc, the phase I practitioner readjusted the occlusion to the current position, using a full-coverage mandibular splint (Fig. 30–22B).

The patient was asymptomatic; however, any attempt at weaning her from the splint initiated a recurrence of symptoms. It was decided that orthodontic treatment would be instituted to finalize the new maxillomandibular relationship.

What is interesting about patients who have successfully completed regimens of splint therapy is that they acquire the position dictated by the splint as their new functional or therapeutically derived position. As in this case, a cephalometric x-ray film taken without the splint represents not the pre-phase I centric occlusion but the post-phase I therapeutically derived occlusion (Fig. 30–22C). The goal of orthodontic treatment in this case would not be to change the maxillomandibular relationship but rather to move the teeth into the therapeutically derived maxillomandibular position.

The pretreatment occlusion was a Class I with satisfactory interdigitation and good working movements. The teeth were bracketed from second molar on the right to first molar on the left, using bracket slots of 0.022 × 0.028, according to Roth.[97] Because of the satisfactory alignment of the teeth, only a short period of leveling was necessary before the vertical correction could be started. The phase I splint was employed throughout treatment because of its acceptance by the patient, whose original symptoms are alleviated.

The distal area of the left side of the splint, covering the mandibular left second bicuspid and first molar, was removed (Fig. 30–22D),

and ³⁄₁₆-inch vertical elastics were placed by the patient and changed daily (Fig. 30–22E). The elastics were removed only for meals and oral hygiene procedures.

Approximately 8 weeks later, the first molars and second bicuspids are in occlusion with the splint in place. The left first bicuspid and cuspid are now freed from the splint (Fig. 30–22F), and similar vertical elastics are employed. Intermaxillary elastics are continued on the molars to maintain their correction (Fig. 30–22G).

This process is continued until full occlusion is established in the left buccal segments (Fig. 30–22H), and it is repeated on the right side (Fig. 30–22I–M). This patient originally exhibited a normal overbite, which, when the splint was inserted, was changed to an open bite (Fig.

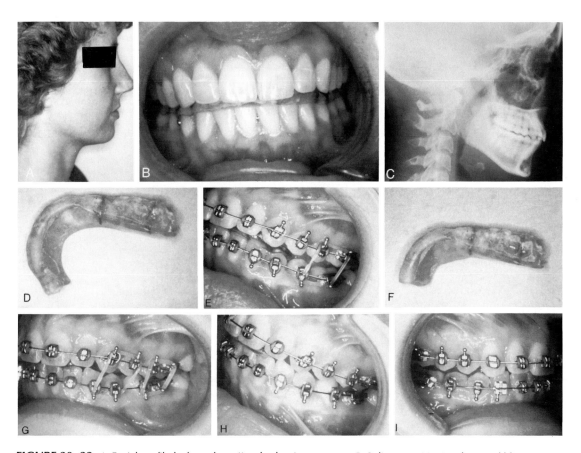

FIGURE 30–22. A, Facial profile before phase II orthodontic treatment. B, Splint repositioning the mandible in a comfortable position in regard to the temporomandibular joint. C, Following phase I cephalostat depicting the therapeutically derived occlusion. D, Splint cut back to expose the lower left second bicuspid and first molar. E, Vertical intermaxillary elastics to occlude first molars and second bicuspids. F, Splint further reduced to expose the lower left cuspid and first bicuspid. G, Vertical intermaxillary elastics applied to left cuspids and first bicuspids and continued on second bicuspids and first molars. H, Left buccal segment closed. Teeth are in occlusion. I, Untreated right buccal segment remains open.

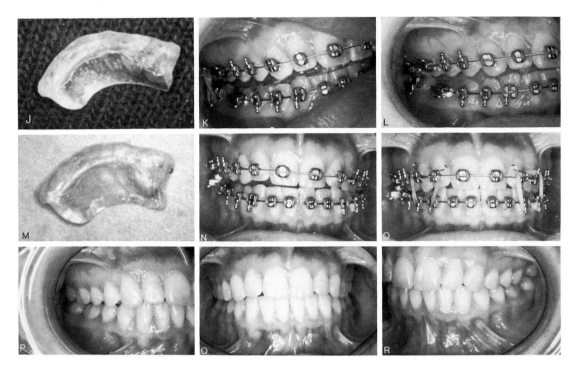

FIGURE 30–22 *Continued J,* Splint reduced in right second molar region. *K,* Vertical elastic traction applied to right second molars. *L,* Right second molars occluded. *M,* Splint reduced to final size to allow remaining teeth in the right buccal segment to be moved together. *N,* Both buccal segments occluded, but anterior teeth are still open. *O,* Intermaxillary elastics applied to cuspids and lateral incisors for final closure. *P, Q,* and *R,* Occlusion at completion of treatment.

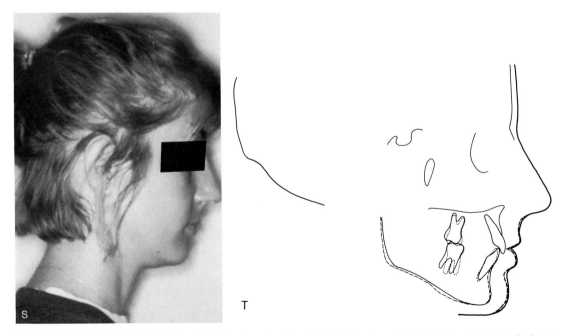

FIGURE 30–22 *Continued S,* Facial profile following phase II orthodontic treatment. *T,* Cephalometric preorthodontic (solid line) and postorthodontic (broken line) cephalometric tracings.

30–22N). After the posterior occlusion was established, vertical closure, using anterior intermaxillary elastics, was necessary (Fig. 30–22O). Following completion of the vertical closure, a period of finishing was necessary to correct any changes brought about by the previous tooth movements. Releveling was instituted, first with more flexible arch wires and finally with heavier and stiffer arch wires to obtain the final tooth positions.

When the fixed appliances were removed (Fig. 30–22P to R), a maxillary full-coverage splint with full occlusal contact was inserted. The patient was instructed to wear the splint at home and while sleeping. The splint was to act as a retainer and to protect against nocturnal parafunctional habits. Any gross occlusal adjustment would have been performed at this time; however, none was required in this case.

It is advisable to delay any fine-tuning of the occlusion until a period of settling occurs, when the teeth achieve their final positions consistent with the musculoskeletal arrangement. Mandibular retention consisted of a Hawley's-type retainer.

Because the objective of treatment was to maintain the maxillomandibular relationship as defined by the splint, little change in the pre-

and postorthodontic treatment facial photographs (Fig. 30–22A, S) or in the cephalostats (Fig. 30–22T) is noted. A small clockwise rotation of the mandible is observed; it resulted from an increase in vertical height.

The reader must realize that cure is measured in degrees, and a return to full health, especially in a case of internal derangement, is not always possible.

Figure 30–23 shows a patient with degenerative joint disease. The reduction of symptoms, primarily the pain, and the stabilization of occlusion in a more comfortable position were the main treatment objectives. To achieve these goals, the phase I practitioner advanced the mandible to reduce the loading of the condyle on the inflamed retrodiscal tissue. This step also produced an opening of the bite.

This patient had a Class I occlusion and a well-developed mandible. When she was an adolescent, her dentist removed a mandibular incisor to relieve a crowded condition. The maxillary left cuspid was labially locked as the result of an arch length deficiency, and some interproximal stripping was necessary to move the tooth into proper alignment without straining the arch.

As was depicted in Figure 30–12A,B, ad-

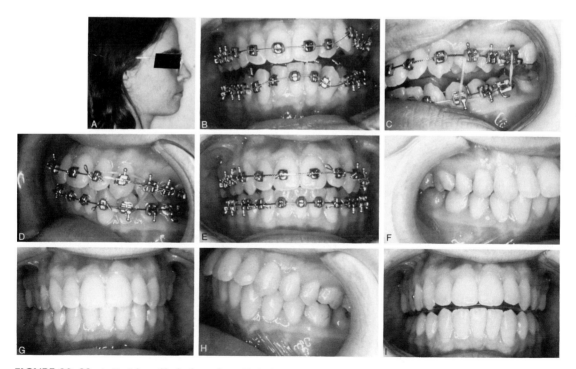

FIGURE 30–23. *A,* Facial profile before phase II. *B,* Repositioning splint in place, and leveling process initiated. *C,* Vertical closure of posterior teeth. *D,* Posterior occlusion established, and anterior bite closure in progress. *E,* Final alignment. *F, G,* and *H,* Completed case. *I,* Full coverage flat plane support and retention splint inserted.

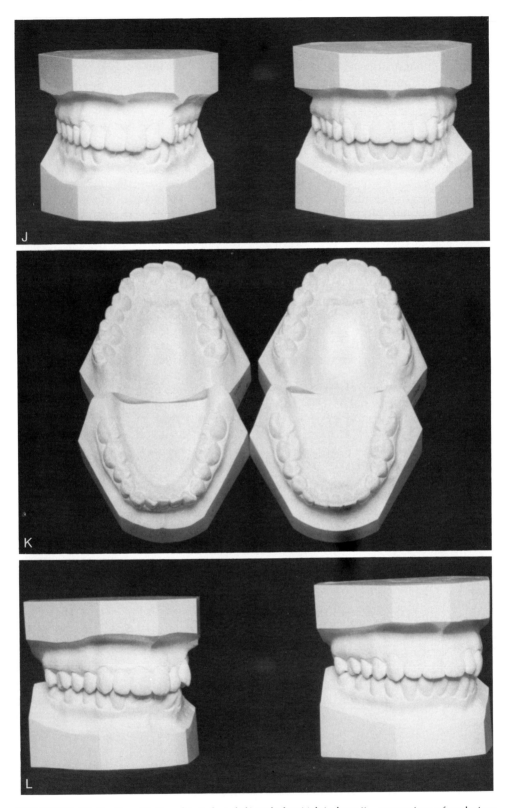

FIGURE 30–23 *Continued J*, K, and *L*, Before (left) and after (right) phase II—comparison of occlusions.

vancing a mandible from a Class I position produces some degree of mesiorelationship of the occlusion (Class III) and more prominence of the chin (Fig. 30–23A). The previously extracted mandibular incisor had allowed the maxillary arch to accommodate the added tooth structure created by the more forward mandibular position. Some reduction of tooth structure would have been necessitated if the incisor had not already been removed.

A lower Gelb appliance[57] established and maintained proper mandibular position throughout treatment. The teeth were bracketed with edgewise appliances (Fig. 30–21B) and leveled. The splint was cut back to free various teeth and allow them to be approximated, using vertical elastics (Fig. 30–23C). After the posterior segments were closed (Fig. 30–23D), the anterior sections were brought into contact (Fig. 30–23E). The work was completed and the appliances removed 21 months after appliance insertion (Fig. 30–23F–H). A full-coverage maxillary stabilization splint was inserted (Fig. 30–23I), along with a bonded wire lingual mandibular splint from cuspid to cuspid. The change both in the occlusion and in the maxillomandibular relationship, as well as increased vertical opening, is seen in Figure 30–23J to L.

When phase I splint therapy necessitates the forward positioning of the mandible and a patient presents with a Class II, division 1 malocclusion, phase II orthodontic treatment serves both the TMD and the occlusal disharmony.

Figure 30–24A portrays in profile the malocclusion just described. This is compared with the post-treatment profile (Fig. 30–24B), in which a more prominent chin is in evidence. Study casts comparing the original occlusal relationship with the proclined splint position are seen in Figure 30–24C.

With the splint in position, the amount of vertical closure is apparent and is commensurate with the thickness of the splint (Fig. 30–24D). As in previous cases, reduction of the acrylic overlying the teeth proceeds in conjunction with the vertical closure of the teeth (Fig. 30–24E,F).

The initial deep overbite was corrected to a normal overbite with the insertion of the splint, and this relationship was stabilized by the extrusion of the posterior teeth. Thus, no anterior vertical elastics were necessary in this case. A maxillary full-coverage (stabilization) splint was chosen for retention and as a TMJ appliance, because the patient had a history of bruxism.

Following orthodontic treatment (Fig. 30–24G–L), some minor flare-ups of muscle soreness occurred during periodic recall examination. Increasing the number of hours of splint wear helped to dissipate the symptoms. The original symptoms of anterior disc displacement, pain, and occasional locking did not recur.

A comparison of the pre- and post-phase II orthodontic cephalograms reveals a forward repositioning of the mandible and an increase in the vertical dimension (Fig. 30–24M).

Class II, division 2 type malocclusions contain all the ingredients that can produce pernicious reactions from the supporting soft tissue. The mandibular arch is virtually locked within the confines of the maxillary arch. The severe upright or lingual inclination of the upper incisors, coupled with a deep overbite, greatly restricts the forward movement of the mandible, which must rotate downward and backward to free itself from the lingual surface of the maxillary incisors.

The Class II, division 2 malocclusion presented in Figure 30–25 depicts a concave profile, caused by a lack of incisal support (Fig. 30–25A). Lingual compression of both arches, both buccally and labially, is evident (Fig. 30–25B–D).

The patient originally presented to the phase I practitioner with acute myofascial pain dysfunction and tenderness of the joints. During phase II orthodontic therapy, recurrence of these symptoms was common. Nevertheless, through close cooperation between the phase I and phase II practitioners and continuous reassurances by both, the patient was treated successfully.

The original splint, containing only an anterior occluding surface (Fig. 30–25E), was modified by removal of the labial bow to allow for edgewise appliance insertion. The object of treatment was to apply lingual root torque to the maxillary incisors and to allow the crowns to move labially (Fig. 30–25F). This accomplishment would unlock the mandible and allow for forward repositioning.

Through the uprighting of the posterior segment, more posterior support can be achieved at a higher occlusal level. The result would be an increase in vertical dimension and an opening of the bite.

To facilitate buccal expansion of the lower

arch, a Wilson's lingual arch with recurved springs[99] was used as an adjunct to the edgewise appliance (Fig. 30–25G). Some vertical elastic traction was necessary to enhance cuspal inter- digitation (Fig. 30–25H,I). When appliances were removed (Fig. 30–25J–L), it appeared that a bonded occlusal overlay would be nec- essary on the maxillary right first molar to es-

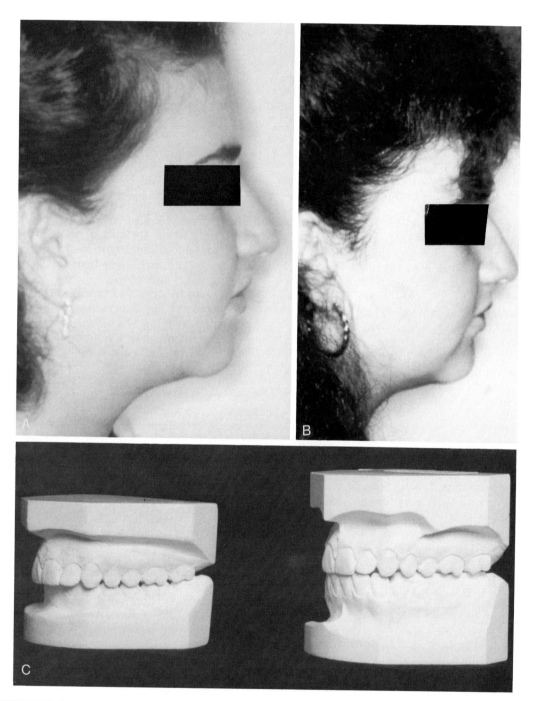

FIGURE 30–24. *A,* Pretreatment facial profile. *B,* Post-treatment facial profile. *C,* Study casts comparing original class II, division 1 malocclusion (left) with the occlusion as established with the forward repositioning splint (right).

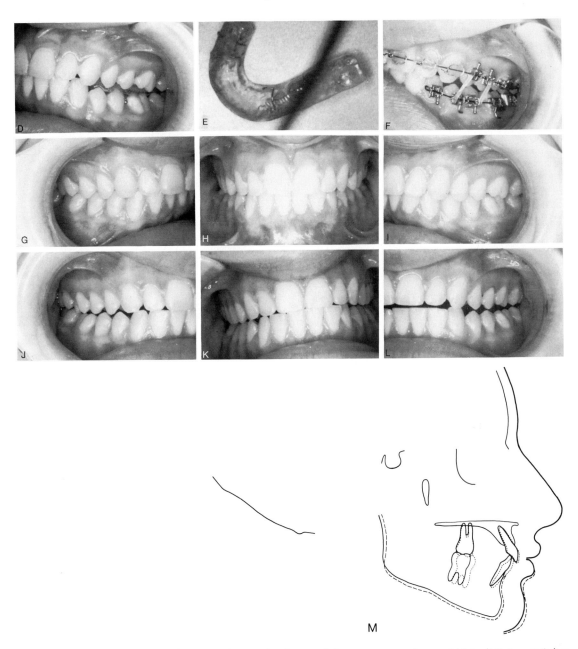

FIGURE 30–24 *Continued D*, Splint inserted. Note the degree of closure necessary for cuspid interdigitation. *E*, Splint reduced for vertical closure. *F*, Vertical elastic traction in progress to be repeated on opposite side. *G, H,* and *I*, Completed case. *J, K,* and *L*, Occlusion in lateral and anterior function. *M*, Cephalometric preorthodontic (solid line) and postorthodontic (broken line) treatment.

tablish better contact. The profile was improved by the phase II treatment (Fig. 30–25M).

Retention consisted of a mandibular Hawley's type appliance without a labial bow, because only lingual support was needed, and a maxillary full-coverage flat plane splint was used, mainly for night wear. The patient has remained remarkably stable and symptom free, considering the eventful TMJ history and recurrent flare-ups.

Cephalometric comparison between the pre- and post-phase II orthodontic treatment bears out our clinical results (Fig. 30–25N). Consid-

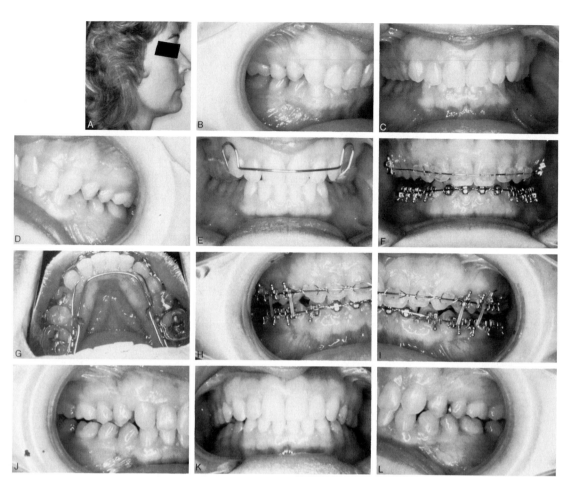

FIGURE 30–25. *A,* Pretreatment facial profile. *B, C,* and *D,* Pretreatment intraoral views. *E,* Phase I splint with anterior incisal contact. *F,* Maxillary incisors torqued, and mandible advanced. *G,* The Wilson lingual expansion arch. *H* and *I,* Vertical intermaxillary elastic to effect cuspid interdigitation. *J, K,* and *L,* Following phase II orthodontic treatment.

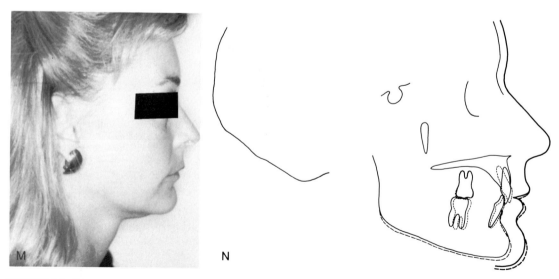

FIGURE 30–25 *Continued M,* Post-treatment facial profile. *N,* Cephalometric preorthodontic (solid line) and postorthodontic (broken line) cephalometric tracings.

erable lingual root torquing of the maxillary incisors is evident, along with a forward repositioning of the mandible.

CONCLUSION

As the practitioner observes, orthodontics for the phase II treatment of TMDs does not require a new line of appliances or further postgraduate courses in new techniques for experienced orthodontists. Some degree of inventiveness is necessary at times, but rigid dedication is always needed to achieve the proper tooth positions consistent with the blueprint, as established by the splint.

Communication with the patient and other members of the professional team contributes to the successful completion of phase II therapy. This is usually the final step in the long series of treatment modalities that constitute the multidisciplinary approach to TMDs.

One needs to plan therapy well, through proper diagnosis and treatment planning procedures, to avoid indecision and confusion along the way. Patients should be informed of their progress and allowed to be participants in their own therapy.

Most important, one must be informed of the patient's status at each appointment. When you ask questions instead of waiting to be asked, patients will feel your concern and develop confidence, which can only produce a better clinician-patient relationship.

Success can be measured in many ways. One is to observe the plaster casts on the table, with the teeth perfectly aligned. Another is to look at a patient's smile and satisfaction with a result that you have achieved through your expertise and your caring.

REFERENCES

1. Roth, R.H.: Temporomandibular pain dysfunction and occlusal relationships. Angle Orthod. 43:136–153, 1973.
2. Helkimo, M.: Studies on function and dysfunction of the masticatory system. II. Index for anamnestic and clinical dysfunction and occlusal state. Swed. Dent. J. 67:101, 1974.
3. Helkimo, M.: Studies on function and dysfunction of the masticatory system. III. Analysis of anamnestic and clinical recordings of dysfunction with the aid of indices. Swed. Dent. J. 67:165, 1974.
4. Helkimo, M.: Studies of function and dysfunction of the masticatory system. An epidemiological investigation of symptoms of dysfunction in Lapps in the North of Finland. Acta Odontol. Scand. 32:255, 1974.
5. Green, C.S. and Marbach, J.J.: Epidemiologic studies of mandibular dysfunction: A critical review. J. Prosthet. Dent. 48:184–190, 1982.
6. Solberg, W.K., Woo, M., and Houston, J.: Prevalence of mandibular dysfunction in young adults. J. Am. Dent. Assoc. 98:25–34, 1979.
7. Hansson, T. and Nilner, M.: A study of the occurrence of symptoms of disease of the temporomandibular joint, masticatory musculature, and related structures. J. Oral Rehabil. 2:313–324, 1975.
8. Agerberg, G. and Osterberg, T.: Maximal mandibular movements and symptoms of mandibular dysfunction in 70 year-old men and women. Swed. Dent. J. 67:147–164, 1974.
9. Hansson, T. and Oberg, T.: En Klinisk bettfysiologisk undersokining AV 67-Aringar i Dalby. Tandlakartidningen 18:650–655, 1971.
10. Grosfeld, O. and Czarneka, B.: Musculo-articular disorders of the stomatognathic system in school children examined according to clinical criteria. J. Oral Rehabil. 4:193–200, 1977.
11. Williamson, E. H.: Temporomandibular dysfunction in pretreatment adolescent patients. Am. J. Orthod. 72:429–433, 1977.
12. Nilner, M. and Lassing, S.A.: Prevalence of functional disturbances and diseases of the stomatognathic system in 7–14 year olds. Swed. Dent. J. 5:173–187, 1981.
13. Egermark-Eriksson, I.: The dependence of mandibular dysfunction in children with functional and morphological malocclusion. Am. J. Orthod. 83:187–194, 1983.
14. Nilner, M.: Prevalence of functional disturbances and diseases of the stomatognathic system in 15–18 year olds. Swed. Dent. J. 5:189–197, 1981.
15. Mohlin, B.: Prevalence of mandibular dysfunction and the relation between malocclusion and mandibular dysfunction in a group of women in Sweden. Eur. J. Orthod. 4:115–123, 1983.
16. Agerberg, G. and Carlsson, G.E.: Functional disorders of the masticatory system. Distribution of symptoms according to age and sex as judged from investigation by questionnaire (abstract). Acta Odontol. Scand. 30:597–613, 1972.
17. Ingervall, B. and Hedegard, B.: Subjective evaluation of functional disturbances of the masticatory system in young Swedish men. Community Dent. Oral Epidemiol. 2:149, 1974.
18. Molin, C., Carlsson, E.E., Friling, B., and Hedegard, B.: Frequency of symptoms of mandibular dysfunction in young Swedish men. J. Oral Rehabil. 3:9–18, 1976.
19. Angle, E.H.: *Treatment of Malocclusion of the Teeth and Fractures of the Maxilla, Angle's System*, 6th ed. S.S. White Dental Manufacturing Co., Philadelphia, 1900.
20. Thompson, J.R.: Differentiation of functional and structural dental malocclusion and its implication to treatment. Angle Orthod. 42:252–262, 1972.
21. Stuart, C.E.: Good occlusion for natural teeth. J. Prosthet. Dent. 41:435–441, 1964.
22. Rickets, R.M.: Abnormal function of the temporomandibular joint. Am. J. Orthod. 41:435–441, 1985.
23. Lieberman, M.A., Gazit, E., Fuchs, C., and Lilos, P.: Mandibular dysfunction in 10–18 year olds as related to morphologic malocclusion. J. Oral Rehabil. 12:209–214, 1985.
24. Roberts, C.A., Tallents, R.H., Katzberg, R.W., et al: Comparison of internal derangements of the TMJ with occlusal findings. Oral Surg. Oral Med. Oral Pathol. 63:645–650, 1987.
25. de Boever, J.A. and van de Berghe, L.: Longitudinal study of functional conditions in the masticatory sys-

tem in Flemish children. Community Dent. Oral Epidemiol. 15:100–103, 1987.

26. Wanman, A.: Craniomandibular disorders in adolescents. A longitudinal study in an urban Swedish population. Swed. Dent. J. (Suppl.) 44:1–61, 1987.

27. Bush, F.M.: Malocclusion, masticatory muscle and temporomandibular joint tenderness. J. Dent. Res. 64:129–133, 1985.

28. Helm, S., Kreiberg, S., and Solow, B.: Malocclusion at adolescence related to self-reported tooth loss and functional disorders in adulthood. Am. J. Orthod. 85:393–400, 1984.

29. Pullinger, A.G., Seligman, D.A., and Solberg, W.K.: Temporomandibular disorders. II. Occlusal factors associated with temporomandibular joint tenderness and dysfunction. J. Prosthet. Dent. 59:363–367, 1988.

30. Riolo, M.L., Brandt, D., and Tenhave, T.R.: Associations between occlusal characteristics and signs and symptoms of TMJ dysfunction in children and young adults. Am. J. Orthod. 92:467–477, 1987.

31. Mohlin, B., Ingervall, B., and Thilander, B.: Prevalence of symptoms of functional disturbances of the masticatory system in Swedish men. J. Oral Rehabil. 7:185–197, 1980.

32. Solberg, W.K., Bibb, C.A., Nordstram, B.B., and Hansson, T.L.: Malocclusion associated with temporomandibular joint changes in young adults at autopsy. Am. J. Orthod. 89:326–330, 1986.

33. Franks, A.S.T.: The dental health of patients presenting with temporomandibular joint dysfunction. Br. J. Oral Surg. 5:157–166, 1967.

34. Berry, D.C. and Watkinson, A.C.: Mandibular dysfunction and incisor relationship. Br. Dent. J. 144:74–77, 1978.

35. Dibbets, J.M.H. and Van der Weele, L.Th.: Orthodontic treatment in relation to symptoms attributed to dysfunction of the temporomandibular joint. Am. J. Orthod. 91:193–199, 1987.

36. Larsson, E. and Ronnerman, A.: Mandibular dysfunction symptoms in orthodontically treated patients 10 years after the completion of treatment. Eur. J. Orthod. 3:89–94, 1981.

37. Janson, M. and Hasund, A.: Functional problems in orthodontic patients out of retention. Eur. J. Orthod. 3:173–179, 1981.

38. Sadowsky, C. and Polson, A.M.: Temporomandibular disorders and functional occlusion after orthodontic treatment: Results of two long-term studies. Am. J. Orthod. 86:386–390, 1984.

39. Perry, H.T.: Relation of occlusion to temporomandibular joint dysfunction: The orthodontic viewpoint. J. Am. Dent. Assoc. 79:137–141, 1969.

40. Sadowski, C. and Be Gole, E.A.: Long term status of temporomandibular joint dysfunctions and functional occlusion after orthodontic treatment. Am. J. Orthod. 78:201–212, 1981.

41. Helkimo, M.: Epidemiologic survey of dysfunction of the masticatory system. In temporomandibular joint function and dysfunction. Oral Sci. Rev. 1:54–59, 1976.

42. Jamsa, T., Alanen, P., and Kirveskari, P.: Orthodontic treatment, interferences and signs of TMJ dysfunction (abstract). J. Dent. Res. (Special edition) 68:937, 1989.

43. Pullinger, A.G., Solberg, W.K., Hollender, L., and Petersson, A.: Relationship of mandibular condyle position to dental occlusion factors in an asymptomatic population. Am. J. Orthod. 91:200–206, 1987.

44. Gianelly, A.A., Hugher, H.M., Wohlgemuth, P., and Gildea, G.: Condylar position and extraction treatment. Am. J. Orthod. 93:201–205, 1988.

45. Farrar, W.B. and McCarty, W.L.: *A Clinical Outline of Temporomandibular Joint Diagnosis and Treatment.* Walker Printing Co., Montgomery, AL, 1983.

46. Pullinger, A.: Natural history and pathologic progression of internal derangement with persistent closed lock. In *Diagnostic and Surgical Arthroscopy of the Temporomandibular Joint.* B. Sanders, K. Murakami and G.T. Clark (eds.). W.B. Saunders Co., Philadelphia, 1989.

47. Graber, T.M. and Swain, B.F.: *Orthodontics—Current Principles and Techniques.* C.V. Mosby, St. Louis, 1985.

48. Rakosi, T.: *An Atlas and Manual of Cephalometric Radiography.* Lea & Febiger, Philadelphia, 1982.

49. Proffit, W.R.: *Contemporary Orthodontics.* C.V. Mosby, St. Louis, 1986.

50. McNamara, T.A.: A method of cephalometric analysis. In *Craniofacial Growth Series No. 14.* T.A. McNamara, K.A. Ribbens, and R.H. Howe (eds.). Center for Human Growth and Development, University of Michigan, Ann Arbor, 1983.

51. Ricketts, R.M.: Perspective in the clinical application of cephalometrics. Angle Orthod. 51:115, 1981.

52. Ricketts, R.M.: The value of cephalometrics and computerized technology. Angle Orthod. 42:177–199, 1972.

53. Jarabak, J.R. and Fizzel, J.A.: *Light Wire Edgewise Appliance.* C.V. Mosby, St. Louis, 1986.

54. Garliner, D.: *Myofunctional Therapy in Dental Practice.* Bartel Dental Book Co., New York, 1971.

55. Ackerman, J.L. and Proffit, W.R.: The characteristics of malocclusion: A modern approach to classification and diagnosis. Am. J. Orthod. 56:443, 1969.

56. Owen, A.H.: Orthodontic/orthopedic treatment of craniomandibular pain dysfunction. IV. Unilateral and bilateral crossbite. J. Craniomandib. Pract. 2:344–349, 1986.

57. Gelb, H.: *Clinical Management of Head, Neck, Facial Pain and TMJ Disorders.* W.B. Saunders Co., Philadelphia, 1986.

58. Haas, A.J.: Rapid palatal expansion of the maxillary dental arch and nasal cavity by opening the midpalatal suture. Angle Orthod. 31:73–90, 1961.

59. Isaacson, R.J., Wood, J.L., and Ingram, A.H.: Forces produced by rapid palatal expansion. Angle Orthod. 34:256–270, 1964.

60. Teuscher, U.: An appraisal of growth and reaction to extraoral anchorage. Am. J. Orthod. 89:113–121, 1986.

61. Harvold, E.P.: Altering craniofacial growth: Force application and neuromuscular bone interaction. In *Clinical Alteration of the Growing Face, Craniofacial Growth Series No. 14.* J.A. McNamara, K.A. Ribbens, and R.P. Howe (eds.). Center for Human Growth and Development, The University of Michigan, Ann Arbor, 1983.

62. Bassett, C.A.L.: Biophysical principles affecting bone structure. In *The Biochemistry and Physiology of Bone,* Vol. III. G.H. Bourne (ed.). Academic Press, New York, 1971.

63. McNamara, J.A.: Functional determinants of craniofacial size and shape. Eur. J. Orthod. 2:131–159, 1980.

64. Stutzmann, J. and Petrovic, A.: Intrinsic regulation of the condylar cartilage growth rate. Eur. J. Orthod. 1:41–54, 1979.

65. McNamara, J.A. and Ribbens, K.A.: Malocclusion and the periodontium. In *Craniofacial Growth Series No. 15*. J.A. McNamara and K.A. Ribbens (eds.). Center for Human Growth and Development, University of Michigan, Ann Arbor, 1984.

66. Petrovic, A., Stutzmann, J.J., and Gasson, N.: The final length of the mandible: Is it genetically predetermined? In *Craniofacial Growth Series No. 10*. D.S. Carlson (ed.). Center for Human Growth and Development, University of Michigan, Ann Arbor, 1981.

67. Woodside, D.G., Metaxes, A., and Altuna, G.: The influence of functional appliance therapy on glenoid fossa remodeling. Am. J. Orthod. 92:181–198, 1987.

68. McNamara, J.A.: Functional adaptations in the temporomandibular joint. Dent. Clin. North Am. 19:457–471, 1975.

69. Graber, L.W.: Chincup therapy for mandibular prognathism. Am. J. Orthod. 72:23–41, 1977.

70. Mitani, H. and Fukazawa, H.: Effects of chincup force on the timing and amount of mandibular growth associated with anterior reversed occlusion (class III malocclusion) during puberty. Am. J. Orthod. 90:454–463, 1986.

71. Wyatt, W.E.: Preventing adverse effects on the temporomandibular joint through orthodontic treatment. Am. J. Orthod. 91:493–499, 1987.

72. Andresen, V.: The Norwegian system of functional gnatho-orthopedics. Acta Gnathol. 1:5, 1936.

73. Häupl, K.: *Gewebumbau und Zahnveränderung in der Funktions—Kieferorthopädie.* Herman Meusser, Leipzig, 1938.

74. Schwarz, A.M. and Gratzinger, M.: *Removable Orthodontic Appliances.* W.B. Saunders Co., Philadelphia, 1966.

75. Balters, W.: *Eine Einführung in die Bionatorheilmethode: Ausgewählte Shriften und Vorträge.* K. Herrmann Verlag, Heidelberg, 1973.

76. Fränkel, R.: A functional approach to orofacial orthopedics. Br. J. Orthod. 7:41, 1980.

77. Angle, E.H.: *Treatment of Malocclusion of the Teeth*, 7th ed. S.S. White Dental Manufacturing Co., Philadelphia, 1907.

78. Angle, E.H.: The latest and best in orthodontic mechanism. D. Cosmos. 70:1143–1158, 1928.

79. Case, C.S.: *Dental Orthopedia.* C.S. Case and Co., Chicago, 1921.

80. Tweed, C.W.: *Clinical Orthodontics.* C.V. Mosby, St. Louis, 1966.

81. Begg, P.R. and Kesling, P.C.: *Begg Orthodontic Theory and Technique.* W.B. Saunders Co., Philadelphia, 1977.

82. Björk, A.: Sutural growth of the upper face studied by metallic implant method. Acta Odontol. Scand. 24:109, 1966.

83. Björk, A.: Variations in the growth of the human mandible: Radiographic study by the implant method. J. Dent. Res. 42:2, 1963.

84. Moss, M.L.: The functional matrix. In *Vistas in Orthodontics.* B.C. Kraus and R.A. Riedal (eds.). Lea & Febiger, Philadelphia, 1962.

85. Graber, T.M., Rakosi, T., and Petrovic, A.G.: *Dentofacial Orthopedics with Functional Appliances.* C.V. Mosby, St. Louis, 1985.

86. Frankel, R.: The functional matrix and its practical importance in orthodontics. Eur. Orthod. Soc. Congr. 18:207, 1969.

87. Frankel, R.: The functional matrix and its practical importance in orthodontics. Eur. Orthod. Soc. Congr. 45:207, 1969.

88. Weinmann, J.P. and Sicher, H.: *Bone and Bones: Fundamentals of Bone Biology.* C.V. Mosby, St. Louis, 1955.

89. Scott, J.: Cartilage of the nasal system. Br. Dent. J. 95:37, 1953.

90. Graber, T.M.: Extrinsic factors influencing craniofacial growth. In *Determinant of Mandibular Growth. Craniofacial Growth Series No. 4.* J.A. McNamara (ed.). Center for Human Growth and Development, University of Michigan, Ann Arbor, 1975.

91. Williamson, E.H.: Removable Herbst treatment of anterior disk dislocations. Fac. Orthop. Temporomand. Arthrol. 2:2–11, 1985.

92. McNamara, J.A., Hinton, R.J., and Hoffman, D.L.: Histological analysis of temporomandibular joint adaptation to protrusive function in young adult rhesus monkeys *(Macaca mulatta).* Am. J. Orthod. 82:288, 1982.

93. Schneiderman, E.D. and Carlson, D.S.: Cephalometric analysis of condylar adaptations to altered mandibular positions in adult rhesus monkeys, *Macaca mulatta.* Arch. Oral. Biol. 30:49, 1985.

94. Graber, L.W. (ed.): *Orthodontics: State of The Art, Essence of The Science.* C.V. Mosby, St. Louis, 1986.

95. Roth, R.H.: Five year clinical evaluation of the Andrews straight wire appliance. J. Clin. Orthod. 10:866, 1976.

96. Roth, R.H.: Treatment mechanics for the straight wire appliance. In *Orthodontics: Current Principles and Techniques.* T.M. Graber and B.F. Swain (eds.). C.V. Mosby, St. Louis, 1985.

97. Roth, R.H.: Roth straight wire appliance philosophy (brochure). "A" Company Inc., San Diego, 1979.

98. Reitan, K.: Tissue rearrangement during retention of orthodontically rotated teeth. Angle Orthod. 29:105–113, 1959.

99. Wilson, R. and Wilson, W.: *Enhanced Orthodontics.* Rocky Mountain Orthodontics, Denver, 1988.

100. Alpern, M.C. and Hyden, L.: A multifunctional orthopedic appliance. J. Clin. Orthod. 20:688–689, 1986.

SECTION V

SURGICAL THERAPY

Leslie B. Heffez

CHAPTER 31

Arthroscopy

Arthroscopy of the temporomandibular joint (TMJ) is a relatively new and exciting field that promises to revolutionize the surgical approach to the treatment of TMJ pathology. The word *arthroscopy* is derived from the Greek language and means "to examine within a joint." The history of arthroscopy can be traced to 1806, when Bozzini[1] examined deeply seated visci using a wax candle mounted in a tin tube. Desormeaux[2] realized the importance of a lens system to concentrate light and used such a system to examine the genitourinary tract more closely. Anecdotal reports dating as early as 1870 describe Kussmaul's[3] attempts at esophagogastroscopy on a professional sword swallower. The development of the first cystoscope in 1879 laid the groundwork for the development of the first arthroscope (1920).[4] Takagi[5,6] is credited with providing the scientific world with a flurry of significant engineering achievements. Watanabe,[7-10] one of Takagi's pupils, employed improved lens systems and more reliable lighting systems to produce a functional arthroscope, the Watanabe's #21 arthroscope.

Although 68 years have passed since Bircher's[11] original description of knee arthroscopy with a Jacobaeus' laparascope, TMJ arthroscopy remains in its infancy. The invention of the Hopkins rod lens system in 1960 and the fiberoptic light system in 1967 would prove to be the two most notable historical events for TMJ arthroscopy. In 1970 and 1975, Ohnishi[12,13] reported on arthroscopy of the cadaveric and live TMJ. In 1978, Hilsabeck and Laskin[14] successfully examined the rabbit TMJ without histologic evidence of serious iatro-

genic damage. Later, in 1980, the arthroscope was used to examine experimentally induced pathologic conditions, including steroid-induced arthropathy, chronic synovial inflammatory change, acute inflammatory disease, and gross damage to the condyle and disc.[15] According to Murakami and Hoshino[16] (1982), Kino (1980) and Kino and colleagues (1981) reported on the arthroscopic and macroscopic findings of fresh human cadaver specimens. The synovial membrane was investigated microscopically as well. Murakami and associates[17] described the arthroscopic findings of infectious arthritis and performed irrigation of the joint cavity under direct vision. Diagnostic arthroscopic parameters were established.[18-20] Surgical treatment for closed lock was pioneered in North America by Sanders and Buoncristiani.[21-22] Since then, several arthroscopic surgical techniques have been described. As the long-term studies of arthroscopic surgery are published, a repertoire of procedures for distinct pathologic entities will emerge. The entire field of arthroscopy is undergoing great and rapid metamorphosis. Fortunately, a solid groundwork has been laid, and it serves as the basis of much of our discussion.

ARTHROSCOPIC ANATOMIC NOMENCLATURE

Several nomenclatures have been proposed to describe the arthroscopic anatomic features of the normal and pathologic joint.[16,18,19] One such nomenclature is described later.[18,19] Because an international nomenclature has yet to be proposed, terms from other classifications are mentioned.

In the normal condyle-disc-fossa relationship, the following arthroscopic anatomic terms are used: *posterior incline, crest,* and *anterior incline of the posterior band, flexure, medial and lateral sulcus,* and *synovial plica* (Fig. 31–1).

The posterior incline is the upward sloping of the posterior band (Fig. 31–1 and Plate 31–1). The crest or the peak of the posterior band marks the point at which its downward slope, the anterior incline (Plate 31–2), begins.

In the arthroscopic description of the normal condyle-disc-fossa relationship, the flexure is the junction of the tympanic portion of the retrodiscal tissue and the posterior incline of the posterior band (see Fig. 31–1 and Plate 31–1). It takes the form of a V- or U-shaped structure. The flexure is the chief orientation landmark

---

Plates were obtained with a 30° forward-oblique rod lens with 2.4-mm Karl Storz telescopes (Karl Storz Endoscopy America Inc.).

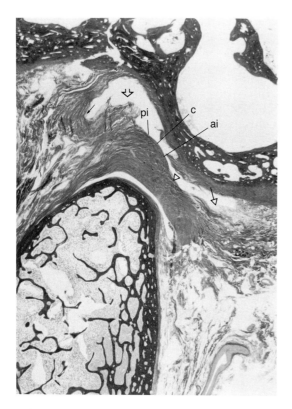

FIGURE 31–1. Sagittal microscopic section of the right temporomandibular joint demonstrating a normal condyle-disc-fossa relationship. Note the arthroscopic anatomic landmarks: posterior incline (pi), crest (c), and anterior incline (ai) of the posterior band and synovial plica (double arrow). The flexure (arrow) in the normal disc relationship represents the junction of the tympanic portion of the retrodiscal tissue and the posterior incline of the posterior band. Anterior attachment (open arrow) and intermediate zone (arrowhead) are indicated. Synovium lines anterior and posterior recesses of joint spaces.

for superior joint space arthroscopy. In the disc displacement, the flexure is the junction of the tympanic portion of the retrodiscal tissue and the remodeled retrodiscal tissue (Fig. 31–2 and Plate 31–3). Joint space distention and manipulation of the telescope accentuate the flexure.

The sulci describe the region of reflection of the retrodiscal tissue or disc onto the lateral capsule (see Plate 31–3). Murakami and Hoshino[16] have employed the terms *medial* and *lateral paradiscal grooves.* Others used the term *gutters.*

A synovial plica is an outpocketing of synovium. One such plica is commonly found in the posterior medial regions of the superior joint space (Plate 31–4).

In the arthroscopic description of the disc displacement, the following anatomic terms are used: *flexure* (defined earlier), *adhesion, corrugations, depression, fibrillations, fold, remodeled posterior band (remodeled disc),* and *remodeled retrodiscal tissue (remodeled posterior attachment).*[20,21]

An adhesion is a band of fibrous connective tissue fixed at both ends. An adhesion may be qualified by the terms *linear* (Plate 31–5) or *web-like* (Plate 31–6). Corrugations are small surface foldings within a tissue. These typically appear in the remodeled retrodiscal tissue near the site of the flexure (Plate 31–7). With simulated mandibular movements, the tissue appears at times compressed and at times effaced.

A depression is an interruption in the normal topography of a structure. The medial capsular ligament may be iatrogenically depressed

FIGURE 31–2. Sagittal microscopic section of the right temporomandibular joint demonstrating disc displacement with considerable deformation and remodeling of the posterior band (double arrow). The anterior band appears folded upon itself (curvilinear arrow). Note the flexure (fx), which marks the junction of the tympanic portion of the retrodiscal tissue and remodeled retrodiscal tissue (series of small arrows).

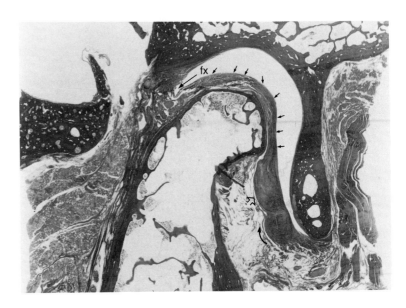

by the trocar. Fibrillations are the splitting of a tissue surface into fibrils. Remodeled retrodiscal tissue often appears fibrillated (Plate 31–8). A fold (pleat) is the thickened cord-like structure within the tympanic portion of the retrodiscal tissue (Plate 31–9). Medial and lateral folds are separated by a depression. The presence of folds within the normal retrodiscal tissue has not been ascertained. *Remodeled posterior band* or *remodeled disc* is the term used to describe the displaced disc (Plate 31–10). The altered morphology is the result of deformation, resorption of its internal fiber architecture, and displacement. The conformation of the disc to the convex eminence and infratemporal articulating surface is an example of disc remodeling. Remodeled retrodiscal tissue (remodeled posterior attachment) is that tissue originating as retrodiscal tissue, which progressively stretches forward over the condyle and is loaded with disc displacement (Plate 31–11). The tissue displays various degrees of superficial vascularity.

To facilitate communication and recording of arthroscopic findings, the superior joint space may be subdivided by osseous landmarks into a glenoid and a pre-eminence region (see Fig. 31–3).[20] That portion immediately under the concavity of the glenoid fossa is the glenoid region. It is bounded anteriorly by an imaginary perpendicular dropped from the apex of the eminence and posteriorly by the origin of the tympanic portion of the retrodiscal tissue.

The glenoid region is further subdivided into anterior and posterior regions by an imaginary perpendicular dropped from the region of maximum concavity. The posterior glenoid region constitutes the posterior recess of the superior joint space. The pre-eminence region is bounded anteriorly by the capsular attachments and posteriorly by the perpendicular at the apex of the eminence. The pre-eminence region constitutes the anterior recess of the superior joint space. Both the apex of the eminence and the region of maximum concavity of the glenoid fossa are readily recognized arthroscopically. Alternatively, Murakami and Hoshino[16] proposed regional anatomic nomenclature based on soft-tissue landmarks. The terms *anterior and posterior pouches (anterior and posterior recesses,* by others), and *higher* and *lower intermediate spaces* were used. The classification based on osseous landmarks may be more reliable, because soft tissues appear to be subject to displacement and remodeling at a faster rate. Furthermore, such a classification permits preoperative radiography to be utilized as a basis for communication.

ARTHROSCOPIC INSTRUMENTATION

Arthroscopic instrumentation includes the telescopes (arthroscopes), solid instruments for capsule penetration and surgery, and external illumination mechanisms.

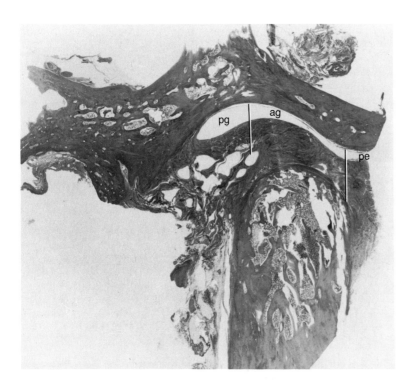

FIGURE 31–3. The superior joint space is divided into glenoid (ag and pg) and pre-eminence regions (pe) by an imaginary perpendicular line drawn from the apex of the eminence. The glenoid region is the area under the concavity of the glenoid fossa. This region is further divided into anterior (ag) and posterior (pg) regions by an imaginary line drawn from the point of maximum concavity of the fossa.

Telescopes

The telescope (arthroscope) is a rigid cylinder that conducts light into a cavity and transmits an image back to the viewer. There are essentially three major components to a telescope: an ocular lens or an eyepiece, a rigid tube containing illumination and transmitting mechanisms, and a prism and an objective at the working end (Fig. 31–4).

The arthroscope belongs to a larger class of instruments employed in rigid arthroscopy. Another instrument of this class is the sinuscope for examination and treatment of paranasal sinus disease. Rigid endoscopy should be distinguished from fiberoptic endoscopy (Figs. 31–5 and 31–6). The last is used in esophagoscopy, sigmoidoscopy, and colonoscopy. The difference lies in the manner in which the image is transmitted to the eyepiece. In rigid endoscopy, a series of lenses mounted within a hollow, rigid cylinder transmit the image (see Fig. 31–6).[4] In fiberoptic endoscopy, a precise arrangement of fiberoptic cables within a flexible tube transmits the image (see Fig. 31–5).[4] The precise arrangement of transmission fiber cables is called *coherence*. Coherence prevents scrambling of the image. The illuminating fiber cables for both the rigid endoscope and fiberscope are similar. The arrangement of these fiber cables is not important and is therefore described as *incoherent*. The fiberscope is flexible because all the transmission and illuminating mechanisms are made of fiberglass.

Two technical terms are frequently selected in discussing the virtues of one telescope over another. These terms are *direction of view* and *field of view*. Direction of view is the direction off the horizontal optical axis from which one obtains an image. Telescopes are often described according to their directions of view. These vary according to manufacturer and can be, for example, 0°, 10°, 25°, 30°, 70°, or 120°. The 0° lens permits viewing of objects directly in front of the lens (Fig. 31–7). This is not advantageous to arthroscopists because they are unable to obtain adequate reference points with a single view. Viewing anatomy through a 0° lens would be equivalent to walking into a room without seeing the ceiling or floor. A 30° lens or its equivalent is the most versatile telescope. It permits the operator to view objects directly in front of the telescope and to gain oblique views superior and inferior to the telescope. Rotation of a 30° telescope about its axis greatly improves the viewing field (Fig. 31–8). The other directions of view are less commonly employed in TMJ arthroscopy.

The field of view (viewing angle) is the outer visual limits of what the operator sees (see Fig. 31–7). The field of view is described in terms of degrees. The arthroscopist can observe the field of view by turning the arthroscope on in a dark room, placing the arthroscope parallel against a paper, and tracing the outer limits of light. In this case, because light transmission is through air and not a fluid medium, the field of view recorded is slightly greater than that obtained in the joint cavity.

The telescopes currently marketed by manufacturers may be classified into three lens systems based on the transmitting mechanism housed within the rigid tube: traditional, Selfoscope type (Olympus Selfoscope or Dyonics Needlescope), and rod lens. The traditional optical system consists of a series of glass lenses

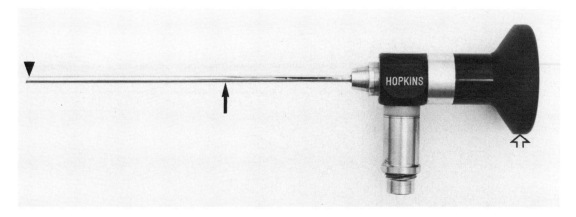

FIGURE 31–4. The three major components to the telescope are the eyepiece containing the ocular lens, the rigid tube containing the illumination and transmission elements, and the working end containing the prism and objective.

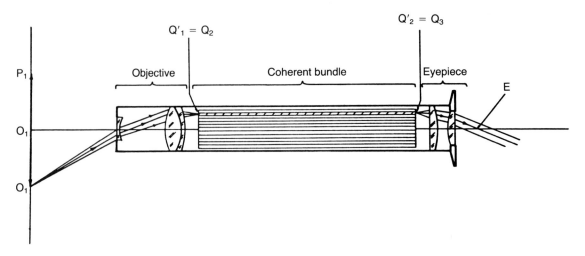

FIGURE 31–5. Compare the fiberscope with the rigid endoscope (Fig. 31–6). In the fiberscope, the fiber bundles are used for illuminating the cavity and transmitting the image back. The fiber bundles for transmission are precisely arranged (coherence) to prevent scrambling of the image. (Reprinted with permission from Berci, G.: *Endoscopy*. Appleton-Century-Crofts, New York, 1976.)

FIGURE 31–6. In the rigid endoscope, the joint cavity is illuminated with fiber bundles. However, the image is transmitted back to the eye via a series of lenses (open arrows). Both the fiber bundles and lenses are housed within a hollow rigid tube.

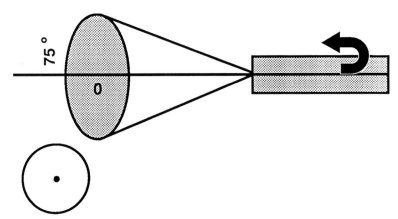

FIGURE 31–7. Direction of view represents the direction off the horizontal optical axis from which the operator obtains an image. The field of view represents the outer limits of what the operator can see (shaded area). This diagram represents the field of view (75 degrees) of a 0-degree lens. There is no effect on the field of view with rotation of the telescope.

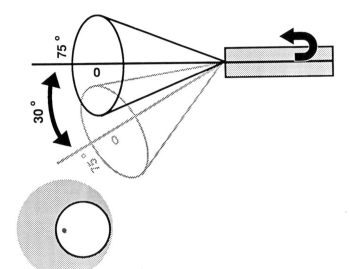

FIGURE 31–8. This diagram represents the field of view (75 degrees) of a 30-degree lens. Note the effective increase in the field of view with rotation of the telescope.

separated by air spaces (Fig. 31–9A). The Selfoscope lens system utilizes a single image-transmitting fiber tube instead of a series of lenses. It is contained within a rigid hollow tube, differentiating it from a fiberscope. In the rod lens system, the functions of air and glass are opposite those in the traditional lens system (see Fig. 31–9B). Air lenses and glass spaces, instead of glass lenses and air spaces, significantly improve light transmission. The diagnostic ca-

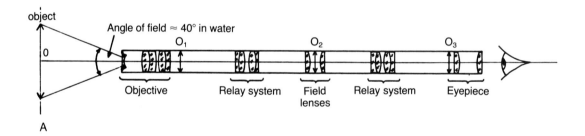

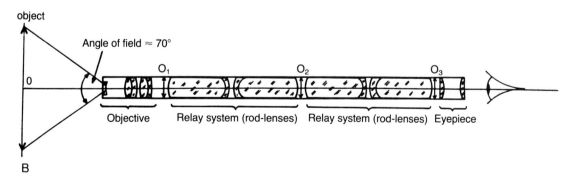

FIGURE 31–9. *A,* Traditional lens system. Note the air spaces between the glass field lenses and the relay systems. *B,* Rod lens system. Note the air lenses between the long glass spaces. Light conduction and image transmission is improved with this system. (Reprinted with permission from Berci, G.: *Endoscopy.* New York, Appleton-Century-Crofts, 1976.)

pability of the rod lenses surpasses that of the other systems because they afford a brighter field with a wider viewing angle.[4,25,26]

Solid Instruments

The solid instruments are those instruments chosen for capsule penetration, joint exploration, and surgery of the joint.

Capsule Penetration Instruments

The lateral ligament/capsule is penetrated with a sharp trocar mounted to an external sheath (Fig. 31–10). The trocar and sheath are held together by either a locking or spring mechanism. The external sheath serves to protect the surrounding tissues, increase the rigidity of the trocar, and provide a pathway for inserting instruments into the joint cavity. Once the joint is penetrated, the arthroscopist may exchange the sharp trocar for a blunt one while maintaining the external sheath within the joint space. The blunt trocar serves to complete the penetration procedure and explore the intra-articular components. The external

sheaths are available in various diameters and lengths to accommodate exploratory and surgical instruments. The external sheath is slightly wider in diameter than the arthroscope itself to permit passage of irrigant into the joint cavity. For example, the 2.7-mm Karl Storz external sheath corresponds to the 2.4-mm 30° forward oblique telescope (Karl Storz Endoscopy America Inc.). An inlet post is attached to the external sheath for the irrigating connecting tube.

Surgical Instruments

Surgical instruments are classified as hand held or motorized.

HAND-HELD INSTRUMENTS

A pediatric resectoscope may be adapted for operative arthroscopy (Fig. 31–11). A 0° telescope is inserted onto a hand-held mechanism, which permits the simultaneous mounting of cutting instruments. The cutting instrument appears in the middle of the field of view. When the trigger mechanism on the hand-held portion is depressed, the cutting instrument

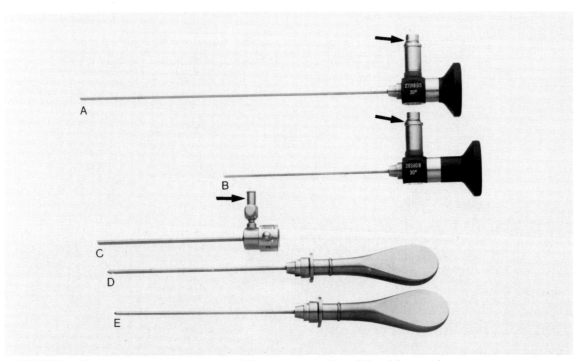

FIGURE 31–10. The 30-degree forward oblique 2.4 mm telescopes (*A* and *B*) and the capsule-penetrating instruments: external sheath (*C*) and dull (*D*) and sharp (*E*) trocars. Note the inlet post on the external sheath (arrow) for attachment of the irrigation fluid. Note the inlet post on the telescopes (arrows) for coupling of the fiberoptic cable.

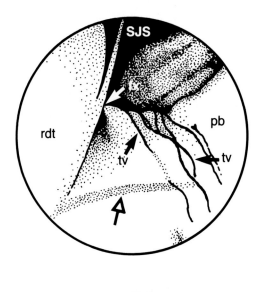

PLATE 31-1. *Right temporomandibular joint. Normal condyle-disc-fossa relationship (slight reducing disc displacement with reduction). Transverse examination phase, posterior-lateral field.* Note the vertically oriented tympanic portion of the retrodiscal tissue (rdt). The flexure (fx) in the normal condyle-disc-fossa relationship is formed grossly by the junction of the retrodiscal tissue and the posterior incline of the posterior band (pb). Note the stark white color of the disc. In this case, a slight disc displacement was present, as noted by the horizontal extension of the retrodiscal tissue (posterior attachment) (open arrow). A few superficial transverse vessels (tv, arrows) course near the posterior incline of the posterior band. The superior joint space (SJS) is in the background.

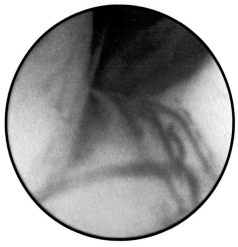

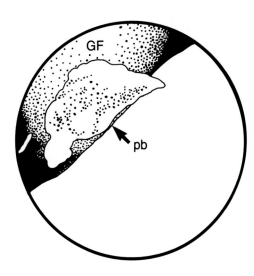

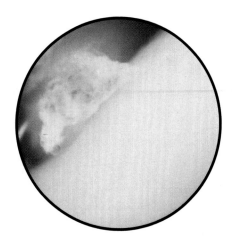

PLATE 31-2. *Right temporomandibular joint. Normal condyle-disc-fossa relationship. Transverse examination phase, anterior-middle field.* Note the stark white color of the anterior incline of the posterior band (pb). The surface of this tissue is dense and compact. In the background, the fibrous connective tissue lining the glenoid fossa (GF) is evident. Compare the color of this tissue to that of the disc. In the center of the field, some debris (arrow) has been introduced by the trocar.

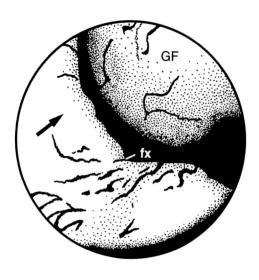

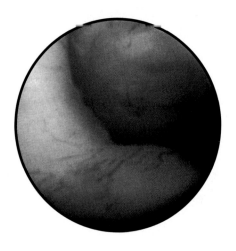

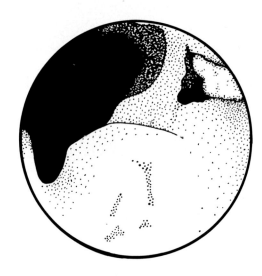

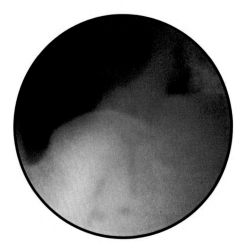

PLATE 31–3. *Right temporomandibular joint. Nonreducing disc displacement. Transverse examination phase, posterior-middle field.* The flexure (fx) is in view. There appears to be multiple folds within the flexure. A small portion of the tympanic portion of the retrodiscal tissue (arrow) is visible. Most of the visible superficial vessels course through the horizontally oriented portion of the remodeled retrodiscal tissue (class II vascularity). Compare the yellow or ivory color of remodeled retrodiscal tissue with that of the disc in Plates 31–1 and 31–2. The tissue changes in the tympanic portion of the retrodiscal tissue appear similar to those in the remodeled retrodiscal tissue, suggesting that the changes in this tissue should be considered as a continuum. The fibrous connective tissue lining the glenoid fossa (GF) is in the background.

PLATE 31–4. *Left temporomandibular joint. Nonreducing disc displacement. Transverse examination phase, posterior-middle field.* Remodeled retrodiscal tissue in the area of the flexure. Note the marked decrease in superficial vascularity (class III vascularity).

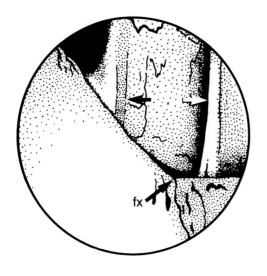

PLATE 31–5. *Left temporomandibular joint. Nonreducing disc displacement. Transverse examination phase, middle-central field.* The condyle and disc are slightly translated, owing to positioning and distention of the superior joint space. In the background, the medial capsule/ligament is visible. Immediately lateral to the capsule, two linear bands (arrows) are visible, probably representing adhesions. Synovial vessels may be seen coursing on the medial capsule. Superficial transverse vessels are present in the region of the flexure (fx). Note the dull, white color of remodeled retrodiscal tissue. The disc was located in the pre-eminence region.

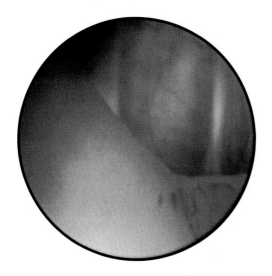

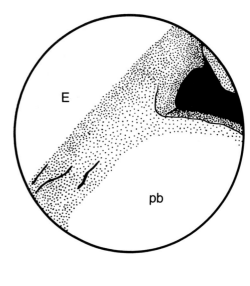

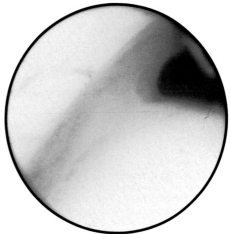

PLATE 31–6. *Left temporomandibular joint. Normal condyle-disc-fossa relationship. Transverse examination phase, anterior-central field.* A dense thick adhesion is located between the posterior slope of the eminence (E) and the anterior incline of the posterior band (pb). The glare from the flash has caused the disc and the fibrous connective tissue lining the eminence to appear stark white.

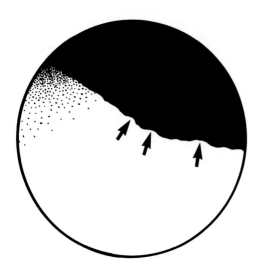

PLATE 31–7. *Right temporomandibular joint. Nonreducing disc displacement. Transverse examination phase, middle-central field.* Note the corrugations on the surface of the ivory-colored remodeled retrodiscal tissue. There are no superficial vessels in this field of view (class IV vascularity).

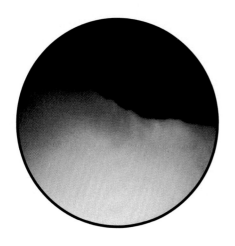

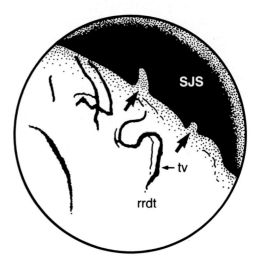

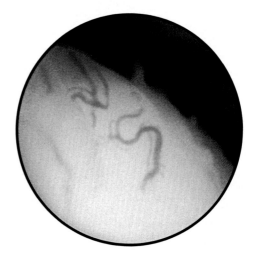

PLATE 31–8. *Right temporomandibular joint. Nonreducing disc displacement. Transverse examination phase, middle-lateral field.* Remodeled retrodiscal tissue (rrdt) is in the foreground. Note the fibrillations (arrows) and the superficial transverse vessels (tv, class III vascularity). The black space above this tissue is the superior joint space (SJS). The fibrous connective tissue lining the glenoid fossa is visible.

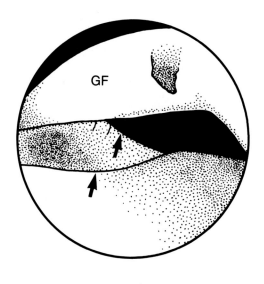

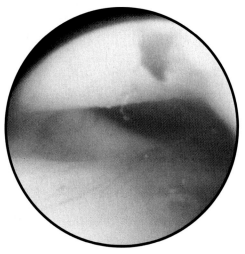

PLATE 31–9. *Left temporomandibular joint. Reducing disc displacement. Transverse examination phase, posterior-central field.* Two folds (arrows) are present in the remodeled retrodiscal tissue. The depression between the folds corresponds to the projection from the glenoid fossa (GF). A few superficial vessels are present in the remodeled retrodiscal tissue.

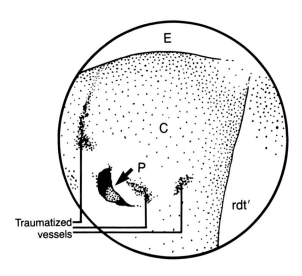

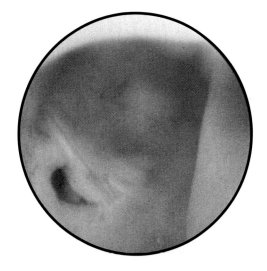

PLATE 31–10. *Left temporomandibular joint. Nonreducing disc displacement. Longitudinal examination phase, lateral field.* Remodeled retrodiscal tissue (rdt') (class IV vascularity) is to the right of the field. Note the surface irregularity of this tissue. Superiorly lies the fibrous connective tissue lining the eminence (E). A small perforation (p) is present in the anterior capsule (C).

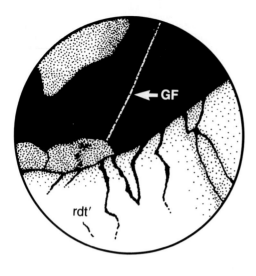

PLATE 31–11. *Right temporomandibular joint. Nonreducing disc displacement. Transverse examination phase, middle-central field.* Superficial transverse vessels course on the remodeled retrodiscal tissue (rdt') (class II vascularity). Debris and clot are found to the left of the field. The fibrous connective lining of the glenoid fossa (GF) is partly obscured by clot. A mucin strand (arrow) is found extending from the roof of the glenoid fossa to the remodeled retrodiscal tissue.

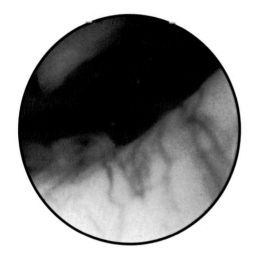

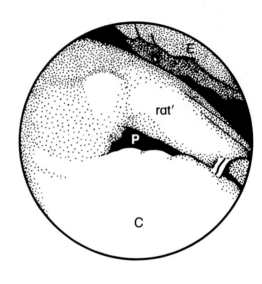

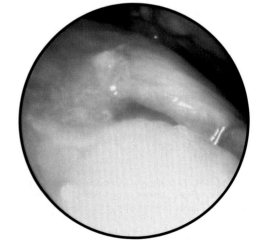

PLATE 31–12. *Right temporomandibular joint. Disc displacement. Transverse examination phase, anterior-lateral field.* Photograph obtained with halogen light source. A perforation (p) is present in the remodeled retrodiscal tissue (rdt'). The superficial vascularity of the remodeled retrodiscal tissue cannot be adequately evaluated in fresh-frozen cadaver specimens. The fibrous, connective tissue–covered condyle (C) is protruding through the perforation. The posterior slope of the eminence (E) is visible to the right and above.

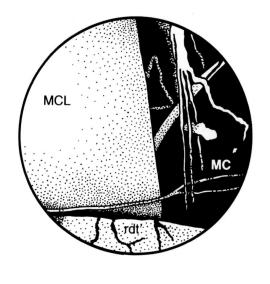

PLATE 31–13. *Right temporomandibular joint. Reducing disc displacement. Transverse examination phase, middle-medial field.* The termination of the medial capsule ligament (MCL) is apparent. The color and appearance of the ligament in this case are unusual. It usually appears grey and more fibrous. The unsupported medial capsule (MC) has been displaced medially by the pressure of the irrigant. The remodeled retrodiscal tissue (rdt') is found in the bottom of the field. Note the superficial transverse vessels (class II vascularity). Some debris is present in the superior joint space.

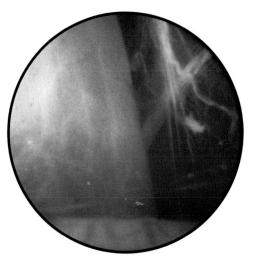

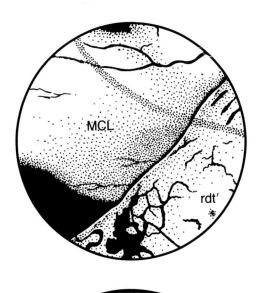

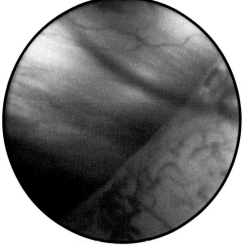

PLATE 31–14. *Left temporomandibular joint. Reducing disc displacement. Transverse examination phase, middle-central field.* Numerous superficial vessels may be seen coursing on the remodeled retrodiscal tissue (rdt', class I vascularity). The grey fibers of the medial capsular ligament (MCL) are present in the background. The black demilune crossing the field of view represents a scratch on the lens.

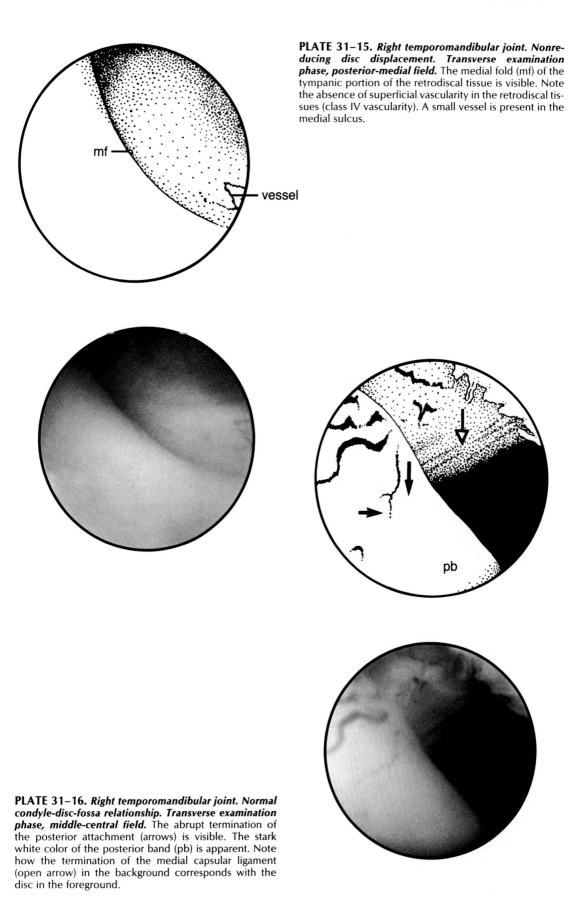

PLATE 31–15. *Right temporomandibular joint. Nonreducing disc displacement. Transverse examination phase, posterior-medial field.* The medial fold (mf) of the tympanic portion of the retrodiscal tissue is visible. Note the absence of superficial vascularity in the retrodiscal tissues (class IV vascularity). A small vessel is present in the medial sulcus.

PLATE 31–16. *Right temporomandibular joint. Normal condyle-disc-fossa relationship. Transverse examination phase, middle-central field.* The abrupt termination of the posterior attachment (arrows) is visible. The stark white color of the posterior band (pb) is apparent. Note how the termination of the medial capsular ligament (open arrow) in the background corresponds with the disc in the foreground.

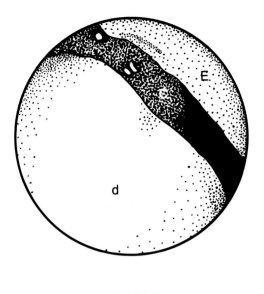

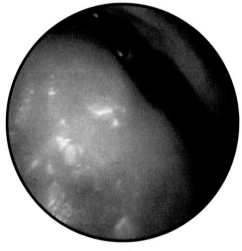

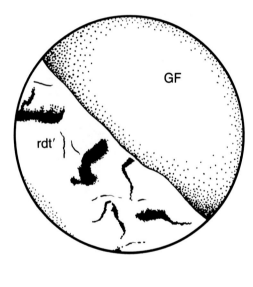

PLATE 31–17. Left temporomandibular joint. Normal condyle-disk-fossa relationship. Longitudinal examination phase, medial (M) field. Photograph obtained with halogen light source. Note the compact white disk (d) that matches the curvature of the fibrous, connective tissue–lined eminence (E). The anterior capsule is in the background.

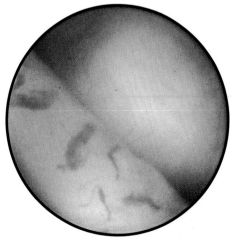

PLATE 31–18. Right temporomandibular joint. Nonreducing disc displacement. Transverse examination phase, middle-central field. The color of the remodeled retrodiscal tissue (rdt') (class III vascularity) is similar to that of the fibrous, connective tissue–lined glenoid fossa (GF). Some of the vessels appear traumatized (arrows). In some areas, the tissue appears fibrilla.

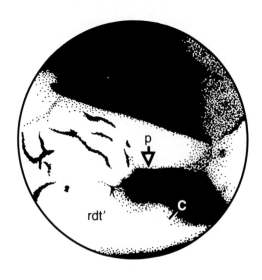

PLATE 31–19. *Left temporomandibular joint. Nonreducing disc displacement. Transverse examination phase, posterior-central field.* A perforation (p) is present in the remodeled retrodiscal tissue (rdt', class III vascularity). Note how the superficial vessels do not extend to the margin of the perforation. The fibrous connective tissue covering the condyle (C) may be seen through the perforation (arrow).

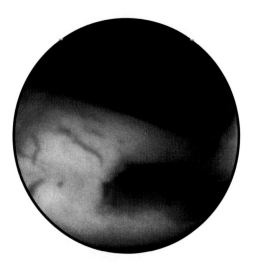

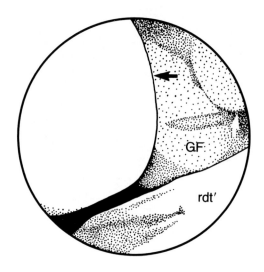

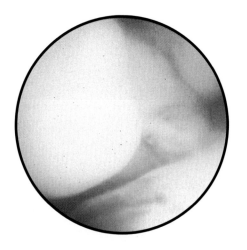

PLATE 31–20. *Right temporomandibular joint. Nonreducing disc displacement. Transverse examination phase, posterior-lateral field.* Note the stark white, loose chondroid body (arrow) in close apposition to the remodeled retrodiscal tissue (rdt'). Additional smaller bodies appear to be extruding from the fibrous, connective tissue–lined glenoid fossa (GF). A diagnosis of synovial chondromatosis was made.

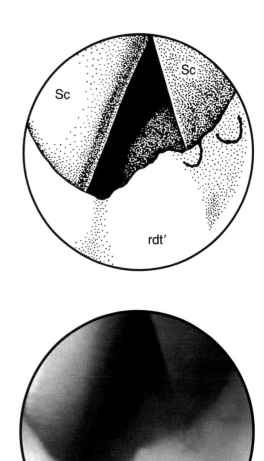

PLATE 31–21. *Right temporomandibular joint. Reducing disc displacement. Transverse examination phase, middle-central field.* A retrodiscotomy is being performed. A microscissor (Sc) is cutting a superficially avascular portion of the remodeled retrodiscal tissue (rdt′).

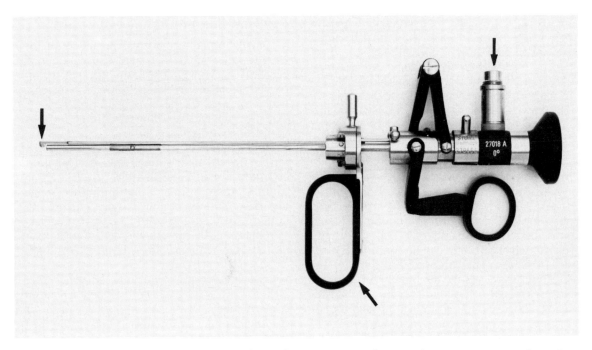

FIGURE 31–11. A pediatric resectoscope may be used as an operating telescope. The instrument is passed into the superior joint space through an elliptically shaped external sheath (not shown). A cutting instrument is mounted in tandem with a 0-degree lens telescope. A trigger mechanism allows for forward and backward movement of the cutting instrument. Triangulation is therefore unnecessary. Note the inlet post for coupling of the fiberoptic cable.

moves away from the lens. In this manner, an arthroscopist can, through a single puncture site, incise tissue under direct vision. Rosette, straight, sickle, and retrograde knives may be utilized. (The difficulty involved with a 0° lens was described earlier.)

Various scissors and knives with long working arms are available (Fig. 31–12). Instruments are manipulated into the joint space through a second part and visualized from within the joint using the telescope. Punch, blunt-nosed, sharp-nosed, up-biting, and down-biting scissors are some of the more common varieties. Myringotomy knives may be adopted for arthroscopic applications, although they require shorter and larger diameter external sheaths. The diameters of the shafts of these instruments must satisfy two require-

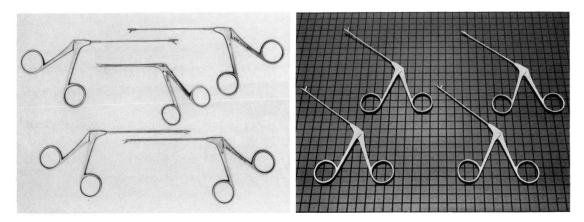

FIGURE 31–12. A variety of scissors and knives. These instruments are passed independent of the telescope through the external sheath of the second port. The operator then triangulates using these instruments.

ments: they must be rigid enough to permit the cutting of tissues, and they must be small enough to pass through the external sheath selected. Orthopedic arthroscopic knives may also be used for their additional rigidity. No external sheath is needed with these instruments. The knives are available in various configurations, including straight, straight offset to the right or left, and rosette.

MOTORIZED INSTRUMENTS

The shaver is a motorized instrument with a pistol grip (Fig. 31–13). It is employed for abrading and incising small amounts of tissue. This instrument consists of a hollow, distally fenestrated sheath that can accommodate a series of blades. The motor within the unit rotates the blades within the hollow tube, essentially pinching off tissue at the site of the fenestration. Suction is applied through the instrument to immediately remove the tissue from the joint space. The joint space must be adequately distended to prevent its collapse by the sucking of the synovium into the fenestrated aperture.[25] The shaver has proven efficacy in removing fibrillated or fragmented knee cartilage and hypertrophied synovium. It is less effective in cutting remodeled retrodiscal tissue.

External Illumination Mechanisms

Illumination mechanisms include both the light source (Fig. 31–14) and light-conducting cables (Fig. 31–15). The term *external* is employed because only the illuminating mechanisms external to the telescope are described. The fiberglass cables housed within the telescope are not discussed here.

Halogen (150-watt) and xenon (6000-Kelvin, 300-watt) light sources are the two most common. The illumination from xenon sources provides images that are closer to the natural color. When still photographs are obtained, a through-the-lens (TTL) cable connection between the camera and light source is essential to regulate the amount of light discharged.

Light-conducting cables may be either fiber or fluid cables (see Fig. 31–15). The fiber cables contain many incoherent fiberglass guides for conducting light to the fiber cables in the telescope and then on to the joint cavity. Light may be internally reflected more than 15,000 times per meter in a single fiberglass guide. Fiber cable lengths and diameters vary among manufacturers. Increasing the diameter increases the conduction of light. However, the number of fiberglass guides within the telescope is the limiting factor to joint cavity illu-

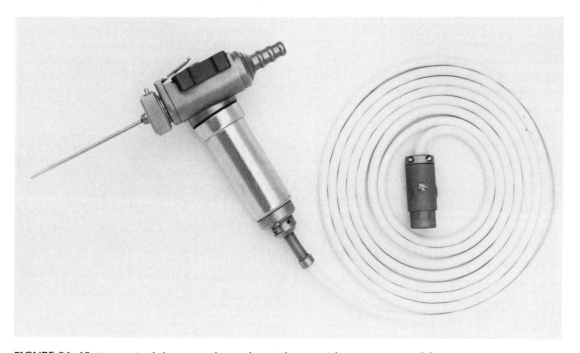

FIGURE 31–13. A motorized shaver may be used to perform partial synovectomies of the superior joint space. The shaver would be inserted through an external sheath.

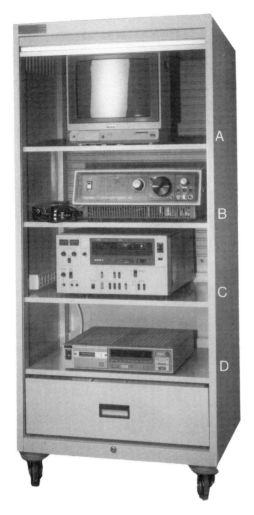

FIGURE 31–14. The mobile cart contains a monitor (*A*), xenon light source (*B*), ¾-inch video recorder (*C*), and ½-inch video recorder (*D*)

lens system. The fiber cable must not be tightly coiled or bent to avoid breakage of the individual fiberglass guides. The operator can check the integrity of the cable by inspecting for dark voids at its distal end.

Ultrasonic cleaning of arthroscopic instruments is avoided because it may loosen soldered joints. However, adapters should be unscrewed and the surfaces cleaned with a mild detergent and water and a cotton-tipped applicator. Stainless steel instruments can be soaked in a water-soluble "milk" bath and the joints lubricated to avoid surface corrosion and increase longevity.

Telescopes are preferably gas sterilized because steam sterilization causes differential thermal expansion and contraction of glass and metallic parts. With gas sterilization, most hospitals insist on an aeration period of 12 to 24 hours, even though the residual ethylene oxide content falls immediately below the 250-ppm maximum recommended level for devices contacting mucosa or skin (Fed. Reg. vol 43, No. 122, Fri. June 23, 1978, Part 5, pp. 27474–27483). As a last resort, telescopes can be cold sterilized in 2% glutaraldehyde solution for 20 minutes. Johnson and colleagues[26] noted an infection rate of 0.04% when this sterilization technique was selected. Repeated cold sterilization may cause deterioration of the seals around the ocular and objective lenses. Fiber and fluid light cables are only gas sterilized. Sterilizing caps are available for the video camera, which can be immersed in glutaraldehyde solution. Optical teaching attachments (articulating arms) cannot be sterilized and are therefore draped in sterile sleeves.

PHOTOGRAPHY

Arthroscopic procedures are routinely documented either on video or in still photography (Fig. 31–16). Documentation provides adequate material for clinical studies, medicolegal protection, and teaching aids. With increasing experience, arthroscopists usually find that they rely on still photographs only for the record. The reason is that with time, unedited videos accrue rapidly and are cumbersome when a synopsis of the case is required. The dynamic arthroscopic view is more suited to demonstration purposes.[25,27,28]

The essentials for still photography include a rod lens telescope, a 35-mm single reflex camera, a lens with focal length of 60 to 130 mm, Ektachrome 400 ASA (Eastman Kodak Com-

mination. The fluid light cables conduct light through a fluid medium. The stiffness of these cables may make them too unwieldy for some operators. However, color reproduction is better than that obtained with the fiber light cables. Compare Plates 31–1 and 31–12. Plate 31–1 was obtained with a fluid cable, and Plate 31–12 with a fiber cable.

STERILIZATION AND MAINTENANCE

The operator always carefully inspects the telescopes before and after use. With incident light, the ocular and objective lenses are checked for scratches or chips. A decrease in clarity of view may indicate damage to the rod

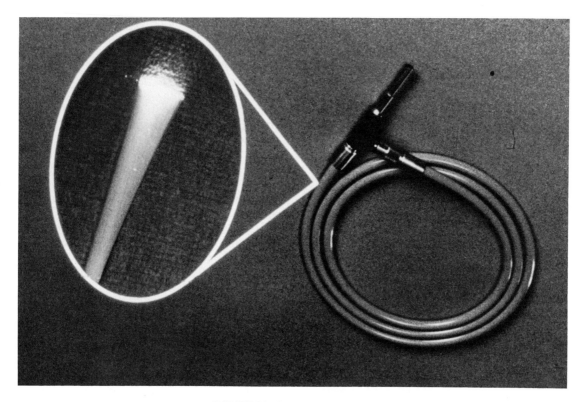

FIGURE 31–15. Fiber light cable.

pany, Rochester, New York) for slides and Kodacolor 400 ASA (Eastman Kodak Company) for prints, xenon or halogen light source, a tripod or stabilizing arm for the camera, and an optical teaching attachment to connect the telescope ocular to the camera (two-, three-, four-joint articulating arms) (Fig. 31–17). A databack system and motorized drive are optional accessories.

The essentials for video photography include

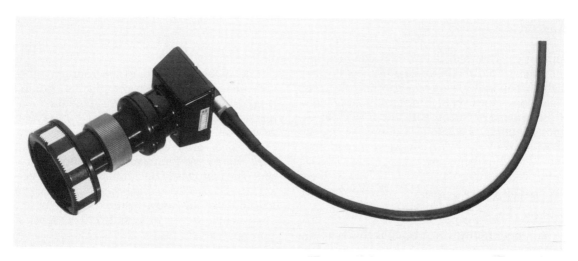

FIGURE 31–16. Lightweight video camera (approximately 50.2 gm or 1.77 oz) can fit into the palm of the operator. It is directly attached to the telescope. The operator can then manipulate the telescope and observe the monitor directly. This is the usual modus operandi.

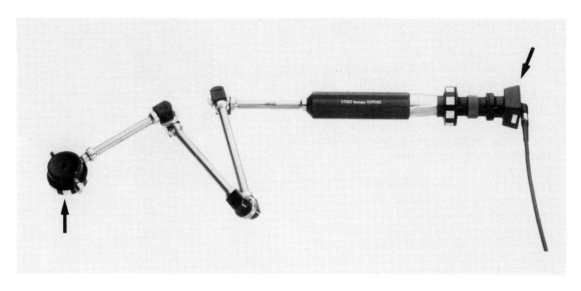

FIGURE 31–17. A four-joint optical teaching instrument may be attached directly to the telescope. (Site of attachment indicated by the arrow.) This permits the operator and assistant to view simultaneously the examination and to obtain photographs. The video camera (arrow) has been attached to the viewing end.

a lightweight video camera (beam splitter to also permit viewing through the telescope) (see Fig. 31–16), a video recorder (¾ inch for optimal resolution and reproducibility), and a high-resolution viewing monitor. An arthroscopist typically learns to work while viewing the television monitor and obtains still photographs of key diagnostic and surgical aspects.

ARTHROSCOPIC TECHNIQUE

Diagnostic arthroscopy may be performed using local anesthesia,[18,24] local anesthesia with sedation, or general anesthesia with single- or two-port systems. Surgical arthroscopy is performed using general anesthesia with the two-port system. Only the superior joint space typically is penetrated and examined. Techniques for inferior joint space arthroscopy have been described.[29] Generally, a reluctance to penetrate the inferior joint space has been noted, because the tight attachments of the medial and lateral ligaments make it difficult to insert the trocar without damaging the fibrous connective tissue and hyaline coverings of the condyle. According to Murakami and colleagues[31] the indications for performing arthroscopy are limitation of motion or locking not responsive to nonsurgical management, symptomatic arthritic conditions not responsive to nonsurgical management, and inability to obtain a diagnosis on imaging. Most clinicians believe that

diagnostic arthroscopy should be performed only when surgical arthroscopy or arthrotomy would be indicated because of lack of response to nonsurgical therapy.[18] Arthroscopy is contraindicated with local infection or neoplasm, because of the risk of dissemination.

Arthroscopy is always performed with the joint space distended employing a fluid or gas medium. The pressure created by either medium increases the joint space to permit the manipulation of instruments and provides hemostasis by sealing off injured vascular channels. Although normal saline can be used, lactated Ringer's solution is the preferred irrigant. The pH of normal saline is variable and acidic at pH 5.3. Reagen and associates[30] demonstrated that normal saline in volumes greater than 500 ml reduced proteoglycan synthesis by chondrocytes. Irrigation can be administered intermittently or continuously with flushes. When the continuous method is selected, a bag of irrigant is suspended above the patient and the flow of irrigant is by gravity. A three-way valve permits the intermittent delivery of lactated Ringer's flushes. Gas distention with carbon dioxide and nitrogen has been described.[32,33] The gas medium provides a greater field of view but carries the risk of embolism. Joint cavity distention has also been accomplished with iced heparinized lactated Ringer's solution (2000 IU heparin per liter of solution)[58] or hyaline fluid (an elastoviscous solution of cross-linked sodium hyaluronate).[36] The concept of administering viscoelastic substances to protect tissues (viscosurgery) has been applied for many years by ophthalmologists[34] and lately by arthroscopists.[35,36] McCain and colleagues[36] concluded from a randomized, controlled study that hyaline fluid (Synvisc, Biomatrix, Inc., Ridgefield, New Jersey) was as safe as standard irrigating fluid. Visibility was improved, the need for pressure irrigation was reduced, and the incidence of scuffing of the fibrous connective tissue covering the fossa/eminence was less.

Arthroscopy is begun with the patient positioned supine on the operating table. In most cases, the operator is able to approach both joints from the same side of the table. The anesthesiologist can tilt the operating table to approximate the joint of interest to the horizontal plane. When a patient has limited cervical range of motion or is obese, the operator may choose to change sides to perform the contralateral arthroscopy. The field is prepared in the usual sterile manner. Special attention is paid to the preparation of the pinna.

The instruments and photography equipment are positioned around the operating table in the interest of comfort and efficiency. In unilateral arthroscopies, a cart containing a television monitor, a light source, and a video recorder is positioned directly opposite the operator (Figs. 31–14 and 31–18). In bilateral cases, the cart may be positioned at the foot of the table (Fig. 31–19). In this instance, the fiber optic, TTL photographic connection, and

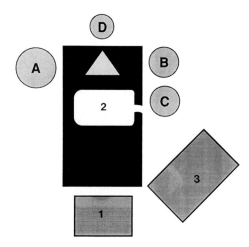

FIGURE 31–19. Alternate positioning around the operating room table. Operator (A), surgical assistant (B), nurse assistant (C), anesthesiologist and photographer (D), patient (triangle), cart containing video and light source equipment (1), Mayo stand (2), and accessory instrument table (3).

video cables must be of sufficient length to reach the patient. A Mayo's stand with arthroscopic instruments (telescopes, trocars, surgical instruments, irrigating syringe, connecting tube) is positioned over the patient. A tripod or still camera holding device is positioned at or over the head of the table. The camera is operated by an unscrubbed assistant who remains at the head of the table.

DIAGNOSTIC ARTHROSCOPY
Single-Port System

Single-port arthroscopy does not provide an avenue for outflow of the irrigation (closed system). As a result, there is greater resistance to joint distention. When debris from a traumatic entry or pathology clouds the field of view, the operator can remove the telescope and insert a Frazier's-tip suction or insert a second port to flush the debris out of the space.

The two-port system for diagnostic arthroscopy can crowd the field and may cause additional iatrogenic damage before a diagnosis is obtained. Placement of the anterior second port increases the risk of facial nerve damage, because the facial zygomatic nerve is located only 8 to 32 mm anterior to the anterior margin of the bony external auditory canal.[37]

A small towel clamp is placed at the angle of the mandible to assist in distraction of the condyle. The location of the condyle is noted by

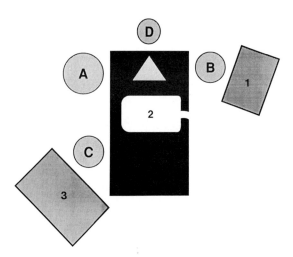

FIGURE 31–18. Positioning around the operating room table. Operator (A), surgical assistant (B), nurse assistant (C), anesthesiologist and photographer (D), patient (triangle), cart containing video and light source equipment (1), Mayo stand (2), and accessory instrument table (3).

moving it back and forth. Next, the following landmarks are traced: the lateral pole of the condyle, the lateral aspect of the glenoid fossa, and the anterior tubercle (Fig. 31–20). A vertical incision about 2 to 3 mm in length is traced at the height of the greatest concavity of the glenoid fossa. When the condyle is manipulated anteriorly, the index finger should fall into a depression immediately posterior to it. Holmlund and Hellsing[23] noted that the punc-ture site was located less than or equal to 3 mm below a tragal-canthal line in 93% of cases. Puncture sites are best selected utilizing palpable landmarks, however.

Once the incision is made, the subcutaneous tissues are undermined. Next, the lateral ligament/condyle is approached through blunt dissection. When these tissues are appreciated at the tip of the hemostat, the mandible is manipulated to assess the proximity of the instrument to the joint space. With anterior traction of the mandible, the hemostat falls posterior to the condyle. This technique of blunt dissection of the lateral ligament/capsule ensures safety and protection of the external auditory canal. Next, a 19-gauge needle attached to a 10-ml syringe of lactated Ringer's solution is directed through the incision toward the lateral tip of the glenoid fossa. An inferosuperior and anterior direction is selected to avoid the external auditory canal, which inclines medially at approximately 45° to the skin surface. When the lateral lip of the glenoid fossa is contacted, the needle is walked around the lateral lip to enter the superior joint

space and contact the roof of the glenoid fossa. The superior joint space is distended with 1 to 2 ml of solution.

The sharp trocar and 2.7-mm external sheath are next assembled. The unit is grasped within the palm of the hand and with the index finger guiding the distal end. The trocar/sheath unit contacts the lateral lip of the glenoid fossa and then is walked around the lip, to contact the roof of the glenoid fossa (Figs. 31–21 and 31–22). Three factors facilitate penetration of the superior joint space: gravity, due to skeletal muscle relaxation and horizontal positioning of the head; distention of the joint space by the lactated Ringer's solution; and active anterior-inferior distraction of the mandible by the assistant. All three factors are needed when there is a bulbous condyle or when the joint space is protected by a prominent lateral lip on the glenoid fossa. Fortunately, the incidence of bulbous condyles in randomly selected dried skull specimens has been reported to be only 3%.[38]

The trocar is unlocked from the external sheath. The sheath is grasped between the index finger and thumb at the skin surface, and the sharp trocar is removed. The 2.4-mm telescope is inserted through the sheath and locked into position. Alternatively, some researchers do not make an incision and puncture the skin directly with the sharp trocar. The blunt trocar then completes the entry into the space.[39]

The fiber or fluid cable is attached to the inlet post on the telescope, and the connecting

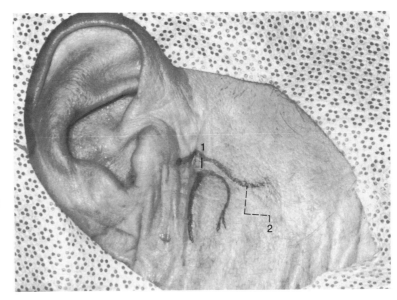

FIGURE 31–20. Landmarks drawn for incisions for single and two port systems. Condyle, lateral rim of the glenoid fossa, and anterior tubercle are drawn. The incision for the posterior port lies at the area of maximum concavity of the glenoid fossa, immediately posterior to the condylar head, when the mandible is translated forward. The incision for the second port lies approximately 1 cm anterior and 1.5 cm inferior to the anterior tubercle. In establishing the second port, the operator envisions an angle of approximately 150 to 160 degrees, which would form between instruments in the posterior and anterior ports.

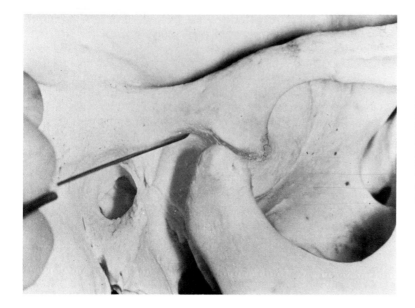

FIGURE 31–21. A needle is used to demonstrate the proper trajectory of the trocar and sheath for establishment of the posterior port. The trocar contacts the lateral lip of the glenoid fossa and is "walked around" this structure to contact the roof of the glenoid fossa.

tube of the irrigant is attached to the inlet post on the external sheath (Fig. 31–23).

Once a joint space has been identified, the operator sweeps the telescope backward and forward in the glenoid region to appreciate the anatomy. The flexure is the principal orientation landmark (see Plate 31–1). To locate the flexure, the operator directs the telescope toward the ear. Six parameters are employed to judge arthroscopic pathology: color, surface morphology, texture, orientation of structures,

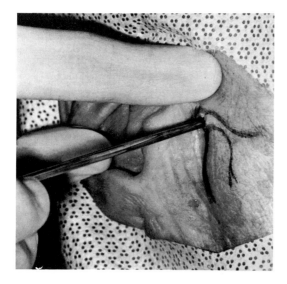

FIGURE 31–22. The trocar has been inserted into the superior joint space. Note the anterior inclination of the trocar to avoid entry into the external auditory canal.

joint space configuration, and topographic relationships. For example, the color of the disc is stark white (see Plates 31–1, 31–2, and 31–6), whereas some areas of remodeled retrodiscal tissue may be ivory to yellow-white (see Plates 31–7 and 31–8). Normal retrodiscal tissue is pink, and the medial and lateral ligaments are grey. Superficial vascularity is present on remodeled retrodiscal tissue and absent over most of the disc. The disc has a smooth, compact, regular surface (see Plates 31–1, 31–2, and 31–6), compared with the fibrillar surface of some areas of remodeled retrodiscal tissue (see Plates 31–7 and 31–8). The tympanic portion of the retrodiscal tissue is vertically oriented (see Plate 31–1). This vertical orientation is most prominent in the lateral and central fields. The joint space configuration is determined by the soft tissues. Thus, the normal posterior band causes the space to be oriented posteroinferiorly to anterosuperiorly up to its crest and posterosuperiorly to anteroinferiorly to the intermediate zone (Fig. 31–24). The abrupt termination of the medial capsular ligament at the posterior half to two thirds of the joint serves as a convenient landmark for topographic relationships (Plates 31–13 and 31–14).[18,19] Normal and pathologic arthroscopic anatomy is described later.

The examination is performed in three phases: transverse, longitudinal, and dynamic transverse (Figs. 31–25 and 31–26).[18,19] The transverse phase examines the surface anatomy of the superior joint space directly beneath the

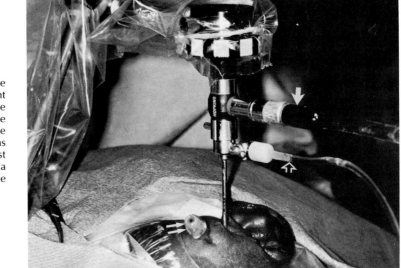

FIGURE 31–23. The telescope is positioned in the superior joint space. The fiberoptic cable (white arrow) has been connected to the inlet post on the telescope. The irrigation tube (open arrow) has been connected to the inlet post on the external sheath. Note a second anterior port (double arrow) has been established.

glenoid fossa, that is, the glenoid regions (see Fig. 31–20). It is called the transverse phase because the telescope is directed along the transverse axis of the space. The transverse phase is the least difficult to approach. The arthroscopist assembles a composite picture of the anatomy by obtaining multiple fields of view by sweeping the telescope under the glenoid regions. The operator may need to look into another field of view or overlap fields to confirm certain impressions. The medial fields are first examined posteroanteriorly, followed by the central and then the lateral fields. This method prevents premature withdrawal of the telescope from the joint space. Rotation of the

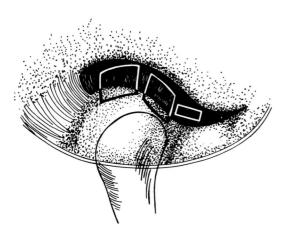

FIGURE 31–24. In the normal condyle-disc-fossa relationship, joint space configuration is determined by the firm, relatively unyielding disc.

30° forward oblique telescope greatly improves the field of view (see Fig. 31–8). In this examination phase, the operator can determine the vascularity pattern on the normal and remodeled retrodiscal tissues, identify the medial capsular ligament and its abrupt termination, and begin to suspect disc displacement.[18,19]

The longitudinal phase examines the pre-eminence region by placing the telescope along the longitudinal axis of the joint space (Fig. 31–26). This is the most difficult phase to perform because the tight lateral ligament attachment resists the insertion of an instrument from the glenoid regions. During this portion of the examination, the operator can identify the stark white displaced disc, the junction of remodeled retrodiscal tissue and disc, the anterior capsule, and the fibrous connective tissue lining of the eminence. In the disc displacement, the remodeled disc, adhesions, termination of the remodeled retrodiscal tissue, and synovial irregularities may be noted. The assistant can manipulate the mandible posteriorly to help in the passage of the telescope. In some cases, the pre-eminence region can be examined only through a second anterior part.[18,19]

The final examination phase is the dynamic transverse phase. It is performed while holding the telescope along the transverse axis of the superior joint space and manipulating the joint backward and forward. In this manner, the operator may acquire a sense of what region of the tissue is loaded during function.[18,19]

When the arthroscopic examination is completed, the arthroscopic log is recorded as a part

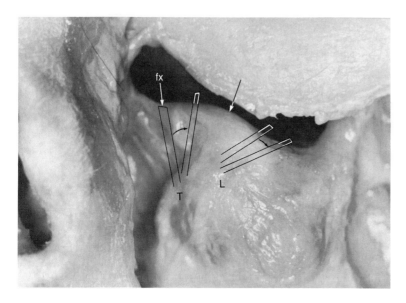

FIGURE 31–25. Fresh cadaver specimen. Right TMJ. The transverse (T) and longitudinal (L) examination phases are demonstrated in a normal condyle-disc-fossa relationship. The lateral capsule/ligament has been partially removed, exposing the superior joint space. Note the flexure (fx) and the posterior band (arrow).

of the medical record (Fig. 31–27). A grid system records the findings of the transverse examination phase (Fig. 31–28). A grid is formed on the roof of the glenoid fossa by the intersection of three transverse regions (anterior, middle, posterior) and three parasagittal regions (lateral, central, medial). The glenoid fossa is thus divided into nine regions. A field of view corresponds to each of the nine regions. A field is named utilizing the transverse-parasagittal coordinate, for example, posterior medial field (Plate 31–15). In small joints, there may be only seven to eight fields of view in the glenoid

region. The arthroscopic findings observed in the longitudinal examination phase are logged according to lateral, central, and medial fields (Fig. 31–29).[18,19]

Diagnostic arthroscopy can be completed in 10 to 15 minutes with 30 to 50 ml of irrigant, depending on an operator's ability to examine all aspects of the joint space. Volumes exceeding 250 ml have been used with single-port arthroscopy with no permanent side effects. Experience with computed tomography and double-contrast arthrography has shown that non-recovered fluid passes along the neck of

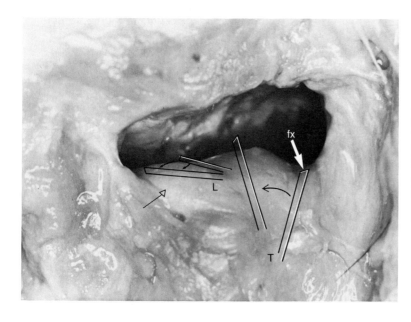

FIGURE 31–26. Fresh cadaver specimen. Left TMJ. The transverse (T) and longitudinal (L) examination phases are demonstrated in a disc displacement. The lateral capsule/ligament is partially removed, exposing the superior joint space. Note the flexure (fx) and the posterior band (open arrow).

the condyle and into the pterygomandibular space.[40] This phenomenon may explain some of the cases of temporary inferior alveolar and lingual paresthesias that do occur following arthroscopy. At the conclusion of the procedure, the joint space is suctioned by way of the external sheath. Some operators choose to deposit a steroid preparation into the space or directly into the retrodiscal tissue. A suture or Steri-Strip (3M Surgical Product Division, St. Paul, Minnesota) is placed over the surgical site. Blood clots are removed from the external auditory meatus with normal saline irrigant, utilizing an angiocatheter and a 10-ml syringe. A codeine-acetaminophen compound is prescribed. Antibiotics have not been routinely provided.

Diagnostic arthroscopy through a transmeatal approach has also been described.[39,40] This technique begins with the traditional lateral puncture. Next, the telescope is directed from within the superior joint space toward the tragus to transilluminate the external auditory meatus. Guided by the light source, the sharp trocar/unit punctures the meatus to enter the superior joint space. The telescope is removed from the lateral port and inserted into the sheath of the meatal port. The operator has the option of examining the topographic anatomy of the superior joint space along the sagittal or coronal planes, by switching the telescope between external sheaths.

Two-Port System

The second port assists in diagnostic arthroscopy when debris obstructs the field of view or when probing of structures is important. The port is placed anterior and inferior to the anterior tubercle. The landmarks are approximately 1 cm anterior to the tubercle and 1.5 cm inferior to the tubercle (see Fig. 31–20). In deciding the location of the second port, the operator attempts to create a 150° to 160° angle, which would form between anterior and posterior sheaths. This method facilitates triangulation (see Fig. 31–23). When the operator selects a location too close to the anterior tubercle, there is the danger of scuffing the fibrous connective tissue lining of the tubercle. An incision of 1 to 2 mm is made with a #11 blade. A sharp trocar and sheath of adequate diameter and length to permit the passage of instruments are directed posterosuperiorly toward the anterior tubercle (Fig. 31–30). Once this structure is contacted laterally, the unit is backed off and directed medioposterosuperiorly to penetrate the pre-eminence region or anterior recess of the superior joint space. When an open system has been determined, irrigation through a posterior inflow port should exit from the anterior port. The establishment of this port may be done under direct vision.

Triangulation is the technique by which the telescope and instrument are manipulated

Date _____

Patient Name _____

Hospital Number _____

Address _____

Telephone _____ business

_____ home

	KEY
mf/lf	medial/lateral folds
v	vessels
rdt	remodeled retrodiscal tissue
rdt	retrodiscal tissue
d	disc
p	perforations
A_w	adhesions: weblike
A_l	linear bands
sp	synovial plica
fb	foreign body
t	tears of fibrous connective tissue
f	fibrillation
——	other findings

FIGURE 31–27. The arthroscopic log.

I. *TRANSVERSE EXAMINATION PHASE*

Flexure identified   yes/no

ORIENT ARTHROSCOPIC MAP BELOW AND INDICATE FINDINGS USING KEY

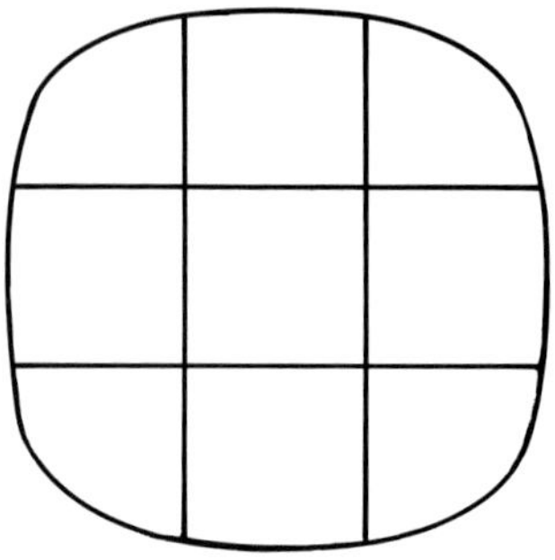

Comments: _____
_____
_____
_____

II. *LONGITUDINAL EXAMINATION PHASE*

Junction of remodeled retrodiscal tissue and disc identified   yes/no

ORIENT ARTHROSCOPIC MAP BELOW AND INDICATE FINDINGS USING KEY

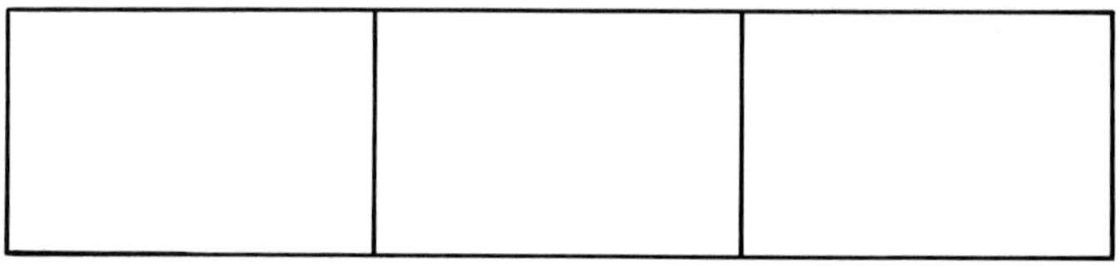

Comments: _____
_____
_____

III. *DYNAMIC TRANSVERSE PHASE*

Condyle pressing on remodeled retrodiscal tissue?   yes/no

Comments: _____
_____
_____

ARTHROSCOPIC DIAGNOSIS _____
_____

FIGURE 31–27 *Continued*

from outside the joint space so that the instrument may be visualized within the joint space.[41] Some workers use the terms *triangulation* and *biangulation* to describe the number of instruments being manipulated into the field of view.[41] This technique is important when an exploratory probe is applied in diagnostic arthroscopy or when performing surgical arthroscopy.

Inferior Joint Space Arthroscopy

The primary focus of arthroscopy has been directed toward examination and surgery of

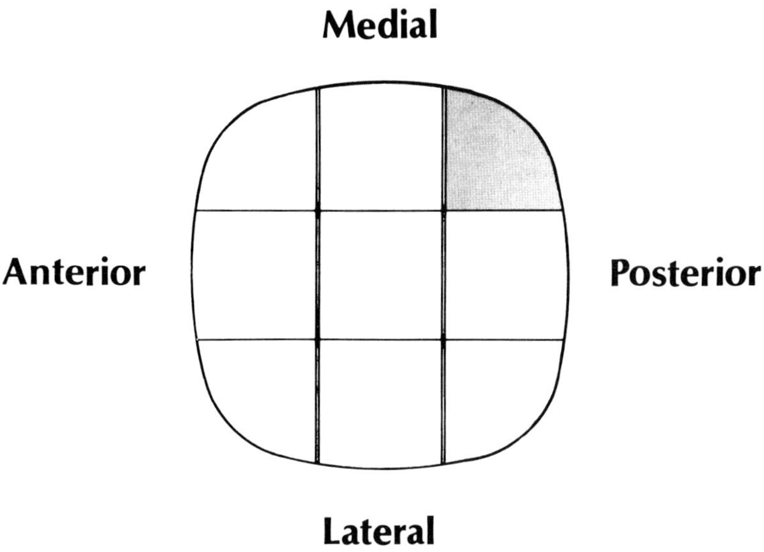

Medial

Anterior

Posterior

Lateral

FIGURE 31–28. A grid system is used to record the findings of the transverse examination phase. The grid is formed by the intersection of three transverse and three parasagittal regions. The result is nine fields of view. The posterior medial field is shaded.

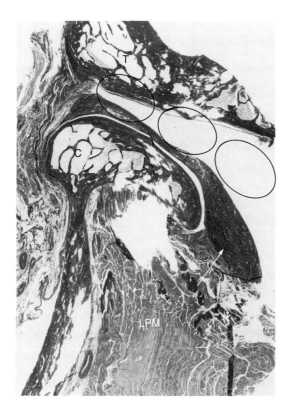

FIGURE 31–29. Coronal microscopic section of the temporomandibular joint demonstrating the fields of view observed in the longitudinal examination phase. Note the anteromedially displaced disc (arrow), lateral pterygoid muscle (LPM), condyle (C), and temporal bone (T).

the superior joint space. However, some investigators have reported that most of the pathosis occurs within the inferior joint space.[42–44] This finding has obvious implications concerning the arthroscopic treatment of internal derangements. Experience with inferior joint space arthroscopy remains in its infancy.[29] A brief description of the inferolateral technique follows.

Capsule-penetrating instruments are identical to those used for superior joint space arthroscopy. The joint space is dilated with lactated Ringer's solution to facilitate penetration of the space by the trocar. The sharp trocar and sheath are directed toward the lateral pole of the condyle, where contact is made. The clinician contacts the lateral pole of the condyle from an inferolateral approach rather than directly lateral (Fig. 31–31). (In this way, the operator can manipulate the telescope without hindrance from the extra-articular soft tissues.) The trocar/sheath unit is pulled back somewhat, and the trocar is directed superoposteriorly as the condyle is distracted anteriorly.

Penetration of instruments into the inferior space is difficult because the attachments of the ligaments limits superior distraction of the disc. Murakami and Ono[29] had difficulty in examining the anterior recess and lateral sulcus. They suggested that an anterolateral approach might facilitate examination of the anterior recess but questioned its diagnostic value. In some instances, a large perforation in the re-

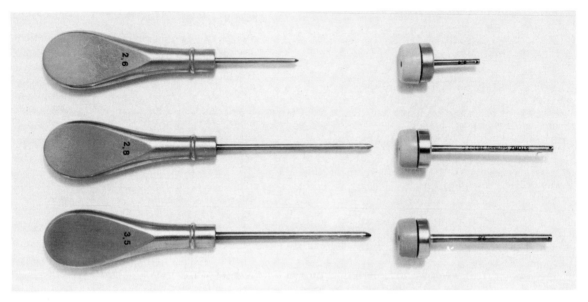

FIGURE 31–30. Selected trocars and sheaths used for the establishment of the second port.

modeled retrodiscal tissue permits the passage of instruments into the inferior joint space by way of the superior joint space.

NORMAL ARTHROSCOPIC ANATOMY

Arthroscopic criteria for normal condyle-disc-fossa relationships have been established primarily through the examination of fresh and fresh-frozen cadaver specimens.[18] In rare instances, because of misdiagnosis, a normal joint has been arthroscoped, and the information obtained has been extremely helpful. Arthroscopic findings are described according to the examination phase in which they are found. Each field is meticulously checked for color, surface morphology, texture, joint space

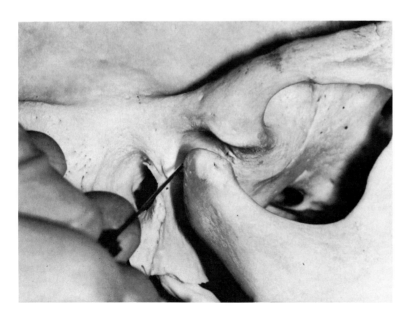

FIGURE 31–31. A needle is used to demonstrate the proper trajectory of the trocar and sheath for entry into the inferior joint space.

configuration, and topographic relationships and orientation of structures. At this time, the limitations of inferior joint space arthroscopy prohibit a detailed discussion of normal and pathologic anatomy. The findings are discussed separately later (see Inferior Joint Space Anatomy).

Transverse Examination Phase Findings

Posterior Fields

In the posterior fields, the tympanic portion of the retrodiscal tissue, posterior attachment, posterior incline of the posterior band, synovium of the glenoid fossa, posterior aspect of the medial sulcus, synovial plicae, and medial capsule are visible. When the mandible drifts forward during examination, the posterior incline of the posterior band may not be visible (see Plate 31–1).

The tympanic portion of the retrodiscal tissue is oriented vertically, is pink, and has a few superficial vessels (see Plate 31–1). The vertical orientation of this structure is more obvious in the lateral fields. The synovium overlying the posterior attachment characteristically contains a few superficial transverse vessels. The underlying posterior attachment appears pink. The demarcation between the synovium of the posterior attachment and the posterior incline of the posterior band is abrupt (Plate 31–16). Sagittal histologic specimens corroborate this finding. The posterior band is avascular and stark white, differentiating it from the more vascular posterior attachment. The ivory or yellow-white color of the fibrous connective tissue lining the glenoid fossa contrasts with the color of the disc and retrodiscal tissue. Vascularity is present in the medial and lateral sulci and not on the roof of the glenoid fossa. The vessels course superiorly from the medial sulcus, arborizing and terminating not far from the sulcus. Medial and lateral folds within the tympanic portion of the retrodiscal tissue have been observed in cadaver specimens. The existence of folds in live, normal patients has yet to be determined.

The grey fibers of the medial capsular ligament are visible (see Plate 31–14). This structure should not be mistaken for an adhesion. The orientation of these fibers depends on the degree of mandibular translation. A synovial plica may be seen in the posterior medial field.

Middle Fields

The posterior incline of the band, the crest of the posterior band, the medial capsular ligament, and the fibrous connective tissue lining of the glenoid fossa are visible here.

The posterior band, as the remainder of the disc, is stark white. Vascularity is only noted at the medial sulcus. The yellow-white color of the fibrous connective tissue lining the glenoid fossa can be differentiated from the color of the disc. When there are surface irregularities or fibrillations on the disc, the operator is alerted to the possibility that this tissue represents remodeled retrodiscal tissue. The mobility of the disc can be tested by gently moving the telescope over its surface. The firm consistency of the disc can be compared with the soft, pliable consistency of the tympanic portion of the retrodiscal tissue. The joint space above the posterior incline of the posterior band is trapezoidal and oriented as demonstrated in Figure 31–24. The medial capsular ligament is more clearly visible than in the posterior fields.

Anterior Fields

The anterior incline of the posterior band, the medial capsule, the termination of the medial capsular ligament, the synovium of the glenoid fossa, and the intermediate zone are visible (see Plate 31–2).

As the glenoid fossa tapers medially, the medial fields may overlap somewhat. The anterior incline of the posterior band slopes inferiorly, matching that of the posterior slope of the eminence. The joint space configuration is trapezoidal and oriented as shown in Figure 31–24. The medial capsular ligament terminates abruptly. Anterior to this structure lies the medial capsule, noted by its fibrillar makeup (see Plate 31–13). The irrigation may cause a ballooning out of the medial capsule and thus create the impression of a separation between the ligament and capsule. The edge of the ligament is somewhat thickened. The termination of the ligament is topographically related laterally to the posterior band. The anterior incline of the posterior band blends upward into the intermediate zone. As the telescope is withdrawn laterally, the operator can acquire a sense of how the disc conforms to the convexity of the eminence. The anterior band cannot be visualized in the superior joint space, because it represents a convexity on the inferior surface of the disc.

Longitudinal Examination Phase Findings

Lateral Field

The disc, the fibrous connective tissue lining the eminence and infratemporal articulating surface, the lateral sulcus, the lateral capsule/ligament, and the anterolateral aspect of the capsule are visible. The firmness of the disc prevents its displacement by the shaft of the telescope. As a result, the curvature of the disc appears to parallel the convexity of the eminence. The blending of the lateral capsule/ligament onto the superior surface of the disc is obvious (Plate 31–17).

Central Field

The relationship of the disc to the apex of the eminence is appreciated.

Medial Field

The disc and the anterior and medial capsule are visualized. The delicate interlacing fibers of the medial capsule contrast with the dense fibers of the medial capsular ligament seen in the glenoid regions. Once the telescope passes into the pre-eminence region, the relationship of the disc to the temporal bone is no longer appreciated. The cul-de-sac of the anterior recess can be noted.

Dynamic Transverse Phase Findings

When the assistant gently distracts the mandible backward and forward, the condyle appears to press on stark white tissue (disc). The tympanic portion of the retrodiscal tissue appears to alternately stretch and collapse like an accordion. Video photography is necessary to record these findings.

Inferior Joint Space Anatomy

Visibility is limited with this technique. The avascular concave surface of the disc matches the convexity of the smooth fibrous connective tissue–covered condyle. Synovial vessels are observed in the posterior and anterior regions. These vessels correspond to the posterior and anterior attachments. Lateral fields are particularly difficult to observe.

PATHOLOGIC ARTHROSCOPIC ANATOMY

Pathology observed arthroscopically has been correlated with findings on corrected lateral cephalometric arthrotomograms, uncorrected magnetic resonance images, cadaveric dissections, and surgical experience.[19,23,35] In cadaveric studies, Liedberg and Westesson[45] noted the tendency toward underdiagnosis (high specificity, low sensitivity). Perforations and disc position were difficult to assess. Similar findings regarding the sensitivity for detecting remodeling changes were reported by Holmlund and Hellsing.[24] Moreover, Goss and colleagues[46] found a high specificity when arthroscopic and gross surgical findings were compared in live patients.

A clear understanding of pathologic gross anatomy is imperative for an understanding of pathologic arthroscopic anatomy. Specific arthroscopic changes in the internally deranged joint are described here.

The findings are recorded according to the phase of the examination in which they are discovered: transverse, longitudinal, and dynamic transverse. The operator must always remember that the telescope magnifies the anatomy. At a distance of 1 mm, an object is magnified approximately ten times. At a 1 cm distance, no magnification occurs. Thus, clinicians should exercise caution when relating the significance of a single pathologic finding to a patient's symptoms.

Specific pathologic changes are described further.

Tympanic Portion of Retrodiscal Tissue

In the transverse phase of the examination, the diagnosis of disc displacement is supported by the presence of a dull white or ivory-colored tympanic portion of the retrodiscal tissue. The flexure in the pathologic condition is represented by the junction of the tympanic portion of the retrodiscal tissue and the remodeled retrodiscal tissue draped over the condyle. The retrodiscal tissue no longer appears pink. The color disparity may be seen by comparing the tympanic portion of the retrodiscal tissue in the slight disc displacement (see Plate 31–1) with that in the chronic displacement (see Plates 31–3 and 31–15). The flexure is more easily distorted by the telescope and the fluid distention because the remodeled retrodiscal tissue is more pliable and softer than the disc.

Joint Space Configuration

The joint space configuration changes as the disc is displaced forward. In the normal condyle-disc-fossa relationship, the posterior band of the disc forces the operator to move the telescope up and over this structure to examine the glenoid regions (see Plate 31–2). In the displaced disc condition, the remodeled retrodiscal tissue does not provide the same obstruction to examination (Plate 31–18).

Some workers choose to describe the percentage of disc coverage of the condyle as *roofing*.[20] Vascularity changes in the remodeled retrodiscal tissue are then related to the glenoid fossa to describe the degree of roofing (see Vascularity Changes, next).

Vascularity Changes

Remodeled retrodiscal tissue exhibits various degrees of superficial vascularity in the glenoid regions. Several distinct zones of vascularity may be noted from field to field. A composite picture of the vascularity can be assembled by logging the vascularity.[47]

In the normal condyle-disc-fossa relationship, synovium normally covers these tissues and extends over the posterior incline of the posterior band, the posterior aspect of the glenoid fossa, and the medial and lateral sulci (see Fig. 31–1). The disc and much of the surface of the glenoid fossa and eminence are devoid of superficial vascularity.

Currently, some disc displacements are hypothesized to progress from a point of reduction to one of absence of reduction and eventual perforation of the remodeled retrodiscal tissue. The increased loading of this structure presumably results in the progressive diminution of its vascularity. The end product of loading is a dense fibrous structure that may be confused for disc on gross and even microscopic examination. Meticulous inspection of the tissue under arthroscopy may reveal its fibrous, fibrillar makeup and its yellow-white (ivory, off-white) appearance, differentiating it from the stark white disc. As remodeling proceeds, the lateral arthroscopic fields tend to show less vascularity than the medial. This finding concurs with the work by Hansson and Oberg,[48] who found greater arthrotic changes in the lateral third of the condyles that they examined.

In the normal condyle-disc-fossa relationship, the synovium overlying the posterior attachment terminates on the posterior incline of the posterior band.[18] In the pathologic disc relationship, this demarcation as well as the demarcation between remodeled retrodiscal tissue and disc is also usually clear. The vessels maintain their transverse orientation under the glenoid regions. The presence of superficial transverse vascularity in and beyond the middle glenoid regions indicates an internally deranged joint.[18,19]

A classification of vascularity has been proposed based on a study of extensive material from arthroscopic video and magnetic resonance sources.[47,49] In this classification, vascularity is classified according to arthroscopic field of view. The same systematic approach to the recording of general arthroscopic findings is used in the recording of the vascularity of the remodeled retrodiscal tissue. The superficial vascularity observed in each arthroscopic field is assigned a classification number, according to the classification described hereafter. The number is then inserted into the grid. The classification system proposed is a grading system of decreasing vascularity:

I. Large number of transverse vessels with some anastomosing vessels. There is minimal to no superficial avascular remodeled retrodiscal tissue present (see Plates 31–1 and 31–14).

II. Intermediate number of transverse vessels present. Few anastomosing vessels are noted. Zones of vascularity juxtapose areas of superficial vascularity (see Plates 31–3 and 31–11).

III. Only occasional vessels noted. Avascular regions predominate. The orientation of the vessels is not clear (see Plates 31–4, 31–8, and 31–18).

IV. Absence of superficial vessels. The tissue appears fibrillated and yellow white (see Plates 31–7, 31–10, and 31–15).

The locations of the disc and perforations of the remodeled retrodiscal tissue are labeled on the arthroscopic map using the qualifying letters *d* and *p*, respectively. The qualifiers do not preclude labeling of the vascularity of the remodeled retrodiscal tissue when it appears within the arthroscopic field. Those fields of view not recorded are indicated by a bar. The vascular assessment of the tympanic portion of the retrodiscal tissue is recorded as a separate line item.[47,49]

Assignment of a global vascularity value to the remodeled retrodiscal tissue is essentially meaningless, because the tissue shows areas of varying vascularity. However, assignment of a global vascularity value to the tympanic portion of the retrodiscal tissue appears to be appropriate. The distention medium is standardized as lactated Ringer's solution. The intracapsular injection of epinephrine-containing solutions is avoided in an effort not to interfere with the assessment of vascularity. Observations are recorded as soon as the clinician confirms accurate positioning of the telescope, to minimize the influence of iatrogenic trauma on the grading of vascularity.[47,49]

Certain difficulties are encountered in the clinical application of the classification previously described. Some overlap in the arthroscopic fields is almost unavoidable. Opening causes the retrodiscal tissue to engorge with blood. The amount of condylar translation may influence the amount of blood channeled to the superficial vessels and therefore may indirectly influence the grading of the vascularity. Opening of the condyle by active distraction causes emptying of the superficial vessels. This may have occurred because of rerouting of blood to deeper vessels or may be inherent in an arthroscopic examination. Clinicians should recognize the importance of evaluating the vascularity as soon as they become oriented to the anatomy. With increasing duration of the examination, the fibrous connective tissue lining the glenoid fossa and eminence is iatrogenically damaged. As a result, the prominence of the superficial vascularity of the remodeled retrodiscal tissue is increased, as well as the color of the tissue. An increase in the number of surface vessels has not been apparent.[47,49]

Vascularity changes within the joint represent a continuum, from the tympanic portion of the retrodiscal tissue to the anterior extent of the remodeled retrodiscal tissue. Vascular areas sometimes appear anterior to avascular areas. This may occur as a result of differential rates of disc slippage, which prohibit progressive equal degrees of remodeling in the tissues; abnormal joint mechanics, causing shunting of blood to collapsed, nonobliterated vessels; and restriction in condylar translation. The source of vascularity is subject to discussion; although it may be innate to the retrodiscal tissue, it may represent ingrowth of synovium from the periphery.[47,49] McCain and colleagues[20] appeared to attribute the vascularity to synovium ingrowth and classified vascularity as (1) mild hypervascularity with large capillaries and pink basement tissue; (2) moderate hypervascularity, with a deeper pink basement tissue and spreading of synovial tissue onto articulating surfaces; and (3) severe hypervascularity with blood-red tissue and loss of distinct individual capillaries and spread of synovium onto articulating tissues.*

Although the vascularity changes within the remodeled retrodiscal tissue may be hypothesized to be secondary and mechanical in origin, nonloading changes may be responsible for the predominant changes in the tympanic portion of the retrodiscal tissue. The variability of the vascularity in the normal tympanic portion of the retrodiscal tissue has not been established. Heffez and Jordan[49] demonstrated that reducing disc displacements demonstrated more vascularity than nonreducing disc displacements.

A classification of vascularity is a step toward diversification of the current classification system of internal derangements. One can begin to monitor treatment results and develop criteria for specific arthroscopic procedures according to the degree of superficial vascularity. This approach is predicated on acceptance of the hypothesis that decreased tissue vascularity is associated with extreme disc remodeling and that disc displacements follow a common evolution. Further studies may shed light on the correlation of degree of superficial vascularity to deeper vascularity and to disc morphology. In addition, the importance of vascularity changes in groups of fields (e.g., all lateral fields) may reveal itself as being more significant than the individual fields.

Fibrillations

Changes in the surface of the remodeled retrodiscal tissue may be due to fibrillations (see Plate 31–8). These changes have also been observed in the fibrous connective tissue lining of the glenoid fossa and eminence. When fibrillation changes are advanced, underlying bone may become exposed.

Sanders[21] described and Indresano[50] confirmed the presence of an abrasion on the anterior slope of the articular eminence ("kissing

---

*The term *synovitis* has been used to describe inflammatory changes associated with the superficial vessels. The clinical distinction between synovial hyperplasia and inflammation is not always clear.

lesion"). McCain and colleagues[20] described a redundancy of synovium, that is, a bogginess or bloating. Some of these findings may be iatrogenic in origin.

Medial Capsular Ligament Relationships

The medial capsular ligament is a convenient landmark for the extension of remodeled retrodiscal tissue (Plates 31–13 and 31–14). The fibers of the ligaments are grey and typically oriented posteroinferior to anterosuperior when the condyle is depressed and only slightly translated. The medial capsular ligament should not be confused with an adhesion.

Perforations

Perforations may rarely occur in the disc proper. They are most typically found in the lateral and central regions of the remodeled retrodiscal tissue (Plates 31–12 and 31–19).[19,45] In the closed-mouth position, remodeled retrodiscal tissue and hence the perforations do not extend into the pre-eminence region, even in the most severe disc displacements.[51] Perforations have not been found in remodeled retrodiscal tissue with superficial vascularity grades I and II. In my experience, perforations diagnosed on fluoroscopy during arthrography have not always been identified arthroscopically.[19] This finding may be explained in part by the tendency for the operator to avoid examination of the lateral fields in an effort not to exit from the space prematurely. During the dynamic transverse phase of the examination, the head of the condyle can be seen protruding through the larger perforations.

Medial and Lateral Folds (Pleats)

These folds appear prominent in an internally deranged joint (see Plate 31–9). Because of the low numbers of live, normal human joints examined, one should be cautious in ascribing any major significance to their appearance.

Lack of Congruity of Structures

In the pre-eminence region, there is a lack of congruity or parallelism between the remodeled retrodiscal tissue below and the eminence above (see Plate 31–10). The reason for this finding is that the telescope displaces the soft retrodiscal tissue. The dense fibrous connective tissue disc prevents this displacement of tissues, hence, the parallelism noted between eminence and disc in the normal condyle-disc-fossa relationship (see Plate 31–17).

Adhesions

Adhesions have been noted in varying frequency by several researchers. Sanders and Buoncristiani[22] reported the frequent finding of adhesions. Heffez and Blaustein[18] and McCain and colleagues[20] have infrequently observed adhesions.

Small web-like bands have been observed in the medial sulci and in the pre-eminence region (see Plate 31–5). These adhesions span a small distance and sometimes appear translucent. Thick linear bands have been observed extending between the posterior slope of the eminence to the disc or remodeled retrodiscal tissue (see Plate 31–6). Adhesions have been noted in the normal condyle-disc-fossa relationship. In Indresano's series,[50] adhesions were not the principal pathologic finding of reducing disc displacements. Some adhesions have been described as creating pseudowalls within the joint space. The walls may hinder a complete examination of the glenoid regions. As a result, the operator may perceive that the glenoid fossa is significantly reduced in volume.

Synovial Bodies

Synovial chondromatosis rarely affects the TMJ.[52–55] In this disease, the synovium proliferates to form cartilaginous nodules that obliterate the joint space and interfere with normal function. The disease usually manifests with pain, swelling, stiffness in the jaw muscles, joint noise, intermittent locking, and recurrent dislocation.[56] Milgram[57] classified the pathogenesis histologically into three stages: (1) synovial metaplasia without detached synovial bodies; (2) synovial metaplasia with detached synovial bodies; and (3) absence of synovial disease with the presence of detached synovial bodies. Arthrotomy has traditionally been used to perform various procedures, including removal of the synovial bodies, synovectomy, discectomy, or high or total condylectomy. Most cases affecting the TMJ have been treated with discectomy, with various degrees of synovectomy.

Arthroscopy may assist an operator in obtaining a diagnosis and staging the disease process. Various sizes and shapes of loose white bodies may be seen within the joint space, partly extruded from the synovial membrane or embedded within the synovium overlying the disc (Plate 31–20).

SURGICAL ARTHROSCOPY

Surgical arthroscopy has principally been used to treat pain and dysfunction associated with internal derangements. Arthroscopy's effectiveness in the management of arthritic conditions and hypermobility has yet to be defined. The indication for gross and arthroscopic surgical intervention for treatment of internal derangements is the same: moderate to severe pain and dysfunction that interfere with a patient's daily routine and are refractory to a reasonable course of nonsurgical therapy.

ARTHROSCOPIC SURGERY
Lysis, Manipulation, and Lavage

Lysis and lavage of the superior joint space and manipulation of the mandible currently constitute the most commonly performed and reported arthroscopic surgical procedure (Fig. 31–32). The technique appears to work most effectively for the management of acute and chronic closed lock.[50]

According to Sanders,[21] Murakami and Ito (1984) described the treatment of closed lock employing a technique to sweep surface adhesions in the superior joint space. The goal was to increase disc mobility and thus eliminate the closed lock. Sanders[21] popularized the procedure in North America. He ascribed closed

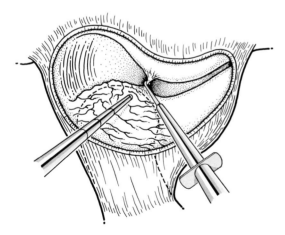

FIGURE 31–32. The lysis, lavage, and manipulation technique as performed in the superior joint space. An arthroscopic knife is used to incise an adhesion between the posterior slope of the eminence and the remodeled retrodiscal tissue. The lysis is demonstrated under direct vision.

lock to disc and fossa "stickiness" ("suction cup effect"), fibrillations, and superior joint space adhesions. The adhesions were most commonly located between the posterior slope of the eminence and the central aspect of the posterior attachment. The technique involves the establishment of a two-port system, diagnostic examination of the superior joint space, resection (lysis) of the adhesions with a blunt trocar, lavage of the joint space, and instillation of a steroid solution. Postoperatively, joint mobility is rapidly gained. Since the original description of the technique, lysis of adhesions has been performed with direct visualization using microscissors and knives or pediatric resectoscopes.

Indresano[50] reported followup of 9 to 30 months in 64 patients (100 joints), following a superior compartment sweep and lavage. Postoperative betamethasone injections were administered. He noted that the greatest success (83%) was with patients with displaced discs and pain and hypomobility, that is, the group with closed lock. A popping noise was noted on initial distention of the joint space with lactated Ringer's solution. This was attributed to release of the adhesion. Response to therapy in categories of internal derangements other than closed lock was poor.

Montgomery and colleagues[58] described their results in 19 subjects followed for 6 to 12 months. Although 90% of patients reported an improvement, 50% still had some residual pain emanating from the region of the joint. Joint sounds showed an initial decrease and then subsequently returned to preoperative levels by weeks 24 and 52. They acknowledged that because postoperative therapy in many of these patients was complex and variable, it was impossible to determine the precise benefit from arthroscopy.

Moses and Poker[59] reported a 92% reduction in pain and restoration of function in 92 patients monitored for a mean of 19 months. The presence of bilaminar zone perforations and degenerative joint disease (degree not defined) did not seem to affect the result. "Condylar osteophytes" and central disc perforations did appear to lead to poorer prognoses.

White[60] reported 85.7% improvement in the condition of 66 patients monitored for 19.4 months. The majority of patients underwent lysis, lavage, and manipulation. Cases were divided into three diagnostic categories: nonreducing disc displacements, severe adhesive capsulitis, and degenerative joint disease. Electrocautery was utilized to scar the posterior ligament in selected cases.

Although Sanders'[21] study presumed the immediate increase in opening was secondary to disc repositioning over the condyle, postoperative magnetic resonance imaging studies subsequently showed minimal to no change in the disc position.[58,61–63] Hellsing and colleagues[64] suggested that the closed lock symptom was resolved by increasing the mobility of the disc complex, rather than by repositioning the disc. Capsule denervation may explain some temporary results. Lavage of the joint space may produce relief by removal of inflammatory products and debris.[24,65] Similar relief of symptoms has been reported following knee joint arthroscopy.[66]

Kondoh and associates[67] believed that the results of arthroscopic lysis, lavage, and manipulation were unstable. They produced more satisfactory results by coagulating the surface of the posterior attachment of the disc with a neodymium:yttrium-aluminum-garnet (Nd:YAG) laser following lysis and repositioning. The purpose of the posterior coagulation was to promote scarring of the tissues to prevent disc displacement after presumed repositioning. Bradrick and colleagues[68] studied the effects of the Nd:YAG laser beam in the mongrel dog TMJ. They noted that the tissue was affected by the laser power output (watts), delivery system, exposure (joules), fluid medium, tissue characteristics, and degree of local circulation. Dense, healthy fibrocartilaginous surfaces tended to reflect laser energy; inflamed tissue absorbed the energy. Fibrocartilage contracted rather than vaporized when the tissue was not contacted. The workers noted greater damage with the Nd:YAG laser than the carbon dioxide laser. Zones of tissue damage consistent with coagulation necrosis enlarged with time. They also postulated on the benefits of scar contracture in the posterior attachment.

Moses and Poker[59] combined the lysis, lavage, and manipulation procedure with a lateral capsule stretch procedure (lateral release). Some 237 patients (419 joints) were monitored for 10.5 months (range, 1 to 33 months). A total of 92% of patients reported a decrease in pain and 97% of patients thought that the procedure was successful. At least 73% of patients were able to achieve a maximum interincisal opening of 40 mm or greater.

Disc-Repositioning Techniques

Some workers have concentrated their efforts on arthroscopic repositioning of discs.

These procedures attempt to mimic gross surgical procedures. The repositioning of the disc is believed to reduce pain and dysfunction. For a complete description of gross-disc repositioning procedures, see Chapter 32.

The anterior release procedure for repositioning of discs has been described by McCain.[69] The procedure involves electrocautery of the medial capsule and external pterygoid fibers and blunt posterior manipulation of the disc (Fig. 31–33). In other cases, all that is performed is the anterior release without disc repositioning. One of the main concerns with electrocautery is the generation of heat in the vicinity of the middle cranial fossa. McCain[70] found that a constant flow of irrigant maintained lower intra-articular temperatures than a pulsated flow. Artificially cooled irrigants were not found to reduce temperatures appreciably. Distilled water is the preferred irrigant because it is not electrolytic.

Tarro[71] combined the lysis of adhesions and partial lateral pterygoid myotomy procedures with a suturing technique to reposition the disc. The suturing was performed blindly and confirmed arthroscopically. In a select group of

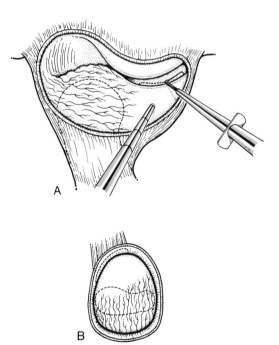

FIGURE 31–33. The arthroscopic anterior release of the lateral pterygoid muscle. *A,* Sagittal view, superior joint space exposed. Electrocautery probe is passed through a second anterior port. *B,* View from above demonstrating the incisions in the anteromedial portion of the capsule.

patients, the posterior attachment was electro-cauterized to promote scar contraction and, hence, a posterior disc position. Length of followup extended from 9 weeks to 12 months. No postoperative imaging studies were done to confirm the change in disc position.

Histology of disc displacements indicates, however, that disc deformation is not uniform. Differential loss of disc substance may result in greater atrophy, deformation, and displacement laterally than medially.[72] Surgical disc repositioning appears to be a viable procedure when disc length is nearly normal and disc deformation minimal.

Retrodiscotomy and Posterolateral Release

The purpose of the retrodiscotomy and posterolateral release procedures is to return patients to a regular diet with minimal restrictions by promoting disc displacement and remodeling.[51] The procedures have been performed with the arthroscope or with fluoroscopic guidance (Fig. 31–34). Transection of the scarred, advanced remodeled retrodiscal tissue presumably accelerates the host's capability of adapting to the pathologic condition without addressing the displaced disc.

Eriksson and Westesson[73] surmised that with time and no intervention, opening in closed lock situations would slowly increase by elongation of the posterior attachment and further anterior displacement and deformation of the disc. The progression may lead further to perforation of the remodeled retrodiscal tissue. Osteoarthrosis may be present histologically and radiographically, without significant symptoms. Support for retrodiscotomy and posterolateral release procedures comes from epidemiologic studies indicating the existence of internal derangements in the asymptomatic or minimally symptomatic general population.[74] This observation strongly suggests that patients are able to adapt to various disc positions and disc shapes.

Toller[75] appears to have described an open lateral release procedure in capsular rearrangement. The procedure was devised to achieve free range of motion of the disc. He believed that capsule denervation minimized reflex muscular effects. The lateral capsule was reconstructed by means of an anteriorly based temporal flap. A total of 14 patients were observed for periods of 6 months to 4 years. All symptoms were relieved in eight patients, and the

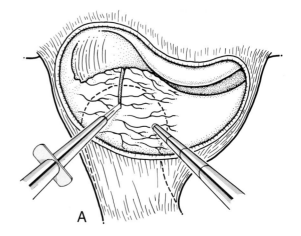

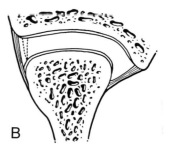

FIGURE 31–34. The retrodiscotomy and posterolateral release procedures. *A,* Sagittal view, superior joint space exposed. An arthroscopic knife is passed through the posterior port. The incision is performed under direct vision. *B,* Coronal view. Ideal location of the lateral limb of the incision (posterolateral release).

chief complaint in four patients. One patient showed improvement, but results were not completely normal. One patient returned one year postoperatively for management of recurrent pain. Joint noise was relieved in all cases, however.

Heffez and Jordan[51] reported on their results in 14 patients found to have internal derangements with or without muscle dysfunction, who were monitored over a mean period of 18 months (range 2 to 48 months). The patients were selected because of refractoriness to nonsurgical therapy.

In the arthroscopic technique, routine single-port superior joint space arthroscopy is first performed to establish the diagnosis and vascularity pattern of the remodeled retrodiscal tissue.[49,50] A second outflow port is next established. The telescope is removed and then inserted through the second, more anterior, port. The telescope is directed toward the flexure to visualize an arthroscopic knife inserted through the posterior port. This instrument performs the retrodiscotomy. The incision is made in a relatively avascular region of the remodeled retrodiscal tissue. Microscissors have also been used (Plate 31–21). In the posterolateral release, a second connecting incision is made to separate the attachment of the remodeled retrodiscal tissue from the lateral capsule. This part of the incision is best made by passing the arthroscopic knife directly through the cartilaginous portion of the external auditory canal. This trajectory permits the proper angulation of the instrument.

When the procedure is performed fluoroscopically, only local anesthesia is used. The inferior joint space is hyperdilated (approximately 0.5 ml) with Reno-M-60 (diatrizoate meglumine 282 mg/ml bound iodine), under fluoroscopy. The needle is withdrawn from the space, and pressure is placed over the preauricular site to prevent extravasation. Next, a myringotomy or arthroscopic knife is inserted into the superior joint space without an external sheath. Blade location is verified on fluoroscopy. The knife is drawn inferolaterally across the remodeled retrodiscal tissue. The operator verifies the penetration of dye into the superior joint space, confirming transection of the tissue.

Preliminary results appear promising. The immediate (0 to 1 month) result appears to be an accurate predictor of the long-term result, unless contralateral quiescent disease is activated necessitating additional surgery. Patients who underwent the fluoroscopic procedure generally remarked on immediate improvement in freedom of joint motion. In most circumstances, this comment was unsolicited. Patients experienced some soreness immediately after the arthroscopic procedure and noted an improvement by 1 to 2 weeks. Of the 14 patients, seven were enjoying a regular diet with minimal restrictions and were not dependent on appliance therapy for relief of symptoms. Two patients wore the appliance intermittently. Five patients continued to wear an appliance at night. A total of ten patients demonstrated eradication of all complaints or significant improvement in their condition by the last followup visit.

The retrodiscotomy and posterolateral release procedures intentionally create a perforation. Experimentally created perforations have been shown to rarely heal spontaneously in primates.[76-78] Incisions in the retrodiscal TMJ tissue of normal rabbits and primates have been shown to heal uneventfully.[79] The vascularity of the cut edges determines the potential for synovial proliferation and, hence, healing.[80] This has been observed in the laboratory, where surgery of the medial meniscus of the canine knee heals only when the peripheral synovial tissues contact the sites of transection.[81]

Healing of the arthroscopic transection site may not be pivotal to a successful result, because the effect of transection is immediate, with presumably minimal separation of the tissue edges. Postoperative imaging in selected cases has failed to demonstrate changes in disc displacement despite improvement in clinical symptoms.

Retrodiscotomy and posterolateral release appear to be most beneficial in cases of chronic restriction in joint motion concurrent with a severely atrophic disc and scarred posterior attachment. Heffez and Jordan[51] have conjectured that the superficial vascularity may be a marker for the disease process. Moreover, it is unlikely that the entire process of disc remodeling and degeneration can be accelerated from its earliest stages using these procedures.

Retrieval of Foreign Bodies

Foreign bodies rarely become dislodged in the region of the TMJ. In rare cases, gunshot debris may need to be removed to restore normal range of motion. With the proliferation of arthroscopic techniques, we can expect an increased incidence of foreign bodies iatrogenically as a result of fracture of instruments. In general, if the foreign body can be localized arthroscopically, it can be removed. Tarro[83] reported on the retrieval of fractured instruments from the superior joint space. Protocols for retrieval of fractured arthroscopic instruments have been established.[83,84] McCain and de la Rua[85] described a "switch stick" technique in which sheaths of increasing external diameters were progressively slipped over trocars of increasing diameter to gain access to the joint space. They outlined the importance of having an extra set of each hand-held instrument to retrieve any fractured segment. A patient should always be prepared preoperatively for the need to perform an arthrotomy. Instruments made of ferromagnetic materials are used so that magnetic retrievers may be employed.[82] As a routine, the integrity of all instruments should be checked before and after the procedure.

Synovectomy

There are no long-term data on the arthroscopic treatment of stage 1 or 2 rheumatoid arthritis. It currently appears that a total synovectomy, the preferred treatment for this condition, may be more expeditiously and effectively completed with open surgical techniques. The microshaver may be selected to perform a partial synovectomy (see Fig. 31–13). A two-port system is utilized. Care must be taken to adequately distend the joint space to avoid sucking tissues into the aperture of this instrument.

Milgram believed that synovectomy was the treatment of choice in stages 1 and 2 of synovial chondromatosis and only removal of nodules in stage 3. He classified the pathogenesis histologically into three stages: (1) synovial metaplasia without detachment of particles, (2) synovial metaplasia with detached particles, (3) no evidence of intrasynovial disease with only detached intra-articular particles present.[57] Arthroscopy may assist an operator in determining the stage of the disease process.

POSTOPERATIVE CARE

Postoperatively, patients are informed that there will be oozing of blood-tinged fluid from the surgical site. A temporary decrease in hearing may be experienced secondary to clotted blood within the external auditory canal. When this is a major complaint or is accompanied by tympanic pain, the clots may be irrigated with diluted hydrogen peroxide.

Patients are encouraged to follow a regimen of passive range of motion exercises at home. As with any other surgical procedure, patients' cooperation is pivotal. In the regimen that I use, an exercise program is begun by the fifth postoperative day. Gentle opening exercises, 20 repetitions at a time, two to three times a day, are initially prescribed. By the third postoperative week, a protrusive exercise is added; by the fourth week, a combination opening-protrusive exercise is added. Patients' progress and cooperation dictate the frequency and duration of these exercises. Active range of motion exercises by the patient or by a physical therapist are sometimes required. Some operators routinely employ the services offered by a physical therapist. After diagnostic arthroscopy, most patients gradually return to the preoperative opening by the second postoperative week. Response to surgical therapy is dependent on the pathology, the procedure, and the duration of the procedure.

Some clinicians place patients on appliance therapy postoperatively to reduce the loading of the joint. Moses and Poker[59] advocated the wearing of an appliance for at least 1 month postoperatively. In the absence of a parafunctional habit, the wearing of the appliance was gradually reduced to evenings and discontinued altogether, within several months.

Criteria to measure postoperative success have varied among clinicians. Some depend primarily on the degree of patients' satisfaction, whereas others depend on precise measurements, such as maximum interincisal opening and protrusive and lateral function.[59]

COMPLICATIONS

Complications associated with arthroscopy may be classified as immediate (within the first 24 hours postoperatively) or delayed.

Immediate complications include hemorrhage, nerve injuries, auricular damage, perforation of the middle cranial fossa, damage to the articular surfaces, fracture of instruments, and tissue emphysema.

Hemorrhage from a branch of the superficial temporal vessels may occur. Bleeding can be well controlled with local pressure and occasionally with placement of a hemostatic clip.

Nerve injuries to the fifth and seventh nerves have occurred. Injury of the inferior alveolar and lingual nerves may occur from towel clamp placement at the angle of the mandible. Single-port arthroscopy may cause long buccal, inferior alveolar, lingual paresthesias through distention of the pterygomandibular space. The intracranial portion of the seventh nerve may be damaged if the arthroscope perforates the tympanic membrane and the middle ear is accidentally instrumented. Westesson and colleagues[86] suggested that the risk of damage to the extracranial portion of the seventh nerve from a properly executed posterior puncture was small.

Auditory complications may result from inadvertent instrumentation of the external auditory canal. Incomalleolar dislocation may result in conductive hearing loss and damage to the petrous portion of the facial nerve (Fig. 31–35).[87] Sanders and Buoncristiani[22] stated that one of their patients undergoing the lysis and lavage procedure developed a severe postoperative middle ear infection, resulting in some permanent hearing loss. Moreover, proper ar-

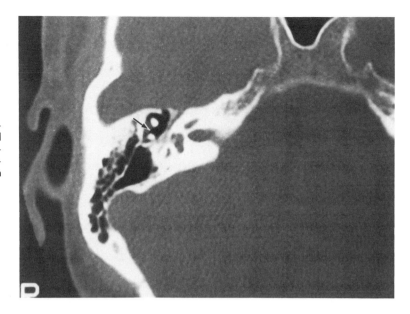

FIGURE 31–35. Axial computerized tomogram of left temporal bone demonstrating incomallealar dislocation (arrow) subsequent to improper manipulation of arthroscopic instruments.

throscopic instrumentation within the articular space does not produce audiometric changes.[88,89] Similar results were reported by McKenna and colleagues[90] following arthrotomy. Perforation of the middle cranial fossa has occurred.[39]

Iatrogenic damage to the contents of the superior joint space includes scuffing or perforation of the fibrous connective tissue–lining of the glenoid fossa/eminence, introduction of pericapsular debris into the joint space, laceration of synovial vessels, perforation of the medial capsule/ligament, inadvertent perforation of the anterior capsule, and perforation of the remodeled retrodiscal tissue. With increasing operator experience, iatrogenic damage is less likely. Synovial vessels that have been torn may be temporarily sealed by raising the pressure of the irrigation fluid. Physical therapy is important in regaining joint mobility and preventing fibrous ankylosis. Operators must remember the degree of magnification achieved with the telescope to accurately evaluate the damage created. At 1 mm from the tissue, there is 10× magnification. When damage is minor, tissues appear clinically to have repaired themselves. Some surgical procedures, such as the anterior release, intentionally interrupt the integrity of the anteromedial capsule.

Delayed complications include infection, hypomobility of the condyle-disc complex, and local subcutaneous atrophy. Infection rarely occurs with diagnostic arthroscopy, presumably because of the large volumes of fluid that are constantly flushed through the joint space and the abundant vascularity of the facial region. Johnson and associates[26] reported an infection rate of 0.04% in diagnostic knee arthroscopy. A reducing disc displacement may occasionally be temporarily or permanently converted to a nonreducing displacement as a result of inflammatory changes. Fibrous ankylosis may develop if a patient's cooperation with postoperative physical therapeutic exercises is poor. Goldberg and colleagues[91] reported the development of local subcutaneous atrophy 1 month after orthroscopy. They postulated that the triamcinolone acetonide instilled in the joint cavity may have leached out into the surrounding tissues.

FUTURE DIRECTION

Arthroscopy of the TMJ is an evolving field that is beginning to challenge many of the basic tenets of open joint surgery. Arthroscopic techniques can be developed and perfected on primate and sheep models. Sheep provide an inexpensive and readily available model.[92] Their TMJ is similar in size and anatomy to the TMJ in humans, though it is situated more laterally from the glenoid fossa. However, the lack of a disease animal model for internal derangements continues to restrict developments in open surgical and arthroscopic treatments. In the future, considerable emphasis will likely be placed on the development of such an animal model.

Diagnostic and surgical arthroscopy are adding to our understanding of the pathogenesis of internal derangements. The results of such procedures as lysis, lavage, and manipulation bring into question the value of joint space lavage with local anesthesia and without arthroscopy. Institutionally controlled studies need to be performed. Hope exists that disorders such as rheumatoid arthritis (stages 1 and 2) and other arthritic conditions, as well as chronic, persistent, and recurrent condylar dislocation, may ultimately be treated arthroscopically. As we move forward, clinicians should proceed with caution and healthy skepticism as they evaluate treatment results under the pressure of such a technological innovation.

REFERENCES

1. Bozzini, P.H.: In *Endoscopy*. G. Berci (ed.). Appleton-Century-Crofts, New York, 1976.
2. Desormeaux, A.J.: In *Endoscopy*. G. Berci (ed). Appleton-Century-Crofts, New York, 1976.
3. Kussmaul, J.: Uber Magenspiegelung. Verh. Naturforsch. Ges. Freiburg 5:112, 1870.
4. Berci, G. (ed.): *Endoscopy*. Appleton-Century-Crofts, New York, pp. 3–63, 74–82, 1976.
5. Takagi, K.: Practical experience using Takagi's arthroscope. J. Jpn. Orthop. Assoc. 8:132, 1933.
6. Takagi, K.: The arthroscope. J. Jpn. Orthop. Assoc. 14:359, 1939.
7. Watanabe, M., Takeda, S., and Ikeuchi, H.: *Atlas of Arthroscopy*. Igaku Shoin, Tokyo, 1957.
8. Watanable, M. and Takeda, S.: The number 21 arthroscope. J. Jpn. Orthop. Assoc. 34:1041, 1960.
9. Watanabe, M. (ed.): *Arthroscopy of Small Joints*. Igaku Shoin, Tokyo, 1985.
10. Watanabe, M.: Arthroscopic diagnosis of the internal derangements of the knee joint. J. Jpn. Orthop. Assoc. 42:993, 1968.
11. Bircher, E.: Die Arthroendoskopie. Zentralbl. Chir. 48:1460, 1921.
12. Ohnishi, M.: Clinical studies on the intrarticular puncture of the temporomandibular joints and its application (in Japanese). Jpn. J. Oral Surg. 22:436–442, 1970.
13. Ohnishi, M.: Arthroscopy of the temporomandibular joint (in Japanese). J. Jpn. Stomat. 42:207–213, 1975.
14. Hilsabeck, R.B. and Laskin, D.M.: Arthroscopy of the temporomandibular joint of the rabbit. J. Oral Surg. 36:938–943, 1978.
15. Williams, R.A. and Laskin, D.M.: Arthroscopic examination of experimentally induced pathologic conditions of the rabbit temporomandibular joint. J. Oral Surg. 38:652–659, 1980.
16. Murakami, K. and Hoshino, K.: Regional anatomical nomenclature and arthroscopic terminology in human temporomandibular joints. Okajimas Folia Anat. Jpn. 58:745–760, 1982.
17. Murakami, K.I., Matsumoto, K., and Iizuka, T.: Suppurative arthritis of the temporomandibular joint. J. Maxillofac. Surg. 12:41–45, 1984.
18. Heffez, L. and Blaustein, D.: Diagnostic arthroscopy of the temporomandibular joint. I. Normal arthroscopic findings. Oral Surg. 64:653–678, 1987.
19. Blaustein, D. and Heffez, L.: Diagnostic arthroscopy of the temporomandibular joint. II. Pathological arthroscopic findings. Oral Surg. 66:135–141, 1988.
20. McCain, J.P., de la Rua, H., and LeBlanc, W.G.: Correlation of clinical, radiographic and arthroscopic findings in internal derangements of the TMJ. J. Oral Maxillofac. Surg. 47:913–921, 1989.
21. Sanders, B.: Arthroscopic surgery of temporomandibular joint: Treatment of internal derangement with persistent closed lock. Oral Surg. 62:361–372, 1986.
22. Sanders, B. and Buoncristiani, R.: Diagnostic and surgical arthroscopy of the temporomandibular joint: Clinical experience with 137 procedures over a 2 year period. J. Craniomand. Dis. Facial Oral Pain 1:202–213, 1987.
23. Holmlund, A. and Hellsing, G.: Arthroscopy of the temporomandibular joint. An autopsy study. Int. J. Oral Surg. 14:169–175, 1985.
24. Holmlund, A., Hellsing, G., and Wredmark, T.: Arthroscopy of the temporomandibular joint. A clinical study. Int. J. Oral Maxillofac. Surg. 15:715–721, 1986.
25. Shahriaree, H. and Erichsen, C.: Arthroscopic instrumentation. In *O'Connor's Textbook of Arthroscopic Surgery*. H. Shahriaree (ed.) JB Lippincott, Philadelphia, 1984.
26. Johnson, L.L., Schneider, D.A., Austin, M.D., et al: Two-percent glutaraldehyde: A disinfectant in arthroscopy and arthroscopic surgery. J Bone Joint Surg. [Am.] 64:237–239, 1982.
27. Jackson, D.W.: Videoarthroscopy: A permanent medical record. Am. J. Sports Med. 6:213–225, 1978.
28. Erikson, E.: Problems in recording arthroscopy. Orthop. Clin. North Am. 10:735, 1979.
29. Murakami, K. and Ono, T.: Temporomandibular joint arthroscopy by inferolateral approach. Int. J. Oral Maxillofac. Surg, 15:410–417, 1986.
30. Reagen, B.F., McInerny, V.K., Trewell, B.V., et al: Irrigating solutions for arthroscopy. J. Bone Joint Surg. [Am.] 65:629–631, 1983.
31. Murakami, K., Matsuki, M., Iizuka, T., and Ono, T.: Diagnostic arthroscopy of the TMJ: Differential diagnoses in patients with limited jaw opening. J. Craniomand. Pract. 4:117, 1986.
32. Ohnishi, M.: Clinical application of arthroscopy in the temporomandibular joint diseases. Bull. Tokyo Med. Dent. Univ. 27:141–150, 1980.
33. Eriksson, E. and Sebik, A.: Arthroscopy and arthroscopic surgery in a gas versus a fluid medium. Symposium on arthroscopic knee surgery. Orthop. Clin. North Am. 13:293–298, 1982.
34. Pape, L.G. and Balazs, E.A.: The use of sodium hyaluronate (Healon) in human anterior segment surgery. Ophthalmology 87:699, 1980.
35. Weiss, C. and Balazs, E.A.: Arthroscopic viscosurgery. Arthroscopy 3:138, 1987.
36. McCain, J.P., Balazs, E.A., and de la Rua, H.: Preliminary studies on the use of viscoelastic solution in arthroscopic surgery of the temporomandibular joint. J. Oral Maxillofac. Surg. 47:1161–1168, 1989.
37. Al-Kayat, A. and Bramley, P.: A modified pre-auricular approach to the temporomandibular joint and malar arch. Br. J. Oral Surg. 17:91, 1979–80.
38. Yale, S.H., Allison, B.D., and Hauptfuehrer, J.D.: An epidemiological assessment of mandibular condyle morphology. Oral Surg. 21:169–177, 1966.
39. McCain, J.P.: Arthroscopy of the human temporomandibular joint. J. Oral Maxillofac. Surg. 46:648–655, 1988.
40. Heffez, L., Mafee, M., Langer, B., and Rosenberg, H.: Double contrast arthrography of the temporomandib-

ular joint: Role of direct sagittal CT. Oral Surg. 65:511–514, 1988.

41. DeHaven, K.: Principles of triangulation for arthroscopic surgery. Symposium on arthroscopic knee surgery. Orthop. Clin. North Am. 13:329–336, 1982.

41. Moses, J.J.: Presentation at International Study Club on Arthroscopy of the TMJ, New York, December, 1988.

42. Farrar, W.B. and McCarty, W.L. Jr.: Inferior joint space arthrography and characteristics of condylar paths in internal derangement of the TMJ. J. Prosthet. Dent. 41:548–555, 1979.

43. Westesson, P.L., Bronstein, S.L., and Leidberg, J.L.: Internal derangement of the temporomandibular joint: Morphologic description with correlation to function. Oral Surg. 59:323–331, 1985.

44. Mizukawa, J.H., Comstock, B., and Hagan, B.: A comparative study of temporomandibular joint pathosis: Upper compartment vs. lower compartment. Educational Summaries and Outlines. Seventy-first Annual Meeting and Scientific Sessions, American Association of Oral & Maxillofacial Surgeons, American Association of Oral and Maxillofacial Surgeons, San Francisco, September 20–24, 47:78, 1989.

45. Liedberg, J. and Westesson, P.L.: Diagnostic accuracy of upper compartment arthroscopy of the temporomandibular joint. Correlation with postmortem morphology. Oral Surg. 62:618–624, 1986.

46. Goss, A.N., Bosanquet, P., and Tideman, H.: The accuracy of temporomandibular joint arthroscopy. J. Craniomaxillofac. Surg. 15:99–102, 1987.

47. Heffez, L. and Jordan, S.: An arthroscopic classification of the superficial vascularity of remodeled retrodiscal tissue. Presentation at International Study Club on Arthroscopy of the TMJ, New York, December, 1988.

48. Hansson, T. and Oberg, T.: Arthrosis and deviation in form in the temporomandibular joint. A macroscopic study on a human autopsy material. Acta Odontol. Scand. 35:167–174, 1976.

49. Heffez, L. and Jordan, S.: Superficial vascularity of TM joint retrodiscal tissue is an element of the internal derangement process. J. Oral Maxillofac. Surg. (Submitted, 1991.)

50. Indresano, A.T.: Arthroscopic surgery of the TMJ. J. Oral Maxillofac. Surg. 47:439–441, 1989.

51. Heffez, L. and Jordan, S.: Retrodiscotomy. A preliminary (1 to 48 months) report on arthroscopic and fluoroscopic guided procedure. J. Oral Maxillofac. Surg. (Submitted, 1991.)

52. Ballard, R. and Weiland, L.H.: Synovial chondromatosis of the temporomandibular joint. Cancer 30:791, 1972.

53. Akhtar, M., Mahajan, S., and Kott, E.: Synovial chondromatosis of the temporomandibular joint. J. Bone Joint Surg. [Am.] 59:266, 1977.

54. Dolan, E., Vogler, J.B., and Angelillo, J.C.: Synovial chondromatosis of the temporomandibular joint diagnosed by magnetic resonance imaging: Report of a case. J. Oral Maxillofac. Surg. 47:411, 1989.

55. Takagi, M. and Ishikawa, G.: Simultaneous villonodular synovitis and synovial chondromatosis of the temporomandibular joint. J. Oral Surg. 39:699, 1981.

56. Silver, C.M., Motamed, M., and Moonan, D.E.: Chondromatosis of the temporomandibular joint arising in the meniscus. J. Oral Maxillofac. Surg. 44:70, 1986.

57. Milgram, J.W.: Synovial chondromatosis. A histopathologic study of thirty cases. J. Bone Joint Surg. 59:792, 1977.

58. Montgomery, M., Van Sickels, J., Harms, S., and

59. Thrash, W.J.: Arthroscopic TMJ surgery. Effects on signs, symptoms and disc position. J. Oral Maxillofac. Surg. 47:1263–1271, 1989.

59. Moses, J.J. and Poker, I.D.: TMJ arthroscopy: An analysis of 237 patients. J. Oral Maxillofac. Surg. 47:790–794, 1989.

60. White, R.D.: Retrospective analysis of 100 consecutive surgical arthroscopies of the temporomandibular joint. J. Oral Maxillofac. Surg. 47:1014–1021, 1989.

61. Gatler, M., Perry, H., Schwartz, R., et al: Effects of arthroscopic TMJ surgery on articular disk position. AADR, 18th Annual Session. J. Dent. Res. (Special Issue) 68:310, 1027, 1989.

62. Moses, J.J., Sartoris, D., Glass, R., et al: The effect of arthroscopic surgical lysis and lavage of the superior joint space on TMJ disc position and mobility. J. Oral Maxillofac. Surg. 47:674, 1989.

63. Perrot, D.H., Alborzi, A., Guerrera, A., and Kaban, L.B.: A prospective study evaluating effectiveness of TMJ arthroscopy. Educational summaries and outlines. Seventy-first annual meeting and scientific sessions, American Association of Oral & Maxillofacial Surgeons, September 20–24, 47:92, 1989.

64. Hellsing, G., Holmlund, A., Nordenram, A., and Torsten, W.: Arthroscopy of the temporomandibular joint. Examination of 2 patients with suspected disc derangement. Int. J. Oral Surg. 13:69–74, 1984.

65. Quinn, J.H. and Bazan, N.G.: Identification of prostaglandin E_2 and leukotriene B_4 pain mediators in dysfunctional TMJ synovial fluid. Educational summaries and outlines. Seventy-first Annual Meeting and Scientific Sessions, American Association of Oral and Maxillofacial Surgeons, San Francisco, September 20–24, 47:79, 1989.

66. Jayson, M.I.V. and Dixon, A.St.I.: Arthroscopy of the knee in rheumatic diseases. Ann. Rheum. Dis. 27:503–511, 1968.

67. Kondoh, T., Norihiko, T., Yutaka, S., and Kanichi, S.: Arthroscopic laser surgery for persistent closed-locking of the TMJ, accompanied with intracapsular fibrous adhesion. Educational summaries and outlines. Seventy-first annual meeting and scientific sessions, September 20–24, 47:94, 1989.

68. Bradrick, J.P., Eckhauser, M.L., and Indresano, A.T.: Morphologic and histologic changes in canine temporomandibular joint tissues following arthroscopic guided neodymium:YAG laser exposure. J. Oral Maxillofac. Surg. 47:1177–1181, 1989.

69. McCain, J.P.: Arthroscopic surgery of the TMJ. Presentation at international study club on arthroscopy of the TMJ, New York, December, 1988.

70. McCain, J.: Electrothermal heat generation during arthroscopic surgery. J. Oral Maxillofac. Surg. (Submitted, 1990.)

71. Tarro, A.W.: Arthroscopic treatment of anterior disc displacement. A preliminary report. J. Oral Maxillofac. Surg. 47:353–358, 1989.

72. Heffez, L. and Jordan, S.: A classification of temporomandibular joint disk morphology. Oral Surg. Oral Med. Oral Pathol. 67:11, 1988.

73. Eriksson, E. and Westesson, P.L.: Clinical and radiological study of patients with anterior disc displacement of the temporomandibular joint. Swed. Dent. J. 7:55–64, 1983.

74. Akerman, S., Kopp, S., and Bohlin, M.: Histological changes in temporomandibular joints from elderly individuals. Acta Odontol. Scand. 44:231–239, 1986.

75. Toller, P.A.: Temporomandibular capsular rearrangement. Br. J. Oral Surg. 11:207, 1974.

76. Helmy, E., Bays, R., and Sharawy, M.: Osteoarthrosis of the temporomandibular joint in *Macaca fascicularis*. J. Oral Maxillofac. Surg. 46:979, 1988.

77. Helmy, E.S., Bays, P., and Sharawy, M.: Microscopic alterations in the temporomandibular joint of adult monkeys following surgical disc perforations. Case reports and outlines of scientific sessions, 66th annual meeting AAOMS, New York, p. 56, 1984.

78. Helmy, E.S., Mercer, J.E., and Sharawy, M.: Histopathological study of human TMJ perforated discs with emphasis on synovial membrane response. Case reports and outlines of scientific sessions, 68th annual meeting AAOMS, New Orleans, p. 27, 1986.

79. Wallace, D.W. and Laskin, D.M.: Healing of surgical incisions in the disc and retrodiscal tissue of the rabbit temporomandibular joint. J. Oral Maxillofac. Surg. 44:965, 1986.

80. Kim, J.M. and Moon, M.S.: The effect of synovectomy upon regeneration of the meniscus in rabbits. Clin. Orthop. 141:287, 1979.

81. Arnoczky, S.P. and Warren, R.F.: The microvasculature of the meniscus and its response to injury. An experimental study in the dog. Am. J. Sports Med. 11:131, 1983.

82. Johnson, L.: *Arthroscopic Surgery, Principles and Practice*, 3rd ed. C.V. Mosby, St. Louis, 1986.

83. Tarro, A.W.: Instrument breakage associated with arthroscopy of the temporomandibular joint: Report of a case. J. Oral Maxillofac. Surg. 47:1226–1228, 1989.

84. McGinty, J.B. and Mapza, R.A.: Evaluation of an outpatient procedure under local anesthesia. J. Bone Joint Surg. 60:787, 1978.

85. McCain, J.P., and de la Rua, H.: Foreign body retrieval: A complication of TMJ arthroscopy. Report of a case. J. Oral Maxillofac. Surg. 47:1221–1225, 1989.

86. Westesson, P.L., Eriksson, L., and Liedberg, J.: The risk of damage to facial nerve, superficial temporal vessels, disc, and articular surfaces during arthroscopic examination of the TMJ. Oral Surg. Oral Med. Oral Pathol. 2:124–127, 1986.

87. Jones, J.L. and Horn, K.L.: The effect of temporomandibular joint arthroscopy on ear function. J. Oral Maxillofac. Surg. 47:1022–1025, 1989.

88. Van Sickels, J.E., Nishioka, G.J., Hegewald, M.B., and Neal, G.P.: Middle ear injury resulting from temporomandibular joint arthroscopy. J. Oral Maxillofac. Surg. 45:962–965, 1987.

89. McCain, J., Goldberg, H.M., and de la Rua, H.: Preoperative and postoperative audiologic measurements in patients undergoing arthroscopy of the TMJ. J. Oral Maxillofac. Surg. 47:1026–1027, 1989.

90. McKenna, S.J., Hall, H.D., and Yallourakis, S.: Failure of audiometry to change following TM surgery. Educational summaries and outlines. Seventy-first Annual Meeting and Scientific Sessions. American Association of Oral and Maxillofacial Surgeons, San Francisco, September 20–24, 47:81, 1989.

91. Goldberg, J.S., Julian, J.B., and Dachille, R.: Local subcutaneous atrophy following arthroscopy of the TMJ. J. Oral Maxillofac. Surg. 47:986–987, 1989.

92. Goss, A.N. and Bosanquet, A.G.: An animal model for TMJ arthroscopy. J. Oral Maxillofac. Surg. 47:537–538, 1989.

SUGGESTED READINGS

Burke, R.: Temporomandibular joint diagnosis. Arthroscopy. J. Craniomand. Pract. 3:233–236, 1985.

Finkelstein, H. and Mayer, L.: The arthroscope: A new method of examining joints. J. Bone Joint Surg. [Am.] 13:583, 1931.

Burman, M.S.: Arthroscopy. The direct visualization of joints: An experimental cadaver study. J. Bone Joint Surg. [Am.] 13:669, 1931.

DeHaven, K.E. and Collins, H.R.: Diagnosis of internal derangements of the knee: Their role in arthroscopy. J. Bone Joint Surg. [Am.] 57:802, 1975.

Goss, A. and Bosanquet, A.: Temporomandibular joint arthroscopy. J. Oral Maxillofac. Surg. 45:962, 1986.

Jackson, R.W. and Dandy, D.J.: *Arthroscopy of the Knee.* Grune & Stratton, New York, 1976.

Kino, K., Ohnishi, M., Shioda, S., and Ichijo, T.: Morphological observation on the inner surface of the temporomandibular joint. Histological investigations relating to the arthroscopic findings in the upper cavity (in Japanese). Jpn. J. Oral Surg. 27:1379, 1981.

Kino, K.: Morphological and structural observation of the synovial membranes and their folds relating to the endoscopic findings in the upper cavity of the human temporomandibular joint (in Japanese, English abstract). J. Jpn. Stomat. 47:98–134, 1980.

Lutz, D., Schwipper, V., and Fritzemeier, C.U.: Die Endoskopie des Kiefergelekes—eine neue Untersuchungsmethode. Dtsch. Zahnaerztl. Z. 36:183–186, 1981.

Miki, M.: Influence of the temperature and pressure of the medium on the arthroscopic findings of the blood vessels of the synovial membrane (in Japanese). J. Jpn. Orthop. Assoc. 16:405–439, 1941.

Murakami, K. and Ito, K.: Arthroscopy of the temporomandibular joint, 3rd report: Clinical experience (in Japanese). Arthroscopy 9:49–59, 1984.

Murakami, K.I. and Hoshino, K.: Histological studies on the inner surfaces of the articular cavities of human temporomandibular joints with special reference to arthroscopic observations. Anat. Anz. 160:167–177, 1985.

Nuelle, D., Alpern, M.C., and Ufema, J.W.: Arthroscopic surgery of the temporomandibular joint. Angle Orthod. 56:118–141, 1986.

Ohnishi, M.: Diagnostic application of arthroscope to ankylosis of the temporomandibular joint (in Japanese). Jpn. J. Oral Surg. 22:436–442. 1976.

Tarro, A.: Arthroscopic diagnosis and surgery of the temporomandibular joint. J. Oral Maxillofac. Surg. 46:282, 1988.

Leon A. Assael

CHAPTER 32

Arthrotomy for Internal Derangements

Surgery is an invasive means of altering the anatomy and functional relationship of biologic structures. Surgery has been of particular interest to those treating temporomandibular disorders (TMDs) because internal derangements are seen most simplistically as anatomic defects requiring anatomic repair. Although this repair may be attempted nonsurgically by means of long-term therapy, little doubt exists that open visualization with repair of a structure is an attractive way of assuring correction of pathology. Surgery can also provide alternatives to the diseased structures by removing, replacing, or finding functional alternatives to body parts.

For some of the public and some health-care providers other than surgeons, surgery has the connotation of being a last resort for a grave illness. Because of anesthetic morbidity, risk of postoperative infection, and undeveloped techniques, it has been only in the later part of this century that surgeons have had the realistic opportunity to afford improvement for a wider range of pathology.

For the surgical treatment of temporomandibular joint (TMJ) pathology, the anatomic defects associated with disc displacement have been well delineated in living individuals since the arthrography work of Norgaard in 1947. Operative intervention for internal derangements of the TMJ occurred sporadically throughout the postwar era. Meniscectomy was reintroduced in the modern era by Dingman and Moorman[1] in 1951. It was not until 1979 that comprehensive operative repair of internal derangements was considered rational by a wide range of oral and maxillofacial surgeons

in the United States.[2-4] In that year, McCarty and Farrar[2] presented their clinical program for joint repair to the first large group of surgeons at the Southeastern Association of Oral and Maxillofacial Surgeons meeting in Knoxville. Much interest immediately ensued in academic centers about the scientific merit of surgical disc repair. This movement toward TMJ surgery was made possible in large part by the strong economic climate in the United States, the decreased risk of surgery, the development of more effective techniques, and the greater willingness of the public and health-care providers to supply surgical services for the less than grave maladies.

As the result of improved understanding of anatomic defects that contribute to TMDs, surgeons have developed techniques that repair, remove and replace, or produce reconfiguration of the diseased site. For example, the understanding of anterior disc displacement as a cause of TMJ pain has led to surgical techniques that include disc plication (repair), discectomy with graft (removal and reconstruction), and condylotomy (reconfiguration). This chapter addresses the spectrum of open surgical management of internal derangements. Arthroscopy is a surgical modality reviewed separately in Chapter 31.

ANATOMIC RATIONALE FOR ARTHROTOMY

As described elsewhere, internal derangement of the TMJ is an abnormal functional anatomic relationship between the condyle, disc, and glenoid fossa. This abnormal relationship may be present during all or part of the range of motion of the joint. It causes abnormal functional movements of the mandible. Internal derangement may produce dysfunction of related structures including the muscles of mastication and the teeth. Intrinsic joint pain may result from inflammation and direct pressure on sensory nerves of the retrodiscal tissues. Joint pain does not occur in normal function because forces within the joint are directed across the intermediate zone of the articular disc. Pain fibers are not present in the intermediate zone. When anterior disc displacement occurs, functional loads are directed across the highly innervated and vascularized retrodiscal tissues. In some individuals, disc displacements thus result in painful functional movements of the jaw. Muscle pain subsequently occurs from guarding and alternation of function jaw movements. Myofascial pain dysfunction syndrome with its cycle of hyperactivity, fatigue, spasm, and pain is the eventual course for many patients.[5]

Internal derangements may be divided into anterior medial disc displacement with reduction, disc displacement without reduction (locking), and disc displacement with perforation (see Chapter 9). Degenerative changes in disc morphology are progressive throughout this process. Early adhesions of the disc to other joint structures occur. The disc may be folded over anteriorly; it may be thickened or have areas of severe thinning. Perforation of the disc is often the expression of end-stage internal derangement or severe acute macrotrauma. The retrodiscal tissues are often inflamed and friable. A loss of elasticity of the retrodiscal tissues may be a factor in the redundancy and impingement of this area.

Each of these pathologic conditions may be associated with osseous changes including degeneration of cartilage, erosion, osteophyte formation, or severe resorption of bone. Bone apposition and degeneration may progress to include the condylar head, glenoid fossa, articular eminence, and tympanic plate. These osseous changes appear more frequently in disc displacements of long duration and in association with disc perforation.

Establishing an anatomic rationale for surgery must include adequate clinical evidence for an internal derangement and imaging evidence that correlates and qualifies the clinical diagnosis.[6] Imaging of the internal derangement can be accomplished with computerized tomography (CT), magnetic resonance imaging (MRI), arthrograms, or diagnostic arthroscopy. Imaging is indicated in order to confirm the clinical diagnosis, qualify its nature, and establish the patient's record.

The anatomic rationale for surgical correction of internal derangement is that repositioning of the disc and correction of ancillary abnormalities of the joint reconstitute a functional moiety and thereby restore health. With the structures of the reconstituted joint in a physiologic position, loading forces are no longer transmitted across the retrodiscal tissues. Hence, intrinsic joint pain is eliminated.

CLINICAL RATIONALE FOR ARTHROTOMY

Arthrotomy is indicated for internal derangement when there is anatomic rationale and sufficient clinical rationale. Patients should have pain in the joint that has produced a significant disability. Intra-articular pain should be refractory to adequate nonsurgical treatment.[7] Advocates of arthroscopy would say that the pain should have as well been refractory to arthroscopic treatment, but this point of view is still debated. Dysfunction may be a coindicator for surgery if hypomobility or annoying joint noise is a problem. Only rarely is dysfunction alone a sufficient indication for arthrotomy for the treatment of internal derangement.

If the pain in the joint can be markedly reduced by nonsurgical means, there is no clear clinical indication for surgery. The only remaining rationale for performing surgery is anatomic correction when pain is not a factor. Advocates of surgery for these cases state that future disease will be prevented by performing arthrotomy. Some opinions have been presented to indicate that osteoarthrosis is a sequela of untreated disc displacement.[3,4,8-10] However, a large body of evidence also suggests that a surgically treated joint also may undergo further degeneration.[11-13]

If surgery could be performed without any morbidity or cost, then anatomic correction would appear to make sense if methods of repair that obviated subsequent degenerative changes could be used. However, the known sequelae of arthrotomy include facial scar, lateral ligament scarring, and sensory denervation of the area. Arthrotomy is also an expensive procedure that produces a period of postsurgical disability. Furthermore, it exposes patients to many potential operative and postoperative complications. For these reasons, TMJ surgery is reserved for those who have both documented anatomic and clinical rationale[3] for surgery.

PRESURGICAL DIAGNOSIS

A complete history should be taken and patient evaluation performed as described in Chapter 17. The clinical evaluation should reveal symptoms directly referable to the TMJ. These include pain, clicking, locking, and crepitation. Tenderness of the lateral ligament and retrodiscal tissues (palpated transaurally) is usually present. Visible or palpable edema of the joint may be noted.

Auscultation may reveal joint noise. Early opening clicks indicate possible minimal disc displacement with reduction. Late opening

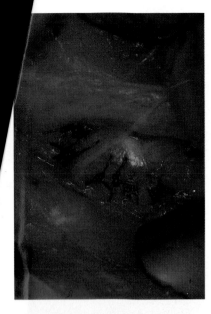

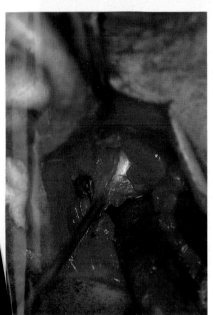

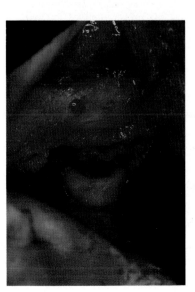

FIGURE 32-10. Suturing of the disc. Once the disc has been sutured into its new position, it is closely adapted to the condyle and moves with it during translation.

B

FIGURE 32-12. Meniscectomy. *A* and *B*, Clinical view demonstrates freeing the meniscus and the specimen.

E 32-14. High condylectomy. Resection of the r portion of the head of the condyle is performed se the joint space.

clicks indicate more extensive disc displacement. In anterior disc displacement without reduction, no joint noise may be evident. Crepitation is a sign of extensive inflammation or perforation of the disc. Joint noise may also be the result of osseous abnormalities and abnormalities of functional movement (see Chapter 9).

Because so many patients with symptoms of a TMD do not have disc displacement, the presurgical workup must confirm the presence of a disc displacement. The workup must include visualization of the disc to establish its anatomic position during function. This may be accomplished using arthrography, arthroscopy, MRI, or CT. The simple presence of joint noise does not establish the diagnosis of disc displacement.

Imaging also offers additional descriptive information on the clinical diagnosis and can help assess the results of therapy. Determining the extent of disc displacement and the direction of displacement permits a more precise surgical treatment plan. The surgical procedure for disc repair does not offer a precise view of disc position and morphology during function. Preoperative imaging, particularly MRI or double-contrast arthrography, assists in the design of disc surgery. Preoperative imaging can also be used to assess the result of surgery if accompanied by intraoperative or postoperative imaging.

PRESURGICAL CARE

The treatment of internal derangements usually consists of a period of initial nonsurgical therapy. Nonsurgical treatment is designed to alleviate symptoms. One of the clinician's goals should always be to decrease the muscular component of symptoms as much as possible before surgery. Another goal should be to improve jaw function and decrease jaw pain sufficiently to avoid the need for surgical repair. This is done with splint therapy, rest, heat, and nonsteroidal anti-inflammatory analgesics. Sufficient time should be given to each modality to assess its effect. The extension of supportive therapy to eliminate the need for surgical repair is controversial, particularly for those who believe that the persistence of disc displacement alone, even if asymptomatic, is rationale enough to perform surgical repair. No clear evidence supports the need for disc repair in minimally symptomatic disc displacement.

The results of surgical therapy following the mitigation of myofascial pain dysfunction symptoms have been shown to be superior to surgical therapy in the absence of presurgical care. Disc displacement is only one of the irritants that may result in myofascial pain dysfunction. Hence, disc repair alone may not alleviate all symptoms related to jaw function. Proper presurgical evaluation in this regard helps a clinician establish a realistic prognosis.

SURGICAL PROCEDURES: REPAIR, REMOVAL AND RECONSTRUCTION, OR RECONFIGURATION

Contemporary repair of disc displacement is reliably performed through open arthrotomy. The structures of the joint are revealed through a transcutaneous surgical approach. These structures may be altered to reproduce more closely the condition of a normal joint. Alternatively, the abnormal structure may be removed and replaced or reconfigured into a new functional relationship.

Surgical access is designed to gain complete exposure of all important joint structures in an aesthetic fashion while preserving all surrounding vital structures from damage. Vital structures include the temporal and frontal branches of the facial nerve. These branches provide motor activity to the muscles of facial expression of the upper face, including the frontalis and the orbicularis oculi. The parotid capsule, external and middle ear, superficial temporal and internal maxillary artery, middle cranial fossa, and trigeminal nerve are additional structures that must be protected from injury during arthrotomy.[14]

The scalp hair must often be shaved sufficiently to keep it out of the wound. The skin incision is most commonly made in the preauricular crease (Figs. 32–1 and 32–3). This is the most common location because it is a natural tension line with access to the joint. The curvilinear nature of the incision limits reflection, however, so some surgeons extend the incision anteriorly above the hairline in a hockey stick–like fashion. Alternatively, some surgeons extend the incision superiorly to produce a hemicoronal flap. The disadvantages of both of these approaches are increased dissection and the risk of alopecia. Elevation of a skin flap as performed in rhytidectomy offers further ease of reflection for those cases in which the skin incision is not extended (Figs. 32–2 and 32–3). Young individuals often do not have a

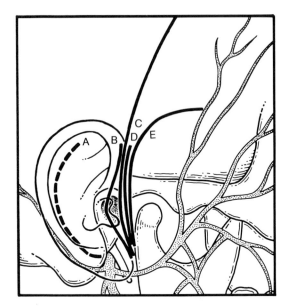

FIGURE 32-3. Surgical approaches to the capsule. The posterior auricular (A), endaural (B), hemicoronal (C), preauricular (D), and extended preauricular (E) incisions offer alternative means to enter the joint capsule.

clear preauricular crease. In these patients, the incision can be made endaurally in the external ear along the cartilage in order to hide the incision (see Fig. 32–3). All preauricular incisions place portions of the auriculotemporal nerve at risk for transection.

A retroauricular skin incision further hides the incision and protects the auriculotemporal nerve (see Fig. 32–3).[15,16] This approach requires an arc-shaped incision behind the ear. The external auditory canal is transected, and the ear is reflected forward to gain access to the joint. Possible problems with this incision include stenosis of the external auditory canal, change of the ear position, and atrophy of the external ear.[8] As a result, it has not gained popularity.

Once the skin incision is made, anterior, inferior, and superior reflection is performed to reveal the superficial temporal fascia and a small portion of its contiguous parotidomasseteric fascia (Fig. 32–4). During this reflection, the superficial temporal artery may be ligated or retracted anteriorly. Retraction is recommended because of the theoretic role that changes in superficial temporal artery vascularity have been known to play in facial pain.

Contained within the superficial fascial layer (superficial temporal fascia, parotidomasseteric fascia) now revealed the temporal and frontal branches of the facial nerve (see Fig. 32–4). These branches were frequently injured in the past when surgeons performed horizontal incisions into the capsule at this point. The temporal and frontal branches course anteriorly and cephalad across the glenoid fossa between 0.8 and 3.5 cm in front of the tympanic plate[17] (Fig. 32–5). Not only are the fibers contained within the superficial temporal fascia, but the fascia is closely apposed to the periosteum of the glenoid fossae and the connective tissue of the lateral ligament[17] (see Fig. 32–4). In a particular patient, the temporal and frontal branches of the facial nerve may lie precisely over the portion of the joint requiring repair.

For these reasons, protection of the nerve requires that an oblique incision be made in the superficial temporal fascia above the zygomatic arch caudad to where the fascia splits into its superficial and deep portions (see Fig. 32–4). This incision reveals the fatty layer cephalad to the zygomatic arch-glenoid fossa. A longitudi-

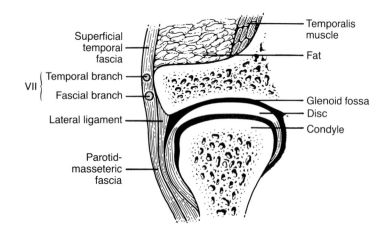

FIGURE 32-4. Location of the facial nerve and capsule. The frontal and temporal branches of the facial nerve are closely adapted to the superficial temporal fascia. The lateral ligament of the capsule is just deep to this fascia.

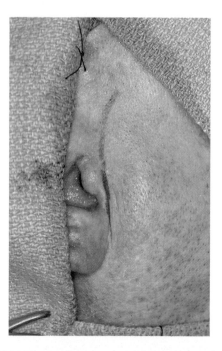

FIGURE 32-1. Skin incision. The standard preauricular skin incision provides simple and aesthetic access to the temporomandibular joint.

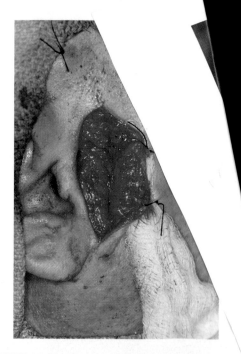

FIGURE 32-2. Skin flaps. A skin flap as performed rhytidectomy improves access and visualization.

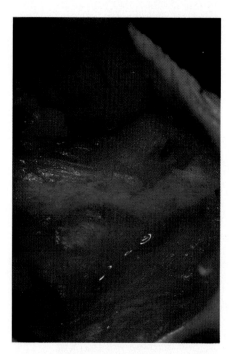

FIGURE 32-6. Surgical access to the capsule. After the superficial temporal fascia is dissected anteriorly and inferiorly and after an oblique incision is made cephalad to the glenoid fossa, the capsule is revealed.

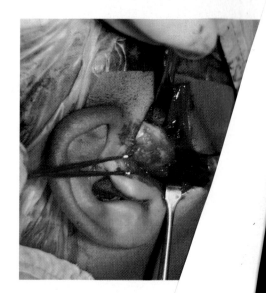

FIGURE 32-7. Arthrotomy approach permits free access to joint.

FIGU
superio
to incre

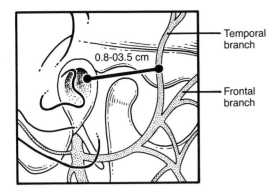

FIGURE 32–5. Facial nerve in relation to the capsule. The temporal ramus is between 0.8 and 3.5 cm anterior to the tympanic plate.

nal incision can then be safely made in the periosteum of the glenoid fossa superior and medial to where the lateral ligament and investing fascia are so closely apposed. This incision is accompanied by a vertical incision over the middle root of the zygomatic arch directly in front of the tympanic plate. Inferior-anterior reflection of periosteum and superficial fibers of the lateral ligament describes a safe and complete access to the capsule of the TMJ (Fig. 32–6).

Before the capsule is entered, it is useful to carry the mandible through its excursions so that the functional derangements, such as clicking or locking, can be duplicated. Mandibular movement is often assisted by placing a towel clip at the angle of the mandible. Alternatively, a mouth prop or pin at the angle of the mandible has been utilized. None of these methods precisely replicates mandibular excursions in an awake patient. Hence, preoperative physical findings may not be repeatable in the operating room.

A horizontal incision is first made in the superior joint space because it is more lateral for simpler access. Direct observations of disc position can now be made. Before the inferior joint space is entered, the position of the disc is identified. This is accomplished by inferiorly distracting the condyle and identifying the posterior band. The band is seen as a thickening of the avascular component of the disc just anterior to the vascular retrodiscal tissues. The posterior band should sit directly cephalad to the condylar head when inferior distraction is obtained with the clip at the angle of the mandible in the closed position. In severe disc displacement, the retrodiscal tissues are identified without difficulty. Perforations are also identi-

fied simply through the superior joint space view. Most disc perforations are seen laterally. Dissection of the glenoid fossa and articular eminence is accomplished in a plane that does not disturb the articular surface. Examination of the glenoid fossa and articular eminence is made through the superior joint space. Abnormalities of contour and degenerative changes can be identified.

A horizontal incision is then made in the inferior joint space. If this incision is made low in the capsule, excess tissue is released for repair and suturing. A low capsular incision also prevents damage to the cartilage of the condylar head. After the inferior joint space is entered, further understanding of the disc morphology can be gained. Thickenings and adhesions are identified. The disc is freed from its lateral ligament constraints and can now be repositioned as it is examined. If only the most lateral portion of the disc is clamped during this repositioning, damage to tissue planned for retention can be avoided.

The condylar head is examined through the inferior joint space for abnormalities of the cartilage and bone. Fibrillation of the condylar head cartilage is often present in osteoarthrosis and disc perforation. Distracting the condyle inferiorly reveals the medial pole of the condyle and often assists in disc repositioning. Hinge axis and translation of the condyle at this stage offer a sense of the condyle-fossa interaction and reveal abnormalities of bone contour. Some of these include a steep eminence and degenerative changes due to osteoarthrosis (Fig. 32–7).

Repair

In patients undergoing capsular repair, a complete assessment of the existing abnormalities is made after dissection of the capsule. Repair is attempted when the disease has not progressed to the point of destruction of the hard- and soft-tissue components of the joint. Direct repair is not possible when disc perforation has resulted in the loss of a large portion of the disc. Repair is also not possible when there has been excessive resorption of the condyle or glenoid fossa. In these cases, replacement of parts of the joint is necessary.

Capsular repair is designed to restore the normal position and shape of all of the hard and soft tissues of the joint. The goal is to establish ideal morphology and structural relationships. Alterations in the shape of the condylar head and glenoid fossa are performed before disc repair. Osteophytes, adhesions, and contour defects are repaired with rotary and hand instruments. Osseous recontouring is also performed to permit the better accommodation of movements of the disc during translation. Advocates of eminectomy often propose this to permit movement of the disc without impingement.[18–20] Similarly, condylar head shave is advocated by some in order to increase the joint space, thereby limiting disc impingement.[21]

All osseous surgery permanently alters the nature of the articulating surface. The condylar head cartilage will not reform after condylar shave.[20] Further degenerative changes after osseous recontouring may occur. For these reasons, many surgeons believe that osseous recontouring should be minimized when capsular repair is attempted. The majority of cases may require no osseous surgery.

Disc repositioning with fixation is accomplished in capsular repair in order to prevent anterior and medial displacement of the disc in function (Fig. 32–8). The disc is positioned to place the posterior band at the superior pole of the condylar head in the closed position. In addition, disc repositioning is designed to permit the articulating surface of the disc to be the intermediate zone. This biconcave alignment puts the convex anterior slope of the condylar head against the inferior concave surface of the intermediate zone and the superior concave surface of the intermediate zone against the convex posterior slope of the articular eminence. The disc is also positioned to cover the entire lateral surface of the condylar head (see Fig. 32–10). In order to produce this position, the disc is draped to adapt closely to the condylar head where it will be sutured to the lateral ligament.

Soft-tissue resection and redraping are usually necessary to produce physiologic disc morphology and position because of alterations in form that occur in discs that are chronically displaced.[22–24] These maneuvers may include reshaping and thinning of the disc, resecting and closing the retrodiscal tissues, suturing the retrodiscal tissues alone, resecting the lateral portion of the disc, and freeing the disc from its attachments to the lateral pterygoid muscle and environs.

Reshaping and thinning the disc are performed to correctly fill the joint space.[24] This procedure is done after review of thickening of the disc and assessment of disc impingement during translation. Areas of folding and adhesion may make recontouring vital but difficult. Because excessive thinning may result in perforation, this procedure is best performed with a beaver-tail blade under microscopic visualization.

Resection of retrodiscal tissues may be necessary to remove redundancy caused by long-standing disc displacement.[7,19] In this technique, an appropriate wedge of tissue is removed to permit suturing the posterior portion of the disc to the retrodiscal tissues. The resected wedge is typically wider on the lateral portion than on the medial, allowing for posterior and lateral repositioning of the disc. Suturing of the disc posteriorly is accomplished with interrupted sutures (see Fig. 32–8).

Suturing of retrodiscal tissues alone has been described as a means of repositioning the disc without entering the inferior joint space[25,26] (Fig. 32–9). This procedure involves oversewing the retrodiscal tissues posteriorly. It may be combined with an eminectomy to increase the freedom of the disc to move with the condylar head. Although this procedure allows for the alteration of retrodiscal position, it does not allow alteration of the relationship of the disc to the lateral ligament.

Resection of the lateral portion of the disc can be performed in order to permit the close lateral adaptation of the disc to the condylar head. This procedure is done in conjunction with posterior repositioning of the disc. Suturing the disc to the lateral ligament thus results in a more secure posterior repositioning (Fig. 32–10). This technique helps ensure that the disc will continue to move with the condylar head during translation. This step is vital because any adhesion of the disc to the glenoid fossa anteriorly prevents posterior movement of the disc as the condyle returns to the fossa after translation. The result is anterior disc displacement. If the disc is properly positioned and closely adapted to the lateral pole of the condyle, anterior displacement of the disc is impossible.

Freeing the disc from the lateral pterygoid muscle and environs is often necessary to permit free movement of the disc posteriorly and laterally. This maneuver may be done by incising the anterior margin of the capsule through the inferior joint space. As previously discussed, the lateral pterygoid muscle probably has only a minimal role in disc position.[27] Scarring and folding over of the anterior disc may change this premise, however. Hence, lysis of

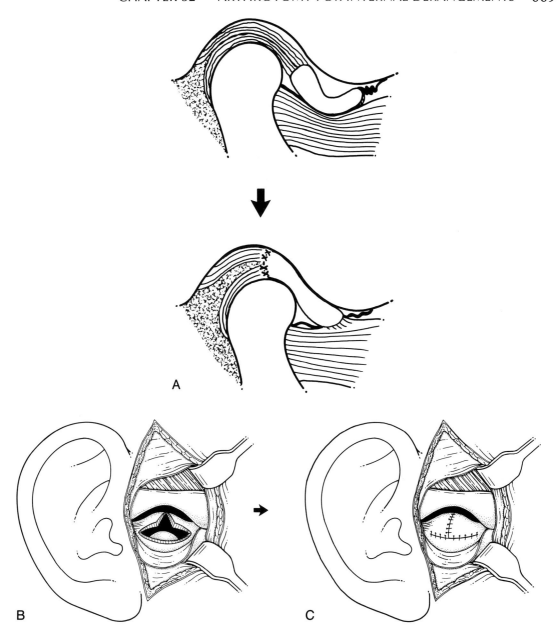

FIGURE 32–8. *A,* Disc plication. The disc may be repositioned posteriorly by resection and repair of retrodiscal tissues. *B,* The wedge removed permits posterior and lateral movement of the disc. *C,* The disc is sutured to the retrodiscal tissues and lateral ligament.

anterior disc attachments should be considered when simple release of the lateral disc attachments does not permit posterior movement of the disc.

Removal and Replacement

Removal of the disc (discectomy or meniscectomy) is generally performed when the disc does not appear to be repairable (Fig. 32–11). Inability to repair the disc may be the result of perforation, adhesion, hypertrophy, and scarring. Discectomy is also utilized for simple disc displacement without perforation. Under these circumstances, the rationale for removal of the disc is to eliminate the displacement of the disc and disc impingement.[1,11,12,28,29]

Removal of the disc is accomplished by com-

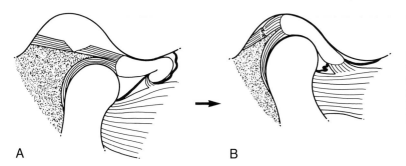

A   B

FIGURE 32–9. Disc plication without entering the inferior joint space. *A* and *B*, resection of retrodiscal tissues via the superior joint space permits posterior repositioning of the disc.

pletely freeing the disc from its ligamentous attachments (Fig. 32–12). The avascular articulating portion of the disc is usually all that is removed. In this circumstance, the condyle is left to function directly against the glenoid fossa. The biconcave nature of the joint is lost. A compound joint with two compartments is converted into a simple joint with one compartment.

The goal of disc replacement is to reconstruct the functional defect created by discectomy. Autogenous, allogeneic, and alloplastic materials have been utilized to replace the disc (Fig. 32–13). Autogenous materials include fascia lata, temporalis fascia, muscle, dermis,

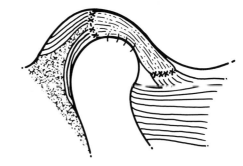

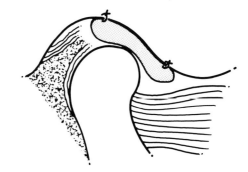

FIGURE 32–13. Disc replacement. The disc may be repaired with autogenous material sutured to the condylar head or allogeneic material fixed to the glenoid fossa.

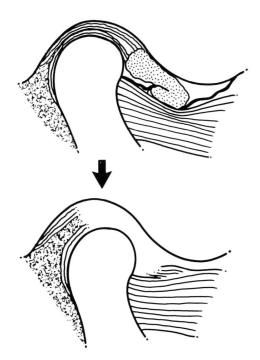

FIGURE 32–11. Meniscectomy. Removal of the central avascular portion of the disc is performed when scarring, adhesion, or perforation does not permit repair.

and cartilage.[30–35] A similar grouping of allogeneic materials has been used, including dura, fascia, collagen sheeting, and cartilage.[8,9] Autogenous material has the advantage of eliminating the possibility of antigenicity or disease transmission. The risk of viral transmission has eliminated the use of allogeneic dura.[8,9]

Alloplastic disc replacements may be made of acrylic, Silastic (silicone) sheeting, Teflon (polytetrafluoroethylene), [PTFE]-coated Proplast 1 and 2 (PTFE and vitreous carbon or aluminum oxide), and Gore-Tex.[13,36–39] Silastic and Gore-Tex replacements have been used as temporary implants.[40] These implants are retained long enough for a fibrous capsule to form. Subsequent to their removal, the dense fibrous connective tissue remains and becomes disc-like in function.

Tightening the lateral capsule follows the resection of the lateral portion of the disc and capsule. Reconstruction of the lateral capsule can be accomplished with temporal fascia flaps,[41] temporalis muscle flaps,[30] and Gore-Tex.[42] Reconstruction of the capsule helps prevent the ingrowth of scar tissue and helps stabilize the condyle-fossa relationship.

Removal of the condylar head has also been advocated as a means of correcting internal derangements, although its use in end-stage destructive lesions of the condyle is much more frequent.[43] Replacement of the condylar head is often then accomplished with costochondral grafting[44] or with alloplastic replacement.[45,46] The most common joint prosthesis utilized in the United States in the 1980s was the Vitek Kent prosthesis.[45] Prostheses have been developed for both the condylar head and fossa. Fossa implants alone have been utilized in the surgical management of arthrosis.[47,48] Developments in precise preoperative imaging have permitted the construction of custom prostheses. One current method produces a glenoid fossa of titanium and polyethylene and a condyle of titanium with a chromium cobalt molybdenum cap.[49]

Reconfiguration

Alteration of the functional anatomy of the TMJ from its existing state is utilized as a means of managing internal derangements without providing true surgical correction. These reconfigurations provide alternate means of producing pain-free function of the joint. Techniques that treat internal derangements in this manner include capsular rearrangement, condylotomy, high condylectomy, eminectomy, and auriculotemporal neurectomy.

Capsular rearrangement is a technique in which the lateral ligament is freed from the disc and the disc is detached from adhesions within the joint spaces.[41] The lateral ligament is reconstructed with a pedicled temporalis fascia flap. The technique is designed to permit free movement of the disc. Reconstruction of the capsule with fascia may prevent the reinnervation of the capsule by the auriculotemporal nerve.

Condylotomy provides a means of increasing the joint space and creating a new func-

tional condyle-disc-fossa relationship without performing an intra-articular procedure[50,51] (Fig. 32–14). A subcondylar osteotomy is created in the coronoid notch, either transorally or through a retromandibular approach. The condyle finds a new articulating surface more anterior-inferior and medial to its presurgical position. In addition, the lateral pterygoid muscle becomes shortened. Impingement on retrodiscal tissues is reduced. No attempt is made to identify or alter disc position during surgery.[51]

High condylectomy is the removal of 1 to 4 mm of the condylar head (Fig. 32–15).[21] Once the condylar head is reduced, it is recontoured to prevent impingement. The disc is then reattached to the condyle with the assistance of holes drilled into the residual condylar head.[21] This procedure is thought to increase the joint space, thereby permitting freer movement of the disc. The condyle is left to function in a new position. No regrowth of the articular cartilage occurs.

Eminectomy is a procedure that removes a portion of the posterior slope of the articular eminence,[2,10,20,25] producing a changed relationship between the disc and fossa during translation. The increased joint space produced is thought to reduce disc impingement and hypermobility of the condyle.

Auriculotemporal neurectomy is performed by neurotmesis or open cryosurgical technique to eliminate sensation to most of the structure of the capsule. An asymptomatic joint usually results from this technique, but no change occurs in the position of joint structures. Most auriculotemporal neurectomies provide only temporary relief of intractable joint pain.[52]

Condylar head plication is utilized to limit the translation of the condyle anteriorly (Fig. 32–16). In this method, suturing the condylar head to the glenoid fossa or placing an obstruction on the articular eminence limits translation. Alloplasts, bone grafts, and osteotomies have been used for this purpose.[10] By limiting mobility of the condyle, the return of disc displacement is thought to be less likely.

POSTSURGICAL CARE

The goals of postsurgical care are to rehabilitate patients from the procedure without morbidity and to adapt patients to the changes in TMJ function. Although repair, removal and reconstruction, and reconfiguration might seem to offer different avenues toward success-

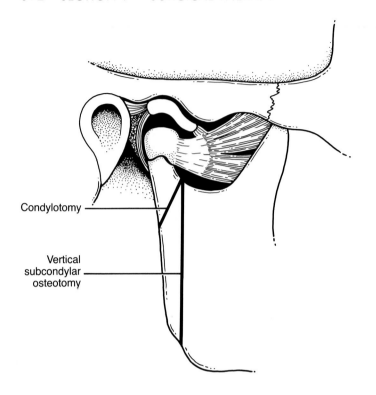

FIGURE 32–15. Condylotomy. A subcondylar osteotomy is performed either high or low to permit increased joint space.

Condylotomy

Vertical subcondylar osteotomy

ful postoperative management, the care of these patients is remarkably similar.

Rehabilitation following surgery always has the features of prevention of infection, pain control, incremental controlled loading of the joint, progressive mobilization of the joint, and physical therapy.

Careful attention to sterile surgical technique, hemostasis, irrigation, and closure of the wound to prevent dead space decreases the risk of infection. Perioperative antibiotics active against skin organisms are widely used. Pain control is usually accomplished with parenteral narcotics during hospitalization. A narcotic-acetaminophen combination is helpful after discharge. Nonsteroidal anti-inflammatory medication is often stopped before surgery and not continued for several days afterward be-

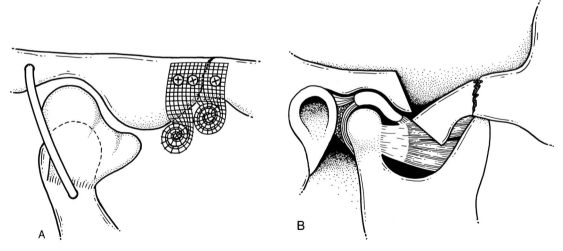

A   B

FIGURE 32–16. Treatment of hypermobility. Suturing the condyle to the glenoid fossa implant (*A*) or osteotomy (*B*) of the articular eminence can be performed to reduce hypermobility.

cause of the platelet function disorder that it may produce.

Joint loading during mastication is incrementally increased in the postoperative period. Although many surgeons keep their patients on a soft diet for many weeks following surgery, others advocate early and complete return to a normal diet.[21,45] In specific instances, early loading may be harmful. Temporary Silastic implants in particular are not subjected to loading.

Progressive mobilization of the joint is necessary to prevent fibrous adhesion and fibrous ankylosis. Physical therapy is the means to ensure progressive mobilization. Patients who receive physical therapy gain early motion with less pain.[53] Mobilization can be divided into active and passive motion.

In active motion, patients are given exercises in which maximum range of motion (opening, excursions, and protrusion) is performed, often several times an hour. These motions are best made in front of a mirror so that patients can assess their own movements. The goal is to achieve an opening of 35 mm and symmetric, adequate, mandibular excursions in the initial weeks following surgery.

Passive motion is a form of physical therapy in which an external method provides the motion of the joint. Among the most effective means of applying this method in postoperative physiotherapy is by continuous passive motion (CPM), which has been utilized to restore joint function by applying sustained low-force movement.[54] A powered device applied to the jaws continuously opens and closes the mouth passively. Passive motion can also be applied manually (see Chapter 24).

RESULTS OF ARTHROTOMY FOR INTERNAL DERANGEMENT

Interpreting the results of TMJ surgery can be difficult. When reviewing the results of a particular clinical report in a peer-reviewed journal, clinicians are presented with variables that far exceed the intrinsic health of the joint. Some of these variables affecting clinical results are patient selection, indications for surgery, patient-physician rapport, other adjunctive therapy, and reporting criteria.[55] Individual review of these factors assists clinicians in the critical analysis of arthrotomy procedures.

Patient Selection. Patients are asked to be excellent historians. They must report on subtle variations of symptoms over time. They must serve as partners in their rehabilitation. They are the final arbiters on the results of their surgery. Hence, the type of patient presenting for surgical treatment may have a significant effect on the reported results.

Indications for Surgery. Do all patients who proceed to arthrotomy meet the same diagnostic criteria? For example, the results of arthrotomy in patients in whom muscle pain has not been mitigated before surgery may be different from results in patients in whom there is no muscle component. Results of surgery for early disc displacement with minimal pain might be different from results for advanced osteoarthrosis. If a surgeon operates on patients with destructive disc pathology and bruxism, results might be adversely affected. Only if patients are in comparable diagnostic groups can the results of surgery be accurately assessed.

Patient-Physician Rapport. Patients who see their surgeon as a kind healer report more favorable postoperative symptoms than patients who perceive their surgeon to be unsympathetic and self-motivated. Continuous and long-term postoperative involvement by the surgeon in care may also positively influence patients' reporting of their symptoms.

Adjunctive Therapy. Patients who are receiving physical therapy, splint therapy, or psychosocial counselling, for example, may report results different from other groups, regardless of the procedure performed.

Reporting Criteria. Self-reporting of surgical results is a notoriously poor way of assessing the results of care. Patients may not wish to offend a surgeon by adverse reporting. Surgeons may gloss over findings in order to color the results in favor of a procedure they believe in. Conversely, a more in-depth search for problems may be the result of a surgeon's becoming dissatisfied with a procedure or material.

In view of all of these reporting problems, it is remarkable that such a large volume of information is available in peer-reviewed journals with regard to arthrotomy of the TMJ. These problems reflect the importance of obtaining multiple views that are carefully analyzed before becoming an advocate or a detractor of a particular procedure.

Results of Disc Repair

The results of disc repair are widely reported. Central to the debate over results is whether the repaired disc will heal. Much evidence indicates that the avascular portion of the disc will not heal,[56] although some investigators have reported successful healing.[57] The junction of the posterior band and retrodiscal tissues is clearly capable of healing after surgical repair, however.[58] Hall[26] produced evidence of good disc repair in experimental animals that had plication in conjunction with osseous surgery. Because many reports of disc repair do not clearly describe the location of resected tissues, some variability in reported results might be expected.

Correlation of disease states identified in the diagnostic phase with operative findings is important in planning disc repair properly. Bronstein and colleagues[59] demonstrated close correlation between operative and arthrographic findings. Westesson demonstrated close anatomic correlation with MRI.

A large body of evidence indicates that disc repair is a successful clinical procedure. The first report of a large series of patients' undergoing disc plication was published by McCarty and Farrar[2] in 1979. They reported a 94% success rate in 327 cases, although the criteria for success became better defined in later reports. The use of objective measurements, postoperative imaging, and clinical pain scales has assisted in improving the quality of data with regard to disc repair. Elias and Weber[18] reported on 81 patients who underwent disc repair and eminectomy. Pain was alleviated in all but three joints, and clicking persisted in eight.

Partial-thickness disc plication and eminectomy without entering the inferior joint space were reported by Hall[26] in 149 joints. Of these patients, 94% indicated elimination or improvement of pain, whereas 23% had persistent joint noise. Stern[60] reported on the results of surturing the disc to the condyle without resection. He reported complete success in all 25 patients, with a significant reduction in pain.

Maximum velocity during opening is sharply decreased in patients with symptomatic internal derangements.[61] Assessment of the results of disc repair indicates that velocity during opening that was less than 50% of normal preoperatively had returned to 85% of normal 1 year postoperatively.

Long-term followup of disc repair continues to indicate that this is a successful modality for surgical management. Not all joints can successfully undergo repair. As osseous changes and disc destruction associated with late internal derangements increase, simple repair becomes impossible.

Results of Removal and Replacement
Results of Discectomy

Removal of the disc is a time-honored means of managing internal derangement.[62,63] Dingman and colleagues[1] reported on discectomy as a comprehensive means of surgical management of all painful TMJs. Degenerative changes in the joint after discectomy are universally reported since presented by Agerberg and Lundberg[64] in 1971. In experimental animals, these changes include dullness and roughening of the articular surface and hyperplasia of the surface cartilage, as well as fibroankylosis.[65,66] Eriksson and Westesson[11] reported structural bony changes 1 year after surgery in all 26 patients who underwent discectomy.

Evidence still exists that replacement of the disc after discectomy may not be necessary. Hall[28] reported on 53 patients who underwent discectomy without replacement 5 years after surgery. Only minimal changes in joint morphology were noted. Of these patients, 72% were free of pain, and 92% had normal mastication.[28] Review of articular surface changes after discectomy in primates revealed that discectomy without replacement maintained joint architecture as well as dermis, Proplast laminates, and temporalis muscle flaps.[67] It remains clear, however, that the loss of disc continuity results in degenerative changes.[68,69]

Bessete[61] reported that patients had achieved 100% of normal mandibular velocity during opening within 1 year after meniscectomy alone. Eriksson and Westesson[12] reported on 15 patients with a remarkable 29-year mean followup after meniscectomy. All of the patients were pain free, although ten had crepitant joints. Tolvanen and colleagues[70] reported similar results in five meniscectomy patients, 30 to 40 years after surgery. These investigators indicate that meniscectomy should remain a useful modality in the treatment of internal derangement.

Results of Discectomy with Replacement

Placement of an autogenous material in the discectomy site remains a popular means of reconstruction.[71] Temporalis fascia grafts have been utilized in both a free and pedicled fashion.[72] Evaluation of temporalis muscle flaps and auricular cartilage grafts for disc replacement has revealed strong improvement in pain and function for both groups.[73,74] Purdy[75] reported a 2-year followup on his first nine temporalis patients with a muscle flap; all nine had a marked decrease in pain and increase in range of motion. In 26 cases of temporalis muscle flap for disc replacement, Pogrel and Kaban[75] reported adequate range of motion in all patients and no need for reoperation. Herbosa and Rotskoff[31] reported on 15 patients who received pedicled temporalis muscle flaps for disc replacement. All patients had improvement of pain and range of motion; however, a reduction of translation was noted.

Autologous auricular cartilage for disc replacement was introduced by Witsenberg and Freihofer[77] and reviewed by Matukas and Lochner[78] in 22 patients. Pain relief and good function were reported at 3 to 24 months in 20 of these individuals. Ionnides and Freihofer[79] demonstrated success in 14 of 17 paitnets who underwent auricular cartilage grafts. Kent[74] compared auricular cartilage replacement with temporalis muscle and found superior function and pain relief with the cartilage grafts.

Dermal grafts have gained wide acceptance since they were introduced by Georgiade[80] in 1962. The results of dermal grafts for disc replacement were reported by Meyer.[33] Of 58 patients, 51 had a successful return to pain-free function after this procedure. Tucker and colleagues[81] showed a return of disc continuity in discs repaired with dermis but no repair in nongrafted experimental perforations.

Disc replacement with reinforced silicone sheeting has gained wide use. Sanders and colleagues[46] utilized it in high condylectomy as well. Problems with this method of disc replacement were soon recognized. Foreign body giant cell reaction and material degeneration were found by Dolwick[19] in all reoperated cases. Synovitis was demonstrated after Silastic degeneration by Worsing and associates.[82] Fixation of these implants and delayed loading were found to be important factors in sustaining success.[83,84]

Temporary Silastic implants have been shown to recreate disc architecture by the fibrous capsule that forms around them.[40] Deterioration of even these temporary implants remains a problem, however.[40,71,85] The results have been inflammation and synovitis. The use of Silastic implants in contemporary practice is widespread, however.

Replacement of the disc with Proplast-Teflon implants was a widely chosen modality in the 1980s,[49] although Gallagher and Wolford[37] demonstrated no superior clinical results over Silastic. Numerous reports of condylar degeneration and symptoms resulted in its discontinuation as an implant material.[71,86–88]

Wagner and Mosby[89] reported on 31 cases in which pain, malocclusion, hypomobility, and condylar degeneration resulted. Severe erosion of the glenoid fossa has resulted in perforation of the middle cranial fossa by a Teflon-Proplast implant.[90] Florine and colleagues[13] compared findings in Proplast disc replacements with disc repair and found joint destruction in only the Proplast group.

Good clinical results in six cases have been reported by Kondoh and colleagues[39] for Gore-Tex (EPTFE) as a disc replacement. Feinberg and Smilak[42] employed Gore-Tex as a reconstructive implant of the lateral ligament in 15 patients, with good functional results. No large series or long-term followup results have thus far been presented for Gore-Tex to date.

Fossa prostheses of Proplast have demonstrated significant wear on the order of 1 mm/year.[91] Rooney and colleagues[92] reported three cases of rapid condylar resorption after placement of Proplast fossa implants. The survival of glenoid fossa prostheses was reported by Kent and Block[93] to be 60.9%.

Condylar head replacement has presented many difficulties when alloplasts are used, with many cases failing and requiring removal. Complications include infection, resorption, hypomobility, and implant failure. Kent and associates,[45] however, reported successful joint replacement in 87% of cases when the Vitek implant was used. Jungels[48] presented 57 cases of cast vitallium-acrylic joint replacements with good results. Costochondral grafting has also been utilized for end-stage internal derangements, with a high degree of success.[44]

Results of Reconfiguration
Capsular Rearrangement

Toller[41] reported on 14 patients who underwent capsular rearrangement; there was one failure. Although this procedure held early promise for success, its use was supplanted in the late 1970s by disc repositioning and repair. Much of the success of capsular rearrangement may have been due to denervation of the auriculotemporal nerve, because no reduction of disc displacement was obtained.

High Condylectomy

High condylectomy with disc repair was reported on by Walker and Kalamichi.[21] Nearly all patients obtained improved function and pain relief with active postoperative physical therapy. Eppley and Delfino[32] reported on 47 high condylectomies with disc repair; 28% of patients had persistent joint pain, and 60% had deviation to the operated side at 24 months. Dolwick[19] studied 68 joints treated with high condylectomy and disc repositioning. Although an 88% success rate was reported, a preference for disc repair without high condylectomy has subsequently developed. Politis and colleagues[94] reported long-term followup of 14 cases of high condylectomy in which eight cases had unsatisfactory results requiring additional surgery. The poor results may be secondary to the irreversible destruction of the articular cartilage that is a necessary result of high condylectomy. Use of this technique might best be reserved for those joints that have already undergone articular cartilage destruction.

Eminectomy

Eminectomy is usually performed in combination with disc repair. Kerstens and associates[95] observed 30 patients who underwent eminectomy and discoplasty for internal derangements; 87% of patients had symptomatic relief. Kerstens and associates[95] used eminectomy alone when the disc position was corrected by the increased joint space. Eppley and Delfino[32] noted less deviation to the operated side than in high condylectomy on 63 patients who received eminectomy and disc repair for internal derangements.

Weinberg and Consens[96] emphasized the importance of disc repositioning and suturing to the condylar head when eminectomy was performed. Prevention of adhesion of the disc to the condylar head permits free function without disc impingement. The workers reported a 90% success rate with this procedure.

Merrill[10] stated that hypermobility was occasionally the cause of disc displacement. As a result, eminoplasty by means of zygomatic arch osteotomy, implant, or eminectomy can be utilized to reduce hypermobility. This procedure can be done in combination with disc repair with good results.

Condylotomy

Ward and colleagues[97,98] reported initial results of excellent success with condylotomy for treatment of TMDs. In 1975, Banks and Mackenzie[50] presented 211 patients treated with condylotomy with a 91% success rate. Merrill[10] reported that condylotomy was a procedure that had 100% success in reducing pain and dysfunction. Nickerson and Boering[23] reported on 29 patients who underwent condylotomy. This study indicated that in 29 patients receiving a questionnaire at 5 years, 24% believed that they needed further treatment. Symptoms of muscle pain were persistent in 50% of patients. Bell and Yamaguchi[99] studied nine patients who had anterior disc displacement and who underwent vertical subcondylar osteotomy. Resolution of TMJ symptoms occurred in all patients, and skeletal malocclusion was also corrected.

Problems with condylotomy that persist include loss of vertical dimension, occlusal prematurity, and open bite.[9] Degenerative changes in the condyle have also been noted.

Neurectomy

Neurectomy has been shown to be an effective means of temporary relief of joint pain. Goss[52] observed six patients who underwent cryoneurectomy of the capsule. All patients had complete pain relief for 1 year, but pain eventually recurred in four patients.

DISCUSSION OF RESULTS OF ARTHROTOMY

A review of the results of procedures advocated for arthrotomy reveals a high rate of success for many modes of surgery. Problems that affect long-term health of the joint are also reported with many of these procedures. By understanding results, surgeons develop an evolving philosophy of therapy. Some of my own conclusions follow.

Surgical repair of the disc seems to offer a high degree of success without any of the features of long-term morbidity that removal and replacement or reconfiguration seem to show. Hence, discs that can be repaired should be repaired and not removed.

At some point, the retention of an untreatable disc will not resolve clinical pathology. Discectomy is indicated. Because of degenerative changes, I believe that replacement is desirable although not necessary.

Every alloplastic replacement for which there is long-term data indicates destructive pathology.[100,101] Hence, I do not currently employ alloplasts for disc replacement or for joint replacement, either permanent or temporary. Allogeneic materials introduce a range of medical problems that are not completely understood. Therefore, I do not believe that allogeneic disc replacement offers any advantages. Autogenous auricular cartilage, temporalis flaps, and dermis all seem to offer satisfactory long-term results without operative morbidity. They are currently the best materials for replacing the disc. Costochondral grafts do not appear to undergo late failure. As a result, they are preferable to any alloplastic replacement of the joint.

Reconfiguration of the joint is utilized when an identifiable geometric problem is present, such as osteophytes or a steep eminence. I have not continued to employ condylotomy because of the lack of control of the occlusal result.

SUMMARY

Surgical treatment of internal derangements of the TMJ offers the opportunity to relieve patients' pain and dysfunction. It should be reserved for conditions that are not amenable to nonsurgical treatment. Options for surgical intervention include those procedures that repair structures present, those that require the removal and possible replacement of structures, and those that offer functional alternatives to natural joint function. The results of surgery on the TMJ have been generally good in contemporary practice. Defining optimal procedures for given joint conditions awaits further careful scientific investigation.

REFERENCES

1. Dingman, R. and Moorman, W.: Menisectomy in the treatment of lesions of the temporomandibular joint. J. Oral Surg. 10:141, 1952.
2. McCarty, W. and Farrar, W.: Surgery for internal derangements of the temporomandibular joint. J. Prosthet. Dent. 42:191, 1979.
3. Farrar, W.B.: Diagnosis and treatment of anterior dislocation of the articular disk. N.Y. J. Dent. 41:348, 1971.
4. Farrar, W.B. and McCarty, W.: *A Clinical Outline of Temporomandibular Joint Diagnosis and Treatment.*

Normandie Publishers, Montgomery, Alabama, 1982.
5. Laskin, D.: Etiology of the pain-dysfunction syndrome. J. Am. Dent. Assoc. 79:147, 1969.
6. Shellhas, K.: Imaging and temporomandibular joint surgery. Oral and Maxillofacial Surgery Clinics of North America 1:221, 1989.
7. Dolwick, M., Reid, R., Sanders, B., et al: 1984 criteria for TMJ meniscus surgery. American Association of Oral and Maxillofacial Surgeons, 1984.
8. Braun, T.: Temporomandibular joint surgery. I. Surgical treatment of internal derangement. Selected Readings in Oral and Maxillofacial Surgery 1:3, 1989.
9. Braun, T.: Temporomandibular joint surgery, part 2. Selected Readings in Oral and Maxillofacial Surgery 1:4, 1990.
10. Merrill, R.: Mandibular dislocation and hypermobility. Oral and Maxillofacial Surgery Clinics of North America 1:399, 1989.
11. Eriksson, L. and Westesson, P.: Discectomy in the treatment of anterior disk displacement of the temporomandibular joint: clinical and radiologic one year follow up study. J. Prosthet. Dent. 55:106, 1986.
12. Eriksson, L. and Westesson, P.: Long-term evaluation of meniscectomy of the temporomandibular joint. J. Oral Maxillofac. Surg. 43:263, 1985.
13. Florine, B., Gatto, D., Wade, M., and Waite, D.: Tomographic evaluation of temporomandibular joints following diskoplasty or placement of PTFE implants. J. Oral Maxillofac. Surg. 46:183, 1988.
14. Howerton, D. and Zysset, M.: Anatomy of the temporomandibular joint and related structures with surgical anatomic considerations. Oral and Maxillofacial Surgery Clinics of North America 1:229, 1989.
15. Alexander, R. and James, R.: Postauricular approach for surgery of the temporomandibular articulation. J. Oral Surg. 33:346, 1975.
16. Walters, P. and Geist, E.: Correction of temporomandibular joint internal derangements by post auricular approach. J. Oral Maxillofac. Surg. 41:616, 1983.
17. Al Kayat, A. and Bramley, P.: A modified preauricular approach to the temporomandibular joint and malar arch. Br. J. Oral Surg. 17:91, 1979.
18. Elias, A. and Weber, W.: Surgical resolution of internal derangement of the temporomandibular joint. J. Oral Maxillofac. Surg. 48S:147, 1990.
19. Dolwick, F.: Surgical treatment of chronic anterior displacement of the TMJ meniscus. Abstract 62, Annual Meeting of American Association of Oral and Maxillofacial Surgeons, New Orleans, September, 1980.
20. Hall, M., Bdaughman, R., Ruskin, J., and Thompson, D.: Healing following meniscoplasty, eminectomy, and high condylectomy in the monkey temporomandibular joint. J. Oral Maxillofac. Surg. 44:177, 1986.
21. Walker, R. and Kalamichi, S.: A surgical technique for management of internal derangement of the temporomandibular joint. J. Oral Maxillofac. Surg. 45:299, 1987.
22. Hansson, T. and Nordstrom, B.: Thickness of soft tissue layers and articular disc in temporomandibular joint with deviations in form. Acta Odontol. Scand. 35:281, 1977.
23. Nickerson, J. and Boering, G.: Osteoarthrosis and internal derangement of the TMJ. Oral and Maxillofacial Surgery Clinics of North America 1:47, 1989.

24. Piper, M.: Microscopic disc preservation surgery of the temporomandibular joint. Oral and Maxillofacial Surgery Clinics of North America 1:279, 1989.

25. Hall M.: Meniscoplasty of the displaced temporomandibular joint meniscus without violating the inferior joint space. J. Oral Maxillofac. Surg. 42:788, 1984.

26. Hall, M.: Partial thickness plication of the TMJ disk in 149 joints. J. Oral Maxillofac. Surg. 47S:140, 1989.

27. Carpentier, P., Young, J., et al: Insertions of the lateral pterygoid muscle: An anatomic study of the human temporomandibular joint. J. Oral Maxillofac. Surg. 46:477, 1988.

28. Hall, H.D.: Evaluation of patients 5 years after diskectomy for TMJ pain. Educational Outlines and Summaries, American Association of Oral and Maxillofacial Surgeons, p. 208, 1988.

29. Hall, H.D. and Link, J.: Diskectomy alone and with ear cartilage interposition grafts in joint reconstruction. Oral and Maxillofacial Surgery Clinics of North America 1:329, 1989.

30. Feinberg, S. and Larsen, P.: The use of a pedicled temporalis muscle-pericranial flap for replacement of the TMJ disc. J. Oral Maxillofac. Surg. 47:142, 1989.

31. Herbosa, E. and Rotskoff, K.: Composite temporalis pedicle flap as an interpositional graft in temporomandibular joint arthroplasty. J. Oral Maxillofac. Surg. 48:1049, 1990.

32. Eppley, B. and Delfino, J.: Surgical treatment of internal derangements of the temporomandibular joint. J. Oral Maxillofac. Surg. 46:721, 1988.

33. Meyer, R.: Autogenous dermal grafts in reconstruction of the temporomandibular joint. Oral and Maxillofacial Surgery Clinics of North America 1:351, 1989.

34. Meyer, R.: The autogenous dermal graft in temporomandibular joint disk surgery. J. Oral Maxillofac. Surg. 46:948, 1988.

35. Narang, R. and Dixon, R.: Temporomandibular joint arthroplasty with fascia lata. Oral Surg. Oral Med. Oral Pathol. 39:45, 1975.

36. Howe, D.: Preformed Silastic temporomandibular joint implant. J. Oral Surg. 37:59, 1979.

37. Gallagher, D. and Wolford, L.: Comparison of Silastic and Proplast implants in the TMJ after condylectomy for osteoarthritis. J. Oral Maxillofac. Surg. 40:627, 1982.

38. Bee, D. and Zeitler, D.: The Proplast-Teflon implant in TMJ reconstruction following meniscectomy. Case Reports and Outlines American Association of Oral and Maxillofacial Surgeons, Annual Meeting, p. 24, 1986.

39. Kondoh, T., Norihiko, T., and Yutaka, S.: The arthroplasty of the TMJ employing Gore-Tex implants. J. Oral Maxillofac. Surg. 47:S94, 1989.

40. Eriksson, L. and Westessen, F.: Deterioration of temporary silicone implant in the temporomandibular joint: A clinical arthroscopic follow-up study. Oral Surg. Oral Med. Oral Pathol. 62:2, 1986.

41. Toller, P.: Temporomandibular capsular rearrangement. Br. J. Oral Surg. 2:157, 1964.

42. Feinberg, S. and Smilack, M.: Lateral capsular ligament reconstruction in temporomandibular joint surgery. J. Oral. Maxillofac. Surg. 46:6, 1988.

43. Henny, F. and Baldridge, O.: Condylectomy for the persistently painful TMJ. J. Oral Surg. 15:214, 1957.

44. MacIntosh, R.: Costochondral and dermal grafts in temporomandibular joint reconstruction. Oral and Maxillofacial Surgery Clinics of North America 1:363, 1989.

45. Kent, J., Misiek, D., and Akin, R.: Temporomandibular joint condylar prosthesis: A ten year report. J. Oral Maxillofac. Surg. 41:245, 1983.

46. Sanders, B., Brady, F., and Adams, D.: Silastic cap temporomandibular joint prosthesis. J. Oral Surg. 35:933, 1977.

47. Christensen, R.: Mandibular joint arthrosis corrected by insertion of a cast vitallium glenoid fossa prosthesis. Oral Surg. Oral Med. Oral Pathol. 17:712, 1964.

48. Jungels, B.: Total joint reconstruction utilizing the Christensen prosthesis. J. Oral Maxillofac. Surg. 48S:136, 1990.

49. Wolford, L.: Customized total temporomandibular joint prosthesis. J. Oral Maxillofac. Surg. 48S:76, 1990.

50. Banks, P. and Mackenzie, I.: Condylotomy: A clinical and experimental appraisal of a surgical technique. J. Maxillofac. Surg. 3:170, 1975.

51. Nickerson, J. and Veaco, N.: Condylotomy in surgery of the temporomandibular joint. Oral and Maxillofacial Surgery Clinics of North America 1:303, 1989.

52. Goss, A.: Cryoneurectomy for intractable temporomandibular joint pain. Br. J. Oral Maxillofac. Surg. 26:26, 1988.

53. Sommers, J. and Walters, P.: Comparison of range of motion in patients having immediate physical therapy after TMJ surgery to patients having delayed physical therapy. J. Oral and Maxillofac. Surg. 47S:141, 1989.

54. Fontenot, M. and Kent, J.: Continuous passive motion following total temporomandibular joint arthroplasty. J. Oral Maxillofac. Surg. 47:S138, 1989.

55. Sanders, B. and Buonocristiani, R.: Temporomandibular joint arthrotomy, management of failed cases. Oral and Maxillofacial Surgery Clinics of North America 1:443, 1989.

56. Zeitler, D.: Healing of meniscus surgery in cynomolgus monkey temporomandibular joints. Case Reports and Outlines of Scientific Sessions, American Association of Oral and Maxillofacial Surgeons, p. 49, 1984.

57. Stith, H., Walters, P., and Akin, R.: Surgical treatment of internal derangements of the temporomandibular joint. Review of 198 joints. Case Reports and Outlines of Scientific Sessions, American Association of Oral and Maxillofacial Surgeons, p. 59, 1984.

58. Wallace, D. and Laskin, D.: Healing of surgical incisions in the disk and retrodiskal tissues of rabbit TMJ. J. Oral Maxillofac. Surg. 44:965, 1986.

59. Bronstein, S., Tomasetti, B., and Ryan, D.: Internal derangements of the temporomandibular joint: Correlation of arthrography with surgical findings. J. Oral Surg. 39:572, 1981.

60. Stern, N.: An alternative procedure for repositioning the anteriorly displaced TMJ disc. J. Craniomand. Pract. 3:46, 1984.

61. Bessette, R.: Role of mandibular tracking in temporomandibular joint surgery. Oral and Maxillofacial Surgery Clinics of North America 1:205, 1989.

62. Annandale, T.: On displacement of the interarticular cartilage of the lower jaw and its treatment by operation. Lancet 1:411, 1887.

63. Silver, C.: Long term results of meniscectomy of the temporomandibular joint. J. Craniomand. Pract. 3:46, 1984.

64. Agerberg, G. and Lundberg, M.: Changes in the tem-

poromandibular joint after surgical treatment. A radiologic followup study. Oral Surg. Oral Med. Oral Pathol. 32:865, 1971.

65. Yaillen, D., et al: TMJ meniscectomy effects on joint structure and masticatory function in *Macaca fascicularis*. J. Maxillofac. Surg. 7:255, 1979.

66. Kwon, P.: Bony changes of the condyle following discectomy in the rabbit temporomandibular joint. J. Oral Maxillofac. Surg. 47S:77, 1989.

67. Block, M., Kent, J., and Walters, P.: Comparison of 5 discectomy treatments in primates. J. Oral Maxillofac. Surg. 47S:76, 1989.

68. Helmy, E., Bays, R., and Sharawy, M.: Osteoarthritis in the monkey TMJ following surgical disk perforation. J. Dent. Res. 4Z:281, 1985.

69. Laskin, D., Wheat, P., and Evaskus, D.: Effects of temporomandibular joint meniscectomy in adult and juvenile primates. American Association for Dental Research, Abstract, p. 350, 1977.

70. Tolvanen, M., Oikarinen, V., and Wolf, J.: A 30 year follow up study of temporomandibular joint meniscectomies: A report on five patients. Br. J. Oral Maxillofac. Surg. 26:311, 1988.

71. Wei Yung Yih and Merrill, R.: Pathology of alloplastic interpositional implants in the temporomandibular joint. Oral and Maxillofacial Surgery Clinics of North America 1:415, 1989.

72. Miller, T.: Temporalis fascia grafts. Plast. Reconstr. Surg. 65:236, 1980.

73. Albert, T., and Merrill, R.: Temporalis myofascial flap for reconstruction of the temporomandibular joint. Oral and Maxillofacial Surgery Clinics of North America 1:341, 1989.

74. Kent, J.: Evaluation of temporalis muscle flap and auricular cartilage grafts for temporomandibular joint reconstruction. J. Oral Maxillofac. Surg. 48S:148, 1990.

75. Purdy, W.: Long term performance of temporalis muscle flap when used as a disc replacement. J. Oral Maxillofac. Surg. 47S:80, 1989.

76. Pogrel, M. and Kaban, L.: The role of the temporalis fascial and muscle flap in temporomandibular joint surgery. J. Oral Maxillofac. Surg. 47S:78, 1989.

77. Witsenberg, B. and Freihofer, P.: Replacement of the pathological temporomandibular disk using autogenous cartilage of the external ear. Int. J. Oral Maxillofac. Surg. 13:401, 1984.

78. Matukas, V. and Lachner, J.: The use of autologous auricular cartilage for temporomandibular joint disc replacement. J. Oral Maxillofac. Surg. 48:348, 1990.

79. Ionnides, G. and Freihofer, H.: Replacement of the damaged intra-articular disk of the TMJ. J. Craniomaxillofac. Surg. 16:273, 1988.

80. Georgiade, N.: The surgical correction of temporomandibular joint dysfunction by means of autogenous dermal grafts. Plast. Reconstr. Surg. 30:412, 1962.

81. Tucker M., Jacoway, J., and White, R.: Autogenous dermal grafts for repair of temporomandibular joint disk perforations. J. Oral Maxillofac. Surg. 44:781, 1986.

82. Worsing, R., Engber, W., and Lange, T.: Reactive synovitis from particulate Silastic. J. Bone Joint Surg. [Am.] 64:581, 1982.

83. Rippert, E.: New design for Silastic implants in TMJ surgery. J. Oral Maxillofac. Surg. 44:163, 1986.

84. Gingrass, D., Ryan, D., Messer, E., and Sewall S.: Fixation of flexible implants in the temporomandibular joint. J. Craniomand. Pract. 4:313, 1986.

85. Westesson, F., Eriksson, L., and Lindstrom, C.: Destructive lesions of the mandibular condyle following diskectomy with temporary silicone implant. Oral Surg. Oral Med. Oral Pathol. 63:143, 1987.

86. Ryan, D.: Alloplastic implants in the temporomandibular joint. Oral and Maxillofacial Surgery Clinics of North America 1:427, 1989.

87. Schellas, K., Wilkes, C., El Deeb, M., et al: Permanent Proplast temporomandibular joint implants: MR imaging of destructive complications. AJR 151:731, 1988.

88. Morgan, J.: Evaluation of alloplastic TMJ implants. J. Craniomand. Pract. 6:224, 1988.

89. Wagner, J. and Mosby, E.: Assessment of Proplast Teflon disc replacements. J. Oral Maxillofac. Surg. 48:1140, 1990.

90. Baraducci, J., Thompson, D., and Scheffer, R.: Perforation into middle cranial fossa as a sequel to use of a Proplast-Teflon implant for TMJ reconstruction. J. Oral Maxillofac. Surg. 48:496, 1990.

91. Fontenot, M. and Kent, J.: Biomechanics of articular surface wear of retrieved fossa prostheses for the TMJ. J. Oral Maxillofac. Surg. 48S:133, 1990.

92. Rooney, T., Haug, R., Toor, A., and Indresano, A.: Rapid condylar degeneration after glenoid fossa prosthesis insertion. J. Oral Maxillofac. Surg. 46:240, 1988.

93. Kent, J. and Block, M.: Five year follow-up of the polymer glenoid fossa prosthesis for partial and total TMJ reconstruction. Educational Summaries and Outlines, American Association of Oral and Maxillofacial Surgeons, p. 156, 1988.

94. Politis, C., Stoelinga, P., Gerritsen, G., and Heyboer, A.: Long term results of surgical intervention on the TMJ. J. Craniomand. Pract. 7:319, 1989.

95. Kerstens, H., Tuinzing, D., and van der Kwast, W.: Eminectomy and discoplasty for correction of the displaced temporomandibular joint disc. J. Oral Maxillofac. Surg. 47:150, 1989.

96. Weinberg, S. and Cousens, G.: Menscocondylar plication: A modified operation for surgical repositioning of the ectopic temporomandibular joint meniscus. Oral Surg. Oral Med. Oral Pathol. 63:393, 1987.

97. Ward, T., Smith, D., and Sommar, M.: Condylotomy for mandibular joint arthroplasty. Plast. Reconstr. Surg. 38:179, 1966.

98. Ward, T.: Surgery of the mandibular joint. Anr. R. Col. Surg. Engl. 28:139, 1961.

99. Bell, W. and Yamaguchi, Y.: Treatment of TMJ dysfunction by intraoral vertical ramus osteotomies. Int. J. Adult Orthod. Orthog. Surg. 5:9, 1990.

100. Chase, D. and McCoy, M.: Histologic staging of internal derangement of the temporomandibular joint. Oral and Maxillofacial Surgery Clinics of North America 1:249, 1989.

101. Dolwick, M. and Aufdemorte, T.: Silicone induced foreign body reaction and lymphadenopathy after temporomandibular joint arthroplasty. Oral. Surg. Oral Med. Oral Pathol. 59:449, 1985.

102. Westesson, P., Katzberg, R., Tallents, R., et al: CT and MR of the temporomandibular joint: Comparison with autopsy specimens. AJR 148:1165, 1987.

Mark A. Piper

CHAPTER 33

A Rationale for Microsurgery

Surgical procedures on the temporomandibular joint (TMJ) have been proposed when alternative forms of noninvasive management have not proven successful.[1,2] This lack of success is generally measured in terms of pain or mechanical instability. Furthermore, documented imaging of structural pathology through arthrography[3-5] or magnetic resonance imaging[6-8] is used to confirm the type of discal displacement, and a surgical treatment plan is then formulated.

Although this may seem to be a logical approach to problems of disc displacement, in reality, the choice between invasive and noninvasive modalities is not always obvious.[9,10] In choosing between these alternatives, one must take into consideration the impact that pain or mechanical problems may have on an individual. Certainly there are patients who may have end-stage pathology on imaging, but these same patients may have been able to adjust to the pain so that they perceive no functional incapacitation. Other patients may have significant pain with only minimally demonstrable pathology on imaging. These individuals are often maintained indiscriminately on noninvasive modalities under the assumption that they will respond and adapt. This approach places a great deal of faith on the predictability of the progression or adaptability of the diseases of the TMJ, whereas in reality there are few documented studies that show that adaptation is always a truly positive event.[2,11,12]

The approaches to most problems of the TMJ are often aimed primarily at reversing discal displacement, whether through splints that prevent occlusal prematurities, splints that reposition the mandible, restorative or orthodontic procedures, arthroscopic surgery, or open joint surgery. The basic problem with all of these approaches, however, is a general lack of proof either before or after treatment that the position of the disc has been altered back to normal alignment.[4,13] The concept of TMJ treatment is thus left open to criticism because of lack of documentation of pathology, diagnosis, and outcome. In essence, without clear documentation through specific diagnostic imaging, the array of modalities for TMJ management becomes empirical at best.

Perhaps disc displacement deserves a second look as it relates to both TMJ pain and mechanical abnormality. Historically, emphasis has been placed on the relative position of the disc, because it became the standard by which we measured clicking, locking, and joint discomfort.[5,12,14] As imaging techniques became more sophisticated, the position of the disc relative to the condyle became the standard to either confirm or rule out TMJ pathology.[13] At the same time, however, it became apparent that in some patients the position of the disc did not correlate with pain levels. Argument thus mounted again over the choice of invasive or noninvasive approaches. Conceptually at least, we may have missed the various other forms of pathology that occur in response to discal displacement, such as pterygoid muscle impingement, retrodiscal attachment compression (loading), and joint effusion; and we may have slowed our diagnoses of other entities of primary joint pathology, such as marrow space avascular necrosis.[15,16] When these other types of pathology are included in the differential diagnosis of TMJ pain and mechanical abnormality, it may become clearer why approaches aimed primarily at disc displacement can have unpredictable results.

The choice of invasive vs. noninvasive management is also dependent on the availability of surgical procedures and a skillful surgeon. The complexity of the TMJ warrants precision in the selection of reconstruction techniques. Arthroscopic surgery and open joint arthrotomy are currently offered when invasive management is chosen. In arthroscopic surgery, proof is lacking on exactly what is being reversed pathophysiologically, and arthroscopic techniques are proliferating without clear documentation of their efficacy.[4] Furthermore, in open joint surgery, choices include disc repair, disc removal, alloplastic or autogenous replacement of the disc, condylectomy, condylotomy, total condylar replacement with alloplastic or autogenous techniques, and eminectomy. The

technique that is employed may depend primarily on the preference of the surgeon and less on a selection based on pathologic mechanisms. Skill levels of surgeons vary widely, and election for noninvasive management may sometimes reflect that.

In this chapter, the surgical techniques of open arthrotomy are presented. Specifically, emphasis is placed on microscopic TMJ surgery, and the various structural details of tissue pathology are discussed. The scope of abnormalities accounting for pain and mechanical abnormalities, in addition to the disc, includes the condylodiscal ligaments, TMJ capsule, lateral pterygoid muscle, retrodiscal attachment, synovium, joint space, surface fibrocartilage, nutrient blood supply, and adjacent bone.[15] After defining the exact tissue abnormalities, the indications for open arthrotomy are then outlined, and a rationale for selection of either disc repair and repositioning or disc removal is given. Although it is not in the scope of this chapter to consider the various noninvasive techniques and arthroscopy, these modalities also warrant a place in the treatment of patients with temporomandibular disorders. However, in reading this chapter, comparisons should be made regarding the relative merits of all techniques—invasive or noninvasive—in accomplishing pain reduction, reversal of pathology, and prevention of progressive disease in the TMJ. With the added advantage of direct observation of pathology through open microscopic arthrotomy, the relative weaknesses and strengths of all techniques can be better understood.

NORMAL AND ABNORMAL ANATOMY

Structurally, the various tissues of the TMJ lie in immediate juxtaposition to one another. Thus, when the anatomy of one tissue is distorted, the adjacent structures are also altered. It is this interrelationship between tissues that accounts for the complexity of TMJ pathology. In diagnosing or treating TMJ problems, the influence that one tissue such as the displaced disc has on adjacent structures must be understood. Furthermore, when treating TMJ pathology, each tissue must be structurally changed back to a more normal anatomy, or alternatively, if this is not possible, the distortion that one tissue may have against an adjacent tissue must be minimized.

Disc

Malposition of the disc relative to the mandibular condyle was first cited in 1918 as the cause of TMJ pain and mechanical dysfunction.[9] As the disc displaced, the condyle either translated forward beneath the anteriorly displaced disc (reduction) or, alternatively, when translated forward, the condyle simply pushed against the posterior band of the disc (closed lock). A closer look at normal and abnormal anatomy of the disc clarifies the difference in the two states.[17]

The normal TMJ disc is a biconcave structure composed primarily of dense fibrous connective tissue. For structural purposes, the disc can be divided into three zones. At the posterior is a relatively thick area referred to as the *posterior band.* The middle of the disc, which generally overlies the head of the condyle, is referred to as the *intermediate zone,* and this is usually about one third to one half the thickness of the posterior band. Anteriorly, the disc thickens again at the anterior band. Thus, the disc assumes a biconcave shape. Functionally, this shape allows the disc to stabilize on top of the condyle during rotatory and translatory movement. Compression of the condyle against the disc occurs in the thinner, or intermediate, zone. The disc is vascularized at the posterior and anterior bands but not in the intermediate zone, allowing for a change in thickness at the anterior and posterior bands as a result of vascular shunting during condyle movement. Hence, the disc can immediately change the thickness of the posterior and anterior bands in response to the relative space between the osseous surfaces.

The concept of spatial relationships is particularly important with regard to disc alignment. The disc has a precise functional zone between the condyle and fossa in a superior position and between the condyle and eminence in an anterior position, into which it must be moved. Therefore, through either a reduction in this space for the disc or an impingement on this space by another structure, the disc may become and remain displaced. Hence, if the disc should change shape or thickness in any of its three zones, the joint may be set up for discal displacement. Likewise, if a structural change occurs in the surface conformity of an adjacent bony structure, the disc may be displaced from uneven compressive forces during function. Alternatively, if other tissue impinges on the disc space, the disc may become displaced. For example, if the volume of the retrodiscal tissue expands, a hydraulic force from the retrodiscal tissue will be placed against the posterior band of the disc, and this force may displace the disc.

The position of the disc relative to the condyle can be altered by either pushing or pulling the disc to a different position. As in the previous example, expanded retrodiscal tissue can herniate anteriorly against the disc. The disc may also be displaced by anterior pulling or tethering from the capsule, muscle, or epimysial tissues. The net result of either mechanism is to force the disc into a more forward or medial functional zone. The retrodiscal tissue thus occupies the space that was originally available for the posterior band of the disc, and the disc herniates to take up the space normally occupied by the lateral pterygoid muscle. In turn, the lateral pterygoid muscle must herniate into adjacent tissue, compress vascular spaces, or reduce in volume from atrophy. The degree of disc displacement dictates to what extent adjacent tissues are distorted.

Once a disc becomes partially displaced anteriorly, the condyle shifts loading from the intermediate zone to the posterior band. The blood is shunted out of the posterior band, and chronic compression is shifted to this area. Because the posterior band is thicker than the intermediate zone, compression does not tend to lock the disc onto the condyle. The disc sits precariously on top of the condyle, and during compression of the condyle against the disc, the disc may completely displace into the area of least resistance, either anteriorly or medially. Successful reduction of the disc in partial displacement thus depends on reduction in volume of the retrodiscal tissue, restoration of normal blood flow mechanics to the posterior band, relocking of the condyle beneath the thinner intermediate zone, and release of contraction or tethering of the lateral pterygoid muscle or capsule.

If reversal of pathology is not accomplished, a higher probability exists of complete disc displacement. In this situation, the posterior band of the disc lies completely anterior to the condyle when the condyle is in a superior position. The condyle functions completely against displaced retrodiscal tissue in a superior position. The shunt of blood flow into the posterior and anterior bands increases because of lack of compression.

The disc then herniates farther anteriorly into the lateral pterygoid muscle. The intermediate zone, being thinner, is prone to buck-

ling and foreshortening. The capsule and collateral ligaments are then stretched beyond their normal functional lengths. Reduction of the disc in this stage is increasingly more difficult; however, the TMJ may continue to click because the condyle may still be able to translate into a forward position beneath the disc.

After a disc has been displaced for a prolonged period, tissue becomes more distorted. In particular, if the posterior band thickens or if the intermediate zone becomes markedly foreshortened, the ability of the condyle to translate beneath the disc may become impossible. This would explain the progression to a closed lock. A TMJ that is in a closed lock develops continuous compression against the retrodiscal tissue. The disc impinges on the lateral pterygoid muscle regardless of condyle position, and in fact, as the condyle is translated forward, the disc is pressed farther into the lateral pterygoid muscle. Important considerations must be given to the compression of the disc against the lateral pterygoid and those structures that course through this muscle.

The consistency of the disc is such that it is pliable yet firm enough to withstand compressive forces. This property is important in maintaining synovial nutrition to adjacent articular surfaces. In essence, the synovial fluid is driven into nonvascularized joint surfaces by compression. The consistency of the disc must be firm enough to squeeze synovial fluid into the surface fibrocartilage and cortex. No other intra-articular structures have the same pliability and firmness as the disc, and when the disc is displaced, normal joint nutrition is interrupted. Likewise, when the disc is lost, it is difficult to find a substitute autogenous graft or alloplastic implant that has similar compressive properties.

The nonvascularized intermediate zone of the disc is dependent on the synovial fluid for nutrition. Proper positioning of the disc during function is necessary to ensure that synovial fluid is compressed into the intermediate zone. That part of the intermediate zone that may become displaced lacks normal nutrition and may degenerate. Furthermore, during normal compression, synovial fluid generally can penetrate to a certain level into the disc. Because the disc is about 2 mm thick at the intermediate zone, synovial fluid must penetrate only 1 mm from the superior and inferior sides. In chronic disc displacement, the intermediate zone thickens, and if the disc can be repositioned, nutrition may be inadequate because of incomplete penetration of synovial fluid. This consideration has implications for how much a disc should be thinned at the time of surgical repair.

Condylodiscal Ligaments

The condylodiscal (collateral) ligaments are located medially and laterally to the condylar head. They help to maintain the disc at each respective pole. Both condylodiscal ligaments blend with the inferior stratum of the retrodiscal tissue. These ligaments attach to the fibrous connective tissue of the corresponding portions of the disc. Although these are not weight-bearing ligaments, they do play a vital role in maintaining the disc in alignment just proximal to midfossa in the superior condyle position. During forward translation of the condyle, these ligaments allow the disc to rotate more posteriorly over the head of the condyle. As in all joints in the body, when ligaments are hyperextended, they are prone to tearing and laxity. In the TMJ, a lax collateral ligament may allow for displacement of that corresponding part of the disc.

The lateral ligament generally develops laxity more readily than the medial. Thus, the lateral half of the disc may displace while the medial half remains normally aligned. This partial disc displacement results in degenerative changes only in that part of the joint where the disc is displaced. Furthermore, the loss of synovial nutrition may occur only in the lateral part of the joint. The problems associated with retrodiscal tissue compression and pterygoid muscle impingement are generally less serious than in complete disc displacement. This partial disc displacement could remain stable for a lifetime, or alternatively, if the medial collateral ligament also breaks down, the disc may become completely displaced. Surgical procedures are not usually necessary when only half of the disc is displaced, even though that part of the disc clicks or locks.

Lateral Pterygoid Muscle

The lateral pterygoid muscle has two bellies. All muscles have a point of origin and a point of insertion. The upper belly of the lateral pterygoid muscle originates from the infratemporal fossa of the greater wing of the sphenoid. The lower belly originates from the lateral portion of the lateral pterygoid plate. The insertion of the upper belly is partially into the disc through an opening of the anterior capsule and partially into the condylar neck beneath the level of the capsule. In magnetic resonance images, the amount of muscle insertion into the disc is variable. The lower belly inserts entirely into the condylar fovea.

The upper and lower bellies have different electromyographic activity.[18] Upon translation, the lower belly is active while the upper belly is inactive. Alternatively, on closure of the mandible, the inferior belly goes to resting potential while the upper belly becomes active. Functionally, then, it is the superior belly of the lateral pterygoid muscle that may influence discal position. Hence, during chronic clenching, the activity of the superior belly creates a constant forward force against the anterior band of the disc. If the collateral ligaments and retrodiscal attachment tissues are lax, the disc may become displaced through this mechanism.

Three potential problems may develop within a muscle to influence the relative length of that muscle. Each muscle generally has a set resting length defined as the distance that the point of insertion is held relative to the point of origin. Essentially, the resting length is determined by the average number of myofibrils in contraction at any time, as well as by the length of connective tissue in the muscle. The first problem that contributes to foreshortening is hypercontraction or spasm. This results from an increase in the number of myofibrils in contraction, with higher electromyographic activity.

The second factor that leads to a change in resting length is alteration of the connective tissue of a muscle. All muscles have connective tissue linings. Individual muscle fibers are surrounded by a reticulum of endomysium. Perimysium collagenous septa divide the muscle fascicles, and epimysium is an outer connective tissue layer that surrounds the belly of a muscle. These connective tissue layers are prone to develop foreshortening when the muscle is not allowed to stretch to its full mechanical length. Thus, in the TMJ, when the condyle has been held in a forward position, these connective tissue layers tighten. This generally does not present a problem for those fibers of the lateral pterygoid that insert into the condyle, for by simply repositioning the condyle more posteriorly from the slope of the eminence to the fossa, these fibers can be stretched.

Difficulties may arise from those parts of the superior belly that insert into the disc, for if these are to be stretched, the condyle must pull against the collateral ligaments. The medial and lateral collateral ligaments must tether the disc, and the disc must likewise pull against the connective tissue of the upper belly. Therefore, success in stretching the upper belly connective tissue depends on the degree of foreshortening, the quantity of connective tissue, and the integrity of the collateral ligaments.

The third factor that alters the resting length of a muscle is the composition of the internal muscle tissue. The relative resting length of a muscle is influenced by atrophic changes that may occur within the belly of the muscle. Muscle atrophy may develop for various reasons, including neurologic disorders, primary muscle disease, and disuse atrophy. In particular, when the TMJ has restricted movement due to mechanical problems in the joint or due to forward positioning of the mandible, disuse atrophy may occur. Histologically, the muscle tissue undergoes both fatty as well as fibrous atrophy. Just as with other causes of fibrous connective tissue foreshortening, this pathology may result in chronic forward disc displacement, and it may be extremely difficult to reposition the disc into more normal alignment in the fossa.

The relative function of a muscle to move adjacent bone is dependent on stable attachments through tendinous structures. Tendons are composed of longitudinally arranged connective tissue that has sparse fibrocytes interspersed throughout. Because this tissue is relatively inert, it requires little nutrition and has a very low blood flow requirement. However, by having low blood flow, tendinous tissue also has diminished repair capacity. Tendons gain their firm attachment to bone through deep penetration of the cortex by collagen fibers called *Sharpey's fibers.* In order to course from an extra-articular to an intra-articular environment, where the tendon of the superior belly inserts into the disc, it must pass through a synovial sheath at the anteromedial capsular wall. A structurally intact pterygoid tendon is taut at both the insertion into the disc and at the insertion into the condyle.

It was mentioned previously that a functional space must exist within TMJ structures, and when one structure becomes malpositioned, the adjacent tissues are impinged. The lateral pterygoid muscle thereby has a functional space between the greater wing of the sphenoid and lateral pterygoid plate and the anterior portions of the disc and condyle.

The lateral pterygoid may be impinged by several mechanisms. When the disc is displaced, it usually assumes a position anterior and medial to the mandibular condyle. In this displaced position, the disc is impinging upon the lateral pterygoid muscle. It is at this level that many types of discal contortions may occur. For example, if the tendon of the pterygoid muscle is firmly tethered to the condyle and to the disc, the disc tends to fold over on itself as it assumes a displaced position. The anterior band of the disc is therefore tethered closely to the insertion point of the tendon to the anterior condyle. Alternatively, if the tendinous insertion of the pterygoid muscle into the condyle is lax, the disc tends to displace without folding, and the anterior band of the disc displaces away from the anterior of the condyle. In both situations, the disc displaces into space that is normally occupied by the lateral pterygoid muscle. Impingement of the displaced disc into the pterygoid muscle accounts for muscle pain and spasm. Furthermore, when the upper belly of the lateral pterygoid is cramped for space, it tends to contract into itself, setting up the potential for fibrosis, fatty atrophy, and foreshortened resting length. Failure to appreciate this pathophysiologic mechanism may account for both nonsurgical and surgical failures, because to reposition the disc into normal alignment in the TMJ, the atrophied muscle must be restretched. Incising the muscle may assist this stretching, as will become clearer later.

A second mechanism to impinge upon the functional space of the lateral pterygoid muscle is movement of the point of insertion toward the point of origin. Thus, if the condyle is translated anteriorly, the muscle must once again contract into itself, and in order for the muscle to occupy a smaller space, blood must flow out of it. For a brief period, such as during normal talking or chewing, this is acceptable and may actually aid in shunting blood through the muscle. However, as in any joint in which movement has been restricted, constriction of connective tissue and muscular elements ensues, and the resting length of the muscle changes as it undergoes fibrous and fatty atrophy. The portions of the muscle that are thus affected alter the relative position of the structures into which they insert. Thus, both the condyle and the disc become more anteriorly situated. When the condyle and the disc are restricted from returning to their normal terminal location within the TMJ, profound foreshortening of the lateral pterygoid muscle may occur within a few days.

One further consideration in muscle foreshortening is the relative reversibility of this pathologic change. If the point of insertion is moved away from the point of origin, the muscle certainly can be stretched. However, the unique anatomic relationships of TMJ structures present a dilemma even when the condyle is repositioned at its normal posterior location, because it is extremely difficult to stretch those fibers of the lateral pterygoid muscle that insert into the disc. In order to lengthen the superior belly fibers that insert into the disc, the collateral ligaments must be stronger than the fibrotic muscle tissues. That is, in order for the disc to be pulled posteriorly, it must be firmly tethered to the mandibular condyle. Unfortunately, when the condyle has been maintained anteriorly and the pterygoid muscle foreshortens, the collateral ligaments are frequently torn or stretched as the condyle moves posteriorly and the fibrotic muscle tethers the disc anteriorly. Therefore, modalities that restrict the condyle and disc from assuming their normal posterior and superior positions might lead to collateral ligament breakdown and eventual disc displacement.

When the TMJ disc is displaced, it not only impinges upon the lateral pterygoid muscle, but it also may compress any structures that pass through the pterygoid. Perhaps of most importance here is the blood supply of adjacent structures. Branches of the maxillary artery course around and through the lateral pterygoid muscle. Crossing inferiorly and then medially to the lateral pterygoid is the middle meningeal artery on its way to the foramen spinosum at the medial part of the articular eminence of the TMJ. Disc displacement can be attended by impingement of the middle meningeal artery, leading to ischemia of the periauricular portion of the middle cranial fossa. This phenomenon raises interesting possibilities about potential pain referral patterns in TMJ disc displacement.

Similarly, branches of the maxillary artery must also eventually penetrate the mandibular condyle at its anterior portion.[19] The head of the condyle is perfused by branches that pass through the superior belly of the lateral pterygoid, and the neck of the condyle receives its blood supply from vessels that penetrate the inferior belly. A critical part of the blood supply

to the mandibular condyle comes from the feeder vessels that must course through the lateral pterygoid muscle. In discal displacement, these vessels may become occluded, and the condylar blood supply may become critically compromised.[15] It is important that surgeons reverse this mechanism of blood supply occlusion by properly removing the disc from a pathologic position that is anterior and medial to the condyle.

Retrodiscal Tissue

The retrodiscal tissue occupies a space confined to the functional zone between the posterior portions of the disc and mandibular condyle and the anterior parts of the bony and cartilaginous ear canal. This tissue has two strata. Within the upper stratum, the retrodiscal tissue must make rapid changes in volume secondary to condylar and discal translation. To accomplish this, the retrodiscal tissue has a rich blood supply and a vascular shunt that is contained within loosely organized fat, collagen, and elastin. The volume in this area must precisely match the positioning of the condyle and disc for mechanical stability. The inferior stratum is composed of inelastic and tightly packed collagen fibers. This layer blends medially and laterally with the collateral ligaments and is responsible for maintaining the disc in a functional relationship over the mandibular condyle.

With structural change of either of the strata, disc displacement may result. For example, if the disc is traumatically displaced anteriorly, the inferior stratum of collagen fibers is stretched or torn. This generally would occur with similar damage to the collateral ligaments. If the lateral pterygoid muscle is also atrophic or fibrotic, the disc is not likely to be returned to normal alignment. During the trauma, it is likely that the upper straum will simultaneously develop edema or a hematoma, resulting in an increase in the volume of the retrodiscal tissue and a compromise in the ability of this tissue to undergo normal shunting. Because the posterior border of the retrodiscal attachment is made up of bone and ear cartilage, the direction of impingement of this expanded tissue tends to be anteriorly against the disc and condyle. Thus, it is not uncommon to observe forward positioning of the condyle and even slight posterior open bite after trauma. It is noteworthy that if the retrodiscal tissue is pathologically expanded in volume, it will create a compressive force against the posterior band of the disc. If laxity simultaneously develops in the inferior stratum or in the collateral ligaments, the disc is pushed and displaced anteriorly by the retrodiscal tissue.

Mechanisms other than macrotrauma may expand the volume of the retrodiscal tissue. For example, if the condyle and disc are chronically positioned anteriorly, the fatty and collagenous elements in the upper stratum expand. Thus, the blood shunt is replaced by expansion of the quantity of fat and connective tissue. After the volume of the retrodiscal tissue has expanded, if the condyle is repositioned more posteriorly, the expanded retrodiscal tissue compresses more forcefully against the posterior band of the disc. Over time, through this mechanism, the collagen of the inferior stratum and collateral ligaments loosens and the disc displaces anteriorly. The fact that forward positioning of the mandible is generally of equal degree bilaterally may explain the high incidence of bilateral discal displacement.

In the event that the disc becomes displaced from anterior pulling by the lateral pterygoid muscle, the retrodiscal tissue develops similar pathologic changes. The inferior stratum stretches, and the superior stratum expands in volume. Although this pathology is a result and not a cause of disc displacement, the mechanical abnormality eventually becomes equal in each mechanism. Any surgical treatment modality that does not properly reduce the volume of the retrodiscal tissue inhibits the ability to recapture the disc.

Capsule and Synovium

The external capsule and synovium constitute the lining of the TMJ. These structures have importance in the surgical reconstruction of the TMJ, and their normal function must be understood.

The capsule of the TMJ helps to define the spaces within which all other tissue elements must function. The capsule is primarily a medial and lateral joint structure. In the medial fossa, the capsule originates along the squamosphenoid suture line, and laterally it originates from the inferolateral edges of the eminence and fossa. On the lateral aspect, the capsule is reinforced by the lateral TMJ ligament, which limits translation and distraction of the condyle. If the lateral ligament is loose, all joint tissues are at risk for hypermobility.

Anteriorly, the capsule is penetrated by the tendon of the lateral pterygoid muscle. Posteriorly, the capsule is an incomplete structure, and this part of the joint is bounded by the ear canal.

The synovial tissue of the TMJ lines the inner capsule and is found at the perimeter of the joint. Synovial tissue does not normally line the compressive portions of joint structures, although synovial fluid does nourish these areas. Synovial fluid functions to lubricate and nourish joint surfaces, which do not have a blood supply. Within the TMJ, the articular cartilage and the intermediate zone of the disc are dependent on synovial fluid for their nutrition. Compression of the disc against adjacent articular cartilage supplies synovial nutrition to these tissues. The consistency of the disc is firm yet pliable enough to allow for the synovial fluid to be driven into the fibrocartilage and intra-articular cortical bone layer. Likewise, the middle portion of the disc derives its nutrition from absorption of synovial fluid, which is driven into the disc by the adjacent bony structures.

This mechanism of nutrition of nonvascularized tissues by compression of synovial fluid is dependent on precise alignment of the disc and condyle. When the disc is displaced, nutrition is altered through several factors. First, the disc and articular bony surfaces may continue to be bathed in synovial fluid, but unless these structures are properly compressed against each other, synovial fluid does not effectively penetrate. Furthermore, as the disc displaces anteriorly, the joint space is constricted by the formation of adhesions. This particularly occurs in the upper joint space as a result of the development of adhesions anterior to the tympanic fissure. The farther forward the disc displacement, the farther forward the formation of adhesions can be detected between the articular fossa and the retrodiscal attachment. Likewise, in the inferior joint space, adhesions develop between the posterior part of the mandibular condyle and the inferior stratum of the retrodiscal attachment. Adhesions limit the access of synovial fluid to articular surfaces. Abnormal production of synovial fluid may also result from disc displacement with the development of joint space effusions. Effusion is in turn a factor in the further development of joint space adhesions.

In the attempt to surgically treat TMJ pathology, strict attention must be paid to re-establishing the normal mechanisms of synovial nutrition if degenerative arthritis is to be avoided. Surgical procedures thus must completely ablate all scar tissue to allow for complete access of synovial fluid to the perimeter of the original joint spaces. The disc must be precisely realigned to the condylar surface to restore mechanisms of compression of synovial fluid into the nonvascularized articular surfaces. The synovial lining must be preserved in normal quantity to allow for production and reabsorption of synovial fluid without leading to a dry joint, devoid of adequate synovial fluid, or a wet joint, with chronic effusion.

Bone

The osseous elements of the TMJ may be the least understood structures, yet they have a profound role in maintaining the stability of the occlusion and facial profile. As marrow physiology is better understood, some of the most important concepts relating to chronic facial pain can be defined. Proper nutrition of the bone, particularly of the mandibular condyle, is critical for maintaining the structural integrity of the TMJ.

As in all synovial joints, the TMJ has a concave member and a convex member. The fossa is the concave portion of the joint, and most functional movement of the condyle takes place within the confines of the fossa. Anterior to the fossa is the articular eminence, which is part of the temporal bone. The eminence is convex from anterior to posterior. Both the fossa and the eminence are richly vascularized by periosteum, and their articular surfaces are nourished by synovium. As a convex surface, the eminence is not generally an area where the opposing convex condyle can function in a stable relationship for prolonged periods. In fact, when two convex articular surfaces remain in prolonged contact, hypercompression of small areas of the surface occurs because of uneven distribution of forces.[16] This hypercompression results in articular surface collapse and deformity, and subarticular marrow edema may develop. Because the marrow is within the closed space of the condyle cortical bone, edema leads to a build-up of marrow pressure with resultant pain. Furthermore, edema compromises the ability for blood to traverse that area of the condyle, and venous stasis develops. Frank subcortical necrosis in the form of osteochondritis dissecans may occur.

The mandibular condyle is the convex inferior articular structure of the TMJ. Complex marrow pathology can occur in the mandibular condyle as a result of marrow ischemia. In order to fully comprehend this pathology, the types of condylar nutrition must be understood.[15]

The mandibular condyle receives nutrition from three sources. Two of these are intracapsular, and one source is extracapsular. The insertion line of the capsule demarcates the types of nutrition. In the extracapsular part of the mandibular condyle, both the cortical bone and the underlying marrow are nourished by the periosteum and penetrating vessels from the periosteum. Because of a large supply of blood from the periosteum, this bone is generally well vascularized and nourished.

The intracapsular nutrition, by comparison, is much more vulnerable. Mechanisms of synovial nutrition have been discussed. The synovial fluid nourishes the articular cartilage and the underlying cortical bone if the condyle and disc are in proper alignment. With the development of disc displacement, intracapsular adhesions, or joint effusion, this nutrition is compromised. The condylar head, which is surrounded by capsule and synovial fluid, does not have periosteum on its articular surface, and this critical source of blood supply and nutrition is not present.

The deeper marrow of the intracapsular mandibular condyle is nourished by the penetrating branches of the maxillary artery, which traverse the lateral pterygoid muscle. Because this blood supply has a limited source and because there is no periosteum on the part of the condyle that is contained within the capsule, the marrow of the condylar head is particularly vulnerable to disruption of blood flow from the penetrating maxillary artery branches.

The blood flow to the mandibular condyle may be compromised by two mechanisms. First, if the displaced disc impinges on the lateral pterygoid muscle in a way that occludes the penetrating vessels, the major source of blood flow to the entire intracapsular portion of the condyle may be lost. Similarly, through hypercompression of the condyle as a result of either trauma or chronic bruxism, edema may develop within the marrow. In this closed space, the build-up of edema is the equivalent of a compartmental syndrome, and the increase in marrow fluid pressure limits the inflow of blood. The net result again is the development of marrow ischemia due to venous sludging.

Intra-articular bone can generally tolerate

partial ischemia for a period of several days before marrow elements such as fat and hematopoietic cells begin to undergo frank necrosis. The onset of this process of necrosis may be followed by resolution and healing, but if the inciting factors of disc displacement or hypercompression persist, progressive stages of avascular necrosis may develop. In this scenario, the marrow undergoes necrosis, hypervascularity, fibrosis, collapse, and sclerosis during a period of several years. Pain develops in the TMJ secondary to marrow space pathology, and despite correction of the discal pathology, the marrow may continue to be necrotic and produce symptoms.

Of great clinical significance is the development of an unstable condyle in the presence of active necrosis and collapse of the condylar head.[11,20,21] This is generally expressed in the occlusion and the facial skeleton. From collapse of the mandibular condyle, patients develop posterior occlusal prematurities, and if the breakdown from avascular necrosis is rapid, they also acquire an anterior open bite. Long-term structural changes can be seen in the facial skeleton. As the condyle degenerates, the mandible and chin point become retrognathic, and the ramus height of the mandible shortens. Furthermore, if the mandibular condyles degenerate at different rates, patients may develop facial asymmetry.

INDICATIONS FOR SURGICAL INTERVENTION

From the previous discussion, it is obvious that pathology of the TMJ is a complex subject. Because of the variability of abnormalities in each of the joint structures, thresholds must be defined for each to demarcate indications for noninvasive or invasive management. However, these guidelines are very general, because as was previously pointed out, an individual's response takes precedence over the mechanical abnormality. Therefore, if pain, locking, progressive occlusal change, or facial distortion is a significant problem for a particular individual, and if the response to these symptoms as a result of noninvasive techniques is inadequate, surgery should then be considered. If surgery is selected, patients should be advised that symptomatic relief may not be complete or permanent. Patients must consider the merits of surgical intervention and have reasonable expectations.

Most pathology that is managed with surgery is related to TMJ discal displacement. However, not all displaced discs need surgical intervention. In fact, it is not the disc that hurts when it is displaced. Instead, a combination of disc displacement and other forms of pathology increases pain levels to a point where patients consider surgery. Hence, pain usually results from progression of pathology in the other TMJ structures. Let us consider a few examples of the thresholds of deformity for each structure.

Depending on the integrity of the collateral ligaments, it is possible for the disc to displace from only part of the mandibular condyle. If the medial ligament is normal and the lateral collateral ligament is lax, the disc is likely to displace only from the lateral pole of the condyle. The joint may have clicking or even locking due to this lateral pole disc displacement, yet a patient may have no associated pain. Furthermore, breakdown may not progress to the medial pole in any particular individual, and pain may never develop in the TMJ.

Alternatively, if the medial ligament also tears and if the inferior stratum of the retrodiscal attachment becomes lax, the disc may displace from both the lateral and medial poles of the mandibular condyle. If this should happen, the clicking or locking TMJ will also have pain associated with either tissue compression or tissue impingement.

Tissue compression is a function of loading of the articular portion of the condyle against structures other than the disc and fossa. If the disc is displaced anteriorly and medially, the condyle compresses directly against redundant retrodiscal tissue. Because this tissue is richly innervated, patients have associated pain. When the convex surface of the condyle remains in function at a forward position against a convex eminentia, compression may lead to underlying marrow edema and pain. In some forms of pathology, the condyle is maintained in a forward position secondary to pterygoid muscle foreshortening or retrodiscal attachment redundancy. The other type of compression is a result of effusion or overproduction of synovial fluid. In this situation, the compression of innervated structures is mediated through the excessive fluid pressure of the intracapsular spaces.

Tissue impingement may cause pain as a result of herniation into a structure or occupation of the functional space of one tissue by another. The obvious example of this is herniation of the displaced disc into the belly of the lateral pterygoid muscle. Not only does this create muscle pain, but it also may lead to compression of the middle meningeal artery and feeder vessels to the condylar head. The displaced disc can thereby cause claudication pain in the distribution of the middle meningeal artery, and it can cause ischemic pain from the condylar head with the development of avascular necrosis. Tissue impingement pain may also come from hydraulic pressure of redundant retrodiscal tissue against the posterior band of the disc. This pain may result from retrodiscal impingement even if the disc is maintained in relatively good alignment.

Other mechanical factors may favor surgical resolution as opposed to noninvasive modalities. If a TMJ click is so loud that it is socially unacceptable and if other forms of therapy do not resolve it, surgery can be considered. Mandibular locking of the condyle behind the posterior band of the disc sometimes severely limits opening range of motion. If the locking persists, surgery can alleviate it.

Some patients develop rather significant chin recession or occlusal change as a result of avascular necrosis of the mandibular condyle. If the diagnostic magnetic resonance scan shows condylar marrow edema due to disc displacement, the patient may be at risk for progressive avascular necrosis of the condyle, and stronger consideration may be given to surgical intervention.[16]

The decision to proceed with surgery on the TMJ is therefore based on the level of individual pain, the type of mechanical dysfunction, the response to noninvasive modalities, the prevention of progressive pathology, and the reasonable certainty with which the abnormalities can be addressed with reconstruction. In general, surgical procedures are most successful when the joint structures are not at an end stage of breakdown. Thus, the period of non-surgical management should be limited if the joint symptoms are not successfully alleviated.

TYPES OF SURGICAL PROCEDURES

Surgical intervention in the TMJ has two primary goals. The first is to restore normal anatomy, and the second is to decompress joint structures. Both goals have an end point of lower levels of pain, and both attempt to restore lost function. Various techniques are available to accomplish these goals, and a surgeon often has to select what may be best for a particular patient.

The technique that is used to restore normal anatomy is the disc repair.[15] This type of surgery is outlined step by step later in this chapter. Philosophically, this approach is based on the premise that the more normal the anatomy of the joint, the less pain there should be and the better the function of the tissues. However, to achieve this successfully, all of the various types of tissue pathology must be recognized. Thus, it would be futile to reposition the disc but not to position it far enough back over the condyle. Surgical repair must take into account the degree of pterygoid muscle foreshortening and the quantity of retrodiscal redundancy to effectively reposition the disc. Furthermore, the disc should be precisely reshaped in order to occupy its original space, or else the compressive forces of the condyle will result in further displacement. Precise disc repair requires magnification, and a microscopic procedure is described later in this chapter.

Several techniques have been developed to decompress joint structures. All of these reduce tissue impingement. All but one, however, result in the loss of one or more joint structures.

Mandibular condylotomy has been developed to take an extra-articular approach to internal derangements of the TMJ. Through either an intraoral or a preauricular approach, the mandibular condylar neck is cut to allow forward and medial drifting of the mandibular condyle. Thus, the articular surface of the condyle is decompressed, and the pressure of the condyle against the retrodiscal attachment is diminished. The condyle sometimes also drifts beneath the disc, although both are anteriorly displaced. This procedure spares all of the original joint structures, but the alignment of these structures is not normal. One further advantage of condylotomy is that it decompresses any edema that may be present in the condylar head. However, the disadvantages of the technique include unpredictable occlusal changes, and the procedure generally must be limited to one side at a time, even in patients with bilateral symptoms.

The next two techniques are considered together because they accomplish similar objectives in decompression of the joint. Eminectomy has been performed in order to decrease the steepness of the articular eminence. High condylectomy is advocated to reduce the overall height of the condyle. Each technique may be done in conjunction with either disc repair or disc removal. Both are rationalized to diminish the loading of the articular bone against the intra-articular soft tissues. The condylectomy may have an additional advantage of decompressing the marrow space of the condyle. The structure that is sacrificed in this operation is the bone, and alterations in the occlusion with development of posterior dental prematurities and changes in the facial skeleton are expected, with development of open bite deformities and chin recession. These techniques destroy the articular cartilage and may predispose the patient to fibrous ankylosis and degenerative arthritis of these joints.[21]

The most common type of decompression technique is simply disc removal, or discectomy.[22,23] This procedure is generally carried out when the TMJ disc cannot be moved surgically to a more normal position. Removal of the disc accomplishes several objectives. The mechanical barrier that restricts condylar movement is removed with discectomy, and clicking and locking are eliminated. Pterygoid muscle pain that is secondary to disc herniation is reduced. To the extent that the disc has been occluding the maxillary artery branches to the condylar head, avascular necrosis may be avoided. The redundant retrodiscal attachment is usually excised with the disc, decreasing the pain of compression on this tissue. Adhesions are lysed, and because the condyle is free to mobilize maximally, they are less likely to recur. The disadvantage of this procedure is that the distribution of joint forces by the disc is lost, and normal synovial nutrition is compromised. Exacerbation of degenerative changes may be the result.

Controversy exists about the need to replace the ablated structures of the TMJ. For discectomy, eminectomy, and condylectomy, both alloplastic and autogenous replacements are available. Alloplastic materials include Silastic interpositional sheets, Proplast interpositional implants, metallic fossae, and metallic condyles. An advantage of these materials is that they are readily available. However, alloplastic materials may present problems unless used in older patients, as is done with other joints. The relatively young age of patients with TMJ problems puts them at higher risk of subsequent alloplastic implant failures because of the number of years of service that these implants would be required to provide.[24] In general terms, these should not be selected as permanent replacements except in rare circumstances, and if they are, patients need continual observation for possible alloplast failure. Autologous replacements include muscle

transfer flaps,[25-27] dermis, fat, conchal cartilage, and rib or iliac bone. Except for the reconstruction of severely destroyed bone, there is no strong indication for using these tissues. The belief of many surgeons that something must replace the disc after it is removed has not been supported by clinical evidence or research.[2,13,15,28] In initial discectomy surgery, there certainly is no evidence that autologous replacement has any advantage over simple disc removal without replacement.[2] The general disadvantage of all of these techniques is that they substitute intra-articular tissues with tissues that originate from an extra-articular source. In so doing, the normal intra-articular mechanisms of synovial and vascular nutrition cannot be realized. Furthermore, although they separate the articular surface, these tissues may actually adhere to either the condyle or fossa and thereby obliterate the normal joint space.

Microsurgical Disc Repair

It is apparent that the TMJ disc may be displaced for various reasons. In order to successfully reduce this disc surgically, all of the pathologic processes in each of the various structures must be addressed. Both the tissue abnormalities that caused the disc displacement and the tissue abnormalities that resulted from the disc displacement must be reversed. This statement implies that adequate preoperative imaging must be performed to diagnose pathology as it exists in the disc, the lateral pterygoid muscle, the retrodiscal attachment, the joint space, the articular surfaces, and the marrow spaces. Magnetic resonance scanning is the only diagnostic technique that can provide this complete perspective of joint pathology.[8] Other diagnostic modalities including transcranial radiographs, tomograms, computed tomographic scans, nuclear medicine scans, arthrograms, and arthroscopy present a less complete perspective of TMJ pathology.

The overall goals of the microscopic repair technique are to preserve joint structures and to return the anatomy to as near to normal as possible.[15] Obviously, the objective of reaching a normal state of anatomy is diminished in proportion to the extent of tissue pathology at the time of the surgical repair. The microsurgeon must reconstruct the TMJ after it is apparent that noninvasive techniques will not be successful and before the tissues distort to the point where repair is not possible. To understand that TMJ structural abnormalities are progressive and that only a certain amount of disc, muscle, bone, and ligament breakdown is tolerable enhances timely referral for surgery to allow for tissue repair and preservation.

Successful surgical repair is dependent on meeting certain minimum objectives for each tissue. For example, the disc must have sufficient length to allow it to interpose between the articular surfaces and must be able to function interpositionally in all movements. Impingement of the disc upon the lateral pterygoid muscle must be relieved to reduce any distortion of the middle meningeal artery and the arterial branches to the condylar head. Furthermore, the disc must be thinner in the intermediate zone so that it locks onto the condylar surface during compression of the articular surfaces, and it must be thinned enough to allow for nutrition by synovial fluid. The joint spaces need to be cleared of adhesions to allow for access of synovial fluid to the periphery of the joint. The synovial lining is preserved to maintain the normal production and reabsorption of synovial fluid. The collateral ligaments and the inferior stratum of the retrodiscal attachment are shortened precisely to tether the disc in normal alignment. The superior stratum of the retrodiscal tissue must be debulked appropriately at both the medial and lateral poles to minimize hydraulic force against the posterior band of the disc. The capsule is released where it has undergone fibrous contracture from disc displacement, and it is repositioned more posteriorly, along with the intra-articular structures. The epimysium and the fibrotic fibers of the lateral pterygoid muscle that insert into the disc must be partially released to increase the length of the muscle. The original muscle resting length is restored in order to reposition the disc at its normal location. The articular cartilage must be preserved by avoiding scuffing and abrasion during the operation. When marrow pathology is present in the mandibular condyle, consideration is given to decompression of the marrow edema.

Because of the minute size of the TMJ, the objectives outlined would be impossible to realize without the aid of enhanced illumination and magnification.[15,29–31] The advantage of using a microscope in reconstructing the TMJ is that it has multiple fiber-optic light sources that are positioned at the end of the lenses, directly above the surgical field. Magnification can be controlled by the operator from a range of 2.5× to 10×. Furthermore, with dual objectives, an assistant can view the operative field, and with a video interface, the operation can be projected onto a monitor for the scrub nurse and anesthesiologist.

With the advantages of improved illumination, magnification, and assistance, it follows that the objectives of reconstruction can be realized and the technical skills of the operator can be improved. Hemostatis throughout the operation is increased, and postoperative hemarthrosis is reduced. Similarly, operators can make a greater effort to avoid mutilating soft tissues, and their attempts to precisely return each of the various joint structures to as near normal anatomy as possible will be enhanced.

Technique

Microsurgical disc repair is most effectively accomplished by dividing the surgery into specific steps. Not only does this approach aid in learning the technique, but it also certifies that each tissue abnormality is specifically addressed. A stepwise approach reduces operator time by maintaining efficiency during the operation, and it allows for early recognition during the operation of a nonrepairable disc.[15]

STEP 1: ARTHROSCOPY

Before the microscopic repair, it is beneficial to preview the intra-articular structures with an arthroscope. This will confirm some of the other diagnostic findings and aid in localizing adhesions in the anteromedial recess, an area that is difficult to visualize with the surgical microscope.

Prearthrotomy arthroscopy aids surgeons in maintaining technical skills for subsequent procedures in which arthroscopy alone may be used. One further advantage of performing these techniques simultaneously is to allow surgeons to appreciate the relative strengths and weaknesses of arthroscopic surgery. In comparison with open microscopic arthrotomy, it is more difficult to judge the degree of disc displacement, the quantity of adhesions in the lateral half of the joint, and the bulk of the retrodiscal attachment. For obvious reasons, the lateral pterygoid muscle and the condylar marrow are not visualized by the arthroscope. When these techniques are compared for relative efficacy in the treatment of different types of joint pathology, the limited benefits of arthroscopic surgery are better appreciated.

STEP 2: SKIN INCISION

The incision for microscopic arthrotomy can be confined to the endaural tragus and to the skin fold anterior to the ascending helix of the ear (Fig. 33–1). Placement in this region ensures an excellent cosmetic closure. Microscopic illumination and magnification allows for a total incision length of no more than 25 to 30 mm, and because of the limited incision, intraoperative facial nerve damage and postoperative edema are minimized. An incision adjacent to the ear cartilage has the further advantage of allowing a clean plane of dissection along the external ear cartilage down to the temporalis fascia. When temporary interpositional implants are used as a part of the surgical repair, that part of the incision anterior to the helix can be reopened to gain access to the implant (see Step 18: Space Maintenance).

STEP 3: CAPSULAR EXPOSURE

After the temporalis fascia is exposed, it is incised horizontally along the fossa to approximately 8 mm anterior to the external bony ear canal. The temporalis fascia is then lifted from the eminence and lateral capsule with blunt dissection. In disc displacement, it is not unusual to find hypertrophied retrodiscal tissue herniating through the posterior 50% of the fossa. The posterior margin of the capsule is displaced anteriorly along with the disc and many times it is found as far forward as mid-

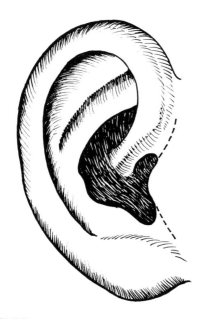

FIGURE 33–1. Skin incision (see text for details).

fossa. Care must be exercised during the dissection of the capsule to avoid cutting into the highly vascular retrodiscal attachment. Enough lateral capsule must be exposed so that the subsequent arthrotomy can be through capsular tissue and not hypertrophied retrodiscal attachment.

STEP 4: SUPERIOR SPACE ARTHROTOMY

An arthrotomy is an opening into a joint space. In the TMJ, there are two joint spaces to be opened. The primary access to the intra-articular structures is through the superior space arthrotomy (Fig. 33–2). The superior joint space incision is made through the capsule along the lateral lip of the fossa and eminence, extending from the tympanic fissure posteriorly to the prominence of the eminence anteriorly. When the incision is kept along the lateral lip, excessive bleeding from the retrodiscal tissue can be avoided. This exposure of the posterior part of the joint allows for removal of adhesions and for retrodiscal attachment reconstruction. The anterior extension of the incision allows for anterior or medial capsulotomy and for access to the lateral pterygoid muscle fibers.

STEP 5: LATERAL CAPSULOTOMY

On completion of the superior space arthrotomy, the degree of disc displacement can be seen. The lateral capsule is generally distorted and displaced anteriorly by the same degree of the disc. Therefore, the lateral capsule can be located lateral to the displaced disc, and in this area it is incised vertically. Placing the incision in this area avoids inadvertent cutting of the retrodiscal attachment. The anterior and posterior flaps of the capsule are then peeled back and sutured out of the way. When the capsulotomy is properly performed, the dissection should be free of any bleeding, and all intra-articular structures should be well visualized (Fig. 33–3).

STEP 6: LYSIS OF ADHESIONS IN THE SUPERIOR SPACE

At this point in the dissection, all adhesions anterior to the tympanic fissure and in the anterior and medial portions of the upper space should be well visualized (see Fig. 33–3). More adhesions are usually encountered in the posterior and lateral joint recesses. Adhesions usually are confined to the nondiscal structures, except where previous surgery has been performed. Utilizing a microblade, all adhesion bands anterior to the squamotympanic and pe-

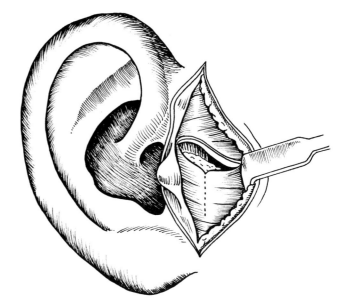

FIGURE 33–2. Superior space arthrotomy (see text for details).

trotympanic sutures are removed (Fig. 33–3). Care must be taken to avoid cutting into the ligament of the tympanic fissure. The attachments posterior to the tympanic fissure also should be avoided. In the midfossa, hypertrophied synovial tissue may line the surface fibrocartilage, and this should be curetted and excised without scuffing the underlying fibrocartilage. Working anteriorly in the joint, further scar bands are encountered along the medial and anterior margins of the internal capsule. As these are divided, any hypertro-

phied synovium is removed. However, the synovial layer directly lining the capsule is preserved.

STEP 7: INFERIOR SPACE ARTHROTOMY

On peeling the flaps of the capsulotomy anteriorly and posteriorly, the lateral collateral ligament is exposed. This ligament will have been stretched by the forward displacement of the disc. The inferior space arthrotomy is made posterior to the collateral ligament (Fig. 33–4). If the collateral ligament is incised, it is difficult

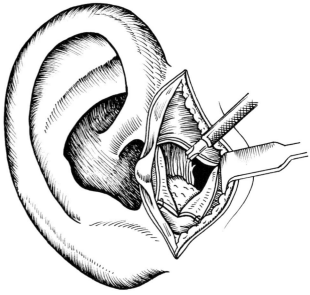

FIGURE 33–3. Lysis of adhesions in the superior space (see text for details).

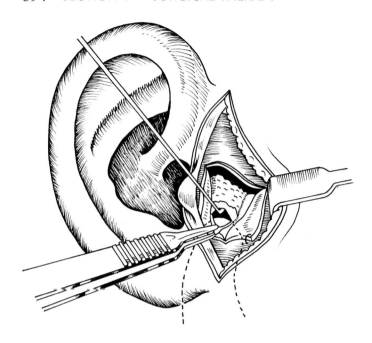

FIGURE 33–4. Interior space arthrotomy (see text for details).

to suture, particularly when it is markedly attenuated. The inferior space arthrotomy incision is placed 3 to 7 mm into the retrodiscal attachment, extending posteriorly from the lateral collateral ligament. The condyle is distracted inferiorly and anteriorly during the incision to avoid damage to the articular cartilage. Most of the inferior space pathology is in the posterior portion of the joint; therefore, the inferior space arthrotomy can be confined as described.

STEP 8: LYSIS OF ADHESIONS IN THE INFERIOR SPACE

After the inferior space arthrotomy is complete, the adhesions are usually seen along the posterior part of the condyle, extending toward the medial pole. These adhesions are usually not as dense as those of the superior joint space. A curette can be used to break apart these adhesions, and the articular cartilage should not be scuffed. In general, adhesions should be released to open the joint space posterior to the condyle to a level that is approximately 10 mm below the most superior part of the condylar head.

STEP 9: ANTERIOR AND MEDIAL CAPSULOTOMY

After the adhesions have been divided from the internal perimeter of both joint spaces, there still may be some capsular distortion secondary to fibrosis of the capsule. These areas can be detected by gently probing the inner capsular wall. When fibrotic areas are found, the disc is seen to move as these are probed. The inner capsular fibrotic areas are sequentially probed and divided, starting from the posterior medial and extending to the anterior lateral. All bands are superficially divided until they no longer tend to displace the disc anteriorly or medially when probed.

STEP 10: PTERYGOID MYOTOMY

After lysis of adhesions and capsular fibrous bands, the only structure that can tether the disc anteriorly is the lateral pterygoid muscle. The tightness of the lateral pterygoid can be checked by placing a hemostat across the retrodiscal attachment and pulling the disc posteriorly. When resistance is met, the position of the posterior band of the disc should be checked relative to the fossa. If the posterior band is not passively resting just proximal to the midfossa, the resting length of the muscle is decreased. If anterior tethering is confirmed, the anterior capsular wall is opened to develop a tissue plane between the periosteum of the anterior eminence and the epimysial layer of the muscle (Fig. 33–5). This is sometimes all that is required to reposition the disc. Alternatively, the epimysium and the uppermost fibers of the lateral pterygoid muscle may need to be divided. It is important not to divide the branches of the maxillary artery that enter the mandibular condylar head.

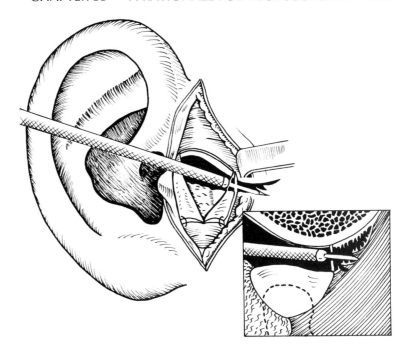

FIGURE 33–5. Pterygoid myotomy (see text for details).

STEP 11: DISC ROOFING

After the anterior release is complete, the disc should lie passively over the condyle with the posterior band just proximal to midfossa. If the disc is anterior to this location, additional release of either the inner capsule or the muscle is required. If further division of the muscle would injure the blood supply to the condyle or if the disc is just too short to cover the condyle, a decision should be made at this time to proceed with discectomy. (If discectomy is performed, the arteries to the condyle must be preserved during the dissection.)

STEP 12: REDUCTION OF RETRODISCAL TISSUE

With the anterior release completed, the disc can be positioned over the condyle, and the amount of redundant retrodiscal tissue can be estimated. This redundant tissue is clamped between two hemostats, and a wedge of appropriate size is removed (Fig. 33–6). It is particularly important to extend the wedge to the medial pole. To fail to do so would maintain too much bulk of retrodiscal attachment at the medial pole, possibly resulting in discal displacement at the medial pole, even if the lateral pole is properly repaired. The wedge of excised tissue usually measures 8 to 12 mm at the lateral pole and 4 to 10 mm at the medial pole. This wedge should be approximately 20 to 25 mm long from lateral to medial. More tissue should be excised from the superior stratum than from the inferior stratum. The inferior stratum will need to be tightened, but it must be left sufficiently long to reconstruct the normal tension of this band on closure.

STEP 13: CONDYLAR COMPRESSION TEST

Once it is established that the disc can rest passively on top of the condyle, it can be tested in loading function, much as might be done by the patient during clenching. By placing a clamp at the angle of the mandible, the operator can apply vertical compression (Fig. 33–7). If there is a mismatch in the fit of the disc against the articular surfaces, the disc will displace anteriorly or medially during compression. The direction of displacement helps to localize areas of abnormal disc thickness. For example, if the disc subluxes more in a medial direction, generally increased thickness will be found toward the medial pole. This test also allows the operator to check that the tethering from the muscle and capsule is completely released. Furthermore, as the condyle and disc are slowly elevated superiorly, it will be obvious if too much bulk remains in the retrodiscal attachment.

STEP 14: DISCOPLASTY

The condyle compression test generally reveals a mismatch in fit for the disc in the space

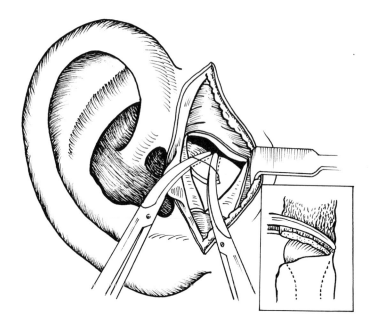

FIGURE 33–6. Reduction of retrodiscal tissue (see text for details).

that is available for it between the mandibular condyle and fossa. The disc is usually thickened in the intermediate zone, although it can have distortion anywhere. The disc is less pliable than normal. The objective of discoplasty is to thin the disc so that it locks on top of the condyle and to decrease its thickness sufficiently to restore synovial nutrition. The more precisely the disc fits the articular surfaces, the better the synovial nutrition will be postoperatively, and the less dead space there will be for the development of scar. The intermediate zone is thinned first to an overall thickness of 2 mm (Fig. 33–8). The anterior and posterior bands are recontoured appropriately to maximize the total surface area in contact between condyle and disc and between disc and fossa. Technically, discoplasty is performed from the superior surface. By confining the recontouring to the superior surface, postoperative adhesions can be managed better with the temporary interpositional implant (see Step 18). Multiple vertical compression tests are carried out during discoplasty to confirm the proper fit of the disc.

STEP 15: ARTHROPLASTY

On occasion, small osteophytes may project from the superior surface of the condyle. These bony projections may have to be reduced to decrease the risk of perforating the disc during the discoplasty. To gain a match in contour between the disc and condyle, it may be necessary to remove part of the condylar bone on the articular surface. This condyloplasty is done by raising a flap of fibrocartilage from the condylar surface (Fig. 33–9). After condyloplasty is completed, the flap is closed with 9-0 nylon suture. The incision line for the flap should be placed posterior to the functional weight-bearing surface of the condyle. A similar fibrocartilaginous flap can be used to obtain a biopsy specimen of the condyle when osteochondritis dissecans is suspected.

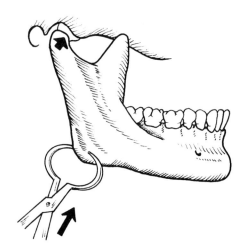

FIGURE 33–7. Condylar compression test (see text for details).

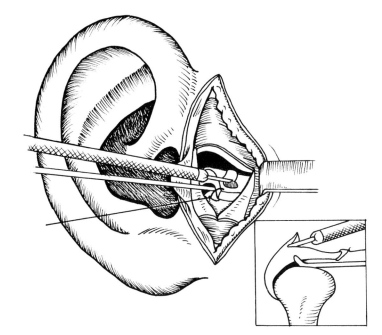

FIGURE 33–8. Discoplasty (see text for details).

STEP 16: REPAIR OF DISCAL-RETRODISCAL TISSUE

If the previous steps are followed closely, the disc will stay on top of the condyle during compression in all functional movements. By establishing a precise fit, the repair of the disc to the retrodiscal tissue can be tension free. Sutures are placed in an interrupted vertical mattress, with the first suture placed on the medial pole of the condyle (Fig. 33–10). If this depth of suturing is not reached, the medial pole of the disc will be at risk for postoperative displacement. Suturing is continued to the lateral pole in an interrupted fashion. Most repairs re-

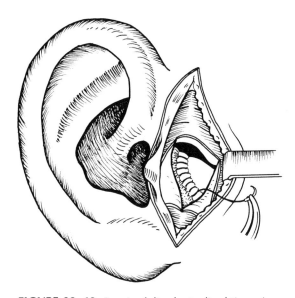

FIGURE 33–10. Repair of discal-retrodiscal tissue (see text for details).

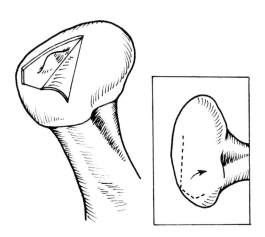

FIGURE 33–9. Arthroplasty (see text for details).

quire that the individual sutures be placed 2 mm apart, and 10 to 12 sutures are placed. During the repair, the sutures should reapproximate superior stratum to superior stratum and inferior stratum to inferior stratum. I prefer to use a nonresorbable tendon suture. Before complete closure of the inferior joint space, total hemostasis must be obtained, and the spaces must be irrigated copiously with lactated Ringer's solution.

STEP 17: CAPSULAR CLOSURE

The flaps of the capsule are identified, and these are reapproximated with a 4-0 chromic suture. Likewise, the anterior and posterior parts of the capsule are closed in the horizontal part of the incision. A small opening is left for insertion of the temporary interpositional implant.

STEP 18: SPACE MAINTENANCE

Adhesions are likely to redevelop in the superior joint space for two reasons. The articular surfaces of the superior joint are more irregular because of the lysis of the original adhesions. Similarly, the superior surface of the disc is roughened by the discoplasty procedure. The functions of the interpositional implant are to prevent redevelopment of adhesions and to restore a smoother surface to the fossa and superior side of the disc. A Silastic interpositional implant is custom trimmed to the contour of the internal perimeter of the joint space (Fig. 33–11). The better the match in fit, the more effectively the implant functions. While the implant is in place, fibrous connective tissue forms in the areas of roughened articular surface. A tail is left on the implant, and this is brought through the capsule. The tip of the implant is sutured in the subcutaneous tissue above the ear tragus with a silk suture so that it can be subsequently identified for retrieval.

The implant is left in place until interincisal opening is 35 mm. The patient must be instructed not to chew while the implant is in place so that particulation of the implant can be mitigated.

STEP 19: DRAINAGE

Postoperative effusion of the TMJ may be several milliliters. Therefore, for the first 24 to 48 hours, the superior joint space is drained until the effusion subsides to less than 5 ml in an 8-hour period. The drain is placed under suction and exits the skin beneath the earlobe. Postoperative drainage of the TMJ helps to reduce swelling and pain, and mobilization is improved.

STEP 20: CONDYLAR CORTICOTOMY

Avascular necrosis and condylar edema are readily demonstrated on magnetic resonance imaging.[16] Decompression of the marrow space of the condyle not only reduces TMJ pain, but it may also enhance critical blood flow to the marrow. The posterosuperior portion of the condyle seems most vulnerable to avascular necrosis; therefore, this area can be decompressed by opening the cortical bone at the lateral condylar neck (Fig. 33–12). This corticotomy is generally placed inferior to the capsular attachment in the extra-articular condyle. However, channels may be cut more superiorly within the marrow to allow for venting of edema from more remote areas. Condylar corticotomy should reduce venous sludging and

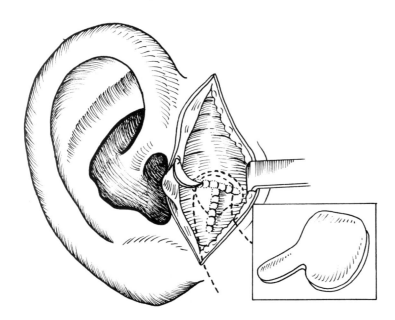

FIGURE 33–11. Space maintenance (see text for details).

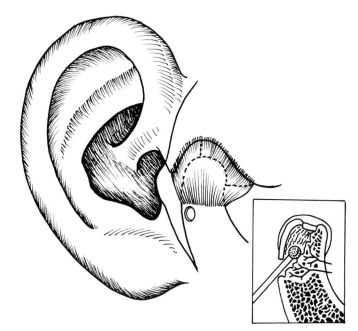

FIGURE 33-12. Condylar corticotomy (see text for details).

improve the flow of blood through the marrow space. When the entire condylar head is sclerotic as a result of avascular necrosis, this approach also allows access for placement of an autogenous cancellous bone graft.

SUMMARY

The TMJ is a highly complex area of the body, and for such a small area, it plays perhaps the major role in the production of facial pain. Fortunately, for the majority of TMJ problems, management can be confined to nonsurgical options. However, for individuals afflicted with the more complex types of TMJ pathology, pain from the TMJ can become totally consuming and can alter virtually every aspect of life. For some, TMJ pathology may also mean a lifetime of occlusal change and facial disfigurement due to condylar degeneration. Choices for these patients are not easy, and in fact, because of the array of nonsurgical and surgical treatment options, decisions on management may seem almost impossible.

It is hoped that a formal discussion of the various types of tissue distortion in the disc, lateral pterygoid muscle, retrodiscal attachment, capsule, joint spaces, and condylar marrow will aid in the choice of nonsurgical and surgical management options. Furthermore, by reviewing the complexities of TMJ reconstruction through the technique of microsurgery,

perhaps all other surgical and nonsurgical techniques can be put to critical inquiry in terms of their roles in alleviating internal derangements and in preventing progressive pathology.

REFERENCES

1. Henny, F.A.: Surgical treatment of the painful temporomandibular joint. J. Am. Dent. Assoc. 79:171, 1969.
2. Wilkes, C.: Internal derangements of the temporomandibular joint: Pathological variations. Arch. Otolaryngol. Head Neck Surg. 115:469, 1989.
3. Bronstein, S.L., Tomasetti, K.I., and Ryan, D.E.: Internal derangement of the temporomandibular joint: Correlation of arthrography with surgical findings. J. Oral Maxillofac. Surg. 39:572, 1981.
4. Piper, M.A. and Chuong, R.: Intraoperative assessment of discal position using C-arm arthrography during arthroscopic surgery. Presented at the 69th Annual Meeting of the American Association of Oral-Maxillofacial Surgeons. Anaheim, California, September, 1987.
5. Schellhas, K.P., Wilkes, C.H., Omlie, M.R., et al: The diagnosis of temporomandibular joint disease: Two compartment arthrography and MR. A.J.N.R. 9:579, 1988.
6. Katzberg, R.W., Schenck, J.F., Roberts, D., et al: Magnetic resonance imaging of the temporomandibular joint meniscus. J. Oral Maxillofac. Surg. 59:332, 1985.
7. Schellhas, K.P., Wilkes, C.H., Heithoff, K.B., et al: Temporomandibular joint: Diagnosis of internal derangement using magnetic resonance imaging. Minn. Med. 69:516, 1986.
8. Schellhas, K.P., Wilkes, C.H., Omlie, M.R., et al: Temporomandibular joint imaging: Practical application of available technology. Arch. Otolaryngol. Head Neck Surg. 113:744, 1987.

9. Pringle, J.: Displacement of the mandibular meniscus and its treatment. Br. J. Surg. 6:385, 1918.

10. Roberts, C.A., Tallents, R.H., Katzberg, R.W., et al: Comparison of internal derangements of the TMJ with occlusal findings. Oral Surg. Oral Med. Oral Pathol. 63:645, 1987.

11. De Bont, L.G.M., Boering, G., Liem, R.S.B., et al: Osteoarthritis and internal derangement of the temporomandibular joint: A light microscopic study. J. Oral Maxillofac. Surg 44:634, 1986.

12. Scapino, R.P.: Histopathology associated with malposition of the human temporomandibular joint disc. Oral Surg. 55:382, 1983.

13. Schellhas, K.P., Wilkes, C.H., Fritts, H.M., et al: Temporomandibular joint: MR imaging of internal derangements and postoperative changes. A.J.N.R. 1093, 1987.

14. Wilkes, C.: Structural and functional alteration of the temporomandibular joint. Northwest Dentistry 57:287, 1978.

15. Piper, M.A.: Microscopic disk preservation surgery of the temporomandibular joint. In *Oral and Maxillofacial Surgery Clinics of North America,* Vol 1, No. 2, p. 279. R.G. Merrill (ed.). 1989.

16. Schellhas, K.P., Wilkes, C.H., Fritts, H.M., et al: MR of osteochondritis dissecans and avascular necrosis of the mandibular condyle. A.J.N.R. 10:3, 1989.

17. Westesson, P.L., Bronstein, S.L., Liedberg, J.: Internal derangement of the temporomandibular joint: Morphologic description with correlation to joint function. Oral Surg. Oral Med. Oral Pathol. 59:323, 1985.

18. McNamara, J.A. Jr.: The independent functions of the two heads of the lateral pterygoid muscle. Am. J. Anat. 138:197, 1973.

19. Boyer, C.C., Williams, T.W., Stevens, F.H.: Blood supply of the temporomandibular joint. J. Dent. Res. 43:224, 1964.

20. Westesson, P.L.: Structural hard-tissue changes in temporomandibular joints with internal derangements. Oral Surg. Oral Med. Oral Pathol. 59:220, 1985.

21. Westesson, P.L., and Rohlin, M.: Internal derangement related to osteoarthrosis in temporomandibular joint autopsy specimens. Oral Surg. 57:17, 1984.

22. Bowman, K.: Temporomandibular joint arthrosis and its treatment by extirpation of the disc. Acta Chir. Scand. (Suppl.)95:118, 1947.

23. Kiehn, C.L.: Meniscectomy for internal derangement of temporomandibular joint. Am. J. Surg. 83:364, 1952.

24. Schellhas, K.P., Wilkes, C.H., El-Deeb, M., et al: Permanent Proplast temporomandibular joint implants: MR imaging of destructive complications. A.J.R. 151:731, 1988.

25. Bessette, R., Katzberg, R., Natiella, J.R., et al: Diagnosis and reconstruction of the human TMJ after trauma of internal derangement. Plast. Reconstr. Surg. 75:192, 1985.

26. Dingman, R.O., Grabb, W.C.: Intra-capsular temporomandibular joint arthroplasty. Plast. Reconstr. Surg. 38:179, 1966.

27. Georgiade, N.: The surgical correction of temporomandibular joint dysfunction by means of autogenous dermal grafts. Plast. Reconstr. Surg. 30:68, 1962.

28. McCarty, W.L. Jr. and Farrar, W.: Surgery for internal derangements for the temporomandibular joint. J. Prosthet. Dent. 42:2, 1979.

29. Kreutziger, K.L.: Microsurgical approach to the temporomandibular joint. Arch. Otolaryngol. 108:422, 1982.

30. Ibid.

31. Kreutziger, K.L.: Surgery of the temporomandibular joint. II. Microsurgery. Oral Surg. 58:647, 1984.

David C. Hoffman

CHAPTER 34

Orthognathic Surgery and Temporomandibular Surgery

Establishing a functional relationship between the temporomandibular joint (TMJ) and the facial skeleton has become a most challenging problem. Largely unanswered questions include, Do patients with class II skeletofacial deformity (SFD) present with an increased incidence of temporomandibular disorders (TMDs)? And, Which is addressed first, a SFD or TMD? The purpose of this chapter is to discuss the interrelationship between TMD and SFD and their surgical correction.

Others chapters have described the pathology of the TMJ. Arthrotomy and arthroscopic treatment have also been discussed and will be mentioned only briefly. However, several definitions should be clarified so that consistency can be maintained throughout this discussion. Furthermore, if the terms *skeletofacial deformity* and *orthognathic surgery* are used, it should be understood that they can imply many different entities. For example, orthognathic surgery encompasses a group of procedures ranging from simple chin augmentation or genioplasty to complicated combinations of maxillary and mandibular osteotomies. Skeletofacial deformities can also include a wide range of acquired and developmental deformities ranging from simple to complex. This discussion is based on rules that govern the interaction of SFDs and TMDs and their surgical treatment.

Rule 1: The TMJ provides skeletal support

for the lower third of the facial skeleton and provides mandibular movement.

The facial skeleton can assume normal and abnormal types. Although normalcy is difficult to define, generally accepted classifications of SFDs exist. For the most part, these groupings are based on the interrelationship of the mandible, maxilla, and cranium. The TMJ is an integral part of this relationship because it connects the mandible to the rest of the facial skeleton and allows for articulated movements. Accordingly, problems that affect the facial skeleton have the potential to affect the TMJ. The corollary is also true: Changes in the TMJ can alter the facial skeleton. The most striking example is the secondary occlusal changes caused by rheumatoid arthritis resulting in a class II open bite (Fig. 34–1).

Although the interrelationship of TMDs and SFDs might seem obvious to most clinicians, it is difficult to find studies that support a cause-and-effect relationship between SFDs and TMDs[1,2] Certainly, it is even more difficult to justify correction of a deformity in an attempt to treat a TMD.

A study at the Free University Hospital of Amsterdam by Kersten and colleagues followed 480 patients undergoing orthognathic surgery over a 3-year period and evaluated them by facial types, surgical procedures, and incidence of preoperative and postoperative TMD symptoms.[45] Results showed a 16.2% incidence of symptoms preoperatively compared with a reported 26% incidence of symptoms in the young adult population studied by Solberg and associates.[2] Kersten's study also showed that two thirds of this symptomatic group reported improvement after surgery, but 11.5% of the asymptomatic group reported postoperative symptoms. This research illustrates the dilemma that clinicians find themselves in when choosing a treatment plan. These reports should stimulate clinicians to investigate more closely the general disease process and its overall effect on patients. Many well-documented indications for both TMJ and orthognathic surgery exist that, when correctly recognized, can be effectively addressed with operative therapy.[3-6]

When orthognathic surgery results in a postoperative TMJ problem, many questions arise. Condylar position, muscle adaptability, and rigid fixation merit consideration. The following discussion reviews such considerations and, when possible, offers guidelines for treatment. If we understand the underlying principles of

701

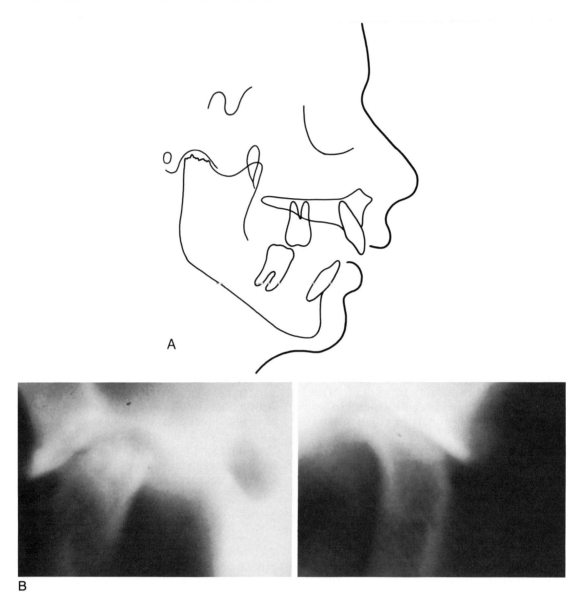

FIGURE 34–1. *A,* Cephalometric illustration of a patient with rheumatoid arthritis. The open bite deformity is caused by the loss of vertical height because of resorption of the condylar head. *B,* Right and left temporomandibular tomograms indicating severe degenerative changes and loss of condylar height.

orthognathic surgical decision making, the chosen treatment plan will afford a sensible clinical rationale.

CLASSIFICATIONS AND DEFINITIONS OF SKELETOFACIAL DEFORMITIES

An SFD may be a congenital, a developmental, or an acquired abnormality.[7] Norms for the facial skeleton, originally defined by analysis of

a small series of cephalometric studies by a group of orthodontists,[8] became more formalized by Broadbent and Broadbent[9] (Fig. 34–2). Today, cephalometric radiographs are only part of the records obtained to analyze a skeletofacial relationship. A complete set of records includes cephalometric and craniofacial radiographs, facial photographs, study casts, and TMJ imaging. A complete history, aesthetic soft-tissue analyses, and a thorough head and neck examination play equally important parts in this assessment. With this information,

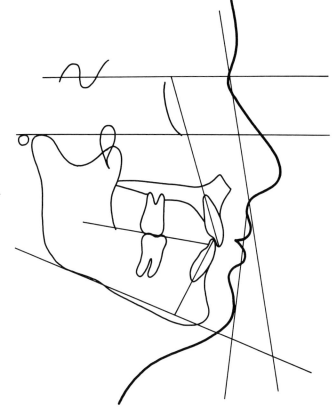

FIGURE 34–2. Normal cephalometric illustration.

clinicians classify a presenting SFD using the following diagnostic groups:

1. Asymmetry: Patients have a difference in the right and left halves of the face in hard tissue, soft tissue, or both, often associated with unilateral TMJ size difference.
2. Hypoplasia: Patients have a deficiency in size, shape, or structure of the bone and possibly of the associated soft tissue.
3. Hyperplasia: Patients have an enlargement in size, shape, or structure of the bone, possibly associated with soft-tissue hyperplasia.

The combined dentofacial skeletal relationship has been traditionally divided into three classes of deformity: Angle's classes I, II, and III. This scheme is based on the first molar and canine relationship and describes the occlusion more than the facial type. Deep bite and open bite may be added to describe the bite more specifically (Fig. 34–3). Class II often is assumed to indicate a deficient or hypoplastic mandible with either flared (division 1) or anterior inverted dentition (division 2) (Fig. 34–4). Class III assumes a prognathic mandible. In reality,

both class II and class III may be due to variations in the mandible or maxilla.[3] Because these classes can be misleading, it is more accurate to describe SFD in the following terms:

1. *Mandibular hypoplasia or hyperplasia with or without asymmetry:* The asymmetry is often a unilateral expression of a hyperplastic situation. This subgroup is limited to deformities in which the abnormal structure is located in the mandible relative to the rest of the facial skeleton.
2. *Maxillary hypoplasia or hyperplasia with or without asymmetry:* This subgroup includes patients in whom the disorder lies in the maxilla. The vertical, transverse, or anterior/posterior vectors can be either bilateral or unilateral.
3. *Combined maxillary and mandibular deformities:* This subgroup includes patients with a combination defect of both the mandible and maxilla. Included are patients with maxillary vertical problems with combined mandibular retrognathia. Rotation of the mandible due to maxillary vertical excess accentuates the associated mandibular hypoplasia. This is consid-

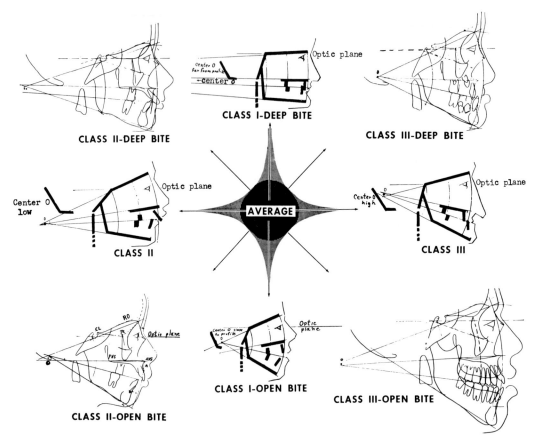

FIGURE 34–3. Classification of facial types as described by Sassouni. (Reprinted with permission from Sassouni, V.: *The Face in Five Dimensions,* 2nd ed. West Virginia University Press, Morgantown, W. Va., 1962.)

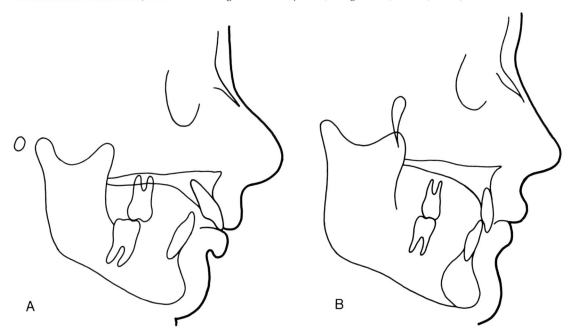

FIGURE 34–4. Cephalometric illustrations of a patient with a Class II, division 1 (*A*) and a patient with a class II, division 2 (*B*) occlusion. Note the variation of the inclination of the maxillary central incisors.

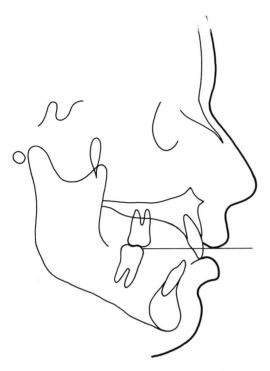

FIGURE 34-5. Cephalometric illustrations of a patient with a vertical maxillary excess. In this instance, a relative mandibular hypoplasia is appreciated. The mandible is in a retrognathic position because of the clockwise autorotation of the mandible. Although the deformity appears to be in the mandible, the true deformity is the vertical posterior maxillary excess.

ered a relative and absolute mandibular hypoplasia with vertical maxillary excess (also called *hyperplasia*) (Fig. 34-5).

4. *Facial asymmetry:* As previously described, this subgroup includes patients with a notable difference between the two halves of the face, either in the soft or hard tissues or both.

5. *Nasal-orbital-zygomatic deformity:* A combination of multiple bones of the face often collectively expressing the same disfigurement.

6. *Craniofacial deformity:* A combination of facial and cranial bones collectively expressing the same disfigurement.

Some individual characteristics of these SFDs are apparent in particular clinical settings. These include the following:

1. *Congenital deformities:* This subgroup includes patients with birth defects expressed in a repeatable pattern (syndromes) that has associated skeletal deformities (e.g., cleft lip and palate, hemifacial microsomia, Pierre Robin anomaly).

2. *Open bite:* Also called *skeletal apertognathia,* open bite is usually a result of vertical maxillary hyperplasia, which limits autorotation of the mandible. It should be differentiated from dental or acquired open bites.

3. *Deep bite:* This subgroup includes patients with an associated overclosure of the mandible, usually with an excess overjet and overbite relationship. It is usually caused by mandibular hypoplasia.

4. *Acquired open bite:* This form of apertognathia is secondary to loss of condylar or vertical ramus height. It should be distinguished from a true open bite secondary to maxillary vertical excess. Acquired open bites are often due to resorption of the TMJ. They may occur independent of pain, dysfunction, or limited range of motion in the TMJ (Fig. 34-6).

5. *Traumatic deformities:* SFDs due to facial trauma can manifest in various problems not necessarily encountered as a specific pattern. Condylar fractures can cause a change in vertical ramus height, provoking a combined TMJ and open bite problem. The same problem combined with a symphysis fracture can cause splaying of the mandibular angles. The resulting deformity is often complex, combining a loss of form and function without routine treatment options. Symptoms can be a direct result of the trauma or secondary to changes in structure and function of the TMJ.[10]

6. *Ankylosis:* Ankylosis can be either a fibrous or bony fusion of the TMJs. It can result in not only decreased range of motion but also a secondary growth disturbance when it occurs before growth is complete (Fig. 34-7 A, B, C). Ankylosis is not always a skeletal problem and can be considered strictly a TMD if growth is complete (Fig. 34-7 D, E, F).

Rule 2: The TMJ is an integral part of the facial skeleton, and diseases that affect one may affect the other.

The diagnostic terms defined earlier illustrate the many forms of dentofacial and skeletofacial deformities. Fortunately, many of the problems are isolated or do not affect the TMJ. Unfortunately, a number of problems can affect the TMJ and facial skeleton.

Rule 3: Treatment of a SFD does not guarantee or imply improvement of an existing TMJ problem.

Although there can be an interrelationship between certain SFDs and TMDs, successful

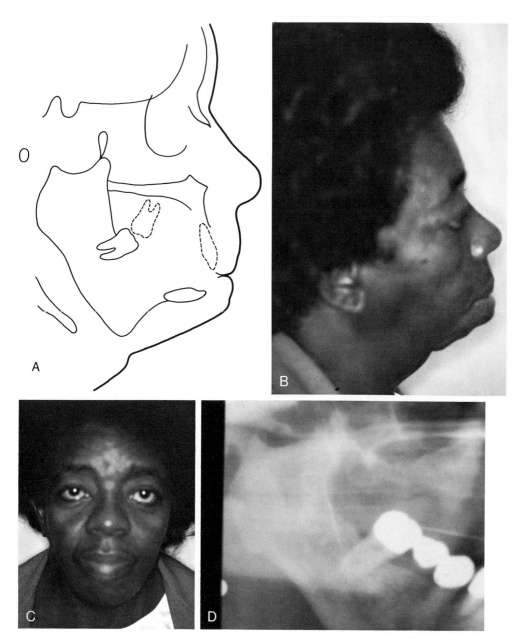

FIGURE 34–6. *A,* This cephalometric illustration shows a patient with an acquired open bite secondary to idiopathic lysis of the condyles. As a result of the clockwise autorotation and a severe open bite, the patient has a retrognathic appearance (*B* and *C*). *D,* Panoramic view of half of the mandible illustrating the destruction found in this patient's condyle.

treatment of the SFD offers only moderate hope for the alleviation of symptoms. Evaluating the symptoms and identifying the cause are essential in developing an appropriate treatment plan for patients with a SFD and TMD.

Rule 4: The TMJ and the masticatory muscles must be evaluated during the initial assessment of a patient with a SFD.

Temporomandibular disorders of the joint can be arbitrarily divided into two categories, intracapsular disorders and extracapsular disorders.

Intracapsular disorders include disease processes of the condylar head and articulating surfaces, the disc and associated ligaments, the eminence, and the temporal fossa. The most common intracapsular disorders are internal derangements and osteoarthrosis.[11,12] Associated SFDs in the early stage of a TMD are variable but sometimes include mandibular hypoplasia and vertical maxillary hyperplasia. In later stages, bony changes may produce a loss of posterior facial height and an acquired open bite.

Extracapsular disorders include a group of problems that affect the surrounding structures that support the TMJ. These include the muscles of mastication and facial expression, as well as the cervical spine and supporting muscles of the cervical collar. Extracapsular disorders may also be associated with SFDs. For example, in patients with facial asymmetries and pseudoprognathism with a large centric slide, a SFD might contribute to an extracapsular disorder.

The distinction between the categories can be surprisingly puzzling at times and plainly obvious at other times. The clinical signs often help the clinician to diagnose the problem.

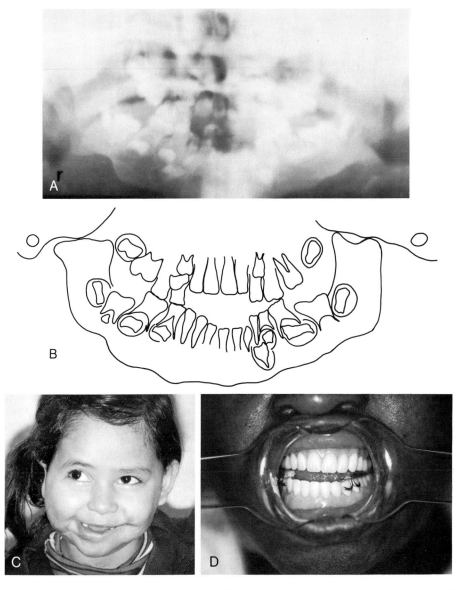

FIGURE 34–7. Panoramic radiograph (*A*) and illustration (*B*) showing condylar destruction and ankylosis. The patient's mandible has deviated owing to growth in an asymmetric pattern. The young patient (*C*) has an obvious facial deformity and inability to open her mouth. *D* to *G*, An adult form of ankylosis. On maximal opening, the patient demonstrates hypomobility (*D*). Because growth was complete prior to the pathologic process in the temporomandibular joint, the patient does not exhibit a facial deformity.

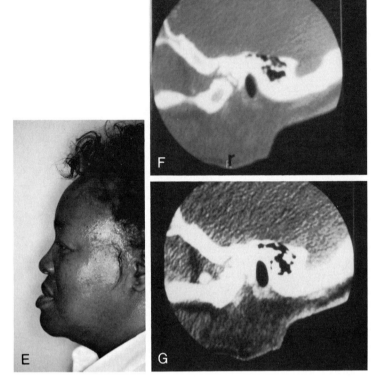

Figure 34–7 *Continued* (*E*). The computerized tomograms (*F* and *G*) clearly illustrate the presence of bony ankylosis.

Taking a careful history and performing a thorough examination of the patients with SFD should be directed at evaluating the following parameters:

1. *Pain.* The clinician should evaluate the source, location, and quantity of any pain and what provokes or eliminates pain.

2. *Range of motion:* The movements of the mandible and cervical spine must be measured. Changes in maximum interincisal distance after diagnostic blocks in the joint and muscles distinguish intracapsular from extracapsular pathology.

3. *Painful dysfunction:* If a patient has a combination of pain and limited movement, the source of pain is often identifiable. For example, patients can be asked, Where does it hurt when you chew? Or, When does your jaw lock?

4. *Unstable joints:* Patients who have multiple occlusions or who complain of a changing bite often have unstable TMJs. Positive or negative imaging studies help direct attention to intra-articular or extracapsular pathology.

5. *Arthritis:* The presence of systemic or localized arthritis may also be the source of a TMD. Inflammatory arthritis leads to a high index of suspicion for an intracapsular disorder. Unfortunately, there may be a strong secondary muscle component of intracapsular pain associated with movement. Accordingly, what may seem to be a classic case of osteoarthrosis of the TMJ may have its major pain component in the facial musculature (Fig. 34–8).

6. *SFD/TMD relationship:* Evaluation of an existing SFD helps provide supporting evidence for the presumed cause of the disorder.

Ultimately, when trying to distinguish between an intracapsular or extracapsular origin of pain, a "chicken and egg" story may develop, and a clinician may mistakenly treat the x-ray findings instead of the patient's problem. On one hand, the use of a "pain picture" in establishing an etiology may be helpful (Fig. 34–9). On the other hand, it may be impossible to treat muscle pain effectively if the etiology is an SFD.

CLASSIFICATION OF SURGICAL PROCEDURES

Surgical procedures can be divided into two main categories: TMJ surgery and orthognathic surgery. Orthognathic surgical procedures are osteotomies of the facial skeleton;

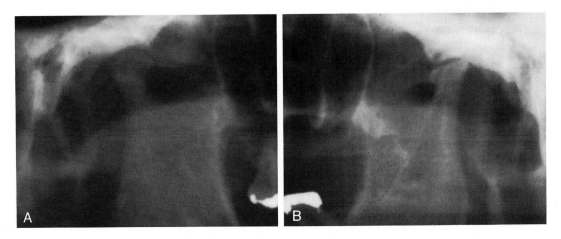

FIGURE 34–8. Right (*A*) and left (*B*) tomograms of a patient with a severe degenerative joint disease and an unstable occlusion. The patient complained of multiple areas of pain including the entire cervical area, temporomandibular joints (TMJs), and muscles of the face and neck. Although the patient had degenerative joint disease, the pain was not specific to the TMJ region.

their primary purpose is to create or restore normal occlusion or facial form. Temporomandibular joint surgery includes procedures that restore function and form.

Certain surgical procedures have dual purposes. For example, a costochondral rib graft allows for repositioning of the mandibular dentition into a new relationship with the maxilla and rebuilds the joint. For the most part, the reason a certain type of procedure is being performed is clear. The following questions are often asked: If both TMJ and orthognathic surgery are indicated, which procedure should be done first? Will orthognathic surgery cause or exacerbate a TMD? Can orthognathic surgery improve an existing TMD?

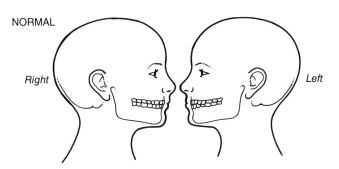

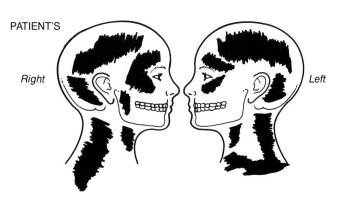

FIGURE 34–9. Pain questionnaire as filled out by the patient described in Figure 34–8.

For purposes of discussion, the following can be considered a representative list of orthognathic and TMJ surgical procedures:

1. Orthognathic surgery
   a. Mandibular ramus osteotomies including sagittal splits, vertical ramus, or other ramus procedures
   b. Genioplasty
   c. Subapical osteotomies and mandibular body or symphysis osteotomies
   d. Maxillary osteotomies, including LeForte's I, II, and III
2. TMJ surgical procedures
   a. Arthroscopic examination and surgery
   b. Disc plication or other disc-related procedures or discoplasties
   c. Meniscectomy
   d. Joint reconstruction with alloplastic or autogenous grafting, including implants, muscle, dermis, fascia, and cartilage grafts
   e. Costochondral rib or other related bony grafts
   f. Total joint prostheses

The last set of terms that are useful to define before a discussion on orthognathic and TMJ surgery relate to occlusion. Besides centric relation and centric occlusion (intercuspal position), there are three other useful groupings: stable occlusion, functional occlusion, and normal occlusion. Although an understanding of centric occlusion and relation is important, these other three terms have a greater significance when speaking about surgical treatment.

A stable occlusion designates any bite relationship that is not changing over a period of time. This is an important concept when the clinician is staging procedures of both orthognathic and TMJ surgery. A change in the bite may indicate a structural change in the joint (bone or disc), a facial skeletal growth or surgical relapse, or an orthodontic change secondary to eruption or dental compensation. An observation period of 2 to 6 months after a major surgical procedure seems logical for watching for changes in the occlusion before it can be considered stable.

A functional occlusion allows for adequate speech and mastication and provides skeletal support. The occlusion can be considered functional even if there is a "malocclusion," as long as there is adequate function. A functional occlusion does not contribute to the cause of a TMD and must be in harmony with the TMJ. A skeletal open bite with occlusion on only the first molars might not be considered a functional occlusion if mastication or speech were impaired.

An ideal occlusion is the traditional concept of a class I occlusion with a normal overbite/overjet relationship and a normal condyle-discfossa relationship. Before guidelines can be delineated for combined orthognathic and TMJ surgery, accepted indications are summarized for each area as an isolated entity.

Diagnostic arthroscopy can be used to do the following[5]:

1. Assess the degree of intracapsular disease as a result of pain or hypomobility, whether acute or chronic
2. Rule out organic disease in patients who present diagnostic dilemmas
3. Assess intra-articular implants
4. Assess significant radiographic or pathologic changes
5. Evaluate the TMJ after arthrotomy
6. Evaluate the TMJ before planned arthrotomy
7. Assess postoperative problems
8. Evaluate suspected arthritis.

Operative or surgical arthroscopy can be used for the following[5]:

1. Treatment of hypomobility disorders
2. Treatment of osteoarthrosis or perforations
3. Treatment of internal derangement
4. Treatment of hypermobility disorders
5. Evaluation and treatment after open joint surgery or previous arthroscopy
6. Treatment of acute injury or trauma.

Open TMJ surgery can be used for the following[6]:

1. Treatment of intracapsular disorders
2. Removal or placement of implants
3. Reconstruction of a structurally debilitated joint
4. Replacement of growth centers with rib grafts
5. Treatment of hypomobility disorders
6. Treatment of hypermobility disorders
7. Treatment of traumatic injuries of the joint.

Indications for total joint replacement whether by autogenous grafts or prostheses are less specific. Most surgeons agree that these procedures are secondary and indicated for a structural loss of the condyle or for replacement of a failed pre-existing total system.[15]

A presentation of specific indications for orthognathic surgery is beyond the scope of this book. The reader is directed to the many textbooks that offer excellent guidelines.[4,13,14] Some of the general indications for orthognathic surgery are as follows:

1. Correction of maxillary SFDs
2. Correction of mandibular SFDs
3. Correction of combined maxillary and mandibular deformities
4. Correction of facial asymmetries
5. Correction of facial syndromes or traumatic injuries
6. Establishment of a functional occlusion.

When the indications for TMJ surgery and orthognathic surgery are compared, very little overlap is noted. Only during restoration of structure to a joint can a surgeon broach changing the facial skeleton. However, subtle changes can affect the function of the TMJ following orthognathic surgery. The work of Finn and colleagues,[18] Boyd,[16] Bell and others[17] clearly demonstrates changes in facial muscle type, direction, and function following these surgical procedures.

Rule 5: When planning and performing orthognathic surgery, every attempt should be made to avoid causing secondary TMJ problems.

Although most orthognathic surgery is well tolerated, it always poses a possibility of causing positive or negative effects on the TMJ. Of major concern is the postsurgical relationship of the condyle, disc, and fossa. With the advent of rigid fixation, condylar position and function have become even more important. Muscle change and condylar placement can be either beneficial or deleterious to TMJ function. Obviously, surgeons should maximize the benefits and avoid unwarranted adverse effects.

DEFINING THE PROBLEM

Most patients present with a fairly specific chief complaint in describing a TMD or an SFD. As previously described, pain, decreased range of motion, inability to chew, malocclusion, or aesthetic concerns encompass the majority of such complaints. Unfortunately, the treatment plan cannot always be straightforward, especially in the case of a patient with a combined joint and skeletal problem. Hence, for this patient, the idiom "for each problem let there be a solution" becomes somewhat elusive.

As previously discussed, the first step in diagnosis is obtaining a careful history and performing a clinical examination. Interpretation of the information obtained and the selective use of imaging techniques can change a patient's chief complaint into a meaningful differential diagnosis. It is important to distinguish which problems (either TMJ or orthognathic) are primary and which are secondary or at least can be delegated to a second stage of care. There are five possibilities in this regard:

1. TMJ pathology as a primary problem, SFD as secondary
2. SFD as a primary problem, TMJ pathology as secondary
3. Combined TMJ pathology and SFD—both primary
4. TMD secondary to orthognathic surgery
5. SFD secondary to TMJ surgery.

When TMJ pathology is a primary problem and SFD is a secondary problem, the patient's chief complaint is the most helpful piece of information.

Problems related to joint function, such as pain on chewing, joint noise, and an inability to open the mouth are more likely to reflect primary TMJ pathology. In this instance, a coexisting SFD may be observed on examination or imaging but is not of major concern to the patient.

When SFD is a primary problem and TMJ pathology is a secondary problem, patients present with complaints and clinical findings of malocclusion or a desire to have aesthetic facial changes. In this instance, patients generally have good range of motion, mild-to-moderate complaints about the joint or masticatory muscles, and possibly concomitant radiographic evidence of TMJ pathology.

Combined TMJ pathology and SFD, both primary, include the most interesting and complex group of cases. Patients often have clear complaints and clinical findings of TMD and SFD, and both problems are almost equal in magnitude. In this instance more than others, the surgeon must include the patient in formulating the treatment plan and must be aware that TMD can be progressive. This subgroup includes patients with active degenerative lesions of the TMJ and resulting changes in the facial skeleton. Patients who have panfacial trauma and both SFD and TMJ pathology often have these combined problems.

Patients with TMJ complaints secondary to orthognathic surgery are the least difficult to classify because, like the first group, their complaints center on the TMJ. However, a patient's history should reveal onset of the symptoms after orthognathic surgery. It is important to confirm that there were no symptoms before surgery. An asymptomatic click often has the potential to become a burden if not well documented and discussed preoperatively.

Rule 6: Evaluate and diagnose hypomobility disorders before surgery.

Postoperative hypomobility after orthognathic surgery is of major concern because of the multiple possible causes following maxillary and mandibular osteotomies.[20] If the mandible has a decreased range of motion before orthognathic surgery, there is no reason to believe that this range will improve unless the restriction was caused by a mechanical locking of bone that was removed during surgery. Inherent in facial bone osteotomies is an early postoperative reduction in mandibular opening, especially with mandibular sagittal split osteotomies.[21] The most common preoperative cause of hypomobility is internal derangement or muscle spasm. The most common cause of postosteotomy hypomobility is scarring of the surgical site. Without a proper preoperative assessment, this distinction becomes cloudy.

More TMDs may be associated with orthognathic surgery since the advent of rigid fixation. Surgeons must effectively evaluate condyle placement with rigid fixation.[22–25] Cases of condylysis have also been reported with mandibular sagittal split osteotomies (Fig. 34–10).[26]

Figure 34–10 shows preoperative and postoperative changes in the condyle following

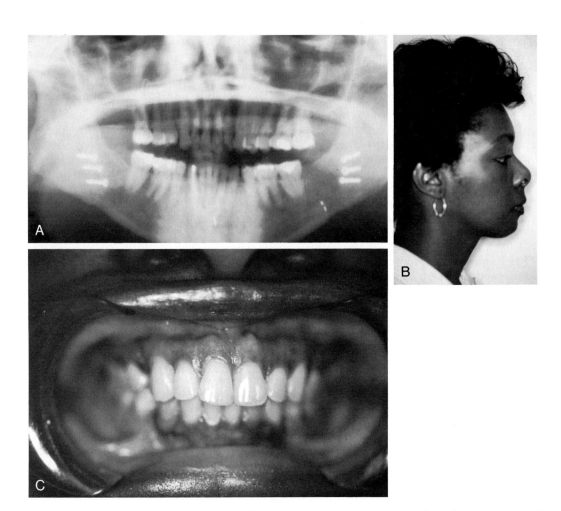

FIGURE 34–10. Panoramic radiograph (*A*) and facial photographs (*B* and *C*) of a patient who had undergone a maxillary and mandibular osteotomy. The 2-year followup revealed severe idiopathic lysis of the condyle, generating a light open bite deformity. Although the patient was asymptomatic, the skeletal deformity was becoming apparent.

maxillary-mandibular osteotomies. An idiopathic loss of condylar height and shape known as *osteochondritis* or *idiopathic lysis* of the condyle is seen. If an unfavorable occlusion results from relapse or progressive loss of condylar height, the potential for a TMD can be appreciated.[27,28]

Rule 7: An SFD after TMJ surgery may be due to the surgery or the disease.

In SFD secondary to TMJ surgery or pathology, determining that an SFD resulted from TMJ surgery is not as easy as one might suspect. The most likely clinical scenario is a postoperative open bite or asymmetry due to a loss of vertical height of the condyle in a patient who has had TMJ surgery. Surgical removal of tissue or the disease state itself may be responsible.

A cause-and-effect relationship with the surgery may be established for the untoward effect. However, the skeletal change may be due to the surgical correction of the pre-existing TMJ pathology or the TMJ problem itself. Figure 34–11 shows a film of a patient who had a destructive lesion in the left condyle. After surgical removal of the degenerated bone, there is a shift in occlusion secondary to the loss of the left condylar height despite attempts to hold the occlusion in place. The problem in this situation is the disease process, and the surgery was an attempt to correct it.

TREATMENT PLANNING AND SURGICAL SEQUENCING

Several options are available to oral and maxillofacial surgeons for formulating a treatment plan. The advent of both TMJ arthroscopy and rigid fixation has had a major impact in this arena. The indications for TMJ and orthognathic surgery were previously described.

Five additional guidelines should be considered before scheduling a patient for surgery:

1. Open or arthroscopic surgical procedures of the joint usually require a period of nonsurgical care. This may include medication, diet modification, appliance therapy, physical therapy, and joint rest. Bony ankylosis and fractures of the TMJ may be exceptions to this rule.[14]

2. Before and after surgery, orthodontic care is necessary in the presence of combined TMD and SFD.

3. When a new maxillomandibular relationship to be established with orthognathic surgery can be duplicated with appliance therapy, it is often advantageous to do so. For example, a repositioning splint can be used in a patient with a maxillary vertical deficiency (short face syndrome) or in a patient with unilateral open bite.[29–31] Clinicians must realize, however, that a sagittal split osteotomy advancement cannot duplicate the condyle position of a repositioning appliance (Fig. 34–12).

4. Treat the patient's chief complaint as the primary problem when possible.

5. It is best to perform TMJ surgery on a patient with a stable and functional occlusion.

Rule 8: When staging procedures, operations that can negatively change the occlusion should precede those that do not have this potential (e.g., a condylectomy would normally precede a maxillary or mandibular osteotomy).

Rule 9: It is difficult and often impossible to correct an occlusal problem with a surgical procedure to the TMJ.

Rule 10: A functional and stable occlusion achieved through orthognathic surgery may not improve the TMD but should enhance the postoperative result of TMJ surgery.

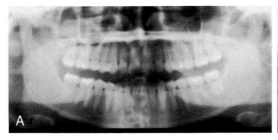 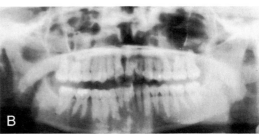

FIGURE 34–11. Preoperative (*A*) and postoperative (*B*) panoramic radiographs of a patient who had undergone open joint surgery to remove a destructive lesion. She experienced changes in occlusion as a result of the loss of the vertical height of the condyle. The patient developed unilateral posterior open bite causing occlusal instability.

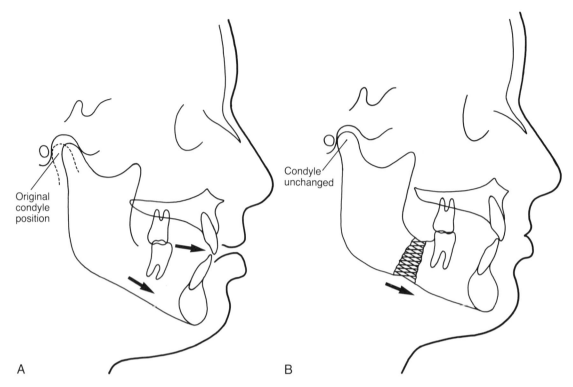

FIGURE 34-12. *A,* Condylar movement with an anterior repositioning appliance. *B,* Lack of condylar movement with a sagittal split osteotomy. These two diagrams illustrate that moving the mandible forward with a sagittal split osteotomy effectively changes the occlusion but not the condylar position. A repositioning appliance will change both the occlusion and the condylar position.

Now that some guidelines have been developed and indications for surgery have been listed, the possible treatment options can be explored. In general, it is my opinion that TMJ surgery should be preceded by arthroscopy and an evaluation period of 1 to 2 months before considering any open joint surgery. Patients with bony ankylosis or TMJ implant failure are some exceptions to this rule.

Treatment Sequencing Options for TMJ Disorders and SFD

Five possibilities exist for sequencing combined TMJ and orthognathic surgical procedures:

1. Arthroscopy; orthognathic surgery
2. Arthroscopy; open joint surgery; orthognathic surgery
3. Orthognathic surgery; open joint surgery
4. Simultaneous procedures
5. Orthognathic surgery; arthroscopy; open joint surgery.

Arthroscopy followed by orthognathic surgery is a logical approach for patients with combined problems. Arthroscopy can both diagnose and adequately treat many surgical TMJ problems. It can often preclude or eliminate the need for open joint surgery and yet allow the clinician to address the TMD.[32-35] Arthroscopy is especially helpful when there is a component of pain or decreased range of motion. It also has a major impact on treatment planning for patients with degenerative lesions, such as perforation or osteoarthrosis. In this situation, further treatment can be planned with respect to rules 8, 9, and 10.

In this first option, orthognathic surgery can be performed with the confidence that the joints have good function, and there is not planned open joint surgery, thereby minimizing the chance of a change in occlusion. This option also allows room for treating both mild and severe TMJ complaints should the patient continue to have symptoms after arthroscopy. It also leaves open the possibility for an open joint procedure, as described in the next option.

Arthroscopy, followed by open joint surgery, followed by orthognathic surgery is used when arthroscopy confirms intracapsular pathology but does not improve it satisfactorily. If needed, a decision must be made about whether open joint surgery or orthognathic surgery should be performed first. Arthrotomy allows for improving the form, function, and stability of the joint. This advantage is extremely important in patients who have had a decreased range of motion or severe pain.[36–38]

If establishing a functional occlusion is indicated, orthognathic surgery should be considered first. The literature suggests that orthognathic surgery will improve TMJ function, but a positive result in a given patient is unpredictable.[22,25]

Rule 11: Employ as few surgical procedures as possible.

When combining orthognathic surgery and TMJ surgery, there is no absolute rule about which procedure to do first in a given patient. The decision must be based on the severity of the pathology, the chief complaint, and most of all on the ability of the surgery to meet the intended goal. If the primary goal is to correct the aesthetic, dental, or functional skeletal pattern, orthognathic surgery might be performed first. Should the alleviation of pain or the increase in range of motion be the primary goal, the sequences discussed as options one or two may be preferable.

Orthognathic surgery as an initial procedure may be appealing after a review of the literature. This type of surgery can enhance neuromuscular adaptation, change the direction of condylar loading, and modify the skeletofacial type. Most parafunctional habits diminish during the first 6 weeks of postoperative rehabilitation.[16–19,35,39] All of these factors may account for the impressive decrease in symptoms that Kersten described as a result of orthognathic surgery.

The ability of orthognathic surgery to treat an internal derangement seems questionable. Many surgeons report that clicking disappears postoperatively, but some studies[40] show that clicking is not a reliable indicator of disc position. This has been confirmed with arthroscopy; preoperative and postoperative magnetic resonance imaging may show no change in disc displacement, but loss of clicking is appreciated (Fig. 34–13).[35]

No studies on preoperative and postoperative orthognathic surgery have so far been published to support the premise that the disc can be reduced. However, a changed condylar position and orientation may account for clinical but not radiographic resolution of an apparent internal derangement. This effect seems most apparent in a patient with an open bite secondary to vertical maxillary excess. Figure 34–14 illustrates severe posterior vertical maxillary excess and apertognathia in a patient who showed a significant anterior disc displacement and clicking before surgery. Postoperatively, the TMJ symptoms were resolved and occlusion was stable.

Many patients with signs and symptoms of TMDs do not need open joint surgery after orthognathic surgery. Temporomandibular joint surgery should not be performed before orthognathic surgery unless clinical signs and symptoms are severe. In that case, the opportunity to avoid a second surgical procedure would appear to be remote.

Combined procedures using rigid fixation have been advocated by some surgeons who plan simultaneous TMJ and orthognathic surgery. The proponents of this approach argue for the single hospital surgical admission, the overall adaptability of the facial skeleton, and the fewer inconveniences for the patient. The issue of which procedure to do first is also resolved. The problem with simultaneous procedures is the need to have very rapid mobilization of the joint and yet provide a stable environment without muscle tension for the osteotomy sites to heal. On a routine basis, simultaneous procedures without rigid internal fixation should be discouraged when immediate postoperative mobilization is indicated, as would be with arthroscopy. If rigid internal fixation is used, immediate function postoperatively is permitted, facilitating rehabilitation of the joint. Simultaneous procedures place the patient at a significant disadvantage in that any postoperative problems are more difficult to analyze. As a result of their high level of complexity, simultaneous procedures are still of limited use.

Certain situations mandate simultaneous orthognathic surgery and joint reconstruction. Unilateral joint reconstruction can require a contralateral mandibular osteotomy to return the occlusion to a normal relationship. In Figure 34–15, the patient had a condylar fracture with a secondary change in mandibular posi-

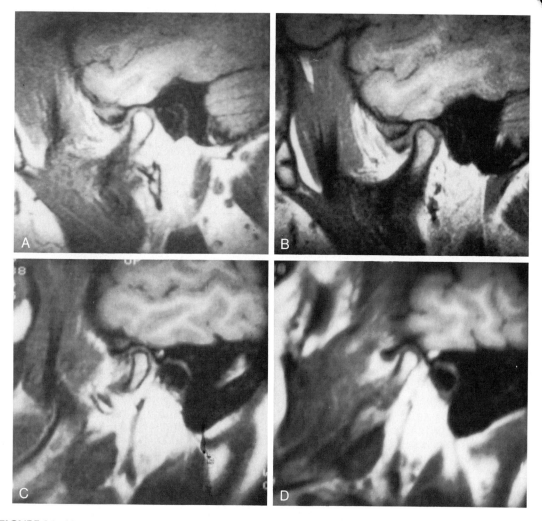

FIGURE 34–13. *A* to *D*, Prearthroscopic and postarthroscopic magnetic resonance images (MRIs). Presurgical (*A*) and postsurgical (*B*) MRIs of the right temporomandibular joint (TMJ). No change occurred in disc position. Presurgical (*C*) and postsurgical (*D*) MRIs of the left TMJ. Note the correction of the disc to a relatively normal position.

tion. Surgery included sagittal split osteotomy and joint reconstruction.

The best approach, however, is to evaluate the risk vs. the benefits. The surgeon and patient must evaluate the advantages of fewer procedures against more involved and often less predictable procedures. The lack of substantial literature in this area speaks for itself.

Orthognathic surgery followed by arthroscopy, followed by open joint surgery is similar to orthognathic surgery combined with TMJ surgery, the only difference being the use of arthroscopy before opening the joint. It is my opinion that arthroscopy should precede open joint surgery in almost all cases. The only possible benefit to this option is that of being able to evaluate the TMJ after the orthognathic surgery.

Rigid fixation has caused concern about superior and posterior positions of the condyle (Fig. 34–16). Postoperative evaluation and treatment of the TMJ after orthognathic surgery have been very successful with arthroscopy.[41] Figure 34–17 shows the use of TMJ arthroscopy following successful orthognathic surgery. The patient's primary complaints were malocclusion and facial appearance. Preoperative evaluation revealed intermittent clicking and a mildly painful right joint. Postoperatively, the patient did well until 9 months after surgery. She then began to experience pain and discomfort and decreased range of motion in

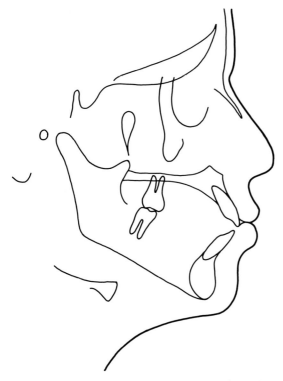

FIGURE 34–14. Cephalometric illustration of a patient with an open bite deformity. Computerized tomographic scans were taken (not shown), indicating an anterior disc displacement preoperatively. The patient's pain resolved after orthognathic surgery. A normal pain-free range of motion returned.

the right TMJ. Arthroscopy revealed the presence of adhesions and fibrosis with small perforations. The patient showed resolution and no need for an open joint procedure.

A need exists to direct treatment toward the chief complaint and to establish a contingency plan, based on possible expected or unexpected changes. A common problem is the loss of an acceptable surgical result because of occlusal changes. The injudicious use of a splint in postorthognathic surgery can often interfere with the intended results and must be carefully monitored.

Establishing a Complete Treatment Plan

Regardless of the sequence that is established, a surgeon must first develop a complete treatment plan. The plan should be made in consultation with the other clinicians treating the patient. The following should be considered when formulating a treatment plan:

Patient's Concerns and Chief Complaint. A list that clearly describes the chief complaints and the patient's concerns should be made. All ambiguous terms should be clarified. During the postoperative visits, this list can be used to evaluate the effectiveness of the treatment plan.

Complete History and Physical Examination. This includes the collection of historical and diagnostic data, including radiographs and photographs. Cephalometric analysis and TMJ radiographs are desirable. Position of the condyles after maxillary-mandibular osteotomies is extremely important. Laboratory tests, such as rheumatoid factor, sedimentation rate, erythrocyte sedimentation rate, and other rheumatologic assessments, may be included when indicated.

Proper Patient Education and Consent. The importance of patients' understanding of the disease and the surgical procedures along with their participation in formulation of the treatment plan does more than imply informed consent. It allows for rapport between patients and clinicians that puts them on the same team and thus working together.

Recognizing Stable and Changing Situations. Unstable occlusion, growing patients, and deteriorating joints all have a common denominator: Active change is taking place. It is preferable first to establish stable parameters and build from that base.

Recognize Pain as a Factor unto Itself. Pain, especially if chronic, can change personalities, dispositions, and appreciation of surgical outcomes. Possible problems with pain control and drug abuse should be recognized, appreciated, and managed.

Rigid Fixation vs. Intermaxillary Fixation (IMF). Rigid fixation allows for early mobilization of the TMJ, compared with immobilization for 6 weeks with IMF. The potential for abuse with rigid fixation vs. the potential for lost range of motion with IMF needs to be carefully considered. No clear evidence supports one technique over the other.

Number and Sequencing of Surgical Procedures. A balance must be maintained among the surgeon's skills, the patient's well-being, and the patient's response to surgery.

Postoperative Care. Postoperative care must be part of the initial treatment plan. It may be modified during surgery or in response to unexpected sequelae. Appropriate physical therapy cannot be overemphasized.

Postoperative Stability. Patients must be carefully monitored for changes after orthognathic

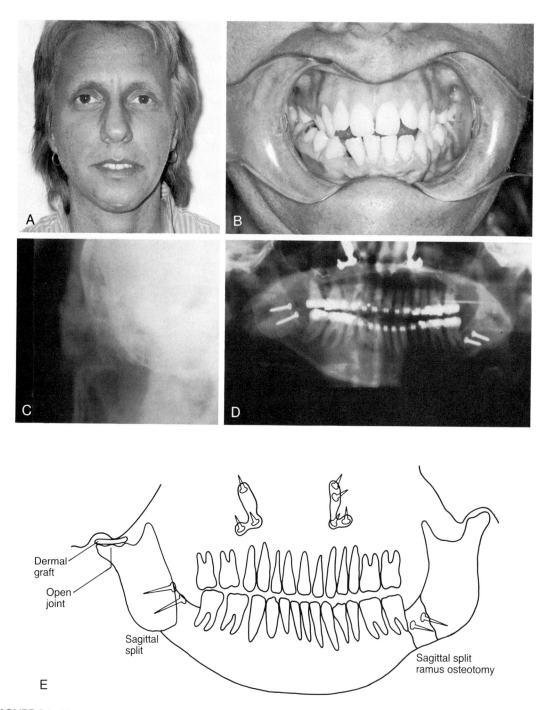

FIGURE 34–15. A patient with a condylar fracture and resulting facial asymmetry. *B,* The change in condylar height resulted in an open bite as seen in the occlusal view and coronal radiograph (*C*). The patient was treated with a maxillary and mandibular osteotomy as shown in the postoperative panoramic film (*D*) and the illustration of the film (*E*). In this case, the displaced condyle was not corrected but the facial skeleton and adequate function were restored with orthognathic surgery.

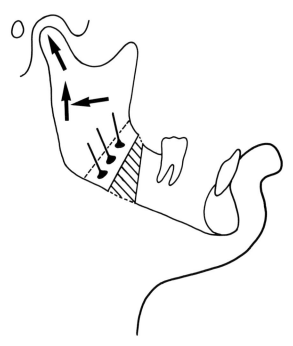

FIGURE 34–16. Diagram of the placement of screws in a sagittal split osteotomy and the possible posterior and superior repositioning of the condyle that could occur from exessive force on the proximal segment.

surgery. Changes in skeletal form may arise from either condylar changes or skeletal relapse (Fig. 34–18).

Range of Motion. Postsurgical scarring may present as a limitation of mandibular movement and must be distinguished from restrictions due to intra-articular disorders. Difficulty in making this distinction may be the major argument against simultaneous surgical procedures. A proper diagnosis of preoperative and postoperative restricted range of motion is essential.

Rule 12: The surgeon should try to divide a complex problem into a series of several simple problems.

Rule 13: Do not operate on a patient when you cannot manage a potential untoward result.

Rule 14: In surgery, better is the enemy of good.

CORRECTION OF DENTAL FACIAL DEFORMITIES WITH MAJOR JOINT RECONSTRUCTION

Rule 9 states that it is difficult to correct an occlusal problem with joint surgery. There are exceptions to this rule, however, especially when performing major joint reconstruction. Major joint reconstruction includes rib graft and total joint replacement. These procedures restore structure and function to the TMJ. Severe destruction of the TMJ may occur as a result of trauma, infection, degenerative joint disease, implant or foreign body rejection, and neoplasia.

Major surgical TMJ reconstruction should address the following goals:

1. It should provide structure and support for the mandible between the remaining segments and the fossa.

2. It should restore vertical height.

3. It should allow for articulation and movement.

4. It should forestall infection, rejection, and further deterioration.

5. It should avoid damage to surrounding structures.

6. It should be durable with respect to time and function.

Total joint reconstruction, regardless of the specific type of surgery, requires placing the dentition in IMF and rebuilding the bony and articulating elements to this position. Although the control of occlusion is not as accurate as in orthognathic surgery, results can often be very acceptable.

Procedures commonly used for joint reconstruction include the following:

1. Costochondral rib grafts (Fig. 34–19)

2. Extraoral vertical ramus osteotomies with superior repositioning (Fig. 34–20). This procedure is often performed with an autogenous graft such as dermis, fascia, or cartilage over the articulating surface.

3. Total joint prostheses (Fig. 34–21)

4. A combination of autogenous grafting procedures to a condylar stump

5. Intermaxillary fixation without restoration of condylar height. (This is not considered to be a true reconstruction procedure and is less predictable, but it can often maintain an occlusion as scar tissue and the muscles stabilize the joint.)

Autogenous grafting material has always been the first choice for reconstuctive material. The benefit of costochondral rib grafts is that they are biologically suited for joint replacement. In a growing child, they can provide a growth center transplant, and in an adult, they

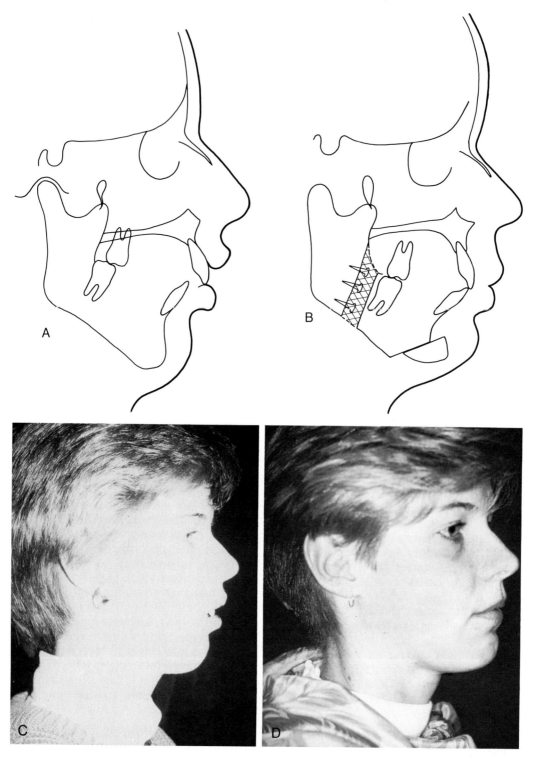

FIGURE 34–17. Preoperative (A) and postoperative (B) cephalometric illustrations of a patient who had severe vertical maxillary excess and mandibular retrognathia with a history of temporomandibular joint (TMJ) pain. The orthognathic surgery established a satisfactory occlusion and an exceptionally favorable change in the profile. Unfortunately, the TMJ symptoms were not improved and had to be treated postoperatively, with arthroscopy that resulted in a functioning joint in a stable facial skeleton. C and D show preoperative and postoperative facial views, respectively.

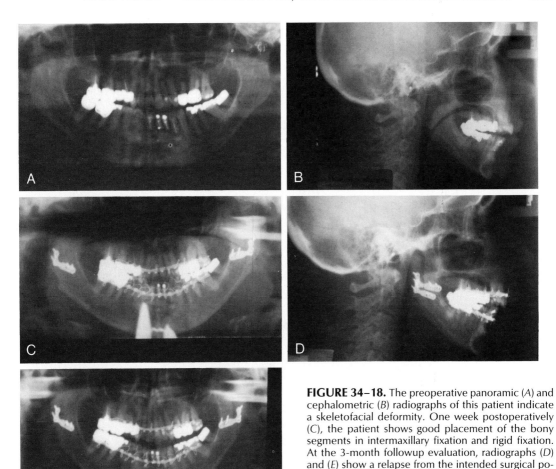

FIGURE 34–18. The preoperative panoramic (A) and cephalometric (B) radiographs of this patient indicate a skeletofacial deformity. One week postoperatively (C), the patient shows good placement of the bony segments in intermaxillary fixation and rigid fixation. At the 3-month followup evaluation, radiographs (D) and (E) show a relapse from the intended surgical positioning and a relapse back to an open bite. This case illustrates the need for careful followup to avoid the need for additional procedures on an unstable occlusion.

provide the missing osseous structure and cartilage for articulating surfaces. Biologically, they are almost 100% compatible, and they remodel as active or living tissue, with little incidence of infection or rejection. Although the masticatory muscles adapt to the transplant, they are generally limited to rotational movement only,[42] because of the absence of a lateral pterygoid attachment to the graft.

In general, the ribs can be harvested as vascularized or free grafts, usually leaving the cartilage perichondrium intact, allowing for preservation of the cartilage end of the rib. Fifth and seventh ribs are the most popular because of size, shape, and access from an inframammary incision line (Figs. 34–22, 34–23, 34–24).[13,43]

The facial incisions are submandibular and preauricular. Careful attention must be directed toward the location of the facial nerve. The ribs can be placed with the cartilage contoured to the fossa and then shaped along the posterior or lateral aspect of the ramus (see Fig. 34–19). The disc, if present, may be left intact.

Rigid fixation allows for early mobilization. Most cases do not require vascular anastomosis, but there are several options to obtain a blood supply if needed.[44] Postoperatively, patients are left in intermaxillary fixation (IMF) from 1 to 6 weeks, and training elastics are used as the patient begins mobilization.

Indications for this procedure include the following:

1. Ankylosis, especially in a growing child
2. Severe osteoarthrosis

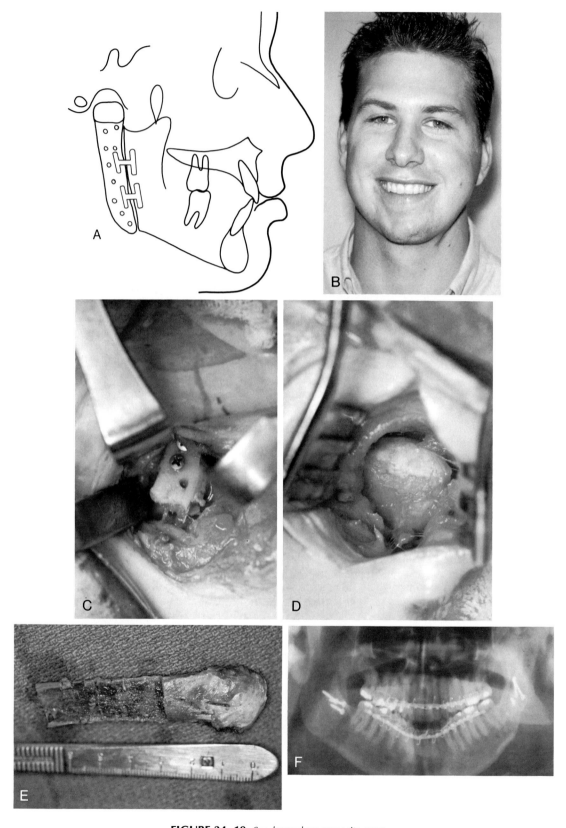

FIGURE 34–19. *See legend on opposite page.*

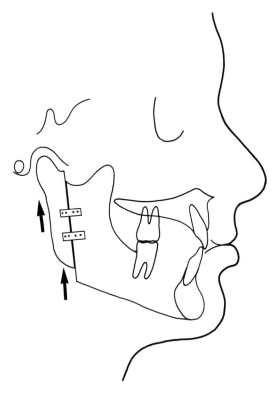

FIGURE 34–20. Diagram of a vertical ramus osteotomy used to restore mandibular posterior height. The posterior vertical ramus is repositioned superiorly, and rigid fixation secures its position.

3. Congenital deformities such as hemifacial microsomia
4. Replacement of the condyles due to severe destruction associated with infection, arthritis, trauma, or iatrogenic damage to the joint
5. As a growth center transplant
6. Replacement of a joint prosthesis.

Three remaining issues are discussed as follows:

1. Rigid vs. nonrigid fixation
2. TMJ problems secondary to orthognathic surgery
3. SFDs secondary to TMJ surgery.

Familiarity with these topics is essential to treatment management of a patient through the postoperative course.

RIGID VS. NONRIGID FIXATION

The introduction of rigid fixation to oral and maxillofacial surgery was met with high anticipation and excitement. It was hoped that the use of mini-plates and small screws would put an end to surgical relapse and a host of other problems. Once the technique was introduced and the procedures were put into routine use, the advantages and disadvantages became

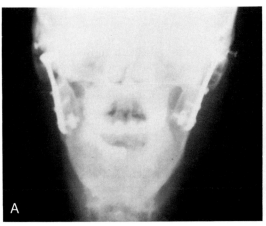
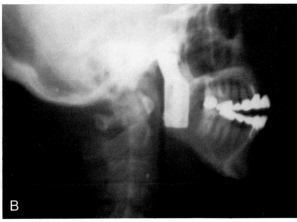

FIGURE 34–21. *A* and *B.* Kent condyle and fossa—one of the more common total joint implant systems available.

FIGURE 34–19. *A,* Diagram illustrating rib graft placement in the posterior vertical ramus. The costochondral junction is secured into the fossa, and the rib is placed in rigid fixation. *B,* Postoperative facial photograph of a patient who underwent this procedure. *C,* Clinical picture of the rib graft in place as seen through the submandibular incision. *D,* The cartilaginous portion of the rib graft placed in the fossa. *E,* The harvested rib. *F,* Panoramic radiograph showing the position of the segments.

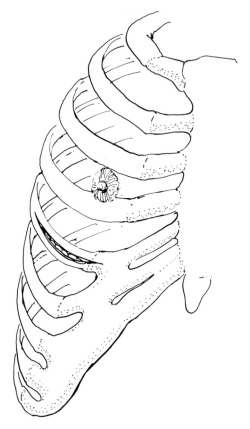

FIGURE 34–22. Illustration of the rib cage showing the fifth rib at the junction of the costochondral margin that will be used for grafting. (Reprinted with permission from Epker, B.N. and Wolford, L.M.: *Dentofacial Deformities— Surgical Orthodontic Correction.* C.V. Mosby Co., St. Louis, 1980.)

more obvious. As described, rigid fixation allowed a surgeon to decrease or eliminate the time of IMF. Patients had previously been placed on IMF for 6 or more weeks following surgery. With rigid fixation, IMF generally is unnecessary, allowing for immediate mobilization. An obvious gain is an increase in the number and variety of surgical procedures that can be performed on a patient at one time.

There are a number of potential negative outcomes, however, but most can be avoided with careful surgical technique and attention to detail. Because rigid fixation holds the condyle in a set position, there is limited room for adaptability of condylar position as seen in routine IMF.[22,24,28] A second concern is the postsurgical position of the condyle in relationship to the fossa. If placed too posterior or superior, the condyle will have no potential for adaptation because of the rigidity associated

with the fixation. Postoperative movement of the segments may be limited because of the rigidity of the skeletal fixation.

Severe limitations may also exist for the use of postoperative elastics and extraoral headgear. Therefore, the surgery itself requires precise attention to positioning of the segments and the condyle. Should the condyle-disc relationship be impaired, little room is allowed for correction.

TEMPOROMANDIBULAR DISORDERS SECONDARY TO ORTHOGNATHIC SURGERY

Any orthognathic surgical procedure has the potential to create a TMD or exacerbate an existing one. Among the possible problems are the following:

1. Unacceptable condylar position
2. Disc displacement
3. Malocclusion secondary to condylar sag or built-in dental relapse (a failure to allow for orthodontic relapse before orthognathic surgery)
4. The need to use excessive force in postoperative care
5. Hypomobility secondary to intraoral scarring
6. Idiopathic condylar lysis with secondary open bite
7. A progressive TMD after orthognathic surgery.

Rule 14: It is less difficult to treat a postoperative orthognathic surgical problem initially after surgery than later. (You will not be the first surgeon to unturn a rigid fixation screw.)

Once the surgical hardware is removed, the dentition can relapse to a pretreatment state. Although these problems can appear, they are for the most part not common and are often eliminated with careful technique and conscientious surgery. Furthermore, postoperative follow-up care often arrests these problems at their onset and allows ample opportunity to correct them.

SKELETOFACIAL DEFORMITIES SECONDARY TO TEMPOROMANDIBULAR JOINT SURGERY

Rule 15: It is less difficult to build working bites than working joints.

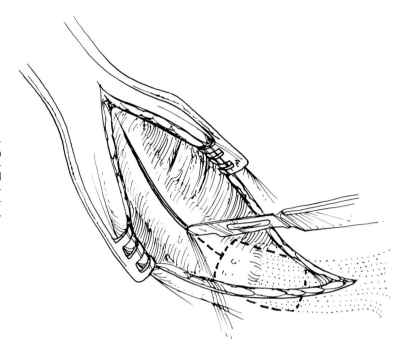

FIGURE 34–23. Surgical technique used to remove rib through an incision. (Reprinted with permission from Epker, B.N. and Wolford, L.M.: *Dentofacial Deformities—Surgical Orthodontic Correction.* C.V. Mosby Co., St. Louis, 1980.)

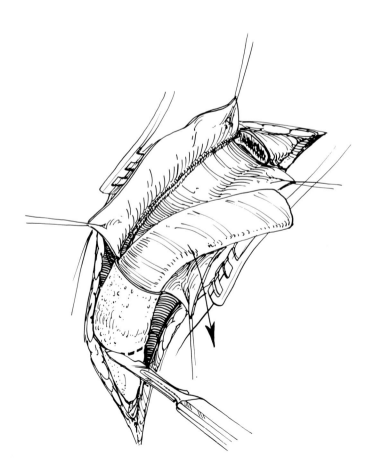

FIGURE 34–24. The rib being removed from its bed, preserving the periosteum and the cartilage. (Reprinted with permission from Epker, B.N. and Wolford, L.M.: *Dentofacial Deformities—Surgical Orthodontic Correction.* C.V. Mosby Co., St. Louis, 1980.)

Surgery on the TMJ can have unforeseen sequelae or can fail to arrest underlying disease. Problems such as avascular necrosis, foreign body rejection, and osteoarthrosis can continue endlessly for some unfortunate patients. I have been consulted in regard to patients who have had as many as 14 surgical procedures, and I have been told about one patient who had as many as 22 open joint procedures.

Rule 16: Know when to recognize that a patient has had his or her last TMJ surgical procedure.

SUMMARY

The available literature on the relationship of orthognathic and TMJ surgery is at best limited. As debate continues on the etiology of TMD and the suggested treatment modalities, to what extent one can subscribe the effects of occlusion in the genesis of TMD is still largely unknown. However, it would be hard to find a dentist who does not believe that a functional occlusion is a healthy occlusion. There is also strong belief among the dental community in the need to have a functional, stable, and normal occlusion. Orthognathic surgery is one method of obtaining that result. Whether orthognathic surgery improves TMJ function or not remains a complex problem, and the results are at best unpredictable in many patients. Alternatively, choosing TMJ surgery as a primary procedure provides a working and articulating foundation for the remaining facial skeleton to be built on.

The literature so far indicates two basic responses that occur in patients with this combined problem. Approximately 50% to 75% of patients who have TMD symptoms and undergo orthognathic surgery show improvement in symptoms. A smaller percentage experience an increase in symptom severity or develop a TMD. Furthermore, the higher incidence of symptoms of TMD in the general population is similar to the incidence in patients with SFDs.[25,45]

This chapter has delineated general guidelines for treating patients with combined TMJ and SFD. There are no absolute or "cookbook" recipes for success. Clinicians are obliged to recognize an SFD and TMD and to formulate a treatment plan with both an understanding of the facts and an appreciation for the probable effectiveness of treatment. The essential components of surgical decision making require a diagnosis, treatment plan, and the ability to vary applications from patient to patient.

REFERENCES

1. Solberg, W.K., Woo, M.W., and Houston, J.B.: Prevalence of mandibular dysfunction in young adults. J. Am. Dent. Assoc. 98:25–34, 1979.
2. Carlsson, G.E., Egermark-Erikson, I., and Magnusson, T.: Intra- and inter-observer variation in functional examination of the masticatory system. Swed. Dent. J. 4:187–194, 1980.
3. Epker, B.N., and Fish, L.C.: Dentofacial Deformities, vols. I and II. Integrated Orthodontic and Surgical Correction. C.V. Mosby Co., St. Louis, 1986.
4. Bell, W.H., Profitt, W.R., and White, R.P.: *Surgical Correction of Dentofacial Deformities,* vol. II. W.B. Saunders Co., Philadelphia, 1980.
5. International Temporomandibular Joint Arthroscopy Study Club Guidelines.
6. Red Book on TMJ Surgery. AAMOS, 1984.
7. Gorlin, R.J., Pindborg, J.J., and Cohen, M.M., Jr.: Syndromes of the Head and Neck, 2nd edition. McGraw-Hill, New York, 1976.
8. Graber, T.M. and Swain, B.F.: *Orthodontics, Current Principles and Techniques.* C.V. Mosby Co., St. Louis, 1985.
9. Broadbent, Sr., B.H. and Broadbent, Jr., B.H.: *Bolton Standards of Dentofacial Developmental Growth.* C.V. Mosby Co., St. Louis, 1975.
10. Bell, W.E.: *Orofacial Pains: Classification Diagnosis Management,* 3rd ed. Year Book Medical Publishers, Chicago, 1985.
11. Dolwick, M.F., Reid, R., Sanders, B., et al: Dolwick standards, criteria for TMJ meniscus surgery. AAOMS, 1984.
12. DeBont, L.M.: *TMJ. Articular Cartilage and Structure and Function.* Riejte Sunier Siteit. Grounger, 1985.
13. Epker, B.N. and Wolford, L.M.: *Dentofacial Deformities. Surgical—Orthodontic Correction.* C.V. Mosby, St. Louis, 1980.
14. Deleted in print.
15. Kent, J.N., Misick, D.J., Akin, R.K., et al: Temporomandibular joint condylar prosthesis: A ten-year report. J. Oral Maxillofac. Surg. 41:245, 1983.
16. Boyd, S., et al: Masseter muscle adaption following surgical correction of VME. J. Oral Maxillofac. Surg. 47:953–962, 1989.
17. Bell, W., et al: *Neuromuscular Aspects of Vertical Maxillary Dysplasia, vol. II.* Surgical Correction of D.F.D., W.B. Saunders Co., Philadelphia, 1712–1731, 1980.
18. Finn, R.A., et al: Biochemical considerations in surgical correction of mandibular deficiency with oral surgery. J. Oral Maxillofac. Surg. 38:257–264, 1980.
19. Throckmorton, G.S., et al: Biomedical differences in lower facial height. temporomandibular joint orthodontics. Am. Orthodont. 77:410–420, 1980.
20. Storum, K.A. and Bell, W.H.: Hypomobility after maxillary and mandibular osteotomies. Oral Surg. 57:7–12, 1984.
21. Aragon, S.B., Van Sickels, J.E., Dolwick, M.F., and Flanary, C.M.: The effects of orthognathic surgery on mandibular range of motion. J. Oral Maxillofac. Surg. 49:938–943, 1985.
22. Sund, G., Eckerdal, O., and Astrand, O.: Changes in the temporomandibular joint after oblique sliding os-

teotomy of the mandibular rami. J. Maxillofac. Surg. 11:87, 1973.

23. Van Sickels, J.E. and Flanary C.M.: Stability associated with mandibular advancement treated by rigid osseous fixation. J. Oral Maxillofac. Surg. 43:338, 1985.

24. Hollander, L. and Ridell, A.: Radiography of the temporomandibular joint after oblique sliding osteotomy of the mandibular rami. Scand. J. Dent. Res. 82:466–469, 1974.

25. Karabouta, I. and Martis, C.: The TMJ dysfunction syndrome before and after sagittal split osteotomy of the rami. J. Oral Maxillofac. Surg. 13:185–188, 1985.

26. Phillips, R.M. and Bell, W.H.: Atrophy of mandibular condyles after sagittal ramus split osteotomy: Report of case. J. Oral Surg. 36:45, 1978.

27. Moblin, B., Ingervall, B., and Thilander, B.: Relation between malocclusion and mandibular dysfunction in Swedish men. Eur. J. Orthod. 2:229, 1980.

28. Wisth, P.J.: Mandibular function and dysfunction in patients with mandibular prognathism. Am. J. Orthod. 85:193–198, 1984.

29. Tucker, M.R. and Thomas, P.M.: Temporomandibular pain and dysfunction in the orthodontic surgical patient: Rationale for evaluation and treatment sequencing. Int. J. Adult Orthod. Orthog. Surg. 1:11–22, 1986.

30. Piecuch, J., Tideman, H., and DeKoomen, H.: Short-face Syndrome: Treatment of Myofascial Pain Dysfunction by Maxillary Disimpaction. C.V. Mosby Co., St. Louis, 112–116, 1980.

31. Van Sickels, J.E. and Ivey, D.W.: Myofacial pain dysfunction: A manifestation of the short-face syndrome. J. Prosthet. Dent. 42:547–550, 1979.

32. White, R.D.: Retrospective analysis of 100 consecutive surgical arthroscopies of the temporomandibular joint. J. Oral Maxillofac. Surg. 47:1014–1021, 1989.

33. McCain, J.P., De La Rua, H., and Le Blanc, W.G.: Correlation of clinical, radiographic, and arthroscopic findings in internal derangements of the TMJ. J. Oral Maxillofac. Surg. 47:913–921, 1989.

34. Moses, J.J. and Poker, I.D.: TMJ arthroscopic surgery: An analysis of 237 patients. J. Oral Maxillofac. Surg. 47:790–794, 1989.

35. O'Ryan, F. and Epker, B.N.: Temporomandibular joint function and morphology: Observations on the spectra of normalcy. Oral Surg. 58:272–279, 1984.

36. International Study Group on TMJ Arthroscopy. Effect of TMJ Arthroscopy on Arthrotomy. Third International TMJ Arthroscopy Symposium, New York. December, 1988 [Abstract.]

37. Tarro, A.W.: Arthroscopic treatment of anterior disc displacement: A preliminary report. J. Oral Maxillofac. Surg. 47:353–358, 1989.

38. Moses, J.J., Sartoris, D., Glass, R. et al: The effect of arthroscopic surgical lysis and lavage of the superior joint space on TMJ disc position and mobility. J. Maxillofac. Surg. 47:674–678, 1989.

39. Wessberg, G.A., O'Ryan, F.S. Washburn, M.C., and Epker, B.N.: Neuromuscular adaption to surgical superior repositioning of the maxilla. J. Oral Maxillofac. Surg. 117–122, 1981.

40. Tallents, R.H., Katzberg, R.W., Miller, T.L., et al: Evaluation of arthrographically assisted splint therapy in treatment of TMJ disk displacement. Pain and Dysfunction, Fifth Annual Meeting, 275–277, 1987.

41. Sanders, B.: Arthroscopic lysis and lavage for closed lock perforations, arthrosis, salvaging arthrotomies and osteotomies. Fourth Annual International Symposium of TMJ Arthroscopy, Hawaii, December, 1989.

42. MacIntosh, B. et al: Surgical Correction of Skeletofacial Deformities, vol. 3. pp. 355–410, 1989.

43. Skouteris, C.A. and Sotereanos, G.C.: Bone complications of rib graft donor sites: donor site morbidity following harvesting of autogenous rib grafts. J. Oral Maxillofac. Surg. 47:808–812, 1989.

44. Obeid, G., Guttenberg, S.A., and Connole, P.W.: Costochondral grafting in condylar replacement and mandibular reconstruction. J. Oral Maxillofac. Surg. 48:177–182, 1988.

45. Kerstens, H.C.J., Tuinzing, D.B., and van der Kwast, W.A.M.: Temporomandibular joint symptoms in orthognathic surgery. J. Craniomaxillofac. Surg. 5:215–218, 1989.

Mohan Thomas
Christopher Lane

CHAPTER 35

Future Directions in Temporomandibular Joint Surgery

A rapid technologic advance in the surgical management of several conditions has occurred in the last decade. For example, neurosurgical advances include the management of seizure disorders with image control and brain mapping. Advances in endoscopy have made the diagnosis and treatment of the gastrointestinal tract less difficult. Lithotripsy has made possible the percutaneous removal of kidney and gallstones. Endoscopic cholecystectomy and nonendoscopic nephrectomy with the use of lasers seem to have greatly advanced general surgery. Orthopedists are utilizing robots and computer-guided surgery to optimally reconstruct the skeleton.

Although these advances in technology are noteworthy, perhaps their widespread clinical application may be premature because of inadequate evaluation. Furthermore, these technologic advances are often incorporated into medical and surgical practices without the support of clinical trials to indicate whether they have a greater value than existing methods. The time to test the value and efficacy of these advances is before they are incorporated into daily medical and surgical practice.

APPLICATION OF TECHNOLOGY TO TEMPOROMANDIBULAR JOINT DISORDERS

In the evaluation and treatment of temporomandibular disorders (TMDs), we are often fascinated by "new gadgets," and we hope that

these will become "quick fixes." Once these gadgets have been incorporated into our practices, it may be more difficult to test their value from a scientific and ethical standpoint. Even if the research community disproves the value of a modality, practitioners may have great hesitation in giving it up, particularly when they have been utilizing it for years.

Our efforts should be directed toward understanding the epidemiology and the natural history of conditions that are included in the broad category of "jaw joint dysfunctions." Scientific scrutiny is hampered by a lack of uniformity as far as diagnostic criteria. The measurement of outcome is of concern. It is extremely difficult for clinicians to repeat the recorded work or make direct comparisons.[1] To address these issues, the American Academy of Craniomandibular Disorders has published a document to provide health professionals with a current review of the evaluation, diagnosis, and management of patients with craniomandibular disorders.[2]

An increase in the number of patients seeking care for myofascial pain dysfunction has been noted in the recent past. Many of these patients are very young. In addition, many dentists who treat young patients are correctly referring them for TMD evaluation. Invasive and noninvasive therapy for TMD has not been adequately examined in the young patient. Pharmacologic management may include tricyclic compounds or nonsteroidal anti-inflammatory drugs.[2] Long-term usage should be discouraged because many of these patients are young females, who may be on the threshold of reproductive life.[3] The effects of surgery on growth and later function are still not well understood. The majority of young patients do get better in the long term, with simple reversible and noninvasive methods.

A segment of patients, however, do present with chronic pain with no relief in sight and are miserably disabled because of a lack of intervention or misdirected intervention. The future of therapy requires a thorough understanding of the course of the illness and a complete knowledge of the results of therapy. As young patients age, we will answer many of these questions.

Future directions can be examined under the broad categories of basic science and technical advances. Researchers are now studying the physiology of the TMJ, including the synovial apparatus and the production of synovial fluid, the histologic characteristics of pathologic

728

23. Kent, J.N. and Misiek, D.J.: Biomaterials for cranial, facial, mandibular and TMJ reconstruction. In *Oral and Maxillofacial Trauma,* vol. 2. R. Fonseca and R. Walker (eds.). 1991.

24. Grande, D.A. and Pitman, M.I.: The use of adhesives in chondrocyte surgery: Preliminary studies. Br. Hosp. Joint Dis. 48:140–148, 1988.

25. Barnett, C., Davies, D. and MacConaill, M.: Synovial joints: Their structure and mechanics. *Synovial Joints.* Thurgood. Charles C Thomas. Springfield, Ill., 1961.

26. Brower, T.D. and Akohos, Y.: The diffusion of dyes through articular cartilage in vivo. J. Bone Joint Surg. 44:456–463, 1962.

27. McCarthy, W.L. and Farrar, W.B.: Surgery for derangements of the TMJ. J. Prosthet. Dent. 42:191–196, 1979.

28. Meyer, R.A.: The autologous dermal graft in temporomandibular joint disc surgery. J. Oral Maxillofac. Surg. 46:948–954, 1988.

29. Tucker, R.M., Kennedy, M.C., and Jacoway, J.R.: Autogenous articular cartilage implantation following discectomy in the primate temporomandibular joint. J. Oral Maxillofac. Surg. 48:38–44, 1990.

30. Raveh, J., Vallemin, T., and Ladrach, K.: Temporomandibular joint ankylosis: Surgical treatment and long-term results. J. Oral Maxillfac. Surg. 47:900–906, 1989.

31. Bronstein, S.L.: Retained alloplastic TMJ disc implants: A retrospective study. Oral Surg. Oral Med. Oral Pathol. 64:135–145, 1987.

32. Pitman, M.I., Menche, D., Song, E.K., Ben-Yishay, A., Gilbert, D., and Grande, D.A.: The use of adhesives in chondrocyte transplantation surgery: In vivo studies. Br. Hosp. Joint Dis. Orthop. Inst. 49:213–220, 1989.

33. Kurita, K., Westesson, P.L., Eriksson, L., and Sternby, N.H.: Osteoplasty of the mandibular condyle with preservation of the articular soft tissue cover. Oral Surg. Oral Med. Oral Pathol. 69:661–667, 1990.

34. Hartog, J.M., Slavin, A.B., and Klein, S.: Reconstruction of the TMJ with cryopreserved cartilage and freeze-dried dura: A preliminary report. J. Oral Maxillofac. Surg. 48:919–925, 1990.

35. Spivak, J.M., Grande, D.A., Grelsamer, R.P., Menche, D.S., and Pitman, M.I.: The effect of low level Nd:YAG laser energy on adult canine cartilage. Presented at the 36th Annual Meeting, Orthopedics Research Society. New Orleans, 1990.

36. Indresano, A.T., Braderick, J.P., and Eckhauser, M.L.: *The Nd:YAG Laser Trilogy.* Metro Health Medical Center, Case Western Reserve University, Cleveland, OH, 1989.

37. Schellhas, K.P., Wilkes, C.H., and Heithoff, K.B.: Temporomandibular joint: Diagnosis of internal derangements using magnetic resonance imaging. Minn. Med. 69:516–519, 1986.

38. Schellhas, K.P., Wilkes, C.H., Hollis, H.M., Omlie, M.K., and Lagrotteria, L.B.: MR of osteochondritis dissecans and avascular necrosis of the mandibular condyle. Am. J. Nucl. Radiol. 10:3–12, 1989.

39. Sanchez-Woodworth, R.E., Tallents, R.H., Katzberg, R.W., and Guay, J.A.: Bilateral internal derangements of TMJ: Evaluation by MRI. Oral Surg. Oral Med. Oral Pathol. 65:281–285, 1988.

40. Schellhas, K.P.: TMJ pathology and MRI. Presented at the 5th Annual Symposium on Arthroscopy of the Human TMJ. New York, 1990.

41. Poremba, E.P. and Moffett, B.C.: The effects of continuous passive motion on the TMJ after surgery. Part I. Oral Surg. Oral Med. Oral Pathol. 67:490–498, 1989.

42. Sebastian, M.H. and Moffett, B.C.: The effects of continuous passive motion on the TMJ after surgery. Part II. Oral Surg. Oral Med. Oral Pathol. 67:644–653, 1989.

43. Chuong, R. and Piper, M.: Open reduction of condylar fracture on the mandible in conjunction with discal injury: A preliminary report. J. Oral Maxillofac. Surg. 46:257–263, 1988.

44. Hilsabeck, R. and Laskin, D.: Arthroscopy of the TMJ of the rabbit. J. Oral Surg. 36:938–943, 1978.

45. Williams, R. and Laskin, D.: Arthroscopic examination of experimentally induced pathologic conditions of the rabbit TMJ. J. Oral Surg. 38:652–659, 1980.

46. Murakami, K. and Ito, K: Arthroscopy of the TMJ. Arthroscopic anatomy and arthroscopic approaches in the human cadaver. Arthroscopy 6:1–13, 1981.

47. Oshinishi, M.: Arthroscopy of the TMJ. Jpn. Stomatol. Soc. 42:207–213, 1975.

48. Murakami, K. and Hoshino, K.: Regional anatomical nomenclature and arthroscopic terminology in the human TMJ. Okajimas Folia Anat. Jpn. 58:745–760, 1982.

49. McCain, J.: Arthroscopic technique. Second International Symposium on TMJ Arthroscopy. New York, December, 1987.

50. Sanders, B., Kaminishi, R., Buoncristiani, R., et al: Arthroscopic surgery for treatment of TMJ hypomobility after mandibular sagittal osteotomy. Oral Surg. Oral Med. Oral Pathol. 69:45–47, 1990.

51. Moses, J., Sartoris, D., Glass, R., et al: The effect of arthroscopic surgical lysis and lavage of superior joint space on TMJ disc position and mobility. J. Oral Maxillofac. Surg. 47:674–678, 1989.

52. Israel, H.: Techniques for placement of a discal traction suture during TMJ arthroscopy. J. Oral Maxillofac. Surg. 47:311, 1989.

53. Mikhael, M.: Presentation at the Proceedings of the Radiology Society of North America Scientific Session, Chicago, Illinois, 1990.

Index

Note: Page numbers in *italics* refer to illustrations; page numbers followed by t refer to tables.